handbook

Clinical

Drug Data

handbook of

Clinical

Drug Data

tenth edition

EDITORS

Philip O. Anderson, PharmD, FASHP, FCSHP
Director, Drug Information Service, Department of Pharmacy
University of California Medical Center, San Diego, California
Clinical Professor of Pharmacy
University of California, San Francisco
San Diego Program, San Diego, California

James E. Knoben, PharmD, MPH
Drug Information Officer
Special Assistant to Associate Director for Specialized Information Services
National Library of Medicine
National Institutes of Health
Baltimore, Maryland

William G. Troutman, PharmD, FASHP
Regents' Professor of Pharmacy, College of Pharmacy
University of New Mexico, Albuquerque, New Mexico

McGraw-Hill
Medical Publishing Division

New York Chicago San Francisco Lisbon London Madrid
Mexico City Milan New Delhi San Juan Seoul Singapore Sydney
Toronto

McGraw-Hill

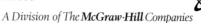

A Division of The McGraw·Hill Companies

HANDBOOK OF CLINICAL DRUG DATA, 10TH EDITION

1 2 3 4 5 6 7 8 9 0 DOC DOC 0 9 8 7 6 5 4 3 2 1

ISBN 0-07-136362-9

This book was set in Times Roman at Pine Tree Composition, Inc.
The editors were Stephen Zollo and Nicky Panton.
The production supervisor was Richard Ruzycka.
The cover designer was Janice Bielawa.
The index was prepared by Jerry Ralya.

R.R. Donnelley and Sons Company was printer and binder.

This book is printed on acid-free paper.

Library of Congress Cataloging-in-Publication Data
Handbook of clinical drug data.—10th ed. / [edited by] Philip Anderson, James Knoben, William Troutman.
   p.; cm.
  Includes index.
  ISBN 0-07-136362-9
  1. Pharmacology—Handbooks, manuals, etc. 2. Drugs—Handbooks, manuals, etc. I. Title: Handbook of Clinical drug data. II. Anderson, Philip O. III. Knoben, James E. IV. Troutman, William G.
  [DNLM: 1. Pharmaceutical Preparations—Handbooks. 2. Pharmacology, Clinical—Handbooks. QV 39 H2358 2001]
RM301.12.H36 2001
615′.1—dc21

00-054887

INTERNATIONAL EDITION ISBN 112445-4
Copyright © 2002. Exclusive rights by the McGraw-Hill Companies, Inc., for manufacture and export. This book cannot be reexported from the country to which it is consigned by McGraw-Hill. The International Edition is not available in North America.

Contents

Contributors

Brian K. Alldredge, PharmD
Professor of Clinical Pharmacy; Clinical Professor of Neurology, UCSF Department of Clinical Pharmacy, University of California, San Francisco, California

Philip O. Anderson, PharmD, FASHP, FCSHP
Director, Drug Information Service, Department of Pharmacy, University of California San Diego Medical Center; Clinical Professor of Pharmacy, University of California, San Francisco, San Diego Program, San Diego, California

Danial E. Baker, PharmD, FASHP, FASCP
Professor of Pharmacy Practice; Director, Drug Information Center; Director, Continuing Education Program, College of Pharmacy, Washington State University at Spokane, Spokane, Washington

Craig R. Ballard, PharmD, FCSHP
HIV Pharmacotherapy Specialist, University of California Medical Center, San Diego, California; Assistant Clinical Professor of Pharmacy, University of California, San Francisco, San Diego Program, San Diego, California

Jerry L. Bauman, PharmD, FACC, FCCP
Professor and Head, Department of Pharmacy Practice, University of Illinois at Chicago, Chicago, Illinois

Blaine E. Benson, PharmD, DABAT
Assistant Professor of Pharmacy, College of Pharmacy; Director, New Mexico Poison and Drug Information Center, University of New Mexico, Albuquerque, New Mexico

Toy S. Biederman, PharmD
Clinical Research Fellow in Neurology, The Ohio State University College of Pharmacy, Columbus, Ohio

R. Keith Campbell, BSPharm, MBA, CDE, FASHP
Associate Dean and Professor of Pharmacy Practice, College of Pharmacy, Washington State University, Pullman, Washington

Juliana Chan, PharmD
Research Assistant Professor of Pharmacy Practice, Department of Pharmacy Practice, University of Illinois at Chicago, Chicago, Illinois

Paul G. Cuddy, PharmD
Associate Professor, School of Medicine, University of Missouri-Kansas City, Kansas City, Missouri

Robert J. DiDomenico, PharmD
Clinical Assistant Professor, Department of Pharmacy Practice, University of Illinois at Chicago; Cardiovascular Pharmacotherapist, University of Illinois at Chicago Medical Center, Chicago, Illinois

Betty J. Dong, PharmD
Professor of Clinical Pharmacy and Family and Community Medicine, Department of Clinical Pharmacy, University of California School of Pharmacy, San Francisco; Clinical Pharmacist, Thyroid Clinic, University of California, San Francisco, California

Robert T. Dorr, PhD
Professor of Pharmacology, Pharmacology Department, College of Medicine, Arizona Cancer Center, University of Arizona, Tucson, Arizona

David G. Dunlop, PharmD, MPA
Inpatient Pharmacy Flight Commander, Wilford Hall Medical Center, Lackland AFB, San Antonio, Texas

Allison E. Einhorn, PharmD
Clinical Associate, Department of Pharmacy Practice, University of Illinois at Chicago, Chicago, Illinois

Raymond W. Hammond, PharmD, FCCP, BCPS
Associate Dean for Practice Programs and Clinical Associate Professor of Pharmacy, University of Houston, College of Pharmacy, Houston, Texas

Philip D. Hansten, PharmD
Professor of Pharmacy, School of Pharmacy, University of Washington, Seattle Washington

Mark T. Holdsworth, PharmD, BCPS, BCOP
Associate Professor of Pharmacy and Pediatrics, College of Pharmacy, University of New Mexico, Albuquerque, New Mexico

Polly E. Kintzel, PharmD, BCPS, BCOP
Clinical Pharmacist Specialist, Barbara Ann Karmanos Cancer Institute, Harper University Hospital, Detroit, Michigan

James E. Knoben, PharmD, MPH
Drug Information Officer, Special Assistant to Associate Director for Specialized Information Services, National Library of Medicine, National Institutes of Health, Bethesda, Maryland

James R. Lane, Jr., PharmD
Pharmacist Specialist, Coordinator of Applied Pharmacokinetics, Department of Pharmacy, University of California San Diego Medical Center; Assistant Clinical Professor of Pharmacy, University of California, San Francisco, San Diego Program, San Diego, California

Patricia L. Marshik, PharmD
Assistant Professor of Pharmacy, College of Pharmacy, University of New Mexico Health Sciences Center, Albuquerque, New Mexico

Gary R. Matzke, PharmD, FCP, FCCP
Professor of Pharmaceutical Sciences and Medicine, Department of Pharmaceutical Sciences and Medicine, School of Pharmacy, University of Pittsburgh, Pittsburgh, Pennsylvania

Renée-Claude Mercier, PharmD, BCPS
Assistant Professor of Pharmacy, College of Pharmacy, University of New Mexico, Albuquerque, New Mexico

William E. Murray, PharmD
Pharmacokinetics Service Coordinator, Pharmacy Department, Children's Hospital, San Diego, California; Assistant Clinical Professor of Pharmacy, University of California, San Francisco, San Diego Program, San Diego, California

James J. Nawarskas, PharmD, BCPS
Assistant Professor of Pharmacy, College of Pharmacy, University of New Mexico, Albuquerque, New Mexico

Robert E. Pachorek, PharmD, BCPS
Clinical Pharmacist, Mercy Hospital, San Diego, California; Adjunct Assistant Professor of Pharmacy Practice, University of Southern California, Los Angeles, California; Assistant Clinical Professor of Pharmacy, University of California, San Francisco, San Diego Program, San Diego, California

Stephen M. Setter, PharmD, CGP, DVM
Assistant Professor of Pharmacy Practice, College of Pharmacy, Washington State University, Spokane, Washington

Fred Shatsky, BSPharm, BCNSP
Nutrition Support Pharmacist, Department of Pharmacy, University of California Medical Center, San Diego, California; Assistant Clinical Professor of Pharmacy, University of California, San Francisco, San Diego Program, San Diego, California

Glen L. Stimmel, PharmD, BCPP
Professor of Clinical Pharmacy and Psychiatry, Schools of Pharmacy and Medicine, University of Southern California, Los Angeles, California

Anna Taddio, BSPharm, MS, PhD
Clinical Specialist, Neonatal Intensive Care and Associate Scientist, Research Institute, The Hospital for Sick Children; Assistant Professor, Faculty of Pharmacy, University of Toronto, Toronto, Ontario, Canada

Dianne E. Tobias, PharmD
President, Tobias Consulting Services, Davis, California

William G. Troutman, PharmD, FASHP
Regents' Professor of Pharmacy, College of Pharmacy, University of New Mexico, Albuquerque, New Mexico

John R. White, Jr., PA-C, PharmD
Associate Professor of Pharmacy Practice, Washington State University, Spokane, Washington; Director, Washington State University/Sacred Heart Medical Center Drug Studies Unit, Spokane, Washington

James M. Wooten, PharmD
Assistant Professor, School of Medicine, Section of Clinical Pharmacology, University of Missouri-Kansas City; Adjunct Assistant Professor, School of Pharmacy, University of Missouri-Kansas City, Kansas City, Missouri

Preface

The Tenth Edition of the *Handbook of Clinical Drug Data* continues a long tradition of providing clinically relevant, well-referenced drug information compiled by expert clinicians and presented in a compact format. The formats of all sections should be familiar to users of the ninth edition. As with recent editions, information in the *Handbook* is divided into three parts.

Drug Monographs in **Part I** have been updated to include numerous newly marketed and promising investigational drugs. Areas with extensive revisions include the Antivirals reflecting the many new agents for HIV infection, Immunosuppressants, Anticonvulsants, and the Hematologic Drugs. Three new subsections have been added to reflect the growing number of agents for rheumatoid arthritis, glaucoma and osteoporosis: Antiarthritic Drugs in the Analgesic and Anti-inflammatory Drugs section, Ophthalmic Drugs for Glaucoma in the Central Nervous System section, and Bisphosphonates in the Renal and Electrolytes section.

Clinical Drug Information in **Part II** continues to provide clinically useful information that helps the reader to decide which drug(s) are most likely to have caused adverse reactions or which are the best choices for patients in special populations. All drug-induced diseases sections have been extensively updated, as have the Cytochrome P450 Interactions, Pregnancy, Breastfeeding, Renal Disease, Immunization, and Cardiac Arrest sections. **Drug-Laboratory Test Interferences** in **Part III** has also been updated.

In this edition, we welcome several new authors: Dan Baker, Jess Benson, Toy Biederman, Juliana Chan, Paul Cuddy, Rob DiDomenico, Allison Einhorn, Ray Hammond, Patty Marshik, Gary Matzke (a returning author), Renée Mercier, and Anna Taddio (our first "international" author). We would also like to thank the previous authors whose work in most cases served as the basis for revisions of the chapters that appear in this edition by new authors: Andrea Anderson (Drugs and Pregnancy), Lisa Ashton (Respiratory Drugs), Arasb Ateshkadi (Renal and Electrolytes), Rosemary Berardi (Gastrointestinal Drugs), Larry Borgsdorf (anaphylaxis) Larry Davis (NSAIDs and Hematologic Drugs), John Flaherty (Aminoglycosides and β-Lactams), John Gambertoglio (Renal Disease), Millie Gottwald (Antimigraine Drugs and Neurodegenerative Diseases), Amy Guenette (Inotropic Drugs and Nitrates), Brian Kearney (Renal Disease), and Carolyn Zaleon (Gastrointestinal Drugs). We are saddened to report the deaths of Drs. Ateshkadi and Gambertoglio since our last edition. Both will be remembered for their professional dedication and the quality of their work. John Gambertoglio had long-time personal and professional ties to the editors and will be particularly missed.

This edition also marks another major change, being the first edition produced with our new publisher, McGraw-Hill and new editors, Stephen Zollo and

Nicky Panton. We thank them for their efforts to maintain the high quality of the *Handbook* that we desire and our readers have come to expect.

Philip O. Anderson
James E. Knoben
William G. Troutman
August 2001

How to Use This Book

Part I of this book is organized around 10 major drug categories, which have been subdivided into common therapeutic groups. Within these therapeutic groups, drug information is alphabetically presented in three formats: *Monographs, Minimonographs,* and *Comparison Charts.* Monographs and Comparison Charts are *grouped together* to ensure that related drugs are easy to *compare* and *contrast*. Charts are located after the monographs to which they relate. Drug antagonists are grouped together with agonists to simplify organization and accessibility.

Monographs are used for drugs of major importance and prototype agents.

Minimonographs are used for drugs similar to prototype drugs, those of lesser importance within a therapeutic class, and promising investigational agents. Minimonographs contain only selected subheadings of information rather than all subheadings contained in the full monographs.

Comparison Charts are used to present clinically useful information on members of the same pharmacologic class and different drugs with a similar therapeutic use, as well as to present clinically relevant information on certain other topics.

The preferred method to gain access to complete information on a *particular brand* or *generic drug* is to use the index at the end of the book. The index may also direct the user to *other pertinent information* on the drug.

MONOGRAPH FORMAT

CLASS INSTRUCTIONS

This is an optional heading at the beginning of each drug class. It consists of patient instructions that apply to more than one of the drug monographs in this subcategory. If all drugs are not identical in their instructions, only the common information is found here. The Patient Instructions section of each monograph that is affected states, *"See Class Instructions"* as the opening phrase.

GENERIC DRUG NAME   Brand Name(s)

The *nonproprietary (generic)* name is listed on the left, followed by common brand names listed on the right. Brand-name products listed are not necessarily superior or preferable to other brand-name or generic products; *"Various"* indicates the availability of additional brand and/or generic products.

Pharmacology. A description of the chemistry, major mechanisms of action, and human pharmacology of the drug in clinical application.

Administration and Adult Dosage. Route of administration, indications, and usual adult dosage range are given for the most common labeled uses. Dosages correspond to those in the product labeling or in standard reference sources. "Dose" refers to a single administration and "dosage" to a cumulative amount (eg, daily dosage).

Special Populations. Dosages in patient populations other than the typical adult are listed:

Pediatric Dosage (given by age or weight range)

Geriatric Dosage (given by age range)

Other Conditions (renal failure, hepatic disease, obesity, etc.)

Dosage Forms. The most commonly used dosage forms and available strengths are listed, as well as popular combination product dosage forms. Prediluted IV piggyback or large-volume parenteral containers are not listed unless this is the only commercially available product.

Patient Instructions. Key information that should be provided to the patient when prescribing or dispensing medication is presented. When introductions apply to an entire drug category, see "Class Instructions" at the beginning of that subcategory.

Missed Doses. What the patient should do if one or more doses are missed.

Pharmacokinetics. Data are presented as the mean ± the standard deviation. Occasionally the standard error of the mean (SE) is the only information available on variability, and it is identified as such.

Onset and Duration (time course of the pharmacologic or therapeutic effect)

Serum Levels (therapeutic and toxic plasma concentrations are given)

Fate (The course of the drug in the body is traced. Pharmacokinetic parameters are generally provided as total body weight normalized values. The volume of distribution is either a V_d in a one-compartment system or V_c and $V_{d\beta}$ or V_{dss} in a two-compartment system.)

$t_{1/2}$ (terminal half-life is presented)

Adverse Reactions. Reactions known to be dose related are usually given first, then other reactions in decreasing order of frequency. Reaction frequency is classified into three ranges. However, percentages of reactions may be provided for reactions that occur more frequently than 1%.

frequent	(>1/100 patients)
occasional	(1/100 to 1/10,000 patients)
rare	(<1/10,000 patients)

Contraindications. Those listed in product labeling are given. "Hypersensitivity" is not listed as a contraindication because it is understood that patients should usually not be given a drug to which they are allergic or hypersensitive—exceptions are noted.

Precautions. Warnings for use of the drug in certain disease states and/or patient populations, together with any cross-sensitivity with other drugs. Part II, Chapter 3, "Drug Use in Special Populations," should be consulted for more information, particularly regarding pregnancy and breastfeeding.

Drug Interactions. The most important drug interactions are listed.

Parameters to Monitor. Important clinical signs and/or laboratory tests to monitor to ensure safe and effective use are presented. The frequency of monitoring may also be given; however, for many drugs the optimal frequency has not been determined.

Notes. Distinguishing characteristics, therapeutic usefulness, or relative efficacy of the drug are presented, as well as unique or noteworthy physicochemical properties, handling, storage, or relative cost.

handbook of
Clinical
Drug Data

PART I

Drug Monographs

Principal Editor: Philip O. Anderson, PharmD

- Analgesic and Anti-inflammatory Drugs
- Antimicrobial Drugs
- Antineoplastics, Chemoprotectants, and Immunosuppressants
- Cardiovascular Drugs
- Central Nervous System Drugs
- Gastrointestinal Drugs
- Hematologic Drugs
- Hormonal Drugs
- Renal and Electrolytes
- Respiratory Drugs

Analgesic and Anti-inflammatory Drugs

Antimigraine Drugs

DIHYDROERGOTAMINE MESYLATE

D.H.E. 45, Migranal

Pharmacology. Dihydroergotamine (DHE) is a semisynthetic ergot alkaloid that is hypothesized to exert its antimigraine effect via its agonist activity at the serotonin $5\text{-}HT_{1D}$ receptor, resulting in vasoconstriction of intracranial blood vessels and inhibition of inflammatory neuropeptide release.[1] The drug also binds with high affinity to adrenergic and dopamine receptors; however, the antimigraine effect of these events is unknown. Compared with ergotamine, DHE is a weaker vasoconstrictor, is less active as an emetic, and is less oxytocic.

Administration and Adult Dosage. **IM** 1 mg initially, then 1 mg q 1 hr prn, to a maximum of 3 mg/day or 6 mg/week. **IV** (for rapid effect) 0.5–1 mg, may repeat in 1 hr to a maximum of 2 mg/day or 6 mg/week. Consider administering metoclopramide 10 mg IV before DHE to treat nausea due to migraine and prevent nausea due to the drug.[2] **Intranasal** one spray (0.5 mg) into each nostril; may repeat in 15 min to a maximum of 2 mg over 24 hr.

Special Populations. *Pediatric Dosage.* Safety and efficacy not established.

Geriatric Dosage. Same as adult dosage.

Dosage Forms. **Inj** 1 mg/mL; **Nasal Spray** 4 mg/mL.

Patient Instructions. This drug can cause numbness and tingling in fingers, toes, or face. Notify your physician if you are pregnant or have heart disease or high blood pressure. Do not exceed the maximum dosage. The nasal spray can cause local irritation. Do not reuse the applicator; use the solution right after opening. Review training materials with your health care provider and report the use of all cold or allergy medications and all over-the-counter medications.

Pharmacokinetics. Onset and Duration. Onset under 5 min IV, within 15–30 min after IM or intranasal spray; duration 3–4 hr. Intranasal 50–70% of patients respond in 4 hr.

Fate. The drug is absorbed directly into the systemic circulation when administered intranasally, but it undergoes extensive first-pass metabolism if given orally. Bioavailability of the nasal spray is $38 \pm 16\%$, variable depending on self-administration technique.[3] Protein binding is 93%. After administration of 1 mg, peak levels are 1 ± 0.4 μg/L (intranasal) and 4.4 μg/L (IM), occurring at 0.9 ± 0.6 hr (intranasal) and 0.4 ± 0.3 hr (IM).[3] After IM administration, V_c is 12 ± 4 L/kg, and $V_{d\beta}$ is 33 ± 0.2 L/kg, suggesting distribution into deep tissue compartments. Cl is 1.6 ± 0.17 L/hr/kg. The drug is metabolized to at least 5 metabolites, 3 of which are active. The major route of excretion for DHE and its metabolites is in the feces via the bile.[1,3]

$t_{1/2}$. α phase (intranasal) 1 ± 0.5 hr, (IM) 0.9 ± 0.3 hr; β phase (intranasal) 7.9 ± 4 hr, (IM) 7.2 ± 2.2 hr.[3]

Adverse Reactions. The most frequently reported adverse events with intranasal administration are rhinitis, pharyngitis, altered sense of taste, application site reactions, nausea, vomiting, and dizziness. With all routes of administration, nausea, vomiting, diarrhea, and localized edema occur frequently.[4,5] Numbness and tingling of fingers and toes, muscle pain in extremities, weakness in legs, pruritus, rash, and infection occur occasionally. Pleural and retroperitoneal fibrosis occur rarely with prolonged use.

Contraindications. Pregnancy and lactation; peripheral vascular disease; coronary artery disease; ischemic heart disease; hemiplegic or basilar migraine; sepsis; recent history of vascular surgery; severely impaired hepatic or renal function; hypersensitivity to ergot alkaloids.

Precautions. Use caution to avoid overuse by patients with chronic vascular headaches. Patients with risk factors for coronary artery disease should undergo periodic cardiovascular evaluation.

Drug Interactions. (*See* Ergotamine Tartrate.) DHE can antagonize the antianginal effects of nitrates. The risk of bleeding with warfarin (eg, wound hematoma, anemia, hematuria) is worsened with co-administration of DHE. Macrolides including erythromycin can increase the risk of ergot toxicity. Sumatriptan can exacerbate coronary artery vasospasm and should not be taken within 24 hr of DHE. SSRIs can cause weakness, hyperreflexia, or incoordination.

Notes. IV DHE is used when oral agents have failed to abort migraine and for terminating cluster or migraine headache in an emergency setting. It is not intended for prophylaxis or the management of hemiplegic or basilar migraine. The intranasal preparation is a noninvasive option for outpatients. Intranasal administration also results in improved bioavailability over the oral form because it does not undergo a first-pass effect in the liver. DHE does not cause physical dependence and is associated with a more favorable side effect profile than ergotamine, especially with regard to GI and peripheral vascular effects. In one study, subcutaneously administered **sumatriptan** appeared to be more effective than DHE nasal spray; however, DHE was better tolerated.[6]

ERGOTAMINE TARTRATE
Ergomar, Ergostat, Various

Pharmacology. Ergotamine is an ergot alkaloid that is hypothesized to exert its antimigraine effects via its agonist activity at the serotonin 5-HT$_{1D}$ receptor, resulting in vasoconstriction of intracranial blood vessels and inhibition of inflammatory neuropeptide release. The drug also binds with high affinity to adrenergic receptors; however, the antimigraine effect of this binding is unknown. The mechanism in migraine is thought to be vasoconstriction of cranial blood vessels, with a concomitant decrease in the amplitude of pulsations as well as depression of serotonergic neurons that mediate pain.

Administration and Adult Dosage. PO for migraine 2 mg initially, then 1 mg each ½ hr prn, to a maximum of 6 mg/day or 10 mg/week; **PR** 2 mg initially, may repeat in 1 hr prn, to a maximum of 4 mg/attack or 10 mg/week; **SL** 2 mg initially, then 2 mg q 30 min as needed, to a maximum of 6 mg/day or 10 mg/week.[7] Titrate the dosage during several attacks gradually, then administer the minimum effective dosage with subsequent attacks. Patients who routinely require over 2 mg/headache can be given the total effective dosage at the onset of the headache.

Special Populations. *Pediatric Dosage.* Safety and efficacy not established. (>12 yr) 1 mg initially, then 1 mg q 30 min prn, to a maximum of 3 mg/attack.

Geriatric Dosage. No specific data are available.

Other Conditions. Decrease dosage by 50% in patients receiving methysergide as prophylaxis.

Dosage Forms. SL Tab 2 mg; **Tab** 1 mg with caffeine 100 mg (Cafergot, Ercaf, various); **Supp** 2 mg with caffeine 100 mg (Cafergot, Wigraine).

Patient Instructions. Initiate therapy at the first signs of an attack. Take only as directed and do not exceed recommended dosages. Report tingling or pain in extremities immediately.

Pharmacokinetics. *Onset and Duration.* Onset (oral) 5 hr; (rectal) 1–3 hr.[7]

Serum Levels. 200 ng/L (176 pmol/L) or greater appears to be therapeutic; a high frequency of adverse reactions has been associated with levels >1.8 µg/L (1.5 nmol/L).[7]

Fate. Bioavailability 1–2% orally, 5% rectally; relative bioavailability decreases in the following order: PR > PO > SL.[7,8] Peak serum level after 2 mg rectally is 454 ± 407 ng/L (390 ± 350 pmol/L), 50 ± 43 min after the dose. Peak serum level after 2 mg with caffeine 100 mg orally is 21 ± 12 ng/L (18 ± 11 pmol/L), 69 ± 191 min after the dose.[8] V_d is 1.9 ± 0.8 L/kg; Cl is 0.68 ± 0.24 L/hr/kg.[9] The drug is extensively metabolized in the liver, with 90% of metabolites excreted in the bile.

$t_{1/2}$. 1.9 ± 0.3 hr; apparent half-life is 3.4 ± 1.9 hr after rectal administration because of slow absorption.[7,8]

Adverse Reactions. Nausea and vomiting occur frequently. Signs and symptoms of ergotamine intoxication include weakness in legs, coldness and muscle pain in extremities, numbness or tingling of fingers and toes, precordial pain, transient tachycardia or bradycardia, and localized edema; these rarely develop with recommended dosages. Frequent or worsening headaches can occur with frequent, long-term, or excessive dosages. Ergotamine dependence can result in withdrawal symptoms occurring within 24–48 hr after drug discontinuation.[7,10] Rectal or anal ulceration can occur with suppository use.

Contraindications. Pregnancy; peripheral vascular disease; coronary artery disease; hypertension; hepatic or renal impairment; sepsis; severe pruritus.

Precautions. Lactation; avoid excessive dosage or prolonged administration because of the potential for ergotism and gangrene.

Drug Interactions. β-Blockers, dopamine, and epinephrine can cause increased vasoconstriction and increased risk of peripheral ischemia or hypertension. The macrolides (especially erythromycin and troleandomycin) can inhibit the metabolism of ergot alkaloids.

Notes. The stimulant action of preparations containing **caffeine** can keep patients from the beneficial effects of sleep. Caffeine, however, can improve dissolution of the oral formulation. Ergotamine is commonly used for abortive therapy of migraine and provides relief in 50–90% of patients.[7] **Aspirin** (650 mg) or **naproxen** (750–1250 mg/day) might be effective in aborting migraine headache in mild cases or in patients who cannot take ergotamine. OTC products containing aspirin, **acetaminophen**, and caffeine (Excedrin Migraine) or **ibuprofen** (Advil Migraine, Motrin Migraine) have FDA approval for mild to moderate migraine. Prescription combination products such as **Midrin** and **Fiorinal** might be useful, but overuse of any antimigraine combination product can lead to rebound headache. **NSAIDs** are useful for prophylaxis against menstrual-related migraines when taken during the perimenstrual period. **Butorphanol** spray might be beneficial for patients with infrequent, severe headaches who cannot tolerate ergot products or triptans, but frequent use can cause dependency. The β-**blockers propranolol** and **timolol** are approved by the FDA for migraine prophylaxis, but other β-blockers without intrinsic sympathomimetic activity (eg, **atenolol, nadolol**) are also useful. **Verapamil** can prevent migraines in some patients but can take several months to reach maximum effectiveness. **Tricyclic antidepressants** (eg, **amitriptyline, nortriptyline**) have been more successful in migraine prophylaxis than SSRIs. **Divalproex** has been used successfully for prophylaxis. Consider frequency of attacks (more than 2/month), co-morbid conditions, and side effects when choosing prophylactic therapy. Effective doses for migraine prophylaxis drugs are usually lower than those used for other indications.[11]

METHYSERGIDE MALEATE   Sansert

Pharmacology. Methysergide is a semisynthetic ergot alkaloid, thought to act centrally as a serotonin agonist and to inhibit blood vessel permeability to humoral factors that affect pain threshold. Unlike other ergots, methysergide does not inhibit reuptake of norepinephrine and has minimal oxytocic, vasoconstrictor, and α-adrenergic blocking effects. Because of its toxicity, methysergide is usually used only after other prophylactic measures have failed.

Adult Dosage. PO for migraine or cluster headache prophylaxis 4–8 mg/day with food. A drug-free interval of 3–4 weeks must follow each 6-month course; however, reduce the dosage gradually to avoid rebound headache.

Dosage Forms. Tab 2 mg.

Pharmacokinetics. Methysergide undergoes extensive liver metabolism to **methylergonovine**, a compound with greater activity and a longer elimination half-life than the parent drug (3.5 hr vs 1 hr). About 56% of an oral dose is eliminated in the urine as unchanged drug and metabolites.

Adverse Reactions. Insomnia, postural hypotension, nausea, vomiting, diarrhea, and peripheral ischemia occur frequently. Occasionally, heartburn, peripheral edema, rash, or arrhythmias occur. Rarely, mental depression occurs. Long-term (>6 months) therapy can cause retroperitoneal and pleuropulmonary fibrosis and thickening of cardiac valves. The drug is contraindicated in peripheral vascular, cardiovascular, or pulmonary disease; phlebitis; pregnancy; and impaired liver or kidney function. Precautions and drug interactions are similar to those of ergotamine.[12]

SUMATRIPTAN SUCCINATE   Imitrex

Pharmacology. Sumatriptan is a serotonin (5-HT) analogue and a selective agonist at 5-HT_{1D} receptors in cerebral vascular smooth muscle. Receptor activation results in migraine relief by vasoconstriction of intracranial blood vessels and attenuation of the release of vasoactive peptides responsible for inflammation of sensory nerves.[13,14] (*See also* Selective Serotonin Agonists Comparison Chart.)

Administration and Adult Dosage. **PO for migraine** 25–100 mg; a second dose of up to 100 mg may be administered in 2 hr if response is unsatisfactory. A 100 mg dose might not provide any greater effect than a 50 mg dose. If headache returns, additional doses may be given q 2 hr, up to 200 mg in a 24-hr period. **SC for migraine** 6 mg; a second 6 mg injection may be administered 1 hr after the initial dose, but limited to no more than 2 injections within a 24-hr period. Controlled studies have not verified a beneficial effect of a second dose. **Intranasal** 5–20 mg in one nostril or 5 mg in each nostril; may repeat in 2 hr to a maximum of 40 mg/day.

Special Populations. *Pediatric Dosage.* (<18 yr) safety and efficacy not established.

Geriatric Dosage. Same as adult dosage. Consider the possibility of undiagnosed heart disease in the elderly.

Dosage Forms. **Tab** 25, 50 mg; **Inj** 6 mg/0.5 mL; **Nasal spray** 5, 20 mg.

Patient Instructions. Sumatriptan is used for relief of migraine and not for the prevention of a migraine attack. Do not take this drug if you are pregnant without consulting with your physician. Inform your physician if you have high blood pressure, diabetes, seizures, or heart, liver, or kidney disease. Report pain or tightness in chest, shortness of breath, wheezing, or rash immediately. **Oral.** Do not take more than 200 mg within 24 hours and allow at least 2 hours after the first tablet. **SC injection.** Do not take more than 2 injections within 24 hours and allow at least 1 hour between injections. Pain or redness at injection site lasts less than 1 hour. **Nasal spray.** If 1 dose does not provide adequate relief, you may take another dose after 2 hours. Do not take more than 40 mg in 1 day.

Pharmacokinetics. *Onset and Duration.* PO 50% of patients respond in 2 hr; peak 1.5 hr. SC 70% of patients respond within 1 hr and 90% within 2 hr;[15] peak 10–15 min.[16] **Intranasal** 50–60% of patients respond in 2 hr.

Fate. Oral bioavailability is $14 \pm 3\%$ owing to presystemic metabolism and erratic absorption. Absorption is delayed by about 0.5 hr if taken with food. After a 100 mg oral dose, a peak of 54 μg/L (180 nmol/L) occurs in about 1.5 hr. SC bioavailability is $97 \pm 16\%$; a peak of 74 μg/L (250 nmol/L) occurs in 12 min after a 6 mg SC dose. After a 20 mg intranasal dose, the mean peak is 16 μg/L (54 nmol/L). Plasma protein binding is 14–21%. V_d is 2.7 L/kg; Cl is 0.96 ± 0.12 L/hr/kg. Hepatic metabolism is by MAO-A to an indole acetic acid, followed by glucuronidation and renal elimination. About 40% is found in the feces and 60% is excreted renally, 22% unchanged, and 40% as the active indole acetic acid metabolite.[17-19]

$t_{1/2}$. 1.9 ± 0.3 hr.[19]

Adverse Reactions. Frequent side effects are pain and redness at SC injection site, tingling, hot flushes, dizziness, and chest tightness or heaviness. With the nasal spray, throat discomfort and unusual taste occur frequently. With all routes of administration, occasional weakness, myalgia, burning sensation, tightness in chest, transient hypertension, drowsiness, headache, numbness, neck pain, abdominal discomfort, mouth/jaw discomfort, and sweating occur. Rarely, cardiac arrhythmias, myocardial ischemia, polydipsia, dehydration, dyspnea, skin rashes, dysuria, and dysmenorrhea occur. The drug can accumulate in melanin-rich tissues such as the eye with long-term use. Several cases of ischemic colitis have been reported after sumatriptan use.

Contraindications. IV administration; ischemic heart disease; Prinzmetal's angina; uncontrolled hypertension; concurrent administration of MAO inhibitors or within 2 weeks of discontinuation; within 24 hr of an ergotamine-containing drug or ergot derivative such as methysergide or dihydroergotamine; hemiplegic or basilar migraine.

Precautions. Pregnancy. Use with caution in those with impaired hepatic function, seizure disorder, neurologic lesion, or cardiovascular disease; postmenopausal women; or men >40 yr.

Drug Interactions. Nonselective MAO inhibitors or MAO-A inhibitors can increase the systemic availability of sumatriptan (especially after oral administration). Theoretically, ergot alkaloids and sumatriptan can cause prolonged vasospastic reactions if used together. (*See* Contraindications.) SSRIs can cause weakness, hyperreflexia, and incoordination when given with sumatriptan and other triptans.

Parameters to Monitor. Renal, hepatic, and cardiovascular status initially and q 6 months.

Notes. Subcutaneous sumatriptan is much more expensive than alternatives. It is effective in the treatment of cluster headache and appears to be more effective than ergotamine/caffeine in aborting migraine.[20] (*See* Selective Serotonin Agonists Comparison Chart.)

SELECTIVE SEROTONIN AGONISTS COMPARISON CHART

DRUG	DOSAGE FORMS	ADULT DOSAGE	ONSET (HR)	HALF-LIFE (HR)	COMMENTS
Almotriptan Axert	Tab 6.25, 12.5 mg.	PO 12.5 mg.	1–2	3–3.7	Low headache recurrence rate. Similar efficacy to oral sumatriptan, but better tolerated. No propranolol interaction.
Eletriptan Relpax (Investigational—Pfizer)	—	PO 20–80 mg.	1–2	4–7	An 80 mg dose is superior to 100 mg of oral sumatriptan. Does not induce CYP3A4.
Frovatriptan (Investigational—Elan)	—	PO 2.5 mg.	2–4	25	Lowest recurrence rate.
Naratriptan Amerge	Tab 1, 2.5 mg.	PO 1–2.5 mg, may repeat in 2 hr; may repeat sequence once in 4 hr, to a maximum of 5 mg/day.	1–3	6	Low headache recurrence rate. More specific than other agents for $5HT_{1B}$. Smoking increases and oral contraceptives decrease clearance.
Rizatriptan Maxalt Maxalt-MLT	Tab 5, 10 mg (conventional and rapidly dissolving).	PO 5–10 mg; may repeat in 2 hr, to a maximum of 30 mg/day.	0.5–2	2–3	Onset of rapidly dissolving tablet is slightly *slower* than conventional. Reduce dose when used with propranolol.
Sumatriptan Imitrex	Inj 6 mg Tab 25, 50 mg Nasal Spray 5, 20 mg/spray.	SC 6 mg, may repeat once in 1 hr, to a maximum of 12 mg/day. PO 25–100 mg, may repeat q 2 hr to a maximum of 200 mg/day. Nasal 5–20 mg, may repeat once in 2 hr to a maximum of 40 mg/day.	0.2 (SC) 0.5–1 (PO) <1 (Nasal)	2.5	Headache recurrence rate of 40%; relatively high (5%) frequency of chest pain and tightness.
Zolmitriptan Zomig Zomig-ZMT	Tab 2.5, 5 mg. Tab (rapidly dissolving) 2.5 mg.	PO 2.5–5 mg, may repeat once in 2 hr to a maximum of 10 mg/day.	0.5–2	3	Cimetidine or oral contraceptives increase AUC by 50%.

From references 13, 14, and 21–29 and product information.

9

Antirheumatic Drugs

ETANERCEPT
Enbrel

Pharmacology. Etanercept is a dimeric fusion protein that binds to tumor necrosis factor (TNFα and β) and blocks its interaction with TNF receptors on the cell surface. This reduces the signs and symptoms of rheumatoid arthritis and delays joint damage in adults with moderate to severe rheumatoid arthritis. It is indicated for patients with inadequate response to one or more disease-modifying drugs.

Administration and Adult Dosage. SC for rheumatoid arthritis 25 mg twice weekly (72–96 hr apart).

Special Populations. *Pediatric Dosage.* (<4 yr) safety and efficacy not established; (4–17 yr) **SC for juvenile rheumatoid arthritis** 0.4 mg/kg twice weekly, not to exceed 25 mg per dose.

Geriatric Dosage. Same as adult dosage.

Dosage Forms. Inj 25 mg.

Patient Instructions. This drug may be self-administered. Instruct patient on proper injection preparation and subcutaneous injection technique along with appropriate syringe and needle disposal methods. Rotate the injection sites and give injections at least 1 inch from an old site; avoid tender, bruised, red, or hard areas. Inform your physician immediately of any persistent fever, bruising, bleeding, or pallor. (*See also* Notes.)

Missed Doses. Injections should be given 72–96 hours apart. Give a missed dose as soon as possible and resume usual schedule.

Pharmacokinetics. *Fate.* Bioavailability with SC injection is 58%, with peak plasma concentrations achieved within 48–96 hr. Median clearance is 52 mL/hr/m^2.

$t_{1/2}$. 115 hr.

Adverse Reactions. Injection site reactions that involve mild to moderate erythema, itching, pain, or swelling occur in about 37% of patients. Upper respiratory infections, headache, rhinitis, dizziness, pharyngitis, and cough occur frequently. Etanercept is well tolerated in children with juvenile rheumatoid arthritis, with adverse reactions similar to those experienced by adults.[30] Rare cases of CNS demyelinating disorders and pancytopenia have been reported.

Contraindications. Sepsis.

Precautions. Do not administer to patients with active infections or children with significant exposure to varicella virus. In patients with juvenile rheumatoid arthritis exposed to varicella zoster, temporarily discontinue etanercept and give varicella zoster immune globulin. Update vaccinations before initiating etanercept therapy. Do not give live vaccines during etanercept therapy. The needle cover provided with the diluent syringe contains latex and should not be handled by those with latex allergy. Administer with caution to patients with recent history of CNS demyelinating disorders.

Parameters to Monitor. Monitor patients closely for infection and hematologic abnormalities during therapy. Discontinue treatment if serious infection, sepsis, or hematologic abnormality develops.

Drug Interactions. None known.

Notes. Etanercept sterile powder must be refrigerated at 2–8°C (38–46°F); do not freeze. Reconstitute 25 mg vial with 1 mL of bacteriostatic sterile water (included); inject diluent slowly to avoid foaming. Administer the solution as soon as possible after reconstitution; however, the solution may be stored under refrigeration for up to 6 hr in the vial. Etanercept may be used concurrently with other rheumatoid arthritis therapies such as analgesics, corticosteroids, or methotrexate. Etanercept is also being studied for the treatment of CHF, endometriosis, organ transplantation, and cachexia.[31]

INFLIXIMAB   Remicade

Pharmacology. Infliximab is a chimeric monoclonal antibody that binds to soluble and transmembrane forms of TNFα, thereby neutralizing the activity of TNFα and inhibiting TNFα binding to its receptor sites. It has no effect on lymphotoxin (TNFβ).[32,33] Infliximab induces pro-inflammatory cytokines including interleukins 1 and 6 and increases endothelial cell permeability by enhancing leukocyte migration.

Administration and Adult Dosage. **IV infusion for rheumatoid arthritis** 3 mg/kg, with repeat infusions at weeks 2 and 6, then q 8 weeks thereafter. For rheumatoid arthritis, infliximab is indicated to be used with methotrexate. **IV for moderately to severely active Crohn's disease** 5 mg/kg as a single IV infusion. Some patients might benefit from treatment q 8 weeks after the single infusion.[34] **IV for fistulizing Crohn's disease** 5 mg/kg at weeks 0, 2, and 6. (*See* Notes.)

Special Populations. *Pediatric Dosage.* Safety and efficacy not established.

Geriatric Dosage. Same as adult dosage.

Dosage Forms. **Inj** 100 mg.

Patient Instructions. Infliximab is administered intravenously by your health care professional. Notify your physician if chest pain, fever, chills, facial flushing, itching, hives, or difficult breathing occurs within a few hours of administration.

Pharmacokinetics. *Fate.* Infliximab is distributed primarily within the vascular compartment. Direct and linear relationship between dose, maximum serum concentration, and AUC. Age and weight do not affect Cl or V_d. No systemic accumulation of infliximab occurs.

$t_{1/2}$. 8–9.5 days.

Adverse Reactions. Serious infections have been reported. Infusion-related reactions such as fever, chills, pruritus, urticaria, chest pain, hypotension, hypertension, and dyspnea have occurred during or within the 2-hr postinfusion period. If these reactions occur, slow the infusion rate. Reactions occurring in ≥5% of patients include headache, nausea, abdominal pain, fatigue, fever, pharyngitis, vomiting, pain, dizziness, bronchitis, rash, rhinitis, chest pain, coughing, pruritus, sinusitis, myalgia, and back pain. Hypersensitivity reactions to infliximab can occur and antibodies to infliximab develop in about 13% of patients. Patients most likely to experience infusion-related reactions are those who developed antibodies.[35] Have medications (eg, acetaminophen, antihistamine, corticosteroid, and epinephrine) available for immediate use in the event of a hypersensitivity reaction. Lupus-like syndrome (1 in 340 patients)[36] and lymphoproliferative disorders occur rarely.

Contraindications. Hypersensitivity to murine proteins; presence of serious infection.

Precautions. Women should use adequate contraception for the duration of and at least 6 months after therapy.[32] Use caution when infliximab is administered with immunosuppressive therapy or to patients who have a history of infections. Avoid use in patients with known GI luminal strictures.[32]

Parameters to Monitor. Monitor patients closely for adverse effects, especially for infusion-related reactions during or within the 2-hr postinfusion period and for infection during therapy. (Crohn's disease) Observe for improvement in abdominal cramping and in bowel consistence and rectal bleeding.

Drug Interactions. None known.

Notes. Dilute the total volume of the reconstituted infliximab solution dose to 250 mL with 0.9% NaCl. Gently mix. Administer over at least 2 hr through a non-pyrogenic, low protein-binding filter with a pore size of $\leq 1.2 \, \mu$.

Infliximab has been reported to be effective in the treatment of severe esophageal Crohn's disease[37] and refractory perineal cutaneous Crohn's disease.[38]

LEFLUNOMIDE Arava

Pharmacology. Leflunomide's active metabolite (M1) inhibits dihydro-oratate dehydrogenase, thereby inhibiting pyrimidine biosynthesis. M1 exhibits immunomodulating and anti-inflammatory effects.

Administration and Adult Dosage. **PO for rheumatoid arthritis** 100 mg/day for 3 days, then 20 mg/day. Reduce dose to 10 mg if 20 mg is not tolerated.

Special Populations. *Pediatric Dosage.* Safety and efficacy not established.

Geriatric Dosage. Same as adult dosage.

Dosage Forms. **Tab** 10, 20, 100 mg.

Patient Instructions. Do not use if you are pregnant or planning to become pregnant. Men should use condoms because leflunomide can cause birth defects. Also, men planning on fathering children should discontinue leflunomide therapy and consult with their physicians. If you experience any major medical problems while on therapy, notify your physician. Avoid alcohol because this medication with alcohol can increase the risk of liver damage. Avoid immunizations unless approved by your physician.

Missed Doses. Take a missed dose as soon as you remember; if it is near the time for next dose, skip the dose; do not take a double dose.

Pharmacokinetics. *Fate.* Leflunomide is 80% bioavailable, with peak plasma levels achieved in 6–12 hr. Because of its long half-life, an oral loading dosage is given over 3 days. Leflunomide is metabolized to a primary active metabolite (M1), with the parent drug rarely detectable in plasma. The specific site of metabolism is unknown; however, hepatic cytosolic and microsomal cellular fractions have been identified. V_{dss} of M1 is 0.13 L/kg; 99.3% is bound to albumin. M1 is eliminated by renal and biliary routes. Approximately 45% is eliminated as glucuronide and oxanilic acid metabolites in the urine and 48% as M1 in the feces.

$t_{1/2}$. (M1) 18 ± 9 days.

Adverse Reactions. Diarrhea, dyspepsia, hypertension, headache, rash, alopecia, and elevated liver function tests occur frequently. (*See* Notes.)

Contraindications. Immunocompromised patients; those positive for hepatitis B or C; pre-existing hepatic impairment; women planning to conceive.

Precautions. Caution in patients with renal insufficiency. Do not give live vaccines to patients receiving leflunomide.

Drug Interactions. Potentially hepatotoxic medications such as methotrexate can increase risk of hepatotoxicity. Rifampin increases peak plasma levels of M1. M1 inhibits CYP2C9. Plasma-free fraction of NSAIDs and tolbutamide levels might be increased. Co-administration with cholestyramine or activated charcoal decreases M1 levels.

Parameters to Monitor. Monitor ALT at baseline and then monthly. If ALT levels are stable, monitor per clinical judgment.

Notes. If toxicity develops or if plasma levels must be decreased quickly, follow this drug elimination protocol: administer cholestyramine 8 g tid for 11 days. Verify that plasma levels are <0.02 mg/L by 2 separate tests at least 14 days apart. Without this procedure, drug elimination can take up to 2 yr. Leflunomide is equally or more effective than traditional antirheumatic agents such as methotrexate, sulfasalazine, injectable gold, and cyclosporine.[39]

ANTIRHEUMATIC DRUGS COMPARISON CHART

DRUG	DOSAGE FORMS	ADULT DOSAGE	ADVERSE EFFECTS	LABORATORY MONITORING
Auranofin Ridaura	Cap 3 mg.	PO 3–9 mg/day (3 mg as a single dose and 6 and 9 mg/day as 2 and 3 divided doses, respectively).	Loose stools, diarrhea, abdominal pain or cramping, rash, pruritus, stomatitis.	CBC, platelets, urine dipstick for protein q 4–12 weeks.
Aurothioglucose Solganal	Inj 50 mg/mL.	IM 25–50 mg at 3–4 week intervals.	Cutaneous reactions, stomatitis, gingivitis, glossitis, hematologic toxicity, nephrotoxicity, hepatotoxicity.	CBC, platelets, urine dipstick q 1–2 weeks for first 20 weeks, then q 1–2 months.
Azathioprine Imuran	Tab 50 mg.	PO 1–2.5 mg/kg/day.	Myelosuppression, nausea, vomiting, anorexia, diarrhea, hepatotoxicity.	CBC, platelets q 1–2 weeks with changes in dosage and q 1–3 months thereafter.
Cyclosporine Neoral[a]	Cap 25, 100 mg. Soln 100 mg/mL.	PO 1.2–7.5 mg/kg/day in divided doses.	Nephrotoxicity, hypertension, tremor, hirsutism, gingival hyperplasia, diarrhea, nausea, vomiting.	C_rs q 2 weeks until stable dosage, then monthly; periodic CBC, K^+, and LFTs.
Etanercept Enbrel	Inj 25 mg.	IV 25 mg twice weekly.	Erythema, itching, pain, swelling at inj site; headache, rhinitis, dizziness, cough.	None.
Gold Sodium Thiomalate Aurolate	Inj 10, 25, 50 mg/mL.	IM 25–50 mg q 2 weeks for 2–20 weeks (may increase interval to 3–4 weeks if stable).	See aurothioglucose.	See aurothioglucose.
Hydroxychloroquine Sulfate Plaquenil	Tab 200 mg.	PO 200–400 mg/day.	Retinopathy, nausea, vomiting, diarrhea, pruritus.	None.

(continued)

14

ANTIRHEUMATIC DRUGS COMPARISON CHART (*continued*)

DRUG	DOSAGE FORMS	ADULT DOSAGE	ADVERSE EFFECTS	LABORATORY MONITORING
Infliximab[b] Remicade	Inj 100 mg.	IV 3 mg/kg, repeat at weeks 2 and 6, then q 8 weeks. Can be given to patients on methotrexate.	Infusion reactions, headache, nausea, fatigue, myalgia, rhinitis, pain, pruritus, urticaria, hypo- or hypertension, chest pain, vomiting, dyspnea.	None.
Leflunomide Arava	Tab 10, 20, 100 mg.	20 mg once daily.	Diarrhea, respiratory infection, headache, nausea, rash, liver enzyme elevations, dyspepsia, alopecia, hypertension, teratogenicity.	ALT monthly during initial therapy, then periodically.
Methotrexate Mexate-AQ Rheumatrex Various	Tab 2.5 mg Inj 2.5 mg/mL.	PO 7.5–25 mg (as a single dose or 3 divided doses) once weekly; or SC or IM 7.5–25 mg once weekly.	Myelosuppression, stomatitis, abdominal distress, diarrhea, nausea, vomiting, hepatotoxicity, pulmonary toxicity.	CBC, platelets, AST, serum albumin, Cr$_S$ q 4–8 weeks.
Penicillamine Cuprimine Depen	Cap 125, 250 mg Tab 250 mg.	PO 500–750 mg/day as a single daily dose (up to 500 mg) or in divided doses if >500 mg.	Sensitivity reaction with skin rash, renal and hematologic toxicity.	CBC, urine dipstick for protein q 2 weeks until dosage is stable, then q 1–3 months.
Sulfasalazine Azulfidine Various	Tab 500 mg.	PO 2 g/day in 2 divided doses.	Nausea, vomiting, heartburn, dizziness, headache, hypersensitivity, skin rash, leukopenia.	CBC q 2–4 weeks for first 3 months, then q 3 months.

[a]Neoral, a nonaqueous liquid formulation forms an emulsion in aqueous fluids and has a higher oral bioavailability than conventional formulations (ie, Sandimmune, which is not indicated for rheumatoid arthritis). Do not use these products interchangeably.
[b]FDA-approved for use in patients taking methotrexate.
Adapted from references 40–44.

Nonsteroidal Anti-inflammatory Drugs

ACETAMINOPHEN   Various

Pharmacology. Acetaminophen possesses analgesic and antipyretic activities with few anti-inflammatory effects. It has the same effectiveness as aspirin in inhibiting brain prostaglandin synthetase but very little activity as a peripheral prostaglandin inhibitor. This difference from aspirin and other NSAIDs might explain its relative lack of effectiveness as an anti-inflammatory, antirheumatic agent. Acetaminophen does not inhibit normal platelet action, prothrombin activity, or adversely affect GI mucosal health.

Administration and Adult Dosage. **PO for pain or fever** (non-SR) 325–1000 mg q 4–6 hr, to a maximum of 4 g/day; (SR Tab) 1300 mg q 8 hr. **PR for pain or fever** 650 mg q 4–6 hr, to a maximum of 4 g/day.

Special Populations. *Pediatric Dosage.* **PO for pain or fever** 10–15 mg/kg q 4–8 hr, may repeat dose q 4 hr, not to exceed 5 doses per day; or (up to 3 months) 40 mg/dose, (4–11 months) 80 mg/dose, (12–23 months) 120 mg/dose, (2–3 yr) 160 mg/dose, (4–5 yr) 240 mg/dose, (6–8 yr) 320 mg/dose, (9–10 yr) 400 mg/dose, (11 yr) 480 mg/dose, (12–14 yr) 640 mg/dose, (>14 yr) 650 mg/dose. **PR for pain or fever** (3–11 months) 80 mg q 6 hr, (1–3 yr) 80 mg q 4 hr, (3–6 yr) 120 to 125 mg q 4–6 hr, to a maximum of 720 mg/day; (6–12 yr) 325 mg q 4–6 hr, to a maximum of 2.6 g/day; (>12 yr) same as adult dosage.

Geriatric Dosage. Same as adult dosage.

Dosage Forms. **Cap** 325, 500 mg; **Gelcap** 500 mg; **Chew Tab** 80, 160 mg; **SR Tab** 650 mg; **Tab** 160, 325, 500, 650 mg; **Drp** 48, 100 mg/mL; **Elxr** 16, 24, 26, 32, 65 mg/mL; **Syrup** 32 mg/mL; **Supp** 80, 120, 125, 300, 325, 650 mg.

Patient Instructions. Do not exceed the maximum recommended daily dosage of 4 g (2 g in alcoholics). Report unresponsive fever or continued pain persisting for more than 3–5 days to your physician. Do not use with other anti-inflammatory agents unless directed by your physician.

Missed Doses. If you take this drug on a regular schedule, take a missed dose as soon as you remember. If it is about time for the next dose, take that dose only; do not double the dose or take extra.

Pharmacokinetics. *Serum Levels.* (Analgesia, antipyresis) 10–20 mg/L (66–132 μmol/L). Serum concentrations >300 mg/L (2 mmol/L) at 4 hr or 45 mg/L (300 μmol/L) at 12 hr after acute overdosage are associated with severe hepatic damage, whereas toxicity is unlikely if levels are <120 mg/L (800 μmol/L) at 4 hr or 30 mg/L (200 μmol/L) at 12 hr.[21] (*See* Notes.)

Fate. Rapid absorption from the GI tract, with peak plasma concentrations being achieved within 0.5–2 hr. Absorption of liquid preparations is more rapid. Unbound to plasma proteins at therapeutic doses; 20–50% bound in overdose. Extensively metabolized in the liver to inactive conjugates of glucuronic and sulfuric acids and cysteine (saturable) and to a hepatotoxic intermediate metabolite (first-order) by CYP1A2 and CYP2E1. The intermediate is detoxified by glutathione (saturable). V_d is 0.95 ± 0.12 L/kg; Cl is 0.3 ± 0.084 L/hr/kg, decreased in hepatitis and increased in hyperthyroidism, pregnancy, and obesity; 2–3% excreted unchanged in urine.[21]

$t_{1/2}$. 2 ± 0.5 hr, decreased in hyperthyroidism and pregnancy, and increased in hepatitis and neonates.[21]

Adverse Reactions. Nontoxic at therapeutic doses. In acute overdose (single dose equaling or exceeding 10 g or 7.5–10 g daily for 1–2 days), potentially fatal hepatic necrosis and possible renal tubular necrosis can occur, but clinical and laboratory evidence of hepatotoxicity might be delayed for several days. (*See* Serum Levels.) Toxic hepatitis also has been associated with long-term ingestion of 5–8 g/day for several weeks or 3–4 g/day for a year. Occasionally, maculopapular rash or urticarial skin reactions occur; methemoglobinemia, neutropenia, and thrombocytopenic purpura are rarely reported. Analgesic nephropathy has been associated with the consumption of 1–15.3 kg of acetaminophen over 3–23 yr.[45]

Contraindications. G6PD deficiency.

Precautions. Use with caution in chronic alcoholics (not to exceed 2 g/day) and patients with phenylalanine hydroxylase deficiency (phenylketonuria) or G6PD deficiency. Some formulations contain aspartame, which is metabolized to phenylalanine; therefore do not use these products in patients with phenylketonuria. Also, some products contain sulfites.

Drug Interactions. Chronic alcoholics might be at increased risk for hepatic toxicity.[46] The risk of hepatotoxicity also is increased by long-term use of other enzyme inducers (eg, barbiturates, carbamazepine, phenytoin, rifampin, sulfinpyrazone) and acetaminophen's efficacy also can be decreased by these agents. Co-administration with isoniazid increases the risk of hepatotoxicity; therefore, avoid acetaminophen in persons on isoniazid. Acetaminophen occasionally increases the anticoagulant effect of warfarin; therefore, monitor INR closely when adding or discontinuing long-term acetaminophen use.[47]

Notes. Management of acute overdosage includes emesis and/or gastric lavage, if no more than a few hours have elapsed since ingestion. Supportive measures such as respiratory support and fluid and electrolyte therapy are recommended in addition. Administration of activated charcoal is not recommended because it can interfere with the absorption of acetylcysteine, which is used in the treatment of severe acute overdosage. Potentially dangerous acetaminophen levels (*see* Serum Levels) can be managed by the administration of 140 mg/kg acetylcysteine diluted 1:3 in a soft drink or plain water; follow with 70 mg/kg q 4 hr for 17 doses. If administered within 8–16 hr of ingestion, this therapy has been shown to minimize the expected hepatotoxicity, but treatment is still indicated as late as 24 hr after ingestion, with some data showing effectiveness up to 36 hr postingestion.[48]

For the short-term treatment of osteoarthritis of the knee, acetaminophen 2.6 and 4 g/day are comparable to **naproxen** 750 mg/day and **ibuprofen** 1.2–2.4 g/day, respectively.[49]

ASPIRIN Various

Pharmacology. Aspirin is an analgesic, antipyretic, and anti-inflammatory agent. Anti-inflammatory properties are related to the inhibition of prostaglandin biosynthesis. Aspirin nonselectively inhibits cyclo-oxygenase-1 (COX-1), which is associated with GI and renal effects and inhibition of platelet aggregation, and cyclo-oxygenase-2 (COX-2), which is associated with the inflammatory response. Unlike other NSAIDs, its antiplatelet effect is irreversible and permanent (because of transacetylation of platelet COX) for the life of the platelet (8–11 days). Salicylates without acetyl groups (eg, **sodium salicylate**) have essentially no antiplatelet effect but retain analgesic, antipyretic, and anti-inflammatory activities. Low dosages (1–2 g/day) decrease urate excretion; high dosages (>5 g/day) induce uricosuria.[50]

Administration and Adult Dosage. **PO or PR for fever or minor pain** 325–1000 mg q 4-6 hr, to a maximum of 4 g/day. **PO for arthritis and rheumatic conditions** 3.6–5.4 g/day in 3–4 divided doses. **PO for acute rheumatic fever** 5–8 g/day in divided doses. **PO for prevention of TIAs or stroke** 81–325 mg/day.[51] **PO for myocardial infarction risk reduction** (primary prevention in healthy men >50 yr with at least one major cardiovascular risk factor) 81–325 mg/day; (secondary prevention) 162–325 mg/day.[52] **PO for unstable angina** 162–325 mg/day.[52] **PO for prevention of coronary artery bypass graft occlusion** 325 mg/day started 6 hr postoperatively and continued for 1 yr.[53] **PO for nonrheumatic atrial fibrillation** (patients who are poor candidates for, or decline, oral anticoagulants) 325 mg/day; (patients <75 yr with no risk factors for stroke) 325 mg/day.[53] The optimum dosage for platelet inhibition has not been determined; doses as low as 50 mg/day inhibit platelet aggregation and provide effective protection against thrombosis.[54]

Special Populations. *Pediatric Dosage.* **PO for juvenile rheumatoid arthritis** 60–110 mg/kg/day in divided doses. **PO for acute rheumatic fever** 100 mg/kg/day in divided doses initially for 2 weeks, then 75 mg/kg/day in divided doses for 4–6 weeks. **PO for Kawasaki disease** 80–120 mg/kg/day; decrease to 10 mg/kg/day after fever resolves. (*See* Precautions.) **PO as an analgesic/antipyretic** 10–15 mg/kg/dose q 4 hr, to a maximum of 60–80 mg/kg/day. Alternatively, (2–3 yr) 162 mg q 4 hr; (4–5 yr) 243 mg q 4 hr; (6–8 yr) 325 mg q 4 hr; (9–10 yr) 405 mg q 4 hr; (11 yr) 486 mg q 4 hr; (≥12 yr) 650 mg q 4 hr. (*See* Precautions.)

Geriatric Dosage. Use minimal effective dosages; elderly are more susceptible to GI bleeding and acute renal insufficiency. **PO for MI risk reduction** (healthy men >50 yr for primary prevention with cardiovascular risk factors) 81–325 mg/day.[52]

Other Conditions. Uremia or reduced albumin levels are likely to produce higher unbound drug levels that can increase pharmacologic or toxic effects. Dosage reduction might be required in these patients (eg, kidney disease, malnutrition).

Dosage Forms. **Chew Tab** 81 mg; **EC Tab** 81, 165, 325, 500, 650, 975 mg; **SR Tab** 650, 800 mg; **Tab** 81, 325, 500 mg; **Supp** 120, 200, 300, 600 mg.

Patient Instructions. Children and teenagers (<16 yr) should not use aspirin-containing medications for chickenpox or flu symptoms because of the association with Reye's syndrome, a rare but serious illness. Take this drug with food, milk, or a full glass of water to minimize stomach upset; report any symptoms of gastrointestinal ulceration or bleeding. Contact your physician if ringing in the ears or gastrointestinal pain occurs. Do not crush or chew enteric-coated or sustained-release preparations. Avoid other products containing aspirin or nonsteroidal anti-inflammatory drugs.

Missed Doses. If you take this drug on a regular schedule and you miss a dose, take it as soon as you remember. If it is about time for the next dose, take that dose only. Do not double the dose or take extra.

Pharmacokinetics. *Onset and Duration.* PO onset of analgesia 30 min.[21]

Serum Levels. (Salicylate) 150–300 mg/L (1.1–2.2 mmol/L) for rheumatic diseases, often accompanied by mild toxic symptoms. Tinnitus occurs at 200–400 mg/L (1.5–2.9 mmol/L), hyperventilation at >350 mg/L (2.6 mmol/L), acidosis at >450 mg/L (3.3 mmol/L), and severe or fatal toxicity at >900 mg/L (6.6 mmol/L) 6 hr after acute ingestion.[55,56]

Fate. Rapidly absorbed from the GI tract; oral bioavailability of aspirin is 80–100%. Enteric coating does not adversely affect absorption.[57] A single analgesic/antipyretic dose produces peak salicylate levels of 30–60 mg/L (0.22–0.44 mmol/L). Aspirin is 49% plasma protein bound, decreased in uremia; V_d is 0.15 ± 0.03 L/kg; Cl is 0.56 ± 0.07 L/hr/kg. Aspirin is rapidly hydrolyzed to salicylate, which also is pharmacologically active. Salicylate is metabolized primarily in the liver to 4 metabolites (salicyluric acid, phenolic and acyl glucuronides, and gentisic acid). Salicylate plasma protein binding is dose dependent, 95% at 15 mg/L and 80% at 300 mg/L, and decreased in uremia, hypoalbuminemia, neonates, and pregnancy; V_d is 0.17 ± 0.03 L/kg; Cl is dose dependent, 0.012 L/hr/kg at 134–157 mg/L, and decreased in hepatitis and neonates. Only 1% of a dose of aspirin is excreted unchanged in the urine.

$t_{1/2}$. (Aspirin) 0.25 ± 0.03 hr.[21] (Salicylate) dose dependent: 2.4 hr with 0.25 g, 5 hr with 1 g, 6.1 hr with 1.3 g, 19 hr with 10–20 g.[58]

Adverse Reactions. Hearing impairment, GI upset, and occult bleeding are frequent, with acute hemorrhage from gastric erosion also likely. As with other NSAIDs, aspirin can cause renal dysfunction, particularly in those with pre-existing renal disease or CHF. Rare hepatotoxicity occurs, primarily in children with rheumatic fever or rheumatoid arthritis and adults with SLE or pre-existing liver disease;[59] the syndrome of asthma, angioedema, and nasal polyps can be provoked in susceptible patients.[60] A single analgesic dose can suppress platelet aggregation and prolong bleeding time for up to 1 week; large dosages can prolong PT.[61]

Contraindications. Bleeding disorders; asthma; hypersensitivity to other NSAIDs or tartrazine dye.

Precautions. Use with caution in patients with renal disease, gastric ulcer, bleeding tendencies, hypoprothrombinemia, or history of asthma, or during anticoagulant therapy. Because of the association with Reye's syndrome, the use of salicylates in children and teenagers with flu-like symptoms or chickenpox is not recommended.[62,63] Those developing bronchospasm with aspirin can develop similar reactions to other NSAIDs.[60] Sodium salicylate and other nonacetylated salicylates (except diflunisal) are usually well tolerated in these patients.[62,64]

Drug Interactions. Alkalinizing agents (eg, acetazolamide, antacids) can reduce salicylate levels; acetazolamide also can enhance CNS penetration of salicylate. Corticosteroids can reduce serum salicylate levels. Large doses of salicylates can increase oral anticoagulant effect; even small doses can increase risk of bleeding with oral anticoagulants or heparin because of the antiplatelet effect of aspirin. Alcohol and salicylate increase the risk of GI blood loss. Salicylates can cause an increased response to sulfonylureas, especially chlorpropamide. Salicylate decreases the uricosuric effect of uricosuric agents (eg, probenecid, sulfinpyrazone). Salicylate, especially in large doses, can decrease renal elimination of methotrexate and displace it from plasma protein binding sites.

Parameters to Monitor. Monitor for abnormal bleeding or bruising and occult GI blood loss (periodic hematocrit) in patients who ingest salicylates regularly. Serum salicylate level determinations are recommended with higher dosage regimens because of the wide variation among patients in serum levels produced. Monitor renal function and hearing changes (tinnitus); however, using tinnitus as an index of maximum salicylate tolerance is *not* recommended.[55]

IBUPROFEN   Advil, Motrin, Nuprin, Various

Pharmacology. Ibuprofen is an NSAID with analgesic and antipyretic properties. It is a nonselective inhibitor of cyclo-oxygenase-1 (COX-1) and cyclo-oxygenase-2 (COX-2) and reversibly alters platelet function and prolongs bleeding time.

Administration and Adult Dosage. **PO for mild to moderate pain** 400 mg q 4–6 hr prn. **PO for primary dysmenorrhea** 400 mg q 4 hr prn. **PO for rheumatoid arthritis and osteoarthritis** 400–800 mg tid or qid, to a maximum of 3.2 g/day.

Special Populations. *Pediatric Dosage.* **PO for fever** (6 months–12 yr) 5 mg/kg for fever <102.5°F or 10 mg/kg for fever >102.5°F given q 6–8 hr, to a maximum of 40 mg/kg/day. **PO for pain** (6 months–12 yr) 10 mg/kg q 6–8 hr prn, to a maximum of 40 mg/kg/day. **PO for juvenile arthritis** 30–40 mg/kg/day in 3 or 4 divided doses; 20 mg/kg/day in milder disease.

Geriatric Dosage. Use minimal effective dosages because the elderly are more susceptible to GI bleeding and acute renal insufficiency.

Dosage Forms. **Cap** 200, 400 mg; **Chew Tab** 50, 100 mg; **Tab** 100, 200, 400, 600, 800 mg; **Drp** 40 mg/mL; **Susp** 20, 40 mg/mL.

Patient Instructions. This drug may be taken with food, milk, or antacid to minimize stomach upset. Report any symptoms of gastrointestinal ulceration or bleeding, skin rash, weight gain, or edema. Dizziness can occur; until the extent of this effect is known, use appropriate caution.

Missed Doses. If you take this drug on a regular schedule and you miss a dose, take it as soon as you remember. If it is about time for the next dose, take that dose only. Do not double the dose or take extra.

Pharmacokinetics. *Serum Levels.* 10 mg/L (48 μmol/L) for antipyretic effect.[21] Serum concentrations over 200 mg/L (971 mmol/L) 1 hr after acute overdosage may be associated with severe toxicity (apnea, metabolic acidosis, and coma).[65]

Fate. Rapidly absorbed from the GI tract with bioavailability over 80%.[21] Peak serum levels in children of 17–42 mg/L (82–204 μmol/L) after a dose of 5 mg/kg and 25–53 mg/L (121–257 μmol/L) after a dose of 10 mg/kg are achieved in 1.1 ± 0.3 hr.[66] Greater than 99% plasma protein bound; metabolized to at least 2 inactive metabolites; V_d is 0.15 ± 0.02 L/kg, increased in cystic fibrosis; Cl is 0.045 ± 0.012 L/hr/kg, increased in cystic fibrosis. Less than 1% is excreted unchanged in the urine.[21]

$t_{1/2}$. 2 ± 0.5 hr.[21] **Adverse Reactions.** Gastric distress, blood loss, diarrhea, vomiting, dizziness, and skin rash occur occasionally; GI ulceration (for all NSAIDs there is a greater risk in the elderly and with higher dosages) and fluid retention have been reported.[67] Ibuprofen occasionally causes renal dysfunction, particularly in those with pre-existing renal disease, CHF, or cirrhosis.[68] A slight rise in the bleeding time, elevation of liver enzymes, lymphopenia, agranulocytosis, aplastic anemia, and aseptic meningitis have been reported rarely.[69,70]

Contraindications. Syndrome of nasal polyps; angioedema; bronchospastic reactivity to aspirin or other NSAIDs.

Precautions. Avoid during pregnancy. Use with caution in patients with pre-existing renal disease, CHF, or cirrhosis;[68] a history of ulcer disease or bleeding; or risk factors associated with peptic ulcer disease (eg, advanced age).

Drug Interactions. NSAIDs may inhibit the antihypertensive response to ACE inhibitors, β-blockers, diuretics, and hydralazine, and the natriuretic effect of diuretics. Possible GI bleeding and the antiplatelet effect of NSAIDs can increase the risk of serious bleeding during anticoagulant therapy. NSAIDs can decrease renal lithium clearance. Some NSAIDs (especially indomethacin and ketoprofen) reduce methotrexate clearance. Indomethacin (and probably other NSAIDs) can reduce renal function.

Parameters to Monitor. Monitor for blood loss, weight gain, and renal function during long-term use.

Notes. Misoprostol is effective in preventing NSAID-associated GI ulceration; H_2-receptor antagonists, however, prevent duodenal but not gastric ulcerations and may mask the signs and symptoms of NSAID-induced GI ulceration. Proton-pump inhibitors (eg, omeprazole) are effective in treating NSAID-related dyspepsia and preventing NSAID-induced ulcers.[71]

INDOMETHACIN   Indocin, Various

Pharmacology. Indomethacin is an indoleacetic acid NSAID that is one of the most potent nonselective inhibitors of cyclo-oxygenase available. In addition to its anti-inflammatory effects, indomethacin has prominent analgesic and antipyretic properties. It also has been used to suppress uterine activity and prevent premature labor.

Adult Dosage. **PO for rheumatoid arthritis, rheumatoid (ankylosing) spondylitis, and osteoarthritis of the hip** 25 mg bid or tid initially. Increase in 25 mg/day increments at weekly intervals until satisfactory response or to a maximum of 150–200 mg/day. Alternatively, up to 100 mg of the daily dosage may be given hs for persistent night or morning stiffness. **PO for acute gouty arthritis** 100 mg, followed by 50 mg tid until resolved. **SR Cap** 75 mg 1–2 times/day can be substituted for all uses except gouty arthritis, based on the non-SR dosage.

Pediatric Dosage. **IV for pharmacologic closure of persistent patent ductus arteriosus in premature infants** 0.2 mg/kg, followed by 2 additional **IV** doses of 0.1–0.25 mg/kg (depending on age) at 12- to 24-hr intervals. Alternatively, give 0.3 mg/kg as a single dose, or 1 or more doses of 0.1 mg/kg as a retention enema or via orogastric tube.[21,61]

Dosage Forms. **Cap** 25, 50 mg; **SR Cap** 75 mg; **Supp** 50 mg; **Susp** 5 mg/mL; **Inj** 1 mg.

Pharmacokinetics. Indomethacin is rapidly and well absorbed from the GI tract, with a bioavailability of 98%. Peak serum levels are reached within 2 hr with effective concentrations in the range of 0.3–3 mg/L (0.8–8 µmol/L). It is 90% plasma protein bound and has extensive O-demethylation and N-deacylation to inactive metabolites; V_d is 0.29 ± 0.04 L/kg; Cl is 0.084 ± 0.012 L/hr/kg, lower in premature infants, neonates, and the aged; $15 \pm 8\%$ is excreted unchanged in the urine. The half-life of the drug is 2.4 ± 0.4 hr, higher in premature infants, neonates, and the aged.

Adverse Reactions. Adverse effects are frequent, and about 20% of patients cannot tolerate the drug. Frontal lobe headache, drowsiness, dizziness, mental confusion, and GI distress are frequent, especially with dosages >100 mg/day; occasional peripheral neuropathy, occult bleeding, and peptic ulcer occur. Pancreatitis, corneal opacities, hepatotoxicity, aplastic anemia, agranulocytosis, thrombocytopenia, aggravation of psychiatric disorders, and allergic reactions are reported rarely. The syndrome of asthma, angioedema, and nasal polyps may be provoked in susceptible patients. Precautions, drug interactions, and monitoring are similar to other NSAIDs. (*See* Ibuprofen.)

NAPROXEN	Naprosyn
NAPROXEN SODIUM	Anaprox

Pharmacology. (*See* Ibuprofen.)

Administration and Adult Dosage. **PO for mild to moderate pain, dysmenorrhea, or acute tendinitis or bursitis** (naproxen) 500 mg, followed by 250 mg q 6–8 hr, to a maximum of 1250 mg/day; (naproxen sodium) 550 mg, followed by 275 mg q 6–8 hr, to a maximum of 1375 mg/day. **PO for rheumatoid arthritis, osteoarthritis, and ankylosing spondylitis** (naproxen) 250–500 mg bid initially, to a maximum of 1500 mg/day for limited periods; (naproxen sodium) 275–550 mg bid or 275 mg q morning and 550 mg q evening initially, to a maximum of 1650 mg/day for limited periods. If no improvement has occurred after 4 weeks of therapy, consider other drug therapy. **PO for acute gout** (naproxen) 750 mg, followed by 250 mg q 8 hr until resolved; (naproxen sodium) 825 mg, followed by 275 mg q 8 hr until resolved.

Special Populations. *Pediatric Dosage.* **PO for juvenile arthritis** 10 mg/kg/day in 2 divided doses.

Geriatric Dosage. Use minimal effective dosages because the elderly are more susceptible to GI bleeding and acute renal insufficiency.

Dosage Forms. **Tab** (naproxen) 250, 375, 500 mg; (naproxen sodium) 220, 275, 550 mg; **EC Tab** (naproxen) 375, 500 mg; **SR Tab** (naproxen sodium) 375, 500, 750 mg; **Susp** (naproxen) 25 mg/mL.

Patient Instructions. (*See* Ibuprofen.)

Pharmacokinetics. *Serum Levels.* Trough concentrations >50 mg/L (>217 μmol/L) are associated with response in rheumatoid arthritis.[21]

Fate. Rapidly absorbed from the GI tract with a bioavailability of about 99%. Greater than 99.7% plasma protein bound, saturable with increasing dosage, increased with uremia, cirrhosis, and in the elderly, and decreased in rheumatoid arthritis and hypoalbuminemia; V_d is 0.16 ± 0.02 L/kg, increased in uremia, cirrhosis, and rheumatoid arthritis. Cl is 0.0078 ± 0.0012 L/hr/kg, increased in rheumatoid arthritis, and decreased in uremia; less than 1% is excreted unchanged in urine.[21]

$t_{1/2}$. 14 ± 1 hr, increased in the elderly.[21]

Adverse Reactions. Naproxen can occasionally cause renal dysfunction, particularly in those with pre-existing renal disease, CHF, or cirrhosis. Interstitial nephritis and nephrotic syndrome have been reported.72,73 (See also Ibuprofen.) Contraindications, precautions, drug interactions, and monitoring are similar to other NSAIDs. (*See* Ibuprofen.)

SELECTIVE COX-2 INHIBITORS:

CELECOXIB	Celebrex
ROFECOXIB	Vioxx

Pharmacology. Inhibition of the COX-2 enzyme isoform is thought to be responsible for the anti-inflammatory effects of NSAIDs, whereas inhibition of COX-1 results in GI and possibly other side effects. A relatively selective COX-2 inhibitor should combine anti-inflammatory, analgesic, and antipyretic efficacies equivalent to older, nonselective NSAIDs with improved safety.[74]

Administration and Adult Dosage. (Celecoxib) **PO for osteoarthritis** 100 mg bid or 200 mg daily; **PO for rheumatoid arthritis** 100–200 mg bid; **PO for familial adenomatous polyposis** 400 mg bid. (Rofecoxib) **PO for osteoarthritis** 12.5–25 mg once daily; **PO for acute pain and primary dysmenorrhea** 50 mg/day prn, to a maximum of 5 days of consecutive use.

Special Populations. *Pediatric Dosage.* (<18 yr) Safety and efficacy not established for either agent.

Geriatric Dosage. (Celecoxib) Dosage adjustment is usually not necessary; however, use the lowest effective dose; (<50 kg) initiate therapy at the lowest recommended dose. (Rofecoxib) dosage adjustment is not necessary; however, initiate with the lowest recommended dose.

Dosage Forms. (Celecoxib) **Cap** 100, 200 mg. (Rofecoxib) **Tab** 12.5, 25, 50 mg; **Susp** 2.5, 5 mg/mL.

Patient Instructions. This drug can cause headache, upset stomach, or diarrhea. Report edema, rash, unusual weight gain, or signs and symptoms of gastrointestinal bleeding to your physician. Avoid products that contain aspirin and nonsteroidal anti-inflammatory drugs unless otherwise directed. Take without regard to meals (except take with food if taking celecoxib 400 mg bid).

Missed Doses. If you take this drug on a regular schedule, take a missed dose as soon as you remember. If it is about time for the next dose, take that dose only; do not double the dose or take extra.

Pharmacokinetics. *Fate.* (Celecoxib) Absolute bioavailability not studied. Peak plasma levels occur in 3 hr. With high-fat meals, peak levels are delayed 1–2 hr with accompanying increases in total absorption of 10–20%; 97% plasma protein bound. Predominantly metabolized hepatically by CYP2C9 to inactive metabolites with <3% excreted unchanged in urine or feces. (Rofecoxib) Rapidly absorbed from the GI tract with bioavailability of 93%. Peak plasma level occurs in 2–3 hr and is delayed 1–2 hr when taken with a high-fat meal, with no effect on peak plasma concentration or extent of absorption; 87% plasma protein bound. Metabolism is predominantly by cytosolic enzymes with minor P450 involvement. Inactive metabolites. Predominantly eliminated via hepatic metabolism with <1% unchanged drug excreted in urine.

$t_{1/2}$. (Celecoxib) 11 hr; (rofecoxib) 17 hr.

Adverse Reactions. COX-2 inhibitors can cause GI toxicity, dyspepsia, abdominal pain, nausea, vomiting, and diarrhea at a rate similar to placebo and less than conventional NSAIDs. Renal and liver effects are equivalent to other NSAIDs.[75,76]

Contraindications. (Celecoxib, rofecoxib) History of aspirin- or NSAID-induced asthma, urticaria, or allergic type reactions. (Celecoxib) allergy to sulfonamides.

Precautions. Use celecoxib and rofecoxib cautiously in patients with pre-existing asthma, renal or hepatic compromise, fluid retention, hypertension, or CHF.

Drug Interactions. NSAIDs can diminish the effects of ACE inhibitors, furosemide, and thiazide diuretics and increase lithium plasma levels. Concurrent use with anticoagulants can increase the risk of bleeding. (Celecoxib) Inhibitors of CYP2C9 (eg, fluconazole) can increase serum concentrations of celecoxib. (Rofecoxib) Increased serum concentrations (23%) and reduced renal clearance of methotrexate. Rifampin decreases rofecoxib serum levels by 50%.

Parameters to Monitor. Monitor for weight gain, renal function during long-term use, and occult blood loss if on concomitant aspirin or anticoagulant therapy.

Notes. Celecoxib 100 or 200 mg bid is as effective as **naproxen** 500 mg bid for the treatment of osteoarthritis and produces fewer gastroduodenal ulcers than naproxen, **dicolfenac**, or **ibuprofen**.[76] Likewise, rofecoxib 12.5 or 25 mg is as effective as ibuprofen 800 mg tid and diclofenac 50 mg tid for the treatment of osteoarthritis and produces fewer gastroduodenal ulcers than ibuprofen.[75] **Parecoxib** (Pharmacia) is an injectable COX-2 inhibitor being studied for the treatment of acute pain. Doses of 20 and 40 mg have been used in clinical trials. It appears to be as effective as injectable **ketorolac**, but with improved safety. Parecoxib is a water-soluble prodrug of **valdecoxib** (Pharmacia) which is also pending FDA approval as an oral drug.

NONSTEROIDAL ANTI-INFLAMMATORY DRUGS COMPARISON CHART

CLASS AND DRUG	DOSAGE FORMS	ADULT DOSAGE	HALF-LIFE (HR)	COMMENTS
ACETIC ACIDS				
Diclofenac Cataflam Voltaren Various	Tab (diclofenac potassium) 50 mg Tab (diclofenac sodium) 50, 75 mg plus misoprostol 200 µg (Arthrotec). SR Tab (diclofenac sodium) 25, 50, 75, 100 mg	PO (pain, dysmenorrhea) (Cataflam) 50 mg tid; PO (arthritis) 100–200 mg/day in 2 doses. PO SR 100 mg once or twice daily (dosages expressed as diclofenac).	1.1 ± 0.2	Although it is unclear whether the risk of hepatotoxicity is any greater than with other NSAIDs, careful monitoring of symptoms and liver function tests is recommended.
Etodolac Lodine Various	Cap 200, 300, mg Tab 400, 500 mg SR Tab 500, 600 mg.	PO (pain) 200–400 mg q 6–8 hr; PO (arthritis) 600–1200 mg/day in 2–3 divided doses.	7.3 ± 4	Recommended for treatment of osteo-arthritis; not as effective as other NSAIDs for rheumatoid arthritis.
Indomethacin Indocin Various	Cap 25, 50 mg SR Cap 75 mg Susp 5 mg/mL Supp 50 mg Inj 1 mg.	PO (gouty arthritis) 100 mg, then 50 mg tid; PO or PR (arthritis) 50–200 mg/day in 3 divided doses. SR in 1–2 doses, can substitute for equal daily dosage of non-SR.	2.4 ± 0.4	*See monograph.* Associated with a high frequency of CNS effects such as drowsiness, dizziness, mental confusion, and frontal lobe headache.
Ketorolac Toradol Various	Tab 10 mg Inj 15, 30, 60 mg.	PO (pain, short term) 10 mg q 4–6 hr prn, to a maximum of 40 mg/day for 5 days (including IM/IV). IM or IV (short-term management of pain) 30 or 60 (IM only) mg once, then 15–30 mg q 6 hr.	4.5	For short-term (up to 5 days) use only. Do not exceed 60 mg/day parenterally in patients 65 yr or older, under 50 kg, or with elevated Cr_s.

(continued)

NONSTEROIDAL ANTI-INFLAMMATORY DRUGS COMPARISON CHART (*continued*)

CLASS AND DRUG	DOSAGE FORMS	ADULT DOSAGE	HALF-LIFE (HR)	COMMENTS
Sulindac Clinoril	Tab 150, 200 mg.	PO (arthritis) 300–400 mg/day in 2 divided doses.	15 ± 4 (active sulfide metabolite)	Purported "renal-sparing" effect has been questioned. Because the active sulfide metabolite has a relatively long half-life, renal effects may not be observed for several days.
Tolmetin Tolectin Various	Cap 400 mg Tab 200, 600 mg.	PO (arthritis) 0.6–1.8 g/day in 3–4 divided doses.	4.9 ± 0.3	Higher frequency of anaphylactoid reactions than other NSAIDs.
ANTHRANILIC ACIDS (FENAMATES)				
Meclofenamate Meclomen Various	Cap 50, 100 mg.	PO (pain) 50 mg q 4–6 hr; PO (arthritis) 200–400 mg/day in 3–4 divided doses.	3	The fenamates as a group are more toxic than other NSAIDs and associated with headache, dizziness, and hemolytic anemia.
Mefenamic Acid Ponstel	Cap 250 mg.	PO (pain, dysmenorrhea) 250 mg q 6 hr for up to 1 week.	3	Not recommended; *see* Meclofenamate Comments.
NONACIDIC COMPOUNDS				
Nabumetone Relafen	Tab 500, 750 mg.	PO (arthritis) 1–2 g/day in 1–2 doses.	23 ± 4 (active 6-MNA metabolite)	Reported to have less GI toxicity than other NSAIDs; however, additional well-controlled, double-blind studies are needed.

(continued)

27

NONSTEROIDAL ANTI-INFLAMMATORY DRUGS COMPARISON CHART (*continued*)

CLASS AND DRUG	DOSAGE FORMS	ADULT DOSAGE	HALF-LIFE (HR)	COMMENTS
OXICAMS				
Meloxicam Mobic	Tab 7.5 mg.	PO (arthritis) 7.5–15 mg once daily.	20	Less mucosal damage than with piroxicam.
Piroxicam Feldene Various	Cap 10, 20 mg.	PO (arthritis) 20 mg/day in 1–2 doses.	48 ± 8	Based on postmarketing surveillance data, reported to cause about 12 times more GI adverse effects than ibuprofen. High frequency of phototoxic cutaneous eruptions.
PROPIONIC ACIDS				
Fenoprofen Nalfon	Cap 200, 300 mg Tab 600 mg.	PO (pain) 200 mg q 4–6 hr; PO (arthritis) 1.2–2.4 g/day in 3–4 divided doses.	2.5 ± 0.5	Similar to ibuprofen.
Flurbiprofen Ansaid	Tab 50, 100 mg.	PO (arthritis) 200–300 mg/day in 2–4 divided doses.	3.8 ± 1.2	Similar to ibuprofen.
Ibuprofen Advil Motrin Nuprin Various	Cap 200, 400 mg Chew Tab 50, 100 mg Tab 100, 200, 400, 600, 800 mg Drp 40 mg/mL Susp 20, 40 mg/mL.	PO (pain, dysmenorrhea) 400 mg q 4–6 hr; PO (arthritis) 1.2–3.2 g/day in 3–4 divided doses.	2 ± 0.5	*See monograph.*
Ketoprofen Orudis Oruvail Various	Cap 25, 50, 75 mg Tab 12.5 mg. SR Cap 100, 150, 200 mg.	PO (pain) 25–50 mg q 6–8 hr; PO (arthritis) 150–300 mg/day in 3 divided doses. PO SR 200 mg/day in 1 dose.	1.8 ± 0.3	Similar to ibuprofen.

(*continued*)

NONSTEROIDAL ANTI-INFLAMMATORY DRUGS COMPARISON CHART (*continued*)

CLASS AND DRUG	DOSAGE FORMS	ADULT DOSAGE	HALF-LIFE (HR)	COMMENTS
Naproxen Aleve Anaprox Naprelan Naprosyn Various	Tab (naproxen sodium) 220, 275, 550 mg Tab (naproxen) 250, 375, 500 mg EC Tab (naproxen) 375, 500 mg SR Tab (naproxen) 375, 500, 750 mg Susp (naproxen) 25 mg/mL.	PO (pain) 500 mg, then 250 mg q 6–8 hr; PO (arthritis) 0.5–1.5 g/day in 2 divided doses. PO (acute gout) 750 mg, then 250 mg q 8 hr. (Doses expressed as naproxen.)	14 ± 1	*See* monograph. Equal in efficacy and safety to ibuprofen
Oxaprozin Daypro	Tab 600 mg.	PO (arthritis) 1.2 g/day in 1 dose.	50–60	Similar to other NSAIDs.
SALICYLATES				
Aspirin Various	*See* monograph.	PO (pain) 325–1000 mg q 4 hr; PO (arthritis) 3.6–5.4 g/day in 3–4 divided doses.[a]	0.25 ± 0.03 (aspirin) 2–19 (salicylate, dose dependent)	*See* monograph.
Choline Magnesium Trisalicylate Trilisate	Tab 500, 750 mg, 1g Liquid 100 mg/mL.	PO (pain, arthritis) 1.5–3 g/day in 1–2 divided doses.[a]	2–19 (salicylate, dose dependent)	Salicylate is only a weak inhibitor of cyclo-oxygenase. It therefore has no antiplatelet effect and can usually be administered safely to individuals with aspirin sensitivity. *See also* Aspirin monograph.
Diflunisal Dolobid Various	Tab 250, 500 mg.	PO (arthritis) 250–500 mg bid.	11 ± 2 (dose dependent)	Not converted to salicylate; similar to other NSAIDs.

(continued)

29

NONSTEROIDAL ANTI-INFLAMMATORY DRUGS COMPARISON CHART (*continued*)

CLASS AND DRUG	DOSAGE FORMS	ADULT DOSAGE	HALF-LIFE (HR)	COMMENTS
Magnesium Salicylate Doan's Various	Tab 500, 545, 600 mg.	PO (pain, arthritis) 3.6–4.8 g/day in 3–4 divided doses.[a]	2–19 (salicylate, dose dependent)	*See* Choline Magnesium Trisalicylate comments and Aspirin monograph.
Salsalate Disalcid Various	Cap 500 mg Tab 500, 750 mg.	PO (arthritis) 3 g/day in 2–3 divided doses.[a]	2–19 (salicylate, dose dependent)	*See* Choline Magnesium Trisalicylate comments and Aspirin monograph.
SELECTIVE COX-2 INHIBITORS				
Celecoxib Celebrex	Cap 100, 200.	PO for osteoarthritis 100 mg bid or 200 mg/day; PO for rheumatoid arthritis 100–200 mg bid; PO for familial adenomatous polyposis 400 mg bid with food.	11.2	Equal efficacy to other NSAIDs with improved GI safety profile. (*See* monograph.)
Rofecoxib Vioxx	Tab 12.5, 25, 50 mg Susp 2.5, 5 mg/mL.	PO for osteoarthritis 12.5–25 mg/day PO for acute pain, primary dysmennorhea 50 mg/day, not to exceed 5 days.	17	Equal efficacy to other NSAIDs with improved GI safety profile. (*See* monograph.)

[a]Long-term dosage for arthritis should be guided by serum salicylate levels; *see* Aspirin monograph.
Adapted from references 21, 61, 72, 73, and 77–85, and product information.

Opioids

Class Instructions. This drug can cause drowsiness. Until the extent of this effect is known, use caution when driving, operating machinery, or performing other tasks requiring mental alertness. Avoid excessive concurrent use of alcohol and other drugs that cause drowsiness. Prolonged use of this drug can cause constipation, and concurrent use of a stool-softening or stimulant laxative may be helpful.

For moderate to severe pain (pain rating >5 on a 0–10 scale), you must take doses at regular intervals around the clock to anticipate and prevent pain. When the drug is taken at the correct interval and pain relief does not last for this period, use additional "rescue" doses of a short-acting drug to maintain pain relief. When more than 4 rescue doses are used in a day, contact the prescriber for a dosage increase. Addiction does not occur when these drugs are used for legitimate painful conditions. Dependence, a condition in which the body may go through withdrawal when the drug is stopped suddenly, can occur with prolonged usage but can be managed by slowly decreasing the dosage when the drug is no longer needed.

Missed Doses. If you miss a dose, take it as soon as you remember. If it is about time for the next dose, take that dose only. Do not double the dose or take extra. Take subsequent doses at the same interval previously established for pain relief.

CODEINE SALTS
Various

Pharmacology. Codeine is 3-methoxymorphine, a phenanthrene opioid with very low affinity for opioid receptors. Its analgesic activity appears to result from conversion to morphine. Poor metabolizers of debrisoquine/sparteine (approximately 7% of the Caucasian population) cannot convert appreciable amounts of codeine to morphine or obtain analgesia from codeine but are still subject to the same adverse effects.[86–89] (*See* Morphine Sulfate.)

Administration and Adult Dosage. **PO, SC, or IM for analgesia** 15–60 mg q 4–6 hr. **PO or SC for antitussive action** 10–20 mg q 4–6 hr, to a maximum of 120 mg/day. **IV** not recommended. (*See* Precautions.)

Special Populations. *Pediatric Dosage.* **PO, SC, or IM for analgesia** ($\geq$1 yr) 0.5 mg/kg q 4–6 hr. **PO for antitussive action** (2–6 yr) 2.5–5 mg q 4–6 hr, to a maximum of 30 mg/day; (7–12 yr) 5–10 mg q 4–6 hr, to a maximum of 60 mg/day; (>12 yr) same as adult dosage. (*See* Notes.)

Geriatric Dosage. Same as adult dosage.[90]

Other Conditions. Reduce initial dosage in debilitated patients or those with hypoxia or hypercapnia.

Dosage Forms. **Tab** 15, 30, 60 mg; **Inj** 15, 30, 60 mg/mL; **Oral Liquid** 2, 2.4, 3 mg/mL in various combinations. Formulated as phosphate or sulfate salt.

Patient Instructions. (*See* Opioids Class Instructions.)

Pharmacokinetics. *Onset and Duration.* PO, SC onset 15–30 min; IM peak analgesia 0.5–1 hr; duration (all routes) 4–6 hr.[91]

Fate. Systemic availability averages 40% but with a wide range (12–84%), reflecting large variability in hepatic enzyme activity.[92] A single PO 15 mg dose produces serum levels of 26–33 µg/L (82–104 nmol/L) in 2 hr and 13–22 µg/L (41–69 nmol/L) in 5 hr.[93] The drug is 7% plasma protein bound. V_d is 2.6 ± 0.3 L/kg; Cl is 0.66 ± 0.12 L/hr/kg.[19] Metabolized in the liver to codeine-6-glucuronide, N-demethylated to norcodeine, and O-demethylated to morphine by genetic polymorphic CYP2D6. Codeine-6-glucuronide is the major metabolite, and norcodeine and morphine are minor metabolites, each accounting for approximately 10% of the dose.[88] Accumulation of morphine occurs with repeated administration, resulting in a morphine:codeine AUC ratio of 0.29:1.[94] Variation in the reported rates of codeine conversion to morphine may be related to the assays used, with much higher concentrations of morphine reported with radioimmunoassays than with HPLC or GC-MS.[92] Primarily urinary excretion of inactive forms; 3–16% is excreted unchanged in urine.[95]

$t_{½}$. 2.9 ± 0.7 hr.[19]

Adverse Reactions. Sedation, dizziness, nausea, vomiting, constipation, and respiratory depression occur frequently. Dose-related signs of intoxication are miosis, drowsiness, decreased rate and depth of respiration, bradycardia, and hypotension. Dose-related adverse reactions in children are somnolence, ataxia, miosis, and vomiting at 3–5 mg/kg/day and respiratory depression at >5 mg/kg/day. Because hepatic glucuronidation is incomplete in infants, they are at particular risk for dose-related adverse effects.[96]

Precautions. Because it can cause severe hypotension, do not administer codeine phosphate IV.[97,98]

Drug Interactions. Potent CYP2D6 inhibitors (eg, quinidine, fluoxetine) can abolish the conversion to morphine and the pharmacologic effects of codeine.[90,99]

Notes. Codeine is no more effective than placebo in suppressing nighttime cough in children. The American Academy of Pediatrics recommends that parents be educated about the lack of proven antitussive effects and the potential risks of codeine-containing products because overdosage has been reported.[96]

FENTANYL   Duragesic, Fentanyl Oralet, Sublimaze, Various

Pharmacology. Fentanyl is a phenylpiperidine opioid agonist with predominant effects on the mu opioid receptor and is about 50–100 times more potent as an analgesic than morphine. Other related compounds are **sufentanil** (Sufenta), which is 5–7 times more potent than fentanyl; **alfentanil** (Alfenta), which is less potent than fentanyl but acts more rapidly and has a shorter duration of action; and **remifentanil** (Ultiva), which is more potent than fentanyl and is extremely short acting because of its rapid ester hydrolysis.[86,87] (See Morphine Sulfate.)

Administration and Adult Dosage. **IV patient-controlled analgesia (PCA)** 20–100 µg per activation with 3–10-min lockout period, both titrated to patient response. (See Patient-Controlled Analgesia Guidelines Chart, page 44.) **Epidurally for analgesia** 25–150 µg as an intermittent bolus dose or 25–150 µg/hr as a continuous infusion, titrated to patient response.[91] (See Notes and Intraspinal Narcotic Administration Guidelines Chart, page 44.) **Transdermal for analgesia** calculate the previous 24-hr analgesic requirement and convert this amount to the equal analgesic oral morphine dosage from the Opioid Analgesics Comparison Chart. A short-acting opioid or the fentanyl lozenge (Actiq) must be used for control of breakthrough pain until sufficient transdermal fentanyl is absorbed to achieve adequate analgesia. Use the following table to determine the fentanyl transdermal dosage from the daily equivalent oral morphine dosage:

TRANSDERMAL FENTANYL COMPARISON CHART

24-HR ORAL MORPHINE DOSAGE[a] (MG/DAY)	FENTANYL TRANSDERMAL DOSAGE (μG/HR)
45–134	25
135–224	50
225–314	75
315–404	100
405–494	125
495–584	150
585–674	175
675–764	200
765–854	225
855–944	250
945–1034	275
1035–1124	300

[a]Assumes morphine 10 mg IM is equivalent to morphine 60 mg orally; however, because of individual variability, equivalent dosages can vary among patients. These conversion dosages are conservative, and approximately 50% of patients are likely to require a dosage increase after initial application. (*See* Opioid Analgesics Comparison Chart.)

Initiate treatment using the recommended transdermal fentanyl dosage and increase based on response no more frequently than q 3–6 days. Multiple transdermal patches can be used to achieve appropriate dosage (do not cut patches for a partial dosage). To change treatment to another opioid, discontinue the transdermal patch for 12–18 hr and start treatment with the new opioid at about one-half the equianalgesic dosage. **IV for induction and maintenance anesthesia** (loading) 4–20 μg/kg, (maintenance) 2–10 μg/kg/hr, (additional bolus) 25–100 μg.[100] **IV for postoperative (recovery room) pain control** 50–100 μg q 1–2 hr as needed; **Lozenge (Oralet) for anesthesia premedication or induction of conscious sedation** 5 μg/kg (provides effects similar to 0.75–1.25 μg/kg given IM), to a maximum of 400 μg. **Lozenge for the management of breakthrough cancer pain (Actiq) in patients already receiving >60 mg of oral morphine/day or >50 μg/hr of transdermal fentanyl** initial dose of 200 μg. Until the appropriate dose is reached, an additional dose can be used to treat an episode of breakthrough pain. Re-administration can start 15 min after the previous lozenge has been completed. Do not give >2 units for a breakthrough pain episode while a patient is in the titration phase. Evaluate each new dose in the titration period over several breakthrough pain episodes. If >4 units/day are needed, increase the dosage of the long-acting opioid.

Special Populations. *Pediatric Dosage.* **IV for sedation in neonates** 9–20 µg/kg/hr; tolerance limits its usefulness for prolonged sedation.[101] **IV for induction and maintenance anesthesia** (2–12 yr) 2–3 µg/kg initially, followed by 1–5 µg/kg/hr.[100] **Lozenge for anesthesia premedication or induction of conscious sedation** (<15 kg) contraindicated; (≥15 kg) 5–15 µg/kg, to a maximum of 400 µg.

Geriatric Dosage. **Lozenge for anesthesia premedication or induction of conscious sedation** (>65 yr) 2.5–5 µg/kg, to a maximum of 400 µg. Altered pharmacodynamics rather than pharmacokinetics appear to be responsible for increased sensitivity in elderly patients.[102]

Other Conditions. In patients with head injury, cardiovascular, pulmonary, or hepatic disease, consider a lower dosage of 2.5–5 µg/kg, to a maximum of 400 µg.

Dosage Forms. **Inj** 50 µg/mL; **SR Patch** 25, 50, 75, 100 µg/hr; **Lozenge for anesthesia (Oralet)** 100, 200, 300, 400 µg; **Lozenge (on a stick) for breakthrough cancer pain (Actiq)** 200, 400, 600, 800, 1200, 1600 µg.

Patient Instructions. (*See* Opioids Class Instructions.) (Fentanyl Actiq) once an effective dosage is determined, limit consumption to ≤4 units/day.

Pharmacokinetics. *Onset and Duration.* IM onset 7–15 min; duration 1–2 hr. Epidural onset 5 min; duration 4–6 hr.[91] Transdermal onset 6–8 hr; peak 24–72 hr; duration after a single application 72 hr.[103,104] More than 17 hr is required for serum levels to fall by one-half after patch removal.

Serum Levels. (Analgesia) 1–3 µg/L (3–9 nmol/L);[103,104] (balanced anesthesia) 6–20 µg/L (18–60 nmol/L).[100]

Fate. Bioavailability is 52% with lozenge. Of the fentanyl released by the transdermal system, 92% is absorbed, but overall systemic bioavailability of the transdermal preparation is approximately 30%. The drug is 84 ± 2% plasma protein bound; it is metabolized rapidly primarily by the liver to norfentanyl and other inactive metabolites; V_d is 4 ± 0.4 L/kg; Cl is 0.78 ± 0.12 L/hr/kg, decreased in the elderly and increased in neonates and children. Pharmacokinetics are not altered in renal insufficiency or compensated hepatic cirrhosis. Less than 10% is excreted unchanged in the urine.[86,102–105]

$t_{1/2}$. 6.1 ± 2 hr;[105] 7.1–11 hr during cardiopulmonary bypass surgery.[100]

Adverse Reactions. (*See* Morphine Sulfate.) Unlike other opioids, fentanyl, alfentanil, remifentanil, and sufentanil are not associated with histamine release and may be preferable when cardiovascular stability is an issue.[100] The frequency of pruritus is lower than that of morphine but not as low as that of meperidine.[106,107] PCA fentanyl produces less depression of postoperative cognitive function in elderly patients than does PCA morphine.[108] Development of withdrawal reactions after use for sedation in neonates and infants is likely with a total dosage >2.5 mg/kg or duration of infusion >9 days.[109]

Contraindications. (*See* Morphine Sulfate.) (Fentanyl SR patch) acute or postoperative pain, including outpatient surgery; patients <12 yr or <50 kg; pain that can be managed by conventional analgesics; and doses >25 μg/hr at the initiation of opioid therapy. (Oralet) management of acute and chronic pain. (Actiq) management of acute or postoperative pain.

Precautions. (*See* Morphine Sulfate.) Analyses of fentanyl transdermal systems after 3 days of continuous application demonstrated a considerable amount of remaining drug (28–84%), which is a potentially lethal dose (1036 μg) for a 70-kg individual.[110] Cutting the membrane-controlled fentanyl transdermal system to achieve a different dosage is not recommended because it can damage the integrity of the semipermeable membrane. Placing a piece of impermeable material (eg, adhesive bandage) on the skin proportionate in surface area to the intended reduction in dosage may be effective.[111]

Drug Interactions. (*See* Morphine Sulfate.) The effects of fentanyl may be potentiated by other CNS depressant drugs (eg, barbiturates, general anesthetics, narcotics, and tranquilizers) and ritonavir, the latter by inhibition of CYP2D6.[112] Carbamazepine may decrease fentanyl's effect during anesthesia for craniotomy.

Parameters to Monitor. Monitor vital signs and pain ratings routinely.

Notes. Epidural administration has not been shown to be more advantageous than IV administration during surgery.[113] Lack of rapid titratability precludes the usefulness of the transdermal fentanyl system for pain control in patients with rapidly changing analgesic requirements. Transdermal fentanyl for cancer pain causes a lower frequency of constipation than SR morphine.[114] IV is the parenteral route of choice after major surgery. This route is suitable for titrated bolus or continuous administration but requires close monitoring because there is a great risk of respiratory depression with inappropriate dosage.[115]

MEPERIDINE HYDROCHLORIDE   Demerol, Various

Pharmacology. Meperidine is a phenylpiperidine opioid agonist with important antimuscarinic activity and negative inotropic effects on the heart. Its major metabolite, normeperidine, has excitant effects that can precipitate tremors, myoclonus, or seizures. Meperidine's antimuscarinic activity might negate the miosis that occurs with other opioids.[87] (*See* Morphine Sulfate.)

Administration and Adult Dosage. **PO, IV, or SC for analgesia** 50–150 mg q 3–4 hr. (*See* Notes.) Oral doses are about one-half as effective as parenteral doses. Reduce dosage when given concomitantly with a phenothiazine or other drugs that potentiate the depressant effects of meperidine. **IV for shaking caused by general anesthesia or amphotericin B** 25–50 mg. (*See* Notes.) **IM** not recommended.[115]

Special Populations. *Pediatric Dosage.* **PO, IV, or SC for analgesia** 1–1.8 mg/kg q 3–4 hr, to a maximum of 100 mg/dose. **IM** painful and should not be used in children.[116] (*See* Notes.)

Geriatric Dosage. Same as adult dosage.

Dosage Forms. **Syrup** 10 mg/mL; **Tab** 50, 100 mg; **Inj** 10, 25, 50, 75, 100 mg/mL.

Patient Instructions. (*See* Opioids Class Instructions.)

Pharmacokinetics. *Onset and Duration.* PO onset about 15 min; duration 2–3 hr. SC or IM onset about 10 min; peak analgesia 0.5–1 hr; duration 2–3 hr.[19,91]

Serum Levels. 500–700 µg/L (2–2.8 µmol/L) appear to be required for analgesia.[103]

Fate. Oral bioavailability is about 52 ± 3%, increasing to 80–90% in cirrhosis caused by decreased first-pass metabolism.[19,117] After a single 100 mg IM dose, mean serum levels of 670 µg/L (2.7 µmol/L) and 650 µg/L (2.6 µmol/L) are attained in 1 and 2 hr, respectively[118,119]; 58 ± 9% plasma protein bound, largely to α_1-acid glycoprotein; decreased in the elderly and in uremia.[19,120] V_d is 4.4 ± 0.9 L/kg, increased in the elderly and premature infants; Cl is 1.02 ± 0.3 L/hr/kg, reduced by 25% in surgical patients and 50% in cirrhosis, and reduced in acute viral hepatitis.[19] Hydrolyzed and metabolized in the liver to normeperidine (an active metabolite), which is also hydrolyzed. An average of 2% unchanged drug and 1–21% (average 6%) normeperidine are excreted in urine.[120]

$t_{1/2}$. (Meperidine) α phase 12 min, β phase 3.2 hr, increasing to 7 hr in patients with cirrhosis or acute liver disease and 14–21 hr in patients with moderate to severe renal dysfunction.[119,121,122] (Normeperidine) 14–21 hr in normals, increasing to 35 hr in renal failure.[123]

Adverse Reactions. (*See* Morphine Sulfate.) Factors that can predispose to normeperidine-induced seizures are dosage >400–600 mg/day, renal failure, history of seizures, long-term administration to cancer patients, and co-administration of agents that increase N-demethylation to normeperidine.[124] (*See* Drug Interactions.) Local irritation and induration occur with repeated SC injection.

Contraindications. MAO inhibitors within the past 14–21 days; chronic pain.

Precautions. (*See* Morphine Sulfate.) Avoid in patients with reduced renal function and avoid continuous administration for more than a few days. The combination of meperidine with promethazine and chlorpromazine (DPT) for painful procedures is not recommended because it has poor efficacy compared with alternative approaches and is associated with a high frequency of adverse effects.[115]

Drug Interactions. (*See* Morphine Sulfate.) Concurrent use with an MAO inhibitor can cause marked blood pressure alterations, sweating, excitation, and rigidity. Barbiturates, chlorpromazine, and phenytoin can decrease meperidine serum concentrations and increase normeperidine, reducing analgesia and increasing the risk of stimulation and seizures.[125] Ritonavir can increase meperidine AUC via CYP2D6 inhibition.[112]

Parameters to Monitor. Monitor vital signs and pain scores at regular intervals. Jerking and twitching movements may be signs of normeperidine accumulation and impending toxicity.[126]

Notes. All opioids including meperidine and morphine increase biliary tract pressure. Sphincter of Oddi spasm may be less with meperidine than with morphine, but there is little evidence that this has clinical relevance. Unlike other opioids, meperidine is useful in treating the shaking and shivering associated with general anesthesia or amphotericin B administration.[124] Because of its low therapeutic index, reserve meperidine for very brief courses in otherwise healthy patients who have demonstrated untoward effects during treatment with other opioids such as morphine or hydromorphone.[115] Because of its unreliable absorption and break-through pain when meperidine is administered IM, more rapid and predictable routes (eg, IV) are recommended.[116,127,128] Oral meperidine is not recommended for cancer pain because the high dosage required to relieve severe pain increases the risk of CNS toxicity.[116]

METHADONE HYDROCHLORIDE   Dolophine, Various

Pharmacology. Methadone is a phenylheptylamine opioid agonist qualitatively similar to morphine but with a chemical structure unrelated to the alkaloid-type structures of the opium derivatives. Analgesic activity of (R)-methadone is 8–50 times that of (S)-methadone, and (R)-methadone has a 10-fold higher affinity for opioid receptors. Methadone is lipophilic and has considerable tissue distribution; plasma concentrations during long-term treatment are sustained by this peripheral reservoir. It does not share cross-tolerance with other opioids, and the dosage required to achieve analgesia in opioid-tolerant patients is much lower than predicted by opioid conversion tables and single-dose studies. Unlike other opioids, methadone does not have active or toxic metabolites that are associated with CNS toxicity (eg, myoclonus, seizures).[129,130] Because methadone is a long-acting narcotic agent, it can be substituted for short-acting narcotic agents for analgesia maintenance and detoxification. Methadone abstinence syndrome is similar to morphine; however, onset is slower and duration is longer. (*See* Morphine Sulfate.)

Administration and Adult Dosage. **PO, IV, or SC for pain** 5–80 mg/day in 1–3 divided doses. Dosage escalation is slower than with other opioids and averages approximately 2%/day.[129] **PO for maintenance and detoxification treatment** the minimum effective dosage for reducing illicit heroin use is approximately 60 mg/day, and the optimum dosage range is 80–120 mg/day. Premature termination of treatment and use of suboptimal dosages remain common problems. If tapering is attempted, taper gradually over 4–12 months or longer.[131] **To convert from another opioid** decrease the previous opioid dosage by one-third over 24 hr and replace it with methadone using a dosage ratio of 1 mg oral methadone = 10 mg oral morphine. During day 2, attempt another one-third decrease in the dosage of the previous opioid; on day 3, the final one-third of the dosage of the previous opioid may be discontinued. Maintain the patient on an q-8-hr schedule with approximately 10% of the daily methadone dosage as an extra dose for breakthrough pain.[129]

Special Populations. *Pediatric Dosage.* **IV for pain** 0.1 mg/kg q 6–8 hr; **PO for pain** 0.2 mg/kg q 6–8 hr.[116]

Geriatric Dosage. Same as adult dosage.

Dosage Forms. **Tab** 5, 10 mg; **Dispersible Tab** 40 mg; **Soln** 1, 2, 10 mg/mL; **Inj** 10 mg/mL; **Pwdr** 50, 100, 500, 1000 g.

Patient Instructions. (*See* Opioids Class Instructions.) Increase dosage cautiously with the assistance of your clinician.

Pharmacokinetics. *Onset and Duration.* (Analgesia) onset SC 10–20 min, PO 30–60 min; peak SC 0.5–1 hr; duration PO, SC, or IV 4–5 hr after a single dose, 8–48 hr with multiple doses.[103,129,130]

Serum Levels. Best rehabilitation in methadone maintenance patients has been associated with serum levels >211 µg/L (682 nmol/L).[132] There is no good correlation between serum levels and analgesia.[130]

Fate. Oral bioavailability is 92 ± 21%; 89% plasma protein bound. Pharmacokinetics are best described by a 2-compartment model. $V_{d\beta}$ is 3.8 ± 0.6 L/kg; Cl is 0.084 ± 0.03 L/hr/kg. Both $V_{d\beta}$ and Cl are greater for (R)-methadone.[130] Extent of metabolism may increase with long-term therapy, resulting in a 15–25% decline in serum levels, although this has also been attributed to poor compliance. Metabolized in the liver to inactive metabolites via N-demethylation; metabolites are excreted in urine and bile.[129] The drug is 24 ± 10% excreted unchanged in the urine, increased by urine acidification.[19,132,133]

$t_{1/2}$. β phase 35 ± 12 hr;[19] (R)-methadone has a longer half-life (37.5 hr) than (S)-methadone (28.6 hr).[130]

Adverse Reactions. (*See* Morphine Sulfate.) Because of its long half-life and lack of cross-tolerance, patients receiving methadone are at greater risk for toxicity when inappropriate dosage increases are made.

Precautions. (*See* Morphine Sulfate.) The process of switching from another opioid to methadone is complex and should only be attempted by an experienced clinician in an inpatient setting over 3–6 days. (*See* Administration and Adult Dosage.)[129]

Drug Interactions. (*See* Morphine Sulfate.) Carbamazepine, phenytoin, rifampin, and other drugs that induce CYP3A4 can decrease methadone serum levels and result in withdrawal symptoms in patients on methadone maintenance programs. Diazepam, erythromycin, fluvoxamine, ritonavir, and possibly other enzyme inhibitors can increase methadone levels and effects.[125,134]

Parameters to Monitor. During analgesia, monitor vital signs and pain ratings routinely. During methadone maintenance, monitor for signs of withdrawal, which include lacrimation, rhinorrhea, diaphoresis, yawning, restlessness, insomnia, dilated pupils, and piloerection.[131]

Notes. For treatment of narcotic addiction in detoxification or maintenance programs, methadone may be dispensed only by approved pharmacies. Maintenance therapy (treatment for longer than 3 weeks) may be undertaken only by approved methadone programs; this does not apply to addicts hospitalized for other medical conditions.

MORPHINE SULFATE	Various

Pharmacology. Morphine and other opioids interact with stereospecific opiate receptors in the CNS and other tissues. (*See* Opioid Receptor Specificity Comparison Chart.) Opioid analgesia is caused by actions at several CNS sites. Morphine and other mu opioid agonists inhibit nociceptive reflexes through inhibition of neurotransmitter release, have inhibitory actions on neurons conveying nociceptive information to higher brain centers, and enhance activity in descending pathways that exert inhibitory effects on the processing of nociceptive information in the spinal cord. Mu receptors are responsible for analgesia, respiratory depression, miosis, decreased GI motility, and euphoria. Stimulation of kappa receptors results in analgesia, less intense miosis and respiratory depression, dysphoria, and psychotomimetic effects. It is unclear what the consequences of delta receptor stimulation are in humans.[86] The relief of pain is fairly specific; other sensory modalities are essentially unaffected, and mental processes are not impaired (unlike anesthetics), except when given in large doses or to opiate-naive individuals. These drugs also have antitussive effects, usually at dosages less than those required for analgesia.

Administration and Adult Dosage. With the exception of transdermal fentanyl, there is no ceiling or maximum dosage for morphine or other opioid agonists, and very large doses may be required for severe pain.[116] **PO for analgesia** 8–20 mg q 4 hr; **SR Tab, 12-hr** (narcotic-naive patients) 30 mg q 8–12 hr initially; (narcotic-tolerant patients) total daily oral morphine dosage equivalent in 2 divided doses q 12 hr; **SR Cap, 24-hr** (narcotic-naive patients) 20 mg q 24 hr initially; (narcotic-tolerant patients) total daily oral morphine dosage equivalent q 24 hr; **SC for analgesia** 5–15 mg q 4 hr (10 mg/70 kg is the optimal initial dose); **PR for analgesia** 10–20 mg q 4 hr. **IV for analgesia** 4–10 mg, dilute and inject slowly over a 2–3-min period. **IV infusion** 1–10 mg/hr;[135] some patients with chronic pain may require a dosage as high as 95 mg/hr or more.[136] **IV PCA** 1 mg per activation initially with 5–20 min lockout period, both titrated to patient response.[137,138] Continuous infusion combined with PCA is effective in chronic cancer pain.[139] **Epidural for analgesia (unpreserved solution)** (intermittent) 5 mg initially, may repeat with 1–2 mg after 1 hr; (continuous infusion) 0.05–0.1 mg/kg loading dose, then 0.005–0.01 mg/kg/hr.[140] **IT for cancer pain (unpreserved solution)** 0.4–8.3 mg/day (average 1–23 mg/day);[141] **IT for cesarean section (unpreserved solution)** 0.1 mg.[142] **Intraventricular (unpreserved solution)** 0.1–2 mg, repeated approximately q 24 hr.[143] **Inhal for dyspnea** 5–15 mg in 2 mL sterile water or NS via nebulizer q 4 hr.[144] **IM** is painful and is not recommended.[116]

Special Populations. *Pediatric Dosage.* **PO** 0.3 mg/kg q 3–4 hr. **IV** 0.05–0.2 mg/kg q 4 hr. **IV infusion** 0.01–0.04 mg/kg/hr. **Epidural** 0.05–0.08 mg/kg. **IT** 0.01–0.03 mg/kg.[116,145,146]

Geriatric Dosage. Reduce initial dosage in elderly patients and make smaller percentage incremental increases in total daily dosage (eg, 25%) than in younger patients.

Other Conditions. Reduce initial dosage in debilitated patients.

Dosage Forms. **Cap** 15, 30 mg; **Soln** 2, 4, 20 mg/mL; **Supp** 5, 10, 20, 30 mg; **Tab** 10, 15, 30 mg; **SR Tab** (8, 12 hr) 15, 30, 60, 100, 200 mg; **SR Cap (24 hr)** 20, 50, 100 mg; **Inj** (unpreserved solution) 0.5, 1, 10, 25, 50 mg/mL; (preserved solution) 2, 3, 4, 5, 8, 10, 15, 25, 50 mg/mL.

Patient Instructions. (*See* Opioids Class Instructions.)

Pharmacokinetics. *Onset and Duration.* (Analgesia) onset IM 10–30 min; peak 0.5–1 hr; duration 3–5 hr.[103]

Serum Levels. It is speculated that moderate analgesia requires serum levels of at least 50 µg/L (88 nmol/L).

Fate. Well absorbed from the GI tract, but first-pass conjugation is extensive, reducing oral bioavailability to 24 ± 12%.[19,147] Nebulized morphine by inhalation has a low bioavailability, 5 ± 3%, but a rapid peak at 10 min.[147] After an IM dose of 10 mg, peak morphine levels of about 56 µg/L (98 nmol/L) are reached within 20 min. The drug is 35 ± 2% plasma protein bound and decreased in acute viral hepatitis, cirrhosis, and hypoalbuminemia.[19] V_d is 2.12 L/kg in young normals and 1.16 L/kg in elderly patients; Cl is 2.02 L/hr/kg in young normals and 1.66 L/hr/kg in elderly patients.[135] Morphine clearance reaches adult level by age 6 months–2.5 yr.[148] Inactivated in the liver, primarily by conjugation to morphine–6–glucuronide (active) and morphine-3-glucuronide (inactive or antagonistic).[19,149] Decreased clearance of glucuronide metabolites has been demonstrated in patients with renal insufficiency.[150] Greater plasma concentrations of morphine–6–glucuronide are present with oral than with parenteral administration.[151] Mostly excreted in urine; 14 ± 7% as the active morphine-6-glucuronide and 3.4% (oral) to 9% (parenteral) of a dose is excreted unchanged.[19,149,152]

$t_{1/2}$. 1.9 ± 0.5 hr, increased in neonates and premature infants.[19]

Adverse Reactions. Respiratory and circulatory depression and constipation are major adverse effects. Patients with renal failure are more prone to develop adverse reactions.[153] Dose-related signs of intoxication are miosis, drowsiness, decreased rate and depth of respiration, bradycardia, and hypotension. Sedation, dizziness, nausea, vomiting, sweating, and constipation occur frequently. Euphoria, dysphoria, dry mouth, biliary tract spasm, postural hypotension, syncope, tachy- or bradycardia, urinary retention, and myoclonus occur occasionally. Myoclonus appears to be somewhat dose related and has been described after large doses via IV or intraspinal routes. Myoclonus can be managed by changing to another opioid or with a **benzodiazepine** or **dantrolene**.[154,155] Frequent adverse effects from epidural administration are urinary retention and pruritus; the latter can be managed with **naloxone** or **butorphanol**.[140] Possible allergic-type reactions are reported occasionally. Most allergic-type reactions consist of skin rash and wheal and flare over a vein, which can occur with IV injection; these are caused by direct stimulation of histamine release, are not allergic, and are not a sign of a more serious reaction. True allergy is rare. Confusion and disorientation have been linked to phenol and formaldehyde preservatives in epidural infusions, and seizures have been associated with high-dose IV infusions containing sodium bisulfite.[156,157]

Precautions. Use with caution and in reduced dosage when giving concurrently with other CNS-depressant drugs. Use with caution in pregnancy; the presence of head injury, other intracranial lesions, or pre-existing increase in intracranial pressure; patients having an acute asthmatic attack; COPD or cor pulmonale; decreased respiratory reserve; pre-existing respiratory depression, hypoxia, or hypercapnia; patients whose ability to maintain blood pressure is already compromised; patients with atrial flutter or other supraventricular tachycardias; patients with prostatic hypertrophy or urethral stricture; elderly or debilitated patients; and patients with acute abdominal pain, when administration of the drug might obscure the diagnosis or clinical course. Use with caution in the elderly and neonates and in patients with renal dysfunction or elevated bilirubin or LDH levels.[148,150,151,153] Infants >1 month eliminate morphine efficiently and are unlikely to be unusually sensitive to the respiratory depressant effects but may require longer dosage intervals.[148] Do not administer IV, IT, or epidurally to opiate-naive patients unless a narcotic antagonist and facilities for assisted or controlled respiration are immediately available.

Drug Interactions. Concurrent use of opioids with other CNS depressants (eg, alcohol, antipsychotics, general anesthetics, heterocyclic antidepressants, and sedative-hypnotics) can cause respiratory depression. Cimetidine can increase serum concentration and duration of effect of the opioids.[125]

Parameters to Monitor. Monitor for pain control and signs of respiratory or cardiovascular depression.

NALOXONE HYDROCHLORIDE   Narcan, Various

Pharmacology. Naloxone, an N-allyl derivative of oxymorphone, is a narcotic antagonist that competitively binds at opiate receptors. Naloxone is essentially free of narcotic agonist properties and is used to reverse the effects of narcotic agonists and drugs with partial agonist properties.[158]

Administration and Adult Dosage. **IV (preferred) or SC for known or suspected narcotic overdose** 0.1–0.2 mg as a first dose, then progressively double the dose q 2–3 min or 0.4 mg diluted in 9 mL saline and injected in 1-mL increments q 30–60 seconds, until respiration and consciousness have become normal or until 10 mg has been given. If response occurs, to prevent recurrent toxicity due to short naloxone half-life, IV infusion at an hourly rate equal to the initial dose required for arousal, with a possible repeat bolus of 50% required 20–30 min after start of infusion.[159,160] If a total of 10 mg has been given and there is no response, the diagnosis of narcotic overdose should be questioned. The frequency of repeat doses is based on clinical evaluation of the patient. **IV for postoperative narcotic depression** 0.1–0.2 mg initially, may repeat q 2–3 min until desired level of reversal is reached. Subsequent doses might be needed if the effect of the narcotic outlasts the action of naloxone. (*See* Notes.) **IV for epidural opioid-induced pruritus** 0.005–0.01 mg/kg either in incremental doses or as an hourly infusion.[140] **PO for opioid-induced constipation** 4–12 mg not more often than q 6 hr; more frequent administration might precipitate withdrawal. Give at a daily dose of approximately 20% of the 24-hr morphine dose. Initial doses should not exceed 5 mg.[161,162]

Special Populations. *Pediatric Dosage.* **IV for known or suspected narcotic overdose** 0.01 mg/kg, may repeat as needed. **IV for postoperative narcotic depression** 0.005–0.01 mg initially, may repeat q 2–3 min until desired level of reversal is reached. **IV (preferred) or SC for narcotic depression** (neonates) 0.01 mg/kg initially, may repeat q 2–3 min until desired level of reversal is reached.

Geriatric Dosage. Same as adult dosage.

Dosage Forms. **Inj** 0.02, 0.4, 1 mg/mL.

Pharmacokinetics. *Onset and Duration.* Onset IV within 2–3 min, up to 15 min when given IM or SC; duration variable but usually 1 hr or less.[163,164]

Fate. From 59% to 67% metabolized by hepatic conjugation and renal elimination of the conjugated compound.[165] V_d is approximately 2–3 L/kg;[19,166] Cl is about 1.3 L/hr/kg.[19]

$t_{1/2}$. 64 ± 12 min in adults,[167] 71 ± 36 min in neonates.[168]

Adverse Reactions. Naloxone administration has been occasionally associated with life-threatening complications such as pulmonary edema, seizures, hypertension, arrhythmias, and violent behavior within 10 min of parenteral administration.[159,160]

Contraindications. None known.

Precautions. Administration to narcotic-dependent persons (including neonates of dependent mothers) might precipitate acute withdrawal symptoms.

Drug Interactions. None known except for opioid antagonism.

Parameters to Monitor. Respiratory rate, pupil size (might not be useful in mixed-drug or narcotic partial agonist overdoses), heart rate, blood pressure, and symptoms of acute narcotic withdrawal syndrome.

Notes. Naloxone is effective when administered endotracheally to patients with difficult venous access.[169] It is routinely used in the initial treatment of patients with coma of unknown origin. Its use in **clonidine** overdose has produced mixed results; use in septic and hemorrhagic shock has been disappointing.[158]

OPIOID PARTIAL AGONISTS

Pharmacology. These agents can be classified based on their effects on the opioid receptors. Opioid partial agonists have analgesic effects but are characterized by an analgesic ceiling, such that, beyond a certain point, further increases in dosage do not result in additional analgesia but might produce adverse effects.[86,116] **Tramadol** is partly metabolized by CYP2D6, thereby producing an active metabolite (M1) that binds to mu opioid receptors. Patients who are poor metabolizers of debrisoquine and sparteine have negligible M1 production and reduced analgesia, although some pain relief remains because of activation of monoaminergic antinociceptive pathways from tramadol enantiomers.[86,170]

Administration, Dosage, and Dosage Forms. (*See* Opioid Analgesics Comparison Chart.)

Patient Instructions. (*See* Opioids Class Instructions.)

Pharmacokinetics. (*See* Opioid Analgesics Comparison Chart.)

Adverse Reactions. Sedation, sweating, dizziness, nausea, vomiting, euphoria, dysphoria (agents with delta receptor activity), and hallucinations are most frequent. Occasionally, insomnia, anxiety, anorexia, constipation, dry mouth, syncope, visual blurring, flushing, decreased blood pressure, and tachycardia are reported. After parenteral use, diaphoresis, sting on injection, respiratory depression, transient apnea in the newborn from administration to the mother during labor, shock, urinary retention, and alterations in uterine contractions during labor occur rarely. Other rarely reported effects are muscle tremor and toxic epidermal necrolysis. Local skin reactions and ulceration and fibrous myopathy at the injection site have been reported with long-term parenteral use of pentazocine.[86] **Tramadol** adverse reactions include seizures (some after the first dose) with recommended and excessive dosages. Seizure risk is increased in patients taking concomitant medications that can reduce the seizure threshold (eg, heterocyclic antidepressants, selective serotonin reuptake inhibitors, MAO inhibitors, neuroleptics) and with certain medical conditions (eg, epilepsy, head trauma, metabolic disorders, alcohol and drug withdrawal, or CNS infection). In addition, **naloxone** administration for tramadol overdose can increase the risk of seizure. Anaphylactoid reactions also have been described in tramadol postmarketing surveillance.[171–173] Dependence/addiction and major psychological disturbances have been reported with **butorphanol** nasal spray.[174]

Contraindications. (Tramadol) prior allergy to any opiate; acute intoxication with alcohol, hypnotics, centrally acting analgesics, opioids, or psychotropic drugs. (*See* Notes.)

Precautions. (*See* Morphine Sulfate.) Also, use cautiously in MI patients because **pentazocine** and **butorphanol** increase cardiac workload. All of these agents can produce dependence and withdrawal symptoms after extended use.

Drug Interactions. (*See* Morphine Sulfate.) With the possible exception of tramadol, these agents can precipitate acute withdrawal in narcotic-dependent individuals.[175]

Notes. Because of their ceiling effect, risk of precipitating opiate withdrawal, and marked adverse effects, these agents are not recommended for the management of cancer pain.[116] Effects of pentazocine are antagonized by naloxone. Naloxone in Talwin NX tablets is not absorbed orally but theoretically prevents parenteral abuse of the oral dosage form; however, IV abuse of Talwin Nx plus tripelennamine has been reported.[176]

OPIOID RECEPTOR SPECIFICITY COMPARISON CHART

| DRUG | RECEPTOR TYPE | | |
	Mu	Kappa	Delta
Buprenorphine	Partial agonist-antagonist	Unknown	Minimal activity
Butorphanol	Partial agonist-antagonist	Agonist	Unknown
Dezocine	Partial agonist-antagonist	Agonist	Minimal agonist activity
Morphine	Agonist	Minimal agonist activity	Unknown
Nalbuphine	Antagonist	Agonist	Agonist
Pentazocine	Partial agonist-antagonist	Agonist	Unknown
Tramadol[a]	Partial or pure agonist[b]	Minimal activity	Unknown

[a]Also blocks norepinephrine and serotonin reuptake.
[b]Not a classic agonist–antagonist; has little or no antagonist properties but appears to have partial mu receptor agonist activity.

PATIENT-CONTROLLED ANALGESIA (PCA) GUIDELINES CHART[a]

DRUG	IV BOLUS DOSE (MG)	LOCKOUT INTERVAL (MIN)
Buprenorphine	0.03–0.2	10–20
Fentanyl	0.02–0.1	3–10
Hydromorphone	0.1–0.5	3–15
Meperidine[b]	5–30	5–15
Methadone	0.5–3	10–20
Morphine[a]	0.5–3	5–20
Nalbuphine	1–5	5–15
Oxymorphone	0.2–0.8	5–15
Pentazocine	5–30	5–15
Sufentanil	0.003–0.015	3–10

[a]Some clinicians recommend combining PCA with a basal continuous infusion of the narcotic. The hourly dosage is determined by the patient's previous narcotic dose requirements and adjusted q 8–24 hr based on the dose of PCA bolus administered, basal continuous infusion, and pain response. A typical starting hourly basal continuous infusion rate for morphine in a 70 kg adult is 0.5–3 mg/hr.
[b]Use with caution (preferably avoid) for PCA and consider factors that might predispose to seizures, which include dosage over 100 mg q 2 hr for longer than 24 hr, renal failure, or history of seizure disorder.
From references 91, 137, and 139.

INTRASPINAL NARCOTIC ADMINISTRATION GUIDELINES CHART[a]

ROUTE AND DRUG	INTRASPINAL BOLUS DOSE (MG)	ONSET (MIN)	DURATION (HR)
EPIDURAL			
Alfentanil	0.7–2[b]	Rapid	1.5–1.7[c]
Fentanyl	0.025–0.15	5	2–4
Hydromorphone	1–2	15	10–16
Methadone	1–10	10	6–10
Morphine	1–10	30	6–24
Sufentanil	0.015–0.05	15	4–6
INTRATHECAL (SUBARACHNOID)			
Morphine	0.1–0.5	15	8–24

[a]Use only preservative-free preparations for intraspinal narcotic administration.
[b]Based on a 70 kg adult body weight (ie, 10–30 μg/kg).
[c]Very short duration of action; requires epidural infusion to obtain prolonged analgesia. Like fentanyl, prolonged epidural infusions produce high systemic concentrations and appear to have little advantage over IV infusion.
From references 91 and 100.

OPIOID ANALGESICS COMPARISON CHART

DRUG AND SCHEDULE[a]	DOSAGE FORMS	EQUIVALENT PARENTERAL DOSAGE[b] (MG)	EQUIVALENT ORAL DOSAGE[c] (MG)	PARENTERAL/ORAL EFFICACY RATIO	DURATION OF ANALGESIA (HR)	PARTIAL ANTAGONIST ACTIVITY
Alfentanil (C-II) Alfenta	Inj 500 μg/mL.	1	—	—	<1	no
Buprenorphine (C-V) Buprenex Subutex[d]	Inj 0.324 mg/mL SL tab 2, 8 mg.	0.3–0.6 [0.4–0.8][d,e]	—	—	6–8	yes
Butorphanol Stadol (NC) Stadol NS (C-IV)	Inj 1, 2 mg/mL Nasal Spray 10 mg/mL (1 mg/spray).[f]	2	—	1/16	3–4	yes
Codeine (C-II) Various	Inj 30, 60 mg/mL Soln 3 mg/mL Tab 15, 30, 60 mg.	120	30	1/2–2/3	4–6	no
Dezocine (NC) Dalgan	Inj 5, 10, 15 mg/mL.	10–15	—	—	3–4	yes
Fentanyl (C-II) Actiq Sublimaze Various	Inj 50 μg/mL SR Patch 25, 50, 75, 100 μg/hr Lozenge 100, 200, 300, 400 μg Lozenge on a stick 200, 400, 600, 800, 1200, 1600 μg.	0.1	—	1/5	1–2 (patch, 72)	no
Hydrocodone and Acetaminophen (C-III) Vicodin Various	Tab 5, 7.5, 10 mg with acetaminophen 400 mg, 2.5, 5, 7.5 mg with acetaminophen 500 mg, 7.5 mg with acetaminophen 400, 500, 650, 750 mg, 10 mg with acetaminophen 325, 400, 500, 650, 660 mg Cap 5 mg with acetaminophen 500 mg Soln 0.5 mg with acetaminophen 33 mg/mL.	—	5	—	4–6	no

(continued)

OPIOID ANALGESICS COMPARISON CHART (continued)

DRUG AND SCHEDULE[a]	DOSAGE FORMS	EQUIVALENT PARENTERAL DOSAGE[b] (MG)	EQUIVALENT ORAL DOSAGE[c] (MG)	PARENTERAL/ORAL EFFICACY RATIO	DURATION OF ANALGESIA (HR)	PARTIAL ANTAGONIST ACTIVITY
Hydromorphone (C-II) Dilaudid Various	Inj 1, 2, 4, 10 mg/mL Inj 250 mg Tab 1, 2, 3, 4, 8 mg Soln 1 mg/mL Supp 3 mg.	1.5	1	1/5–1/2	3–5	no
Levorphanol (C-II) Levo-Dromoran	Inj 2 mg/mL Tab 2 mg.	2	—	1/2	4–6	no
Meperidine (C-II) Demerol Various	Inj 10, 25, 50, 75, 100 mg/mL Tab 50, 100 mg Syrup 10 mg/mL.	75–100	50	1/3–1/2	2–4	no
Methadone (C-II) Dolophine Various	Inj 10 mg/mL Tab 5, 10 mg Dispersible Tab 40 mg Pwdr 50, 100, 500, 1000 g Soln 1, 2, 10 mg/mL.	g	g	1/2	8–48	no
Morphine (C-II) Various	Inj 0.5, 1, 2, 4, 5, 8, 10, 15, 25, 50 mg/mL Tab 10, 15, 30 mg Cap 15, 30 mg Soln 2, 4, 20 mg/mL SR Cap 20, 50, 100 mg SR Tab 15, 30, 60, 100, 200 mg Supp 5, 10, 20, 30 mg.	10	5	1/3	3–5	no

(continued)

OPIOID ANALGESICS COMPARISON CHART (*continued*)

DRUG AND SCHEDULE[a]	DOSAGE FORMS	EQUIVALENT PARENTERAL DOSAGE[b] (MG)	EQUIVALENT ORAL DOSAGE[c] (MG)	PARENTERAL/ORAL EFFICACY RATIO	DURATION OF ANALGESIA (HR)	PARTIAL ANTAGONIST ACTIVITY
Nalbuphine (NC) Nubain Various	Inj 10, 20 mg/mL.	10	—	1/6	3–6	yes
Oxycodone (C-II) Oxycontin Roxicodone	Cap 5 mg Tab 5 mg Tab 2.5, 5 mg with acetaminophen 325 mg, 5 mg with aceta- minophen 500 mg, 7.5 mg with acetaminophen 500 mg, 10 mg with acetaminophen 650 mg. Soln 1, 20 mg/mL SR Tab 10, 20, 40, 80 mg.	—	5	—	3–4	no
Oxymorphone (C-II) Numorphan	Inj 1, 1.5 mg/mL Supp 5 mg.	1–1.5	—	1/6	4–5	no
Pentazocine (C-IV) Talwin Talwin Nx Various	Inj 30 mg/mL Tab 50 mg with naloxone 0.5 mg. Tab 12.5 mg with aspirin 325 mg, 25 mg with acetaminophen 650 mg.	30–60	25	1/3	2–3	yes
Propoxyphene (C-IV) Darvon Various	Cap (HCl) 65 mg Tab (HCl) 65 mg with acetaminophen 650 mg. Tab (Napsylate) 50, 100 mg Tab (Napsylate) 50 mg with acetaminophen 325 mg, 100 mg with acetaminophen 650 mg. Susp (Napsylate) 10 mg/mL.	—	65 (HCl) 100 (Napsylate)	—	4–6	no

(continued)

OPIOID ANALGESICS COMPARISON CHART (continued)

DRUG AND SCHEDULE[a]	DOSAGE FORMS	EQUIVALENT PARENTERAL DOSAGE[b] (MG)	EQUIVALENT ORAL DOSAGE[c] (MG)	PARENTERAL/ORAL EFFICACY RATIO	DURATION OF ANALGESIA (HR)	PARTIAL ANTAGONIST ACTIVITY
Remifentanil (C-II) Ultiva	Inj 3, 5, 10 mg.	0.1	—	—	< 0.5	no
Sufentanil (C-II) Sufenta	Inj 50 µg/mL.	0.01	—	—	2.5–3.5	no
Tramadol (NC) Ultram	Tab 50 mg. Tab 50 mg with acetaminophen (Ultracet)	—	25	—	4–6	—

[a]Controlled Substance Schedule designated after each drug (in parentheses); NC = not controlled.
[b]Parenteral dose equivalent to 10 mg morphine.
[c]Oral dose equivalent to 30 mg codeine. Not for SR products.
[d]Subutex and Suboxone (buprenorphine plus naloxone) are used in treating addiction.
[e]Equivalent sublingual dose.
[f]Recommended dosage is one spray in one nostril, repeated prn in 60–90 min; this cycle may then be repeated q 3–4 hr prn pain.
[g]See Pharmacology and Notes in Methadone monograph.
From references 86, 91, 100, 103, 104, 117, 177–180 and product information.

REFERENCES

1. Scott AK. Dihydroergotamine: a review of its use in the treatment of migraine and other headaches. *Clin Neuropharmacol* 1992;15:289–96.
2. Ducharme J. Canadian Association of Emergency Physicians guidelines for the acute management of migraine headache. *J Emerg Med* 1999;17:137–44.
3. Humbert H et al. Human pharmacokinetics of dihydroergotamine administered by nasal spray. *Clin Pharmacol Ther* 1996;60:265–75.
4. Dihydroergotamine Nasal Spray Multicenter Investigators. Efficacy, safety, and tolerability of dihydroergotamine nasal spray as monotherapy in the treatment of acute migraine. *Headache* 1995;35:177–84.
5. Gallagher RM. Acute treatment of migraine with dihydroergotamine nasal spray. *Arch Neurol* 1996;53:1285–91.
6. Touchon J et al. A comparison of subcutaneous sumatriptan and dihydroergotamine nasal spray in the acute treatment of migraine. *Neurology* 1996;47:361–5.
7. Perrin VL. Clinical pharmacokinetics of ergotamine in migraine and cluster headache. *Clin Pharmacokinet* 1985;10:334–52.
8. Sanders SM et al. Pharmacokinetics of ergotamine in healthy volunteers following oral and rectal dosing. *Eur J Clin Pharmacol* 1986;30:331–4.
9. Ibraheem JJ et al. Kinetics of ergotamine after intravenous and intramuscular administration to migraine sufferers. *Eur J Clin Pharmacol* 1982;23:235–40.
10. Saper JR. Ergotamine dependency a review. *Headache* 1987;27:435–8.
11. Bartleson JD. Treatment of migraine headaches. *Mayo Clin Proc* 1999;74:702–8.
12. Bredberg U et al. Pharmacokinetics of methysergide and its metabolite methylergometrine in man. *Eur J Clin Pharmacol* 1986;30:75–7.
13. Dechant KL, Clissold SP. Sumatriptan. A review of its pharmacodynamic and pharmacokinetic properties, and therapeutic efficacy in the acute treatment of migraine and cluster headache. *Drugs* 1992;43:776–98.
14. Plosker GL, McTavish D. Sumatriptan. A reappraisal of its pharmacology and therapeutic efficacy in the acute treatment of migraine and cluster headache. *Drugs* 1994;47:622–51.
15. The Subcutaneous Sumatriptan International Study Group. Treatment of migraine attacks with sumatriptan. *N Engl J Med* 1991;325:316–21.
16. Lacey LF et al. Single dose pharmacokinetics of sumatriptan in healthy volunteers. *Eur J Clin Pharmacol* 1995;47:543–8.
17. Fowler PA et al. The clinical pharmacology, pharmacokinetics and metabolism of sumatriptan. *Eur Neurol* 1991;31:291–4.
18. Dixon CM et al. Disposition of sumatriptan in laboratory animals and humans. *Drug Metab Dispos Biol Fate Chem* 1993;21:761–9.
19. Benet LZ et al. Design and optimization of dosage regimens: pharmacokinetic data. In, Hardman JG et al., eds. *Goodman and Gilman's the pharmacological basis of therapeutics.* 9th ed. New York: McGraw-Hill; 1996:1707–92.
20. The Multinational Oral Sumatriptan and Cafergot Comparative Study Group. A randomized, double-blind comparison of sumatriptan and Cafergot in the acute treatment of migraine. *Eur Neurol* 1991;31:314–22.
21. Dahlof C. The ideal 5-HT1D agonist. In, Olesen J, Tfelt-Hansen P, eds. *Headache treatment: trial methodology and new drugs.* Philadelphia: Lippincott-Raven; 1997:243–51.
22. Connor HE et al. Naratriptan: biological profile in animal models relevant to migraine. *Cephalalgia* 1997;17:145–52.
23. Deleu D, Hanssens Y. Current and emerging second-generation triptans in acute migraine therapy: a comparative review. *J Clin Pharmacol* 2000;40:687–700.
24. Ferrari MD. 311C90: increasing the options for therapy with effective acute antimigraine 5HT1B/1D receptor agonists. *Neurology* 1997;48(suppl 3):S21–4.
25. Zagami AS. 311C90: long-term efficacy and tolerability profile for the acute treatment of migraine. *Neurology* 1997;48(suppl 3):S25–8.
26. Diener HC, Klein KB. The first comparison of the efficacy and safety of 311C90 and sumatriptan in the treatment of migraine. Proc 3rd European Headache Conference 1996;10–1.
27. Goadsby PJ et al. Eletriptan in acute migraine: a double-blind, placebo-controlled comparison to sumatriptan. Neurology 2000;54:156–63.
28. Spierings ELH et al. Oral almotriptan versus oral sumatriptan in a double-blind, randomized, parallel-group study of quality of life and health economics in migraine patients. Neurology 2000;54(suppl 3):A266. Abstract.
29. Gomez-Mancilla B et al. A 6-month open-label study of orally administered almotriptan in migraine patients. Neurology 2000;54(suppl 3):A269. Abstract.

30. Lovell DJ et al. Etanercept in children with polyarticular juvenile rheumatoid arthritis. *N Engl J Med* 2000;342:763–9.
31. Cooksey LJ. Enbrel: TNF-receptor blocker for treating patients with refractory rheumatoid arthritis. *Formulary* 1999;34:211–9.
32. Bell SJ, Kamm MA. Review article: the clinical role of anti-TNFalpha antibody treatment in Crohn's disease. *Aliment Pharmacol Ther* 2000;14:501–14.
33. van Deventer SJ. Anti-TNF antibody treatment of Crohn's disease. *Ann Rheum Dis* 1999;58(suppl 1):I114–20.
34. Rutgeerts P et al. Efficacy and safety of retreatment with anti-tumor necrosis factor antibody (infliximab) to maintain remission in Crohn's disease. *Gastroenterology* 1999;117:761–9.
35. Hanauer SB. Review article: safety of infliximab in clinical trials. *Aliment Pharmacol Ther* 1999;13(suppl 4):16–22.
36. Maini R et al. Infliximab (chimeric anti-tumor necrosis factor α monoclonal antibody) versus placebo in rheumatoid arthritis patients receiving concomitant methotrexate: a randomised phase III trial. *Lancet* 1999;354:1932–9.
37. Heller T et al. Treatment of severe esophageal Crohn's disease with infliximab. *Inflamm Bowel Dis* 1999;5:279–82.
38. Geyer AS et al. Effectiveness of infliximab in the treatment of refractory perineal cutaneous Crohn disease. *Arch Dermatol* 2000;136:459–60.
39. Rozman B. Clinical experience with leflunomide in rheumatoid arthritis. *J Rheumatol* 1998;25(suppl 53):27–32.
40. American College of Rheumatology Ad Hoc Committee on Clinical Guidelines. Guidelines for the management of rheumatoid arthritis. *Arthritis Rheum* 1996;39:713–22.
41. American College of Rheumatology Ad Hoc Committee on Clinical Guidelines. Guidelines for monitoring drug therapy in rheumatoid arthritis. *Arthritis Rheum* 1996;39:723–31.
42. Gremillion RB, van Vollenhoven RF. Rheumatoid arthritis: designing and implementing a treatment plan. *Postgrad Med* 1998;103:103–6,110,116–8.
43. Horton S. Use of cyclosporine in rheumatoid arthritis. *Ann Pharmacother* 1993;27:44–6.
44. Schuna AA et al. Rheumatoid arthritis. In, DiPiro JT et al., eds. *Pharmacotherapy: a pathophysiologic approach.* 4th ed. Stamford, CT: Appleton & Lange; 1999:1427–40.
45. Segasothy M et al. Paracetamol: a cause for analgesic nephropathy and end-stage renal disease. *Nephron* 1988;50:50–4.
46. Zimmerman HJ, Maddrey WC. Acetaminophen (paracetamol) hepatotoxicity with regular intake of alcohol: analysis of instances of therapeutic misadventure. *Hepatology* 1995;22:767–73.
47. Shek KL et al. Warfarin-acetaminophen drug interaction revisited. *Pharmacotherapy* 1999;19:1153–8.
48. Buckley NA et al. Oral or intravenous N-acetylcysteine: which is the treatment of choice for acetaminophen (paracetamol) poisoning? *J Toxicol Clin Toxicol* 1999;37:759–67.
49. Towheed TE, Hochberg MC. A systematic review of randomized controlled trials of pharmacological therapy in osteoarthritis of the knee, with an emphasis on trial methodology. *Semin Arthritis Rheum* 1997;26:755–70.
50. Hirsh J et al. Aspirin and other platelet-active drugs. The relationship among dose, effectiveness, and side effects. *Chest* 1995;108:247S–57.
51. Albers GW et al. Antithrombotic and thrombolytic therapy for ischemic stroke. *Chest* 1998;114:683S–98.
52. Cairns JA et al. Antithrombotic agents in coronary artery disease. *Chest* 1998;114:611S–33.
53. Stein PD et al. Antithrombotic therapy in patients with saphenous vein and internal mammary artery bypass grafts. *Chest* 1998;114:658S–65.
54. Patrono C et al. Platelet-active drugs: the relationships among dose, effectiveness, and side effects. *Chest* 1998;114:470S–88.
55. Mongan E et al. Tinnitus as an indication of therapeutic serum salicylate levels. *JAMA* 1973;226:142–5.
56. Done AK. Aspirin-overdosage: incidence, diagnosis, and management. *Pediatrics* 1978;62(suppl):890–7.
57. Lanza FL et al. Endoscopic evaluation of the effects of aspirin, buffered aspirin, and enteric-coated aspirin on gastric and duodenal mucosa. *N Engl J Med* 1980;303:136–8.
58. Levy G. Pharmacokinetics of salicylate elimination in man. *J Pharm Sci* 1965;54:959–67.
59. Tolman KG. Hepatotoxicity on non-narcotic analgesics. *Am J Med* 1998;105(1B):13S–9.
60. Stevenson DD, Mathison DA. Aspirin sensitivity in asthmatics. When may this drug be safe? *Postgrad Med* 1985;78:111–9.
61. Bonica JJ, ed. *The management of pain,* 2nd ed. Philadelphia: Lea & Febiger; 1990.
62. Rahwan GL, Rahwan RG. Aspirin and Reye's syndrome: the change in prescribing habits of health professionals. *Drug Intell Clin Pharm* 1986;20:143–5.
63. Pinsky PF et al. Reye's syndrome and aspirin: evidence for a dose-response effect. *JAMA* 1988;260:657–61.

64. Housholder GT. Intolerance to aspirin and the nonsteroidal anti-inflammatory drugs. *J Oral Maxillofac Surg* 1985;43:333–7.

65. Hall AH et al. Ibuprofen overdose—a prospective study. *West J Med* 1988;148:653–6.

66. Nahata MC et al. Pharmacokinetics of ibuprofen in febrile children. *Eur J Clin Pharmacol* 1991;40:427–8.

67. Hollander D. Gastrointestinal complications of nonsteroidal anti-inflammatory drugs: prophylactic and therapeutic strategies. *Am J Med* 1994;96:274–81.

68. Whelton A et al. Renal effects of ibuprofen, piroxicam, and sulindac in patients with asymptomatic renal failure. *Ann Intern Med* 1990;112:568–76.

69. Stempel DA, Miller JJ. Lymphopenia and hepatotoxicity with ibuprofen. *J Pediatr* 1977;90:657–8.

70. Bernstein RF. Ibuprofen-related meningitis in mixed connective tissue disease. *Ann Intern Med* 1980;92:206–7.

71. Wolfe MM et al. Gastrointestinal toxicity of nonsteroidal antiinflammatory drugs. *N Engl J Med* 1999;340:1888–99.

72. Maniglia R et al. Non-steroidal anti-inflammatory nephrotoxicity. *Ann Clin Lab Sci* 1988;18:240–52.

73. Marsh CC et al. A review of selected investigational nonsteroidal anti-inflammatory drugs of the 1980s. *Pharmacotherapy* 1986;6:10–25.

74. Hawkey CJ. COX-2 inhibitors. *Lancet* 1999;353:307–14.

75. Rozenfeld V. Cyclooxygenase (COX)-2 inhibition: focus on rofecoxib. *P&T* 1999;24:161–6.

76. Clemett D, Goa KL. Celecoxib. A review of its use in osteoarthritis, rheumatoid arthritis and acute pain. *Drugs* 2000;59:957–80.

77. Riendeau D et al. Comparison of the cyclooxygenase-1 inhibitory properties of nonsteroidal anti-inflammatory drugs (NSAIDs) and selective COX-2 inhibitors, using sensitive microsomal and platelet assays. *Can J Physiol Pharmacol* 1997;75:1088–95.

78. Furst DE. Meloxicam: selective COX-2 inhibition in clinical practice. *Semin Arthritis Rheum* 1997;26(suppl 1):21–7.

79. Wallace JL. Nonsteroidal anti-inflammatory drugs and gastroenteropathy: the second hundred years. *Gastroenterology* 1997;112:1000–16.

80. Vane JR, Botting RM. Mechanism of action of aspirin-like drugs. *Semin Arthritis Rheum* 1997;26(suppl 1):2–10.

81. Litvak KM, McEvoy GK. Ketorolac, an injectable nonnarcotic analgesic. *Clin Pharm* 1990;9:921–35.

82. Brooks PM, Day RO. Nonsteroidal anti-inflammatory drugs—differences and similarities. *N Engl J Med* 1991;324:1716–25.

83. Helfgott SM et al. Diclofenac-associated hepatotoxicity. *JAMA* 1990;264:2660–2.

84. Middleton E Jr et al., eds. *Allergy principles and practice.* 3rd ed. St. Louis: CV Mosby; 1988.

85. Quercia RA, Ruderman M. Focus on nabumetone: a new chemically distinct nonsteroidal anti-inflammatory agent. *Hosp Formul* 1991;26:25–34.

86. Reisine T, Pasternak G. Opioid analgesics and antagonists. In, Hardman JG et al., eds. *Goodman and Gilman's the pharmacological basis of therapeutics.* 9th ed. New York: McGraw-Hill; 1996:521–55.

87. Way WL. Opioid analgesics and antagonists. In, Katzung BG, ed. *Basic and clinical pharmacology.* 6th ed. Norwalk, CT: Appleton & Lange; 1995:460–75.

88. Poulsen L et al. Codeine and morphine in extensive and poor metabolizers of sparteine: pharmacokinetics, analgesic effect and side effects. *Eur J Clin Pharmacol* 1995;51:289–95.

89. Eckhardt K et al. Same incidence of adverse drug events after codeine administration irrespective of the genetically determined differences in morphine formation. *Pain* 1998;76:27–33.

90. Özdemir V et al. Pharmacokinetic changes in the elderly. Do they contribute to drug abuse and dependence? *Clin Pharmacokinet* 1996;31:372–85.

91. Bonica JJ, ed. *The management of pain.* 2nd ed. Philadelphia: Lea & Febiger; 1990.

92. Persson K et al. The postoperative pharmacokinetics of codeine. *Eur J Clin Pharmacol* 1992;42:663–6.

93. Schmerzier E et al. Gas chromatographic determination of codeine in serum and urine. *J Pharm Sci* 1966;55:155–7.

94. Guay DRP et al. Pharmacokinetics of codeine after single- and multiple-oral-dose administration to normal volunteers. *J Clin Pharmacol* 1987;27:983–7.

95. Way EL, Adler TK. The pharmacologic implications of the fate of morphine and its surrogates. *Pharmacol Rev* 1968;12:383–446.

96. American Academy of Pediatrics Committee on Drugs. Use of codeine- and dextromethorphan-containing cough remedies in children. *Pediatrics* 1997;99:918–20.

97. Cox RG. Hypoxaemia and hypotension after intravenous codeine phosphate. *Can J Anaesth* 1994;41:1211–3.

98. Parke TJ et al. Profound hypotension following intravenous codeine phosphate. Three case reports and some recommendations. *Anaesthesia* 1992;47:852–4.

99. Caraco Y et al. Pharmacogenetic determination of the effects of codeine and prediction of drug interactions. *J Pharmacol Exp Ther* 1996;278:1165–74.

100. Bowdle TA et al., eds. *The pharmacologic basis of anesthesiology.* New York: Churchill Livingstone; 1994.

101. Arnold JH et al. Changes in the pharmacodynamic response to fentanyl in neonates during continuous infusion. *J Pediatr* 1991;119:639–43.

102. Scholz J et al. Clinical pharmacokinetics of alfentanil, fentanyl and sufentanil. An update. *Clin Pharamacokinet* 1996;31:275–92.

103. Donnelly AJ. Pharmacology of pain management agents. *Anesthesia Today* 1989;1:6–10.

104. Gourlay GK et al. The transdermal administration of fentanyl in the treatment of postoperative pain: pharmacokinetics and pharmacodynamic effects. *Pain* 1989;37:193–202.

105. Varvel JR et al. Absorption characteristics of transdermally administered fentanyl. *Anesthesiology* 1989;70:928–34.

106. Smith AJ et al. A comparison of opioid solutions for patient-controlled epidural analgesia. *Anaesthesia* 1996;51:1013–7.

107. Woodhouse A et al. A comparison of morphine, pethidine and fentanyl in the postsurgical patient-controlled analgesia environment. *Pain* 1996;64:115–21.

108. Herrick IA et al. Postoperative cognitive impairment in the elderly. Choice of patient-controlled analgesia opioid. *Anaesthesia* 1996;51:356–60.

109. Jacqz-Aigrain E, Burtin P. Clinical pharmacokinetics of sedatives in neonates. *Clin Pharmacokinet* 1996;31:423–43.

110. Marquardt KA et al. Fentanyl remaining in a transdermal system following three days of continuous use. *Ann Pharmacother* 1995;29:969–71.

111. Lee HA, Anderson PO. Giving partial doses of transdermal patches. *Am J Health Syst Pharm* 1997;54:1759–60.

112. Michalets EL. Update: clinically significant cytochrome P-450 drug interactions. *Pharmacotherapy* 1998;18:84–112.

113. Guinard J-P et al. Epidural and intravenous fentanyl produce equivalent effects during major surgery. *Anesthesiology* 1995;82:377–82.

114. Ahmedzai S, Brooks D. Transdermal fentanyl versus sustained-release oral morphine in cancer pain: preference, efficacy, and quality of life. *J Pain Symptom Manage* 1997;13:254–61.

115. Acute Pain Management Guideline Panel. *Acute pain management: operative or medical procedures and trauma. Clinical practice guideline.* AHCPR Publication No. 92-0032. Rockville, MD: Agency for Health Care Policy and Research, Public Health Service, Department of Health and Human Services; February 1992.

116. Jacox A et al. *Management of cancer pain. Clinical practice guideline no. 9.* AHCPR Publication No. 94-0592. Rockville, MD: Agency for Health Care Policy and Research, Public Health Service, Department of Health and Human Services; March 1994.

117. Edwards DJ et al. Clinical pharmacokinetics of pethidine: 1982. *Clin Pharmacokinet* 1982;7:421–33.

118. Fochtman FW, Winek CL. Therapeutic serum concentrations of meperidine (Demerol). *J Forensic Sci* 1969;14:213–8.

119. Klotz U et al. The effect of cirrhosis on the disposition and elimination of meperidine in man. *Clin Pharmacol Ther* 1974;16:667–75.

120. Julius HC et al. Meperidine binding to isolated alpha1-acid glycoprotein and albumin. *DICP* 1989;23:568–72.

121. McHorse TS et al. Effect of acute viral hepatitis in man on the disposition and elimination of meperidine. *Gastroenterology* 1975;68:775–80.

122. Chan K et al. Pharmacokinetics of low-dose intravenous pethidine in patients with renal dysfunction. *J Clin Pharmacol* 1987;27:516–22.

123. Tang R et al. Meperidine-induced seizures in sickle cell patients. *Hosp Formul* 1980;15:764–72.

124. Clark RF et al. Meperidine: therapeutic use and toxicity. *J Emerg Med* 1995;13:797–802.

125. Quinn DI, Day RO. Drug interactions of clinical importance. An updated guide. *Drug Saf* 1995;12:393–452.

126. Geller RJ. Meperidine in patient-controlled analgesia: a near-fatal mishap. *Anesth Analg* 1993;76:655–7.

127. Erstad BL et al. Site-specific pharmacokinetics and pharmacodynamics of intramuscular meperidine in elderly postoperative patients. *Ann Pharmacother* 1997;31:23–8.

128. Isenor L, Penny-MacGillivray T. Intravenous meperidine infusion for obstetric analgesia. *J Obstet Gynecol Neonatal Nurs* 1993;22:349–56.

129. Ripamonti C et al. An update on the clinical use of methadone for cancer pain. *Pain* 1997;70:109–15.

130. Kristensen K et al. Stereoselective pharmacokinetics of methadone in chronic pain patients. *Ther Drug Monit* 1996;18:221–7.

131. Moolchan ET, Hoffman JA. Phases of treatment: a practical approach to methadone maintenance treatment. *Int J Addict* 1994;29:135–60.

132. Holmstrand J et al. Methadone maintenance: plasma levels and therapeutic outcome. *Clin Pharmacol Ther* 1978;23:175–80.

133. Berkowitz BA. The relationship of pharmacokinetics to pharmacological activity: morphine, methadone and naloxone. *Clin Pharmacokinet* 1976;1:219–30.

134. Geletko SM, Erickson AD. Decreased methadone effect after ritonavir initiation. *Pharmacotherapy* 2000;20:93–4.

135. Beauclair TR, Stoner CP. Adherence to guidelines for continuous morphine sulfate infusions. *Am J Hosp Pharm* 1986;43:671–6.

136. Holmes AH. Morphine IV infusion for chronic pain. *Drug Intell Clin Pharm* 1978;12:556–7.

137. White P. Use of patient-controlled analgesia for management of acute pain. *JAMA* 1988;259:243–7.

138. Baumann TJ et al. Patient-controlled analgesia in the terminally ill cancer patient. *Drug Intell Clin Pharm* 1986;20:297–301.

139. Kerr IG et al. Continuous narcotic infusion with patient-controlled analgesia for chronic cancer pain in outpatients. *Ann Intern Med* 1988;108:554–7.

140. Lutz LJ, Lamer TJ. Management of postoperative pain: review of current techniques and methods. *Mayo Clin Proc* 1990;65:584–96.

141. Gestin Y et al. Long-term intrathecal infusion of morphine in the home care of patients with advanced cancer. *Acta Anaesthesiol Scand* 1997;41:12–7.

142. Milner AR et al. Intrathecal administration of morphine for elective Caesarean section. A comparison between 0.1 mg and 0.2 mg. *Anaesthesia* 1996;51:871–3.

143. Lobato RD et al. Intraventricular morphine for intractable cancer pain: rationale, methods, clinical results. *Acta Anaesthesiol Scand* 1987;31(suppl 85):68–74.

144. Farncombe M, Chater S. Clinical application of nebulized opioids for treatment of dyspnoea in patients with malignant disease. *Support Care Cancer* 1994;2:184–7.

145. Dews TE et al. Intrathecal morphine for analgesia in children undergoing selective dorsal rhizotomy. *J Pain Symptom Manage* 1996;11:188–94.

146. Pounder DR, Steward DJ. Postoperative analgesia: opioid infusions in infants and children. *Can J Anaesth* 1992;39:969–74.

147. Masood AR, Thomas SHL. Systemic absorption of nebulized morphine compared with oral morphine in healthy subjects. *Br J Clin Pharmacol* 1996;41:250–2.

148. Saarenmaa E et al. Morphine clearance and effects in newborn infants in relation to gestational age. *Clin Pharmacol Ther* 2000;68:160–6.

149. Glare PA, Walsh TD. Clinical pharmacokinetics of morphine. *Ther Drug Monit* 1991;13:1–23.

150. Davies G et al. Pharmacokinetics of opioids in renal dysfunction. *Clin Pharmacokinet* 1996;31:410–22.

151. Tiseo PJ et al. Morphine-6-glucuronide concentrations and opioid-related side effects: a survey in cancer patients. *Pain* 1995;61:47–54.

152. Stanski DR et al. Kinetics of intravenous and intramuscular morphine. *Clin Pharmacol Ther* 1978;24:52–9.

153. Chan GLC, Matzke GR. Effects of renal insufficiency on the pharmacokinetics and pharmacodynamics of opioid analgesics. *Drug Intell Clin Pharm* 1987;21:773–83.

154. Mercadante S. Dantrolene treatment of opioid-induced myoclonus. *Anesth Analg* 1995;81:1307–8.

155. Holdsworth MT et al. Continuous midazolam infusion for the management of morphine-induced myoclonus. *Ann Pharmacother* 1995;29:25–9.

156. Du Pen SL et al. Chronic epidural morphine and preservative-induced injury. *Anesthesiology* 1987;67:987–8.

157. Meisel SB, Welford PK. Seizures associated with high-dose intravenous morphine containing sodium bisulfite preservative. *Ann Pharmacother* 1992;26:1515–7.

158. Chamberlain JM, Klein BL. A comprehensive review of naloxone for the emergency physician. *Am J Emerg Med* 1994;12:650–60.

159. Hoffman RS, Goldfrank LR. The poisoned patient with altered consciousness. Controversies in the use of a 'coma cocktail.' *JAMA* 1995;274:562–9.

160. Osterwalder JJ. Naloxone—for intoxications with intravenous heroin and heroin mixtures—harmless or hazardous? A prospective clinical study. *J Toxicol Clin Toxicol* 1996;34:409–16.

161. Culpepper-Morgan JA et al. Treatment of opioid-induced constipation with oral naloxone: a pilot study. *Clin Pharmacol Ther* 1992;52:90–5.

162. Sykes NP. An investigation of the ability of oral naloxone to correct opioid-related constipation in patients with advanced cancer. *Palliat Med* 1996;10:135–44.

163. Longnecker DE et al. Naloxone for antagonism of morphine-induced respiratory depression. *Anesth Analg* 1973;52:447–53.

164. Evans JM et al. Degree and duration of reversal by naloxone of effects of morphine in conscious subjects. *Br Med J* 1974;2:589–91.

165. Fishman J et al. Disposition of naloxone-7,8-3H in normal and narcotic-dependent men. *J Pharmacol Exp Ther* 1973;187:575–80.

166. Vozeh S et al. Pharmacokinetic drug data. *Clin Pharmacokinet* 1988;15:254–82.

167. Ngai SH et al. Pharmacokinetics of naloxone in rats and in man: basis for its potency and short duration of action. *Anesthesiology* 1976;44:398–401.

168. Stile IL et al. The pharmacokinetics of naloxone in the premature newborn. *Dev Pharmacol Ther* 1987;10:454–9.

169. Tandberg D, Abercrombie D. Treatment of heroin overdose with endotracheal naloxone. *Ann Emerg Med* 1982;11:443–5.

170. Poulsen L et al. The hypoalgesic effect of tramadol in relation to CYP2D6. *Clin Pharmacol Ther* 1996;60:636–44.

171. Spiller HA et al. Prospective multicenter evaluation of tramadol exposure. *J Toxicol Clin Toxicol* 1997;35:361–4.

172. Kahn LH et al. Seizures reported with tramadol. *JAMA* 1997;278:1661. Letter.

173. Nightingale SL. From the Food and Drug Administration. Important new safety information for tramadol hydrochloride. *JAMA* 1996;275:1224. News.

174. Fisher MA, Glass S. Butorphanol (Stadol): a study in problems of current drug information and control. *Neurology* 1997;48:1156–60.

175. Strain EC et al. Precipitated withdrawal by pentazocine in methadone-maintained volunteers. *J Pharmacol Exp Ther* 1993;267:624–34.

176. Reed DA, Schnoll SH. Abuse of pentazocine-naloxone combination. *JAMA* 1986;256:2562–4.

177. Gourlay GK, Cousins MJ. Strong analgesics in severe pain. *Drugs* 1984;28:79–91.

178. Miller RR. Evaluation of nalbuphine hydrochloride. *Am J Hosp Pharm* 1980;37:942–9.

179. Ameer B, Salter FJ. Drug therapy reviews: evaluation of butorphanol tartrate. *Am J Hosp Pharm* 1979;36:1683–91.

180. Dayer P et al. The pharmacology of tramadol. *Drugs* 1994;47(suppl 1):3–7.

Antimicrobial Drugs

Aminoglycosides

AMINOGLYCOSIDES

Pharmacology. Aminoglycosides are aminocyclitol derivatives that have concentration-dependent bactericidal activity against Gram-negative aerobic bacteria via binding to the interface between the 30S and 50S ribosomal subunits; anaerobic bacteria are universally resistant because aminoglycoside transport into cells is oxygen dependent. Dibasic cations (eg, magnesium, calcium) and acidic conditions decrease their in vitro action. Streptomycin and kanamycin have poor activity against some Gram-negative bacteria, especially *P. aeruginosa*. Some Gram-positive organisms (eg, streptococci) are relatively resistant to all aminoglycosides; however, in combination with some penicillins or vancomycin, these organisms are often synergistically inhibited or killed. Aminoglycosides have a postantibiotic effect against Gram-negative bacteria, which can be exploited by using less frequent dosage intervals. Resistance is due to transferable plasmid-mediated enzymatic modification or decreased drug uptake.[1,2] (*See* Notes.)

Administration and Adult Dosage. **IM or IV by slow intermittent infusion over 30–60 min,** although 15-min infusions are safe. Newer dosage regimens combine the usual daily dosage into a **single IV infusion administered over 60 min.**[3,4] This method takes advantage of the concentration-related bactericidal effects and postantibiotic effect of aminoglycosides and may result in less toxicity.[2–4] **IT or intraventricular administration** is usually necessary to achieve therapeutic CSF levels. (*See* Aminoglycosides Comparison Chart.)

Special Populations. *Pediatric Dosage.* (*See* Aminoglycosides Comparison Chart.)

Geriatric Dosage. Same as adult dosage, but adjust for age-related reduction in renal function.

Other Conditions. Use of IBW for determining the mg/kg dosage appears to be more accurate than dosage based on TBW. In morbid obesity, dosage requirement may best be estimated using a dosing weight of IBW + 0.4 (TBW − IBW).[1,2] With conventional dosage methods, serum drug levels should be in the range of 3–10 mg/L; high peaks (>6 mg/L with gentamicin and tobramycin) may be associated with better outcome in bacteremia, pneumonia, and other systemic infections.[1,2] Critically ill patients with serious infections or in disease states known to markedly alter aminoglycoside pharmacokinetics (eg, cystic fibrosis, burns, or major surgery)[1,2] often have variable distribution and excretion of the drugs. When the drug is administered once daily, higher peak concentrations (>10–20 mg/L with gentamicin and tobramycin) are targeted based on the patients's disease state and pharmacokinetic parameters.[3–5] (*See* Aminoglycosides Comparison

Chart.) Adjust dosage based on renal function. Individualization is critical because these agents have a low therapeutic index. In renal impairment, the following guidelines may be used to determine initial dosage (modified from reference 6):

1. Select loading dose in mg/kg (LBW or dosing weight as above) to provide peak serum levels in the range listed below for the desired aminoglycoside.

AMINOGLYCOSIDE	USUAL LOADING DOSE	EXPECTED PEAK SERUM LEVEL
Tobramycin	1–2 mg/kg	3–10 mg/L
Gentamicin	1–2 mg/kg	3–10 mg/L
Amikacin	5–7.5 mg/kg	15–30 mg/L

2. Select maintenance dose (as percentage of chosen loading dose) to continue peak serum levels indicated above, according to desired dosage interval and the patient's corrected Cl_{cr}.

PERCENTAGE OF LOADING DOSE REQUIRED FOR DOSAGE INTERVAL SELECTED

Cl_{CR} (ML/MIN)	HALF-LIFE[a] (HR)	8 HR	12 HR	24 HR
90	3.1	84%	—	—
80	3.4	80	91%	—
70	3.9	76	88	—
60	4.5	71	84	—
50	5.3	65	79	—
40	6.5	57	72	92%
30	8.4	48	63	86
25	9.9	43	57	81
20	11.9	37	50	75
17	13.6	33	46	70
15	15.1	31	42	67
12	17.9	27	37	61
10[b]	20.4	24	34	56
7[b]	25.9	19	28	47
5[b]	31.5	16	23	41
2[b]	46.8	11	16	30
0[b]	69.3	8	11	21

[a]Alternatively, 50% of the chosen loading dose can be given at an interval approximately equal to the estimated half-life.
[b]Use measured serum levels to adjust dosage for patients with Cl_{cr} <10 mL/min. Give supplemental doses of 50–75% of the loading dose after each hemodialysis period.

These guidelines are based on population data; serum levels in individual patients might deviate from guideline estimates. No guidelines have been developed for netilmicin or streptomycin.

Dosage Forms. (*See* Aminoglycosides Comparison Chart.)

Patient Instructions. Report any dizziness or sensations of ringing or fullness in the ears.

Pharmacokinetics. *Serum Levels.* (*See* Parameters to Monitor and Aminoglycosides Comparison Chart.)

Fate. Absorption after oral or rectal administration is about 0.2–2%; absorption across denuded skin can reach 5%. Irrigation of vascularized areas (eg, peritoneal cavity) results in absorption approximating IM use.[7] IM administration is followed by rapid and complete absorption, with peak serum levels occurring after 0.5–1.5 hr. IV infusions over 0.5–1 hr produce serum levels similar to equal IM doses. Binding of aminoglycosides to plasma proteins is low. These agents distribute rapidly into the extracellular fluid compartment with a V_d of about 0.3 ± 0.08 L/kg, which is increased by fever, edema, ascites, and fluid overload, and in neonates.[8] Aminoglycosides accumulate markedly in some tissues, especially the renal cortex, to levels many times those found in the serum,[2,8] particularly with frequent dosage intervals compared with the same dosage given at less frequent intervals.[2,3] Levels in the CSF of patients with meningitis generally do not exceed 25% of serum levels, except in neonates;[2,8] penetration into the eye is inadequate for treatment of intraocular infections. Penetration into lung tissues and sputum is low, and large doses might be necessary to optimally treat pneumonia with relatively insensitive organisms (eg, *P. aeruginosa*). Distribution of aminoglycosides into the peritoneal cavity of patients with peritonitis is therapeutically adequate.[7,8] Elimination is via glomerular filtration of unchanged drug;[1,2] Cl is about 90% of Cl_{cr}. After discontinuation, low levels of aminoglycoside can be detected in the urine for several days caused by excretion of drug that had accumulated in deep tissue compartments.[2,8]

$t_{1/2}$. α Phase 5–15 min; β phase (adults) about 2 ± 0.4 hr with normal renal function (1.5–9 hr in neonates <1 week and 3 hr in older infants); can be more variable in certain groups (eg, obstetric and burn patients) despite normal renal function; 50–70 hr in anuria. A prolonged γ elimination phase is observed when concentrations fall to the lower range of detectability, representing egress from deep tissue compartments and subsequent renal elimination; the half-life of this phase is 60–350 hr (usually 150–200).[2–8] β Phase half-life is most important for use in calculating individualized dosage, but the γ phase may account for the gradual rise of serum levels and apparent increase in half-life with continued therapy, despite stable renal function.[2,8]

Adverse Reactions. Aminoglycoside-induced nephrotoxicity is usually mild and reversible; progression to severe renal disease and dependence on dialysis is rare. Nephrotoxicity is manifested by elevations in Cr_s, BUN, and aminoglycoside concentrations and appearance of renal tubular casts, enzymes, and β_2-microglobulin and occurs in 5–30% of patients, depending on the criteria used and the population risk factors present.[1,2,9] Duration of therapy, prior aminoglycoside therapy, advanced age, pre-existing renal disease, liver disease, volume depletion, and female sex have been identified as risk factors for nephrotoxicity.[1,2] Concomitant use of nephrotoxic drugs also increases the risk of nephrotoxicity. Elevated trough levels are *not* a risk factor but often a result of nephrotoxicity.[2,10] There is no evidence that there are clinically important differences in nephrotoxicity between gentamicin, tobramycin, netilmicin, and amikacin.[9] Depletion of magnesium and other minerals caused by increased renal excretion occurs. Occasional, but often permanent, vestibular toxicity is reported, usually in association with streptomycin. Subclinical vestibular disturbances can be detected in 40% or more of patients receiving aminoglycosides.[1,2,9] Early cochlear damage can be detected only by sequential audiometric examination because hearing loss in conversational frequencies is a sign of advanced auditory impairment. Furthermore, early auditory damage is not as apparent in the elderly or others with pre-existing high-tone deficits. Risk factors for ototoxicity are duration of therapy, bacteremia, hypovolemia, peak temperature, and liver disease.[1,2] Elevated serum concentrations apparently are not associated with increased ototoxicity risk,[10] and there are no apparent clinically important differences between gentamicin, tobramycin, netilmicin, and amikacin.[9] Oral aminoglycosides, primarily neomycin, have been associated with a sprue-like malabsorption syndrome.[1,2] Neuromuscular blockade with respiratory failure is rare, except in predisposed patients. (*See* Precautions.)

Precautions. Pregnancy; pre-existing renal impairment; vestibular or cochlear impairment; myasthenia gravis; hypocalcemia; postoperative or other conditions that depress neuromuscular transmission.

Drug Interactions. Concurrent or sequential use of other nephro- or ototoxic agents can increase the risk of aminoglycoside toxicities. Concurrent use of aminoglycosides with neuromuscular blocking agents can potentiate neuromuscular blockade and cause respiratory paralysis.[2] The action of oral anticoagulants can be potentiated by oral neomycin, presumably via reduced absorption or synthesis of vitamin K. Ticarcillin and acylampicillins can degrade aminoglycosides in vitro, resulting in artificially low levels; the extent of degradation is dependent on time, temperature, and β-lactam concentration.[8,11] Degradation can occur in vivo in patients with renal insufficiency.[12] Amikacin is the aminoglycoside least susceptible to β-lactam inactivation.[8,11]

Parameters to Monitor. Renal function tests before and q 2–3 days during therapy. Audiometry and electronystagmography may be performed in patients able to cooperate. Monitor aminoglycoside serum concentrations carefully, especially in the elderly, those with renal impairment, hemodynamically unstable patients, and those requiring high peak serum concentrations or prolonged (>10 days) therapy. In adults receiving conventional therapy, monitor serum levels after steady state is achieved. With once-daily therapy targeting high peaks and undetectable troughs, obtain levels after the first dose. Obtain follow-up levels if renal function changes.[2–5] In neonates or other patients with rapidly changing renal function, obtain serum drug concentrations initially and q 2–3 days until stable. However, with once- or twice-daily dosage and in pediatric patients, trough serum levels are often undetectable and other sampling strategies are necessary.[3–5,13] (*See also* Special Populations, Other Conditions.)

Notes. Of the available aminoglycosides, gentamicin, tobramycin, netilmicin, and amikacin are the most clinically useful. **Streptomycin** use is largely restricted to the treatment of enterococcal endocarditis (in combination with ampicillin), tuberculosis, brucellosis, plague, and tularemia; it is currently available only for compassionate use from the manufacturer. Amikacin is often used as part of a combination regimen for treatment of *Mycobacterium avium* complex infection. **Neomycin** is much more toxic than the other aminoglycosides when given parenterally; it is restricted to oral use for gut sterilization and topical use for minor infections. Resistance among Gram-negative organisms, especially *P. aeruginosa,* has virtually eliminated the systemic use of **kanamycin. Tobramycin** is roughly equivalent to gentamicin therapeutically, although it is about 2–4 times more active against *P. aeruginosa* than is gentamicin, is often active against gentamicin-resistant *P. aeruginosa,* and might be preferred because of a superior peak-to-MIC ratio.[15] Resistance of Gram-negative bacilli is lowest with amikacin; amikacin use does not appear to result in increased resistance to the drug.[1,2]

AMINOGLYCOSIDES COMPARISON CHART

DRUG	DOSAGE FORMS	ADULT DOSAGE[a]	PEDIATRIC DOSAGE[a]	USUAL THERAPEUTIC SERUM LEVELS (MG/L)[b]	
				Peak[c]	Trough
Amikacin Sulfate Amikin	Inj 50, 250 mg/mL.	IM or IV 15–20 mg/kg/day in 2 equally divided doses; IT 5–20 mg/day.	IM or IV (<1 week) 12–15 mg/kg q 36–48 hr; IM or IV (infants >1 week) 12 mg/kg q 24 hr; IM or IV (children) same as adult mg/kg dosage.	20–35	≤10
Gentamicin Sulfate Garamycin Various	Inj 10, 40 mg/mL IT Inj 2 mg/mL Ophth Oint 3 mg/g Ophth Soln 3 mg/mL Top Crm 0.1% Top Oint 0.1%.	IM or IV 5–6 mg/kg/day in equally divided doses q 8–12 hr or in a single-dose IV q 24 hr;[d] IM or IV for less serious infections[d] 3–5 mg/kg/day in equally divided doses q 8–12 hr or in a single-dose IV q 24 hr; IT 4–8 mg q 24 hr.	IM or IV (<1 week) 4–5 mg/kg q 36–48 hr; IM or IV (infants >1 week) 4 mg/kg q 24 hr; IM or IV (children) 6–7.5 mg/ kg/day (7–10 mg/kg/day in cystic fibrosis) in 3–4 equally divided doses q 6–8 hr; IT 1–2 mg q 24 hr.	6–12	≤2
Netilmicin Sulfate Netromycin	Inj 100 mg/mL.	IM or IV 3[d]–6.5 mg/kg/day in 1–3 equally divided doses q 8–24 hr.	Same as gentamicin.	6–12	≤2

(continued)

AMINOGLYCOSIDES COMPARISON CHART (*continued*)

DRUG	DOSAGE FORMS	ADULT DOSAGE[a]	PEDIATRIC DOSAGE[a]	USUAL THERAPEUTIC SERUM LEVELS (MG/L)[b] Peak[c]	Trough
Streptomycin Sulfate Various	Inj 400 mg/mL.	IM 15–25 mg/kg/day (usually 1–2 g/day) in 2 equally divided doses q 12 hr; IM for TB 12–15 mg/kg/day to a maximum of 1 g or 25–30 mg/kg to a maximum of 1.5 g 2–3 times/week.	IM (neonates) 20–30 mg/kg/day in 2 equally divided doses q 12 hr; IM (children) 20–40 mg/kg/ day in 2 equally divided doses q 12 hr; IM for TB 20–40 mg/kg/ day or 25–30 mg/kg 2–3 times/week.	15–30	≤5
Tobramycin Sulfate Nebcin TOBI Various	Inj 10, 40 mg/mL Inj 1.2 g Ophth Oint 3 mg/g Ophth Soln 3 mg/mL Nebulizer Soln 60 mg/mL.	IM or IV same as gentamicin; IV for cystic fibrosis 10 mg/kg/day; Inhal for cystic fibrosis 300 mg q 12 hr for 28 days; IT 4–8 mg q 24 hr.	IM or IV same as gentamicin; IV for cystic fibrosis 10 mg/kg/day; Inhal for cystic fibrosis 300 mg q 12 hr for 28 days.	6–12	≤2

[a]For systemic infections; UTIs are adequately treated with lower dosages.
[b]Based on divided doses given q 8–12 hr; higher peaks and lower (or undetectable) troughs are seen when less frequent dosage intervals are used.
[c]As seen 30 min after a 30-min IV infusion or approximately 1 hr after IM administration of a usual adult dose. Uncomplicated UTIs can be treated with smaller doses that produce much lower serum levels; however, serious infections, such as Gram-negative bacteremia, pneumonia, or endocarditis might require doses resulting in serum levels in the higher part of the range. Clinical efficacy appears to increase as the ratio of the peak serum level to the MIC of the pathogen increases.[15]
[d]These doses conform to those used in published clinical trials, but higher dosages might be necessary in certain patient populations.

Antifungal Drugs

AMPHOTERICIN B	Fungizone
AMPHOTERICIN B CHOLESTERYL SULFATE	Amphotec
AMPHOTERICIN B LIPID COMPLEX	Abelcet
LIPOSOMAL AMPHOTERICIN B	AmBisome

Pharmacology. Amphotericin B is a polyene macrolide antifungal drug isolated from the bacteria *Streptomyces nodosus*. Drug binding to ergosterol constituents within the cytoplasmic membrane of fungi, with subsequent disruption of membrane integrity and function, is the pharmacologic mechanism of action for amphotericin B. Innate or acquired resistance to amphotericin B is rare. Sensitivity of fungi to amphotericin B is related to the concentration of ergosterol present in the cytoplasmic membrane.[16,17]

Administration and Adult Dosage. Intravenous (*See* Amphotericin B Formulations Comparison Chart.) A **test dose** may be given before the first amphotericin B dose. The greatest utility of a test dose is identification of patients particularly sensitive to infusion-related adverse effects of amphotericin B, or identification of patients with hypersensitivity to an alternative amphotericin B formulation. Conventional amphotericin B 1 mg in D5W 20 mL, or an adequate admixture volume to deliver 2–5% of the initial dose of any amphotericin B formulation, infused over 10–20 min without premedication can be used as a test dose. Monitor patients closely for 30–60 min after the test dose.[16] The manufacturer of amphotericin B lipid complex recommends against a test dose. Initiate therapy with the full treatment dose for patients with life-threatening fungal disease. Some advocate initiation of amphotericin B at a fraction of the therapeutic dose with daily incremental increases to achieve the desired therapeutic dosage. Although it has not been evaluated in a controlled manner, the intent of this approach is improvement of patient tolerance to infusion-related adverse effects.[16,18] **Maintenance therapy** conventional amphotericin B and amphotericin B lipid complex can be given every other day or Monday, Wednesday, and Friday.[16,19] **IV for prophylaxis after bone marrow transplantation** (conventional amphotericin B) 0.1 mg/kg or 5–10 mg daily has been used.[20] **Infusion time** the frequency and severity of infusion-related adverse effects is similar with administration of amphotericin B over 1–2 hr and 4–6 hr. To prevent drug-induced hyperkalemia, amphotericin B must be infused over 4–6 hr in patients with renal failure, pre-existing hyperkalemia, or markedly reduced potassium clearance.[18] **Duration of therapy** with amphotericin B is not well defined. Patients with life-threatening mycotic disease must receive amphotericin B until resolution of clinical and microbiologic evidence of fungal infection, or until unacceptable drug-induced toxicity occurs. Cumulative total dosage of amphotericin B is generally 10–20 mg/kg.[16,18] **PO for oral candidiasis** (amphotericin B suspension) 1 mL qid swished and held in mouth for 1 min, or as long as possible, then swallow. Continue therapy for at least 2 weeks. **Top** apply to affected area 2–4 times daily for 1–4 weeks. **IM or PO administration** is not recommended for injectable amphotericin B.

Alternative routes of administration of extemporaneously prepared amphotericin B for injection are infrequently used to facilitate drug availability to a sanctuary site or minimize systemic toxicity. Use of alternative routes of amphotericin B administration is based primarily on case reports, and the safety and efficacy of extemporaneously prepared amphotericin B administered by alternative routes have not been evaluated in a controlled manner. Subsequently, administration of amphotericin B by an alternative route should *not* replace standard therapy. **Intra-articular for fungal arthritis** 5–50 mg q 2–7 days. The dose of intra-articular amphotericin B is determined by the size of the infected joint.[21] **Intracavitary for pulmonary aspergillomas** 5–50 mg in D5W daily or 2–3 times weekly has been used in patients unable to undergo surgical resection.[22] **Inhalation for prophylaxis against *Aspergillus* sp. after bone marrow transplantation** 0.15% in D5W nebulized to deliver 10 mg/day in 2 divided doses.[23] **Intranasal for prophylaxis in bone marrow transplant recipients** amphotericin B 0.5% in sterile water 10 mg/day in divided doses.[24] **Intraperitoneal for the treatment of fungal peritonitis** has been used in patients receiving peritoneal dialysis.[16] Instillation is problematic because amphotericin B is physically incompatible with ionic solutions such as dialysate. **Intrathecal** administration of conventional amphotericin B 0.5–1 mg 2–3 times/week or 0.3 mg/day has been reported. The intrathecal dosage of conventional amphotericin B is generally started at 0.025–0.05 mg/dose, with subsequent doses increased at 0.025–0.05 mg/day increments to the desired therapeutic or maximum tolerated dosage. **CNS administration** is generally via an Ommaya reservoir. Although an Ommaya reservoir is not mandatory for intrathecal administration of amphotericin B, the device facilitates repeated drug administration with more precise drug delivery, improved patient tolerance, and clarified CSF diagnostic quality. Amphotericin B administration by lumbar puncture and intracisternal injection has been reported.[16] **Bladder irrigation for the treatment of uncomplicated fungal cystitis** infuse 50 mg/L in sterile water over 24 hr.[16] **Topical ocular for the treatment of keratomycosis** amphotericin B 0.15% (0.1–0.25%) in preservative-free sterile water has been given concurrently with atropine ophthalmic drops q 30–60 min for the initial 48–72 hr of treatment; subsequent to subjective improvement and ocular re-epithelization, the dosage interval may be changed to qid for at least 1 month.[16,25] **Intravitreal for fungal keratomycosis** 5 μg/0.1 mL preservative-free sterile water has been used.[26] **Subtenonian injection for the treatment of postoperative fungal endophthalmitis** 500–750 μg/day for 8 doses has been used.[16]

Special Populations. *Pediatric Dosage.* **IV.** Same as adult dosage for conventional amphotericin B, amphotericin B colloidal dispersion, amphotericin B lipid complex, and liposomal amphotericin. **IV for prophylaxis after bone marrow or solid organ transplantation** (liposomal amphotericin B) 1 mg/kg/day has been used.[27] **PO** same as adult dosage. **Top** same as adult dosage for cream, lotion, and ointment.

Geriatric Dosage. Same as adult dosage for conventional amphotericin B, amphotericin B colloidal dispersion, amphotericin B lipid complex, and liposomal amphotericin. Long-term IV administration is more likely to be limited by renal impairment. Comorbid conditions might reduce patient tolerance to ancillary medications used for management of infusion-related adverse effects (eg, corticosteroid-induced sodium retention).

Other Conditions. (All products) With pre-existing chronic renal dysfunction, no dosage adjustment is necessary, but the duration of the infusion must be 4–6 hr to prevent drug-related hyperkalemia. In acute renal dysfunction, interrupt treatment or extend dosage interval or decrease dosage to reduce exacerbation of renal impairment, as patient's clinical condition allows.[18] For patients ≥1.3 times IBW, calculate dose based on IBW or dosing weight of IBW + 0.4 x (TBW − IBW).[28]

Dosage Forms. **Inj** (*see* Amphotericin B Formulations Comparison Chart.) **Oral Susp** 100 mg/mL; **Top Crm** 30 mg/g; **Top Lot** 30 mg/mL; **Top Oint** 30 mg/g.

Patient Instructions. (Injection). Infusion reactions such as shaking, chills, fever, nausea, and other symptoms can occur when this medication is being given. Although uncomfortable, these effects are transient. Certain medications reduce infusion reactions for most people. Amphotericin B might affect your kidneys. If this occurs, you may need to take mineral supplements by mouth. (Oral Suspension). Shake container well before use. Swish and hold the product in your mouth for one minute, or as long as possible, and then swallow. Discontinue if mouth irritation occurs. (Topical). This preparation can stain clothing.

Missed Doses. Take a missed oral or topical dose as soon as it is remembered. If it is time for the next dose, do not double the dose.

Pharmacokinetics. Preclinical and phase 1 testing of conventional amphotericin B preceded development of high-performance liquid chromatography and refinement of pharmacokinetic methodology. Pharmacokinetic parameters quoted in tertiary literature might actually reflect drug concentration analysis using microbiologic assays.

Serum Levels. A correlation between serum levels and therapeutic or toxic drug effects has not been identified or defined for any commercially available amphotericin B formulation.

Fate. (Conventional amphotericin B) poor oral and IM absorption. End of infusion serum concentration was 0.984 ± 0.056 mg/L after 0.25 mg/kg to 8 normal healthy volunteers.[16] V_{dss} is 0.74 ± 0.13 L/kg.[29] Extensively bound (>90%) to plasma lipoproteins.[16] Accumulates in hepatic, splenic, pulmonary, and renal tissue.[28] V_{dss} of 4 ± 0.3 L/kg is derived from bioanalysis of serum from 2 patients completing chronic therapy with amphotericin B.[16] Cl is 0.01 ± 0.001 L/hr/kg.[29] Metabolites of amphotericin B have not been identified.[16] Urinary elimination is 3–8%.[16,29] (Amphotericin B cholesteryl sulfate) V_{dss} is 4.2 ± 1.4 L/kg in adults and 4.6 ± 1.7 L/kg in children; Cl is 0.11 ± 0.03 L/hr/kg in adults and 0.14 ± 0.02 L/hr/kg in children; AUC is 9.6 ± 2.6 mg/L/hr in adults and 7.1 ± 2.6 mg/L/hr in children.[30] (Amphotericin B lipid complex) V_{dss} is 3.9 ± 0.3 L/kg; Cl is 0.08 ± 0.02 L/hr/kg; AUC is 2.76 ± 0.25 mg/L/hr.[29] (Liposomal amphotericin B) V_{dss} is 0.37 L/kg; Cl is 0.023 L/hr/kg; AUC is 423 mg/L/hr.[31]

$t_{1/2}$. (Conventional amphotericin B) β phase 24–50 hr; γ phase 15 days;[16,29] (amphotericin B cholesteryl sulfate) 32 ± 5.6 hr in adults and 32 ± 13 hr in children;[30] (amphotericin B lipid complex) β phase 45 ± 6.3 hr;[29] (liposomal amphotericin B) α phase 1.74 hr; β phase 23.6 hr.[31]

Adverse Reactions. Frequent adverse effects include infusion-related reactions, nephrotoxicity, normochromic normocytic anemia and phlebitis. Infusion reactions ordinarily include rigors, chills, and fever. Less common infusion-related reactions include nausea, tachycardia, tachypnea, hypotension, hypertension, bradycardia, myalgia, and arthralgia. Symptoms generally occur during or within 60–90 min after completion of the infusion. Symptoms decrease with ancillary medications and repeated administration. **Meperidine** 25–50 mg IV reduces the duration and intensity of rigors and chilling. **Acetaminophen** 325–650 mg PO reduces hyperpyrexia, and is often administered as premedication. **Diphenhydramine** 25–50 mg PO or IV is often included as a premedication. **Hydrocortisone**, which reduces fever, chills, and nausea, is reserved for patients with infusion reactions refractory to other ancillary medications. Case reports describe the use of **dantrolene** for refractory rigors and chills. Although premedication with **ibuprofen** reduces the rigors and chills, most patients receiving amphotericin B are at risk for adverse effects from the nephrotoxic and antiplatelet effects of NSAIDs.[16,18] The prevalence of infusion reactions is greater with conventional amphotericin B or amphotericin B cholesteryl sulfate than with amphotericin B lipid complex or liposomal amphotericin. Rapid infusion (<60 min) of amphotericin B can cause hyperkalemia and cardiovascular collapse in anephric or hyperkalemic patients.[18] Amphotericin B cholesteryl sulfate, amphotericin B lipid complex, and liposomal amphotericin are each less nephrotoxic than conventional amphotericin B. However, the lipid-based formulations are not devoid of nephrotoxicity. Nephrotoxicity is generally reversible. Permanent renal impairment can occur, particularly in patients receiving conventional amphotericin B at doses over 1 mg/kg/day or have pre-existing renal impairment, prolonged therapy, sodium depletion, or concurrent nephrotoxic drugs. Signs of nephrotoxicity are increased BUN and Cr_s, hypomagnesemia, hypokalemia, and renal tubular acidosis. Nephrotoxicity can be reduced with infusion of 0.9% NaCl 250–1000 mL over 30–45 min immediately before amphotericin B. The saline infusion may be repeated immediately after amphotericin B administration. The patient's body size and cardiovascular status must be considered when selecting the volume and rate of 0.9% NaCl infusion. Normochromic normocytic anemia, which is secondary to amphotericin B–induced nephrotoxicity, is mild and transient and rarely requires intervention. Phlebitis is secondary to chronic peripheral administration of conventional amphotericin B. Some advocate adding heparin 1 IU/mL to minimize phlebitis.[16,18]

Rare adverse effects reported with amphotericin B are anorexia, emesis, diarrhea, cramping epigastric pain, premature ventricular contraction, bradycardia, dilated cardiomyopathy, hypertension, diffuse alveolar hemorrhage, rhabdomyolysis, and parkinsonian syndrome.[16,18,32–35]Intrathecal administration of amphotericin B causes headache, nausea, vomiting, abdominal pain, urinary retention, tinnitus, visual changes, ventriculitis, paresthesias, numbness, mono- or paraparesis, arachnoiditis, focal neurologic defects, and chemical or bacterial meningitis. Life-threatening brain puncture and hemorrhage can occur with intracisternal injection.[16]

Precautions. Pregnancy. Impaired renal function. Avoid rapid infusions (<4 hr) in patients with Cl_{cr} <20 mL/min, hyperkalemia, or reduced ability to excrete potassium.[18] Separate from neutrophil infusions by at least 6 hr.[36] Complete infusion at least 2 hr before platelet transfusions.[37]

Drug Interactions. Additive nephrotoxicity can occur with cyclosporine, tacrolimus, aminoglycosides, loop diuretics, or other nephrotoxic agents. Corticosteroids can enhance potassium loss.

Parameters to Monitor. Monitor infusion-related adverse effects with first 3 doses, then as indicated by severity of reactions. Monitor serum Cr_s, BUN, magnesium, potassium before therapy, and at least twice weekly during therapy. Monitor patients at great risk for renal dysfunction daily. Monitor Hb at least weekly. Monitor microbiologic, radiographic, and clinical signs of fungal infection. Ancillary use of hydrocortisone, acetaminophen, or aspirin might mask fevers.

Notes. To ensure even lipid complex distribution, invert admixtures of amphotericin B lipid complex several times immediately before starting the infusion and q 2 hr thereafter. Because amphotericin B has a propensity to precipitate, avoid admixture or Y-site administration of all amphotericin B formulations with IV fluids (except dextrose solution), other intravenous drugs, or blood products. Avoid admixture of conventional amphotericin B with lipid emulsion. Physical incompatibility of this admixture evolves >10 μ particles and phase separation.[38] Acronyms for the various amphotericin B formulations are as follows: conventional amphotericin B, DAmB; amphotericin B cholesteryl sulfate, ABCD; amphotericin B lipid complex, ABLC; liposomal amphotericin B, L-AmB. Amphotericin B cholesteryl sulfate is also known as amphotericin B colloidal dispersion and Amphocil.

AMPHOTERICIN B PRODUCTS COMPARISON CHART

	CONVENTIONAL AMPHOTERICIN B	AMPHOTERICIN B CHOLESTERYL SULFATE	AMPHOTERICIN B LIPID COMPLEX	LIPOSOMAL AMPHOTERICIN B
	Fungizone	*Amphotec*	*Abelcet*	*AmBisome*
LIPID CHEMISTRY				
Lipid component	Deoxycholate	Cholesteryl Sulfate	DMPG, DMPC	HSPC, DSPC
Diameter (nm)	50	120–140	1600–11,000	80
Configuration	Micelle	Discoid	Ribbon-like	Spherical liposome
PHARMACEUTICAL CHARACTERISTICS				
Vial size (mg)	50	50, 100	50, 100	50
Storage conditions	2–8°C	15–30°C	2–8°C	2–8°C
ADMINISTRATION AND DOSAGE				
Daily dosage (mg/kg)				
Sensitive fungi	0.5–1	3–4	2.5–5	1–3
Less-sensitive fungi	1–1.5	6	5	3–5
Infusion duration (hr)	1–6 (≤50 mg/hr)	2–4	2	1–2
In-line filter	Not recommended.	Do not filter.	Do not filter.	May use if pore size ≥1 µ.
Compatible IV fluids	D5W	D5W	D5W	D5W
Admixture concentration (mg/mL)	0.5–0.25	0.16–0.83	1–2	1–2
Admixture expiration	Determined by lack of preservative	24 hr at 2–8°C	48 hr at 2–8°C, then an additional 6 hr at room temperature	6 hr at 2–8°C or at room temperature

(continued)

AMPHOTERICIN B PRODUCTS COMPARISON CHART (*continued*)

	CONVENTIONAL AMPHOTERICIN B	AMPHOTERICIN B CHOLESTERYL SULFATE	AMPHOTERICIN B LIPID COMPLEX	LIPOSOMAL AMPHOTERICIN B
	Fungizone	*Amphotec*	*Abelcet*	*AmBisome*
PHARMACOKINETICS				
V_{dss} (L/Kg)	0.74 + 0.13 L/kg	(Adult) 4.2 ± 1.4 (Child) 4.6 ± 1.7	3.9 ± 0.3	0.37
Clearance (L/hr/kg)	0.01 ± 0.001	(Adult) 0.11 ± 0.03 (Child) 0.14 ± 0.02	0.08 ± 0.02	0.023
AUC (mg/L/hr)[a]	—	(Adult) 9.6 ± 2.6 (Child) 7.1 ± 2.6	2.8 ± 0.25	423
Half-life (hr)	24–50	32 ± 5.6	45 ± 6.3	α phase 1.7 β phase 23.6

DMPC = dimyristoylphosphatidyl choline; DMPG = dimyristoylphosphatidyl glycerol; DSPC = distearoylphosphatidyl choline; HSPC = hydrogenated soy phosphatidyl choline.
[a]AUC values normalized to a dosage of 1 mg/kg/day.
From references 16, 28, 29, 30, and 31 and product information.

CASPOFUNGIN ACETATE
Cancidas

Pharmacology. Caspofungin is an echinocandin antifungal that is a specific non-competitive inhibitor of β-(1-3) glucan synthetase in fungal cell membranes. This action leads to a weakened cell wall and eventual cell lysis and death. It is active against *Candida* and *Aspergillus* spp., and *Pneumocystis carinii* with little cross-resistance with the azoles.

Adult Dosage. IV for refractory invasive aspergillosis 70 mg on day 1, then 50 mg/day. Infuse doses over 1 hr. Do not mix with dextrose-containing solutions. Some evidence supports a 70 mg/day dose in patients unresponsive to 50 mg/day. In moderate hepatic impairment, give 35 mg/day after the 70 mg loading dose; no experience exists in severe hepatic impairment. Safety and efficacy not established under 18 yr.

Dosage Forms. Inj 50, 70 mg.

Pharmacokinetics. Caspofungin is about 97% plasma protein bound and extensively distributed in tissues. It is slowly metabolized by hydrolysis and N-acetylation. Less than 2% is excreted unchanged in urine. The principle half-life is 9–11 hr and accounts for most elimination; a longer 40–50 hr half-life is also reported.

Adverse Reactions. Caspofungin has been well tolerated in limited studies, with headache, fever, nausea, vomiting, flushing, pruritus and infusion vein complications most commonly reported. Some effects may be related to histamine release. One case of anaphylaxis has been reported. Elevation of liver function tests has been reported, especially with concurrent cyclosporine.

Drug Interactions. Caspofungin can reduce tacrolimus levels by about 20%. Cyclosporine increases caspofungin AUC by 35% and causes transient increases in ALT and AST. Concomitant use of cyclosporine and caspofungin is not recommended. Caspofungin does not inhibit any P450 enzymes, is not a substrate for these enzymes and does not induce CYP3A4. Some inducers of drug metabolism appear to decrease caspofungin levels; consider using the 70 mg/day dosage in patients who do not respond while on an inducer.

CLOTRIMAZOLE
Gyne-Lotrimin, Lotrimin, Mycelex

Pharmacology. Clotrimazole is an imidazole used for local therapy of fungal infections. The topical formulations are equivalent to other topical antifungals in the treatment of *Candida* spp. or dermatophyte skin infections.[39] (*See* Topical Antifungals Comparison Chart.)

Adult Dosage. Top for tinea infections apply to affected area bid. Vag Tab for vulvovaginal candidiasis 100 mg/day at bedtime for 7 days; or 2 100 mg tablets once daily at bedtime for 3 days; or 1 500 mg tablet once at bedtime. Vag Crm for vulvovaginal candidiasis 1 applicatorful (50 mg) at bedtime for 6–14 days. PO to treat oropharyngeal candidiasis dissolve 10 mg troche in the mouth 5 times/day; PO for prophylaxis of oral candidiasis in patients receiving immunosuppressive drugs dissolve 10 mg troche in the mouth tid.

Pediatric Dosage. **Top** same as adult dosage. **Troche** (<3 yr) safety and efficacy not established; (≥3 yr) same as adult dosage. **Vag Crm, Tab** (<12 yr) safety and efficacy not established; (≥12 yr) same as adult dosage.

Dosage Forms. **Top Crm, Top Lot, Top Soln, Vag Crm** 1%; **Troche** 10 mg; **Vag Tab** 100, 500 mg. **Combination Packages Combination Packages** (Gyne-Lotrimin 3) **Vag Supp** 200 mg (#3) and **Vag Crm** 1%; (Gyne-Lotrimin 7) **Vag Supp** 100 mg (#7) and **Top Crm** 1%.

Adverse Reactions. Nausea, vomiting, bad taste, and mildly abnormal liver function tests have occurred with oral troche. Vulvovaginal burning, itching, and irritation have been reported with vaginal products. Skin rash occurs occasionally with vaginal or topical use.

FLUCONAZOLE
Diflucan

Pharmacology. Fluconazole is a triazole antifungal agent that is highly water soluble and active in vivo against many fungal species (especially *Cryptococcus* spp.). The drug is active against *Candida* sp., *Blastomyces dermatitidis, Coccidioides immitis,* and *Histoplasma capsulatum.* Antifungal effects are caused by inhibition of fungal cytochrome P450-dependent enzymes that prevent conversion of lanosterol to ergosterol.[40-42]

Administration and Adult Dosage. **PO or IV for oropharyngeal or esophageal candidiasis** 200 mg on day 1, then 100 mg/day for 10–14 days. Severe esophageal candidiasis may require up to 400 mg/day.[40,43] **PO or IV for cryptococcal meningitis: short-term therapy** 400 mg/day for 6–10 weeks; **maintenance therapy in patients with AIDS** 200 mg/day indefinitely. Dosages up to 1 g/day have been used for cryptococcal meningitis. **PO for uncomplicated vaginal candidiasis** 150 mg as a single dose.[42] **PO or IV for coccidioidal meningitis** 400 mg/day indefinitely;[44] dosages up to 800 mg/day have been used. **PO or IV for prophylaxis of candidiasis in bone marrow transplantation** 400 mg/day and continued for 7 days after granulocyte count exceeds 1000/μL. Initiate therapy several days before onset of neutropenia.[43]

Special Populations. *Pediatric Dosage.* **PO or IV for candidiasis** 6 mg/kg once, then 3 mg/kg/day for at least 2 weeks for oropharyngeal candidiasis and at least 3 weeks (or 2 weeks after symptom resolution) for esophageal candidiasis; dosages up to 12 mg/kg/day have been used. **PO or IV for systemic candidiasis** 6–12 mg/kg/day. **PO or IV for treatment or prophylaxis of cryptococcal meningitis** 12 mg/kg once, then 6 mg/kg/day; continue treatment for at least 10–12 weeks after CSF cultures become negative. Prophylaxis in HIV-infected children continues indefinitely.

Geriatric Dosage. (>65 yr) although half-life is prolonged, dosage adjustment appears unnecessary, unless renal impairment is severe.[41] (*See* Other Conditions.)

Other Conditions. Reduce dosage in impaired renal function: for Cl$_{cr}$ of 20–50 mL/min, give the usual dose q 48 hr; Cl$_{cr}$ of 10–19 mL/min, 50–200 mg q 48 hr; Cl$_{cr}$ <10 mL/min, 50–100 mg q 48 hr. Give a full dose after hemodialysis on dialysis days. Patients on chronic ambulatory peritoneal dialysis may receive 50–200 mg/day.

Dosage Forms. **Tab** 50, 100, 150, 200 mg; **Susp** 10, 40 mg/mL; **Inj** 2 mg/mL.

Patient Instructions. Take with a meal if stomach upset occurs. Report changes in appetite, dark urine, or light stools.

Missed Doses. Take this drug at regular intervals. If you miss a dose of this medicine, take it as soon as you remember. If it is almost time for your next dose, take that dose only and go back to your regular dosage schedule. Leave at least 12 hours between doses. Do not double the dose or take extra.

Pharmacokinetics. *Fate.* Rapidly and well absorbed (90%) orally, unaffected by gastric pH. Peak concentrations of 1.8–2.8 mg/L (5.9–9 μmol/L) achieved 2–4 hr after administration of 100–150 mg orally. Plasma protein binding is 11–12%; penetrates well into CSF (>60% of simultaneous serum levels). V_d is 0.65 ± 0.2 L/kg; Cl is 0.015 ± 0.006 L/hr/kg. About 64–90% of a dose is excreted unchanged in urine.[41]

$t_{1/2}$. 22 ± 4 hr; 37 hr in patients >65 yr; up to 125 hr in patients with renal impairment.[41]

Adverse Reactions. Occasional nausea, vomiting, diarrhea, abdominal pain, or elevations of liver transaminases occur. Severe hepatitis or exfoliative skin reactions occur rarely.[40,43]

Precautions. Observe patients who develop rash for worsening of the lesions and discontinue the drug if necessary.

Drug Interactions. Rifampin induces the metabolism of fluconazole and can lead to clinical failure. Fluconazole inhibits metabolism of phenytoin, warfarin, and, to a minor extent, cyclosporine. Low dosages have been shown to increase the serum levels of tolbutamide, glipizide, glyburide, and possibly other sulfonylureas. This could lead to a greater hypoglycemic effect, and dosage reduction might be necessary.[43]

Parameters to Monitor. Liver function tests weekly initially, then monthly. Monitor renal function tests weekly if abnormal at outset of therapy. (*See* Precautions). Monitor patients with elevated transaminases more carefully for hepatitis.

Notes. Combination therapy with fluconazole and **flucytosine** for treatment of cryptococcal meningitis appears to be superior to single-agent therapy;[40] further studies of this combination and of fluconazole plus **amphotericin B** are needed. Fluconazole-resistant *Candida albicans* has been clinically demonstrated; increased use of prophylactic fluconazole increases the likelihood of the emergence of resistant strains such as *Candida krusei.*[43]

FLUCYTOSINE
Ancobon

Pharmacology. Flucytosine (5-FC) is a fluorinated cytosine analogue that appears to be deaminated to the cytotoxic antimetabolite fluorouracil by cytosine deaminase, an enzyme present in fungal but not in human cells. It has a narrow spectrum of activity and is used with other antifungals because resistance develops rapidly when used alone in *Candida* and *Cryptococcus* sp. infections.[39]

Administration and Adult Dosage. PO 50–150 mg/kg/day in 4 divided doses; the use of higher dosages has been suggested to prevent the emergence of resistance. Duration of therapy must be guided by the severity of infection and response to therapy.

Special Populations. *Pediatric Dosage.* **PO** same as adult dosage in mg/kg.

Geriatric Dosage. Same as adult dosage but adjust for age-related reduction in renal function.

Other Conditions. Reduce dosage in impaired renal function. An approximate dosage reduction can be determined by administering doses at intervals in hours equal to 4 times the Cr_s in mg/dL. Alternative regimens such as reduced doses at 6-hr intervals have been recommended. In patients on maintenance hemodialysis q 48–72 hr, give 20–50 mg/kg after each dialysis.[39,45] Use normal dosage in liver disease.

Dosage Forms. **Cap** 250, 500 mg.

Patient Instructions. Take the capsules required for a single dose over a 15-minute period with food to minimize stomach upset.

Missed Doses. Take this drug at regular intervals. If you miss a dose of this medicine, take it as soon as you remember. If it is almost time for your next dose, take that dose only and go back to your regular dosage schedule. Leave at least 4 hours between doses. Do not double the dose or take extra.

Pharmacokinetics. *Serum Levels.* Toxicity most likely >100 mg/L (780 μmol/L). (*See also* Precautions.)

Fate. Rapidly and well absorbed (about 90%), with peak about 1–2 hr after administration of a 500 mg dose to adults averaging 8–12 mg/L (62–93 μmol/L) in patients with normal renal function. Negligible binding to plasma proteins; V_d is 0.7 L/kg. Widely distributed throughout the body, including the CSF and eye. Eliminated almost entirely (average 90%) in the urine by glomerular filtration unchanged, with urine levels many times greater than serum levels. Low serum concentrations of **fluorouracil** have been found in patients taking flucytosine and may be responsible for hematologic toxicity.[39,45]

$t_{1/2}$. 6 ± 0.6 hr; up to 100 hr or greater with renal impairment.[39,45]

Adverse Reactions. Occasional nausea, vomiting, diarrhea, bone marrow suppression (often dose limiting in HIV-infected patients), and elevated liver function tests (usually asymptomatic and rapidly reversible). Diarrhea occurs occasionally; ulcerating enteritis occurs rarely.[39,45]

Precautions. Pregnancy; severe renal impairment (elimination is highly variable and monitoring of serum levels is recommended; keep peak concentrations <100 mg/L); impaired hepatic function; hematologic disorders; or history of therapy with myelosuppressive drugs (eg, zidovudine, ganciclovir, cancer chemotherapy) or radiation.[39,45]

Drug Interactions. Amphotericin B can increase the toxicity of flucytosine by increasing its cellular penetration and impairing its elimination secondary to nephrotoxicity.

Parameters to Monitor. Before and, frequently during, therapy, monitor BUN, Cr_s, Cl_{cr}, full hematology, and liver function tests. (*See also* Precautions.)

Notes. Flucytosine may be synergistic with **amphotericin B,** depending on the organism involved; the combination is useful in treating cryptococcal meningitis in AIDS and non-AIDS patients,[46] although the superiority of the combination in

AIDS patients has not been established. Flucytosine might be additive or synergistic with **fluconazole** for the treatment of cryptococcal meningitis; however, further experience in clinical trials is needed before this combination can be recommended.[47]

GRISEOFULVIN
Fulvicin, Grifulvin V, Grisactin

Pharmacology. Griseofulvin is a fungistatic agent that appears to affect mitosis in fungal cells. It is active against dermatophytes and not useful in the treatment of yeast or other fungal infections.[39]

Adult Dosage. PO (microsize) 0.5–1 g/day in a single or 2–4 divided doses; (ultramicrosize) 330–660 mg/day in 1–2 divided doses. Therapy usually must be continued for at least 3 weeks; infections of the palms or soles require 4–8 weeks of therapy; nail infections usually require 6–12 months of therapy. Instruct patients to take the drug with meals to enhance absorption, avoid prolonged sun exposure, and avoid alcohol.

Pediatric Dosage. (Microsize) 11 mg/kg/day; (ultramicrosize) 7.3 mg/kg/day, given as for adults.

Dosage Forms. (Microsize) **Cap** 250 mg; **Tab** 250, 500 mg; **Susp** 25 mg/mL; (ultramicrosize) **Tab** 125, 165, 250, 330 mg.

Adverse Reactions. Adverse reactions include occasional nausea and vomiting. Photosensitivity reactions, peripheral neuritis, and leukopenia are rare. The drug can exacerbate acute intermittent porphyria.

ITRACONAZOLE
Sporanox

Pharmacology. Itraconazole is a synthetic triazole antifungal agent that is more active than ketoconazole or fluconazole against certain fungi, notably *Aspergillus* spp. It also has activity against *Coccidioides, Cryptococcus, Candida, Histoplasma, Blastomyces,* and *Sporotrichosis* spp. Itraconazole inhibits fungal cytochrome P450-dependent enzymes. This inhibition blocks ergosterol biosynthesis, creating disturbances in membrane function and membrane-bound enzymes and affecting fungal cell growth and viability.[43,48]

Administration and Adult Dosage. PO for systemic fungal infections 200–600 mg/day, depending on site and severity of infection. Give dosages over 200 mg/day in 2–3 divided doses. **PO for vulvovaginal candidiasis** 200 mg bid for 1 day or 200 mg/day for 7 days. **PO for dermatomycoses** 100 mg/day for 15 days or 200 mg/day for 7 days. **PO for pityriasis versicolor** 200 mg/day for 7 days. **PO for plantar tinea pedis and palmar tinea manuum** 100 mg/day for 30 days or 200 mg bid for 7 days. **PO for onychomycosis** 200 once daily for 3 months.[49] **IV for blastomycosis, histoplasmosis or aspergillosis** 200 mg bid for 4 doses, then 200 mg/day.

Special Populations. *Pediatric Dosage.* Safety and efficacy not established.

Geriatric Dosage. Same as adult dosage.

Other Conditions. Dosage reduction in patients with hepatic impairment might be necessary, but guidelines are not established. No dosage adjustment is necessary in renal impairment. However, the manufacturer recommends that the injection not be used in patients with Cl_{cr} <30 mL/min.

Dosage Forms. **Cap** 100 mg; **Soln** 10 mg/mL; **Inj** 10 mg/mL.

Patient Instructions. Take this drug with food to ensure maximal absorption. Do not take with medications that decrease stomach acid (eg, antacids, H_2-blockers, omeprazole). Report symptoms of fatigue, loss of appetite, nausea, vomiting, yellowing of the skin, dark urine, or pale stools.

Missed Doses. Take this drug at regular intervals. If you miss a dose of this medicine, take it as soon as you remember. If it is almost time for your next dose, take that dose only and go back to your regular dosage schedule. Leave at least 12 hours between doses. Do not double the dose or take extra.

Pharmacokinetics. *Serum Levels.* Levels <5 mg/L (<7 μmol/L) are associated with treatment failure in *Aspergillus* infections.[50]

Fate. Relative oral bioavailability of the capsules compared with an oral solution is >70%.[43] The solubility of itraconazole is aided by an acidic environment, and food increases absorption. Peak serum concentration occurs in 4–5 hr; peak concentration is 20 μg/L (28 nmol/L) after a single 100 mg oral dose during fasting, increasing to 180 μg/L (0.26 μmol/L) when taken with food.[48] The drug is >99% protein bound, primarily to albumin, with only 0.2% available as free drug.[48] It is highly lipid soluble, and concentrations are much higher in tissues than in serum. Itraconazole is metabolized in the liver and exhibits dose-dependent elimination.[43] One metabolite, hydroxyitraconazole, has antifungal activity, and serum concentrations are double those of itraconazole at steady state.

t½. 24–42 hr; possibly longer with large daily dosages.[43]

Adverse Reactions. Itraconazole is generally well tolerated with long-term use. It has a negative inotropic effect and can worsen CHF. Occasional rash, pruritus, nausea, vomiting, abdominal discomfort, headache, dizziness, decreased libido, and hypertension occur. Mild transient elevations of transaminases occur frequently. Hepatotoxicity is rare, but deaths have occurred. There are no apparent adverse effects on testicular or adrenal steroidogenesis.[43,48]

Contraindications. Coadministration with astemizole, cisapride, oral midazolam, pimozide, quinidine, dofetilide, triazolam or HMGCoA reductase inhibitors metabolized by CYP3A4.

Precautions. Pregnancy; lactation. Treatment of onychomycosis in patients with ventricular dysfunction (eg, CHF).

Drug Interactions. Itraconazole inhibits CYP3A3/4 and inhibits metabolism of certain drugs such as cyclosporine and warfarin. (*See* Contraindications.) Warfarin dosage reduction might be necessary during concurrent use. Cyclosporine dosage might need to be reduced by 50% with itraconazole dosages over 100 mg/day. Avoid concurrent carbamazepine, phenytoin, or rifampin because they can dramatically reduce the serum itraconazole concentration.[50,51]

Parameters to Monitor. Closely monitor prothrombin time in patients on concurrent warfarin and cyclosporine levels in patients taking these drugs. Monitor liver function tests in patients with pre-existing hepatic impairment. Monitoring serum drug concentrations can be helpful if poor absorption or increased metabolism of itraconazole is suspected.

KETOCONAZOLE

Pharmacology. Ketoconazole is an imidazole antifungal agent that exerts its antifungal effects through inhibition of the synthesis of ergosterol (a fungal cell wall component) by inhibiting fungal cytochrome P450. It is used primarily for mucocutaneous fungal infections, including candidiasis, and in tinea versicolor unresponsive to topical therapy. It is used to treat blastomycosis, histoplasmosis, and paracoccidioidiomycosis in immunocompetent patients. It appears to suppress rather than eliminate coccidioidomycosis. Because of its poor CSF penetration, ketoconazole is not recommended for fungal infections of the CNS.[45,48] Because of its effects on steroid synthesis (*see* Adverse Reactions), the drug has been used in prostatic cancer and Cushing syndrome.

Administration and Adult Dosage. **PO** 200–400 mg daily or bid, depending on site and severity of infection. **Top** apply once daily or bid for dermatophytoses, superficial mycoses, or seborrheic dermatitis. **Top for dandruff** apply shampoo twice weekly for 4 weeks.

Special Populations. *Pediatric Dosage.* **PO** (<2 yr) not established; (>2 yr) 3.3–6.6 mg/kg/day in 1 or 2 divided doses. The drug is bioavailable when tablets are crushed and mixed in applesauce or juice. **Top** apply once daily.

Geriatric Dosage. Same as adult dosage.

Other Conditions. Limited data suggest that dosage adjustment is unnecessary in patients with hepatic impairment; however, definitive studies are needed. No adjustment is necessary in renal dysfunction.

Dosage Forms. **Tab** 200 mg; **Crm** 2%; **Shampoo** 1, 2%.

Patient Instructions. This drug may be taken with meals if stomach upset occurs, but do not take with medications that decrease stomach acid (eg, antacids, H_2 blockers, omeprazole). Report symptoms of fatigue, loss of appetite, yellowing of the skin, dark urine, or pale stools. Taking this drug with an acidic beverage (eg, a cola drink) can increase the absorption substantially. In patients receiving the drug in 0.1 N HCl to promote absorption, the solution should be sipped through a straw to avoid damaging the teeth.

Missed Doses. Take this drug at regular intervals. If you miss a dose of this medicine, take it as soon as you remember. If it is almost time for your next dose, take that dose only and go back to your regular dosage schedule. Leave at least 12 hours between doses. Do not double the dose or take extra.

Pharmacokinetics. *Fate.* Bioavailability is about 75% and is dose dependent. An acidic environment is necessary for dissolution and absorption. Bioavailability appears to be decreased by 20–40% when the drug is administered with food and is even more markedly reduced if gastric pH is elevated. Poor absorption can occur in AIDS patients because of achlorhydria and other pathologic changes in the GI track. Peak serum levels of 3.4 ± 0.3 mg/L (6.4 ± 0.6 μmol/L) are attained after a 200 mg dose taken with a meal. The drug is 93–96% plasma protein bound. V_d is estimated to be 0.36 ± 0.1 L/kg with a single dose, increasing to 2.4 ± 1.6 L/kg during long-term therapy; Cl is estimated to be 0.5 ± 0.25 L/hr/kg during long-term therapy. Ketoconazole is extensively metabolized by the liver to inactive metabolites, with only 2–4% of a dose excreted unchanged in urine.[39,52,53]

$t_{1/2}$. 8.7 ± 0.2 hr after a single dose, decreasing to 3.3 ± 1 hr during long-term therapy.[39,52]

Adverse Reactions. Generally well tolerated, with the most frequent side effects being nausea, vomiting, pruritus, and abdominal discomfort. Hepatotoxicity, including massive hepatic necrosis, occurs occasionally, but mild elevations of transaminases occur frequently. Gynecomastia occurs, probably caused by ketoconazole-induced suppression of testosterone synthesis. Ketoconazole also blocks cortisol production; however, clinically apparent hypoadrenalism occurs rarely. Irritation, pruritus, and stinging can occur with topical use.

Contraindications. Co-administration with astemizole or cisapride.

Precautions. Pregnancy; lactation.

Drug Interactions. Ketoconazole inhibits human CYP3A4 and inhibits metabolism of certain drugs such as cyclosporine, methylprednisolone, and warfarin. (*See* Contraindications.) Warfarin dosage reduction may be necessary during concurrent use. H_2-receptor antagonists, antacids, and probably proton-pump inhibitors (eg, omeprazole, lansoprazole) might reduce ketoconazole oral absorption.

Parameters to Monitor. Monitor liver function tests before starting therapy and often during therapy. Closely monitor prothrombin time in patients on concurrent warfarin and cyclosporine levels in patients taking this drug.

Notes. Achlorhydric patients may be given the drug with glutamic acid hydrochloride or 0.1 N HCl (using a drinking straw) to increase absorption.[53] An acidic drink (eg, a cola) also may be used to increase ketoconazole absorption by about 65% in achlorhydria.[54]

MICONAZOLE	Monistat IV
MICONAZOLE NITRATE	M-Zole, Micatin, Monistat, Various

Pharmacology. Miconazole is an imidazole antifungal agent available in topical preparations and as a solubilized IV preparation in a polyethoxylated castor oil (Cremophor EL).[39] (*See* Topical Antifungals Comparison Chart.)

Adult Dosage. IV 1.2–3.6 g/day in 3 divided doses, diluted in at least 200 mL of D5W or NS and infused over 30–60 min. **Top for tinea infections** apply bid. **Vag Tab for vulvovaginal candidiasis** 100 mg at bedtime for 7 days, or 200 mg hs for 3 days. **Vag Crm for vulvovaginal candidiasis** 5 g hs for 7 days.

Pediatric Dosage. IV (<1 yr) 15–30 mg/kg/day; (1–12 yr) 20–40 mg/kg/day. Do not exceed 15 mg/kg/dose. **Top** same as adult dosage; **Vag Crm, Tab** (<12 yr) safety and efficacy not established; (≥12 yr) same as adult dosage.

Dosage Forms. Inj 10 mg/mL; **Top Crm, Top Spray, Top Pwdr, Vag Crm,** 2%; **Vag Supp** 100, 200 mg. **Combination Packages** (Monistat Dual-Pak, M-Zole 3 Combination Pak) **Vag Supp** 200 mg (#3) and **Vag Crm** 2%; (Monistat 7 Combination Pak) **Vag Supp** 100 mg (#7) and **Vag Crm** 2%.

Adverse Reactions. Phlebitis, pruritus, nausea, vomiting, fever, chills, and rash are frequent side effects of IV miconazole.

Notes. Because of the serious toxicity (eg, cardiorespiratory arrest, hyponatremia) of the parenteral preparation (most likely caused by the vehicle) and data challenging the clinical effectiveness of this agent, restrict parenteral use to treating fungal infections known to be resistant to amphotericin B (eg, *Scadosporium apiospermum*). Vaginal and topical effects are similar to those of clotrimazole.

NYSTATIN
Mycostatin, Nilstat, Various

Pharmacology. Nystatin is a polyene antifungal agent very similar to amphotericin B but too toxic for parenteral use. Oral absorption is negligible, and there is no absorption through intact skin or mucous membranes.[39] (*See* Topical Antifungals Comparison Chart.)

Adult Dosage. **PO for oral candidiasis** (Susp) 400,000–600,000 units qid (as a "swish and swallow"); (troches) 200,000–400,000 units 4–5 times/day. Treat for at least 48 hr after oral symptoms have cleared and cultures have returned to normal. Immunocompromised patients require longer therapy (eg, 10–14 days). The vaginal tablet has been successfully used orally in place of the oral suspension; its slow dissolution allows prolonged contact time. **PO for GI candidiasis** 500,000–1,000,000 units tid. **Vag for candidiasis** 100,000 units daily or bid for 2 weeks.

Pediatric Dosage. **PO for candidiasis** (newborns) 100,000 units qid; (older infants and children) 200,000–400,000 units qid. **Top** same as adult dosage.

Dosage Forms. **PO Tab** 500,000 units; **PO Troche** 200,000 units; **Susp** 100,000 units/mL; **Top Crm, Oint, Pwdr** 100,000 units/g; **Vag Tab** 100,000 units.

Adverse Reactions. Nontoxic by oral, topical, and vaginal routes. Allergic sensitization occurs rarely.

Notes. Nyotran (Investigational-Aronex) is an injectable liposomal formulation of nystatin being studied for candidemia, cryptococcal meningitis and aspergillosis.

TERBINAFINE
Lamisil

Pharmacology. Terbinafine is a synthetic allylamine antifungal agent that exerts its activity by inhibiting fungal ergosterol synthesis through inhibition of squalene epoxidase. Terbinafine is active orally and topically. It has demonstrated activity against dermatophyte infections but is less active than azole antifungal against yeast species.[39,55] (*See* Topical Antifungals Comparison Chart.)

Adult Dosage. **PO** 250 mg once daily for 6 weeks for onychomycosis of fingernails or for 12 weeks for onychomycosis of the toenails. Reduce dosage in severe hepatic or renal dysfunction. **Top for tinea corporis or cruris, or cutaneous candidiasis** apply cream bid for 1 week; **Top for tinea pedis** apply solution or spray bid for 1 week, cream may require therapy up to 4 weeks, especially for plantar infections; **Top for tinea versicolor** apply solution or spray bid for 1 week.

Pediatric Dosage. Safety and efficacy not established <12 yr.

Dosage Forms. **Crm** 1%; **Top Spray** 1%; **Top Soln** 1%; **Tab** 250 mg.

Pharmacokinetics. Terbinafine is 70–80% orally absorbed regardless of the presence of food. Peak concentrations after 250 and 500 mg oral doses are 0.9 mg/L (3.1 μmol/L) and 2 mg/L (6.9 μmol/L), respectively, within 2 hr. Terbinafine is highly lipophilic and is widely distributed with a V_d of 13.5 L/kg. It is extensively metabolized to inactive metabolites, and its elimination half-life is 11–16 hr; however, an additional elimination phase of 200–400 hr may reflect the gradual release of terbinafine from adipose tissue.

Adverse Reactions. Frequent adverse reactions during oral therapy are dyspepsia, abdominal pain, diarrhea, skin reactions, malaise, lethargy, and taste disturbance. Hepatic failure has been reported rarely with the treatment of onychomycoses. Avoid in patients with liver disease.

Drug Interactions. Terbinafine can inhibit CYP2D6 and increase levels of drugs metabolized by this route. Its clearance is increased 100% by rifampin and decreased 33% by cimetidine.

Parameters to Monitor. Baseline AST and ALT; repeat if symptoms of hepatotoxicity occur.

VORICONAZOLE (Investigational-Pfizer)   Vfend

Pharmacology. Voriconazole is an azole antifungal that is a derivative of fluconazole, with the same mechanism of action. It has superior activity against *Candida albicans, C. krusei* and *C. glabrata.* Activity against *Aspergillus* sp. is equivalent to intraconazole. Activity also extends to *Pseudalescherii boydii* and *Scedosporium asiosperium.*[56]

Adult Dosage. **PO or IV** 50–400 mg/day has been used investigationally.

Pediatric Dosage. **PO or IV** Little data, but 7–10 mg/kg/day has been used.

Dosage Forms. Not yet available.

Pharmacokinetics. Oral bioavailability is 90%. Steady-state plasma levels are 2.1–4.8 mg/L with an oral dosage of 200 mg bid. The drug is 51–67% plasma protein bound; V_d is 2 L/kg. It is metabolized by the liver, primarily by CYP2C9 and 3A4. Elimination half-life is about 6 hr, but the drug can be detected in urine and feces for several days after prolonged therapy. Less than 5% of unchanged drug appears in urine.[56]

Adverse Reactions. Reversible mild to moderate dose-related visual disturbances occur frequently. Elevations in hepatic enzymes are also frequent. One case of photosensitivity has been reported. Voriconazole may interact with drugs that affect or are metabolized by CYP2C9 and 3A4, but more data are needed.[56]

TOPICAL ANTIFUNGALS COMPARISON CHART

CLASS AND DRUG	DOSAGE FORMS	ADULT DOSAGE[a]	COMMENTS
ALLYLAMINES AND BENZYLAMINES			
Butenafine HCl Mentax	Top Crm 1%.	Top (tinea pedis) apply daily for 1–4 weeks.	A benzylamine similar to the allylamines.
Naftifine HCl Naftin	Top Crm 1% Top Gel 1%.	Top (tinea) apply bid for 4 weeks.	First agent of allylamine class; response is faster than with imidazoles.
Terbinafine HCl Lamisil	Top Crm 1% Top Soln 1% Top Spray 1%.	Top (tinea cruris or corporis) apply daily–bid for 1–4 weeks; (tinea pedis) apply bid for up to 4 weeks.	Allylamine; 10–100 times more potent than naftifine. Response is more rapid than imidazoles, and it has excellent penetration in tinea pedis.
IMIDAZOLES			
Butoconazole Nitrate Femstat Gynazole-1	Vag Crm 2%.	Vag (nonpregnant) 2% crm hs for 3–6 days; or (Gynazole-1) 2% crm 1 applica-torful once (pregnant, 2nd or 3rd trimester) 2% crm hs for 6 days.	Spectrum similar to other imidazoles.
Clotrimazole Lotrimin Mycelex	Top Crm 1% Top Lot 1% Top Soln 1% Vag Tab 100, 200, 500 mg Vag Crm 1%.	Top (*Candida*, tinea) apply bid. Vag 100 mg supp or 1% crm hs for 7 days; 500 mg supp hs once;	Useful for 1st trimester *Trichomonas* vaginitis, but less effective than metronidazole.
Econazole Nitrate Spectazole	Top Crm 1%.	Top (*Candida*) apply bid; (tinea) apply once daily.	Activity similar to other imidazoles.

(continued)

TOPICAL ANTIFUNGALS COMPARISON CHART (*continued*)

CLASS AND DRUG	DOSAGE FORMS	ADULT DOSAGE[a]	COMMENTS
Ketoconazole Nizoral	Top Crm 2% Shampoo 1, 2%.	Top (*Candida*, tinea) apply daily for 2–6 weeks; (seborrhea) apply bid for 4 weeks; (shampoo) twice weekly for 4 weeks, then prn.	
Miconazole Nitrate Micatin, Monistat	Top Crm 2% Top Oint 2% Vag Crm 2%. Vag Supp 100, 200 mg	Top apply bid. Vag 100 mg supp or 2% crm hs for 7 days or 200 mg supp hs for 3 days.	Possibly less effective than some newer topical imidazoles.
Oxiconazole Nitrate Oxistat	Top Crm 1% Top Lot 1%.	Top (tinea) apply daily–bid for 2–4 weeks.	Similar to other imidazoles; superior to tolnaftate in dermatomycoses.
Sulconazole Nitrate Exelderm	Top Crm 1% Top Soln 1%.	Top (tinea) apply daily–bid for 3–4 weeks.	Similar to other imidazoles, but superior to miconazole in dermatomycoses.
Terconazole Terazol	Vag Crm 0.4, 0.8% Vag Supp 80 mg.	Vag 0.4% crm hs for 7 days; 0.8% crm or supp hs for 3 days.	Similar to other imidazoles, but superior to miconazole in vaginal candidiasis.
Tioconazole Vagistat-1	Vag Oint 6.5%.	Vag hs once.	Possibly more effective than older imidazoles; appears effective in vaginal trichomoniasis.
POLYENES			
Amphotericin B Fungizone	Top Crm 3% Top Lot 3%	Top (*Candida*) apply bid–qid for 1–4 weeks.	Inconvenient application schedule.

(continued)

TOPICAL ANTIFUNGALS COMPARISON CHART (continued)

CLASS AND DRUG	DOSAGE FORMS	ADULT DOSAGE[a]	COMMENTS
Nystatin Mycostatin Nilstat	Top. Crm 100,000 units/g Top. Oint 100,000 units/g Top. Pwdr 100,000 units/g Vag. Tab 100,000 units.	Top. (*Candida*) apply bid–tid. Vag. 1 tab hs for 14 days.	Similar to amphotericin B.
MISCELLANEOUS			
Ciclopirox Olamine Loprox Penlac	Top. Crm 1% Top. Lot 1% Nail Lacquer 8%	Top. Crm, Lot (*Candida*, tinea) apply bid. Top. Nail Laquer apply daily.	A hydroxypyridone. More effective than clotrimazole for tinea versicolor. Nail lacquer is inexpensive, but has poor efficacy rate.
Haloprogin Halotex	Top. Crm 1% Soln 1%.	Top. (tinea) apply bid for 2–4 weeks.	Equivalent to tolnaftate.
Tolnaftate Tinactin Ting	Top. Crm 1% Top. Gel 1% Top. Soln 1% Pwdr 1% Spray Liquid 1% Spray Pwdr 1%.	Top. (tinea) apply bid for 2–6 weeks.	A thiocarbamate. Possibly slightly less effective than imidazoles in dermato-mycoses.

[a]The dosage for vaginal creams for candidal infections is one applicatorful at the interval shown. Tinea pedis should be treated at the maximum dosage (usually bid) for the longest time mentioned, usually 4 weeks.
From references 39 and product information.

Antimycobacterial Drugs

CLOFAZIMINE
Lamprene

Pharmacology. Clofazimine is a lipophilic rhimophenazine dye approved for treating leprosy and used in atypical *Mycobacterium* infections, discoid lupus erythematosus, and pyoderma gangrenosum.[57,58]

Adult Dosage. **PO for leprosy, *Mycobacterium avium* complex infections, and discoid lupus erythematosus** 100 mg/day with food; dosages up to 200 mg/day are used for erythema nodosum leprosum. **PO for pyoderma gangrenosum** 300–400 mg/day have induced remission, but the manufacturer states that dosages >200 mg/day are not recommended.

Pediatric Dosage. **PO for leprosy** 1 mg/kg/day; **PO for *M. avium* complex** 1–2 mg/kg/day.

Dosage Forms. **Cap** 50 mg.

Pharmacokinetics. The drug is about 50% bioavailable. A peak serum concentration of 0.5–2 mg/L (1–4 µmol/L) 2 hr after an oral 100 to 200 mg dose is proposed as evidence of adequate absorption. Clofazimine accumulates in fatty tissues and the reticuloendothelial system and is eliminated with a half-life of about 70 days.

Adverse Reactions. Bodily secretions, skin, conjunctivae, cornea, urine, and feces can turn red to brownish black; an orange–pink skin discoloration is common and can take months to years to disappear after stopping the drug. Dose-related GI pain, nausea, vomiting, and diarrhea can occur because of crystalline deposits in GI tissue. Eosinophilic enteritis and splenic infarction occur rarely at dosages >100 mg/day. (*See also* Second-Line Antituberculosis Agents Comparison Chart.)

ETHAMBUTOL
Myambutol

Pharmacology. Ethambutol is a tuberculostatic agent that is only active against mycobacteria, including *Mycobacterium avium* complex. It does not directly enhance short course (6–9 months) regimens of isoniazid, rifampin, and pyrazinamide. Ethambutol is recommended to be included as part of a 4-drug initial regimen if there is a possibility of drug resistance and should be continued for 12 months if isoniazid resistance is demonstrated. Ethambutol is also used in combination with clarithromycin to treat disseminated *M. avium intracellulare* (MAI) infection in patients with AIDS.[58–62]

Adult Dosage. **PO for treatment of active tuberculosis** 15–25 mg/kg/day as a single dose given in combination with isoniazid and/or rifampin and/or pyrazinamide. **PO for MAI** 15 mg/kg/day, to a maximum of 1 g/day as a single dose in combination with clarithromycin or azithromycin.

Pediatric Dosage. Same as adult dosage.

Dosage Forms. **Tab** 100, 400 mg.

Pharmacokinetics. Ethambutol is about 80% absorbed from the GI tract with complex disposition characteristics. A peak serum concentration of 2–6 mg/L (8–25 μmol/L) 2 hr after an oral 15–25 mg/kg dose is proposed as evidence of adequate absorption. Its half-life is 4–6 hr, increasing to 32 hr in severe renal impairment. Approximately 80% is excreted unchanged in urine.

Adverse Reactions. Adverse reactions are rare with the recommended dosage of 15–25 mg/kg/day. Optic neuritis (manifested as blurred vision, color blindness, and restricted visual fields) occurs rarely with dosages of 15 mg/kg/day and is usually reversible with prompt drug discontinuation. Hyperuricemia can occur because of impairment of uric acid excretion.

ISONIAZID
Various

Pharmacology. Isoniazid (INH) is a synthetic hydrazine derivative of isonicotinic acid that inhibits the synthesis of mycolic acid, a component of the mycobacterial cell wall; it probably has other actions. Its activity is limited to mycobacteria; it is tuberculostatic or tuberculocidal depending on concentration and reproductive rate of the organism. Resistance is uncommon in preventive therapy but can develop rapidly if used alone in active tuberculosis. Primary resistance is becoming increasingly common in certain communities and has occurred in a variety of institutional settings (eg, hospitals, prisons). These settings are characterized by a high prevalence of HIV infection.[58,59,61,63,64]

Administration and Adult Dosage. PO for treatment of latent tuberculosis infection 5 mg/kg/day (usually 300 mg) as a single daily dose, to a maximum of 300 mg/day, given as a single agent for 6–9 months.[65] (*See* Notes, and Treatment of Latent Tuberculosis Infection Comparison Chart.) Alternatively, give INH 15 mg/kg/dose (up to 900 mg) twice weekly by directly observed therapy (DOT) for 6–9 months.[65] **PO for treatment of active tuberculosis** same dosage as above combined with rifampin 600 mg/day and pyrazinamide 15–30 mg/kg/day for 8 weeks, followed by 16 weeks of INH and rifampin. Alternatively, give the doses of INH, rifampin, ethambutol, and pyrazinamide for 2 weeks, followed by INH 15 mg/kg (to a maximum of 900 mg), rifampin 600 mg, ethambutol 50 mg/kg (to a maximum of 2.5 g), and pyrazinamide 50–70 mg/kg (to a maximum of 4 g) in 2 or 3 divided doses twice weekly for a total of 6 weeks by directly observed therapy (DOT), then continue INH and rifampin twice weekly for 16 weeks by DOT.[60,61] In 3-times-a-week regimens, ethambutol dosage is 25–30 mg/kg/day (to a maximum of 2.5 g), with INH, rifampin, and pyrazinamide at the same doses as in the twice-weekly regimen, but continued for 6 months by DOT. If pyrazinamide cannot be taken, a 9-month course may be administered in which INH in the above dosage is combined with rifampin 600 mg/day. **IM or IV** (rarely used) same as oral dosage.

Special Populations. *Pediatric Dosage.* **PO for treatment of latent tuberculosis infection** 10–20 mg/kg/day as a single dose, to a maximum of 300 mg/day, given as a single agent for 6–9 months.[65] Alternatively, give INH 20–40 mg/kg/dose (up to 900 mg) twice weekly by directly observed therapy (DOT) for 6–9 months.[65] **PO for treatment of active tuberculosis** same dosage as above, but combine with rifampin 10–20 mg/kg (to a maximum of 600 mg), and pyrazinamide

15–30 mg/kg/day (to a maximum of 2 g) in 2 or 3 divided doses for 8 weeks followed by 16 weeks of INH and rifampin. Alternatively, give the daily doses of INH, rifampin, ethambutol, and pyrazinamide for 2 weeks, followed by INH 20–40 mg/kg (to a maximum of 900 mg), rifampin 10–20 mg/kg (to a maximum of 600 mg), ethambutol 50 mg/kg (to a maximum of 2.5 g), and pyrazinamide 50–70 mg/kg (to a maximum of 4 g) in 2 or 3 divided doses twice weekly for a total of 6 weeks by DOT, then continue INH and rifampin twice weekly for 16 weeks by DOT. In 3-times-a-week regimens, pyrazinamide dosage is 50–70 mg/kg/day (to a maximum of 3 g) in 2–3 divided doses. If pyrazinamide cannot be taken, a 9-month course may be administered in which INH in the above dosage is combined with rifampin 10–20 mg/kg (to a maximum of 600 mg).[60,61] **IM or IV** (rarely used) same as oral dosage.

Geriatric Dosage. Same as adult dosage.

Other Conditions. Acetylator phenotype has not been evaluated as a parameter for dosage individualization; however, some sources recommend a dosage of 150–200 mg/day in slow acetylators with renal impairment.[66] In individuals with HIV infection being treated for tuberculosis, treatment regimens are not altered but should continue for a total of 9 months and at least 6 months beyond culture conversion.

Dosage Forms. **Tab** 50, 100, 300 mg; **Syrup** 10 mg/mL; **Cap** 150 mg with rifampin 300 mg (Rifamate); **Tab** 50 mg with rifampin 120 mg and pyrazinamide 300 mg (Rifater); **Inj** 100 mg/mL.

Patient Instructions. Report any burning, tingling, or numbness in the extremities; unusual malaise; fever; dark urine; or yellowing of the skin or eyes.

Missed Doses. Take this drug at regular intervals. If you miss a dose of this medicine, take it as soon as you remember. If it is almost time for your next dose, take that dose only and go back to your regular dosage schedule. Leave at least 12 hours between doses. Do not double the dose or take extra.

Pharmacokinetics. *Serum Levels.* A peak serum level of 3–5 mg/L (22–36 μmol/L) 2 hr postdose is proposed as evidence of adequate absorption.[58]

Fate. Rapid and nearly complete oral absorption with peak serum concentrations of 1–5 mg/L (7–36 μmol/L) 1 hr after a 5 mg/kg dose.[63] Widely distributed in body tissues including the CSF of normal patients and those with meningitis. V_d is 0.67 ± 0.15 L/kg; Cl is 0.22 ± 0.07 L/hr/kg in slow acetylators and 0.44 ± 0.12 L/hr/kg in rapid acetylators.[52] Eliminated primarily by acetylation in the liver to inactive metabolites that are excreted in the urine. Specific pattern of elimination depends on acetylator phenotype of the individual.[66]

$t_{\frac{1}{2}}$. (Rapid acetylators) 1.1 ± 0.1 hr, (slow acetylators) 2.1 ± 1.1 hr. Increased to 4 hr with renal impairment and 6.7 hr with liver disease.

Adverse Reactions. Pyridoxine-responsive peripheral neuropathy can occur, especially in alcoholics, diabetics, patients with renal failure, malnourished patients, and slow acetylators, and with dosages >5 mg/kg/day.[66] Subclinical hepatitis is frequent (10–20%) and characterized by usually asymptomatic elevations of AST and ALT, which can return to normal despite continued therapy; it might be more frequent with combined INH–rifampin therapy.[67] Clinical hepatitis is rare in those <20 yr, but is strikingly related to age (rising to 2–3% in 50–65 yr-old patients). Rare cases of massive liver atrophy resulting in death usually appear in association with alcoholism or pre-existing liver disease; most severe cases occur within the first 6 months.[67] With acute overdosage (usually 6–10 g), INH can produce severe CNS toxicity including coma and seizures as well as hypotension, acidosis, and occasionally death.[66]

Contraindications. Acute or chronic liver disease; previous INH-associated hepatitis.

Precautions. Pregnancy; lactation. Use with caution in daily users of alcohol, elderly patients, and those with a slow acetylator phenotype.

Drug Interactions. INH can inhibit the metabolism of carbamazepine and phenytoin, increasing the risk of toxicity, particularly of phenytoin in slow acetylators. Mental changes can result from effects of INH and disulfiram on metabolism of adrenergic neurotransmitters; avoid the use of disulfiram in patients who must take INH. Aluminum-containing antacids can interfere with INH absorption. Rifampin can increase the metabolism of INH to hepatotoxic metabolites.

Parameters to Monitor. Question for prodromal signs of hepatitis (eg, fever, malaise) and signs of peripheral neuropathy (eg, burning, tingling, numbness) monthly during therapy. Baseline and monthly AST and ALT are recommended only in high-risk groups (those >35 yr, daily alcohol users, and those with a history of liver dysfunction),[67] although they are not predictive of clinical hepatitis.

Notes. It is generally recommended that all patients receive INH for treatment of latent tuberculosis infection who have had positive reactions to intermediate-strength purified protein derivative (PPD, 5 tuberculin units) and who (1) are household contacts of patients with active tuberculosis; (2) converted their PPD to positive within the past 12–24 months; (3) have radiologic evidence of inactive tuberculosis or a history of inadequately treated active tuberculosis; (4) are foreign-born persons (and their families) from high-prevalence areas who have entered the United States within the past 2 years; (5) are persons with known or suspected HIV infection; (6) are persons with medical or iatrogenic conditions that increase the risk of tuberculosis—silicosis, gastrectomy, jejunoileal bypass, weight of 10% or more below ideal, chronic renal failure, diabetes mellitus, corticosteroid or other immunosuppressive therapy, hematopoietic malignancy, other malignancy, and other conditions in which immunosuppression results from the disease or its treatment. Most sources suggest that the use of INH prophylaxis in patients >35 yr should be further restricted because of the increased risk of fatal hepatotoxicity, although this is controversial.

To prevent peripheral neuropathy, give **pyridoxine** in a dosage of 50 mg/day to adults receiving large dosages of INH (10 mg/kg/day or more) and those who are predisposed to peripheral neuritis (eg, diabetics, HIV-infected, alcoholics). Pyridoxine IV in a dosage equal to the estimated amount of INH ingested is recommended for acute INH overdose.[68]

Add **ethambutol** or **streptomycin** to the initial treatment regimen until drug susceptibility studies are available, or unless there is little possibility of drug resistance (ie, there is <4% primary resistance to INH in the patient's community, and the patient has had no previous treatment with antituberculosis medications, is not from a country with a high prevalence of drug resistance, and has no known exposure to a drug-resistant case).[60,69]

PYRAZINAMIDE   Various

Pharmacology. Pyrazinamide is a synthetic analogue of niacinamide that is only active against mycobacteria. The mode of action is unknown. The drug is most active at acid pH and is active against intracellular organisms. Resistance develops rapidly when used alone, but no cross-resistance with isoniazid is observed.[60–63]

Adult Dosage. PO for treatment of latent tuberculosis infection 15–20 mg/kg/day (to a maximum of 2 g) in combination with rifampin 10 mg/kg/day (to a maximum of 600 mg) as a single daily dose for 2 months. Alternatively, give pyrazinamide 50 mg/kg/dose (to a maximum of 4 g) in combination with rifampin 10 mg/kg/dose (to a maximum of 600 mg) twice weekly for a total of 2–3 months by DOT. (*See* Treatment of Latent Tuberculosis Infection Comparison Chart.) **PO for treatment of active tuberculosis** (*see* Isoniazid Dosage).

Dosage Forms. **Tab** 500 mg; **Tab** 300 mg with isoniazid 50 mg and rifampin 120 mg (Rifater).

Pharmacokinetics. The drug is well absorbed from the GI tract with serum concentrations of 40–50 mg/L (0.3–0.4 mmol/L) achieved about 2 hr after a 1 g dose. A peak serum concentration of 20–60 mg/L (163–488 μmol/L) 2 hr after an oral 1–2 g dose is proposed as evidence of adequate absorption. The parent compound and several metabolites are excreted in urine.

Adverse Reactions. Frequent hyperuricemia, probably caused by prevention of uric acid excretion by one of the metabolites, and occasional dose-dependent hepatotoxicity occur. As many as 1–5% of patients taking regimens including isoniazid, rifampin, and pyrazinamide develop laboratory evidence of hepatic damage.

RIFABUTIN   Mycobutin

Pharmacology. Rifabutin is a rifamycin similar to rifampin chemically and in antibacterial spectrum. Rifabutin is more active against mycobacteria than rifampin, including some rifampin-resistant strains of *Mycobacterium tuberculosis* and atypical mycobacteria, and is particularly active against MAI.[70–73]

Adult Dosage. **PO for prophylaxis of MAI infections in patients with advanced HIV infection** 300 mg/day. **PO for treatment of active tuberculosis** 300 mg/day as a single daily dose in combination with at least one other antitubercular agent. (*See* Notes.)

Dosage Forms. **Cap** 150 mg.

Pharmacokinetics. Well absorbed orally, but rifabutin has a low bioavailability of 12–20% because of first-pass metabolism. Rifabutin is widely distributed in the body and is concentrated intracellularly to a greater extent than rifampin. It is 71 ± 2% plasma protein bound and has an estimated V_d of 45 ± 17 L/kg and Cl of 0.69 ± 0.32 L/hr/kg. The drug is hepatically metabolized to a number of compounds, with about 10% excreted unchanged in urine. It induces its own metabolism; its terminal half-life after long-term use is 45 ± 16 hr.

Adverse Reactions. The most frequent adverse reactions are rash, taste alterations, anorexia, nausea, insomnia, nervous system disorders (facial paralysis, twitching, and peripheral neuritis), leukopenia, and hyperbilirubinemia. Uveitis has occurred with dosages >300 mg/day.

Drug Interactions. Rifabutin induces the metabolism of drugs metabolized via CYP3A4; although the clinical importance of this effect is not clear, it appears to be less than that of rifampin.

Notes. Rifabutin can be substituted for rifampin in antituberculosis regimens.

RIFAMPIN
Rimactane, Rifadin, Various

Pharmacology. Rifampin is a synthetic rifamycin B derivative that inhibits the action of DNA-dependent RNA polymerase. It is highly active against mycobacteria, most Gram-positive bacteria, and some Gram-negative bacteria, most notably *Neisseria meningitidis*. It is also used to enhance bactericidal activity of other antistaphylococcal agents in refractory or chronic infections.[74] Antagonism with vancomycin is observed in vitro but is probably not clinically relevant. Primary resistance is uncommon, but resistance can develop rapidly if used alone.[75]

Administration and Adult Dosage. **PO for treatment of latent tuberculosis infection** 10 mg/kg/day (to a maximum of 600 mg) as a single daily dose for a total of 4 months. Alternatively, rifampin can be combined with pyrazinamide. (*See* pyrazinamide dosage and Treatment of Latent Tuberculosis Infection Comparison Chart.) **PO or IV (rarely used) for treatment of tuberculosis** 600 mg/day as a single daily dose in combination with at least one other antitubercular agent. (*See* Isoniazid.)[60,61] **PO for prophylaxis of meningococcal meningitis** 600 mg/day for 4 days or 600 mg bid for 2 days. **PO for staphylococcal infection** 600 mg/day as a single dose in combination with another antistaphylococcal agent.

Special Populations. *Pediatric Dosage.* **PO for treatment of tuberculosis** (>5 yr) 10–20 mg/kg/day as a single daily dose, to a maximum of 600 mg/day, in combination with at least one other antitubercular agent.[60,61] **PO for prophylaxis of meningococcal meningitis** (<1 month) 5 mg/kg bid for 2 days; (1 month–12 yr) 10 mg/kg/day, to a maximum of 600 mg/day for 4 days, or 10 mg/kg bid, to a maximum of 600 mg bid for 2 days.

Geriatric Dosage. Same as adult dosage.

Other Conditions. Accumulation is expected in patients with hepatic dysfunction or biliary obstruction, but dosage guidelines are not available. No dosage adjustment is necessary in patients with impaired renal function.

Dosage Forms. **Cap** 150, 300 mg; **Cap** 300 mg with isoniazid 150 mg (Rifamate); **Tab** 120 mg with isoniazid 50 mg and pyrazinamide 300 mg (Rifater); **Inj** 600 mg.

Patient Instructions. Take this medication with a full glass of water on an empty stomach (1 hour before or 2 hours after meals) for best absorption. It is important to take this medication regularly as directed because inconsistent use might increase its toxicity. This drug can cause harmless red–orange discoloration of sweat, tears (it can permanently discolor soft contact lenses), saliva, feces, and urine.

Missed Doses. Take this drug at regular intervals. If you miss a dose of this medicine, take it as soon as you remember. If it is almost time for your next dose, take that dose only and go back to your regular dosage schedule. Leave at least 12 hours between doses. Do not double the dose or take extra.

Pharmacokinetics. *Serum Levels.* A peak serum level of 8–24 mg/L (10–29 μmol/L) 2 hr after a 600–750 mg oral dose is proposed as evidence of adequate absorption.[58]

Fate. 100% absorbed orally, with a 600 mg dose producing a peak serum concentration of approximately 10 mg/L (12 μmol/L) 1–3 hr after administration. Food delays absorption but does not affect overall bioavailability. First-pass hepatic extraction is substantial but saturated with doses >300–450 mg; thus, larger doses produce disproportionate increases in serum levels. Widely distributed throughout the body; however, useful amounts appear in the CSF only in the presence of inflamed meninges. About 80% plasma protein bound; V_d is 0.97 ± 0.36 L/kg; Cl is 0.21 ± 0.1 L/hr/kg. Eliminated primarily by deacetylation in the liver to a partially active metabolite that is extensively enterohepatically recirculated, producing very high biliary concentrations. About 50–60% of a dose is eventually excreted in the feces. Urinary excretion is variable and appears to increase with the dose. At usual dosages, 12–15% is excreted unchanged in the urine.[73]

$t_{1/2}$. 3.5 ± 0.8 hr. Half-life increases with higher doses but can become shorter over the first few weeks of treatment. It is not changed by renal impairment but is increased unpredictably by liver disease or biliary obstruction.[73]

Adverse Reactions. Adverse reactions are more frequent and severe with intermittent, high-dose administration. GI symptoms are frequent. Acute, reversible renal failure, characterized as tubular damage with interstitial nephritis, sometimes appearing with concomitant hepatic failure has been reported rarely, especially in association with intermittent administration.[63–66] Asymptomatic elevation of liver enzymes occurs frequently, whereas clinical hepatitis is rare but more common with pre-existing liver disease or alcoholism; the effect of **isoniazid** co-administration on the frequency of hepatitis is unclear.[67] Competition with bile for biliary excretion can produce jaundice, especially with pre-existing liver disease. Intermittent therapy is also associated with thrombocytopenia and a flu-like syndrome (ie, fever, joint pain, muscle cramps).

Contraindications. Hypersensitivity to any rifamycin derivative.

Precautions. Pregnancy; lactation. Use with caution in daily users of alcohol, those with pre-existing liver disease, and those with a history of drug-associated hepatic damage (especially from antituberculars).

Drug Interactions. Rifampin accelerates the metabolism of many drugs such as oral contraceptives, corticosteroids, cyclosporine, enalapril, HIV protease inhibitors, propranolol, methadone, metoprolol, mexiletine, phenytoin, quinidine, theophylline, tolbutamide, oral verapamil, warfarin, and zidovudine because of potent inducing effects on CYP3A.[76] The dosage of these drugs may need to be increased during concurrent use. Rifampin can increase the metabolism of isoniazid to hepatotoxic metabolites.

Parameters to Monitor. Question for prodromal signs of hepatitis (eg, fever, malaise). Baseline and monthly AST and ALT have been recommended, especially for patients with factors predisposing to hepatotoxicity (eg, alcoholism, preexisting liver disease), although they are not predictive of clinical hepatitis in the absence of symptoms.

Notes. Rifampin is a useful drug for tuberculosis but should be used only in combination regimens because of rapid emergence of resistant mutants of *Mycobacterium tuberculosis* when it is used alone. The recent emergence of multiple drug resistance among strains of *M. tuberculosis* in patients with AIDS includes high-level rifampin resistance. The routine use of rifampin in methicillin-resistant *Staphylococcus aureus* (MRSA) endocarditis is not recommended except after failure of conventional therapy and possibly with renal, myocardial, splenic, or cerebral abscess. If rifampin is added to vancomycin for treatment of MRSA, add a third drug (eg, gentamicin) to reduce the likelihood of resistance development. In nonendocarditis infections caused by MRSA, do not use rifampin unless there is inadequate response to vancomycin alone.

RIFAPENTINE
Priftin

Pharmacology. Rifapentine is a rifamycin, similar to rifampin and rifabutin. It is used in the treatment of pulmonary tuberculosis and is similar in efficacy to daily rifampin, although relapse rates can be greater with rifapentine.[77]

Adult Dosage. **PO for tuberculosis** 600 mg twice weekly for 2 months with at least 72 hr between doses, then once weekly for 4 months. It should be used in conjunction with other antitubercular drugs in both phases. The drug may be taken with food to decrease nausea, vomiting, or GI upset.

Dosage Forms. **Tab** 150 mg.

Pharmacokinetics. Peak serum levels occur 5–6 hr after an oral dose. Food increases the bioavailability and peak serum level. Rifapentine is 93% bound to serum albumin. V_d is estimated to be 70 ± 1 L/kg. Cl is 2.5 ± 0.14 L/hr/kg in males and 1.7 ± 0.41 L/hr/kg in females. The drug is hydrolyzed by an esterase to the active metabolite 25-desacetyl rifapentine. Half-lives of the drug and metabolite are each about 13 hr.

Adverse Reactions. The most frequent side effects in combination regimens were neutropenia, leukopenia, increased liver enzymes, dyspepsia, and anorexia, although these appeared to be less frequent than in equivalent rifampin-containing regimens. Pyuria and hematuria occurred more frequently with rifapentine than with rifampin. Obtain baseline liver enzymes, bilirubin, CBC, and platelet count before starting therapy. Routine laboratory monitoring during therapy is not necessary unless clinically indicated.

Contraindications. Hypersensitivity to any rifamycin.

Drug Interactions. Rifapentine induces CYP2C8/9 and 3A4 and can increase the metabolism of drugs metabolized by these isozymes. Rifapentine decreases indinavir peak by 55% and AUC by 70%. Use with great caution in conjunction with protease inhibitors and other drugs metabolized by CYP2C8/9 or 3A4.

TREATMENT OF LATENT TUBERCULOSIS INFECTION

DRUGS	DURATION (MONTHS)	DOSAGE INTERVAL	RATING (EVIDENCE) HIV–	RATING (EVIDENCE) HIV+
Isoniazid	9	Daily	A (II)	A (II)
		Twice weekly	B (II)	B (II)
Isoniazid	6	Daily	B (I)	C (I)
		Twice weekly	B (II)	C (I)
Rifampin-pyrazinamide	2	Daily	B (II)	A (I)
	2–3	Twice weekly	C (II)	C (I)
Rifampin	4	Daily	B (II)	B (III)

Rating: A = preferred; B = acceptable alternative; C = offer when A and B cannot be given. Evidence: I = randomized clinical trial data; II = data from clinical trials that are not randomized or were conducted in other populations; III = expert opinion.
From reference 65.

SECOND-LINE ANTITUBERCULOSIS AGENTS COMPARISON CHART[a]

DRUG	DOSAGE FORMS	ADULT DOSAGE	PEDIATRIC DOSAGE	SERUM LEVELS[b] (MG/L)	HALF-LIFE Normal	HALF-LIFE Renal Impairment	MAJOR ADVERSE EFFECTS
Aminosalicylic Acid Salts[c] Various	Tab 500 mg Gran 4g.	PO 8–12 g/day in 2–4 divided doses (as the acid).	150–300 mg/kg/day in 3–4 divided doses, to a maximum of 12 g/day.	20–60[d] (4 g)	1 hr	—	GI intolerance: hepatitis; lupus-like syndrome. Rarely used.
Capreomycin Sulfate Capastat	Inj 1 g.	Same as streptomycin.	Same as streptomycin.	Same as streptomycin.	2.5 hr	↑	Nephrotoxicity, ototoxicity.
Clofazimine Lamprene	Cap 50 mg.	PO 100–200 mg/day.	Not well established.	0.5–2 (100–200 mg)	70 days	—	Brown–black discoloration of skin and bodily secretions; nausea; vomiting; GI pain because of deposition in GI tissues.
Cycloserine Seromycin	Cap 250 mg.	PO 15–20 mg/kg/day (usually 500 mg) in 2 divided doses, to a maximum of 1 g/day.	PO 10–15 mg/kg/day to a maximum of 1 g/day.	20–35 (250–500 mg)	10 hr	↑	CNS (drowsiness, dizziness, headache, depression, rare seizures, and psychosis).
Ethionamide Trecator-SC	Tab 250 mg.	PO 15–20 mg/kg/day (usually 500–750 mg) as a single daily dose, to a maximum of 1 g/day.	PO 15–20 mg/kg/day to a maximum of 1 g/day.	1–5 (250–500 mg)	3 hr	—	GI intolerance: hepatitis; CNS (drowsiness, dizziness, headache, depression, rare seizures).

(continued)

SECOND-LINE ANTITUBERCULOSIS AGENTS COMPARISON CHART[a] (*continued*)

DRUG	DOSAGE FORMS	ADULT DOSAGE	PEDIATRIC DOSAGE	SERUM LEVELS[b] (MG/L)	HALF-LIFE Normal	HALF-LIFE Renal Impairment	MAJOR ADVERSE EFFECTS
Kanamycin Sulfate Kantrex	Inj 37.5, 250, 333, 500 mg/mL.	Same as streptomycin.	Same as streptomycin.	Same as streptomycin.	2–3 hr	80–90 hr	Nephrotoxicity; ototoxicity.
Rifabutin Mycobutin	Cap 150 mg.	PO 300 mg/day as a single dose.	Not well established. (1 yr) 15–25 mg/kg/day; (2–10 yr) 4–19 mg/kg/day; (14–16 yr) 2.8–5.4 mg/kg/day.	—	45 ± 16 hr	—	See monograph.
Streptomycin Sulfate Various	Inj 400 mg/mL.	IM 12–15 mg/kg/day to a maximum of 1 g, or 22–25 mg/kg to a maximum of 1.5 g 2–3 times/week.	IM 20–40 mg/kg/day to a maximum of 1 g, or 25–30 mg/kg to a maximum of 1.5 g 2–3 times/week.	35–40 (12–15 mg/kg) 65–80 (22–25mg/kg)	2–3 hr	↑	Vestibular ototoxicity.

[a]Use only in combination with other effective antituberculars.
[b]Peak serum level 1 hr (parenteral) or 2 hr (oral) after the adult dose in parentheses that is evidence of adequate absorption.
[c]Sodium salt contains 73% aminosalicylic acid; increase dosage accordingly. Sodium content is 4.7 mEq/g.
[d]Peak serum level 6 hr after a dose of Paser granules.
Adapted from references 58, 60, 63, and 66.

Antiparasitic Drugs

Class Instructions. Pinworms. Purgation, enemas, or special dietary restrictions are unnecessary with this drug, which may be taken with food or beverages. To avoid reinfestation with pinworms, wash the perianal area thoroughly each morning. Change and wash nightclothes, undergarments, and bedclothes daily. Wash hands and under fingernails thoroughly after bowel movements and before eating. Treat all family members simultaneously and clean bedroom and bathroom floors thoroughly at the end of the course of treatment. To demonstrate a cure, no eggs must be found in the anal area at least 5 weeks after the end of treatment.

ALBENDAZOLE   Albenza

Pharmacology. Albendazole is a benzimidazole drug related to mebendazole and has a similar mechanism of action; however, it has a broader range of activity than mebendazole.

Administration and Adult Dosage. PO for hydatid cyst 400 mg bid for 1–6 months; **PO for cysticercosis** 400 mg bid for 8–30 days, repeat prn; **PO for** *Clonorchis sinensis* 10 mg/kg/day for 7 days; **PO for cutaneous larva migrans** 400 mg/day for 3 days; **PO for capillariasis** 400 g/day for 10 days; **PO for ascariasis, eosinophilic enterocolitis, hookworm, trichostrongylus, or trichuriasis** 400 mg once; **PO for pinworms** 400 mg once, then repeat in 2 weeks; **PO for microsporidiosis** 400 mg bid (ocular infections require the addition of **fumagillin**); **PO for trichinosis** 400 mg bid for 8–14 days; **PO for visceral larva migrans (toxocariasis)** 400 mg bid for 5 days.[78]

Special Populations. *Pediatric Dosage.* Safety and efficacy not established. **PO for hydatid cyst** 15 mg/kg/day to a maximum of 800 mg/day for 1–6 months; **PO for cysticercosis** 15 mg/kg/day to a maximum of 800 mg/day in 2 divided doses for 8–30 days, repeat prn; **PO for** *Clonorchis sinensis* 10 mg/kg/day for 7 days; **PO for cutaneous larva migrans** 400 mg/day for 3 days; **PO for capillariasis** 400 g/day for 10 days; **PO for ascariasis, eosinophilic enterocolitis, trichostrongylus, or trichuriasis** 400 mg once; **PO for eosinophilic enterocolitis** 400 mg once; **PO for pinworms** 400 mg once, then repeat in 2 weeks; **PO for trichinosis** 400 mg bid for 8–14 days; **PO for visceral larva migrans (toxocariasis)** 400 mg bid for 5 days.[78]

Geriatric Dosage. Same as adult dosage.

Dosage Forms. Tab 200 mg.

Patient Instructions. Take this drug with a fatty meal to increase absorption and improve effectiveness.

Missed Doses. Take this drug at regular intervals. If you miss a dose of this medicine, take it as soon as you remember. If it is almost time for your next dose, take that dose only and go back to your regular dosage schedule. Do not double the dose or take extra.

Pharmacokinetics. *Fate.* Absorption is poor but enhanced by fat. Oral bioavailability of unchanged albendazole is negligible because of first-pass metabolism to albendazole sulfoxide, the active form of the drug. The sulfoxide has a peak serum level 2–3 hr after a dose. CNS concentrations are 40% of serum levels; concentration in echinococcal cysts is about 25% of serum levels. The absorbed drug is excreted primarily in urine as metabolites.[79]

$t_{1/2}$. (Albendazole sulfoxide) 10–15 hr.[79]

Adverse Reactions. Occasionally, diarrhea, abdominal pain, and migration of roundworms through the mouth and nose occur. Rarely, leukopenia, alopecia, or increased transaminases occur.[78]

Precautions. Pregnancy; liver dysfunction.

Drug Interactions. Concurrent dexamethasone increases serum levels by 50%.[79]

Parameters to Monitor. Monitor hepatic transaminases and WBC count during prolonged therapy.

IVERMECTIN
Stromectol

Pharmacology. Ivermectin is a semisynthetic anthelmintic that binds to glutamate-gated chloride channels in invertebrate nerve and muscle cells, leading to increase cellular permeability, hyperpolarization of nerve cells, paralysis, and death.

Administration and Adult Dosage. PO for strongyloidiasis 200 µg/kg/day for 1–2 days; PO for onchocerciacis 150 µg/kg once, repeat in 3–12 months until asymptomatic; PO for *Mansonella streptocerca* 150 µg/kg once; PO for pediculosis (head or pubic lice) or scabies 200 µg/kg once; PO for cutaneous larva migrans 200 µg/kg/day for 1–2 days.[78] (*See* Notes.)

Special Populations. *Pediatric Dosage.* (<15 kg) safety and efficacy not established; PO for above infestations same as adult dosage.

Geriatric Dosage. Same as adult dosage.

Dosage Forms. Tab 6 mg.

Pharmacokinetics. *Fate.* Ivermectin is absorbed orally. It does not enter the CNS. Most of the drug is metabolized hepatically, and the drug and metabolites are excreted in the feces. Less than 1% is excreted unchanged in urine. Its half-life is about 16 hr.

Adverse Reactions. Fairly well tolerated, with abdominal and chest pain, dizziness, pruritus, rash, urticaria, diarrhea, nausea, and vomiting occurring frequently. In treating onchocerciasis, inflammation caused by dead and dying larvae can cause more severe and frequent cutaneous reactions, fever, lymph node swelling and tenderness, edema, and arthralgia; ocular effects include limbitis and punctate opacity.

Precautions. Pregnancy.

Notes. Ivermectin is the drug of choice for strongyloidiasis and onchocerciasis and an alternative for the other infestations listed.

MEBENDAZOLE
Vermox, Various

Pharmacology. Mebendazole is active against many intestinal roundworms. It binds to helminth tubulin and inhibits glucose uptake in the parasite, with no effect on blood glucose concentrations in the host.[79]

Administration and Adult Dosage. **PO for pinworms** 100 mg once, repeat in 2 weeks; **PO for ascariasis or hookworms** 100 mg bid for 3 days or 500 mg once; **PO for capillariasis** 200 mg bid for 20 days; **PO for eosinophilic enterocolitis** 100 mg bid for 3 days; **PO for roundworms, or whipworms** 100 mg bid for 3 days.[78]

Special Populations. *Pediatric Dosage.* (<2 yr) Safety and efficacy not established. **PO for pinworms, ascariasis, capillariasis, roundworms, whipworms, eosinophilic enterocolitis, or hookworms** same as adult dosage.[78]

Geriatric Dosage. Same as adult dosage.

Dosage Forms. **Chew Tab** 100 mg.

Patient Instructions. (*See* Pinworms Class Instructions.) Chew tablets before swallowing.

Pharmacokinetics. *Fate.* Poorly absorbed orally. Almost all eliminated unchanged in the feces, but up to 10% can be recovered in the urine 48 hr after a dose, primarily as the decarboxylated metabolite.[79]

Adverse Reactions. Occasional abdominal pain and diarrhea in cases of massive infestation and expulsion of worms. Occasionally, migration of roundworms through the mouth and nose occurs. Rarely, leukopenia, agranulocytosis, and hypospermia have been reported.[78]

Precautions. Pregnancy.

Drug Interactions. Carbamazepine and hydantoins can reduce mebendazole serum levels.

Parameters to Monitor. When treating whipworm, take a stool sample for egg count 3 weeks after treatment to detect frequent (about 30%) persistent infestation requiring retreatment.

Notes. Mebendazole is the agent of choice for whipworm, producing about a 70% cure rate with a single treatment; the cure rate is 90–100% with roundworms, hookworms, and pinworms. Particularly useful in mixed infestations.[78,79]

PERMETHRIN   Acticin, Elimite, Nix, Various

Pharmacology. Permethrin is a pyrethroid that acts on arthropod nerve cell membranes to cause delayed polarization and paralysis. It is active against lice (including unhatched eggs) and mites (eg, scabies).

Administration and Adult Dosage. **Top for head lice** apply 1% cream rinse to hair one time after washing hair. Leave on for no longer than 10 min and rinse with water. If live lice are seen after >7 days, reapply as above. **Top for pubic lice** although not FDA-approved, use of topical 5% permethrin has been used (*see also* Ivermectin);[78] repeat application at 10 days has been recommended.[80,81] **Top for scabies** thoroughly massage 5% cream into the skin from the head to the soles of the feet. Remove by showering or bathing after 8–14 hr.

Special Populations. *Pediatric Dosage.* **Top for lice** (<2 months) safety and efficacy not established; (>2 months) same as adult dosage. **Top for scabies** (<2 months) safety and efficacy not established. Neonates have been treated, but remove cream after 6 hr;[82] (>2 months) same as adult dosage.

Geriatric Dosage. Same as adult dosage.

Dosage Forms. Liquid (creme rinse) 1% (Nix, various); **Crm** 5% (Acticin, Elimite).

Patient Instructions. Lice. Wash hair and towel dry. Apply enough creme rinse to saturate hair and scalp, especially behind the ears and on the nape of the neck. Use the comb provided with the product to remove nits. Wash all pillow cases, pajamas, and towels in hot, soapy water and dry using the hot cycle of a dryer for at least 20 minutes. Clothing and bedding that cannot be washed should be sealed in a plastic bag for 2 weeks or dry cleaned. Soak combs in hot water for 5–10 minutes. If infestation of the eyebrows or eyelashes occurs, consult your health care provider. **Scabies.** Itching, mild burning, or stinging can occur after application. Itching usually resolves by 4 weeks. If irritation persists, consult your health care provider.

Pharmacokinetics. *Fate.* Usually <2% absorbed after topical application. Permethrin is rapidly metabolized by ester hydrolysis to inactive metabolites which are excreted in urine.[83]

Adverse Reactions. Adverse reactions are mild and occur only occasionally with the treatment of lice. With the 5% cream for treatment of scabies, mild, transient burning, stinging, or tingling occurs in about 10% of patients. Itching, edema, and erythema are often symptoms of scabies and can be exacerbated temporarily by treatment with permethrin. Intolerable burning and stinging can occur in patients with AIDS and scabies.[83] Itching and skin irritation can persist after successful treatment because of local allergic reactions to the dead mites. Allergic reactions are rare and might be caused by the formaldehyde preservative.

Contraindications. Documented allergy to any pyrethroid or vehicle component.

Precautions. Pregnancy, although animal studies indicate no teratogenicity. During lactation, discontinue nursing temporarily during treatment with 5% cream; use of 1% creme rinse poses little risk during breastfeeding. Avoid contact with eyes and mucous membranes.

Drug Interactions. None known.

Parameters to Monitor. Observe for parasites 7–10 days after treatment of lice infestation or 14 days after treatment of scabies.

Notes. Permethrin is the drug of choice for pediculosis and scabies. **Malathion** 0.5% lotion (Ovide) is an alternative for pediculosis. **Synergized pyrethrins** (pyrethrins and piperonyl butoxide) have efficacies similar to that of permethrin for head lice but are not as persistent as permethrin and require a repeat treatment after 1 week.[78] In scabies, permethrin is safer and more effective than **lindane** and more effective and easier to use than **crotamiton**.[81,83] Lindane is not recommended because resistance occurs frequently and lindane is a persistent environmental contaminant.[81]

PRAZIQUANTEL
Biltricide

Pharmacology. Praziquantel causes a loss of intracellular calcium, resulting in paralysis and dislodgement of worms from sites of attachment. In higher dosages, it damages the parasite's surface membrane, allowing the host's immune response to destroy the worm.[84]

Administration and Adult Dosage. PO for schistosomiasis (*Schistosoma haematobium* or *mansoni*) 40 mg/kg in 2 divided doses the same day, but heavy infestations require 60 mg/kg in 3 divided doses at 4–6 hr intervals;[78,84] (*Schistosoma japonicum* or *mekongi*) 60 mg/kg in 3 doses at 4–6 hr intervals. PO for flukes (eg, clonorchiasis, opisthorchiasis) 25 mg/kg tid for 1 day; (paragonimiasis) 25 mg/kg tid for 2 days.[78,84] PO for tapeworms (beef, dog, fish, pork) 5–10 mg/kg once; (dwarf tapeworm) 25 mg/kg once. PO for neurocysticercosis 50–100 mg/kg/day in 3 doses for 30 days.[78] (*See* Notes.)

Special Populations. *Pediatric Dosage.* (<4 yr) safety and efficacy not established. PO for above infestations same as adult dosage.[78]

Geriatric Dosage. Same as adult dosage.

Dosage Forms. Tab 600 mg.

Patient Instructions. Take with liquid during meals but do not chew tablets. This drug can cause dizziness or drowsiness. Use caution when driving, operating machinery, or performing other tasks requiring mental alertness.

Pharmacokinetics. *Fate.* The drug is 80% absorbed orally, but undergoes extensive first-pass metabolism. CSF concentrations are 14–20% of serum levels. The drug is metabolized and metabolites are excreted primarily in urine.

$t_{1/2}$. 1.1 ± 0.3 hr.

Adverse Reactions. Side effects are usually mild. Dizziness, headache, and malaise occur frequently after large doses. Occasionally, abdominal discomfort, fever, sweating, and eosinophilia occur. Drowsiness or fatigue might occur because of a structural similarity to benzodiazepines. Pruritus and rash occur rarely.[78] In patients treated for cysticercosis, an inflammatory response, presumably caused by dead and dying organisms, occurs that is manifested by headache, seizures, and increased intracranial pressure.

Contraindications. Ocular cysticercosis.

Precautions. Pregnancy; liver disease; avoid breastfeeding for 72 hr after the last dose.

Drug Interactions. Drugs that induce CYP3A3/4 (eg, dexamethasone, carbamazepine, phenobarbital, phenytoin) can increase clearance, decrease bioavailability, and cause treatment failure; drugs that inhibit CYP3A3/4 (eg, cimetidine, ketoconazole, erythromycin) decrease clearance, increase serum levels, and lengthen half-life.[79,84]

Parameters to Monitor. Observe for CNS toxicity when treating cysticercosis.

Notes. Concomitant corticosteroid therapy is recommended for patients treated for neurocysticercosis.

PYRANTEL PAMOATE
Antiminth, Various

Pharmacology. Pyrantel is a depolarizing neuromuscular blocker that produces spastic paralysis of the parasite with no similar effects on the host after oral use. It also inhibits acetylcholinesterases.[79]

Administration and Adult Dosage. PO for pinworms and roundworms 11 mg/kg, to a maximum of 1 g in a single dose; **for pinworms** repeat in 2 weeks; **PO for moniliformis** 11 mg/kg 3 times at 2-week intervals; **PO for hookworms and eosinophilic enterocolitis** 11 mg/kg/day, to a maximum of 1 g for 3 days.[78] Doses are expressed as base equivalent.

Special Populations. *Pediatric Dosages.* (<2 yr) Safety and efficacy not established. **PO for above infestations** same as adult dosage.[78]

Geriatric Dosage. Same as adult dosage.

Dosage Forms. Cap 180 mg (62.5 mg as pyrantel base); **Liq** 50 mg/mL (as pamoate base); **Susp** 50 mg/mL (as pamoate base).

Patient Instructions. (*See* Pinworms Class Instructions.)

Pharmacokinetics. *Fate.* Slight oral absorption. Over 50% is excreted unchanged in feces, and less than 15% of the dose is excreted as parent drug and metabolites in the urine.[79]

Adverse Reactions. Occasional nausea, vomiting, headaches, dizziness, rash, and transient AST elevations.[78]

Contraindications. Liver disease.

Precautions. Avoid during pregnancy.

Drug Interactions. Piperazine and pyrantel might be mutually antagonistic in ascariasis.

Notes. Except for pinworms, for which it is virtually 100% effective, and monilaformis, pyrantel is an alternative to other drugs.[78]

Antiviral Drugs

Class Instructions: HIV Drugs. Underdosage, noncompliance, or partial compliance with drug regimens for these drugs might result in development of a resistant strain(s) of HIV that will not be susceptible to treatment. Do not stop taking this medication unless told to do so by your health care provider. This drug should be used in combination with other anti-HIV medications. Protease inhibitors do not cure or prevent HIV infection. It is possible for a person taking this medication to transmit the virus to another person. Opportunistic infections and other complications associated with HIV infection can continue to develop while you take this medication. Protease inhibitors and nonnucleoside reverse transcriptase inhibitors have a potential for serious interactions with a large number of commonly prescribed drug products. Always check with your health care provider before starting any new medication.

Missed Doses. Missing doses can result in the development of resistance that can lead to treatment failure. If you forget a dose, take it as soon as you remember. If it is almost time for your next scheduled dose (within 4 hours), skip the missed dose. Do not double your dose.

ACYCLOVIR	Zovirax, Various
VALACYCLOVIR	Valtrex

Pharmacology. Acyclovir is an acyclic nucleoside analogue of deoxyguanosine that is selectively phosphorylated by the virus-encoded thymidine kinase to its monophosphate form. Cellular enzymes then convert the monophosphate to the active antiviral acyclovir triphosphate, which inhibits viral DNA synthesis by incorporation into viral DNA, resulting in chain termination. Acyclovir has potent activity against herpes simplex virus (HSV) I and II and herpes zoster virus (varicella-zoster virus [VZV]). Activity against cytomegalovirus, which lacks a specific virus-encoded thymidine kinase, is limited, but resistance can be overcome with high serum concentrations in some patient populations. Acyclovir inhibits Epstein-Barr virus but has not been found clinically useful. Human herpes virus 6 is resistant.[85-87] Valacyclovir is the L-valyl ester of acyclovir, which undergoes extensive first-pass hydrolysis to yield high serum acyclovir concentrations.[88]

Administration and Adult Dosage. **IV for severe localized HSV infection** (acyclovir) 5 mg/kg q 8 hr for 5 days for nonimmunocompromised patients or 7–10 days for immunocompromised patients; **IV for VZV (chickenpox) infection in immunocompromised patients** 10 mg/kg q 8 hr for 7–10 days; **IV for HSV encephalitis** 10 mg/kg q 8 hr for 10–14 days. Dilute to 50–250 mL and infuse over at least 60 min; avoid bolus IV, SC, or IM injections. Maintain minimum urine output of 500 mL/24 hr for each gram of acyclovir administered. **PO for primary or recurrent genital HSV infection** (acyclovir) 200 mg 5 times/day for 10 days; (valacyclovir, immunocompetent patients) 500 mg bid for 5 days. **PO for prevention of recurrent genital HSV infection** (acyclovir) 400 mg bid or 200 mg 3–5 times/day; (valacyclovir in immunocompetent patients) 1 g/day or 500 mg bid; **PO for active VZV (chickenpox) or herpes zoster** (acyclovir) 800 mg q 4 hr 5 times/day for 5 days (chickenpox) or 7–10 days (zoster). **PO for herpes zoster in immunocompetent patients** (valacyclovir) 1 g q 8 hr for 7 days. **Top for initial genital HSV infection and limited non–life-threatening mucocutaneous HSV infections in immunocompromised patients** (acyclovir) 0.5-inch ribbon to cover 4-square-inch affected skin area q 3 hr 6 times/day for 7 days.

Special Populations. *Pediatric Dosage.* (All dosages apply to acyclovir.) **IV for HSV infection** (neonates) 10 mg/kg q 8 hr for 10–14 days;[86] (13 months–11 yr) 750 mg/m^2/day in 3 divided doses for 7 days. **IV for VZV (chickenpox) in immunocompromised children** (13 months–11 yr) 1500 mg/m^2/day in 3 divided doses. **IV for HSV encephalitis** (6 months–11 yr) 1500 mg/m^2/day in 3 divided doses for 10 days. Infuse over at least 60 min; avoid bolus IV, SC, or IM injections. **PO for VZV (chickenpox)** (acyclovir) (>2 yr and <40 kg) 20 mg/kg/dose, to a maximum of 800 mg q 6 hr for 5 days; (>40 kg) same as adult dosage; (valacyclovir) safety and efficacy not established.

Geriatric Dosage. Same as adult dosage, adjusted for renal function.

Other Conditions. (Acyclovir) in obesity, base dosage on IBW. In renal insufficiency, reduce parenteral and oral dosage: (Cl_{cr} 25–50 mL/min) usual dose q 12 hr; (Cl_{cr} 10–25 mL/min) usual dose q 24 hr; (Cl_{cr} 0–10 mL/min) 50% of the usual dose q 24 hr. For patients on hemodialysis, give the usual daily dosage after dialysis. (Valacyclovir) in renal insufficiency, reduce the dosage: (Cl_{cr} 30–49 mL/min) 1 g q 12 hr; (Cl_{cr} 10–29 mL/min) 1 g q 24 hr; (Cl_{cr} <10 mL/min) 500 mg q 24 hr.

Dosage Forms. (Acyclovir) **Cap** 200; **Tab** 400, 800 mg; **Inj** 500 mg, 1 g; **Inj** 50 mg/mL; **Oint** 5%; **Susp** 40 mg/mL. (Valacyclovir) **Tab** 500 mg.

Patient Instructions. Use a finger cot or latex glove when applying acyclovir ointment. The ointment might cause transient burning or stinging.

Missed Doses. Take this (oral) drug at regular intervals. If you miss a dose of this medicine, take it as soon as you remember. If it is almost time for your next dose, take that dose only and go back to your regular dosage schedule. Leave at least 4 hours between doses. Do not double the dose or take extra.

Pharmacokinetics. *Fate.* Oral bioavailability of acyclovir is estimated to be 15–30%; valacyclovir is well absorbed, with a bioavailability of 54%.[89] Valacyclovir is extensively converted to acyclovir after oral administration. After 200–600 mg of acyclovir orally, mean peak steady-state levels are 0.56–1.3 mg/L (2.5–5.9 μmol/L); levels after IV doses of 2.5–15 mg/kg are 5–24 mg/L (23–105 μmol/L). After an oral dose of 1 g of valacyclovir, mean peak steady-state acyclovir level is 5–6 mg/L (22–27 μmol/L).[90] CSF acyclovir concentrations are 25–70% of simultaneous serum level. Decay is biphasic, with V_{dB} of 0.69 ± 0.19 L/kg; Cl is 0.21 ± 0.03 L/hr/kg with normal renal function;[89] 86–92% is excreted unchanged in urine; the remainder is metabolized to 9-carboxy-methoxymethylguanine. Renal clearance is 75–80% of total clearance and is markedly reduced by concomitant probenecid.[91]

$t_{1/2}$. (Acyclovir) α phase 0.34 hr, β phase 2.9 ± 0.8 hr in adult patients, increasing to nearly 20 hr in end-stage renal disease; 5.7 hr on dialysis; about 4 hr in neonates.[91]

Adverse Reactions. (Acyclovir) nephrotoxicity, thought to be caused by precipitation of acyclovir crystals in the nephron, occurs in about 10% of patients if the drug is given by bolus (<10 min) injection. Phlebitis at injection site occurs frequently with IV infusion because of the high pH (9–11) of the product. Other reported side effects are CNS toxicity (eg, headache, lethargy, tremulousness, delirium, seizures), nausea, vomiting, and skin rash. CNS toxicity occurs primarily in patients with underlying neurologic disease or end-stage renal disease, or with cancer chemotherapy and irradiation to the CNS, and might not be primarily caused by the drug. Topical application to herpes lesions can be painful.[85,86] (Valacyclovir) adverse reactions appear comparable to acyclovir. Nausea, vomiting, diarrhea, abdominal pain, and headache have been reported frequently with valacyclovir use. Thrombotic thrombocytopenic purpura/hemolytic-uremic syndrome has been reported in patients with advanced HIV disease and in bone marrow and renal transplant patients. This phenomenon has not been reported in immunocompetent patients.[90]

Contraindications. (Valacyclovir) allergy to the drug or to acyclovir.

Precautions. Use caution in renal impairment, dehydration, or pre-existing neurologic disorders. Valacyclovir not indicated in immunocompromised patients.

Drug Interactions. Zidovudine and acyclovir can result in drowsiness and lethargy. Probenecid can increase oral bioavailability and half-life of acyclovir.

Parameters to Monitor. Monitor renal function and injection site for signs of phlebitis daily. Carefully monitor patients with underlying neurologic diseases for evidence of neurotoxicity. (*See* Adverse Reactions.)

Notes. Acyclovir-resistant strains of virus that are deficient in thymidine kinase have been isolated from patients after treatment. Although thought to be less virulent than sensitive strains, HSV strains resistant to acyclovir have been described in AIDS patients.[86]

CIDOFOVIR
Vistide

Pharmacology. Cidofovir (HPMPC) is a nucleotide analogue with potent in vitro and in vivo activities against cytomegalovirus (CMV) and other herpes viruses. Cidofovir contains a phosphonate group that enables it to bypass initial virus-dependent phosphorylation. Cellular enzymes convert cidofovir to cidofovir diphosphate, the active intracellular metabolite.[92–94]

Adult Dosage. **IV induction for CMV retinitis** 5 mg/kg infused over 1 hr once weekly for 2 weeks, then **IV maintenance** 5 mg/kg once every other week. Reduce dosage to 3 mg/kg if Cr_s increases by 0.3–0.4 mg/dL above baseline or if >2+ proteinuria occurs. It is essential to give the following with cidofovir: 2 g **probenecid PO** 3 hr before administration and 1 L of NS IV over 1 hr just before administration. If tolerated, give another liter of NS with or after cidofovir administration; finally, give PO 1 g probenecid 2 hr and 8 hr after the end of cidofovir infusion. Cidofovir is also being investigated as an intravitreal injection for CMV retinitis.

Dosage Forms. **Inj** 75 mg/mL.

Pharmacokinetics. Peak serum cidofovir concentration averages 26.1 ± 3.2 mg/L (83 ± 10 μmol/L) after a 5 mg/kg IV infusion with concomitant probenecid and hydration. Cidofovir is not appreciably bound to plasma proteins; V_d averages 0.5 L/kg. Cidofovir is excreted almost entirely unchanged in the urine. The elimination half-life of cidofovir is 3–6 hr when administered with probenecid. Cidofovir diphosphate has a prolonged intracellular half-life, with a range of 17–65 hr, which allows infrequent administration schedules of once weekly to once every other week.

Adverse Reactions. Nephrotoxicity is the most frequent adverse reaction, and high-dose probenecid (*see* Adult Dosage) must be used with administration of cidofovir. Probenecid decreases uptake of cidofovir in proximal renal tubular cells, decreasing the risk of nephrotoxicity. Other frequent adverse reactions are proteinuria, elevated Cr_s, nausea, vomiting, fever, asthenia, neutropenia, rash, headache, diarrhea, alopecia, anemia, and abdominal pain. Ocular hypotony and decreased intraocular pressure have been reported occasionally. Nausea, vomiting, fever, rash, and chills are frequent reactions reported with probenecid.

DIDANOSINE
Videx, Videx EC

Pharmacology. Didanosine (dideoxyinosine [ddI]) is a purine nucleoside that undergoes complex metabolism in vivo to dideoxyadenosine (ddA), which ultimately undergoes metabolism to an active triphosphorylated form (ddATP). Incorporation of ddATP into viral DNA leads to chain termination, and ddATP is a competitive inhibitor of HIV reverse transcriptase, which further contributes to the interference of HIV replication.[95,96]

Administration and Adult Dosage. PO for HIV infection (tablets or solution) (≥60 kg) 200 mg (as 2 tablets) q 12 hr, or 400 mg/day (as 2 tablets), or 250 mg (as powder) q 12 hr; (<60 kg) 125 mg (as 2 tablets) q 12 hr, or 250 mg/day (as 2 tablets), or 167 mg (as powder) q 12 hr. Take each dose as 2 whole (not partial) tablets to provide adequate buffering. **PO for HIV infection (EC capsules)** same dosage as above, but as a single daily dose.

Special Populations. *Pediatric Dosage.* PO for HIV infection 120 mg/m^2 bid.

Geriatric Dosage. Same as adult dosage, but not studied in this population.

Other Conditions. Consider dosage reduction in patients with renal or hepatic impairment. (Tablets or solution) Cl_{cr} 30–59 mL/min: (≥60 kg) 200 mg/day (as 2 tablets or EC capsules) or 100 mg (as 2 tablets) bid; (<60 kg) 150 mg/day (as 2 tablets), 75 mg (as 2 tablets) bid or 125 mg /day (as EC capsules). Cl_{cr} 10–29 mL/min: (≥60 kg) 150 mg/day (as 2 tablets) or 125 mg/day (as EC capsules); (<60 kg) 100 mg/day (as 2 tablets). Cl_{cr} <10 mL/min: (≥60 kg) 100 mg/day (as 2 tablets); (<60 kg) 75 mg/day (as 2 tablets)—EC capsules not recommended. Didanosine is removed by hemodialysis, but the quantity removed is low and supplemental doses are not recommended.[97]

Dosage Forms. **Chew/Dispersible Tab** 25, 50, 100, 150, 200 mg; **EC Cap** 125, 200, 250, 400 mg; **Pwdr for Oral Soln** 100, 167, 250 mg; **Pwdr for Oral Soln (pediatric)** 2, 4 g.

Patient Instructions. *(See HIV Drugs Class Instructions.)* Didanosine must be taken on an empty stomach 1 hour before or 2 hours after a meal. It is essential that the 2-tablet dose be taken each time to avoid destruction of the drug by stomach acid. For children >1 year, use the 2-tablet dose; for those <1 year of age, use the 1-tablet dose. Tablets may be chewed and swallowed or dissolved in at least 30 mL of water and swallowed immediately. Do *not* swallow the tablets whole. Reconstituted solution may be stored for up to 30 days when refrigerated. Shake solution thoroughly before administering each dose. Do not crush or chew EC capsule.

Missed Doses. Take this drug at regular intervals. If you miss a dose of this medicine, take it as soon as you remember. If it is almost time for your next dose, take that dose only and go back to your regular dosage schedule. Leave at least 12 hours between doses. Do not double the dose or take extra.

Pharmacokinetics. *Fate.* Didanosine is rapidly degraded at acidic pH. Appreciable interpatient variability and dose-dependent characteristics affect didanosine absorption. Oral bioavailability of the buffered powder for oral solution is 33 ± 11%.[98,99] The chewable/dispersible buffered tablets are 20–25% more bioavailable than the buffered powder for solution. The peak serum concentration is 1.1 ±

0.7 mg/L (4.7 ± 2.9 μmol/L) after a 375 mg oral dose of buffered powder for solution. Protein binding is less than 5%. CSF concentration 1 hr after infusion of didanosine averages 21% of the concurrent serum concentration. $V_{dβ}$ is 1 ± 0.7 L/kg; Cl is 1 ± 0.08 L/hr/kg.[97] Up to 60% of dose is excreted unchanged in the urine; the remainder is extensively metabolized to ddATP, hypoxanthine, and uric acid.[97,100]

$t_½$. 1.75 ± 0.99 hr;[97] in vitro intracellular half-life of ddATP is 8–43 hr.[101]

Adverse Reactions. Pancreatitis has occurred at a frequency of 5–9% in clinical trials at or below current recommended dosages and can be fatal. Peripheral neuropathy occurs in 16–34% of patients, with 12% requiring dosage reduction. Diarrhea has been reported with the buffered powder for oral solution at a frequency of 34%. In children, pancreatitis and peripheral retinal depigmentation have occurred frequently, although the latter has not been associated with visual impairment.[102] Peripheral neuropathy has not occurred in children.

Precautions. Avoid didanosine tablets in patients with phenylketonuria because these contain phenylalanine. Didanosine has been associated with hyperuricemia; use caution in patients with a history of gout or baseline hyperuricemia; avoid in individuals with a history of pancreatitis.

Drug Interactions. Administration with fluoroquinolones can reduce fluoroquinolone serum levels because of buffers in formulation. Avoid concurrent administration with dapsone, indinavir, itraconazole, ketoconazole, or other medications requiring an acidic environment for absorption because of buffers in didanosine formulation. Ganciclovir and trimethoprim-sulfamethoxazole appear to increase didanosine's bioavailability, but the clinical importance is unknown. Use with alcohol, high-dose trimethoprim-sulfamethoxazole, or other pancreatitis-associated drugs can increase the risk of pancreatitis.[103,104]

Parameters to Monitor. Obtain serum amylase, lipase, and triglycerides monthly. Symptoms of abdominal pain, nausea, and vomiting can indicate pancreatitis. Symptoms of distal numbness, tingling, or pain in the feet or hands can indicate neuropathy and might necessitate dosage modification. Monitor clinical signs, symptoms, and laboratory markers for progression of HIV disease to help decide regimen changes in antiretroviral therapy. Baseline CD4 and HIV-1 RNA polymerase chain reaction viral load tests are useful to measure clinical benefit of therapy. Repeat tests after 1 month and q 3–4 months thereafter have been suggested to monitor benefit of antiretroviral therapy.

Notes. As with other nucleoside reverse transcriptase inhibitors, drug-resistant HIV-1 isolates emerge with long-term didanosine therapy (≥12 months).[105] (*See* Antiviral Drugs for HIV Infection Comparison Chart.)

FAMCICLOVIR	Famvir
PENCICLOVIR	Denavir

Pharmacology. Famciclovir is the diacetyl, 6-deoxy ester of the antiviral guanosine analogue penciclovir. Famciclovir is absorbed rapidly and converted to penciclovir in the intestinal wall and liver. Viral thymidine kinase converts penciclovir to its monophosphate form. Cellular enzymes then convert the monophosphate to the active antiviral penciclovir triphosphate. The triphosphate inhibits viral DNA synthesis by incorporation into viral DNA, resulting in termination of the chain. Penciclovir has potent activity against HSV I and II and herpes zoster virus (varicella-zoster). Penciclovir also has some activity against Epstein-Barr virus and CMV but has not demonstrated clinical usefulness against infections with these agents.[106-109]

Adult Dosage. **PO for herpes zoster** (famciclovir) 500 mg q 8 hr for 7 days. In renal insufficiency, reduce the dosage as follows: Cl_{cr} 40–59 mL/min, 500 mg q 12 hr; Cl_{cr} 20–39 mL/min, 500 mg q 24 hr; Cl_{cr} <20 mL/min, 250 mg q 48 hr; with hemodialysis, 250 mg after each dialysis. **PO for recurrent genital HSV infection** (famciclovir) 125 mg bid for 5 days. In renal insufficiency, reduce the dosage as follows: Cl_{cr} 20–39 mL/min, 125 mg q 24 hr; Cl_{cr} <20 mL/min, 125 mg q 48 hr; with hemodialysis, 125 mg after each dialysis. **Top for herpes labialis** (penciclovir) apply to lesions q 2 hr while awake for 4 days, starting as early as possible at the beginning of an outbreak.

Dosage Forms. **Crm** (penciclovir) 1%; **Tab** (famciclovir) 125, 250, 500 mg.

Pharmacokinetics. Topical penciclovir is virtually unabsorbed. The absolute bioavailability of penciclovir is 77% after a 500 mg oral dose of famciclovir. Peak serum concentrations are 0.84 ± 0.22 (3.3 ± 0.9 μmol/L) and 3.34 ± 0.58 mg/L (13 ± 2.3 μmol/L) 45 min after 125 and 500 mg oral doses of famciclovir, respectively. Penciclovir is <20% protein bound, and the V_d is approximately 1 L/kg. Penciclovir is eliminated primarily by renal excretion. The elimination half-life is approximately 2 hr with normal renal function, increasing to over 13 hr in patients with severely impaired renal function.

Adverse Reactions. Nausea, vomiting, diarrhea, and headache occur frequently with famciclovir. Pruritus, paresthesias, and fatigue occur occasionally. Penciclovir causes mild erythema occasionally.

Drug Interactions. Cimetidine might enhance the bioavailability of famciclovir and its conversion to penciclovir.

FOSCARNET SODIUM   Foscavir

Pharmacology. Foscarnet sodium (phosphonoformic acid [PFA]) is a pyrophosphate analogue. Foscarnet actively inhibits viral DNA polymerases in its parent form and does not require phosphorylation for optimal antiviral activity. It has antiviral activity against HSV I and II, human CMV, Epstein-Barr virus, hepatitis B virus, varicella-zoster virus, and some retroviruses including HIV. Foscarnet sodium inhibits DNA synthesis in CMV and other herpes viruses by inhibiting viral DNA polymerase.[110]

Administration and Adult Dosage. **IV induction for CMV retinitis in AIDS patients** 60 mg/kg q 8 hr or 90 mg/kg q 12 hr for 14–21 days.[111] **IV maintenance for CMV retinitis in AIDS patients** 90–120 mg/kg/day in 1 dose. **IV for acyclovir-resistant herpes virus infections** 40 mg/kg q 8 hr or 60 mg/kg q 12 hr until clinical resolution.[111] **IV for acyclovir-resistant varicella-zoster infections**

in immunocompromised patients 40 mg/kg q 8 hr or 60 mg/kg q 12 hr for 10–21 days or until clinical resolution.[87,112]

Special Populations. *Pediatric Dosage.* Safety and efficacy not established.

Geriatric Dosage. Same as adult dosage but adjusted for renal function.

Other Conditions. Reduce dosage in renal impairment. (*See* product information.)

Dosage Forms. **Inj** 24 mg/mL.

Patient Instructions. Foscarnet is not a cure for CMV retinitis, and progression of disease might continue during or after treatment. Regular eye examinations are important to monitor for disease progression. Report symptoms of tingling around the mouth or numbness in extremities, which might indicate a need for temporary discontinuation of foscarnet.

Missed Doses. Take this drug at regular intervals. If you miss a dose of this medicine, take it as soon as you remember. If it is almost time for your next dose, take that dose only and go back to your regular dosage schedule. Leave at least 12 hours between doses. Do not double the dose or take extra.

Pharmacokinetics. *Fate.* After twice-daily infusion of 90 mg/kg over 2 hr, peak serum levels are 98 ± 27 mg/L (577 ± 161 μmol/L) and troughs are 6.4 ± 8.3 mg/L (38 ± 49 μmol/L).[111] Plasma protein binding is 14–17%. CSF concentrations are 35–103% of simultaneous serum levels. V_{dss} is 0.3–0.7 L/kg; Cl is 0.13 ± 0.05 L/hr/kg. Foscarnet is not metabolized and is 70–90% excreted unchanged in the urine.[111]

$t_{1/2}$. α phase 1.4 ± 0.6 hr, β phase 6.8 ± 5 hr in patients receiving continuous or intermittent infusions. A terminal half-life of 36–196 hr might represent release of the drug from binding sites in bone.[111]

Adverse Reactions. Abnormal renal function, including decreased Cl_{cr} and acute renal failure, occurs in about one-third of patients. Electrolyte abnormalities such as hypocalcemia, hypophosphatemia, hyperphosphatemia, hypokalemia, and hypomagnesemia occur in 6–16% of patients. Seizures have been reported in 10% of patients and might be related to electrolyte abnormalities or underlying disease. Other adverse reactions frequently reported are fever 65%, nausea 47%, anemia 33%, diarrhea 30%, vomiting 26%, headache 26%, and granulocytopenia 14%. Local irritation, inflammation, and pain might occur at the injection site with peripheral administration at a frequency of 1–5%.[111,113,114]

Precautions. Use with extreme caution in patients with renal impairment of nephrotoxic drugs, pre-existing cytopenias, pre-existing electrolyte abnormalities, or underlying neurologic disorders.

Drug Interactions. Concurrent use of nephrotoxic drugs such as aminoglycosides or radiologic contrast media can increase risk and severity of nephrotoxicity. IV pentamidine can increase the risk of hypocalcemia; avoid this combination, if possible, although inhaled pentamidine does not seem to be a risk factor.[104]

Parameters to Monitor. Monitor Cr_s 2 or 3 times/week during induction therapy and weekly during maintenance therapy. Monitor serum calcium, magnesium, potassium, and phosphorus at the same frequency as Cr_s. Symptoms of perioral tingling, numbness in extremities, or other paresthesias might indicate electrolyte abnormalities and require more frequent monitoring and a need to obtain ionized calcium levels.

GANCICLOVIR	Cytovene, Vitrasert
VALGANCICLOVIR	Valcyte

Pharmacology. Ganciclovir (DHPG) is a synthetic acyclic nucleoside analogue of guanine. Antiviral activity is a result of its conversion to the triphosphate form, which functions as an inhibitor of and faulty substrate for viral DNA polymerase. Ganciclovir has antiviral activity against HSV I and II, human CMV, Epstein-Barr virus, and varicella-zoster virus.[83,114] Valganciclovir is the valine ester prodrug that is hydrolyzed to ganciclovir after oral administration.

Administration and Adult Dosage. Take all oral doses with food. **IV for CMV retinitis (induction)** 5 mg/kg q 12 hr for 14–21 days, then (**maintenance**) 5 mg/kg once daily for 7 days/week or 6 mg/kg once daily for 5 days/week. **PO for CMV retinitis (induction)** (valganciclovir) 900 mg q 12 hr for 21 days, then (maintenance) 900 mg once daily. Induction may be repeated for patients who experience disease progression. **IV for prevention of CMV disease in transplant recipients** 5 mg/kg q 12 hr for 7–14 days, followed by 5 mg/kg once daily for 7 days/week or 6 mg/kg once daily for 5 days/week. Duration depends on duration and degree of immunosuppression. Dilute IV dose in 100 mL NS or D5W and infuse over 60 min. **PO for CMV retinitis (maintenance after IV induction)** (ganciclovir) 1 g q 8 hr or (valganciclovir) 900 mg once daily. **PO for prophylaxis of CMV disease** (ganciclovir) 1 g q 8 hr indefinitely; (valganciclovir) 900 mg once daily.

Special Populations. *Pediatric Dosage.* The adult dosage in mg/kg has been used.

Geriatric Dosage. Same as adult dosage adjusted for renal function.

Other Conditions. In renal insufficiency (Ganciclovir). *Parenteral induction:* (Cl_{cr} 50–69 mL/min) 2.5 mg/kg q 12 hr; (Cl_{cr} 25–49 mL/min) 2.5 mg/kg q 24 hr; (Cl_{cr} <25 mL/min) 1.25 mg/kg q 24 hr; (hemodialysis) 1.25 mg/kg 3 times/week. On hemodialysis days, give dose after hemodialysis. *Parenteral maintenance:* (Cl_{cr} 50–69 mL/min) 2.5 mg/kg q 24 hr; (Cl_{cr} 25–49 mL/min) 1.25 mg/kg q 24 hr; (Cl_{cr} 10–24 mL/min) 0.625 mg/kg q 24 hr; (hemodialysis) 0.625 mg/kg 3 times/week after hemodialysis. *Oral maintenance:* (Cl_{cr} 50–69 mL/min) 1.5 g once daily or 500 mg tid; (Cl_{cr} 25–49 mL/min) 1 g/day in 1 or 2 doses; (Cl_{cr} 10–24 mL/min) 500 mg/day; (Cl_{cr} <10 mL/min) 500 mg 3 times/week after hemodialysis. (Valganciclovir) *Oral induction:* (Cl_{cr} 40–59 mL/min) 450 mg q 12 hr; (Cl_{cr} 25–39 mL/min) 450 mg/day; (Cl_{cr} 10–24 mL/min) 450 mg q 48 hr; (hemodialysis) use ganciclovir. *Maintenance:* (Cl_{cr} 40–59 mL/min) 450 mg/day; (Cl_{cr} 25–39 mL/min) 450 mg q 48 hr; (Cl_{cr} 10–24 mL/min) 450 mg twice weekly.

Dosage Forms. (Ganciclovir) **Cap** 250, 500 mg; **Inj** 500 mg; **Ocular Implant** 4.5 mg (nominal release). (Valganciclovir) **Tab** 450 mg.

Patient Instructions. This drug is not a cure for CMV retinitis, and progression might continue during or after treatment. Concurrent use with zidovudine can result in severe reduction in white blood cell count; therefore, report any signs or symptoms of infection, such as fever, chills, or sweats. Take oral ganciclovir or valganciclovir with food.

Missed Doses. Take this drug at regular intervals. If you miss a dose of this medicine, take it as soon as you remember. If it is almost time for your next dose, take that dose only and go back to your regular dosage schedule. Leave at least 4 hours between doses. Do not double the dose or take extra.

Pharmacokinetics. *Fate.* Ganciclovir is absorbed poorly from the GI tract; oral bioavailability is 6% when taken with food (about 20% greater than when taken on an empty stomach). Average peak serum concentration of 0.34 ± 0.13 mg/L (1.3 ± 0.5 μmol/L) occurs 1–2 hr after a single 1 g oral dose. Valganciclovir bioavailability is 61%. Mean peak and trough steady-state levels after IV doses of 5 mg/kg q 12 hr in patients with normal renal function are 5.3 ± 2.8 mg/L (21 ± 11 μmol/L) and 1.1 ± 0.4 mg/L (4.3 ± 1.5 μmol/L), respectively. Ganciclovir is 1–2% plasma protein bound; CSF concentration is 24–67% of simultaneous serum level. V_c is 0.26 ± 0.08 L/kg; $V_{d\beta}$ is 1.17 ± 0.54 L/kg; Cl is 0.25 ± 0.13 L/hr/kg with normal renal function. The drug is 90–99% excreted unchanged in the urine. Hemodialysis reduces serum levels by $53 \pm 12\%$. Renal excretion occurs principally via glomerular filtration, although limited renal tubular secretion also can occur.[114,115]

$t_{\frac{1}{2}}$. α phase 0.76 ± 0.67 hr; β phase 3.6 ± 1.4 hr in adult patients, increasing to 11.5 ± 3.9 hr in renal insufficiency.[114,115]

Adverse Reactions. Granulocytopenia (ANC <1000/μL) occurs in 13–67% of patients and is the most frequent dose-limiting adverse effect.[114] Thrombocytopenia (platelets <50,000/μL) occurs in 20% of patients. CNS toxicity (headache, lethargy, dizziness, confusion, seizure, coma) has been reported at a frequency of 5–17%. Phlebitis, inflammation, and pain at the site of IV infusion occur frequently because of the high pH of the solution. Anemia, fever, rash, and abnormal liver function tests occur in about 2% of patients.[114,116]

Contraindications. Hypersensitivity to acyclovir or ganciclovir.

Precautions. Use with caution in renal impairment, pre-existing cytopenias, or concurrent myelosuppressive drug therapy.

Drug Interactions. Didanosine AUC can be increased when given within 2 hr of ganciclovir. Probenecid decreases the renal excretion of ganciclovir. Use extreme caution in combination with zidovudine because of additive myelosuppression. Concurrent nephrotoxic drugs can increase the nephrotoxicity of ganciclovir. Concurrent cytotoxic drugs increase the toxicity of ganciclovir. Seizures have been reported with concurrent use of ganciclovir and imipenem-cilastatin.

Parameters to Monitor. Monitor CBC and platelet counts twice weekly during induction treatment and at least weekly during maintenance. Monitor renal function at least q 2 weeks. Check injection site for phlebitis and infection daily.

Notes. Ganciclovir-resistant CMV strains have been isolated from patients during treatment.[117] Disease progression caused by these strains has been observed and might require changing therapy to an alternative antiviral (eg, foscarnet).

INDINAVIR
Crixivan

Pharmacology. Indinavir is an HIV protease inhibitor with a mechanism of action similar to that of saquinavir.[96,118] (*See* Antiviral Drugs for HIV Infection Comparison Chart.)

Adult Dosage. PO for HIV infection 800 mg q 8 hr. Take each dose on an empty stomach with water or other fat-free liquid or with light, fat-free foods (eg, toast, jelly, skim milk, coffee). **PO for HIV infection with ritonavir** 400 mg q 12 hr with ritonavir 400 mg q 12 hr, or 800 mg q 12 hr with ritonavir 200 mg q 12 hr. In mild to moderate hepatic insufficiency caused by cirrhosis, the dosage is 600 mg q 8 hr. The combination can be taken with food.

Dosage Forms. Cap 200, 333, 400 mg.

Pharmacokinetics. Indinavir is rapidly absorbed in the fasting state. Administration of indinavir with a meal high in calories, fat, or protein decreases oral absorption by about 75%. When indinavir is combined with ritonavir, food does not decrease bioavailability of indinavir. Absolute bioavailability not been determined in humans, but fasting bioavailability is 14–70% in animals. Indinavir is 60% bound to human plasma proteins. It is primarily metabolized by CYP3A4 and <20% is excreted unchanged in the urine; half-life is 1.8 ± 0.4 hr.

Adverse Reactions. Frequent adverse reactions are nausea, vomiting, abdominal pain, diarrhea, headache, asthenia, insomnia, taste perversion, transient elevations of hepatic transaminases, asymptomatic hyperbilirubinemia, and nephrolithiasis. Dizziness, somnolence, anorexia, malaise, and dry mouth occur occasionally. Nephrolithiasis occurred in 4% of patients in clinical trials and can be managed with hydration and temporary drug discontinuation. Patients should drink at least 1.5 L/day of liquids to ensure adequate hydration while taking indinavir.

LAMIVUDINE
Epivir

Pharmacology. Lamivudine (3TC) is a synthetic pyrimidine nucleoside active against HIV-1, HIV-2, and hepatitis B. Lamivudine is metabolized intracellularly to lamivudine triphosphate and acts as a chain terminator of viral DNA and a competitive inhibitor of HIV reverse transcriptase. Lamivudine alone to treat HIV infection leads to rapid emergence of high-level resistance; therefore, it is used in combination with zidovudine. Resistance to zidovudine is markedly delayed when the drug is used with lamivudine, and the combination results in greater and more sustained elevations in CD4 cell counts than zidovudine monotherapy.[97,102,109,119,120] (*See* Antiviral Drugs for HIV Infection Comparison Chart.)

Adult Dosage. PO for HIV infection 150 mg bid. **PO for chronic hepatitis B** 100 mg/day. Reduce dosage in renal impairment. **For HIV co-infection with hepatitis B** use HIV dosage with appropriate combination antiretroviral therapy.

Pediatric Dosage. PO (3 months–12 yr) 4 mg/kg, to a maximum of 150 mg bid with zidovudine.

Dosage Forms. Tab 100, 150 mg; Soln 5, 10 mg/mL.

Pharmacokinetics. Oral bioavailability is 82%. V_d is 1.3 L/kg; elimination half-life is 2.5 hr. Excretion is primarily by the renal route, with 68–71% of drug excreted unchanged in urine.

Adverse Reactions. The most frequently reported adverse effects have been headache, fatigue, nausea, insomnia, neuropathy, and musculoskeletal pain.

NELFINAVIR MESYLATE   Viracept

Pharmacology. Nelfinavir mesylate is an antiviral that inhibits HIV-1 and HIV-2 proteases by binding to the active enzymatic site, preventing cleavage of polyprotein precursors. This cleavage is essential for maturation of infectious virus, and its inhibition results in the formation of immature, noninfectious HIV particles. (*See* Antiviral Drugs for HIV Infection Comparison Chart.)

Administration and Adult Dosage. **PO for HIV disease in combination with nucleoside analogues** 750 mg tid or 1250 mg bid.[121]

Special Populations. *Pediatric Dosage.* **PO for HIV disease in combination with nucleoside analogues** (<2 yr) safety and efficacy not established; (2–13 yr) 20–30 mg/kg tid.

Geriatric Dosage. Not studied but expected to be the same as adult dosage.

Dosage Forms. **Tab** 250 mg; **Pwdr** 50 mg nelfinavir base/level scoopful (1 g).

Patient Instructions. (*See* HIV Drugs Class Instructions.) Each dose must be taken orally with a light snack or meal to increase the amount of the drug absorbed. If you are taking an oral contraceptive, you should use an alternate or additional contraceptive measure. Store nelfinavir in a dry place at room temperature. New onset diabetes mellitus, exacerbation of pre-existing diabetes mellitus, and hyperglycemia have been reported in HIV-infected patients receiving protease inhibitors. Some patients require initiation or dosage adjustments of insulin or oral hypoglycemic agents. Diabetic ketoacidosis has also occurred. Hyperglycemia persisted in some cases after drug discontinuation.

Pharmacokinetics. *Fate.* Bioavailability is unknown in humans, but animal data suggest an oral bioavailability of 20–80%. Nelfinavir absorption is increased 2- to 3-fold when administered with food. Peak serum concentrations occur 2–4 hr after a dose. After multiple oral doses of 750 mg tid, peak serum concentrations average 3–4 mg/L (5.3–7 μmol/L) and trough concentrations average 1–3 mg/L (1.8–5.3 μmol/L). Plasma protein binding is >98%. Nelfinavir is metabolized by cytochrome P450 enzymes, primarily CYP3A4 and to a minor extent by CYP2C9, 2C19, and 2D6. The major oxidative metabolite has in vitro antiviral activity comparable to the parent drug. Less than 2% of nelfinavir is excreted unchanged in urine.

$t_{1/2}$. 3.5–5 hr.

Adverse Reactions. Diarrhea, abdominal pain or discomfort, flatulence, nausea, rash, and difficulty swallowing tablets are frequent. Diarrhea often resolves spontaneously 1–2 weeks after initiation of therapy. Antidiarrheal medications are often beneficial in alleviating or minimizing symptoms. Oral calcium carbonate 500–1000 mg once or twice daily has decreased prevalence of nelfinavir-associated diarrhea in some patients. Occasional reactions include asthenia, headache, and fatigue.

Contraindications. (*See* Drug Interactions.)

Precautions. Do not use nelfinavir as monotherapy. Appropriate use is with other antiretroviral therapy to reduce potential for developing drug resistance. Nelfinavir powder for oral solution contains 11.2 mg phenylalanine/g of powder and should be used cautiously in patients with phenylketonuria.

Drug Interactions. Nelfinavir is an inhibitor of CYP3A and can cause increased serum concentrations of drugs primarily metabolized by CYP3A. It is also a substrate for CYP3A, and nelfinavir concentrations can be affected by the induction or inhibition of CYP3A by other drugs. Do not co-administer nelfinavir with rifampin because it decreases nelfinavir's steady-state AUC by 82%. Co-administration with rifabutin reduces nelfinavir's AUC by 32% and increases rifabutin's AUC by 207%. If administered together, the manufacturer recommends reducing the rifabutin dosage by 50%, although alternatives should be considered. Avoid other drugs (eg, carbamazepine, phenobarbital, phenytoin) that strongly induce CYP3A4 because they can substantially reduce nelfinavir serum concentrations. Avoid co-administration with astemizole or cisapride because of possible prolonged QT intervals and serious cardiovascular adverse events. Co-administration with ethinyl estradiol/norethindrone resulted in a 47% decrease in ethinyl estradiol serum concentration and an 18% decrease in norethindrone serum concentration. Alternative contraceptives need to be used while receiving nelfinavir therapy. Co-administration with indinavir results in an 83% increase in nelfinavir AUC and a 51% increase in indinavir AUC. Co-administration with ritonavir results in a 152% increase in nelfinavir AUC and minimal change in ritonavir AUC. Various protease inhibitor combinations are under study, but safety and efficacy of these combinations have not been established.

Parameters to Monitor. Monitor clinical signs, symptoms, and laboratory markers for progression of HIV disease to help decide regimen changes in antiretroviral therapy. Baseline CD4+ and HIV-1 RNA polymerase chain reaction viral load tests are standard of practice markers to measure clinical benefit of therapy. Monitor adherence to the drug regimen throughout treatment course to help in assessment of effectiveness. Repeat tests after 1 month and q 3–4 months to monitor benefit of antiretroviral therapy.

NEVIRAPINE   Viramune

Pharmacology. Nevirapine is a dipyridodiazepinone nonnucleoside HIV-1 reverse transcriptase inhibitor. Nevirapine and other reverse transcriptase inhibitors are not active against HIV-2 reverse transcriptase. The inhibition by nevirapine is noncompetitive, and the binding site is located near but not directly at the catalytic amino acid residues, which might provide nevirapine activity against HIV-1 mutants that are resistant to nucleoside reverse transcriptase inhibitors. Nevirapine provides added benefit (eg, increased CD4 count, decreased viral load) in combination with zidovudine and didanosine.[122-125] (*See* Antiviral Drugs for HIV Infection Comparison Chart.)

Adult Dosage. PO for HIV 200 mg/day for 2 weeks, followed by 200 mg bid or 400 mg once daily.

Pediatric Dosage. PO (<13 yr) 120 mg/m^2/day for 2 weeks, then bid.

Dosage Forms. Tab 200 mg; Susp 10 mg/mL.

Pharmacokinetics. Oral absorption is not affected by food or antacids; bioavailability is 90%. The median time to peak concentration is 4 hr after a 400 mg dose with average peak concentrations after the first dose of 3.4 ± 1 mg/L. Peak and trough concentrations average 7.2 ± 1.4 mg/L (27 ± 5 μmol/L) and 4 ± 1.2 mg/L (15 ± 4 μmol/L), respectively, after 14 days of therapy. The average elimination half-life is 45 hr in the initial 2-week period and decreases to 25–30 hr thereafter because of metabolic autoinduction mediated by the cytochrome P450 system. Less than 3% of the dose is excreted renally.

Adverse Reactions. A mild to moderate rash occurs in up to 48% of patients. Rash can be associated with liver function test elevations and a low frequency of clinical hepatitis. Severe, occasionally fatal, hepatotoxicity has occurred in those using nevirapine in postexposure prophylactic regimens with various other antiretrovirals. This use is not recommended, but the single-dose use to prevent HIV transmission appears to be safe. The risk of developing rash is highest within 2 weeks of drug initiation or dosage escalation to 400 mg/day and is reduced by following the recommended dosage escalation schedule. Other occasional adverse reactions are arthralgia, fatigue, fever, myalgia, and somnolence.

Parameters to Monitor. Monitor liver function closely for at least the first 12 weeks of therapy and periodically thereafter.

RITONAVIR
Norvir

Pharmacology. Ritonavir is an HIV protease inhibitor with a mechanism of action similar to saquinavir.[126,127] (*See* Antiviral Drugs for HIV Infection Comparison Chart.)

Adult Dosage. PO for treatment of HIV 600 mg q 12 hr with food in combination with nucleoside analogues. Ritonavir might be better tolerated initially if the dosage is initiated at 300 mg q 12 hr and increased to 600 mg q 12 hr over 10–14 days. If the 600 mg q 12-hr dosage is not reached after 2 weeks of therapy, discontinue therapy because the risk of developing viral resistance to ritonavir or cross-resistance to other protease inhibitors is increased with lower dosages. **PO in protease inhibitor combination treatment of HIV** (*see* Antiviral Drugs for HIV Infection Comparison Chart).

Dosage Forms. Cap 100 mg; Soln 80 mg/mL. Capsules must be refrigerated.

Pharmacokinetics. Ritonavir is rapidly absorbed and increased by approximately 15% with food. Absolute bioavailability has not been determined in humans, but bioavailability is 30–70% in animals. Ritonavir is 98–99% protein bound, primarily to albumin and α_1-acid glycoprotein. After a 600 mg oral dose taken with food, a peak serum concentration of 11.2 ± 3.6 mg/L (15.5 ± 5 μmol/L) occurs at 3.3 ± 2.2 hr and the trough is 3 ± 2.1 mg/L (4.2 ± 2.9 μmol/L). Serum concentrations can decrease over time because of autoinduction of the CYP3A and CYP2D isoenzymes responsible for metabolism of ritonavir.

Adverse Reactions. Nausea, vomiting, diarrhea, asthenia, anorexia, abdominal pain, taste perversion, perioral paresthesia, peripheral paresthesia, headache, insomnia, and elevated serum triglyceride concentrations occur frequently. Occasionally, elevations of hepatic transaminases and CPK occur.

Drug Interactions. Ritonavir is a potent inhibitor of several cytochrome P450 enzymes (CYP2C9, 2C19, 2D6, and 3A3/4) and can produce large increases in serum concentrations of highly metabolized drugs. Consult the product information for contraindicated drugs and carefully review the patient's medication list for interactions before starting this therapy.

SAQUINAVIR	Fortovase
SAQUINAVIR MESYLATE	Invirase

Pharmacology. Saquinavir is a synthetic peptide-like substrate analogue that inhibits HIV protease. Inhibition of HIV protease prevents the cleavage of polyprotein precursors, which is essential for maturation of infectious virus.[128,129] Saquinavir mesylate is formulated in a hard gelatin capsule. Saquinavir has been reformulated into a soft gelatin capsule that combines saquinavir base in an oillike substance that allows microdispersion upon contact with gastric fluids enhancing oral bioavailability. (*See* Antiviral Drugs for HIV Infection Comparison Chart.)

Administration and Adult Dosage. PO for advanced HIV disease in combination with other nucleoside analogues (saquinavir mesylate) 600 mg q 8 hr (FDA-approved regimen but achieves inadequate serum concentrations to suppress HIV); (saquinavir) 1200 mg q 8 hr.

Special Populations. *Pediatric Dosage.* (<16 yr) safety and efficacy not established.

Geriatric Dosage. Not studied but expected to be same as adult dosage.

Dosage Forms. (Saquinavir) **Cap** 200 mg; (saquinavir mesylate) **Cap** 200 mg.

Patient Instructions. (*See* HIV Drugs Class Instructions.) Saquinavir mesylate (Invirase) must be taken within 2 hours after a full meal to achieve adequate concentrations of drug to inhibit viral replication. Saquinavir (Fortovase) is better absorbed and requires a snack or some food to help increase the amount of medication getting into the blood. Store saquinavir in the refrigerator. New onset diabetes mellitus, worsening of pre-existing diabetes mellitus, and hyperglycemia have been reported in HIV-infected patients receiving protease inhibitors. Some patients require initiation or dosage adjustments of insulin or oral hypoglycemic agents. Diabetic ketoacidosis also has occurred. Hyperglycemia persists in some cases after drug discontinuation.

Pharmacokinetics. *Fate.* Oral absorption of saquinavir mesylate is erratic and the drug undergoes extensive first-pass metabolism. Approximately 30% of a 600 mg dose is absorbed when given within 2 hr after food; absolute bioavailability averages 4%. Saquinavir bioavailability relative to saquinavir mesylate is

331%. Saquinavir is 98% plasma protein bound; concentrations in the CSF are negligible. Saquinavir undergoes metabolism primarily by CYP3A4; Cl is 1.14 L/hr/kg.[123]

$t_{1/2}$. 12 hr.

Adverse Reactions. Abdominal discomfort or pain, diarrhea, anorexia, and nausea occur frequently. Occasional adverse reactions include asthenia, rash, elevations of transaminases, and headache. Rare reactions include ataxia, confusion, hemolytic anemia, thrombophlebitis, attempted suicide, seizures, and exacerbation of chronic liver disease.

Contraindications. (*See* Drug Interactions.)

Precautions. Do not use saquinavir as monotherapy because of the greater potential for developing resistance.

Drug Interactions. Do not administer saquinavir with rifampin because steady-state AUC of saquinavir decreases by 80%. Administration with rifabutin reduces saquinavir plasma concentrations by 40% and alternatives to this combination should be considered. Avoid other drugs that strongly induce CYP3A4 because they can substantially decrease saquinavir serum concentrations. Avoid co-administration with astemizole or cisapride because of possible prolonged QT intervals and serious cardiovascular adverse events. Concurrent ketoconazole and possibly other inhibitors of CYP3A4 can increase the bioavailability and half-life of saquinavir. (*See* Cytochrome P450 Enzyme Interactions.) Ingesting grapefruit juice with saquinavir has been suggested to increase the bioavailability of saquinavir by inhibition of CYP3A4. However, the grapefruit juice must be concentrated, taken with every dose of saquinavir, and contain flavinoids to have any benefit. This method is not likely to be palatable to most patients because of gastric irritation and appears unnecessary with the soft gelatin capsule formulation of saquinavir.

Parameters to Monitor. (*See* Nelfinavir.)

Notes. Saquinavir (Fortovase) should be refrigerated; once brought to room temperature (≤25°C), use it within 3 months. Fortovase has a dosage of 1200 mg tid to achieve saquinavir plasma concentrations sufficient to inhibit the replication of HIV. The hard gelatin capsule formulation dosage of 600 mg tid does not consistently achieve adequate saquinavir plasma concentrations. The use of **ritonavir** 400 mg bid and saquinavir 400 mg bid in combination has been used to improve concentrations of saquinavir and tolerance of ritonavir.

STAVUDINE
Zerit

Pharmacology. Stavudine (d4T) is a synthetic pyrimidine nucleoside reverse transcriptase inhibitor that is structurally similar to zidovudine and has been shown to inhibit HIV replication in vitro. Stavudine is phosphorylated by cellular enzymes to stavudine triphosphate, which acts as a competitive inhibitor of HIV reverse transcriptase and an alternative nucleoside substrate, which leads to premature elongation of viral DNA.[130,131] (*See* Antiviral Drugs for HIV Infection Comparison Chart.)

Adult Dosage. **PO for HIV** (<60 kg) 30 mg bid; (≥60 kg) 40 mg bid. Dosage can be reduced to 15 mg q 12 hr for patients <60 kg or 20 mg q 12 hr for patients ≥60 kg if they are at risk for peripheral neuropathy. Reduce dosage in renal impairment.

Dosage Forms. Cap 15, 20, 30, 40 mg; **Soln** 1 mg/mL.

Pharmacokinetics. Stavudine is well absorbed with or without food and oral bioavailability is 82%. Average time to peak concentration is 1 hr with serum concentrations of about 1.2 mg/L after a single 0.67 mg/kg dose. V_d is 0.53 L/kg. Limited data suggest that stavudine distributes into the CSF, with concentrations approximately 40% of serum concentration. Renal clearance is about 40% of total clearance, with the remaining drug metabolized to thymine and eventually to β-aminoisobutyric acid.

Adverse Reactions. The most frequent adverse effect is peripheral neuropathy; occasionally, elevated hepatic transaminases occur.

ZIDOVUDINE
Retrovir

Pharmacology. Zidovudine is a thymidine analogue that inhibits HIV replication. It is converted to the active monophosphate form by thymidine kinase and ultimately to zidovudine triphosphate by intracellular enzymes. This form exerts its activity at viral DNA polymerase (reverse transcriptase) by competing with other cellular deoxynucleosides and by acting as a chain terminator of DNA synthesis.[100] (*See* Antiviral Drugs for HIV Infection Comparison Chart.)

Administration and Adult Dosage. **PO for HIV infection with** 300 mg bid or 200 mg tid. **PO for maternal–fetal HIV transmission (maternal)** 300 mg bid, begun after the 14th week of pregnancy and continued throughout the pregnancy, then **IV during labor** 2 mg/kg over 1 hr, followed by a continuous infusion of 1 mg/kg/hr until delivery. (*See also* Pediatric Dosage.) **PO for combination therapy with zalcitabine** 200 mg q 8 hr with zalcitabine 0.75 mg q 8 hr. **PO for post-exposure prophylaxis** 1–1.5 g/day in 4 or 5 divided doses has been used,[132] but the effectiveness of this regimen is not confirmed in humans and informed consent should be obtained. **IV for patients unable to take oral medication** 1–2 mg/kg q 4 hr infused over 1 hr, only until oral therapy can be initiated.

Special Populations. *Pediatric Dosage.* **PO for prevention of maternal HIV transmission** 2 mg/kg/dose q 6 hr for first 6 weeks of life, beginning 8–12 hr after birth.[133] **IV for prevention of maternal HIV transmission if unable to receive PO** 1.5 mg/kg/dose q 6 hr until oral therapy can be initiated. **PO for HIV infection** (0–2 weeks) 2 mg/kg/dose q 6 hr; (2–4 weeks) 3 mg/kg/dose q 6 hr; (4 weeks–13 yr) 180 mg/m²/dose (to a maximum of 200 mg) q 6 hr; (over 13 yr) 100 mg q 4 hr 5 times/day.[105]

Geriatric Dosage. Same as adult dosage but adjust for age-related reduction in renal function.

Other Conditions. Reduce dosage by 50% in patients with Cl_{cr} <25 mL/min[97] and 75% in those with cirrhosis.[134]

Dosage Forms. Cap 100 mg; Tab 300 mg; Syrup 10 mg/mL; Inj 10 mg/mL. (*See* Notes.)

Patient Instructions. (*See* HIV Drugs Class Instructions.) This drug is not a cure for HIV disease. Opportunistic infections and other complications associated with HIV infection can continue to develop. This drug may be taken with food to decrease abdominal discomfort or nausea. It is important to have blood counts followed closely during therapy to monitor for decreases in blood cell counts.

Pharmacokinetics. *Serum Levels.* Not established; intracellular concentrations of zidovudine triphosphate might correlate with therapeutic benefit, but in vivo data are not available.

Fate. Zidovudine (ZDV) undergoes marked presystemic metabolism. Oral bioavailability is 60–70%, possibly reduced with high-fat meals. Peak serum levels are approximately 1.2 mg/L (4.5 μmol/L) after a 250 mg oral dose. Protein binding is less than 25%. CSF concentrations are 24% of serum in children receiving a continuous infusion of the drug. V_{dss} is 1.6 ± 0.6 L/kg; Cl is 1.3 ± 0.3 L/hr/kg in adults and 36.4 ± 11.5 L/hr/m^2 in children. ZDV is rapidly metabolized to the inactive ether glucuronide (GZDV). GZDV formation is reduced, and zidovudine AUC and half-life are increased in patients with cirrhosis. About 60% of an oral dose is excreted as GZDV in urine. GZDV excretion is reduced in patients with renal dysfunction; hemodialysis removes GZDV but not ZDV.[97,134,135]

$t_{\frac{1}{2}}$. (Adults) 1.1 ± 0.2 hr; 2.1 hr in uremia; 2.4 hr in cirrhosis.[97] (Children) 1.5 ± 0.6 hr.

Adverse Reactions. Severe anemia and granulocytopenia occur frequently and might necessitate blood transfusions; epoetin might help alleviate anemia in patients with low serum erythropoietin levels. Other frequent adverse reactions associated with zidovudine in placebo-controlled trials include abdominal discomfort, nausea, vomiting, insomnia, myalgias, and headaches. Adverse reactions that occasionally occur with long-term use (>12 weeks) are myopathy and nail pigmentation.[100]

Contraindications. Life-threatening allergy to the drug or its components.

Precautions. Pregnancy; lactation. Use with caution in liver disease or hepatomegaly, especially in obese women.

Drug Interactions. Several drugs decrease the glucuronidation of zidovudine, including atovaquone, methadone, probenecid, valproic acid, and possibly fluconazole; rifampin increases zidovudine glucuronidation; however, the clinical importance of these interactions is not established.[104] Initial studies showed that prolonged administration of acetaminophen was associated with increased hematologic toxicity from zidovudine, but further study does not support this finding.[136]

Parameters to Monitor. Hemoglobin, hematocrit, MCV, and WBC for hematologic toxicity. Monitor clinical signs, symptoms, and laboratory markers for progression of HIV disease to help decide regimen changes in antiretroviral therapy. Baseline CD4 and HIV-1 RNA polymerase chain reaction viral load tests are useful to measure clinical benefit of therapy. Repeat tests after 1 month and q 3–4 months thereafter have been suggested to monitor benefit of antiretroviral therapy.

Notes. Viral resistance to zidovudine has occurred in vitro with isolates recovered from patients and is associated with prolonged zidovudine use and more advanced disease; correlation between viral resistance in vitro and progression of disease has not been established. Studies with **lamivudine** (3TC) suggest that the combination can delay or prevent HIV-1 viral resistance to zidovudine. **Aztec** (Verex) is an SR dosage form in late-stage testing.

ANTIRETROVIRAL THERAPY FOR HIV

The use of protease inhibitors and/or nonnucleoside reverse transcriptase inhibitors in combination with nucleoside reverse transcriptase inhibitors has dramatically changed the treatment of HIV infection. Regimens containing a protease inhibitor or nonnucleoside reverse transcriptase inhibitor have enhanced the ability to inhibit replication of HIV, affecting immunologic and viral markers, delaying progression of disease, and improving survival. Many formidable hurdles stand in the way of effective treatment, including patient adherence to dosage regimens, adverse effects, and drug–drug interactions. These hurdles interfere with quality of life and control of the viral burden and also contribute to the emergence of resistance. It is essential for health care providers and patients to appreciate the complexity of antiretroviral medication regimens to achieve harmony between goals of antiretroviral therapy and optimal patient care. General principals of treatment that guide contemporary treatment decisions are outlined below:

- Viral load monitoring is essential to guide decision making.
- Attaining and maintaining an undetectable HIV RNA in blood (which can indirectly reflect lymph concentrations) is the goal of therapy.
- Introduce effective antiretroviral therapy *before* extensive immune system damage has occurred.
- Three-drug combination therapy, is the regimen most likely to achieve the goal of an undetectable HIV RNA level and provide a durable response.
- Compliance with the treatment regimen is critical to success and must be considered in initiating and choosing regimens.
- Change most or all drugs in a failing regimen simultaneously; use antiretroviral drug resistance testing to guide new antiretroviral regimen decisions.

For further information and clarification on appropriate uses of antiretroviral therapy, see U.S. Public Health Service guidelines for the use of antiretroviral agents in pediatric HIV infection and HIV-infected adults and adolescents (references 137 and 138).

ANTIVIRAL DRUGS FOR HIV INFECTION COMPARISON CHART

DRUG	DOSAGE FORMS	ADULT DOSAGE	PEDIATRIC DOSAGE	EFFECT ON CYP450 ISOZYMES	ADVERSE REACTIONS	COMMENTS
HIV NUCLEOSIDE REVERSE TRANSCRIPTASE INHIBITORS						
Abacavir Ziagen	Tab 300 mg Soln 20 mg/mL.	PO 300 mg bid.	PO (3 months–16 yr) 8 mg/kg (to a maximum of 300 mg) bid.	No effect.	Rash, asthenia, hypersensitivity reaction.	Patients who have a hypersensitivity reaction must not take the drug; it could be fatal.
Didanosine Videx Videx EC	Chew Tab 25, 50, 100, 150, 200 mg Pwdr for Oral Soln (adult) 100, 167, 250, mg Pwdr for Oral Soln (pediatric) 2, 4 g.	(*See monograph.*)	(*See monograph.*)	No effect.	Neuropathy, pancreatitis, nausea, dysgeusia, diarrhea, hyperuricemia, headache, asthenia, seizures, pruritus.	Cl_{cr} ≤60 mL/min, consider dosage reduction, (*see monograph*).

(continued)

ANTIVIRAL DRUGS FOR HIV INFECTION COMPARISON CHART (*continued*)

DRUG	DOSAGE FORMS	ADULT DOSAGE	PEDIATRIC DOSAGE	EFFECT ON CYP450 ISOZYMES	ADVERSE REACTIONS	COMMENTS
Lamivudine Epivir	Tab 100, 150 mg Soln 5, 10 mg/mL.	PO 150 mg bid.	PO (3 months–12 yr) 4 mg/kg q 12 hr, to a maximum of 150 mg q 12 hr.	No effect.	Nausea, headache, fatigue, rash, anorexia; generally well tolerated, but pancreatitis is a risk in pediatric population, but not in adults.	Reduce dosage in renal impairment: Cl$_{cr}$ 30–49 mL/min, 150 mg/day; Cl$_{cr}$ 15–29 mL/min, 150 mg once, then 100 mg/day; Cl$_{cr}$ 5–14 mL/min, 150 mg once, then 50 mg/day; Cl$_{cr}$ <5 mL/min, 50 mg once, then 25 mg/day.
Stavudine Zerit	Cap 15, 20, 30, 40 mg Soln 1 mg/mL.	PO (≤60 kg) 30 mg bid; PO (>60 kg) 40 mg bid. Reduce dosage for mild to moderate peripheral neuropathy.	PO (≤30 kg) 1 mg/kg q 12 hr.	No effect.	Neuropathy, headache, nausea, asthenia, insomnia, elevated hepatic enzymes.	Reduce dosage in renal impairment: Cl$_{cr}$ 26–50 mL/min, reduce dosage by 50% and give q 12 hr; Cl$_{cr}$ 10–25 mL/min, reduce dosage by 50% and give q 24 hr.
Zalcitabine Hivid	Tab 0.375, 0.75 mg.	PO 0.75 mg tid. Reduce dosage for symptoms of peripheral neuropathy.	Not established.	No effect.	Neuropathy, oral and esophageal ulceration, elevated hepatic enzymes, pancreatitis, rash, pruritus.	Reduce dosage in renal impairment: Cl$_{cr}$ 10–40 mL/min, same dose q 12 hr; Cl$_{cr}$ <10 mL/min, same dose q 24 hr.

(continued)

ANTIVIRAL DRUGS FOR HIV INFECTION COMPARISON CHART (*continued*)

DRUG	DOSAGE FORMS	ADULT DOSAGE	PEDIATRIC DOSAGE	EFFECT ON CYP450 ISOZYMES	ADVERSE REACTIONS	COMMENTS
Zidovudine Retrovir	Cap 100 mg Tab 300 mg Syrup 10 mg/mL Inj 10 mg/mL.	PO 200 mg tid or 300 mg bid. (*See* monograph for other indications.)	PO (neonates) 2 mg/kg q 6 hr; IV (neonates) 1.5 mg/kg q 6 hr (infants and children) 80 mg/m² q 6 hr.	No effect.	Bone marrow suppression (anemia, neutropenia), nausea, abdominal pain, elevated hepatic enzymes, headache, malaise, elevated CPK, myopathy, nail discoloration.	Reduce dosage in renal impairment: $Cl_{cr} \leq 25$ mL/min, reduce recommended dosage by 50%.
Zidovudine and Lamivudine Combivir	Tab 300 mg zidovudine plus 150 mg lamivudine.	PO 1 tablet bid.	Not recommended.	No effect.	(*See* lamivudine and zidovudine.)	Contraindicated in renal impairment.
Zidovudine, Lamivudine and Abacavir Trizivir	Tab 300 mg zidovudine plus 150 mg lamivudine plus 300 mg abacavir.	PO 1 tablet bid.	Not established	No effect	(*See* individual agents.)	Contraindicated in renal impairment.

HIV NUCLEOTIDE REVERSE TRANSCRIPTASE INHIBITORS

DRUG	DOSAGE FORMS	ADULT DOSAGE	PEDIATRIC DOSAGE	EFFECT ON CYP450 ISOZYMES	ADVERSE REACTIONS	COMMENTS
Tenofovir DF Disoproxil Fumarate (Investigational Gilead)	Tab 300 mg.	PO 300 mg/day	Not established.	No effect.	Nausea	Well tolerated in early trials. Activity may be enhanced by concomitant lamivudine.

(continued)

ANTIVIRAL DRUGS FOR HIV INFECTION COMPARISON CHART (*continued*)

DRUG	DOSAGE FORMS	ADULT DOSAGE	PEDIATRIC DOSAGE	EFFECT ON CYP450 ISOZYMES	ADVERSE REACTIONS	COMMENTS
NONNUCLEOSIDE REVERSE TRANSCRIPTASE INHIBITORS						
Delavirdine Rescriptor	Tab 100, 200 mg.	PO 400 mg tid. or 600 mg bid.	Not established.	*Inhibits* CYP2C9 CYP2C19 CYP3A4	Rash, headache, elevated hepatic enzymes.	Tablets may be dispersed in water to allow easier administration.
Efavirenz Sustiva	Cap 50, 100, 200 mg.	PO 600 mg qd.	(10–14 kg) 200 mg/day; (15–19 kg) 250 mg/day; (20–24 kg) 300 mg/day; (25–32.5 kg) 350 mg/day; (32.5–39 kg) 400 mg/day; (≥40 kg) 600 mg/day.	*Induces* CYP3A4 *Inhibits* CYP2C9 CYP2C19 CYP3A4	CNS symptoms, dizziness, rash, dysphoria, anxiety, nausea, insomnia, inability to concentrate.	CNS symptoms frequently resolve within 2–4 weeks of initiating therapy. It may be helpful to take dose at bedtime or to take in 2–3 divided doses to help reduce symptoms. Rash frequent in first 2 weeks, but usually resolves in 2 months.
Nevirapine Viramune	Tab 200 mg Susp 10 mg/mL.	PO 200 mg/day for 14 days, then 400 mg/day in 1 or 2 doses. (*See* comments.)	PO initiate with 120 mg/m^2 once daily for 14 days, then increase to full dosage of 120–200 mg/m^2 q 12 hr.	*Induces* CYP3A4	Rash, hepatitis, fatigue, headache.	To reduce the frequency of rash, it is essential to increase the dosage over 14 days. Increase to full dosage only if no rash or other adverse effects occur.

(*continued*)

ANTIVIRAL DRUGS FOR HIV INFECTION COMPARISON CHART (*continued*)

DRUG	DOSAGE FORMS	ADULT DOSAGE	PEDIATRIC DOSAGE	EFFECT ON CYP450 ISOZYMES	ADVERSE REACTIONS	COMMENTS
PROTEASE INHIBITORS						
Amprenavir Agenerase	Cap 50, 150 mg. Soln 15 mg/mL.	PO 1.2 g bid. *Combination:* PO 600 mg plus ritonavir PO 100 mg bid.[a]	PO 20–22.5 mg/kg bid.	*Inhibits* CYP3A4 CYP2C19 CYP2E1	Rash (frequent), nausea, vomiting, diarrhea, flatulence, perioral paresthesias. Triglycerides, LFTs, and glucose.	Rash usually occurs within 9 days and resolves in 1 week after discontinuation; Stevens-Johnson syndrome has occurred.
Indinavir Mesylate Crixivan	Cap 200, 333, 400 mg.	PO 800 mg q 8 hr. *Combinations:* 1. PO 400 mg bid plus PO ritonavir 400 mg bid. 2. PO 800 mg bid plus PO ritonavir 200 mg bid.[a]	PO 500 mg/m² q 8 hr (under study in clinical trials).	*Inhibits* CYP3A4	Nausea, headache, abdominal pain, hyperbilirubinemia, insomnia, dizziness, nephrolithiasis.	Administer on an empty stomach 1 hr before or 2 hr after a meal (or can take with a light meal). Adequate hydration is required to minimize risk of nephrolithiasis.
Lopinavir and Ritonavir Kaletra	Cap 133.3 mg lopinavir plus 33.3 mg ritonavir.	PO 3 caps bid.	Not established	(*See* ritonavir.)	(*See* ritonavir.)	Generally well tolerated because of lowered ritonavir dosage. Refrigerate but may keep at room temperature for 30 days.

(continued)

ANTIVIRAL DRUGS FOR HIV INFECTION COMPARISON CHART (continued)

DRUG	DOSAGE FORMS	ADULT DOSAGE	PEDIATRIC DOSAGE	EFFECT ON CYP450 ISOZYMES	ADVERSE REACTIONS	COMMENTS
Nelfinavir Mesylate Viracept	Tab 250 mg Pwdr 50 mg nelfinavir free base per level scoopful (1 g).	PO 750 mg tid or 1250 mg bid.	PO 20–30 mg/kg tid.	*Inhibits* CYP3A4	Diarrhea, nausea, dysphagia, rash.	Administer with food or light snack to increase absorption 2- to 3-fold.
Ritonavir Norvir	Cap[b] 100 mg Soln[b] 80 mg/mL.	PO 600 mg q 12 hr.[c] *Combination:* PO 400 mg q 12 hr plus saquinavir PO 400 mg q 12 hr.[a]	PO 400 mg/m^2 q 12 hr.[d]	*Inhibits* CYP3A4 CYP2C9 CYP2C19 CYP2D6	Nausea, vomiting, diarrhea, headache, circumoral and extremity paresthesias, asthenia, taste perversion, elevated serum triglycerides, hepatic transaminases, CPK, uric acid.	Titrate dosage from 300 mg q 12 hr to 600 mg q 12 hr over 10–14 days to reduce adverse events.
Saquinavir Fortovase	Cap 200 mg.	PO 1.2 g tid. *Combination:* 1. PO 400 mg q 12 hr plus ritonavir 400 mg PO q 12 hr. 2. PO 800 mg q 12 hr plus ritonavir PO 200 mg q 12 hr.[a]	Not established.	*Inhibits* CYP3A4	Abdominal cramping, nausea, diarrhea, headache.	Bioavailability relative to Invirase formulation is 331%. Refrigerate capsules, but may keep at room temperature for 90 days.

(continued)

ANTIVIRAL DRUGS FOR HIV INFECTION COMPARISON CHART (*continued*)

DRUG	DOSAGE FORMS	ADULT DOSAGE	PEDIATRIC DOSAGE	EFFECT ON CYP450 ISOZYMES	ADVERSE REACTIONS	COMMENTS
Saquinavir Mesylate Invirase	Cap 200 mg.	PO 600–1800 mg tid. *Combination:* PO 400 mg q 12 hr with ritonavir 400 mg PO q 12 hr.	Not established.	*Inhibits* CYP3A4	Nausea, headache, elevated hepatic transaminases.	Bioavailability is 4% and erratic; use Fortovase if tolerated.

[a]Under study in clinical trials.
[b]Ritonavir capsules must be kept refrigerated. Ritonavir solution must be stored in the original container.
[c]Adult dosage escalation for ritonavir: days 1–2, 300 mg PO bid; days 3–5, 400 mg PO bid; days 6–13, 500 mg PO bid; day 14, 600 mg PO bid.
[d]Pediatric dosage escalation for ritonavir: Initiate therapy at 250 mg/m² q 12 hr and increase stepwise to full dosage over 5 days as tolerated.
From references 137–139 and product information.

OSELTAMIVIR PHOSPHATE   Tamiflu

Pharmacology. Oseltamivir phosphate is the ethyl ester prodrug of oseltamivir carboxylate, which is a selective inhibitor of the enzyme neuraminidase. (*See* Zanamivir.)[140–142]

Administration and Adult Dosage. **PO for treatment of influenza virus A or B (start within 48 hr of onset of symptoms)** 75 mg bid for 5 days.

Special Populations. *Pediatric Dosage.* (<18 yr) Safety and efficacy not established.

Geriatric Dosage. Same as adult dosage.

Other Conditions. In renal insufficiency (Cl_{cr} 10–30 mL/min) reduce dose to 75 mg/day for 5 days. There is no dosage information for Cl_{cr} <10 mL/min.

Dosage Forms. **Cap** 75 mg.

Patient Instructions. Begin treatment with oseltamivir within 2 days of initial flu symptoms. Oseltamivir is not a substitute for influenza vaccination.

Missed Doses. Take this drug at regular intervals. If you miss a dose of this medicine, take it as soon as you remember. If it is almost time for your next dose (within 2 hours), take that dose only and go back to your regular dosage schedule. Leave at least 12 hours between doses. Do not double the dose or take extra.

Pharmacokinetics. *Fate.* Oseltamivir phosphate is extensively absorbed after oral ingestion and converted by hepatic esterases to the active oseltamivir carboxylate. Food does not affect overall systemic exposure to the oseltamivir carboxylate. Oral bioavailability of oseltamivir carboxylate is >75% after a 75 mg dose. The peak serum concentration is 348 ± 63 μg/L within 2–3 hr after a 75 mg dose. Protein binding of oseltamivir carboxylate is approximately 3%. V_d is estimated to be 0.35 ± 0.02 L/kg. Oseltamivir is eliminated (>99%) by renal excretion.[140,141]

$t_{1/2}$. 7.5 ± 0.7 hr.[141]

Adverse Reactions. Nausea and vomiting are the most frequent adverse events, occurring in about 10% of patients. Bronchitis, insomnia, and vertigo occur occasionally.[141,143]

Drug Interactions. Oseltamivir is not a substrate and does not affect cytochrome P450 isoenzymes. There are no known drug interactions.

Parameters to Monitor. Progression of influenza symptoms.

Notes. There are no data to support the safety or efficacy in patients who begin oseltamivir after 48 hr of influenza symptom onset. Patients should continue to receive an annual influenza vaccination according to guidelines on immunization practices.

ZANAMIVIR   Relenza

Pharmacology. Zanamivir is an inhibitor of the enzyme neuraminidase (sialidase), which is essential for the replication of type A and B influenza viruses. Neuraminidase catalyzes the viral cleavage of terminal sialic acid (*N*-acetylneuraminic acid) and this action allows release of budded virus from infected cells, such that virons do not aggregate at the cell surface or with each other, allowing viral spread to occur within the host.[140,143,144]

Administration and Adult Dosage. Inhal for influenza virus A or B (start within 48 hr of onset of symptoms) 10 mg (2 inhalations) bid for 5 days. Give the first dose under the supervision of an informed healthcare professional to observe correct use of the inhalation device.

Special Populations. *Pediatric Dosage.* (<7 yr) Safety and efficacy not established; (≥7 yr) same as adult dosage.

Geriatric Dosage. Same as adult dosage.

Dosage Forms. **Dry Pwdr Inhal** 5 mg.

Patient Instructions. Read and follow carefully the accompanying Patient Instructions for Use with each Diskhaler device. Take 2 doses on the first day of treatment if they are given at least 2 hours apart. Take doses on days 2 through 5 approximately 12 hours apart and at the same time each day. To avoid the spread of infection, do not use the inhaler for more than one person. Zanamivir is not a substitute for influenza vaccination.

Missed Doses. Take this drug at regular intervals. If you miss a dose of this medicine, take it as soon as you remember. If it is almost time for your next dose, take that dose only and go back to your regular dosage schedule. Leave at least 12 hours between doses. Do not double the dose or take extra.

Pharmacokinetics. *Fate.* (Inhal) The peak serum concentration is 39–54 μg/L within 1–2 hr after a 10 mg inhaled dose. Oral bioavailability of inhaled zanamivir is 4–17%. Protein binding is less than 10%. Zanamivir is excreted unchanged in the urine.[144]

$t_{1/2}$. 3.6 ± 1.3 hr.[144]

Adverse Reactions. Nasal and throat discomfort, cough, headache have occurred in 2–3% of patients. This prevalence is similar to placebo and might be related to inhalation of the lactose vehicle. Bronchospasm has occurred occasionally in patients with asthma or COPD.[143]

Precautions. Use with extreme caution in patients with underlying airway diseases such as asthma or COPD because of the potential for causing bronchospasm. Instruct patients who use inhaled bronchodilators concurrently with zanamivir to use their bronchodilators before inhaling zanamivir.

Drug Interactions. Zanamivir is not a substrate and does not affect cytochrome P450 isoenzymes. There are no known clinically relevant drug interactions.

Parameters to Monitor. Inhalation technique, progression of influenza symptoms.

Notes. There are no data to support the safety or efficacy in patients who begin zanamivir treatment after 48 hr of influenza symptom onset. Patients should continue to receive an annual influenza vaccination.

β-Lactams

AMOXICILLIN
Amoxil, Various

Pharmacology. Amoxicillin differs from ampicillin by the presence of a hydroxyl group on the amino side chain. It has activity essentially identical to ampicillin.[145,146] (*See* Ampicillin and β-Lactams Comparison Chart.)

Adult Dosage. PO 250–500 mg q 8 hr or 500-875 mg bid, to a maximum of 4.5 g/day. **PO for endocarditis prophylaxis** 2 g 1 hr before dental or upper airway procedures.

Pediatric Dosage. PO 20–40 mg/kg/day in 3 equally divided doses q 8 hr. **PO for endocarditis prophylaxis** 50 mg/kg 1 hr before dental or upper airway procedures.

Dosage Forms. **Cap** 250, 500 mg; **Chew Tab** 125, 200, 250, 400 mg; **Drp** 50 mg/mL; **Susp** 25, 50 mg/mL; **Tab** 500, 875 mg.

Pharmacokinetics. Amoxicillin is completely absorbed, with about 85% bioavailability because of a small first-pass effect. Serum concentrations are greater than those after equal doses of ampicillin; postabsorptive pharmacokinetics are identical to those of ampicillin.

Adverse Reactions. Adverse effects are similar to those of ampicillin, although diarrhea and rashes are much less frequent with amoxicillin.

AMOXICILLIN AND POTASSIUM CLAVULANATE
Augmentin

Pharmacology. Clavulanic acid has weak antibacterial activity but is a potent inhibitor of plasmid-mediated β-lactamases, including those produced by *Haemophilus influenzae*, *Moraxella (Branhamella) catarrhalis*, *Staphylococcus aureus*, *Neisseria gonorrhoeae*, and *Bacteroides fragilis*. Thus, when combined with certain other β-lactam antibiotics, the combination is very active against many bacteria resistant to the β-lactam alone.[147,148]

Adult Dosage. PO One "250" or "500" tablet q 8 hr or 1 "875" tablet q 12 hr. (*See* Dosage Forms.)

Pediatric Dosage. PO 20–40 mg/kg/day (of the amoxicillin component) in 3 divided doses or 45 mg/kg/day in 2 divided doses. (*See* Dosage Forms.)

Dosage Forms. Do not substitute combinations of lower-dose tablets to make a higher dose because diarrhea is markedly increased. **Tab** (8 hr) 250 mg amoxicillin/125 mg clavulanic acid, 500 mg amoxicillin/125 mg clavulanic acid; (12 hr) 875 mg amoxicillin/125 mg clavulanic acid; **Chew Tab** (8 hr) 125 mg amoxicillin/31.25 mg clavulanic acid, 250 mg amoxicillin/62.5 mg clavulanic acid; (12 hr) 200 mg amoxicillin/28.5 mg clavulanic acid, 400 mg amoxicillin/57 mg clavulanic acid; **Susp** (8 hr) 25 mg amoxicillin/6.25 mg clavulanic acid/mL, 50 mg amoxicillin/12.5 mg clavulanic acid/mL; (12 hr) 40 mg amoxicillin/5.7 mg clavulanic acid/mL, 80 mg amoxicillin/11.4 mg clavulanic acid/mL.

Pharmacokinetics. Peak serum clavulanate concentration is 2.6 mg/L 40–60 min after an oral dose of 250 mg amoxicillin/125 mg clavulanate. Amoxicillin pharmacokinetics are not affected by clavulanic acid. Clavulanic acid half-life is approximately 60 min.

Adverse Reactions. Adverse effects of this preparation include those of amoxicillin; however, diarrhea is more frequent with the combination and depends on the dosage of clavulanate. The 12-hr formulations reduce the frequency of diarrhea. Nausea and diarrhea is less frequent when this preparation is administered with food. (*See* β-Lactams Comparison Chart.)

AMPICILLIN   Various

Pharmacology. Ampicillin has a similar mechanism of action and is comparable in activity to penicillin G against Gram-positive bacteria, but is more active than penicillin G against Gram-negative bacteria.[145,146] (*See* β-Lactams Comparison Chart.)

Adult Dosage. PO 250–500 mg q 6 hr. **IM or IV** 500 mg–3 g q 4–6 hr to a maximum of 12 g/day. Give the same dose q 12 hr with a Cl_{cr} <20 mL/min. **IV or IM for endocarditis prophylaxis** 2 g within 30 min of procedure.

Pediatric Dosage. PO (<20 kg) 50–100 mg/kg/day in 2–4 divided doses; (>20 kg) 100–400 mg/kg/day in 4–6 divided doses. **IV** (neonates) 25–100 mg/kg/dose q 6–12 hr—higher dosages for meningitis; (<20 kg) 50–100 mg/kg/day in 2–4 divided doses; (>20 kg) 400 mg/kg/day in 4–6 divided doses. **IV or IM for endocarditis prophylaxis** 50 mg/kg within 30 min of procedure.

Dosage Forms. **Cap** 250, 500 mg; **Susp** 25, 50, mg/mL; **Inj** 125, 250, 500 mg, 1, 2, 10 g.

Pharmacokinetics. Oral forms are about 50% absorbed in the fasting state; food delays absorption. Plasma protein binding is low, and therapeutic concentrations are attained in most tissues and fluids including CSF (in the presence of inflammation). About 90% is excreted unchanged in urine. Half-life is 1.2 hr, 2 hr in neonates, increasing to 20 hr in anuric patients.

Adverse Reactions. Nausea and diarrhea occur frequently with oral therapy. Other reactions include frequent skin rash (more frequent in patients receiving allopurinol and very frequent in patients with Epstein-Barr virus infection [mononucleosis]). Most of these eruptions probably are not hypersensitivity reactions but immunologically mediated. They are generally dose related (higher frequency at higher dosages), are macular rather than urticarial, and disappear with continued administration of the drug.

ANTISTAPHYLOCOCCAL PENICILLINS

Pharmacology. Methicillin, nafcillin, oxacillin, cloxacillin, and dicloxacillin are similar to other penicillins in their mechanism of action. However, these drugs are not hydrolyzed by staphylococcal penicillinases. Therefore, nearly all isolates of *Staphylococcus aureus* and some isolates of coagulase-negative staphylococci are susceptible to these drugs. Methicillin- (actually β-lactam-) resistant staphylococci have altered penicillin-binding proteins (transpeptidases). Although these drugs are used primarily in staphylococcal infection, they retain good activity against most streptococci, except enterococci.[138,145,149]

Adult Dosage. Oral administration of nafcillin and oxacillin is not recommended because they are poorly absorbed. (*See* β-Lactams Comparison Chart.)

Pediatric Dosage. (*See* β-Lactams Comparison Chart.)

Dosage Forms. (*See* β-Lactams Comparison Chart.)

Pharmacokinetics. Only cloxacillin and dicloxacillin are adequately absorbed from the GI tract. Except for methicillin, these drugs are mostly hepatically eliminated by metabolism and biliary excretion.

Adverse Reactions. Interstitial nephritis is frequent with methicillin but occurs only rarely with the other drugs. Hepatic damage occurs rarely with oxacillin. Nafcillin has a propensity for local irritation at the IV infusion site and causes neutropenia more frequently than other antistaphylococcal penicillins.

AZTREONAM   Azactam

Pharmacology. Aztreonam is a monobactam with activity similar to that of third-generation cephalosporins against most Gram-negative aerobic bacteria (including *P. aeruginosa*) but it is inactive against Gram-positive bacteria and anaerobes.[150–152] (*See* β-Lactams Comparison Chart.)

Adult Dosage. **IM or IV** 500 mg–2 g q 6–12 hr, to a maximum of 8 g/day, depending on severity and site of infection. Reduce maintenance dosage by 50% with a Cl_{cr} of 10–30 mL/min and by 75% with a Cl_{cr} <10 mL/min. Give one-eighth of the initial dose after hemodialysis.

Pediatric Dosage. **IV** (<1 month) 30 mg/kg q 6–12 hr; (1 month–16 yr) 30 mg/kg q 6–8 hr. Dosages as high as 50 mg/kg q 6 hr have been used in children with cystic fibrosis or serious Gram-negative infections (eg, *P. aeruginosa*).

Dosage Forms. **Inj** 500 mg, 1, 2 g.

Pharmacokinetics. Peak serum concentrations of 164 and 255 mg/L occur after 30-min IV infusions of 1 and 2 g, respectively. With inflamed meninges, CSF concentrations are similar to those observed with comparable dosages of third-generation cephalosporins, but experience in treating meningitis is limited. The drug is 60% plasma protein bound and has a V_d of about 0.24 L/kg; 60–70% is excreted in urine unchanged. The half-life is 1.5–2 hr, increasing to 6 hr in renal failure and 3.2 hr in alcoholic cirrhosis.

Adverse Reactions. Adverse effects of aztreonam are minimal. Cross-allergenicity between aztreonam and other β-lactams is low, and aztreonam has been used safely in penicillin- or cephalosporin-allergic patients.

CEPHALOSPORINS

Pharmacology. Cephalosporin antibiotics have broad-spectrum activity against many Gram-positive and Gram-negative pathogens. These agents are generally considered to be bactericidal through binding to various penicillin-binding proteins in bacteria, which results in changes in cell wall structure and function. Members of this class are frequently subdivided into "generations" based on their antimicrobial activity (as well as order of introduction into clinical use).[152–156]

First-generation cephalosporins have activity against Gram-positive bacteria (eg, *Staphylococcus* sp.) and a limited, but important, number of species of aerobic Gram-negative bacilli (eg, *Escherichia coli*, *Klebsiella* sp., *Proteus mirabilis*). *Haemophilus influenzae* and most other aerobic Gram-negative bacilli often indigenous to hospitals (eg, *Enterobacter*, *Pseudomonas* spp.) are resistant to these drugs. Anaerobic bacteria isolated in the oropharynx are generally susceptible to these agents; however, anaerobes such as *Bacteroides fragilis* are resistant.[152,156]

The **second-generation cephalosporins** cefamandole, cefonicid, and cefuroxime differ from first-generation agents in their improved activity against *H. influenzae* and some strains of *Enterobacter*, *Providencia*, and *Morganella* spp.[152,156] The oral second-generation cephalosporins cefuroxime axetil, ceprozil, and loracarbef (a carbacephem) have similar but less potent activity.[157–160] Cefoxitin, cefmetazole, and cefotetan (which are actually cephamycins) have increased activity against anaerobes, including *B. fragilis*;[152,161,162] the other second-generation cephalosporins have poor activity against this organism.[152]

Third-generation cephalosporins are noteworthy for their marked potency against common Gram-negative organisms (eg, *E. coli*, *Klebsiella pneumoniae*) and their activity against Gram-negative bacilli resistant to older agents (eg, *Serratia* sp., *P. aeruginosa*). Although grouped together, some agents have better activity against certain organisms (eg, ceftazidime is better against *P. aeruginosa*), and poorer activity against others (eg, cefixime and ceftazidime are poorer against *Staphylococcus aureus*).[152,153,155,156]

Fourth-generation cephalosporins have a spectrum similar to that of third-generation drugs, plus activity against some Gram-negative strains that are resistant to the third-generation agents, such as *Enterobacter* sp. Their antianaerobic activity is poor. Resistance to cephalosporins is mediated by β-lactamase, reduction in outer cell wall membrane permeability, and alteration of the affinity of these agents for penicillin-binding proteins. Resistance among certain β-lactamase–producing organisms (eg, *Enterobacter* and *Citrobacter* spp.) to third-generation cephalosporins has increased in recent years such that these agents cannot be relied on to provide effective therapy.[156]

Administration and Adult Dosage. (*See* β-Lactams Comparison Chart.)

Special Populations. *Pediatric Dosage.* (*See* β-Lactams Comparison Chart.)

Geriatric Dosage. Same as adult dosage but adjust for age-related reduction in renal function.

Other Conditions. Most agents require dosage modification in renal dysfunction; exceptions are ceftriaxone and cefoperazone, which have biliary and renal or primarily biliary elimination, respectively.[155] Dosage reduction of all agents is required in patients with concomitant hepatic and renal dysfunction. (*See* β-Lactams Comparison Chart.)

Pharmacokinetics. Some of the greatest differences between agents reside in their pharmacokinetic properties. Of note is the improved CSF penetration of certain later-generation agents over the first-generation agents. Therapeutic CSF concentrations are achieved with cefotaxime, ceftriaxone, and ceftazidime; these agents have proven efficacy in the treatment of meningitis caused by susceptible organisms in adults and children.[152,155,156] Adequate CSF concentrations of ceftizoxime also have been observed, although its use in the treatment of meningitis is less well established. Cefuroxime penetrates adequately into CSF but is less effective for meningitis than third-generation agents.[152,163] No data are available on cefepime concentrations in the CNS, but it does cross the blood–brain barrier. (*See* β-Lactams Comparison Chart.)

Adverse Reactions. Most cephalosporins are generally well tolerated, although a few agents have unique adverse reactions. Hypersensitivity reactions can occur in approximately 10% of patients known to be allergic to penicillin; do not administer these agents to patients with histories of an immediate reaction to penicillin.[164] Nausea and diarrhea occur with all agents; however, diarrhea is more common with ceftriaxone and cefoperazone because of high biliary excretion.[152,155,156] Colitis caused by *Clostridium difficile* has been reported with all the cephalosporins but might be more common with ceftriaxone and cefoperazone. Nephrotoxicity is rare, particularly when used without other nephrotoxic agents.[156] All agents with an *N*-methylthiotetrazole (NMTT) moiety in the 3 positions of the cephem nucleus (cefoperazone, cefamandole, cefotetan, and cefmetazole) can produce a disulfiram-like reaction in some patients with ingestion of alcohol-containing beverages. In addition, these agents might be associated with varying degrees with bleeding secondary to hypoprothrombinemia, which is corrected or prevented by vitamin K administration.[152,155,156,165] Although controversial, the mechanism of this reaction appears to involve inhibition of enzymatic reactions requiring vitamin K in the activation of prothrombin precursors by NMTT. However, other factors (eg, malnutrition, liver disease) might be more important risk factors for bleeding than the NMTT-containing cephalosporins.[165] Thus, cautious use (and perhaps even avoidance) of agents with the NMTT side chain is recommended in patients with poor oral intake and critical illness. Administration of vitamin K and monitoring of the prothrombin time are indicated with these agents, particularly when therapy is prolonged. Positive direct Coombs' tests occur frequently but hemolysis is rare.[152,156] Ceftriaxone has been associated with biliary pseudolithiasis (sludging), which can be asymptomatic or resemble acute cholecystitis.[166] This adverse effect occurs most often with dosages of ≥2 g/day, especially in patients receiving prolonged therapy or those with impaired gallbladder emptying. The mechanism is ceftriaxone-calcium complex formation, and it is usually reversible with drug discontinuation.[166] Neonates given ceftriaxone can develop kernicterus caused by displacement of bilirubin from plasma protein binding sites; its use in this population is best avoided. Development of resistance during treatment of infections caused by *Enterobacter* sp., *Serratia* spp., and *P. aeruginosa* has occurred with all these agents.[152,155,156]

Precautions. Penicillin allergy. Use agents with NMTT side chain with caution in patients with underlying bleeding diathesis, poor oral intake, or critical illness. Use with caution in renal impairment and in those on oral anticoagulants (especially NMTT-containing drugs). Avoid use of ceftriaxone in neonates, particularly premature infants.

Drug Interactions. Avoid concomitant ingestion of alcohol or alcohol-containing products with agents containing the NMTT side chain. Probenecid reduces renal clearance and increases serum levels of most agents, except those that do not undergo renal tubular secretion (eg, ceftazidime, ceftriaxone).

Parameters to Monitor. Monitor prothrombin time 2–3 times/week with agents having an NMTT side chain, particularly when using large dosages; monitor bleeding time with high dosages of agents having an NMTT side chain. Obtain antimicrobial susceptibility tests for development of resistance in patients relapsing during therapy. Monitor renal function tests initially and periodically during high-dose regimens or when the drug is used concurrently with nephrotoxic agents. Monitor for diarrhea, particularly with ceftriaxone and cefoperazone; test stool specimen for *C. difficile* toxin if diarrhea persists or is associated with fever or abdominal pain.

CEFAZOLIN SODIUM
Ancef, Kefzol, Various

Pharmacology. Cefazolin is a first-generation cephalosporin with activity against most Gram-positive aerobic organisms except enterococci and some Gram-negative bacilli (eg, *Escherichia coli*, *Klebsiella* sp., *Proteus mirabilis*).[154,156]

Adult Dosage. IM or IV for treatment 250 mg–2 g q 6–12 hr (usually 1–2 g q 8 hr), to a maximum of 12 g/day. Decrease dosage in renal impairment. (See β-Lactams Comparison Chart.) IM or IV for surgical prophylaxis 1 g 30–60 min before surgery. IM or IV for endocarditis prophylaxis 1 g within 30 min before a dental or upper airway procedure.

Pediatric Dosage. IM or IV (≤1 month) 25 mg/kg/dose given q 8–12 hr; (>1 month) 50–100 mg/kg/day in 3 divided doses given q 8 hr, to a maximum of 6 g/day. IM or IV for endocarditis prophylaxis 25 mg/kg within 30 min before a dental or upper airway procedure.

Dosage Forms. Inj 250, 500 mg, 1, 5, 10, 20 g.

Pharmacokinetics. Cefazolin is 75–85% plasma protein bound and widely distributed throughout the body, with high concentrations in many tissues and cavities but subtherapeutic concentrations in the CSF. Virtually 100% is excreted unchanged in the urine via filtration and secretion; the half-life is about 1.8 hr, increasing to 30–40 hr in renal impairment.

Adverse Reactions. (*See* Cephalosporins.)

CEFEPIME HYDROCHLORIDE
Maxipime

Pharmacology. Cefepime is a fourth-generation cephalosporin with a broader spectrum of activity than other cephalosporins. Its activity is similar to that of ceftazidime against Gram-negative bacteria, including *P. aeruginosa*, but it is also active against some isolates resistant to third-generation cephalosporins (eg, *Enterobacter* sp.). Cefepime has greater potency against Gram-positive organisms (eg, staphylococci) than ceftazidime and is similar in activity to ceftriaxone. Its anaerobic activity is poor, particularly against *Bacteroides fragilis*.[167–169]

Administration and Adult Dosage. IM or IV 500 mg–2 g q 12 hr; moderate to severe infections are treated with IV 1–2 g q 12 hr. Higher dosages may be required in pseudomonal infections.

Special Populations. *Pediatric Dosage.* **IM or IV for empiric therapy of febrile neutropenia** (2 months–16 yr) 50 mg/kg q 8 hr; **IM or IV for pneumonia, uncomplicated UTI, skin and soft tissue infections** (2 months–16 yr) 50 mg/kg q 12 hr.

Geriatric Dosage. Same as adult dosage, adjusting for age-related renal impairment.

Other Conditions. In patients with Cl_{cr} of 30–60 mL/min, the usual dose is given q 24 hr; with a Cl_{cr} of 10–29 mL/min, 50% of the usual dose is given q 24 hr; and with a Cl_{cr} <10 mL/min, 25% of the dose (but no less than 250 mg) is given q 24 hr.

Dosage Forms. Inj 500 mg, 1, 2 g.

Pharmacokinetics. *Fate.* After a 30-min IV infusion of 1 g, serum concentrations of 79 mg/L are achieved. It is about 20% plasma protein bound. Cefepime penetrates most tissues and fluids well; CSF concentrations are 3.3–6.7 mg/L after 50 mg/kg q 8 hr. About 85% of a dose is eliminated renally by glomerular filtration. Elderly patients have a slightly lower total clearance, which parallels Cl_{cr}.

$t_{1/2}$. 2.3 hr.

Adverse Reactions. The most common adverse reactions are injection-site reactions, rash, positive direct Coombs' test without hemolysis, decreased serum phosphorus, increased hepatic enzymes, eosinophilia, and abnormal PT and PTT. Encephalopathy has been reported in patients with renal impairment given unadjusted dosages. (*See* Cephalosporins monograph.)

Contraindications. Previous immediate hypersensitivity reaction to any β-lactam.

Precautions. Adjust dosage in patients with impaired renal function. Use with caution in patients with GI disease, especially colitis.

Parameters to Monitor. Obtain renal and hepatic function tests, and PT and PTT periodically.

CEFOTAXIME SODIUM   Claforan

Pharmacology. Cefotaxime is a third-generation cephalosporin with activity against Gram-negative organisms resistant to first- and second-generation cephalosporins (eg, indole-positive *Proteus* sp., *Serratia* spp.). Its desacetyl metabolite (DACM) has good activity and might be synergistic with cefotaxime against certain organisms. The activity of cefotaxime against *P. aeruginosa* is inferior to ceftazidime and against *Staphylococcus aureus* is inferior to cefazolin. Cefotaxime is more active than other cephalosporins (except ceftriaxone) against *Streptococcus pneumoniae* that are intermediately resistant to penicillin G.[152,153,155,156,170]

Adult Dosage. IM or IV 250 mg–2 g q 6–12 hr (usually 1–2 g q 8–12 hr), to a maximum of 12 g/day. Reduce dosage by 50% in patients with a Cl_{cr} <20 mL/min.

Pediatric Dosage. **IV** (newborns up to 1 week of age) 50 mg/kg q 12 hr; (newborns 1–4 weeks) 50 mg/kg q 8 hr; (older infants and children) 50–200 mg/kg/day (200 mg/kg/day for meningitis) given in 3–4 divided doses q 6–8 hr.

Dosage Forms. **Inj** 500 mg, 1, 2, 10 g.

Pharmacokinetics. CSF concentrations range from 0.3 to 0.44 mg/L after a 1 g dose and in higher dosages cefotaxime is effective for treatment of meningitis. About 50% of a dose is excreted unchanged in urine and 50% metabolized to DACM. DACM is metabolized to inactive metabolites and excreted unchanged in urine.

Adverse Reactions. Cefotaxime is well tolerated, with coagulopathies only rarely reported. (*See* Cephalosporins.)

CEFOTETAN DISODIUM   Cefotan

Pharmacology. Cefotetan is a cephamycin, structurally and pharmacologically similar to the cephalosporins, particularly second-generation agents, and it contains an *N*-methylthiotetrazole side chain. It has greater activity against enteric Gram-negative bacteria than first- and second-generation cephalosporins and superior activity against *Bacteroides fragilis* and other anaerobic bacteria (comparable to cefoxitin and cefmetazole). Gram-positive activity is less than that of cefazolin.[152,161,162]

Adult Dosage. **IV or IM for treatment** 500 mg–2 g q 12–24 hr (usually 1–2 g q 12 hr), to a maximum of 6 g/day; **IV or IM for surgical prophylaxis** 1–2 g 30–60 min before surgery, then 1–2 g q 12 hr for up to 24 hr postoperatively. Reconstitute the drug with 0.5% lidocaine for IM administration because IM injection is painful. Give usual dose q 24 hr with a Cl_{cr} of 10–30 mL/min, and q 48 hr in patients with a Cl_{cr} <10 mL/min.

Pediatric Dosage. Safety and efficacy not established. **IV** 40–60 mg/kg/day given in equally divided doses q 12 hr.

Dosage Forms. **Inj** 1, 2, 10 g.

Pharmacokinetics. Cefotetan is excreted primarily unchanged in urine, with an elimination half-life of 3.5 hr.

Adverse Reactions. (*See* Cephalosporins.)

CEFTAZIDIME   Ceptaz, Fortaz, Tazicef, Tazidime

Pharmacology. Ceftazidime is a third-generation cephalosporin with activity generally similar to that of cefotaxime, but having superior activity against *P. aeruginosa* and inferior activity against Gram-positive (particularly against *Staphylococcus aureus* and penicillin-resistant pneumococci) and anaerobic bacteria.[152–156,170]

Adult Dosage. **IM or IV** 500 mg–2 g q 8–12 hr; q 12-hr administration appears to be adequate in the elderly. Reduce dosage by 50% with a Cl_{cr} of 30–50 mL/min; with a Cl_{cr} of 15–30 mL/min, the maximum dosage is 1 g q 24 hr; with a Cl_{cr} <15 mL/min, the dosage is 500 mg q 24–48 hr.

Pediatric Dosage. IV (newborns) 30 mg/kg q 12 hr; (older infants and children) IM or IV 30–50 mg/kg q 8 hr, to a maximum of 6 g/day (225 mg/kg/day for treatment of meningitis).

Dosage Forms. Inj 500 mg, 1, 2, 6, 10 g. Conventional formulations of ceftazidime release carbon dioxide during reconstitution; the lysine formulation (eg, Ceptaz) avoids this problem.

Pharmacokinetics. Ceftazidime is less than 20% plasma protein bound and 80–90% excreted unchanged in urine by filtration, with a half-life of 1.6 hr, which increases to 25–34 hr in renal failure.

Adverse Reactions. The drug is generally well tolerated. (*See* Cephalosporins.)

CEFUROXIME SODIUM	Kefurox, Zinacef
CEFUROXIME AXETIL	Ceftin

Pharmacology. Cefuroxime is a second-generation cephalosporin whose activity is greater than cefazolin but less than cefotaxime, against *Haemophilus influenzae*, including β-lactamase–producing strains. The activity of cefuroxime against *Staphylococcus aureus* is slightly less than that of cefazolin. Its activity against anaerobes is poor, similar to the first-generation cephalosporins.[152,156,163,171]

Adult Dosage. IM or IV for treatment 750 mg–1.5 g q 8 hr (q 6 hr in serious infections); IM or IV for prophylaxis 1.5 g 1 hr before surgery; doses of IM or IV 750 mg may be given q 8 hr for up to 24 hr postoperatively (1.5 g q 12 hr to a total of 6 g for open heart surgery). Reduce parenteral dosage in renal impairment; with a Cl_{cr} of 10–20 mL/min, give the usual dose q 12 hr; with Cl_{cr} <10 mL/min, give the usual dose q 24 hr. PO 125–500 mg q 12 hr.

Pediatric Dosage. IM or IV (newborns) 10–25 mg/kg q 12 hr; (older infants and children) 50–100 mg/kg/day, to a maximum of 250 mg/kg/day for meningitis in 3–4 divided doses. PO 15–20 mg/kg q 12 hr in children (40 mg/kg/day for otitis media); it may be given in applesauce.

Dosage Forms. Inj 750 mg, 1.5, 7.5 g; Susp 25, 50 mg/mL; Tab 125, 250, 500 mg. Do not interchange the tablets and suspension on a mg/kg basis. (*See* β-Lactams Comparison Chart.)

Pharmacokinetics. In adults, oral bioavailability appears to be lower with the suspension than with the tablets, and food increases the bioavailability of the tablets. After absorption of oral cefuroxime axetil, it is hydrolyzed in the bloodstream to cefuroxime. Cefuroxime's pharmacokinetics are similar to cefazolin's, but CSF concentrations are adequate for treatment of meningitis caused by certain organisms; however, the third-generation agents ceftriaxone and cefotaxime are superior in *H. influenzae* meningitis. Over 95% of the drug is excreted unchanged in the urine and the elimination half-life is 1.2 hr.

Adverse Reactions. The drug is generally well tolerated. (*See* Cephalosporins.)

EXTENDED-SPECTRUM PENICILLINS

Pharmacology. The carboxypenicillin ticarcillin and the acylureidopenicillins (mezlocillin and piperacillin) have the same mechanisms of action as other penicillins but are more active against enteric Gram-negative bacteria and *Pseudomonas aeruginosa*. Ticarcillin is not active against *Klebsiella* sp., but the acylureido derivatives have activity and are generally more potent against susceptible isolates. The acylureidopenicillins also have activity comparable to those of ampicillin against enterococci. The combination of clavulanic acid plus ticarcillin is active against *Klebsiella* sp. as well as β-lactamase–producing staphylococci, *Haemophilus influenzae*, and *Bacteroides* sp. The combination of tazobactam plus piperacillin is similar to clavulanic acid plus ticarcillin. These two combination products are not appreciably more active against *P. aeruginosa* or *Enterobacter cloacae* than ticarcillin or piperacillin alone.[145,146,148,172–174]

Adult Dosage. (*See* β-Lactams Comparison Chart.)

Pediatric Dosage. (*See* β-Lactams Comparison Chart.)

Dosage Forms. (*See* β-Lactams Comparison Chart.)

Pharmacokinetics. Usual half-life is 1–1.5 hr, which is prolonged in anuria, although acylureido derivatives are partially metabolized and accumulate to a lesser extent. The acylureidopenicillins are also subject to capacity-limited elimination (ie, increasing dosage results in progressive saturation of elimination pathways, resulting in decreased clearance), which allows administration of higher doses at 6- to 8-hr intervals.

Adverse Reactions. Adverse effects are similar to those of other penicillins. Sodium content of the usual daily dosage of parenteral ticarcillin approaches the equivalent of 1 L of NS. Prolonged bleeding time can occur as a result of binding to platelets and prevention of platelet aggregation.

IMIPENEM AND CILASTATIN SODIUM   Primaxin

Pharmacology. Imipenem is a carbapenem with an extremely broad spectrum of activity against many aerobic and anaerobic Gram-positive and Gram-negative bacterial pathogens. The commercial preparation contains an equal amount of cilastatin, a renal dehydropeptidase inhibitor that has no antimicrobial activity but prevents imipenem's metabolism by proximal tubular kidney cells, thus increasing urinary imipenem concentrations and possibly decreasing nephrotoxicity.[152,174,175] (*See* Notes.)

Administration and Adult Dosage. IV 1–4 g/day in 3 or 4 divided doses (usually 500 mg q 6–8 hr). For severe, life-threatening infections, a dose of 1 g q 6 hr is recommended (not to exceed 50 mg/kg/day or 4 g/day, whichever is less).[174] Infuse 250–500 mg doses over 20–30 min and 1 g doses over 40–60 min; reduce infusion rate if nausea and/or vomiting develops. **IM** 500–750 mg q 12 hr.

Special Populations. *Pediatric Dosage.* (<1 week) 25 mg/kg q 12 hr; (1–4 weeks) 25 mg/kg q 8 hr; (4 weeks–3 months) 25 mg/kg q 6 hr; (3 months–3 yr) 25 mg/kg q 6 hr; (>3 yr) 15 mg/kg q 6 hr.[174,176]

Geriatric Dosage. Same as adult dosage but adjust for age-related reduction in renal function.

Other Conditions. Reduce dosage with renal insufficiency as follows: Cl_{cr} 30–70 mL/min, give 75% of the usual dosage; Cl_{cr} 20–30 mL/min, give 50% of the usual dosage; Cl_{cr} <20 mL/min, give 25% of the usual dosage. Give a supplemental dose after hemodialysis.[174]

Dosage Forms. **Inj (IV)** 250 mg imipenem/250 mg cilastatin, 500 mg imipenem/500 mg cilastatin; **Inj (Susp, IM only)** 500 mg imipenem/500 mg cilastatin, 750 mg imipenem/750 mg cilastatin. (*See* Notes.)

Pharmacokinetics. *Fate.* Peak serum imipenem concentrations are 21–58 mg/L after a 30-min infusion of 500 mg and 1–84 mg/L after a 30-min infusion of 1 g; levels are <1 mg/L at 6 hr. CSF levels are 0.5–11 mg/L with inflamed meninges and appear to be adequate to treat meningitis, but experience in treating meningitis is limited and seizures can occur in such patients. Imipenem is 20% plasma protein bound; V_d is 0.26 L/kg. Probenecid increases imipenem serum levels and prolongs its half-life. About 70% of imipenem is excreted unchanged in urine when given with cilastatin, with the remainder excreted as metabolite; cilastatin is excreted 90% unchanged in urine.[174,175]

$t_{1/2}$. (Imipenem) 0.9 ± 0.1 hr; 3–4 hr in renal failure; (cilastatin) 0.8 ± 0.1 hr; 17 hr in renal failure.[174,175]

Adverse Reactions. Nausea and vomiting occur in 1–2% of patients, sometimes associated with hypotension or diaphoresis, particularly with high doses and rapid infusion.[174,175] Rashes occur occasionally, and cross-allergenicity with penicillins has been documented. Convulsions have occurred, primarily in the elderly, in those with underlying CNS disease, with overdosage in patients with renal failure, or with other predisposing factors.[174,175,177,178]

Precautions. Use with caution in elderly patients or those with a history of seizures or who are otherwise predisposed. Adjust dosage carefully in renal impairment. Imipenem can cause immediate hypersensitivity reactions in patients with a history of anaphylaxis to penicillin.[178]

Drug Interactions. Concomitant administration with probenecid produces higher and prolonged serum concentrations of imipenem and cilastatin. Imipenem has been shown in vitro to antagonize the activity of other β-lactams (eg, acylureidopenicillins, most cephalosporins) presumably via β-lactamase induction; although the clinical relevance is unclear, avoid co-administration.[175] Co-administration of imipenem/cilastatin with ganciclovir has been associated with generalized seizures in a few patients; the mechanism of this interaction is unknown.

Parameters to Monitor. Obtain renal function tests periodically.

Notes. Used alone, emergence of resistance during treatment of *Pseudomonas aeruginosa* infections occurs frequently; however, cross-resistance to other classes (eg, aminoglycosides, cephalosporins) does not occur.[174,175] Addition of an aminoglycoside might prevent development of resistance, but in vitro synergism occurs only infrequently.

    Vials may be reconstituted into a suspension using 10 mL of the infusion solution and then diluted further by transferring the suspension into the infusion container; alternatively, the powder in the 120-mL vials can be diluted initially with 100 mL of solution. The initial dilution must be shaken well to ensure suspension/solution. Do not inject the suspension. The resulting solution ranges from colorless to yellow. Reconstituted solutions are stable in dextrose-containing solutions for 4 hr at room temperature and 24 hr under refrigeration, and in normal saline for 10 hr at room temperature and 48 hr under refrigeration. With IM administration use 2 mL of lidocaine 1% injection to reconstitute a 500 mg vial and give the suspension by deep IM injection into a large muscle mass (eg, gluteal muscle).[175]

MEROPENEM
Merrem

Pharmacology. Meropenem is a carbapenem with a mechanism of action similar to that of imipenem. Unlike imipenem, meropenem is not appreciably degraded by renal dehydropeptidase-I and thus does not require concomitant administration of a dehydropeptidase inhibitor.[175,179,180] (*See* Notes.)

Administration and Adult Dosage. IV for less severe infections 500 mg–1 g q 8–12 hr; **IV for severe or life-threatening infections (eg, meningitis)** 2 g q 8 hr.

Special Populations. *Pediatric Dosage.* IV (<3 months) safety and efficacy not established, but 20 mg/kg q 12 hr has been used; (3 months–12 yr) 10–20 mg/kg q 8 hr; in meningitis 40 mg/kg q 8 hr has been used.[179]

Geriatric Dosage. Same as adult dosage but adjust for age-related reduction in renal function.

Other Conditions. Reduce dosage in renal impairment. With a Cl_{cr} of 26–50 mL/min, give the normal dose q 12 hr; with Cl_{cr} of 11–25 mL/min, the dosage is reduced by 50%; with Cl_{cr} <10 mL/min, give one-half the dose once daily.[179,181]

Dosage Forms. Inj 500 mg, 1 g.

Pharmacokinetics. *Fate.* The pharmacokinetics of meropenem are similar to those of imipenem, although meropenem can be given by IV infusion and bolus.[177,179] After IV infusion of 1 g, the peak serum concentration is 39–68 mg/L; the drug distributes well into most tissues and fluids, including the CSF. Plasma protein binding is low and the V_{dss} is 0.32 ± 0.03 L/kg. Meropenem is primarily eliminated renally by glomerular filtration and tubular secretion. Up to 70% of a dose is recovered unchanged in the urine, with a renal metabolite accounting for the remainder of the dose (up to 30%). Meropenem is appreciably removed by hemodialysis, and a supplemental dose is required after dialysis. Children have pharmacokinetics similar to adults; increased clearance and reduced half-life occur in cystic fibrosis.[181]

$t_{1/2}$. 0.9 ± 0.09 hr, increasing to 6.8–13.7 hr in end-stage renal disease.[181]

Adverse Reactions. Adverse effects are similar to imipenem; the most common are injection-site reactions, rash, nausea, vomiting, and diarrhea.[175,179] Animal studies suggest that meropenem has a lower epileptogenic potential, which has been supported by a low frequency of seizures in clinical trials, including studies in patients with meningitis.[179]

Precautions. Use with caution in patients with hypersensitivity to penicillins because meropenem can cause immediate hypersensitivity reactions in patients allergic to penicillins.[178] Adjust dosage in renal impairment.

Drug Interactions. Probenecid can reduce renal clearance of meropenem and increase its half-life by 38% and AUC by 56%; avoid the combination.

Parameters to Monitor. Obtain renal function tests periodically.

Notes. Meropenem is more active than imipenem against enteric Gram-negative bacilli; the two have equivalent activity against *Pseudomonas aeruginosa* and *Bacteroides fragilis,* and meropenem is slightly less active than imipenem against Gram-positive organisms.[175,179]

PENICILLIN G AND V SALTS   Various

Pharmacology. Penicillins G and V have activity against most Gram-positive organisms and some Gram-negative organisms, notably *Neisseria* sp, by interfering with late stages of bacterial cell wall synthesis; resistance is caused primarily by bacterial elaboration of β-lactamases; some organisms have altered penicillin-binding protein targets (eg, enterococci and pneumococci); others have impermeable outer cell wall layers.[145,146]

Administration and Adult Dosage. **PO** (penicillin V) 125–500 mg q 6-8 hr for mild to moderate infections. **IV** (penicillin G) 2–5 million units q 4-6 hr to a maximum of 24 million units/day, depending on infection. **IM** not recommended (very painful); use benzathine or procaine penicillin G as indicated.

Special Populations. *Pediatric Dosage.* **PO** (penicillin V) (<12 yr) 15–50 mg/kg/day in 3–4 divided doses; (>12 yr) same as adult dosage. **IV (preferably) or IM** (penicillin G) (<1 month) 25,000–50,000 units/kg q 6–12 hr; up to 400,000 units/kg/day has been used in meningitis; (>1 month) 100,000–300,000 units/kg/day in 4–6 divided doses.

Geriatric Dosage. Same as adult dosage but adjust for age-related reduction in renal function.

Other Conditions. With the usual oral dosage, no dosage adjustment is required in patients with impaired renal function; however, in treating more severe infections with larger IV dosages, careful adjustment is necessary.[182]

Dosage Forms. (Penicillin G) **Inj** (as potassium salt) 1, 5, 10, 20 million units; **Inj** 1, 2, 3 million units/50 mL (frozen); **Inj** (as sodium salt) 5 million units. (Penicillin V) **Susp** 25, 50 mg/mL; **Tab** 125, 250, 500 mg (250 mg = 400,000 units).

Patient Instructions. Take this (oral) drug with a full glass of water on an empty stomach (1 hour before or 2 hours after meals) for best absorption; refrigerate solution.

Missed Doses. Take this drug at regular intervals. If you miss a dose, take it as soon as you remember. If it is about time for the next dose, take that dose only. Leave at least 4–6 hours between doses. Do not double the dose or take extra.

Pharmacokinetics. *Fate.* (Penicillin G) A peak of 20 mg/L is achieved with a dose of 12 million units IV. Widely distributed in body tissues, fluids, and cavities, with biliary levels up to 10 times serum levels; 45–68% plasma protein bound. Penetration into CSF is poor, even with inflamed meninges; however, large parenteral dosages (>20 million units/day) adequately treat meningitis caused by susceptible organisms. (Penicillin V) Oral absorption is 60–73%, with a peak concentration of 5–6 mg/L after a 500 mg oral dose. It is about 80% plasma protein bound and has poor CNS penetration. For both drugs, 80–85% of the absorbed dose is excreted unchanged in the urine.[145,146]

$t_{1/2}$. (Penicillins G and V) 30–40 min; 7–10 hr in patients with renal failure; 20–30 hr in patients with hepatic and renal failure.[182]

Adverse Reactions. Occasionally, nausea or diarrhea occurs after usual oral doses. As with all penicillins, CNS toxicity can occur with massive IV dosages (penicillin G 60–100 million units/day) or excessive dosage in patients with impaired renal function (usually >10–20 million units/day of penicillin G in anuric patients); characterized by confusion, drowsiness, and myoclonus, which can progress to convulsions and result in death. Large dosages of the sodium salt form can result in hypernatremia and fluid overload with pulmonary edema, especially in patients with impaired renal function or CHF. Large dosages of the potassium salt form can result in hyperkalemia, especially in patients with impaired renal function and with rapid infusions. Occasional positive Coombs' reactions with rare hemolytic anemia have been reported after large IV doses. Interstitial nephritis has been rarely reported after large IV dosages. Hypersensitivity reactions (primarily rashes) occur in 1–10% of patients. Most serious hypersensitivity reactions follow injection rather than oral administration.[145,178]

Contraindications. History of anaphylactic, accelerated (eg, hives), or serum sickness reaction to previous penicillin administration. (*See* Notes.)

Precautions. Use caution in patients with a history of penicillin or cephalosporin hypersensitivity reactions, atopic predisposition (eg, asthma), impaired renal function (hence neonates and geriatric patients), impaired cardiac function, or pre-existing seizure disorder.

Drug Interactions. Physically and/or chemically incompatible with aminoglycosides leading to drug inactivation; never mix them together in the same IV solution or syringe. Probenecid competes with penicillin for renal excretion, resulting in higher and prolonged serum concentrations.[145,146]

Parameters to Monitor. Obtain renal function tests initially when using high dosages. During prolonged high-dose therapy, monitor renal function tests and serum electrolytes periodically.

Notes. Skin testing with **penicilloylpolylysine** (PPL, Pre-Pen) and **minor determinant mixture** (MDM) can help determine the likelihood of serious reactions to penicillin in penicillin-allergic individuals.[145,183] Availability of MDM is limited; it is locally available in small amounts only at larger medical centers. Desensitization is recommended in pregnant women with syphilis and may be attempted (rarely) in patients with life-threatening infections that are likely to be responsive only to penicillin, but this is a dangerous procedure and many alternative antibiotics are available.[145] (*See* also β-Lactams Comparison Chart.)

β-LACTAMS COMPARISON CHART

DRUG CLASS AND DRUG	DOSAGE FORMS	ADULT DOSAGE	PEDIATRIC DOSAGE	ADULT DOSAGE IN RENAL IMPAIRMENT[a]	PEAK SERUM LEVELS (MG/L)[b]	PERCENTAGE PROTEIN BOUND	COMMENTS
CARBAPENEMS							
Imipenem and Cilastatin Sodium Primaxin	Inj (IV) 250 plus 250 mg, 500 plus 500 mg; (IM) 500 plus 500 mg, 750 plus 750 mg.	IV 1–4 g/day (1–2 g/day preferred) in 3 or 4 divided doses; IM 500–750 mg q 12 hr.	(<3 months) *See* monograph; IV (3 mo–3 yr) 25 mg/kg q 6 hr; (>3 yr) 15 mg/kg q 6 hr.	Cl$_{cr}$ 31–70 mL/min: 75% of usual dosage; Cl$_{cr}$ <20–30 mL/min: 50% of usual dosage; Cl$_{cr}$ <20 mL/min: 25% of usual dosage.	21–58 (IV 500 mg imipenem)	20	Very broad activity against most aerobic and anaerobic bacteria. Frequent nausea and dose-related seizure potential.
Meropenem Merrem	Inj 500 mg, 1 g.	IV 500 mg–1 g q 8–12 hr; 2 g q 8 hr in life-threatening infections.	(<3 months) *See* monograph; IV (3 mo–12 yr) 10–20 mg/kg q 8 hr, 40 mg/kg q 8 hr in meningitis.	Cl$_{cr}$ 26–50 mL/min: usual dose q 12 hr; Cl$_{cr}$ 11–25 mL/min: 50% of usual dose q 12 hr; Cl$_{cr}$ <10 mL/min: 50% of usual dose q 24 hr.	55	2	Less active than imipenem against Gm+ and more active against most Gm− bacteria; equivalent against *P. aeruginosa* and *B. fragilis.* Less seizure potential than imipenem.

(continued)

β-LACTAMS COMPARISON CHART (*continued*)

DRUG CLASS AND DRUG	DOSAGE FORMS	ADULT DOSAGE	PEDIATRIC DOSAGE	ADULT DOSAGE IN RENAL IMPAIRMENT[a]	PEAK SERUM LEVELS (MG/L)[b]	PERCENTAGE PROTEIN BOUND	COMMENTS
CEPHALOSPORINS, FIRST-GENERATION							
Cefadroxil Duricef Various	Cap 500 mg Susp 25, 50, 100 mg/mL Tab 1 g.	PO 1–2 g/day in 1 or 2 divided doses; PO for endocarditis prophylaxis 2 g 1 hr prior to dental procedure.	PO 30 mg/kg/day in 1 or 2 divided doses; PO for endocarditis prophylaxis 50 mg/kg 1 hr prior to dental procedure.	PO 1 g, then 500 mg at intervals below; Cl$_{cr}$ 26–50 mL/min: 12 hr; Cl$_{cr}$ 10–25 mL/min: 24 hr; Cl$_{cr}$ <10 mL/min: 36 hr.	12–16	20	Spectrum similar to cefazolin.
Cefazolin Sodium Ancef Kefzol Various	Inj 250, 500 mg, 1, 5, 10, 20 g.	IM or IV 250 mg–2 g q 6–12 hr; (usually q 8 hr), to a maximum of 12 g/day. IM or IV for surgical prophylaxis 1 g 30–60 min prior to surgery; IM or IV for endocarditis prophylaxis 1 g within 30 min prior to upper airway procedure.	IM or IV (neonates <1 month) 25 mg/kg q 8–12 hr; (infants >1 month) 50–100 mg/kg/day in 3 divided doses to a maximum of 6 g/day. IM or IV for endocarditis prophylaxis 25 mg/kg within 30 min of procedure.	Cl$_{cr}$ 10–30 mL/min: 50% of usual dose q 12 hr; Cl$_{cr}$ <10 mL/min: 50% of usual dose q 24 hr.	185	75–85	Good Gm+ coverage (including *S. aureus*), plus some Gm– activity (*E. coli*, *Klebsiella* spp.). Sodium = 2 mEq/g

(continued)

β-LACTAMS COMPARISON CHART (*continued*)

DRUG CLASS AND DRUG	DOSAGE FORMS	ADULT DOSAGE	PEDIATRIC DOSAGE	ADULT DOSAGE IN RENAL IMPAIRMENT[a]	PEAK SERUM LEVELS (MG/L)[b]	PERCENTAGE PROTEIN BOUND	COMMENTS
Cephalexin Keflex Keftab Various	Cap 250, 500 mg Drp 100 mg/mL Susp 25, 50 mg/mL Tab 250, 500 mg, 1 g.	PO 250 mg–1 g q 6 hr; to a maximum of 4 g/day. PO for endocarditis prophylaxis 2 g 1 hr prior to dental procedure.	PO 25–50 mg/kg/day in divided doses q 6 hr; severe infections may require 50–100 mg/kg/day, to a maximum of 3 g/day. PO for endocarditis prophylaxis 50 mg/kg 1 hr prior to dental procedure.	Cl$_{cr}$ 10–50 mL/min: 50% of usual dosage; Cl$_{cr}$ <10 mL/min: 25% of usual dosage.	18–38	6	Oral absorption is almost complete; spectrum similar to cefazolin.
Cephapirin Sodium Cefadyl Various	Inj 1 g.	IM or IV 500 mg–1 g q 4–6 hr, to a maximum of 12 g/day.	IM or IV (<3 months) not well studied; (children) 40–80 mg/kg/day in divided doses q 6 hr.	Cl$_{cr}$ 10–50 mL/min: usual dose q 6–8 hr Cl$_{cr}$ <10 mL/min: usual dose q 12 hr.	10–20	45–50	Spectrum similar to cefazolin. Sodium = 1.2 mEq/g.

(continued)

β-LACTAMS COMPARISON CHART *(continued)*

DRUG CLASS AND DRUG	DOSAGE FORMS	ADULT DOSAGE	PEDIATRIC DOSAGE	ADULT DOSAGE IN RENAL IMPAIRMENT[a]	PEAK SERUM LEVELS (MG/L)[b]	PERCENTAGE PROTEIN BOUND	COMMENTS
Cephradine Velosef Various	Cap 250, 500 mg Susp 25, 50 mg/mL	PO 250 mg–1 g q 6 hr to a maximum of 4 g/day.	PO same as cephalexin.	PO same as cephalexin.	10–20 (PO)	10–20	Oral form comparable to cephalexin; spectrum similar to cefazolin.
CEPHALOSPORINS, SECOND-GENERATION							
Cefaclor Ceclor Various	Cap 250, 500 mg SR Tab 375, 500 mg Susp 25, 37.5, 50, 75 mg/mL.	PO 250–500 mg q 8 hr SR Tab 375–500 mg q 12 hr.	PO 20–40 mg/kg/ day in divided doses q 8 hr to a maximum of 2 g/day.	Cl_cr 10–50 mL/min: 50% of usual dosage; Cl_cr <10 mL/min: 25% of usual dosage.	10	25	Spectrum similar to cefazolin, but includes some ampcillin-resistant *H. influenzae.*

(continued)

β-LACTAMS COMPARISON CHART (*continued*)

DRUG CLASS AND DRUG	DOSAGE FORMS	ADULT DOSAGE	PEDIATRIC DOSAGE	ADULT DOSAGE IN RENAL IMPAIRMENT[a]	PEAK SERUM LEVELS (MG/L)[b]	PERCENTAGE PROTEIN BOUND	COMMENTS
Cefamandole Natate Mandol	Inj 1, 2, g.	IM or IV 500 mg–1 g q 4–8 hr.; life threatening infections may require 2 g q 4 hr.	IM or IV 50–150 mg/kg/day in divided doses q 4–8 hr.	Cl$_{cr}$ 10–50 mL/min: 50% of usual dose q 8 hr; Cl$_{cr}$ <10 mL/min: 25% of usual dose q 12 hr.	80–90	56	NMTT side chain. Spectrum similar to cefuroxime. Sodium = 3.3 mEq/g.
Cefonicid Sodium Monocid	Inj 1 g.	IM or IV 500 mg–2 g/day as a single dose.	Not established.	IM or IV 7.5 mg/kg, then 25–50% of usual dose given: Cl$_{cr}$ 10–50 mL/min: q 24–48 hr; Cl$_{cr}$ <10 mL/min; q 3–5 days.	220 (IV bolus)	83–98[c]	Poor activity against *Staphylococcus* spp. Unbound drug levels low and excreted rapidly because of saturable protein binding. Sodium = 3.7 mEq/g.
Cefotetan Disodium Cefotan	Inj 1, 2, 10 g.	IM or IV 500 mg–2 g q 12–24 hr.	Not established.	IM or IV give usual dose at intervals below: Cl$_{cr}$ 10–30 mL/min: 24 hr; Cl$_{cr}$ <10 mL/min: 48 hr.	140–180 (IV bolus)	78–91[c]	NMTT side chain. Spectrum similar to cefoxitin. Sodium = 3.5 mEq/g. Reconstitute IM with 0.5% lidocaine.

(continued)

β-LACTAMS COMPARISON CHART (continued)

DRUG CLASS AND DRUG	DOSAGE FORMS	ADULT DOSAGE	PEDIATRIC DOSAGE	ADULT DOSAGE IN RENAL IMPAIRMENT[a]	PEAK SERUM LEVELS (MG/L)[b]	PERCENTAGE PROTEIN BOUND	COMMENTS
Cefoxitin Sodium Mefoxin	Inj 1, 2, 10 g.	IV 1–2 g q 6–8 hr.	IV 80–160 mg/kg/day in divided doses q 4–6 hr.	Cl_{cr} 10–50 mL/min: 50% of usual dose q 6–8 hr; Cl_{cr} <10 mL/min: 25% of usual dose q 12 hr.	110	75	Gm+ activity less than cefazolin, but better Gm– and anaerobic activity. Sodium = 2.3 mEq/g.
Cefprozil Cefzil	Tab 250, 500 mg Susp 25, 50 mg/mL.	PO 500 mg daily–bid.	PO (6 mo–12 yr) 15 mg/kg q 12 hr.	Cl_{cr} ≤30 mL/min: 50% of usual dose at same interval.	10.5	36	Spectrum similar to cefaclor, but more active against *H. influenzae.*
Cefuroxime Sodium Kefurox Zinacef	Inj 750 mg, 1.5, 7.5 g.	IM or IV 750 mg–1.5 g q 6–8 hr; to a maximum of 6 g/day.	IM or IV (neonates) 10–25 mg/kg 12 hr; (children) 50–100 mg/kg/day in divided doses q 6–8 hr.	IM or IV: Cl_{cr} 10–20 mL/min: usual dose q 12 hr; Cl_{cr} <10 mL/min: usual dose q 24 hr.	100 (IV 1.5 g)	33–50	Gm+ activity similar to cefazolin, but better Gm– activity, including *H. influenzae.* Sodium = 2.4 mEq/
Cefuroxime Axetil Ceftin	Susp 25, 50 mg/mL Tab 125, 250, 500 mg.	PO 125–500 mg q 12 hr.	PO 15–40 mg/kg/day in divided doses q 12 hr.	—	3.6 (PO)	33–50	Do not interchange suspension and tablets.

(continued)

145

β-LACTAMS COMPARISON CHART (*continued*)

DRUG CLASS AND DRUG	DOSAGE FORMS	ADULT DOSAGE	PEDIATRIC DOSAGE	ADULT DOSAGE IN RENAL IMPAIRMENT[a]	PEAK SERUM LEVELS (MG/L)[b]	PERCENTAGE PROTEIN BOUND	COMMENTS
Loracarbef Lorabid	Cap 200, 400 mg Susp 20, 40 mg/mL.	PO 200–400 mg q 12–24 hr.	PO (6 mo–12 yr) 7.5–15 mg q 12 hr.	Cl$_{cr}$ 10–49 mL/min: 50% of usual dosage; Cl$_{cr}$ <10 mL/min: usual dose q 3–5 days.	6.8 (PO 200 mg)	25	Carbacephem analogue of cefaclor with similar spectrum; must be taken on an empty stomach.
CEPHALOSPORINS, THIRD-GENERATION							
Cefdinir Omnicef	Cap 300 mg Susp 25 mg/mL.	PO 600 mg/day in 1 or 2 doses.	PO 14 mg/kg/day in 1 or 2 doses.	Cl$_{cr}$ <30 mL/min: 300 mg/day.	2.9 (PO 600 mg)	60–70	Spectrum similar to cefixime, but better Gm+ activity
Cefditoren Spectracef	Tab 200 mg.	PO 200 q 12 hr.	PO (<12 yr) not established.	Cl$_{cr}$ <50 mL/min: reduce dosage.	2.6 (PO 200 mg)	88	Spectrum similar to cefdinir and cefpodoxime but more active.
Cefixime Suprax	Tab 200, 400 mg Susp 20 mg/mL.	PO 400 mg/day in 1 or 2 doses. PO for gonorrhea 400 mg once.	PO 8 mg/kg/day in 1 or 2 divided doses.	Cl$_{cr}$ 20–60 mL/min: 75% of usual dosage; Cl$_{cr}$ <20 mL/min: 50% of usual dosage.	4.9	70	More active than cefuroxime or cefaclor against *H. influenzae*, but less Gm+ activity.

(*continued*)

β-LACTAMS COMPARISON CHART (continued)

DRUG CLASS AND DRUG	DOSAGE FORMS	ADULT DOSAGE	PEDIATRIC DOSAGE	ADULT DOSAGE IN RENAL IMPAIRMENT[a]	PEAK SERUM LEVELS (MG/L)[b]	PERCENTAGE PROTEIN BOUND	COMMENTS
Cefopera- zone Sodium Cefobid Various	Inj 1, 2, 10 g.	IM or IV 2–8 g/day in divided doses q 12 hr.	IM or IV (neonates) 50 mg/kg/dose q 12 hr; (children) 50–75 mg/kg q 8–12 hr.	No change.	125	85–95[c]	Less active than cefta- zidime against *P. aeruginosa.* NMTT side chain. Sodium = 1.5 mEq/g.
Cefotaxime Sodium Claforan	Inj 500 mg, 1, 2, 10 g.	IM or IV 1–2 g q 8–12 hr; life- threatening infec- tions may require 2 g q 6 hr.	IM or IV (neonates) ≤1 week) 50 mg/kg q 12 hr; (neonates 1–4 weeks) 50 mg/kg q 8 hr; (infants >4 weeks) 50–200 (200 in meningitis) mg/ kg/day in divided doses q 4–6 hr.	Cl$_{cr}$ 10–50 mL/ min: usual dose q 8–12 hr; <10 mL/min usual dose q 24 hr.	40–100	37	Good Gm+ and Gm- activity except for *P. aeruginosa*; modest anti-anaerobic activity. Sodium = 2.2 mEq/g.
Desacetylcefo- taxime	—	—		—	1–65		Active metabolite of cefotaxime.

(continued)

β-LACTAMS COMPARISON CHART (continued)

DRUG CLASS AND DRUG	DOSAGE FORMS	ADULT DOSAGE	PEDIATRIC DOSAGE	ADULT DOSAGE IN RENAL IMPAIRMENT[a]	PEAK SERUM LEVELS (MG/L)[b]	PERCENTAGE PROTEIN BOUND	COMMENTS
Cefpodoxime Proxetil Vantin	Tab 100, 200 mg Susp 10, 20 mg/mL.	PO 100–400 mg q 12 hr; PO for gonorrhea 200 mg once.	PO 5 mg/kg q 12 hr.	Cl_{cr} <30 mL/min: usual dose given q 24 hr.	2.9 (PO 200 mg)	18–30	Spectrum similar to cefixime, but better Gm+ activity.
Ceftazidime Ceptaz Fortaz Tazicef Tazidime	Inj 500 mg, 1, 2, 6 g.	IM or IV 500 mg– 2 g q 8–12 hr.	IM or IV (≤1 month) 30 mg/kg/dose q 12 hr; (>1 month) 30–50 mg/kg/dose q 8 hr.	Cl_{cr} 30–50 mL/min: 50% of usual dose q 12–24 hr; Cl_{cr} 15–30 mL/min: 1 g q 24 hr; Cl_{cr} <15 mL/min: 500 mg q 24–48 hr.	70–90	17	Best activity against *P. aeruginosa*; poor Gm+ activity. Sodium = 2.3 mEq/g.
Ceftibuten Cedax	Cap 400 mg Susp 18, 36 mg/mL.	PO 400 mg q 24 hr.	PO 9 mg/kg/day in 1 dose.	Cl_{cr} 30–49 mL/min: 4.5 mg/kg or 200 mg q 24 hr; Cl_{cr} <30 mL/min: 2.25 mg/kg or 100 mg q 24 hr.	11 (PO 200 mg)	60–77	Spectrum similar to cefixime.

(continued)

β-LACTAMS COMPARISON CHART *(continued)*

DRUG CLASS AND DRUG	DOSAGE FORMS	ADULT DOSAGE	PEDIATRIC DOSAGE	ADULT DOSAGE IN RENAL IMPAIRMENT[a]	PEAK SERUM LEVELS (MG/L)[b]	PERCENTAGE PROTEIN BOUND	COMMENTS
Ceftizoxime Sodium Cefizox	Inj 500 mg, 1, 2, 10 g.	IM or IV 1–2 g q 8–12 hr; life-threatening infections may require up to 4 g q 8 hr.	IM or IV (>6 months) 50 mg/kg/dose q 6–8 hr.	Cl_{cr} 10–50 mL/min: 50% of usual dose q 12–24 hr; Cl_{cr} <10 mL/min: 25–50% of usual dose q 24–48 hr.	60–87	31	Spectrum similar to cefotaxime except slightly more active against anaerobes. Sodium = 2.6 mEq/g.
Ceftriaxone Disodium Rocephin	Inj 250, 500 mg, 1, 2, 10 g.	IM or IV 1–2 g/day as a single dose; IV for meningitis 2 g q 12 hr; IM for gonorrhea 250 mg once.	IM or IV 50–100 (100 in meningitis) mg/kg/day in 2 divided doses.	No change. (*See* Comments.)	151	83–96[c]	Spectrum similar to cefotaxime. Reduce dose with concurrent renal and hepatic dysfunction. Sodium = 3.6 mEq/g.

(continued)

β-LACTAMS COMPARISON CHART (continued)

DRUG CLASS AND DRUG	DOSAGE FORMS	ADULT DOSAGE	PEDIATRIC DOSAGE	ADULT DOSAGE IN RENAL IMPAIRMENT[a]	PEAK SERUM LEVELS (MG/L)[b]	PERCENTAGE PROTEIN BOUND	COMMENTS
CEPHALOSPORINS, FOURTH-GENERATION							
Cefepime Maxipime	Inj 500 mg, 1, 2 g.	IM or IV 500 mg–2 g q 12 hr; 2 g q 8 hr may be required for pseudomonal - infections and febrile neutropenia.	IM or IV (2 months–16 yr) febrile neutropenia 50 mg/kg q 8 hr; other infections 50 mg/kg q 12 hr.	Cl$_{cr}$ 30–60 mL/min: usual dose q 24 hr; Cl$_{cr}$ 10–29 mL/min: 50% of usual dose q 24 hr; Cl$_{cr}$ <10 mL/min: 25% of usual dose q 24 hr.	79	16–19	Spectrum similar to ceftazidime; more active against Gm+ organisms; also active against resistant *Enterobacter* spp.
MONOBACTAM							
Aztreonam Azactam	Inj 500 mg, 1, 2 g.	IM or IV 0.5–2 g q 6–12 hr.	Safety and efficacy not established. IV 30 mg/kg q 6–8 hr (50 mg/kg q 6–8 hr in cystic fibrosis, to a maximum of 200 mg/kg/day).	Cl$_{cr}$ 10–30 mL/min: 50% of usual dosage; Cl$_{cr}$ <10 mL/min: 25% of usual dosage.	164	60	Spectrum similar to ceftazidime against aerobic Gm− organisms only. No cross-allergenicity in penicillin-allergic patients.

(continued)

β-LACTAMS COMPARISON CHART (continued)

DRUG CLASS AND DRUG	DOSAGE FORMS	ADULT DOSAGE	PEDIATRIC DOSAGE	ADULT DOSAGE IN RENAL IMPAIRMENT[a]	PEAK SERUM LEVELS (MG/L)[b]	PERCENTAGE PROTEIN BOUND	COMMENTS
PENICILLIN G AND V							
Penicillin G Potassium Various	Inj 1, 5, 10, 20 million units Inj 1, 2, 3 million units/50 mL (frozen).	IV 2–5 million units q 4–6 hr.	IV (neonates) 25,000– 50,000 units/kg q 6–12 hr; (>1 month) 100,000– 300,000 units/ kg/day in divided doses q 4–6 hr.	Cl$_{cr}$ 10–50 mL/min: 75% of dosage; Cl$_{cr}$ <10 mL/min: 25–50% of dosage.	1.5–2.7 (IV 500 mg).	60	Gm+ (except most *Staphylococcus* strains), some Gm– (*Neisseria* spp.), and anaerobes (except *B. fragilis*). Poor oral absorption. Potassium = 1.7 mEq/ million units.
Penicillin G Benzathine Various	Inj 300,000, 600,000, 1.2 million units/mL.	IM for *Strep.* pharyngitis 1.2 million units once; IM for syphilis (early) 2.4 million units once; (late) 2.4 million units/ week for 3 weeks.	IM for *Strep.* pharyngitis (<27 kg) 300,000– 600,000 units once; (>27 kg) 900,000 units once.	No change.	0.063 (IM 600,000 units)	60	Use limited to syphilis and *Strep.* pharyngitis. For IM use only.

(continued)

β-LACTAMS COMPARISON CHART (*continued*)

DRUG CLASS AND DRUG	DOSAGE FORMS	ADULT DOSAGE	PEDIATRIC DOSAGE	ADULT DOSAGE IN RENAL IMPAIRMENT[a]	PEAK SERUM LEVELS (MG/L)[b]	PERCENTAGE PROTEIN BOUND	COMMENTS
Penicillin G *Procaine* Various	Inj 300,000, 600,000 units/mL.	IM 600,000–2.4 million units q 12–24 hr (0.6–4.8 million units/day divided q 12–24 hr).	IM (neonates) 50,000 units/ kg/day in 1–2 divided doses; (>27 kg) 900,000 units once daily.	No change.	0.9 (IM 300,000 units)	60	For IM use only.
Penicillin V *Potassium* Pen Vee K Veetids Various	Tab 125, 250, 500 mg Susp 25, 50 mg/mL.	PO 125–500 mg q 6–8 hr.	PO 15–50 mg/ kg/day in 3–4 divided doses.	No change.	3–8	78	Spectrum similar to penicillin G. About 60% absorbed; pre-ferred oral form of penicillin.
ANTISTAPHYLOCOCCAL PENICILLINS							
Cloxacillin *Sodium* Cloxapen Tegopen Various	Cap 250, 500 mg Susp 25 mg/mL.	PO 250–500 mg q 6 hr.	PO (<20 kg) 50–100 mg/kg/ day in divided doses q 6 hr; (>20 kg) same as adult dosage.	No change.	7–18	94	Used primarily for *S. aureus* infections. Suspension may be better tolerated than dicloxacillin.

(*continued*)

β-LACTAMS COMPARISON CHART (continued)

DRUG CLASS AND DRUG	DOSAGE FORMS	ADULT DOSAGE	PEDIATRIC DOSAGE	ADULT DOSAGE IN RENAL IMPAIRMENT[a]	PEAK SERUM LEVELS (MG/L)[b]	PERCENTAGE PROTEIN BOUND	COMMENTS
Dicloxacillin Sodium Dynapen Pathocill Various	Cap 125, 250, 500 mg Susp 12.5 mg/mL.	PO 125–500 mg q 6 hr.	PO 12.5–25 mg/ kg/day in divided doses q 6 hr.	No change.	7–18	98	Comparable to cloxacillin.
Nafcillin Sodium Unipen	Cap 250 mg Inj 500 mg, 1, 2, 4, 10 g.	IV 500 mg–2 g q 4–6 hr; PO 250 mg–1 g q 4–6 hr.	IV (neonates <7 days) 25 mg/kg q 8–12 hr; (neonates >7 days) 25 mg/ kg q 6–8 hr.	No change.	3.4 (PO) 40–57 (IV)	89	Comparable to oxacillin. Reversible neutropenia may be more common with nafcillin. Poorly absorbed orally; cloxacillin or dicloxacillin preferred. IV sodium = 2.9 mEq/g.

(continued)

153

β-LACTAMS COMPARISON CHART (*continued*)

DRUG CLASS AND DRUG	DOSAGE FORMS	ADULT DOSAGE	PEDIATRIC DOSAGE	ADULT DOSAGE IN RENAL IMPAIRMENT[a]	PEAK SERUM LEVELS (MG/L)[b]	PERCENTAGE PROTEIN BOUND	COMMENTS
Oxacillin Sodium Bactocill Prostaphlin	Cap 250, 500 mg Susp 50 mg/mL Inj 250, 500 mg, 1, 2, 4, 10 g.	IV 250 mg–2 g q 4–6 hr. PO 500 mg–1 g q 6 hr, but not recommended.	IV (≤14 days) 25 mg/kg q 8–12 hr; (15–30 days) 25 mg/kg q 6 hr; (children) same as adult dosage. PO 50–100 mg/kg/ day in 4–6 divided doses.	No change.	2.5 (PO) 40 (IV)	92	Poorly absorbed orally; cloxacillin or dicloxacillin preferred. IV Rare hepatic toxicity. IV sodium = 2.9 mEq/g.
AMPICILLIN DERIVATIVES							
Amoxicillin Amoxil Various	Cap 250, 500 mg Chew Tab 125, 200, 250, 400 mg Drp 50 mg/mL Susp 25, 50 mg/mL Tab 500, 875 mg.	PO 250–500 mg tid, or 500–875 mg bid, to a maximum of 4.5 g/day; PO for endocarditis prophylaxis 2 g 1 hr before procedure.	PO 20–40 mg/ kg/day in 3 divided doses; PO for endocarditis prophylaxis 50 mg/kg 1 hr before procedure.	Cl$_{cr}$ 10–30 mL/min: 250–500 mg bid; Cl$_{cr}$ <10 mL/min: 250–500 mg q 24 hr.	9	20	Spectrum similar to ampicillin, but better bioavailability (85%) and less diarrhea.

(continued)

β-LACTAMS COMPARISON CHART (*continued*)

DRUG CLASS AND DRUG	DOSAGE FORMS	ADULT DOSAGE	PEDIATRIC DOSAGE	ADULT DOSAGE IN RENAL IMPAIRMENT[a]	PEAK SERUM LEVELS (MG/L)[b]	PERCENTAGE PROTEIN BOUND	COMMENTS
Ampicillin Sodium Various	Cap 250, 500 mg Susp 25, 50, mg/mL Inj 125, 250, 500 mg, 1, 2, 10 g.	PO 250–500 mg qid; IM or IV 500 mg–3 g q 4–6 hr, to a maximum of 12 g/day.	PO (<20 kg) 50–100 mg/kg/day in 2–4 divided doses; PO or IV (>20 kg) 100–400 mg/kg/ day in divided doses q 4–6 hr.	Cl$_{cr}$ <20 mL/min: same dose q 12 hr.	4 (PO) 58 (IV)	22	About 50% oral bio-availability; GI side effects and rashes are frequent. IV sodium = 3 mEq/g.
EXTENDED-SPECTRUM PENICILLINS							
Mezlocillin Sodium Mezlin	Inj 1, 2, 3, 4, 20 g.	IV 3–4 g q 4–6 hr.	IV (<7 days) 50–100 mg/kg q 12 hr; (neonates >7 days) 50–100 mg/kg q 6–8 hr; (children) 300 mg/kg/ day in divided doses q 4–6 hr to a maximum of 24 g/day.	Cl$_{cr}$ 10–30 mL/min: 3 g q 8 hr; Cl$_{cr}$ <10 mL/min: 2 g q 8 hr.	263 (IV 4 g)	35	Spectrum similar to ticarcillin, but better enterococcal coverage. Least active drug in this class against *P. aeruginosa*. Sodium = 1.85 mEq/g.

(continued)

β-LACTAMS COMPARISON CHART (continued)

DRUG CLASS AND DRUG	DOSAGE FORMS	ADULT DOSAGE	PEDIATRIC DOSAGE	ADULT DOSAGE IN RENAL IMPAIRMENT[a]	PEAK SERUM LEVELS (MG/L)[b]	PERCENTAGE PROTEIN BOUND	COMMENTS
Piperacillin Sodium Pipracil	Inj 2, 3, 4, 40 g.	IV 3–4 g q 4–6 hr, to a maximum of 24 g/day	Not well established. IV (neonates) 100 mg/kg q 12 hr; (children) 200–300 (350–500 in cystic fibrosis) mg/kg/day in divided doses q 4–6 hr.	Cl_{cr} 20–40 mL/min: 3–4 g q 8 hr; Cl_{cr} <20 mL/min: 3–4 g q 12 hr.	244 (IV 4 g)	15–20	Best activity against *P. aeruginosa.* Sodium = 1.85 mEq/g.
Ticarcillin Disodium Ticar	Inj 1, 3, 6, 20, 30 g.	IV 2–4 g q 4–6 hr, to a maximum of 24 g/day.	IV (neonates ≤7 days and <2 kg) 75 mg/ kg q 12 hr; (neonates >7 days and <2 kg or ≤7 days and >2 kg) 75 mg/kg q 8 hr; (neonates >7 days and >2 kg) 75mg/kg q 6 hr; (children) 200–300 mg/kg/day in divided doses q 6–8 hr.	Cl_{cr} 30–60 mL/min: 2 g q 4 hr; Cl_{cr} 10–30 mL/min: 2 g q 8 hr; Cl_{cr} <10 mL/min: 2 g q 12 hr.	260 (IV 3 g)	50–60	Less active than piperacillin against *P. aeruginosa;* no activity against *Klebsiella* spp. More antiplatelet effect than mezlocillin or piperacillin. Sodium = 5.2–6.5 mEq/g.

(continued)

DRUG CLASS AND DRUG	DOSAGE FORMS	ADULT DOSAGE	PEDIATRIC DOSAGE	ADULT DOSAGE IN RENAL IMPAIRMENT[a]	PEAK SERUM LEVELS (MG/L)[b]	PERCENTAGE PROTEIN BOUND	COMMENTS
PENICILLIN AND β-LACTAMASE INHIBITOR COMBINATIONS							
Amoxicillin and Clavulanate Potassium Augmentin	Chew Tab 125 mg amoxicillin plus 31.25 mg clavulanate, 200 mg amoxicillin plus 28.5 mg clavulanate, 250 mg amoxicillin plus 62.5 mg clavulanate, 400 mg amoxicillin plus 57 mg clavulanate; Susp 25 mg amoxicillin plus 6.25 mg clavulanate/mL, 40 mg amoxicillin plus 5.7 mg clavulanate, 50 mg amoxicillin plus 12.5 mg clavulanate, 80 mg amoxicillin plus 11.4 mg clavulanate/mL. Tab 250 mg amoxicillin plus 125 mg clavulanate, 500 mg amoxicillin plus 125 mg clavulanate, 875 mg amoxicillin plus 125 mg clavulanate.	PO "250" or "500" tablet q 8 hr or "875" tablet q 12 hr.	PO 20–40 mg/kg/day (of amoxicillin) in 3 divided doses or 45 mg/kg/day in 2 divided doses.	CL_{cr} 10–30 mL/min: 250–500 mg bid CL_{cr} <10 mL/min 250–500 mg q 24 hr.	9 (PO 500 mg amoxicillin) 2.6 (PO 125 mg clavulanate)	20 (amoxicillin) 22 (clavulanate)	Active against ampicillin-resistant *S. aureus*, *B. fragilis*, and β-lactamase–producing Enterobacteriacae. More diarrhea than with amoxicillin. Do not substitute 2 "250" tablets for 1 "500" tablet.

(*continued*)

β-LACTAMS COMPARISON CHART (continued)

DRUG CLASS AND DRUG	DOSAGE FORMS	ADULT DOSAGE	PEDIATRIC DOSAGE	ADULT DOSAGE IN RENAL IMPAIRMENT[a]	PEAK SERUM LEVELS (MG/L)[b]	PERCENTAGE PROTEIN BOUND	COMMENTS
Ampicillin Sodium and Sulbactam Sodium Unasyn	Inj 1 g ampicillin plus 500 mg sulbactam/vial, 2 g ampicillin plus 1 g sulbactam/vial, 10 g ampicillin plus 5 g sulbactam/vial.	IM or IV 1.5–3 g of the combination q 6–8 hr, to a maximum of 12 g/day.	IM or IV (3 months–12 yr) 150–300 mg of the combination q 6 hr to a maximum of 12 g/day.	Cl_{cr} 15–30 mL/min: same dose q 12 hr; Cl_{cr} 5–14 mL/min: same dose q 24 hr.	58 (IV 1 g ampicillin) 30 (IV 500 mg sulbactam)	22 (ampicillin) 38 (sulbactam)	Spectrum similar to Augmentin. Sodium = 5 mEq/1.5 g.
Piperacillin Sodium and Tazobactam Sodium Zosyn	Inj 2.25, 3.375, 4.5, 40.5 g (0.5 g tazobactam/ 4 g piperacillin).	IV 3.375–4.5 g q 4–6 hr; 3.375 g q 4 hr or 4.5 g q 6 hr for *P. aeruginosa.*	Safety and efficacy not established.	Cl_{cr} 20–40 mL/min: 2.25 g q 6 hr; Cl_{cr} <20 mL/min: 2.25 g q 8 hr.	400 (IV 4 g piperacillin) 34 (IV 0.5 g tazobactam)	15–20 (piperacillin) 1 (tazobactam)	Similar spectrum to Timentin, but better activity against *P. aeruginosa* and enterococci. Sodium = 2.35 mEq/g of piperacillin.
Ticarcillin Disodium and Clavulanate Potassium Timentin	Inj 3.1, 31 g (100 mg clavulanate/3 g ticarcillin).	IV 3.1 g q 4–6 hr.	IV (≥3 months) <60 kg: 50 mg/kg (of ticarcillin) q 4–6 hr; ≥60 kg: same as adult dosage.	Cl_{cr} 30–60 mL/min: 3.1 g q 6 hr; Cl_{cr} 10–30 mL/min: 3.1 g q 8 hr; Cl_{cr} <10 mL/min: 3.1 g q 12 hr.[d]	260 (IV 3 g ticarcillin) 8 (IV 100 mg clavulanate)	50–60 (ticarcillin) 22 (clavulanate)	Improved activity over ticarcillin against *S. aureus, H. influenzae,* and anaerobes, but not *P. aeruginosa* or *E. cloacae.* Sodium = 4.7 mEq/g of ticarcillin.

[a]Usual dose means individual doses given at the specified interval; usual dosage means total daily dosage.
[b]Average peak serum concentrations following administration of a 500 mg oral dose or a 1 g IV infusion over 30 min, except as noted.
[c]Concentration dependent.
[d]With dosages recommended in marked renal impairment, clavulanate concentrations may provide ineffective synergism with ticarcillin.[173]
From references 172–174 and 184–190 and product information.

Macrolides

AZITHROMYCIN
Zithromax

Pharmacology. Azithromycin is a macrolide with a 15-membered ring (making it an azalide) that is slightly less active than erythromycin against Gram-positive bacteria but substantially more active against *Moraxella (Branhamella) catarrhalis*, *Haemophilus* sp., *Legionella* sp., *Neisseria* sp., *Bordetella* sp., *Mycoplasma* spp., and *Chlamydia trachomatis*. The drug also has activity against aerobic Gram-negative bacilli and *Mycobacterium avium* and is comparable to erythromycin in its activity against *Campylobacter* sp. It is the most active macrolide for *Toxoplasma gondii*, including activity against the cyst form.[191–194]

Administration and Adult Dosage. **PO for mild to moderate acute bacterial exacerbations of COPD, pneumonia, pharyngitis or tonsillitis, and uncomplicated skin and skin structure infections** 500 mg as a single dose on the first day followed by 250 mg/day on days 2–5 for a total dosage of 1.5 g. **PO for nongonococcal urethritis and cervicitis caused by *C. trachomatis* or for chancroid (*Haemophilus ducreyi*)** 1 g as a single dose.[195] **PO for treatment of *M. avium* complex in AIDS patients** 500 mg/day in combination with ethambutol.[196] **PO for prophylaxis of *M. avium* complex in AIDS patients** 1.2 g once weekly alone or in combination with rifabutin 300 mg/day.[197] **PO for endocarditis prophylaxis** 500 mg 1 hr before procedure. **IV for pelvic inflammatory disease** 500 mg/day for 1–2 days, followed by PO 250 mg/day to complete 7 days of therapy. **IV for community-acquired pneumonia** 500 mg/day for at least 2 days followed by PO 500 mg/day to complete 7–10 days of therapy.

Special Populations. *Pediatric Dosage.* **PO for otitis media** (≥6 months) 10 mg/kg as a single daily dose on day 1, followed by 5 mg/kg/day as a single dose on days 2–5. **PO for streptococcal pharyngitis/tonsillitis** (≥2 yr) 12 mg/kg/day as a single dose for 5 days.[198–200] **PO for endocarditis prophylaxis** 15 mg/kg 1 hr before procedure. **IV** (<16 yr) safety and efficacy not established.

Geriatric Dosage. Same as adult dosage.

Other Conditions. Dosage reduction may be needed in severe hepatic impairment, but guidelines are not available.

Dosage Forms. **Tab** 250, 600 mg; **Susp** 20, 40 mg/mL; **Pwdr for Oral Susp** 1 g; **Inj** 500 mg.

Patient Instructions. Take the oral suspension with a full glass of water on an empty stomach (1 hour before or 2 hours after meals) for best absorption. Tablets may be taken without regard to meals. Do not take aluminum- or magnesium-containing antacids with azithromycin.

Missed Doses. Take this drug at regular intervals. If you miss a dose, take it as soon as you remember. If it is about time for the next dose, take that dose only. Leave at least 12 hours between doses. Do not double the dose or take extra.

Pharmacokinetics. *Fate.* Oral bioavailability is 37%. After a 500 mg oral capsule, a peak serum concentration of 0.41 mg/L (0.55 μmol/L) is achieved in 2 hr. Plasma protein binding is 7–50%, primarily to α_1-acid glycoprotein.

Azithromycin penetrates macrophages and polymorphonuclear leukocytes, accounting for intracellular concentrations that are 40-fold extracellular concentrations. Azithromycin is widely distributed throughout the body, and tissue concentrations (including the CNS) range from 10- to 150-fold higher than those in serum. Tissue concentrations peak 48 hr after administration, and high concentrations persist for several days after drug discontinuation. Elimination is polyphasic, reflecting rapid initial distribution into tissues, followed by slow elimination. V_d is 23–31 L/kg; Cl is 38 L/hr in adults. Azithromycin is metabolized in the liver and eliminated largely through biliary excretion; only 6% is excreted unchanged in urine.[192,194,201,202]

$t_{1/2}$. Terminal phase 11–68+ hr.[192,202]

Adverse Reactions. The drug is well tolerated. Frequent adverse effects are mild to moderate diarrhea, nausea, and abdominal pain. Headache and dizziness occur occasionally. Rash, angioedema, hepatomegaly, and cholestatic jaundice are reported rarely.[192]

Contraindications. Hypersensitivity to any macrolide.

Precautions. Use during pregnancy only if clearly needed. Use caution in patients with impaired hepatic function or severely impaired renal function.

Drug Interactions. Azithromycin does not interact with hepatic cytochrome P450 enzymes and, unlike erythromycin and clarithromycin, is not associated with these types of interactions.[203]

Parameters to Monitor. Baseline and periodic liver function tests during prolonged therapy.

CLARITHROMYCIN Biaxin

Pharmacology. Clarithromycin is a semisynthetic macrolide antibiotic that is slightly more active than erythromycin against Gram-positive bacteria, *Moraxella (Branhamella) catarrhalis*, and *Legionella* sp. It is very active against *Chlamydia* sp. and superior to other macrolides in its activity against *Mycobacterium avium* complex (MAC).[192,194,201,204,205]

Administration and Adult Dosage. **PO for respiratory and skin infections** 250–500 mg bid; **PO for MAC in AIDS patients** 500 mg bid. **PO for endocarditis prophylaxis** 500 mg 1 hr before procedure. **PO for eradication of *Helicobacter pylori*** 500 mg tid in combination with proton pump inhibitors and other drugs. (*See* Gastrointestinal Drugs, Treatment of *Helicobacter pylori* Infection in Peptic Ulcer Disease Chart.)[206]

Special Populations. *Pediatric Dosage.* **PO for community-acquired pneumonia** 15 mg/kg q 12 hr for 10 days; **PO for other indications** 7.5 mg/kg bid, to a maximum of 500 mg bid. **PO for endocarditis prophylaxis** 15 mg/kg 1 hr before the procedure.

Geriatric Dosage. Same as adult dosage.

Other Conditions. Reduce dosage by 50% with Cl_{cr} <30 mL/min.

Dosage Forms. **Tab** 250, 500 mg; **Susp** 25, 37.5, 50 mg/mL.

Pharmacokinetics. *Fate.* Clarithromycin is acid-stable and absorbed well with or without food. Bioavailability is 55%, with peak serum concentrations of about 2 mg/L attained after a 400 mg oral dose. The hydroxy metabolite is active and may be synergistic in vitro with the parent drug.[202]

$t_{1/2}$. (Clarithromycin) 4.5 hr; (hydroxy-metabolite) 4–9 hr.[202]

Adverse Reactions. Similar to erythromycin, but clarithromycin has better GI tolerance.

Contraindications. Hypersensitivity to any macrolide antibiotic; concurrent use with certain other drugs. (*See* Drug Interactions.)

Precautions. Use with caution in severe renal or hepatic function impairment; dosage reduction is advised.

Drug Interactions. Clarithromycin has a lower affinity for CYP3A4 than erythromycin and therefore has fewer clinically important drug interactions; however, its use is contraindicated with astemizole or cisapride. Serum concentrations of theophylline and carbamazepine also can be increased by clarithromycin.

ERYTHROMYCIN AND SALTS   Various

Pharmacology. Erythromycin is a bacteriostatic macrolide antibiotic with a spectrum similar to that of penicillin G; it is also active against *Mycoplasma pneumoniae* and *Legionella pneumophila*.[207–209] It acts by binding to the 50S ribosomal subunit, inhibiting protein synthesis. Gram-positive organisms develop resistance via R-factor mediated alteration of the binding site. Gram-negative organisms are resistant because of cell wall impermeability.

Administration and Adult Dosage. (*See* Macrolide Antibiotics Comparison Chart.) **For gastroparesis** 200 mg IV of the lactobionate salt, 250 mg PO of the ethylsuccinate salt or 500 mg PO of the base 15–120 min before meals and at bedtime appear to be effective.[210]

Special Populations. *Pediatric Dosage.* (*See* Macrolide Antibiotics Comparison Chart.)

Geriatric Dosage. Same as adult dosage.

Other Conditions. Dosage adjustment is probably unnecessary in renal impairment.[198,207]

Dosage Forms. (*See* Macrolide Antibiotics Comparison Chart.)

Patient Instructions. Take this drug with a full glass of water on an empty stomach (1 hour before or 2 hours after meals) for best absorption. Refrigerate the suspension.

Missed Doses. Take this drug at regular intervals. If you miss a dose, take it as soon as you remember. If it is about time for the next dose, take that dose only. Leave at least 4–6 hours between doses. Do not double the dose or take extra.

Pharmacokinetics. *Fate.* Oral absorption varies widely with the salt and dosage forms (*see* Macrolide Antibiotics Comparison Chart), with peak serum concentrations occurring from 30 min (suspension) to 4 hr (coated tablet) after administration. However, enteric-coated erythromycin base tablets, stearate tablets, and estolate capsules produce equivalent erythromycin serum levels when administered to fasting subjects. Food or restricted water intake (ie, <20 mL) with a dose dramatically lowers the absorption of the stearate form. The drug is $83 \pm 5\%$ plasma protein bound and widely distributed into most tissues, cavities, and body fluids except the brain and CSF (even with meningeal inflammation). V_d is 0.6 ± 0.1 L/kg; Cl is 0.55 ± 0.25 L/hr/kg. Erythromycin is partially metabolized in the liver by CYP3A3/4 and excreted primarily as unchanged erythromycin with high concentrations in the bile and feces. Only 12–15% of an IV dose is excreted unchanged in urine.[52,207]

$t_{1/2}$. 1.6 ± 0.7 hr; unchanged or slightly prolonged in anuric patients, based on minimal data; prolonged in cirrhosis.[52]

Adverse Reactions. Frequent GI distress. IM form is very painful, despite local anesthetic (butamben) in the product, and might produce sterile abscesses. IV administration frequently produces pain, venous irritation, and phlebitis. Mild elevations of serum hepatic enzymes occur frequently. Transient deafness occurs occasionally with high dosages.[207,211] Rare, but potentially serious, reversible intrahepatic cholestatic jaundice occurs primarily with the estolate and ethylsuccinate forms, usually in adults after 10–14 days of therapy, although it can occur after the first dose if there is a history of previous use. Prodrome includes malaise, nausea, vomiting, fever, and abdominal pain (which can be severe and misdiagnosed as acute surgical abdomen). Symptoms resolve in 1–2 weeks, and serum enzymes return to normal over several months.

Contraindications. Concurrent use with astemizole, cisapride or pimozide; IM form in patients with hypersensitivity to local anesthetics of the para-aminobenzoic acid type (eg, procaine); hepatic dysfunction (estolate and ethylsuccinate forms).

Precautions. Pregnancy. Use with caution in patients with liver disease because of possibly impaired excretion.

Drug Interactions. Erythromycin inhibits CYP3A4 and can reduce hepatic metabolism of some drugs, including astemizole, carbamazepine, cisapride, cyclosporine, theophylline, triazolam, warfarin, and others.[212] (*See* Contraindications.)

Parameters to Monitor. Liver function tests in patients who experience prodromal symptoms (*see* Adverse Reactions) while receiving the estolate or ethylsuccinate form; check daily for vein irritation and phlebitis in patients receiving IV forms. Closely monitor the effects of other drugs that interact with erythromycin during concurrent use.

Notes. Avoid injectable forms if at all possible. Erythromycin is more active in an alkaline environment. Unrelated to its antibacterial effect, erythromycin in low doses binds to motilin receptors in the GI tract to stimulate gastric emptying. It is the most prokinetic macrolide and has been used in gastroparesis and other GI motility disorders.[210,213–216]

MACROLIDE ANTIBIOTICS COMPARISON CHART

DRUG	DOSAGE FORMS	ADULT DOSAGE	PEDIATRIC DOSAGE	COMMENTS
Azithromycin Zithromax	Tab 250, 600 mg Susp 20, 40 mg/mL Pwdr for Oral Susp 1 g Inj 500 mg.	PO 500 mg once, then 250 mg/day for 4 days; PO for urethritis and cervicitis 1 g; PO for MAC treatment 500 mg/day; PO for MAC prophylaxis 1.2 g once/week. IV 500 mg/day.	PO for otitis media or pneumonia, 10 mg/kg once, then 5 g/kg/day for 4 days; PO for pharyngitis/tonsilitis 12 mg/kg/day for 5 days.	Broader spectrum than erythromycin. Less GI intolerance than erythromycin. Little or no P450 inhibition.
Clarithromycin Biaxin	Tab 250, 500 mg Susp 25, 37.5, 50 mg/mL.	PO 250–500 mg bid; PO for MAC 500 mg bid; PO for *H. pylori* 500 mg tid with other agents.	PO for pneumonia 15 mg/kg q 12 hr for 10 days; PO for other uses 7.5 mg/kg bid.	Broader spectrum than erythromycin. Food does not decrease absorption. Less GI intolerance than erythromycin. Less inhibition of CYP3A3/4 than erythromycin.
Dirithromycin Dynabac	EC Tab 250 mg.	PO 500 mg once daily for 7–14 days.	<12 yr not recommended.	Spectrum similar to erythromycin, but less GI intolerance and little or no P450 inhibition.
Erythromycin **Base** E-Mycin Ery-Tab ERYC Various	EC Tab 250, 333, 500 mg EC Tab 333, 500 mg SR Cap 250 mg	PO 1 g/day in 2–4 doses, to a maximum of 4 g/day.	PO 30–50 mg/kg/day in 4 doses; may double in severe infection.[a]	Food interferes with absorption of uncoated products; EC products appear to be among the best tolerated erythromycin formulations.[b]

(continued)

MACROLIDE ANTIBIOTICS COMPARISON CHART (*continued*)

DRUG	DOSAGE FORMS	ADULT DOSAGE	PEDIATRIC DOSAGE	COMMENTS
Erythromycin Estolate Ilosone Various	Cap 250 mg Susp 25, 50 mg/mL Tab 500 mg.	PO 250–500 mg q 6 hr, to a maximum of 4 g/day.	PO 30–50 mg/kg/day in 3–4 doses.[a]	PO well absorbed; unaffected by food and highly resistant to gastric acid hydrolysis; absorbed as propionate ester which predominates in serum (8:1) and might be less active; rare intrahepatic cholestatic jaundice.[b]
Erythromycin Ethylsuccinate E.E.S. EryPed Various	Drp 40 mg/mL Susp 40, 80 mg/mL Chew Tab 200 mg Tab (coated) 400 mg.	PO 400 mg q 6 hr, to a maximum of 4 g/day.	PO 30–50 mg/kg/day in 3–4 doses; may double in severe infection.[a]	Absorbed better than base; intermediate susceptibility to gastric acid hydrolysis. Absorbed as ester, which predominates in serum (3:1) and might be less active. Rare intrahepatic cholestatic jaundice.[b]
Erythromycin Gluceptate Ilotycin	Inj (IV only) 1 g.	IV 15–20 mg/kg/day in 3–4 doses, to a maximum of 4 g/day.	IV same as adult dosage in 2–4 doses; may double in severe infection.[a]	Painful; phlebitis frequent; avoid use if possible. Infuse over 20–60 min.[b]

(continued)

MACROLIDE ANTIBIOTICS COMPARISON CHART *(continued)*

DRUG	DOSAGE FORMS	ADULT DOSAGE	PEDIATRIC DOSAGE	COMMENTS
Erythromycin Lactobionate Erythrocin Various	Inj (IV only) 500 mg, 1 g.	Same as erythromycin gluceptate.	Same as erythromycin gluceptate.[a]	Same as erythromycin gluceptate.[b]
Erythromycin Stearate Erythrocin Various	Tab (film coated) 250, 500 mg.	PO 1 g/day in 2 or 4 doses, to a maximum of 4 g/day.	PO 30–50 mg/kg/day in 4 doses; may double in severe infections.	Absorption about equal to ethylsuccinate, although food interferes markedly with absorption. Hydrolyzed to free base before absorption.[b]

[a]In newborns, data are available for erythromycin estolate only, suggesting an oral dosage of 40 mg/kg/day in 2–4 divided doses.
[b]Despite differences in oral absorption, no clinical studies have shown any salt to be clearly superior in any particular therapeutic use.
From references 217–222 and product information.

Quinolones

CIPROFLOXACIN
Ciloxan, Cipro

Pharmacology. Ciprofloxacin is a fluoroquinolone that inhibits bacterial DNA-gyrase, an enzyme responsible for the unwinding of DNA for transcription and subsequent supercoiling of DNA for packaging into chromosomal subunits. It is highly active against aerobic, Gram-negative bacilli, especially Enterobacteriaceae, with MICs often <0.1 mg/L. It is also active against some strains of *Pseudomonas aeruginosa* and *Staphylococcus* spp., with an MIC_{90} of 0.5–1 mg/L. However, recent reports indicate increasing resistance to this agent in methicillin-resistant *S. aureus*. It has poor activity against streptococci and anaerobes.[223,224]

Administration and Adult Dosage. **PO for uncomplicated UTIs** 250 mg q 12 hr. **PO for moderate to severe systemic infections** 500–750 mg q 12 hr; **PO for gonorrhea** 250–500 mg once. **PO for chancroid** 500 mg q 12 hr for 3 days.[195] **IV** 200–400 mg q 12 hr

Special Populations. *Pediatric Dosage.* (<16 yr) safety and efficacy not established. Use has been limited because of the potential for arthropathy. Ciprofloxacin has been used in children 6–16 yr old in limited situations to treat serious infections. **IV for *P. aeruginosa* infections in cystic fibrosis** 15–30 mg/kg/day in 2–3 divided doses. **PO for *P. aeruginosa* infections in cystic fibrosis** 20–40 mg/kg/day in 2 divided doses.[225]

Geriatric Dosage. Reduce dosage for age-related reduction in renal function, although dosage reduction is not necessary with only minor age-related renal function changes.[226]

Other Conditions. Reduce dosage by 50% or double the dosage interval when Cl_{cr} <30 mL/min; special dosage adjustments in patients with cystic fibrosis are not necessary.[227]

Dosage Forms. **Inj** 200, 400 mg; **Susp** 50, 100 mg/mL; **Tab** 100, 250, 500, 750 mg; **Ophth Drp** (Ciloxan) 3.5 mg/mL (equivalent to 3 mg/mL base); **Otic Susp** 2 mg plus hydrocortisone 10 mg/mL.

Patient Instructions. This drug may be taken with food to minimize stomach upset. Avoid antacid use during treatment; calcium, iron, or zinc supplements can reduce absorption. Avoid excessive exposure to sunlight during ciprofloxacin treatment. Report any tendon pain or inflammation that occurs during therapy.

Missed Doses. Take this drug at regular intervals. If you miss a dose, take it as soon as you remember. If it is about time for the next dose, take that dose only. Leave at least 6–8 hours between doses.

Pharmacokinetics. *Serum Levels.* A peak serum level of 4–6 mg/L (12–18 mmol/L) 2 hr after an oral 750–1000 mg dose is proposed as evidence of absorption adequate for tuberculosis therapy.[58]

Fate. About 70–80% absorbed orally; food decreases the rate but not the extent of absorption. Aluminum-, calcium-, or magnesium-containing antacids or sucralfate markedly decrease the extent of absorption. Peak serum concentrations are

3 ± 0.6 mg/L (9 ± 1.8 mmol/L) after a 750 mg oral dose; a 200 mg IV dose infused over 30 min results in a peak concentration of about 3.2 ± 0.6 mg/L. V_d averages 2 L/kg. Renal clearance averages 0.26 L/hr/kg. Less than 30% is plasma protein bound. Ciprofloxacin attains very high concentrations in many body fluids and tissues, most notably urine, prostate, and pulmonary mucosa. CSF concentrations are <1 mg/L; experience with the drug in the treatment of meningitis is very limited. From 45% and 60% of a parenteral dose is recovered unchanged in urine; the remainder is excreted as four metabolites or eliminated in feces.[202,226-230]

$t_{1/2}$. 4.2 ± 0.63 hr,[229] 6.9 ± 2.9 hr in severe renal impairment.[230]

Adverse Reactions. GI intolerance (nausea, vomiting, diarrhea, abdominal discomfort) occurs frequently. CNS effects such as headaches and restlessness have occurred in 1–2% of patients. Other CNS effects (eg, dizziness, insomnia, anxiety, irritability, and seizures) have been reported in fewer than 1% of patients. Skin rashes and photosensitivity occur occasionally. Anaphylaxis occurs rarely.[202]

Contraindications. Hypersensitivity to any quinolone.

Precautions. Pregnancy; lactation.

Drug Interactions. Aluminum-, calcium-, or magnesium-containing antacids markedly reduce oral absorption. Although there is some information that spacing administration by ≥2 hr might minimize these interactions, it is probably best not to use ciprofloxacin in patients taking long-term antacid therapy. Iron supplements and zinc-containing multivitamins can reduce absorption. Theophylline clearance can be reduced in some patients receiving ciprofloxacin. Patients receiving fluoroquinolones and methylxanthines such as theophylline or caffeine might be at increased risk of CNS toxicity (eg, convulsions). Warfarin metabolism can be impaired by ciprofloxacin, although studies with the fluoroquinolone enoxacin indicate that only the metabolism of the less active (R)-warfarin is affected. Use caution when adding ciprofloxacin in a patient taking warfarin. The solubility of ciprofloxacin is reduced at higher pH values; thus, avoid alkalinization of the urine.[228]

Parameters to Monitor. Monitor serum theophylline levels closely in patients receiving theophylline. Monitor prothrombin time and signs of bleeding in patients on warfarin.

OFLOXACIN	Floxin, Ocuflox
LEVOFLOXACIN	Levaquin, Quixin

Pharmacology. Ofloxacin is a systemic fluoroquinolone similar to ciprofloxacin. Levofloxacin is the active L-isomer of ofloxacin that allows higher dosages of the active form to be given with fewer side effects. Ofloxacin has greater activity against *Chlamydia trachomatis, Ureaplasma urealyticum, Mycoplasma pneumoniae,* and *Mycobacterium tuberculosis* than ciprofloxacin, but less activity against *Pseudomonas aeruginosa.*[58,202,223,224,231] (*See* Fluoroquinolones Comparison Chart.)

Adult Dosage. (Ofloxacin) **IV or PO for systemic infections** 400 mg q 12 hr; **PO for nongonococcal urethritis** 300 mg q 12 hr for 7 days; **PO for acute, un-**

complicated gonorrhea 400 mg once; **IV or PO for urinary tract infections** 200 mg q 12 hr. (Levofloxacin) **IV or PO** 250–500 mg once daily. Reduce the dosage of both drugs in renal impairment. **Ophth** (Ofloxacin) 1–2 drops q 30 min while awake and q 4–6 hr after retiring for 2 days, then q 1 hr while awake for 4–6 days, then qid until cure. (Levofloxacin) 1–2 drops q 2 hr while awake up to 8 times/day for 2 days, then q 4 hr while awake for 5 days. **Otic** (Ofloxacin) 10 drops bid for 14 days. (*See* Fluoroquinolones Comparison Chart.)

Pediatric Dosage. **PO, IV** (<18 yr) safety and efficacy not established. **Ophth** (<1 yr) safety and efficacy not established; (ofloxacin, levofloxacin) same as adult dosage. **Otic** (Ofloxacin) 5 drops bid for 10 days.

Dosage Forms. (Ofloxacin) **Inj** 200, 400 mg; **Tab** 200, 300, 400 mg; **Ophth Drp** (Ocuflox) 3 mg/mL; **Otic Drp** 3 mg/mL. (Levofloxacin) **Inj** 5, 25 mg/mL; **Tab** 250, 500 mg; **Ophth Drp** (Quixin) 5 mg/mL.

Pharmacokinetics. Ofloxacin is >95% bioavailable orally. A peak serum concentration of 8–12 mg/L (22–33 mmol/L) 2 hr after an oral dose of 600–800 mg is proposed as evidence of absorption adequate for tuberculosis therapy. Ofloxacin is predominantly renally excreted with a half-life of 5–7 hr.

Adverse Reactions. (*See* Ciprofloxacin.)

Drug Interactions. Ofloxacin does not alter hepatic metabolism of methylxanthine compounds (eg, caffeine, theophylline). However, like other fluoroquinolones, cations markedly reduce the absorption of this agent.

FLUOROQUINOLONES COMPARISON CHART

DRUG	DOSAGE FORMS	ADULT DOSAGE	DOSAGE IN RENAL IMPAIRMENT	ORAL BIOAVAILABILITY (PERCENT)	PEAK SERUM LEVELS (MG/L)[a]	COMMENTS[b]
Ciprofloxacin Cipro Ciloxan Cipro HC Otic	Tab 100, 250, 500, 750 mg Inj 200, 400 mg Susp 50, 100 mg/mL. Ophth Drp 0.3% (Ciloxan) Otic Susp 2 mg 2.5, 5 mL plus hydrocorti-sone 10 mg/mL.	PO 250–750 mg q 12 hr; PO for gonorrhea 500 mg once; IV 200–400 mg q 12 hr; Ophth 2 drops q 15 min–4 hr.	Cl$_{cr}$ 30–50 mL/min: PO 250–500 mg q 12 hr; IV usual dosage; Cl$_{cr}$ 5–29 mL/min: PO 250–500 mg q 18 hr; IV 200–400 mg q 18–24 hr; Dialysis: PO 250–500 mg q 24 hr after dialysis.	60–80	3 ± 0.6 (PO 750 mg) 3.2 ± 0.6 (IV 200 mg)	Most active against *P. aeruginosa.* Do not use against Gm+ organisms such as *S. aureus.*
Enoxacin Penetrex	Tab 200, 400 mg.	PO 200–400 mg q 12 hr; PO for gonorrhea 400 mg once.	Cl$_{cr}$ <30 mL/min: usual dose q 24 hr.	83–90	5.5 (PO 400 mg)	Most potent inhibitor of theophylline metabolism.

(continued)

FLUOROQUINOLONES COMPARISON CHART (continued)

DRUG	DOSAGE FORMS	ADULT DOSAGE	DOSAGE IN RENAL IMPAIRMENT	ORAL BIOAVAILABILITY (PERCENT)	PEAK SERUM LEVELS (MG/L)[a]	COMMENTS[b]
Gatifloxacin Tequin	Tab 200, 400 mg Inj 2, 10 mg/mL.	PO or IV 200–400 mg q 24 hr.	Cl_{cr} <40 mL/min: 400 mg once, then 200 mg/day.	93	4.3 (PO 400 mg) 4.6 (IV 400 mg)	No effect on theophylline metabolism. Can be taken with or without food. Enhanced Gm+ activity. Prolongs QT_c interval in some patients.
Levofloxacin Levaquin	Tab 250, 500 mg Inj 5, 25 mg/mL.	PO or IV 250–500 mg q 24 hr.	Cl_{cr} 20–49 mL/min: usual dose once, then 250 mg q 24 hr; Cl_{cr} 10–19 mL/min: usual dose once, then 250 mg q 48 hr; Hemodialysis or peritoneal dialysis: 500 mg once, then 250 mg q 48 hr.	95–100	5.7 (PO 500 mg) 6.4 (IV 500 mg)	Active S–(–) enantiomer of ofloxacin. Levofloxacin is not appreciably removed from the body during hemo dialysis or peritoneal dialysis.
Lomefloxacin Maxaquin	Tab 400 mg.	PO 400 mg once daily.	Cl_{cr} <40 mL/min: PO 400 mg once, then 200 mg/day.	95–98	3.5 (PO 400 mg)	No effect on theophylline metabolism. Long half-life of 8 hr. Relatively weak antibacterial. Phototoxic.
Moxifloxacin Avelox	Tab 400 mg.	PO 400 mg once daily.	No change required.	95	4.5 (400 mg)	No effect on theophylline or warfarin metabolism. No food interactions. Enhanced activity against common community-acquired pneumonia pathogens. Prolongs QT_c in some patients.

(continued)

FLUOROQUINOLONES COMPARISON CHART (continued)

DRUG	DOSAGE FORMS	ADULT DOSAGE	DOSAGE IN RENAL IMPAIRMENT	ORAL BIOAVAILABILITY (PERCENT)	PEAK SERUM LEVELS (MG/L)[a]	COMMENTS[b]
Norfloxacin Noroxin Chibroxin	Tab 400 mg Ophth Drp 0.3% (Chibroxin) 5 mL.	PO 200–400 mg q 12 hr; PO for gonorrhea 800 mg once; Ophth 1 or 2 drops q 2 hr–qid.	Cl_{cr} <30 mL/min: PO 400 mg/day.	30–40 (estimated)	1.4–1.6 (PO 400 mg)	Used in urinary and GI tract infections, sexually transmitted diseases and prostatitis only because of poor oral bioavailability.
Ofloxacin Floxin Ocuflox	Tab 200, 300, 400 mg Inj 200, 400 mg Ophth Drp 0.3% (Ocuflox).	PO or IV 200–400 mg q 12 hr. PO for gonorrhea 400 mg once. Ophth 1 or 2 drops q 2–4 hr for 2 days, then qid up to 5 days.	Cl_{cr} 10–50 mL/min: usual dose q 24 hr; Cl_{cr} <10 mL/min: 50% of usual dose q 24 hr.	95–100	3.5–5.3 (PO 400 mg) 5.2–7.2 (400 mg IV)	Most active against *Chlamydia* spp.; little effect on theophylline metabolism.
Sparfloxacin Zagam	Tab 200 mg.	PO 400 mg once, then 200 mg q 24 hr.	Cl_{cr} <50 mL/min: 400 mg once, then 200 mg q 48 hr.	90	0.62–0.71 (PO 200 mg) 0.56–1.60 (PO 400 mg)	Can be taken with or without food. No effect on theophylline metabolism. Pneumococcal activity superior to ciprofloxacin or ofloxacin. Phototoxic.

(continued)

FLUOROQUINOLONES COMPARISON CHART (*continued*)

DRUG	DOSAGE FORMS	ADULT DOSAGE	DOSAGE IN RENAL IMPAIRMENT	ORAL BIOAVAILABILITY (PERCENT)	PEAK SERUM LEVELS (MG/L)[a]	COMMENTS[b]
Trovafloxacin **Alatrofloxacin** **Mesylate** Trovan	Tab 100, 200 mg Inj 5 mg/mL.	PO 200 mg/day[c]; IV 200–300 mg/ day.[c]	No adjustment needed in renal impairment or dialysis.	88	1.1 (PO 100 mg) 3.3 (PO 300 mg)	Broad spectrum of activity. Penetrates into CSF better than other quinolones. May have benefit against resistant organisms.[c]

[a]Peak serum concentrations following administration of the dose shown in parentheses.

[b]All fluoroquinolones are associated with tendon rupture. Discontinue therapy at the first sign of tendon pain or inflammation, and patients should refrain from exercise until the diagnosis of tendinitis can be confidently excluded.[203]

[c]Trovafloxacin has been associated with serious liver injury, leading to liver transplantation or death. Reserve trovafloxacin for patients with serious, life-, or limb-threatening infections who receive their initial therapy in an inpatient facility (eg, hospital, long-term nursing care facility). Do not use trovafloxacin when a safer, alternative antimicrobial regimen will be effective.
From references 202 and 223–239.

Sulfonamides

TRIMETHOPRIM AND SULFAMETHOXAZOLE   Bactrim, Septra, Various

Pharmacology. Sulfamethoxazole (SMZ) is a synthetic analogue of para-aminobenzoic acid (PABA), which competitively inhibits the synthesis of dihydropteric acid (an inactive folic acid precursor) from PABA in microorganisms. Trimethoprim (TMP) acts at a later step to inhibit the enzymatic reduction of dihydrofolic acid to tetrahydrofolic acid. The most important determinant of efficacy is usually the level of susceptibility to TMP; resistance to the combination is uncommon but appears to be increasing worldwide. The combination is active against many bacteria except anaerobes, *Pseudomonas aeruginosa*, and many *Streptococcus faecalis* spp. It is also highly active and effective against the protozoan *Pneumocystis carinii*. TMP/SMZ has in vitro activity against methicillin-resistant *Staphylococcus aureus* (MRSA), but clinical success has been variable and unpredictable.[240–243]

Administration and Adult Dosage. **PO for UTI** 160 mg of TMP and 800 mg of SMZ q 12 hr for 10–14 days. **PO for prophylaxis of recurrent UTI** 40 mg TMP and 200 of SMZ at bedtime 3 times a week. **PO for shigellosis** 160 mg of TMP and 800 of SMZ q 12 hr for 5 days. **IV for severe Gram-negative infections or shigellosis** 8–10 mg/kg/day of TMP and 40–50 mg/kg/day of SMZ, in 2–4 equally divided doses, q 6–12 hr for 5 days for shigellosis and up to 14 days for severe UTI. **PO or IV for** *P. carinii* **pneumonia (PCP)** 12.5–20 mg/kg/day of TMP and 62.5–100 mg/kg/day of SMZ, in 2–4 equally divided doses, for up to 21 days. **PO for PCP infection prophylaxis** 160 mg of TMP and 800 mg of SMZ once daily; intermittent dosage (eg, 3 times a week) is also used. In patients with HIV infection, the drug is indicated if there was a previous episode of PCP or CD4 counts are <200 cells/μL.[241] (*See* Notes.)

Special Populations. *Pediatric Dosage.* **PO for UTI or shigellosis** (2 months–12 yr) 8 mg/kg/day of TMP and 40 mg/kg/day of SMZ (Susp 1 mL/kg/day) in 2 equally divided doses; (>12 yr) same as adult mg/kg dosage. **PO for otitis media** same as UTI dosage. **IV for severe Gram-negative infection or shigellosis** (>2 months) same as adult mg/kg dosage. **PO or IV for PCP** same as adult mg/kg dosage. **PO for** *P. carinii* **infection prophylaxis** 150 mg/m²/day of TMP and 750 mg/m²/day of SMZ, in divided doses, given 3 days a week.[244]

Geriatric Dosage. Reduce dosage for age-related reduction in renal function, although dosage reduction is not necessary with only minor age-related renal function changes. (*See* Precautions.)

Other Conditions. For a Cl_{cr} <30 mL/min, give normal dosage for 1–6 doses; with a Cl_{cr} of 15–30 mL/min, follow with 50% of the usual dosage; with a Cl_{cr} <15 mL/min, follow with 25–50% of the usual dosage in 1 or 2 divided doses. Give patients on hemodialysis a normal dose after each dialysis procedure. For systemic infections treated with higher dosages, monitor serum levels.

Dosage Forms. **Susp** 8 mg/mL of TMP and 40 mg/mL of SMZ; **Tab** 80 mg of TMP and 400 mg of SMZ (single strength), 160 mg of TMP and 800 mg of SMZ (double strength); **Inj** 16 mg/mL of TMP and 80 mg/mL of SMZ.

Patient Instructions. Take this medication with a full 8 fluid ounce glass of water on an empty stomach (1 hour before or 2 hours after meals) for best absorption. Drink several additional glasses of water daily, unless directed otherwise.

Missed Doses. Take this drug at regular intervals. If you miss a dose, take it as soon as you remember. If it is about time for the next dose, take that dose only. If you are taking the drug once a day, leave at least 10–12 hours between doses. If you are taking the drug twice a day, leave at least 5–6 hours between doses. Do not double the dose or take extra.

Pharmacokinetics. *Serum Levels.* Trimethoprim levels >5 mg/L (>17 μmol/L) and SMZ peak levels of about 100 mg/L (396 μmol/L) may be required in PCP.[245]

Fate. TMP and SMZ are 90–100% absorbed orally. In normal adults, peak serum concentrations of 0.9–1.9 mg/L (3.1–6.5 μmol/L) of TMP and 20–50 mg/L (79–198 μmol/L) of SMZ occur about 1–4 hr after 160 mg of TMP and 800 mg of SMZ. An additional 10–20 mg/L of SMZ exists in the serum as inactive metabolites. IV infusion of 160 mg of TMP and 800 mg of SMZ over 1 hr produces peak serum levels of 3.4 mg/L (11.7 μmol/L) of TMP and 46.3 mg/L (183 μmol/L) of SMZ. TMP and SMZ are widely distributed in the body, although TMP is much more widely distributed because of its greater lipophilicity. TMP is 45% plasma protein bound and has a V_d of 1–2 L/kg; SMZ is 60% plasma protein bound and has a V_d of 0.36 L/kg. TMP concentrations in various tissues and fluids (including the prostate, bile, and sputum) are several times greater than concomitant serum concentrations; CSF concentrations in normal adults are approximately 50% of serum concentrations. Nearly all TMP is excreted in the urine within 24–72 hr, 50–75% as unchanged drug. SMZ undergoes extensive liver metabolism, producing N^4-acetylated and N^4-glucuronidated derivatives; 85% is excreted in the urine within 24–72 hr, 10–30% as unchanged drug. The pharmacokinetics of these drugs are essentially unchanged when given in combination. The pH of the urine influences renal excretion of both drugs but does not markedly alter overall elimination.[246]

t½. 11 ± 2.3 hr for TMP and 8 ± 0.4 hr for SMZ in normal adults.[246] 20–30 hr or more for TMP in severe renal failure; 18–24 hr for SMZ in anuria.[243]

Adverse Reactions. GI irritation including nausea, vomiting, and anorexia occurs frequently, and frequency and severity appear to be dose related. Rashes and other hypersensitivity reactions similar to those caused by other sulfonamides occur occasionally. In patients with AIDS, allergic skin reactions, rash (usually diffuse, erythematous or maculopapular, and pruritic) are frequent and might be associated with fever, leukopenia, neutropenia, thrombocytopenia, and increased transaminase levels.[247] Desensitization has been successful. (*See* Notes.) In patients without underlying myelosuppression and treated with conventional dosages, the frequency of megaloblastic anemia and other hematologic disorders is rare but might be higher in folate-deficient patients. Hepatotoxicity and nephrotoxicity are rare; renal dysfunction can occur in patients with pre-existing renal disease, but it is reversible.[243,246] Allergic skin reactions, including toxic epidermal necrolysis, exfoliative dermatitis, Stevens-Johnson syndrome, erythema multiforme, and fixed drug eruptions, occur rarely. Other rare adverse effects are cholestatic jaundice, pancreatitis, pseudomembranous colitis, hyperkalemia, myalgia, headache, insomnia, fatigue, ataxia, vertigo, depression, and anaphylaxis.[243]

Contraindications. Pregnancy; infants <2 months; history of hypersensitivity reaction to sulfonamide derivatives or trimethoprim; megaloblastic anemia caused by folate deficiency. Lactation is stated by manufacturer to be a contraindication, but risk is probably limited to nursing infants <2 months of age.

Precautions. G-6-PD deficiency; impaired renal or hepatic function. Adverse reactions can be more frequent in the elderly, especially with impaired hepatic or renal function or in those taking thiazide diuretics.

Drug Interactions. The effects of methotrexate, sulfonylureas, and warfarin are increased when used with trimethoprim-sulfamethoxazole. Enhanced bone marrow suppression can occur with the combination of trimethoprim/sulfamethoxazole and mercaptopurine. A decreased effect of cyclosporine and an increased risk of nephrotoxicity can occur. High-dose trimethoprim-sulfamethoxazole with didanosine can increase the risk of pancreatitis. Phenytoin clearance can be decreased with concurrent use.

Parameters to Monitor. Baseline and periodic CBC counts for patients on long-term or high-dose treatment. Monitor SMZ serum levels in patients treated for PCP if absorption is questionable or response is poor. In patients with AIDS, monitor for hypersensitivity skin reactions (rash and urticaria).

Notes. Protect all dosage forms from light. The efficacy and safety of TMP and SMZ have been demonstrated in numerous infectious conditions (eg, chronic UTI, chronic bronchitis, sepsis, enteric fever, prostatitis, endocarditis, meningitis, and gonorrhea), and the combination is considered an effective alternative to conventional therapy in most cases.[241,246] Efficacy of TMP and SMZ in the treatment of PCP is equivalent to **pentamidine,** which makes the combination the therapy of choice because of its greater safety and lower cost.[245] Oral desensitization or rechallenge with TMP/SMZ has been successful in permitting continued use in patients with AIDS who experience hypersensitivity reactions.[248]

Tetracyclines

DOXYCYCLINE AND SALTS   Vibramycin

Pharmacology. Tetracyclines are broad-spectrum bacteriostatic compounds that inhibit protein synthesis at the 30S ribosomal subunit. Activity includes Gram-positive, Gram-negative, aerobic, and anaerobic bacteria, as well as spirochetes, mycoplasmas, rickettsiae, chlamydiae, and some protozoa. Many bacteria have developed plasmid-mediated resistance. Most Enterobacteriacae and *P. aeruginosa* are resistant. Doxycycline is somewhat more active than other tetracyclines against anaerobes and facultative Gram-negative bacilli.[249,250]

Administration and Adult Dosage. **PO** 100 mg q 12 hr for 2 doses, then 50–100 mg/day in 1 or 2 doses, depending on the severity of the infection, to a maximum of 200 mg/day. **PO for uncomplicated chlamydial genital infections** 100 mg bid for at least 7 days. **PO for primary and secondary syphilis** 100 mg tid for at least 10 days. **PO for prophylaxis against travelers' diarrhea** 200 mg en route, then 100 mg/day for duration of travel (6 weeks maximum). **PO for malaria prophylaxis in short-term (<4 months) travelers** 100 mg/day beginning 1–2 days before travel to malarious areas and for 4 weeks after leaving the area. **IV** 200 mg in 1 or 2 divided doses for 1 day, followed by 100–200 mg/day, infused at a concentration of 0.1–1 g/L over 1–4 hr; double maintenance dosage in severe infections. **Intrapleural for pleural effusions** 500 mg in 25–30 mL of NS has been used; most patients require 2–4 infusions for maximum efficacy.[251] **Not for SC or IM use.**

Special Populations. *Pediatric Dosage.* **Not recommended ≤8 yr.** PO (>8 yr, <45 kg) 2.2 mg/kg q 12 hr for 2 doses, then 2.2–4.4 mg/kg/day in 1 or 2 divided doses, depending on the severity of the infection; (>45 kg) same as adult dosage. **PO for malaria prophylaxis in short-term (<4 months) travelers** (>8 yr) 2.2 mg/kg/day to a maximum of 100 mg/day beginning 1–2 days before travel to malarious areas and for 4 weeks after leaving the area. **IV** (<45 kg) 4.4 mg/kg in 1 or 2 divided doses for 1 day followed by 2.2–4.4 mg/kg/day in 1 or 2 divided doses, infused at a concentration of 0.1–1 g/L over 1–4 hr; (>45 kg) same as adult dosage.

Geriatric Dosage. Same as adult dosage.

Other Conditions. No dosage adjustment is necessary in renal impairment.

Dosage Forms. **Cap** (as hyclate) 20, 50, 100 mg; **Tab** (as hyclate) 50, 100 mg; **Cap** (as monohydrate) 50, 100 mg; **Susp** (as monohydrate) 5 mg/mL (reconstituted); **Syrup** (as calcium) 10 mg/mL; **Inj** (as hyclate) 100, 200 mg.

Patient Instructions. Take doxycycline by mouth with a full glass of water on an empty stomach; if stomach upset occurs, the drug may be taken with food or milk but not with antacids or iron products. Avoid prolonged exposure to direct sunlight while taking this drug.

Missed Doses. Take this drug at regular intervals. If you miss a dose, take it as soon as you remember. If it is about time for the next dose, take that dose only. Leave at least 6–8 hours between doses. Do not double the dose or take extra.

Pharmacokinetics. *Onset and Duration.* Duration of protection against travelers' diarrhea is about 1 week after drug discontinuation.[252]

Fate. About 93% is orally absorbed, producing a peak of 3 mg/L (6.5 µmol/L) 2–4 hr after administration of a 200 mg dose; antacids and iron can markedly impair oral absorption; milk causes about a 30% decrease in bioavailability and food has little effect. Widely distributed in the body, penetrating most cavities including CSF (12–20% of serum levels). The drug is 88 ± 5% plasma protein bound. V_d is 0.75 ± 0.32 L/kg; Cl is 0.032 ± 0.01 L/hr/kg. About 41 ± 19% is excreted unchanged in the urine in normal adults; the remainder is eliminated in feces via intestinal and biliary secretion.[52,252,253]

$t_{1/2}$. 16 ± 6 hr in normal adults; slightly prolonged in severe renal impairment.[52,252]

Adverse Reactions. IV administration frequently produces phlebitis. Oral doxycycline causes less alteration of intestinal flora than other tetracyclines but can cause nausea and diarrhea with equal frequency. It binds to calcium in teeth and bones, which can cause discoloration of teeth in children, especially during growth; however, doxycycline has a lower potential for this effect than most other tetracyclines. In contrast to other tetracyclines, doxycycline is not very antianabolic and will not further increase azotemia in renal failure. Phototoxic skin reactions occur occasionally.[249,250,252]

Contraindications. Hypersensitivity to any tetracycline.

Precautions. Not recommended in pregnancy or in children ≤8 yr because permanent staining of the child's teeth will occur. Use with caution in severe hepatic dysfunction. The syrup contains sulfites.

Drug Interactions. Antacids containing di- or trivalent cations, bismuth salts, or zinc salts interfere with absorption of oral tetracyclines. Oral iron salts lower doxycycline serum levels, even of IV doxycycline, by interfering with absorption and enterohepatic circulation. Barbiturates, carbamazepine, and phenytoin can enhance doxycycline hepatic metabolism, possibly decreasing its effect. Tetracyclines can interfere with enterohepatic circulation of contraceptive hormones, causing menstrual irregularities and possibly unplanned pregnancies. Combined use of tetracyclines with the bactericidal agents such as penicillins can result in decreased activity in some infections.

Parameters to Monitor. Check for signs of phlebitis daily during IV use.

Notes. Doxycycline is the tetracycline of choice because it is better tolerated than other tetracyclines, although tetracyclines are the drugs of choice for very few infections.[249,250] Each vial contains 480 mg of ascorbic acid per 100 mg of doxycycline hyclate for injection. (*See* Tetracyclines Comparison Chart.)

TETRACYCLINE AND SALTS   Various

Pharmacology. Tetracycline has an antimicrobial spectrum of activity similar to that of doxycycline. Current uses are for treatment of infection caused by *Chlamydia* sp., *Mycoplasma* sp., and *Brucella* spp.[249,250] It is also used as a treatment for acne and in some regimens against *Helicobacter pylori*. (*See* Gastrointestinal Drugs, Treatment of *Helicobacter pylori* Infection in Peptic Ulcer Disease.)

Adult Dosage. PO 1–2 g/day in 2–4 divided doses. Reduce dosage, or preferably use another drug, in severe renal or hepatic impairment.

Pediatric Dosage. **Not recommended ≤8 yr; PO** (>8 yr) 25–50 mg/kg/day in 2–4 divided doses.

Dosage Forms. (*See* Tetracyclines Comparison Chart.)

Pharmacokinetics. Tetracycline is well absorbed from the GI tract. Multivalent cations chelate tetracyclines and inhibit absorption; warn patients to avoid concurrent antacids, dairy products, iron, or sucralfate. The half-life of tetracycline is about 10 hr, increasing to as high as 108 hr in anuria.[52]

Adverse Reactions. GI irritation is frequent and can result in esophageal ulceration if the drug is taken at bedtime with insufficient fluid. Disruption of bowel flora occurs frequently and can result in diarrhea, candidiasis, or rarely pseudomembranous colitis. Antianabolic effects produce elevated BUN, hyperphosphatemia, and acidosis in patients with renal failure. Acute fatty infiltration of the liver with pancreatitis occurs rarely with large (>2 g) IV doses, especially in pregnancy; avoid tetracyclines in pregnancy. Do not give tetracyclines to children <8 yr because of binding of calcium in teeth and resultant discoloration.

Contraindications. (*See* Doxycycline.)

Precautions. (*See* Doxycycline.)

Drug Interactions. Oral absorption is markedly inhibited by di- and trivalent cations (eg, antacids, iron salts). (*See also* Doxycycline Interactions.)

TETRACYCLINES COMPARISON CHART

DRUG	DOSAGE FORMS	ADULT DOSAGE	PERCENTAGE ORAL ABSORPTION	HALF-LIFE (HOURS)		PERCENTAGE EXCRETED UNCHANGED IN URINE	COMMENTS
				NORMAL	ANURIA		
Demeclocycline Hydrochloride Declomycin	Cap 150 mg Tab 150, 300 mg.	PO 600 mg/day in 2–4 divided doses. PO for SIADH 300 mg tid–qid.	66	15	40–60	42	Most phototoxic tetracycline; causes nephrogenic diabetes insipidus rarely.
Doxycycline Calcium **Doxycycline Hyclate** **Doxycycline Monohydrate** Vibramycin Various	Cap 20, 50, 100 mg Tab 50, 100 mg Susp 5 mg/mL Syrup 10 mg/mL Inj 100, 200 mg.	PO 100 mg q 12 hr for 2 doses, then 50–100 mg/day in 1–2 divided doses; IV 200 mg in 1–2 divided doses on day 1, then 100–200 mg/day.	93	16 ± 6	12–22	41	Safest in renal failure because of its lack of accumulation and lack of antianabolic effects. Well tolerated when given IV.
Minocycline Hydrochloride Minocin Various	Cap 50, 75, 100 mg Susp 10 mg/mL Inj (IV only) 100 mg.	PO or IV 200 mg initially, then 100 mg q 12 hr.	95–100	16 ± 2	11–23	11	Very frequent transient vestibular toxicity.

(continued)

179

TETRACYCLINES COMPARISON CHART (*continued*)

DRUG	DOSAGE FORMS	ADULT DOSAGE	PERCENTAGE ORAL ABSORPTION	HALF-LIFE (HOURS) NORMAL	HALF-LIFE (HOURS) ANURIA	PERCENTAGE EXCRETED UNCHANGED IN URINE	COMMENTS
Oxytetracycline *Oxytetracycline Hydrochloride* *Oxytetracycline Calcium* Various	Cap 250 mg Inj (IM only, contains 2% lidocaine) 50, 125 mg/mL.	PO 1–2 g/day in 2–4 divided doses; IM 250 mg once daily to 300 mg/day in 2–3 doses.	58	9	47–66	70	Seldom used. IM produces lower serum levels than oral.
Tetracycline	Cap 100, 250, 500 mg	PO 1–2 g/day in 2–4 divided doses.	77	10.6 ± 5	57–108	60	(See monograph.)
Tetracycline Hydrochloride Various	Tab 250, 500 mg Susp 25 mg/mL Top Soln 2.2 mg/mL Top Oint 3%.	Top (soln) for acne apply in the morning and evening.					

From reference 52 and product information.

Miscellaneous Antimicrobials

ATOVAQUONE
Mepron

Pharmacology. Atovaquone is a highly lipophilic hydroxynaphthoquinone with activity against *Pneumocystis carinii*, *Toxoplasma gondii*, and *Plasmodium* sp. It is a structural analogue of ubiquinone, a small hydrophobic respiratory chain electron carrier molecule found in mitochondria. The mechanism of antipneumocystis activity by atovaquone is unclear but might be inhibition of the mitochondrial electron transport chain, which inhibits pyrimidine synthesis and leads to inhibition of nucleic acid and ATP synthesis.[254,255]

Administration and Adult Dosage. **PO for PCP treatment** 750 mg bid for 21 days; **PO for PCP prophylaxis** 1.5 g once daily. (*See* Notes.)

Special Populations. *Pediatric Dosage.* Safety and efficacy not established.

Geriatric Dosage. (>65 yr) not evaluated, but dosage adjustment appears not to be necessary.

Other Conditions. Dosage alteration is not required with renal or hepatic impairment.

Dosage Forms. **Susp** 150 mg/mL.

Patient Instructions. It is extremely important to take this medication with food to increase absorption; failure to do so might limit response to therapy. Shake the suspension gently before use.

Missed Doses. Take this drug at regular intervals. If you miss a dose, take it as soon as you remember. If it is about time for the next dose, take that dose only. Leave at least 6–8 hours between doses. Do not double the dose or take extra.

Pharmacokinetics. *Serum Levels.* Steady-state serum levels >14 mg/L (>38 μmol/L) are correlated with survival in patients with PCP; serum levels <6 mg/L (<16 μmol/L) might be ineffective.[255]

Fate. Atovaquone exhibits slow, irregular absorption, depending on the formulation. A high-fat meal increases absorption of the suspension 2.3-fold compared with the fasting state. A peak concentration of 11.5 mg/L (31 μmol/L) is achieved with a single 750 mg dose of the suspension. Oral administration of 750 mg bid as the suspension produces a steady-state level of 24 mg/L (65 μmol/L). More than 99.9% is protein bound, and the drug does not appear to cross the blood–brain barrier well. It appears to undergo enterohepatic cycling with >94% excreted over 21 days in the feces, with no metabolite identified and <0.6% renally excreted.[255]

$t_{1/2}$. 67 ± 10 hr.[255]

Adverse Effects. Maculopapular rash occurs frequently, but many patients can continue atovaquone therapy; in most instances, the rash resolves without sequelae. GI disturbances such as abdominal pain, nausea, vomiting, and diarrhea occur in more than 10% of patients. Fever, headaches, and insomnia also have been reported frequently. Elevations of hepatic transaminases and hyponatremia occur frequently (1–10% of patients) but do not require cessation of therapy.

Contraindications. Severe diarrhea or malabsorption syndrome because pre-existing diarrhea is associated with poor outcome, presumably as a result of decreased absorption and serum levels.

Precautions. Lactation. Consider alternative therapy in patients who cannot take the drug with food or with GI disorders that might decrease oral absorption.

Drug Interactions. Rifampin can decrease atovaquone serum levels.

Parameters to Monitor. Baseline and periodic liver function tests for patients on prolonged treatment.

Notes. Use atovaquone only in the treatment of mild to moderate episodes of PCP. Atovaquone has been used for prevention of PCP in patients who cannot tolerate or who have failed other traditional prevention medication; although clinical trials are ongoing the safety, efficacy, and optimal dosage for this indication are not well established.

    Malarone tablets contain atovaquone 250 mg and **proguanil** 100 mg/tablet; Malarone Pediatric Tablets contain atovaquone 62.5 mg and proguanil 25 mg/tablet. Malarone is used for prevention or treatment of chloroquine-resistant malaria.

CHLORAMPHENICOL AND SALTS
Chloromycetin, Various

Pharmacology. Chloramphenicol is a broad-spectrum bacteriostatic antibiotic isolated from *Streptomyces venezuelae* and is particularly useful against ampicillin-resistant *Haemophilus influenzae*, *Salmonella* sp., rickettsial infections such as Rocky Mountain Spotted Fever, typhoid fever, most anaerobic organisms, and many vancomycin-resistant enterococci. It inhibits protein synthesis by binding the 50S ribosomal subunit and might be bactericidal against some bacteria including pneumococci, meningococci, and *H. influenzae*. Resistance occurs because of impermeability of the cell wall or bacterial production of chloramphenicol acetyltransferase, a plasmid-mediated enzyme that acetylates chloramphenicol into a microbiologically inert form.[209,250,256,257]

Administration and Adult Dosage. **PO or IV** 50–100 mg/kg/day in 4 divided doses, depending on severity, location, and organism, to a maximum of 4 g/day. **IM not recommended.**

Special Populations. *Pediatric Dosage.* **PO or IV** (<7 days or <2 kg) 25 mg/kg once daily; (neonates >7 days and >2 kg) 25 mg/kg q 12 hr; (older infants and children) 50–100 mg/kg/day given q 6 hr. These regimens produce unpredictable levels, and serum level monitoring is recommended.[253] **IM not recommended.**

Geriatric Dosage. Same as adult dosage.

Other Conditions. Reduce dosage with impaired liver function as guided by serum levels; no alteration necessary in impaired renal function.[253]

Dosage Forms. **Cap** 250 mg; **Inj** (as sodium succinate) 1 g (100 mg/mL when reconstituted); **Ophth Oint** 10 mg/g; **Ophth Pwdr for Soln** 25 mg/vial; **Ophth Soln** 5 mg/mL.

Pharmacokinetics. *Serum Levels.* Therapeutic peak 10-20 mg/L; therapeutic trough 5–10 mg/L. (*See* Adverse Reactions.)

Fate. Well absorbed orally with 75–90% bioavailability and a peak serum level of 12 mg/L after administration of 1 g to adults. IV 1 g produces levels of 5–12 mg/L (15–37 μmol/L) 1 hr after administration to normal adults. In infants and young children, hydrolysis of succinate to the active form can be slow and incomplete. IM administration produces serum levels of active drugs that are 50% lower than the equivalent oral dose. The drug attains therapeutic levels in most body cavities, the eye, and CSF; it is 53% plasma protein bound. V_d is 0.94 ± 0.06 L/kg; Cl is 0.14 ± 0.01 L/hr/kg. Most of the drug is eliminated by glucuronidation in the liver followed by excretion in the urine; the remainder is excreted in the urine unchanged. The rate of glucuronidation and renal elimination is greatly reduced in neonates; 6.5–80% of succinate can be excreted unhydrolyzed. Urine concentrations can be inadequate to treat UTIs, especially in patients with moderately to severely impaired renal function. A small amount (2–4%) of a dose appears in the bile and feces, mostly as the glucuronide.[52,250]

$t_{½}$. 4 ± 2 hr in healthy adults;[52] extremely prolonged and variable in neonates, infants, and young children. Unpredictable in patients with impaired liver function. Some normal patients and patients with impaired renal function exhibit impaired free drug elimination.

Adverse Reactions. Serum levels >25 mg/L (>77 μmol/L) frequently produce reversible bone marrow depression with reticulocytopenia, decreased hemoglobin, increased serum iron and iron-binding globulin saturation, thrombocytopenia, and mild leukopenia.[253] The drug inhibits iron uptake by bone marrow, and anemic patients do not respond to iron or vitamin B_{12} therapy while receiving chloramphenicol. This anemia most often follows parenteral therapy, large dosages, long duration of therapy, or impaired drug elimination. Complete recovery usually occurs within 1–2 weeks after drug discontinuation. Aplastic anemia occurs rarely (1/12,000 to 1/50,000) and can be fatal. It is not dose related and can occur long after a short course of oral or parenteral therapy;[253] its occurrence after ophthalmic or parenteral use is controversial.[259] Fatal cardiovascular-respiratory collapse (gray syndrome) can develop in neonates given excessive dosages. This syndrome is associated with serum levels of about 50–100 mg/L (155–310 μmol/L).[253] A similar syndrome has been reported in children and adults given large overdoses.

Contraindications. Trivial infections; prophylactic use; uses other than those for which it is indicated.

Precautions. Pregnancy; lactation. Use with caution in patients with liver disease (especially cirrhosis, ascites, and jaundice) or pre-existing hematologic disorders or patients receiving other bone marrow depressants. It can cause hemolytic episodes in patients with G-6-PD deficiency; observe dosage recommendations closely in neonates and infants.

Drug Interactions. Chloramphenicol inhibits CYP2C9 and increases serum concentrations of phenytoin, warfarin, and sulfonylurea oral hypoglycemic agents. Phenytoin, phenobarbital, and rifampin can decrease serum levels of chloramphenicol.

Parameters to Monitor. CBC with platelet and reticulocyte counts before and frequently during therapy; serum iron and iron-binding globulin saturation also might be useful. Liver and renal function tests before and occasionally during therapy. Monitor serum levels weekly because of variability in Pharmacokinetics. More frequent monitoring might be necessary in patient with hepatic dysfunction and during long-term (>2 weeks) therapy.

CLINDAMYCIN SALTS
Cleocin, Various

Pharmacology. Clindamycin is a semisynthetic 7-chloro, 7-deoxylincomycin derivative that is active against most Gram-positive organisms except enterococci and *Clostridium difficile*. Gram-negative aerobes are resistant, but most anaerobes are sensitive. It inhibits bacterial protein synthesis by binding to the 50S ribosomal subunit; it is bactericidal or bacteriostatic depending on the concentration, organism, and inoculum.[260,261]

Administration and Adult Dosage. **PO** 150–450 mg q 6-8 hr; **PO for prevention of endocarditis in patients at risk undergoing dental, oral, or upper respiratory tract procedures and who are allergic to penicillin** 600 mg 1 hr before procedure.[219] **IM or IV** 600 mg–2.7 g/day in 2–4 divided doses, to a maximum of 4.8 g/day. **IV for endocarditis prophylaxis** 600 mg within 30 min before a dental procedure. Single IM doses >600 mg are not recommended; infuse IV no faster than 30 mg/min. **Top for acne** apply bid. **Vag for bacterial vaginosis** 1 applicatorful hs for 7 days.

Special Populations. *Pediatric Dosage.* **PO** (<10 kg) give no less than 37.5 mg q 8 hr; (>10 kg) 8–25 mg/kg/day in 3 or 4 divided doses; **PO for endocarditis prophylaxis** 20 mg/kg 1 hr before a dental procedure. **IM or IV** (<1 month) 15–20 mg/kg/day in 3 or 4 divided doses; the lower dosage may be adequate for premature infants; (>1 month) 15–40 mg/kg/day in 3 or 4 divided doses (not less than 300 mg/day in severe infection, regardless of weight). **IV for endocarditis prophylaxis** 20 mg/kg within 30 min before a dental procedure.

Geriatric Dosage. Same as adult dosage.

Other Conditions. Dosage adjustment is unnecessary in renal impairment or cirrhosis, although the effect of acute liver disease is unknown.[253,260,262]

Dosage Forms. **Cap** (as hydrochloride) 75, 150, 300 mg; **Soln** (as palmitate) 15 mg/mL (reconstituted); **Inj** (as phosphate) 150 mg/mL; **Top Soln** (as phosphate) 1%; **Top Gel** (as phosphate) 1%; **Vag Crm** 2%.

Patient Instructions. Report any severe diarrhea or blood in the stools immediately and do *not* take antidiarrheal medication. Do not refrigerate the reconstituted oral solution because it will thicken.

Missed Doses. Take this drug at regular intervals. If you miss a dose, take it as soon as you remember. If it is about time for the next dose, take that dose only. Leave at least 4–6 hours between doses. Do not double the dose or take extra.

Pharmacokinetics. *Fate.* Absorption is nearly 87% and is the same from the capsule or the solution; food can delay, but not decrease, absorption. The palmitate and phosphate esters are absorbed intact and rapidly hydrolyzed to the active base. Unhydrolyzed phosphate ester usually constitutes <20% of the total peak serum level after parenteral clindamycin but can increase to 40% in patients with impaired renal function. A 500 mg oral dose produces a peak serum level of 5–6 mg/L (12–14 μmol/L) in 1 hr. A 300 mg IM dose produces a peak level of 5–6 mg/L 1–2 hr postinjection. A 600 mg IV dose infused over 30 min produces a peak serum level of 10 mg/L (23 μmol/L). The drug is widely distributed throughout the body except the CSF. It is 94% plasma protein bound; V_d is 1.1 ± 0.3 L/kg; Cl is 0.28 ± 0.08 L/hr/kg. There is hepatic metabolism and excretion of active forms in the bile. From 5% to 10% of the absorbed dose is recovered as unchanged drug and active metabolites in the urine within 24 hr.[52,253,260,263]

$t_{1/2}$. 2.9 ± 0.7 hr; increased in premature infants;[52] unchanged or slightly increased in severe renal disease; might be increased or unchanged in liver disease.[261]

Adverse Reactions. After oral administration, anorexia, nausea, vomiting, cramps, and diarrhea occur frequently.[253,260,262] Oral and rarely parenteral clindamycin can cause severe, sometimes fatal, pseudomembranous colitis (PMC), which might be clinically indistinguishable at onset from non-PMC diarrhea.[260] Antibiotic-associated PMC is secondary to overgrowth of toxin-producing *Clostridium difficile*. Symptoms usually appear 2–9 days after initiation of therapy. PMC has been reported after topical administration.[262] PMC is terminated in many patients by discontinuing the antibiotic immediately; however, if diarrhea is severe or does not improve promptly after discontinuation, treat with oral metronidazole or vancomycin.[260,261] The value of corticosteroids, cholestyramine, and antispasmodics in the management of antibiotic-associated diarrhea and PMC has not been established.[260] Antidiarrheals such as diphenoxylate or loperamide may worsen PMC and should *not* be used.

Precautions. Pregnancy; lactation. Use with caution in neonates <4 weeks of age and in patients with liver disease. Discontinue *immediately* if severe diarrhea occurs. Drug accumulation might occur in patients with severe concomitant hepatic and renal dysfunction, but data are lacking.

Drug Interactions. Clindamycin might enhance the action of nondepolarizing neuromuscular blocking agents. Kaolin-pectin mixture delays but does not decrease oral absorption of clindamycin.

Parameters to Monitor. Observe for changes in bowel frequency.

Notes. Oral solution is stable for 2 weeks at room temperature after reconstitution; do not refrigerate.

LINEZOLID Zyvox

Pharmacology. Linezolid belongs to a new class of anti-infective agents known as oxazolidinones. It inhibits protein synthesis by binding to the bacterial 23S ribosomal RNA of the 50S subunit and prevents the formation of a functional 70S initiation complex inhibiting bacterial translation. It has bacteriostatic activity against staphylococci and enterococci including vancomycin-resistant *Enterococcus faecium* and *faecalis* and bactericidal activity against most streptococcal strains. In vitro the spectrum also includes certain Gram-negative and anaerobic organisms. Linezolid is a reversible, nonselective inhibitor of monoamine oxidase.[264]

Administration and Adult Dosage. PO or IV 400–600 mg q 12 hr.

Special Populations. *Pediatric Dosage.* Safety not established in infants and children. **PO or IV** a dosage of 10 mg/kg q 12 hr has been used.

Geriatric Dosage. Same as adult dosage.

Other Conditions. No dosage adjustment necessary in renal or hepatic insufficiency.

Dosage Forms. **Tab** 400, 600 mg; **Inj** 2 mg/mL; **Susp** 20 mg/mL.

Patient Instructions. This drug may be taken without regard to meals. Avoid concurrent use of diet pills and cough-and-cold remedies and restrict consumption of aged foods high in tyramine. (*See* Foods That Interact with MAO Inhibitors Chart in the Antidepressants chapter.)

Missed Doses. Take this drug at regular intervals. If you miss a dose, take it as soon as you remember. If it is about time for the next dose, take that dose only.

Pharmacokinetics. *Fate.* Rapidly absorbed orally; bioavailability is approximately 100% and not affected by food. A single dose of 600 mg achieves a peak of 12.7 mg/L when administered orally and 12.9 mg/L IV. Plasma protein binding is 31% and linezolid is readily distributed into well-perfused tissues. Linezolid is primarily metabolized by oxidation. Nonrenal clearance accounts for approximately 65% of the total clearance. Children appear to have a higher average clearance.

$t_{1/2}$. 4.7–5.4 hr in adults.

Adverse Reactions. Adverse reactions are usually mild to moderate and the most commonly reported are diarrhea, headache, and nausea. Occasional reactions are oral and vaginal candidiasis, hypertension, dyspepsia, abdominal pain, pruritus, and tongue discoloration. Treatment periods beyond 28 days have not been evaluated and are not recommended.

Precautions. Pregnancy; lactation. Linezolid can lead to pseudomembranous colitis, so it is an important consideration if patients present with diarrhea. Avoid large quantities of food containing tyramine (>100 mg/meal) with linezolid. Use caution with pre-existing myelosuppression, other drugs that cause myelosuppression, or chronic infection with previous or concomitant antibiotic therapy. Myelosuppression (including anemia, leukopenia, pancytopenia and thrombocytopenia) has been reported; consider discontinuing therapy if this occurs or worsens. Myelosuppression is usually reversible after drug discontinuation.

Drug Interactions. Linezolid is not metabolized by cytochrome P450 and does not inhibit or induce the activities of clinically important CYP isoforms. By inhibiting MAO, it can interact with adrenergic and serotonergic agents such as phenylpropanolamine and pseudoephedrine; reduce initial doses of epinephrine and dopamine and titrate to response.

Parameters to Monitor. CBC with platelet counts before and during weekly therapy.

Notes. Although the drug is effective for many types of infections, it should generally be reserved for treating resistant organisms.

METRONIDAZOLE
Flagyl, MetroGel, Various

Pharmacology. Metronidazole is a synthetic nitroimidazole active against *Trichomonas vaginalis* (trichomoniasis), *Entamoeba histolytica* (amebiasis), and *Giardia lamblia* (giardiasis); it is bactericidal against nearly all obligate anaerobic bacteria including *Bacteroides fragilis*. It is inactive against aerobic bacteria and requires microbial reduction by a nitroreductase enzyme to form highly reactive intermediates that disrupt bacterial DNA and inhibit nucleic acid synthesis, leading to cell death.[258]

Administration and Adult Dosage. **PO or IV for anaerobic infections** 15 mg/kg (usually 1 g) initially, followed by 7.5 mg/kg (usually 500 mg) q 6–8 hr, to a maximum of 2 g/day. Infuse each IV dose over 1 hr. **PO for antibiotic-associated colitis** 250 mg qid for 7–10 days.[265] (*See* Notes.) **PO for trichomoniasis** 2 g as a single dose or in 2 doses on the same day, or 500 mg bid for 7 days.[195] **PO for giardiasis** 250 mg tid for 5 days. (*See* Notes.)[265] **PO for symptomatic intestinal amebiasis** (amebic dysentery) 750 mg tid for 10 days. **PO for extraintestinal amebiasis** 750 mg tid for 10 days;[265] some practitioners include a drug effective against the intestinal cyst form because occasional failures with metronidazole therapy have been reported. **PO for bacterial vaginosis** 500 mg bid for 7 days, or 2 g as a single dose.[195] **Vag for bacterial vaginosis** 1 applicatorful (5 g) bid for 5 days. **Top for rosacea** apply bid.

Special Populations. *Pediatric Dosage.* **IV for anaerobic infections** (preterm infants) 15 mg/kg once, then 7.5 mg/kg q 24–48 hr; (term infants) 15 mg/kg once, then 7.5 mg/kg q 12–24 hr; (infants >1 week old and children) same as adult mg/kg dosage. **PO for giardiasis** 15 mg/kg/day in 3 divided doses for 5 days, to a maximum of 750 mg/day. (*See* Notes.) **PO for amebic dysentery or extraintestinal amebiasis** 35–50 mg/kg/day in 3 divided doses for 10 days, to a maximum of 2.5 g/day.

Geriatric Dosage. (>65 yr) decreased clearance can result in accumulation of the drug. Dosage reduction or changing dosage interval to once or twice daily are reasonable modifications to avoid potential adverse reactions.[266]

Other Conditions. No dosage alteration required with renal impairment. Patients with substantial liver dysfunction metabolize metronidazole slowly, with resultant accumulation of metronidazole and its metabolites in the serum. For such patients, it has been suggested that dosage intervals be increased to 12–24 hr, although specific guidelines are not available.[266]

Dosage Forms. **Cap** 375 mg; **SR Tab** 750 mg; **Tab** 250, 500 mg; **Inj** 500 mg; **Crm** 1%; **Top Gel** 0.75%; **Vag Gel** 0.75%.

Patient Instructions. This drug may be taken with food to minimize stomach upset. It can cause a harmless dark discoloration of the urine and metallic taste in the mouth. Nausea, vomiting, flushing, and faintness can occur if alcohol is taken during therapy with this drug.

Missed Doses. Take this drug at regular intervals. If you miss a dose, take it as soon as you remember. If it is about time for the next dose, take that dose only. Leave at least 4–6 hours between doses. Do not double the dose or take extra.

Pharmacokinetics. *Serum Levels.* Not used clinically.

Fate. IV 500 mg q 12 hr over 1 hr produces steady-state peak and trough levels of 23.6 mg/L (138 μmol/L) and 6.7 mg/L (39 μmol/L), respectively. IV 500 mg q 8 hr over 1 hr produces steady-state peak and trough levels of 27.4 mg/L (160 μmol/L) and 15.5 mg/L (91 μmol/L), respectively. Well absorbed orally with levels similar to those after IV infusion; 250 and 500 mg doses produce peak concentrations of 4–6 mg/L (23–35 μmol/L) and 10–13 mg/L (58–76 μmol/L), respectively, at 1–2 hr in adults. Bioavailability of vaginal gel is 53–58%. Less than 20% plasma protein bound; wide distribution with therapeutic levels in many tissues, including abscesses, bile, bone, breast milk, CSF, and saliva. V_d is 0.85 ± 0.25 L/kg; Cl is 0.07 ± 0.02 L/hr/kg. Extensively metabolized in the liver by hydroxylation, oxidation, and glucuronide formation; 44–80% excreted in the urine in 24 hr, about 6–18% as unchanged drug.[265,266]

$t_{\frac{1}{2}}$. 6–10 hr in adults; not increased with impaired renal function; prolonged variably with severe hepatic impairment.[52,265,266]

Adverse Effects. Metallic taste in mouth and GI complaints occur frequently with high dosages. Occasional dizziness, vertigo, and paresthesias have been reported with very high dosages. Reversible mild neutropenia reported occasionally.[209,265] Reversible, rare, but severe peripheral neuropathy can occur with high dosages given over prolonged periods. Antibiotic-associated colitis has been reported rarely with oral metronidazole. The IV preparation is occasionally associated with phlebitis at the infusion site. Experimental production of tumors in some rodent species and mutations in bacteria have raised concern regarding potential carcinogenicity; to date, human epidemiologic research has not detected an appreciable risk, although more data are needed.[265]

Contraindications. First trimester of pregnancy, although there is no direct evidence of teratogenicity in humans or animals.[209]

Precautions. Pregnancy; lactation; active CNS disease or neutropenia; hepatic impairment.

Drug Interactions. Disulfiram-like reactions are reported with concurrent alcohol use but are uncommon. Confusion and psychotic episodes have been reported with concurrent disulfiram; avoid this combination, if possible. Metronidazole inhibits CYP2C9, CYP3A3/4, and CYP3A5-7 and can affect the metabolism of many drugs; the best documented is an enhanced hypoprothrombinemic response to warfarin. Phenytoin metabolism also might be inhibited. It is also a substrate of CYP2C9.

Parameters to Monitor. Before and after the completion of any lengthy or repeated courses of therapy, monitor WBC count. Monitor signs of toxicity in patients with severe liver disease.[266]

Notes. The treatment of *asymptomatic* trichomoniasis is controversial. Signs of endocervical inflammation or erosion on physical examination are considered an indication for treatment. Also, most practitioners treat asymptomatic male consorts because lack of such treatment might be a cause of treatment failure or recurrent infection of the female partner.[195] Metronidazole has been used in combination regimens to treat *Helicobacter pylori*–infected patients with duodenal or gastric ulcers. (*See* Gastrointestinal Drugs, Treatment of *Helicobacter pylori* in Peptic Ulcer Disease Comparison Chart.) Although it is slightly less effective than **vancomycin**, metronidazole is considered by some to be the drug of choice for antibiotic-associated pseudomembranous colitis because of its lower cost[267] and the emergence of vancomycin-resistant enterococci.

NITROFURANTOIN   Macrodantin, Macrobid, Various

Pharmacology. Nitrofurantoin is a synthetic nitrofuran that is active against most bacteria that cause UTIs except *P. aeruginosa, Proteus* sp., many *Enterobacter* sp., and *Klebsiella* spp. The drug is used primarily to prevent recurrent UTIs but is also effective in the treatment of uncomplicated UTIs.[268]

Adult Dosage. PO for UTI (macrocrystals) 50–100 mg qid with meals and hs for treatment; (Macrobid) 100 mg bid for 7 days. **PO for chronic suppression** 50–100 mg hs. The drug should be taken with food.

Pediatric Dosage. PO for treatment of UTI 5–7 mg/kg/day in 4 divided doses, to a maximum of 400 mg/day; **PO for chronic UTI suppression** 1 mg/kg/day in 1–2 doses, to a maximum of 100 mg/day.

Dosage Forms. Cap (macrocrystals) 25, 50, 100 mg; **Susp** 5 mg/mL; **Cap** 100 mg, containing 25 mg as macrocrystals and 75 mg in an SR form (Macrobid).

Pharmacokinetics. Well absorbed orally; however, serum and extraurinary tissue concentrations are subtherapeutic. About 60% of drug is metabolized to inactive metabolites; 25–35% is excreted in urine with a urine concentration of about 200 mg/L from an average dose.

Adverse Reactions. Adverse effects are primarily nausea, vomiting, and diarrhea and are dose related; use of the macrocrystalline form and administration with food can minimize GI distress. Hypersensitivity reactions such as rash occur only rarely. Acute allergic pneumonitis is reversible with discontinuation of therapy. Chronic interstitial pulmonary fibrosis also occurs occasionally with long-term therapy and might be irreversible. Ascending polyneuropathy associated with prolonged high-dose therapy or use of the drug in renal failure is only slowly reversible. Intravascular hemolysis can occur in patients with severe G-6-PD deficiency. Although the drug is mutagenic in mammalian cells, there is no clinical evidence of carcinogenicity or teratogenicity.

PENTAMIDINE ISETHIONATE   Pentam 300, NebuPent

Pharmacology. Pentamidine is an aromatic diamidine used in the treatment of trypanosomiasis and PCP. Pentamidine inhibits dihydrofolate reductase, interferes with anaerobic glycolysis, inhibits oxidative phosphorylation, and limits nucleic acid and protein synthesis, but the mechanism by which pentamidine kills *P. carinii* is unclear.[269]

Administration and Adult Dosage. IV (preferred) or IM 3–4 mg/kg/day as a single dose for 2–3 weeks; infuse IV over 60 min. **Inhal for PCP prophylaxis in high-risk HIV-infected patients** 300 mg q 4 weeks via Respirguard II nebulizer. (*See* Notes.)

Special Populations. *Pediatric Dosage.* Same as adult dosage.

Geriatric Dosage. Same as adult dosage.

Other Conditions. Dosage adjustment does not appear necessary in renal impairment.[270]

Dosage Forms. **Inj** 300 mg; **Inhal** 300 mg.

Pharmacokinetics. *Serum Levels.* Not used clinically.

Fate. Negligible oral absorption. Peak serum levels of 0.5–3 mg/L (1.5–8.8 μmol/L) occur after 4 mg/kg IV infusion. Serum levels are very low after inhalation (<0.1 mg/L). About 70% plasma protein bound; distributed widely in tissues, with highest concentrations found in spleen, liver, kidneys, and adrenal glands. V_c is 3 L/kg; terminal V_d is 190 ± 70 L/kg; Cl is 1.08 ± 0.42 L/hr/kg. There are no data on the effects of liver impairment. Less than 20% of a dose is excreted unchanged in urine.[52,271]

$t_{1/2}$. α phase 1.2 ± 0.6 hr; terminal elimination half-life is up to 29 ± 25 days, suggesting rapid tissue uptake with slow release and subsequent urinary excretion.[270]

Adverse Reactions. With IV administration, nephrotoxicity occurs in up to 25% of patients, hypoglycemia in up to 27%, and hypotension in up to 10% of patients. Fever, rash, leukopenia, and liver damage occur occasionally. Hyperglycemia, type 1 diabetes mellitus, and pancreatitis have been reported. Pentamidine-induced torsades de pointes occurs rarely. IM injection frequently produces pain and abscess formation at the injection site. With aerosolized pentamidine, reversible bronchoconstriction and unpleasant taste occur frequently. Severe adverse reactions are less frequent, but reports of pancreatitis, hypoglycemia, and cutaneous eruptions have occurred rarely, suggesting some systemic absorption.[269]

Precautions. Use with caution in diabetes mellitus.

Drug Interactions. IV pentamidine can increase the risk of hypocalcemia with foscarnet; avoid this combination, if possible, although inhaled pentamidine does not seem to be a risk factor.

Parameters to Monitor. Obtain serum glucose, Cr_s, BUN, liver function tests, electrolytes, and CBC and platelet counts daily. Monitor blood pressure after administration.

Notes. Concomitant therapy with pentamidine and **trimethoprim-sulfamethoxazole** appears to offer no benefit and might be additively toxic. There is concern about occupational exposure with inhalation therapy. No studies have determined the health effects of exposure to pentamidine itself; however, transmission of tuberculosis to health care workers has been attributed in part to the use of aerosolized pentamidine among clinic patients coinfected with HIV and tuberculosis. Health care workers administering aerosolized pentamidine should wear masks and protective eye wear.[269]

QUINUPRISTIN AND DALFOPRISTIN   Synercid

Pharmacology. Quinupristin and dalfopristin are streptogramin antibiotics that are naturally occurring compounds isolated from *Streptomyces pristinaspiralis*. Quinupristin, a derivative of pristinamycin IA, and dalfopristin, a derivative of pristinamycin IIA, are combined in a fixed ratio of 30:70 (w/w). This combination inhibits protein synthesis by sequential binding to the 50S subunit of bacterial ribosomes; its synergistic activity can be caused by binding of dalfopristin, altering conformation of the ribosome such that its affinity for quinupristin is increased. Individually, pristinamycin I and II are bacteriostatic, but in combination they are bactericidal against Gram-positive bacteria, including MRSA. Synergy has been reported with vancomycin against MRSA and multiply resistant enterococci. It also has activity against anaerobic organisms, but most Gram-negative organisms such as the Enterobacteriacae, *Acinetobacter* spp., and *P. aeruginosa* are resistant.[272-274] Although the drug is effective for many types of infections, it should generally be reserved for treating resistant organisms such as vancomycin-resistant *Enterococcus faecium*. It has no activity against *Enterococcus faecalis*.

Adult Dosage. IV 7.5 mg/kg (of the combination) q 8–12 hr infused in D5W over 60 min. Consider reducing dosage in patients with hepatic impairment who do not tolerate the usual dosage. However, specific guidelines have not been established.

Dosage Forms. Inj 500 mg (quinupristin 150 mg and dalfopristin 350 mg)/10 mL vial.

Pharmacokinetics. The pharmacokinetics are complex and not fully elucidated. Peak concentrations are 2.4–2.8 mg/L (2.3–2.7 μmol/L) for quinupristin and 6.2–7.2 mg/L (9–10.4 μmol/L) for dalfopristin after a 7.5 mg/kg dose in healthy volunteers. Quinupristin is about 90% protein bound and dalfopristin is 10–36% bound in vitro. Clearance of both drugs decreases with repeated doses and in obese patients. Dalfopristin might have an active metabolite. Both drugs are eliminated primarily in feces, with only about 15–20% excreted unchanged in urine. Half-lives are about 1 hr for quinupristin and 0.5–1 hr for dalfopristin, both possibly increased in cirrhosis.

Adverse Reactions. Mild to moderate local reactions of itching, pain, and burning at the injection site are frequent and often lead to drug discontinuation. To avoid such side effects, administer the drug through a central venous catheter. Nausea, vomiting, diarrhea, and headache also have been reported frequently. Occasionally, reversible myalgia and arthralgia occur and liver function tests are increased.

Drug Interactions. Quinupristin/dalfopristin inhibits CYP3A4 and markedly impairs cyclosporine clearance, requiring cyclosporine dosage reduction.

TELITHROMYCIN (Investigational—Aventis)   Ketek

Pharmacology. Telithromycin is a ketolide antibiotic, a class similar to macrolides with a similar mechanism of action. It has good activity against Gram-positive organisms, especially respiratory pathogens such as *S. aureus, S. pneumoniae, H. influenzae, M. catarrhalis* and some atypical organisms and anaerobes. It is active against some macrolide-resistant Gram-positive cocci.

Adult Dosage. PO for community-acquired pneumonia 800 mg once daily. No change required in renal or hepatic dysfunction.

Dosage Forms. Tab (investigational).

Pharmacokinetics. Following an 800 mg oral dose, a peak level of 2.3 mg/L occurs in 1 hr. It is primarily metabolized in the liver and about 18% is excreted unchanged in urine. Terminal half-life is about 10 hours with single doses, and about 13 hr with multiple doses.

Adverse Reactions. The most frequent adverse reactions are nausea, diarrhea and GI pain similar to the macrolides. Elevated LFTs and hepatoxicity reported.

TRIMETHOPRIM Proloprim, Trimpex, Various

Pharmacology. Trimethoprim is a synthetic folate-antagonist antibacterial. (*See* Trimethoprim and Sulfamethoxazole.) Trimethoprim is effective in acute UTI. It has a potential advantage over the sulfa-containing combination in patients with allergy or toxicity attributed to sulfonamides; however, the relative potential for trimethoprim alone to permit the development of resistance is undetermined. Used alone, trimethoprim is ineffective against *Pneumocystis carinii*, but in combination with **dapsone** (a sulfone), it is effective in treating mild to moderate PCP.[246,247]

Adult Dosage. **PO for uncomplicated acute UTI** 200 mg/day in 1 or 2 doses for 10 days. **PO for the treatment of mild to moderate (PaO$_2$ >60 mm Hg) PCP** 20 mg/kg/day in 3 or 4 divided doses with dapsone 100 mg once daily.

Dosage Forms. **Tab** 100, 200 mg; **Soln** 10 mg/mL.

Pharmacokinetics. Trimethoprim is rapidly absorbed orally. A 100 mg dose yields a serum concentration of 1 mg/L (3.4 μmol/L) 1–4 hr after the dose. It is 40% plasma protein bound and 50–60% is excreted unchanged in urine. Half-life is 8–10 hr with normal renal function.

Adverse Reactions. Occasional adverse effects are mild thrombocytopenia, nausea, fever, and rash; the frequency appears to be dose related. Methemoglobinemia and dose-related hemolysis have occurred in patients with G-6-PD deficiency receiving dapsone with trimethoprim; it is important to check G-6-PD status before initiating combination therapy.

TRIMETREXATE Neutrexin

Pharmacology. Trimetrexate is a lipophilic analogue of methotrexate that inhibits dihydrofolate reductase, leading to the disruption of purine biosynthesis. It has activity against *Pneumocystis carinii* and *Toxoplasma gondii* and has demonstrated modest efficacy against a number of malignancies. It is approved for the treatment of moderate to severe PCP in immunocompromised patients and has been used investigationally in advanced solid tumors alone or in combination with **fluorouracil** and **leucovorin**.[275–277]

Adult Dosage. **IV for moderate to severe PCP** 45 mg/m^2/day infused over 60–90 min for 21 days. Give IV or PO calcium leucovorin 20 mg/m^2 q 6 hr concomitantly and continue it for 3 days after the end of trimetrexate administration. **IV for colorectal cancer** 110 mg/m^2 on day 1, followed by leucovorin 200 mg/m^2 and a fluorouracil-leucovorin regimen on day 2. **IV for advanced urogenital cancer** 8 mg/m^2/day for 5 days q 3 weeks.[278] Reduce dosage by 50% in patients with Cr$_s$ >1.6 mg/dL.

Dosage Forms. **Inj** 25 mg.

Pharmacokinetics. Trimetrexate has at least 2 metabolites, both of which inhibit dihydrofolate reductase. It is eliminated primarily by hepatic metabolism; less than one-third is excreted unchanged in urine. The elimination half-life is 4–12 hr in patients with AIDS and PCP and 8–26 hr in patients with cancer.

Adverse Reactions. The primary toxicity is myelosuppression (neutropenia, thrombocytopenia, and anemia); myelosuppression is minimized with concurrent administration of calcium leucovorin. Hypoalbuminemia (($\leq$3.5 g/dL) or hypoproteinemia ($\leq$6 g/dL) increase the risk of severe or life-threatening myelosuppression, presumably because of increased unbound drug levels.[279] Elevated liver function tests, fever, rash, peripheral neuropathy, mucositis, and nausea or vomiting occur frequently. Hypersensitivity reactions and seizures are reported rarely.

VANCOMYCIN HYDROCHLORIDE
Vancocin, Various

Pharmacology. Vancomycin is a glycopeptide that binds irreversibly to the cell wall in a manner slightly different from β-lactams. Many Gram-positive cocci and bacilli, including MRSA and *Clostridium difficile*, are inhibited. Most Gram-negative bacteria are resistant, and vancomycin-resistant enterococci have been reported in association with overuse of vancomycin.[243] Glycopeptide intermediately resistant *S. aureus* have been reported.

Administration and Adult Dosage. **IV** 20–30 mg/kg/day (usually 2 g/day) in 2–4 divided doses as a dilute infusion over 1–2 hr. **PO for staphylococcal enterocolitis** 2 g/day in 2–4 divided doses. **PO for antibiotic-associated colitis** 125–500 mg q 6 hr for 7–10 days; retreat with a longer course if relapse occurs. (*See* Notes.) **Not for IM use.**

Special Populations. *Pediatric Dosage.* **IV** (neonates) 20 mg/kg/day; (older infants and children) 40 mg/kg/day in 2–4 divided doses. **PO** 10–50 mg/kg/day in 4 divided doses. **Not for IM use.**

Geriatric Dosage. Same as adult dosage but adjust for age-related reduction in renal function.

Other Conditions. Adjust dosage carefully in renal impairment; Cl is directly related to Cl$_{cr}$. Anuric patients on hemodialysis have been given the usual dose q 3–7 days. Dosage adjustment is unnecessary in liver disease.

Dosage Forms. **Cap** 125, 250 mg; **Susp** 1, 10 g; **Inj** 500 mg, 1, 5, 10 g.

Patient Instructions. Report pain at infusion site, dizziness, or fullness or ringing in ears with intravenous use; nausea or vomiting with oral use.

Missed Doses. (Oral) if you miss a dose, take it as soon as you remember. If it is about time for the next dose, take that dose only.

Pharmacokinetics. *Serum Levels.* Therapeutic range is not well defined. Ototoxicity has been associated with high serum concentrations but has been noted at lower levels.[280,281] Peaks thought to be associated with efficacy are 20–40 mg/L (14–28 μmol/L); troughs >15 mg/L (>10 μmol/L) might be excessive.

Fate. Oral absorption is negligible, although appreciable serum levels can be observed in patients with renal dysfunction receiving oral vancomycin for

C. difficile-induced antibiotic-associated colitis. Fecal concentrations with PO 500 mg q 6 hr reach 3 mg/g. IV 500 mg produces serum levels of 6–10 mg/L (4–7 μmol/L) in 1 hr. Plasma protein binding is 30 ± 10%. The drug is widely distributed, except into the CSF, although some success has been reported in the treatment of meningitis, particularly in children. V_c is 0.1–0.15 L/kg; V_{d_∞} is 0.39 ± 0.06 L/kg; Cl is 0.084 L/hr/kg with normal renal function. In renal impairment, Cl (in mL/min) can be estimated as $[0.79 \times Cl_{cr}$ (in mL/min)$] + 3.5$. Metabolism and biliary excretion are negligible; 80–90% is excreted unchanged in the urine within 48 hr.[52,282]

$t_{\frac{1}{2}}$. β phase 5.6 ± 1.8 hr, 6–10 days with renal impairment. No change with hepatic disease.[52,279]

Adverse Reactions. Chills, fever, nausea, and phlebitis can occur frequently, especially with direct injection of undiluted drug (not recommended). Rapid infusion can cause transient systolic hypotension.[283] The "red man" or "red neck" syndrome of erythema, pruritus, and localized edema is associated with histamine release caused by rapid infusions of doses ≥500 mg; it often does not occur or is less severe with subsequent doses.[284] Extravasation causes local tissue necrosis. Ototoxicity (auditory and vestibular) and possibly nephrotoxicity occur but have not been definitely linked to high serum levels.[281,285] Eosinophilia, neutropenia, and urticarial rashes have been reported frequently. Side effects of vancomycin might not be as prevalent today as in the past, perhaps because of changes in the manufacturing process that eliminated some impurities.[286]

Precautions. Pregnancy. Use with caution in patients with impaired renal function or pre-existing hearing loss or in those receiving other ototoxic or nephrotoxic agents.

Drug Interactions. Administration with an aminoglycoside can increase the risk of nephrotoxicity.[286]

Parameters to Monitor. With IV use, obtain initial renal function tests and repeat twice weekly during therapy. Routine monitoring of serum levels in patients with normal renal function is not recommended because it has questionable value, but is often performed.[285] Check for signs of phlebitis daily.

Notes. An alternative agent for treatment or prophylaxis of staphylococcal or streptococcal infections when a less toxic agent is inappropriate (eg, penicillin or cephalosporin allergy, or resistant organisms) or has not produced an adequate therapeutic response. Use of vancomycin in antibiotic-associated colitis is becoming less desirable because of the emergence of vancomycin-resistant enterococci. Reserve vancomycin for cases refractory to metronidazole.[267]

REFERENCES

1. Lortholary O et al. Aminoglycosides. *Med Clin North Am* 1995;79:761–87.
2. Gilbert DN. Aminoglycosides. In, Mandell GL et al., eds. *Principles and practice of infectious diseases.* 5th ed. Churchill Livingstone: New York; 2000:307–36.
3. Preston SL, Briceland LL. Single daily dosing of aminoglycosides. *Pharmacotherapy* 1995;15:297–306.
4. Nicolau DP et al. Experience with a once-daily aminoglycoside program administered to 2184 patients. *Antimicrob Agents Chemother* 1995;39:650–5.

5. Blaser J et al. Monitoring serum concentrations for once-daily netilmicin dosing regimens. *J Antimicrob Chemother* 1994;33:341–8.
6. Sarubbi FA, Hull JH. Amikacin serum concentrations, predictions of levels and dosage guidelines. *Ann Intern Med* 1978;89:612–8.
7. Walshe JJ et al. Crossover pharmacokinetic analysis comparing intravenous and intraperitoneal administration of tobramycin. *J Infect Dis* 1986;153:796–9.
8. Zaske DE. Aminoglycosides. In, Evans WE et al., eds. *Applied pharmacokinetics. Principles of therapeutic drug monitoring.* 3rd ed. Vancouver, WA: Applied Therapeutics; 1992;14:1–47.
9. Kahlmeter G, Dahlager JI. Aminoglycoside toxicity—a review of clinical studies published between 1975 and 1982. *J Antimicrob Chemother* 1984;13(suppl A):9–22.
10. McCormack JP, Jewesson PJ. A critical reevaluation of the "therapeutic range" of aminoglycosides. *Clin Infect Dis* 1992;14:320–9.
11. Pickering LK et al. Effect of concentration and time upon inactivation of tobramycin, gentamicin, netilmicin, and amikacin by azlocillin, carbenicillin, mecillinam, mezlocillin, and piperacillin. *J Pharmacol Exp Ther* 1981;217:345–9.
12. Thompson MIB et al. Gentamicin inactivation by piperacillin or carbenicillin in patients with end-stage renal disease. *Antimicrob Agents Chemother* 1982;21:268–73.
13. Erdmay SM et al. An updated comparison of drug dosing methods. Part III. Aminoglycoside antibiotics. *Clin Pharmacokinet* 1991;20:374–88.
14. Massey KL et al. Identification of children in whom routine aminoglycoside serum concentration monitoring is not cost-effective. *J Pediatr* 1986;109:897–901.
15. Moore RD et al. Clinical response to aminoglycoside therapy: importance of the ratio of peak concentration to minimum inhibitory concentration. *J Infect Dis* 1987;155:93–9.
16. Gallis HA et al. Amphotericin B: 30 years of clinical experience. *Rev Infect Dis* 1990;12:308–9.
17. Gary-Bobo CM. Polyene-sterol interaction and selective toxicity. *Biochimie* 1989;71:37–47.
18. Kintzel PE et al. Practical guidelines for preparing and administering amphotericin B. *Am J Hosp Pharm* 1992;49:1156–64.
19. Kline S et al. Limited toxicity of prolonged therapy with high doses of amphotericin B lipid complex. *Clin Infect Dis* 1995;21:1154–8.
20. O'Donnell MR et al. Prediction of systemic fungal infection in allogeneic marrow recipients: impact of amphotericin B prophylaxis in high-risk patients. *J Clin Oncol* 1994;12:827–34.
21. Bennett JE. Antifungal drugs. In, Mandell GL et al., eds. *Principles and practice of infectious diseases.* 3rd ed. New York: Churchill Livingstone; 1990:361–76.
22. Varkey B et al. Pulmonary aspergilloma. A rational approach to treatment. *Am J Med* 1976;61:626–31.
23. Schwartz S et al. Aerosolized amphotericin B inhalations as prophylaxis of invasive aspergillus infections during prolonged neutropenia: results of a prospective randomized multicenter trial. *Blood* 1999;93:3654–61.
24. Trigg ME et al. Successful program to prevent aspergillus infections in children undergoing marrow transplantation: use of nasal amphotericin. *Bone Marrow Transplant* 1997;19:43–7.
25. Gordon MA et al. Corneal allescheriosos. *Arch Ophthalmol* 1959;62:758–63.
26. Perraut LE et al. Successful treatment of *Candida albicans* endophthalmitis with intravitreal amphotericin B. *Arch Ophthalmol* 1981;99:1565–7.
27. Ringden O et al. Prophylaxis and therapy using liposomal amphotericin B (AmBisome) for invasive fungal infection in children undergoing organ or allogeneic bone marrow transplantation. *Pediatr Transplant* 1997;1:124–9.
28. Christiansen KJ et al. Distribution and activity of amphotericin B in humans. *J Infect Dis* 1985;152:1037–43.
29. Kan VL et al. Comparative safety, tolerance, and pharmacokinetics of amphotericin B lipid complex and amphotericin B desoxycholate in healthy male volunteers. *J Infect Dis* 1991;164:418–21.
30. Amantea MA et al. Population pharmacokinetics and renal function-sparing effects of amphotericin B colloidal dispersion in patients receiving bone marrow transplants. *Antimicrob Agents Chemother* 1995; 39:2042–7.
31. Heinemann V et al. Pharmacokinetics of liposomal amphotericin B (AmBisome) versus other lipid-based formulations. *Bone Marrow Transplant* 1994;14(suppl 5):S8–9.
32. Levy M et al. Amphotericin B–induced heart rate decrease in children. *Clin Pediatr* 1995;34:358–64.
33. Le Y et al. Amphotericin B–associated hypertension. *Ann Pharmacother* 1996;30:765–7.
34. Manley TJ et al. Reversible parkinsonism in a child after bone marrow transplantation and lipid-based amphotericin B therapy. *Pediatr Infect Dis J* 1998;17:433–4.
35. Rossi MR et al. Severe rhabdomyolysis, hyperthermia and shock after amphotericin B colloidal dispersion in an allogeneic bone marrow transplant recipient. *Pediatr Infect Dis J* 2000;19:172–3.

36. Wright DG et al. Lethal pulmonary reactions associated with the combined use of amphotericin B and leukocyte transfusions. *N Engl J Med* 1981;304:1185–9.

37. Hussein MA et al. Transfusing platelets 2 h after the completion of amphotericin-B decreases its detrimental effect on transfused platelet recovery and survival. *Transfusion Med* 1998;8:43–7.

38. Trissel LA. Amphotericin B does not mix with fat emulsion. *Am J Health Syst Pharm* 1995;52:1463–4. Letter.

39. Hoy JF. Antifungal drugs. In, Kucers A et al., eds. *The use of antibiotics.* 5th ed. Oxford: Butterworth-Heinemann; 1997:1245–505.

40. Powderly WG. Fluconazole. *Infect Med* 1995;12:257, 281–82.

41. Debruyne D, Ryckelynck J-P. Clinical pharmacokinetics of fluconazole. *Clin Pharmacokinet* 1993;24:10–27.

42. Perry CM et al. Fluconazole. An update of its antimicrobial activity, pharmacokinetic properties, and therapeutic use in vaginal candidiasis. *Drugs* 1995;49:984–1006.

43. Como JA, Dismukes WE. Oral azole drugs as systemic antifungal therapy. *N Engl J Med* 1994;330:263–72.

44. Galgiani JN et al. Fluconazole therapy for coccidioidal meningitis. *Ann Intern Med* 1993;119:28–35.

45. Terrell CL, Hughes CE. Antifungal agents for deep-seated mycotic infections. *Mayo Clin Proc* 1992;67:69–91.

46. Bennett JE et al. A comparison of amphotericin B alone and combined with flucytosine in the treatment of cryptococcal meningitis. *N Engl J Med* 1979;301:126–31.

47. Allendoerfer R et al. Combined therapy with fluconazole and flucytosine in murine cryptococcal meningitis. *Antimicrob Agents Chemother* 1991;35:726–9.

48. Lyman CA, Walsh TJ. Systemically administered antifungal agents. A review of their clinical pharmacology and therapeutic applications. *Drugs* 1992;44:9–35.

49. Haria M et al. Itraconazole. A reappraisal of its pharmacological properties and therapeutic use in the management of superficial fungal infections. *Drugs* 1996;51:585–620.

50. Tucker RM et al. Interaction of azoles with rifampin, phenytoin, and carbamazepine: in vitro and clinical observations. *Clin Infect Dis* 1992;14:165–74.

51. Ducharme MP et al. Itraconazole and hydroxyitraconazole serum concentrations are reduced more than tenfold by phenytoin. *Clin Pharmacol Ther* 1995;58:617–24.

52. Benet LZ et al. Design and optimization of dosage regimens: pharmacokinetic data. In, Hardman JG et al., eds. *Goodman and Gilman's the pharmacological basis of therapeutics.* 9th ed. New York: McGraw-Hill; 1996:1707–92.

53. Barriere SL. Pharmacology and pharmacokinetics of traditional antifungal agents. *Pharmacotherapy* 1990;10(suppl):134S–40.

54. Chin TWF et al. Effects of an acidic beverage (Coca-Cola) on absorption of ketoconazole. *Antimicrob Agents Chemother* 1995;39:1671–5.

55. Balfour JA, Faulds D. Terbinafine: a review of its pharmacodynamic and pharmacokinetic properties, and therapeutic potential in superficial mycoses. *Drugs* 1992;43:259–84.

56. Sabo JA, Abdel-Rahman SM. Voriconazole: a new triazole antifungal. *Ann Pharmacother* 2000;34:1032–43.

57. Arbiser JL et al. Clofazimine: a review of its medical uses and mechanisms of action. *J Am Acad Dermatol* 1995;32:241–7.

58. Peloquin CA. Pharmacology of the antimycobacterial drugs. *Med Clin North Am* 1993;77:1253–62.

59. Brausch LM, Bass JB. The treatment of tuberculosis. *Med Clin North Am* 1993;77:1277–90.

60. Bass JB Jr et al. Treatment of tuberculosis and tuberculosis infection in adults and children. *Am J Resp Crit Care Med* 1994;149:1359–74.

61. Initial therapy for tuberculosis in the era of multidrug resistance. *MMWR* 1993;42(RR-7):1–8.

62. Heifets LB. Antimycobacterial drugs. *Semin Respir Infect* 1994;9:84–103.

63. van Scoy RE, Wilkowske CJ. Antituberculous agents. *Mayo Clin Proc* 1992;67:179–87.

64. Prevention and treatment of tuberculosis among patients infected with human immunodeficiency virus: principles of therapy and revised recommendations. *MMWR* 2000;47(RR-20):36–42.

65. Targeted tuberculin testing and treatment of latent tuberculosis infection. *MMWR* 2000;49(RR-6):1–53.

66. Pratt WB, Fekety R. Drugs that act on mycobacteria. In, Pratt WB, Fekety R, eds. *The antimicrobial drugs.* New York: Oxford University Press; 1986:277–316.

67. Alexander MR et al. Isoniazid-associated hepatitis. *Clin Pharm* 1982;1:148–53.

68. Holdiness MR. Neurological manifestations and toxicities of the antituberculosis drugs. A review. *Med Toxicol Adv Drug Exp* 1987;2:33–51.

69. O'Brien RJ. Drug-resistant tuberculosis: etiology, management and prevention. *Semin Respir Infect* 1994;9:104–12.

70. Skinner MH et al. Pharmacokinetics of rifabutin. *Antimicrob Agents Chemother* 1989;33:1237–41.

71. Nightingale SD et al. Two controlled trials of rifabutin prophylaxis against *Mycobacterium avium* complex infection in AIDS. *N Engl J Med* 1993;329:828–33.

72. Masur H. Recommendations on prophylaxis and therapy for disseminated *Mycobacterium avium* complex disease in patients infected with the human immunodeficiency virus. Public Health Service Task Force on Prophylaxis and Therapy for *Mycobacterium avium* Complex. *N Engl J Med* 1993;329:898–904.

73. Blaschke TF, Skinner MH. The clinical pharmacokinetics of rifabutin. *Clin Infect Dis* 1996;(suppl 1):S15–22.

74. Vesely JJK, et al. Rifampin, a useful drug for nonmycobacterial infections. *Pharmacotherapy* 1998;18:345–57.

75. Thornsberry C et al. Rifampin: spectrum of antibacterial activity. *Rev Infect Dis* 1983;5(suppl 3):S412–7.

76. Venkatesan K. Pharmacokinetic drug interactions with rifampicin. *Clin Pharmacokinet* 1992;22:47–65.

77. Temple ME, Nahata MC. Rifapentine: its role in the treatment of tuberculosis. *Ann Pharmacother* 1999;33:1203–10.

78. Anon. Drugs for parasitic infections. *Med Lett Drugs Ther* 2000;(March):1–12. (http://www.medicalletter.com/freedocs/ parasitic.pdf)

79. Jernigan JA, Pearson RD. Antiparasitic drugs. In, Mandell GL et al., eds. *Principles and practice of infectious diseases.* 4th ed. New York: Churchill Livingstone; 1995:458–92.

80. Kalter DC et al. Treatment of pediculosis pubis. *Arch Dermatol* 1987;123:1315–9.

81. Brown S et al. Treatment of ectoparasitic infections: review of the English-language literature, 1982–9. *Clin Infect Dis* 1995;20(suppl 1):S104–9.

82. Quarterman MJ, Lesher LJ Jr. Neonatal scabies treated with permethrin 5% cream. *Pediatr Dermatol* 1994;11:264–6.

83. Meinking TL, Taplin D. Safety of permethrin vs lindane for the treatment of scabies. *Arch Dermatol* 1996;132:959–62. Editorial.

84. Liu LX, Weller PF. Antiparasitic drugs. *N Engl J Med* 1996;334:1178–84.

85. Elion GB. Acyclovir: discovery, mechanism of action, and selectivity. *J Med Virol* 1993;(suppl 1):2–6.

86. Whitley RJ, Gnann JW. Acyclovir: a decade later. *N Engl J Med* 1992;327:782–9.

87. Nikkels AF, Pierard GE. Recognition and treatment of shingles. *Drugs* 1994;48:528–48.

88 Bell AR. Valaciclovir update. *Antiviral Chemother* 1999;5:149–157.

89. Soul-Lawton J et al. Absolute bioavailability and metabolic disposition of valaciclovir, the L-valyl ester of acyclovir, following oral administration to humans. *Antimicrob Agents Chemother* 1995;39:2759–64.

90. Jacobson MA. Valaciclovir (BW256U87): the L-valyl ester of acyclovir. *J Med Virol* 1993;(suppl 1):150–3.

91. Laskin OL. Acyclovir, pharmacology and clinical experience. *Arch Intern Med* 1984;144:1241–6.

92. Cundy KC et al. Clinical pharmacokinetics of cidofovir in human immunodeficiency virus–infected patients. *Antimicrob Agents Chemother* 1995;39:1247–52.

93. Lalezari JP et al. (S)-1-[3-hydroxy-2-(phosphonylmethoxy)propyl]cytosine (cidofovir): results of a phase I/II study of a novel antiviral nucleotide analogue. *J Infect Dis* 1995;171:788–96.

94. Flaherty JF. Current and experimental therapeutic options for cytomegalovirus disease. *Am J Health Syst Pharm* 1996;53(suppl 2):S4–11.

95. Perry CM, Noble S. Didanosine an updated review of its use in HIV infection. *Drugs* 1999;58:1099–135.

96. Moyle G, Gazzard B. Current knowledge and future prospects for the use of HIV protease inhibitors. *Drugs* 1996;51:701–12.

97. Dudley MN. Clinical pharmacokinetics of nucleoside antiretroviral agents. *J Infect Dis* 1995;171(suppl 2):S99–112.

98. Knupp CA et al. Pharmacokinetics of didanosine in patients with acquired immunodeficiency syndrome or acquired immunodeficiency syndrome–related complex. *Clin Pharmacol Ther* 1991;49:523–35.

99. Hartman NR et al. Pharmacokinetics of 2′,3′-dideoxyinosine in patients with severe human immunodeficiency infection. II. The effects of different oral formulations and the presence of other medications. *Clin Pharmacol Ther* 1991;50:278–85.

100. Neuzil KM. Pharmacologic therapy for human immunodeficiency virus infection: a review. *Am J Med Sci* 1994;307:368–73.

101. Stretcher BN. Pharmacokinetic optimisation of antiretroviral therapy in patients with HIV infection. *Clin Pharmacokinet* 1995;29:46–65.

102. van Leeuwen R et al. The safety and pharmacokinetics of a reverse transcriptase inhibitor, 3TC, in patients with HIV infection: a phase I study. *AIDS* 1992;6:1471–5.

103. Moore KHP et al. Pharmacokinetics of lamivudine administered alone and with trimethoprim-sulfamethoxazole. *Clin Pharmacol Ther* 1996;59:550–8.

104. Taburet A-M, Singlas E. Drug interactions with antiviral drugs. *Clin Pharmacokinet* 1996;30:385–401.

105. Johnson VA. Nucleoside reverse transcriptase inhibitors and resistance of human immunodeficiency virus type 1. *J Infect Dis* 1995;17(suppl 2):S140–9.

106. Pue MA et al. Linear pharmacokinetics of penciclovir following administration of single oral doses of famciclovir 125, 250, 500 and 750 mg to healthy volunteers. *J Antimicrob Chemother* 1994;33:119–27.

107. Perry CM, Wagstaff AJ. Famciclovir: a review of its pharmacological properties and therapeutic efficacy in herpesvirus infections. *Drugs* 1995;50:396–415.

108. Sacks SL, Wilson B. Famciclovir/penciclovir. *Antiviral Chemother* 1999;5:135–47.

109. Eron JJ et al. Treatment with lamivudine, zidovudine, or both in HIV-positive patients with 200 to 500 CD4+ cells per cubic millimeter. *N Engl J Med* 1995;333:1662–9.

110. Minor JR, Baltz JK. Foscarnet sodium. *DICP* 1991;25:41–7.

111. Wagstaff AJ, Bryson HM. Foscarnet. A reappraisal of its antiviral activity, pharmacokinetic properties and therapeutic use in immunocompromised patients with viral infections. *Drugs* 1994;48:199–226.

112. Sasadeusz JJ, Sacks SL. Systemic antivirals in herpesvirus infections. *Dermatol Clin* 1993;11:171–85.

113. Jacobson MA et al. Foscarnet-induced hypocalcemia and effects of foscarnet on calcium metabolism. *J Clin Endocrinol Metab* 1991;72:1130–5.

114. Crumpacker CS. Ganciclovir. *N Engl J Med* 1996;335:721–9.

115. Sommadossi J-P et al. Clinical pharmacokinetics of ganciclovir in patients with normal and impaired renal function. *Rev Infect Dis* 1988;10(suppl 3):S507–14.

116. Morris DJ. Adverse effects and drug interactions of clinical importance with antiviral drugs. *Drug Saf* 1994;10:281–91.

117. Erice A et al. Progressive disease due to ganciclovir-resistant cytomegalovirus in immunocompromised patients. *N Engl J Med* 1989;320:289–93.

118. Plosker GL, Noble S. Indinavir. A review of its use in the management of HIV infection. *Drugs* 1999;58:1165–203.

119. Jarvis B, Faulds D. Lamivudine. A review of its therapeutic potential in chronic hepatitis b. *Drugs* 1999;58:101–41.

120. Merrill DP et al. Lamivudine or stavudine in two- and three-drug combinations against human immunodeficiency virus type I replication in vitro. *J Infect Dis* 1996;173:355–64.

121. Peterson A et al. Comparison of bid and tid dosing of nelfinavir (NFV) in combination with stavudine (d4T) and lamivudine (3TC): an interim look. Presented at the 5th Conference on Retroviruses and Opportunistic Infections. February 1–5, 1998; Chicago. Abstract 373.

122. Cheeseman S et al. Phase I/II evaluation of nevirapine alone and in combination with zidovudine for infection with human immunodeficiency virus. *J Acquir Immune Defic Syndr Hum Retrovirol* 1995;8:141–51.

123. Havlir D et al. High-dose nevirapine: safety, pharmacokinetics, and antiviral effect in patients with human immunodeficiency virus infection. *J Infect Dis* 1995;171:537–45.

124. Investigational drug brochure: Viramune (nevirapine) expanded access program. Ridgefield, CT: Boehringer Ingelheim; March 1996.

125. D'Aquila RT et al. Nevirapine, zidovudine, and didanosine compared with zidovudine and didanosine in patients with HIV-1 infection. A randomized, double-blind, placebo-controlled trial. *Ann Intern Med* 1996;124:1019–30.

126. Danner SA et al. A short-term study of the safety, pharmacokinetics, and efficacy of ritonavir, an inhibitor of HIV-1 protease. *N Engl J Med* 1995;333:1528–33.

127. Markowitz M et al. A preliminary study of ritonavir, an inhibitor of HIV-1 protease, to treat HIV-1 infection. *N Engl J Med* 1995;333:1534–9.

128. Kitchen VS et al. Safety and activity of saquinavir in HIV infection. *Lancet* 1995;345:952–5.

129. Vella S. Update on a proteinase inhibitor. *AIDS* 1994;8(suppl 3):S25–9.

130. Sommadossi J-P. Comparison of metabolism and in vitro antiviral activity of stavudine versus other 2_,3_ dideoxynucleoside analogues. *J Infect Dis* 1995;171(suppl 2):S88–92.

131. Murray HW et al. Stavudine in patients with AIDS and AIDS-related complex: AIDS clinical trials group 089. *J Infect Dis* 1995;171(suppl 2):S123–30.

132. Lange JM et al. Failure of zidovudine prophylaxis after accidental exposure to HIV-1. *N Engl J Med* 1990;322:1375–7.

133. Recommendations of the U.S. Public Health Service task force on the use of zidovudine to reduce perinatal transmission of human immunodeficiency virus. *MMWR* 1994;43(RR-11):1–20.

134. Taburet AM et al. Pharmacokinetics of zidovudine in patients with liver cirrhosis. *Clin Pharmacol Ther* 1990;47:731–9.

135. Acosta EP et al. Clinical pharmacokinetics of zidovudine: an update. *Clin Pharmacokinet* 1996;4:251–62.

136. Steffe EM et al. The effect of acetaminophen on zidovudine metabolism in HIV-infected patients. *J Acquir Immune Defic Syndr* 1990;3:691–4.

137. Panel on Clinical Practices for Treatment of HIV Infection. Guidelines for the use of antiretroviral agents in HIV-infected adults and adolescents. *MMWR* 1998;47(RR-5):43–82.

138. Panel on Clinical Practices for Treatment of HIV Infection. Guidelines for the use of antiretroviral agents in pediatric HIV infection. *MMWR* 1998;47(RR-4):1–43.

139. Centers for Disease Control and Prevention. Public Health Service Task Force recommendations for the use of antiretroviral drugs in pregnant women infected with HIV-1 for maternal health and for reducing perinatal HIV-1 transmission in the United States. *MMWR* 1998;47(RR-2):1–30.

140. Colman PM. A novel approach to antiviral therapy for influenza. *J Antimicrob Chemother* 1999;44(suppl B):17–22.

141. Bardsley-Elliot A, Noble S. Oseltamivir. *Drugs* 1999; 58:851–60.

142. Anon. Two neuraminidase inhibitors for treatment of influenza. *Med Lett Drugs Ther* 1999;41:91–3.

143. Long JK et al. Antiviral agents for treating influenza. *Cleve Clin J Med* 2000;67:92–5.

144. Dunn CJ, Goa KL. Zanamivir a review of its use in influenza. *Drugs* 1999;58:761–84.

145. Chambers HF, Neu HC. Penicillins. In, Mandell GL et al., eds. *Principles and practice of infectious diseases.* 5th ed. New York: Churchill Livingstone; 2000:261–74.

146. Barza M. Antimicrobial spectrum, pharmacology and therapeutic use of antibiotics. Part 2: penicillins. *Am J Hosp Pharm* 1977;34:57–67.

147. Weber DJ et al. Amoxicillin and potassium clavulanate: an antibiotic combination. *Pharmacotherapy* 1984;4:122–36.

148. Sutherland R. β-lactam/β-lactamase inhibitor combinations: development, antibacterial activity and clinical applications. *Infection* 1995;23:191–200.

149. Neu HC. Antistaphylococcal penicillins. *Med Clin North Am* 1982;66:51–60.

150. Johnson DH, Cunha BA. Aztreonam. *Med Clin North Am* 1995;79:733–43.

151. Brogden RN, Heel RC. Aztreonam. A review of its antibacterial activity, pharmacokinetic properties and therapeutic uses. *Drugs* 1986;31:96–130.

152. Donowitz GR, Mandell GL. Beta-lactam antibiotics (2 parts). *N Engl J Med* 1988;318:419–26,490–500.

153. Cunha BA. Third-generation cephalosporins: a review. *Clin Ther* 1992;14:616–47.

154. Nightingale CH et al. Pharmacokinetics and clinical use of cephalosporin antibiotics. *J Pharm Sci* 1975;64:1899–927.

155. Barriere SL, Flaherty JF. Third-generation cephalosporins: a critical evaluation. *Clin Pharm* 1984;3: 351–73.

156. Karchmer AW. Cephalosporins. In, Mandell GL et al., eds. *Principles and practice of infectious diseases.* 5th ed. New York: Churchill Livingstone; 2000:274–91.

157. Rodman DP et al. A critical review of the new oral cephalosporins. *Arch Fam Med* 1994;3:975–80.

158. Fassbender M et al. Pharmacokinetics of new oral cephalosporins, including a new carbacephem. *Clin Infect Dis* 1993;16:646–53.

159. Force RW, Nahata MC. Loracarbef: a new orally administered carbacephem antibiotic. *Ann Pharmacother* 1993;27;321–9.

160. Cooper RDG. The carbacephems: a new beta-lactam antibiotic class. *Am J Med* 1992;92(suppl 6A):2S–6.

161. DiPiro JT, May JR. Use of cephalosporins with enhanced anti-anaerobic activity for treatment and prevention of anaerobic and mixed infections. *Clin Pharm* 1988;7:285–302.

162. Ward A, Richards DM. Cefotetan. A review of its antibacterial activity, pharmacokinetic properties and therapeutic use. *Drugs* 1985;30:382–426.

163. Schaad UB et al. A comparison of ceftriaxone and cefuroxime for the treatment of bacterial meningitis in children. *N Engl J Med* 1990;322:141–7.

164. Petz LD. Immunologic cross-reactivity between penicillins and cephalosporins: a review. *J Infect Dis* 1978;137(suppl):S74–9.

165. Lipsky JJ. Antibiotic-associated hypoprothrombinemia. *J Antimicrob Chemother* 1988;21:281–300.

166. Schaad UB et al. Reversible ceftriaxone-associated biliary pseudolithiasis in children. *Lancet* 1988;2: 1411–3.

167. Shiffman ML et al. Pathogenesis of ceftriaxone-associated biliary sludge. *Gastroenterology* 1990;99:1772–8.

168. Cunha BA, Gill MV. Cefepime. *Med Clin North Am* 1995;79:721–32.

169. Barradell LB, Bryson HM. Cefepime. A review of its antibacterial activity, pharmacokinetic properties and therapeutic use. *Drugs* 1994;47:471–505.

170. Friedland IR, McCracken GH Jr. Management of infections caused by antibiotic-resistant *Streptococcus pneumoniae. N Engl J Med* 1994;331:377–82.

171. Smith BR, LeFrock JL. Cefuroxime: antibacterial activity, pharmacology, and clinical efficacy. *Ther Drug Monit* 1983;5:149–60.

172. Drusano GL et al. The acylampicillins: mezlocillin, piperacillin, and azlocillin. *Rev Infect Dis* 1984;6:13–32.

173. Holmes B et al. Piperacillin. A review of its antibacterial activity, pharmacokinetic properties and therapeutic use. *Drugs* 1984;28:375–425.

174. Clissold SP et al. Imipenem/cilastatin. A review of its antibacterial activity, pharmacokinetic properties and therapeutic efficacy. *Drugs* 1987;33:183–241.

175. Norrby SR. Carbapenems. *Med Clin North Am* 1995;79:745–59.
176. Ahonkhai VI et al. Imipenem-cilastatin in pediatric patients: an overview of safety and efficacy in studies conducted in the United States. *Pediatr Infect Dis J* 1989;8:740–7.
177. Calandra GB et al. Review of adverse experiences and tolerability in the first 2,516 patients treated with imipenem/cilastatin. *Am J Med* 1985;78(suppl 6A):73–8.
178. Saxon A. Immediate hypersensitivity reactions to beta-lactam antibiotics. *Ann Intern Med* 1987;107: 204–15.
179. Wiseman LR et al. Meropenem. A review of its antibacterial activity, pharmacokinetic properties and clinical efficacy. *Drugs* 1995;50:73–101.
180. Pryka RD, Haig GM. Meropenem: a new carbapenem antimicrobial. *Ann Pharmacother* 1994;28:1045–54.
181. Mouton JW, van den Anker JN. Meropenem clinical pharmacokinetics. *Clin Pharmacokinet* 1995;28:275–86.
182. Wright AJ. The penicillins. *Mayo Clin Proc* 1999;74:290–307.
183. Weiss ME, Adkinson NF Jr. β-Lactam allergy. In, Mandell GL et al., eds. *Principles and practice of infectious diseases.* 5th ed. New York: Churchill Livingstone; 2000:299–305.
184. Plaisance KI, Nightingale CH. Pharmacology of cephalosporins. In, Queener SF et al., eds. *Beta-lactam antibiotics for clinical use.* New York: Marcel Dekker; 1986:285–347.
185. Dudley MN, Nightingale CH. Effects of protein binding on the pharmacology of cephalosporins. In, Neu HC, ed. *New beta-lactam antibiotics: a review from chemistry to clinical efficacy of the new cephalosporins.* Philadelphia: Francis Clarke Wood Institute for the History of Medicine; 1982:227–39.
186. Carver P et al. Comparative pharmacokinetic study of cefotetan and cefoxitin in healthy volunteers. *Infect Surg* 1986;suppl:11–4.
187. Wise R. The pharmacokinetics of the oral cephalosporins: a review. *J Antimicrob Chemother* 1990;26(suppl E):13–20.
188. Melikian DM, Flaherty JF. Antimicrobial agents. In, Schrier RW, Gambertoglio JG, eds. *Handbook of drug therapy in liver and kidney disease.* Boston: Little, Brown; 1991:14–45.
189. Klepser ME et al. Clinical pharmacokinetics of newer cephalosporins. *Clin Pharmacokinet* 1995;28:361–84.
190. Hardin TC et al. Comparison of ampicillin-sulbactam and ticarcillin-clavulanic acid in patients with chronic renal failure: effects of differential pharmacokinetics on serum bactericidal activity. *Pharmacotherapy* 1994;14:147–52.
191. Bahal N, Nahata MC. The new macrolide antibiotics: azithromycin, clarithromycin, dirithromycin, and roxithromycin. *Ann Pharmacother* 1992;26:46–55.
192. Schlossberg D. Azithromycin and clarithromycin. *Med Clin North Am* 1995;79:803–15.
193. Berry A et al. Azithromycin therapy for disseminated *Mycobacterium avium-intracellulare* in AIDS patients. First National Conference on Human Retroviruses. Washington, DC; 1993. Abstract #292.
194. Zuckerman JM. The newer macrolides: azithromycin and clarithromycin. *Infect Dis Clin North Am* 2000; 14:449–62.
195. 1993 Sexually transmitted diseases treatment guidelines. *MMWR* 1993;42(RR-14):1–102.
196. Centers for Disease Control and Prevention. Recommendations on prophylaxis and therapy for disseminated *Mycobacterium avium* complex for adults and adolescents infected with human immunodeficiency virus. *MMWR* 1993;42(RR-9):14–20.
197. Havlir D et al. Prophylaxis against disseminated *Mycobacterium avium* complex with weekly azithromycin, daily rifabutin, or both. *N Engl J Med* 1996;335:392–8.
198. McLinn S. Double blind and open label studies of azithromycin in the management of acute otitis media in children: a review. *Pediatr Infect Dis J* 1995;14:S62–6.
199. Hopkins SJ, Williams D. Clinical tolerability and safety of azithromycin in children. *Pediatr Infect Dis J* 1995;14:S67–71.
200. Nahata MC. Pharmacokinetics of azithromycin in pediatric patients: comparison with other agents used for treating otitis media and streptococcal pharyngitis. *Pediatr Infect Dis J* 1995;14:S39–44.
201. Piscitelli SC et al. Clarithromycin and azithromycin: new macrolide antibiotics. *Clin Pharm* 1992;11:137–52.
202. Rodvold KA, Piscitelli SC. New oral macrolide and fluoroquinolone antibiotics: an overview of pharmacokinetics, interactions, and safety. *Clin Infect Dis* 1993;17(suppl 1):S192–9.
203. Dunn CJ, Barradell LB. Azithromycin: a review of its pharmacological properties and use as 3-day therapy in respiratory tract infections. *Drugs* 1996;51:483–505.
204. McConnell SA, Amsden GW. Review and comparison of advanced-generation macrolides clarithromycin and dirithromycin. *Pharmacotherapy* 1999;19:404–15.
205. Matsiota-Bernard P et al. Comparison of clarithromycin-sensitive and clarithromycin-resistant Mycobacterium avium strains isolated from AIDS patients during therapy regimens including clarithromycin. *J Infect* 2000;40:49-54.
206. Markham A, Mctavish D. Clarithromycin and omeprazole as *Helicobacter pylori* eradication therapy in patients with *H. pylori*–associated gastric disorders. *Drugs* 1996;51:161–78.

207. Brittain DC. Erythromycin. *Med Clin North Am* 1987;71:1147–54.
208. Washington JA, Wilson WR. Erythromycin: a microbial and clinical perspective after 30 years of clinical use. (2 parts). *Mayo Clin Proc* 1985;60:189–203,271–8.
209. Smilack JD et al. Tetracyclines, chloramphenicol, erythromycin, clindamycin, and metronidazole. *Mayo Clin Proc* 1991;66:1270–80.
210. Weber FH et al. Erythromycin: a motilin agonist and gastrointestinal prokinetic agent. *Am J Gastroenterol* 1993;88:485–90.
211. Eichenwald HF. Adverse reactions to erythromycin. *Pediatr Infect Dis J* 1986;5:147–50.
212. Amsden GW. Macrolides versus azalides: a drug interaction update. *Ann Pharmacother* 1995;29:906–17.
213. Peeters TL. Erythromycin and other macrolides as prokinetic agents. *Gastroenterology* 1993;105:1886–99.
214. Lartey PA et al. New developments in macrolides: structures and antibacterial and prokinetic activities. *Adv Pharmacol* 1994;28:307–43.
215. Kreek MJ, Culpepper-Morgan JA. Constipation syndromes. In, Lewis JH, ed. *A pharmacologic approach to gastrointestinal disorders.* Baltimore: Williams & Wilkins; 1994:179–208.
216. Dive A et al. Effect of erythromycin on gastric motility in mechanically ventilated critically ill patients: a double-blind, randomized, placebo-controlled study. *Crit Care Med* 1995;23:1356–62.
217. Guay DRP. Macrolide antibiotics in paediatric infectious diseases. *Drugs* 1996;51:515–36.
218. Bloomfield G. A comparison of gastrointestinal tolerance to five different forms of erythromycin. *P&T* 1996;April:209–14.
219. Dajani AS et al. Prevention of bacterial endocarditis. Recommendations by the American Heart Association. *JAMA* 1990;264:2919–22.
220. Ginsburg CM. Pharmacology of erythromycin in infants and children. *Pediatr Infect Dis J* 1986;5:124–9.
221. Brogden RN, Peters DH. Dirithromycin. A review of its antimicrobial activity, pharmacokinetic properties and therapeutic efficacy. *Drugs* 1994;48:599–616.
222. Anon. Dirithromycin. *Med Lett Drugs Ther* 1995;37:109–10.
223. Just PM. Overview of the fluoroquinolone antibiotics. *Pharmacotherapy* 1993;13:4S–17.
224. Suh B, Lorber B. Quinolones. *Med Clin North Am* 1995;79:869–94.
225. Schaad UB et al. Use of fluoroquinolones in pediatrics: consensus report of an international society of chemotherapy commission. *Pediatr Infect Dis J* 1995;14:1–9.
226. Schentag JJ, Gross TF. Quinolone pharmacokinetics in the elderly. *Am J Med* 1992;92(suppl 4A):33S–7.
227. Nightingale CH. Pharmacokinetic considerations in quinolone therapy. *Pharmacotherapy* 1993;13:34S–8.
228. Radandt JM et al. Interactions of fluoroquinolones with other drugs mechanisms, variability, clinical significance, and management. *Clin Infect Dis* 1992;14:272–84.
229. Dudley MN et al. Effect of dose on the serum pharmacokinetics of intravenous ciprofloxacin with identification and characterization of extravascular compartments using noncompartmental and compartmental pharmacokinetic models. *Antimicrob Agents Chemother* 1987;31:1782–6.
230. Forrest A et al. Relationships between renal function and disposition of oral ciprofloxacin. *Antimicrob Agents Chemother* 1988;32:1537–40.
231. Davis R. Bryson HM. Levofloxacin. *Drugs* 1994;47:677–700.
232. Balfour JA et al. Fleroxacin. A review of its pharmacology and therapeutic efficacy in various infections. *Drugs* 1995;49:794–850.
233. Wadworth AN, Goa KL. Lomefloxacin. *Drugs* 1991;42:1018–60.
234. Goa KL et al. Sparfloxacin. *Drugs* 1997;53:700–25.
235. Wagstaff AJ, Balfour JA. Grepafloxacin. *Drugs* 1997;53:817–24.
236. Fish DN, Chow AT. The clinical pharmacokinetics of levofloxacin. *Clin Pharmacokinet* 1997;32:101–19.
237. Haria M, Lamb HM. Trovafloxacin. *Drugs* 1997;54:435–45.
238. Hooper DC. Quinolones. In, Mandell GL et al., eds. *Principles and practice of infectious diseases.* 5th ed. New York: Churchill Livingstone; 2000:404–23.
239. Pickerill KE et al. Comparison of the fluoroquinolones based on pharmacokinetic and pharmacodynamic parameters. *Pharmacotherapy* 2000;20:417–28.
240. Foltzer MA, Reese RE. Trimethoprim-sulfamethoxazole and other sulfonamides. *Med Clin North Am* 1987;71:1177–94.
241. Smilack JD. Trimethoprim-sulfamethoxazole. *Mayo Clin Proc* 1999;74:730–4.
242. Markowitz N et al. Trimethoprim-sulfamethoxazole compared with vancomycin for the treatment of *Staphylococcus aureus* infection. *Ann Intern Med* 1992;117:390–8.
243. Lundstrom TS, Sobel JD. Vancomycin, trimethoprim-sulfamethoxazole, and rifampin. *Infect Dis Clin North Am* 1995;9:747–67.
244. Goodwin SD. *Pneumocystis carinii* pneumonia in human immunodeficiency virus–infected infants and children. *Pharmacotherapy* 1993;13:640–6.

245. Davey RT Jr, Masur H. Recent advances in the diagnosis, treatment, and prevention of *Pneumocystis carinii* pneumonia. *Antimicrob Agents Chemother* 1990;34:499–504.

246. Pratt WB, Fekety R. The antimetabolites. In, Pratt WB, Fekety R, eds. *The antimicrobial drugs.* New York: Oxford University Press; 1986:229–51.

247. Masur H. Prevention and treatment of pneumocystis pneumonia. *N Engl J Med* 1992;327:1853–60.

248. Absar N et al. Desensitization to trimethoprim/sulfamethoxazole in HIV-infected patients. *J Allergy Clin Immunol* 1994;93:1001–5.

249. Standiford HC. Tetracyclines and chloramphenicol. In, Mandell GL et al., eds. *Principles and practice of infectious diseases.* 5th ed. New York: Churchill Livingstone; 2000:336–48.

250. Kapusnik-Uner JE et al. Antimicrobial agents: tetracyclines, chloramphenicol, erythromycin and miscellaneous antibacterial agents. In, Hardman JG et al., eds. *Goodman and Gilman's the pharmacological basis of therapeutics.* 9th ed. New York: McGraw-Hill; 1996:1130–5.

251. Fingar BL. Sclerosing agents used to control malignant pleural effusions. *Hosp Pharm* 1992;27:622–8.

252. Francke EL, Neu HC. Chloramphenicol and tetracyclines. *Med Clin North Am* 1987;71:1155–68.

253. Kasten MJ. Clindamycin, metronidazole, and chloramphenicol. *Mayo Clin Proc* 1999;74:825–33.

254. Haile LG, Flaherty JF. Atovaquone: a review. *Ann Pharmacother* 1993;27:1488–94.

255. Spencer CM, Goa KL. Atovaquone. A review of its pharmacological properties and therapeutic efficacy in opportunistic infections. *Drugs* 1995;50:176–96.

256. Norris AH et al. Chloramphenicol for the treatment of vancomycin-resistant enterococcal infections. *Clin Infect Dis* 1995;20:1137–44.

257. Greenfield RA. Symposium on antimicrobial therapy X. Chloramphenicol, clindamycin, and metronidazole. *J Okla State Med Assoc* 1993;86:336–41.

258. Smilack JD. The tetracyclines. *Mayo Clin Proc* 1999;74:729–9.

259. Rayner SA, Buckley RJ. Ocular chloramphenicol and aplastic anemia. Is there a link? *Drug Saf* 1996;14:273–6.

260. Pratt WB, Fekety R. Bacteriostatic inhibitors of protein synthesis. In, Pratt WB, Fekety R, eds. *The antimicrobial drugs.* New York: Oxford University Press; 1986:184–228.

261. Dhawan VK, Thadepalli H. Clindamycin: a review of 15 years of clinical experience. *Rev Infect Dis* 1982;4:1133–53.

262. Klainer AS. Clindamycin. *Med Clin North Am* 1987;71:1169–76.

263. Van Arsdel PP et al. The value of skin testing for penicillin allergy diagnosis. *West J Med* 1986;144:311–4.

264. Anon. Linezolid (Zyvox). *Med Lett Drugs Ther* 2000;42:45–46.

265. Falagas ME, Gorbach SL. Clindamycin and metronidazole. *Med Clin North Am* 1995;79:845–67.

266. Lau AH et al. Clinical pharmacokinetics of metronidazole and other nitroimidazole anti-infectives. *Clin Pharmacokinet* 1992;23:328–64.

267. Wenisch C et al. Comparison of vancomycin, teicoplanin, metronidazole, and fusidic acid for treatment of *Clostridium difficile*–associated diarrhea. *Clin Infect Dis* 1996;22:813–8.

268. Black M et al. Antimicrobial agents: sulfonamides, trimethoprim-sulfamethoxazole, quinolones. In, Hardman JG et al., eds. *Goodman and Gilman's the pharmacological basis of therapeutics.* 9th ed. New York: McGraw-Hill; 1996:1069–70.

269. Wispelwey B, Pearson RD. Pentamidine: a review. *Infect Control Hosp Epidemiol* 1991;12:375–82.

270. Conte JE Jr. Pharmacokinetics of intravenous pentamidine in patients with normal renal function or receiving hemodialysis. *J Infect Dis* 1991;163:169–75.

271. Donnelly H et al. Distribution of pentamidine in patients with AIDS. *J Infect Dis* 1988;157:985–9.

272. Chant C, Rybak MJ. Quinupristin/dalfopristin (RP 59500): a new streptogramin antibiotic. *Ann Pharmacother* 1995;29:1022–7.

273. Bryson HM, Spencer CM. Quinupristin-dalfopristin. *Drugs* 1996;52:406–16.

274. Griswold MW et al. Quinupristin-dalfopristin (RP 59500): an injectable streptogramin combination. *Am J Health Syst Pharm* 1996;53:2045–53.

275. Fulton B et al. Trimetrexate. A review of its pharmacodynamic and pharmacokinetic properties and therapeutic potential in the treatment of *Pneumocystis carinii* pneumonia. *Drugs* 1995;49:563–76.

276. Marshall JL, DeLap RJ. Clinical pharmacokinetics and pharmacology of trimetrexate. *Clin Pharmacokinet* 1994;26:190–200.

277. Blanke CD et al. Phase II study of trimetrexate, fluorouracil, and leucovorin for advanced colorectal cancer. *J Clin Oncol* 1997;15:915–20.

278. Witte RS et al. An Eastern Cooperative Oncology Group phase II trial of trimetrexate in the treatment of advanced urothelial carcinoma. *Cancer* 1994;73:688–91.

279. Grem JL et al. Correlates of severe of life-threatening toxic effects from trimetrexate. *J Natl Cancer Inst* 1988;80:1313–8.

280. Lake KD, Peterson CD. A simplified method for initiating vancomycin therapy. *Pharmacotherapy* 1985;5:340–4.

281. Rybak MJ et al. Nephrotoxicity of vancomycin, alone and with an aminoglycoside. *J Antimicrob Chemother* 1990;25:679–87.
282. Matzke GR et al. Clinical pharmacokinetics of vancomycin. *Clin Pharmacokinet* 1986;11:257–82.
283. Newfield P, Roizen MF. Hazards of rapid administration of vancomycin. *Ann Intern Med* 1979;91:581.
284. Healy DP et al. Vancomycin-induced histamine release and "red man syndrome": comparison of 1- and 2-hour infusions. *Antimicrob Agents Chemother* 1990;34:550–4.
285. Edwards DJ, Pancorbo S. Routine monitoring of serum vancomycin concentrations: waiting for proof of its value. *Clin Pharm* 1987;6:652–4.
286. Farber BF, Mollering RC. Retrospective study of the toxicity of preparations of vancomycin from 1974–1981. *Antimicrob Agents Chemother* 1983;23:138–41.

Antineoplastics, Chemoprotectants, and Immunosuppressants

Antineoplastics

Antineoplastics. The agents included in this section are those having widespread use in cancer chemotherapy. Agents with therapeutic importance in small patient populations are not included.

Information on the dosage of these drugs has largely been determined empirically, and clinical investigations are continually being performed to find safer and more effective dosage regimens. Thus, dosages in this section should only be considered as guidelines based on the most widely accepted usage at the time of this writing. Because space does not permit detailed discussions of the toxicity, dosage regimens, and other aspects of these drugs, the reader should become familiar with specific agents before initiating treatment.[1] References are provided in this section for more detailed information concerning the proper and safe use of these agents. Specific investigational protocols, if available, also can provide information that is unavailable from other sources, especially with regard to dosage and regimens.

Cancer chemotherapeutic agents as a class are the most toxic drugs in use. Adverse reactions listed represent those most likely to occur with the usual doses and methods of use. Infrequent, but serious, reactions are also listed; however, the lists of adverse reactions are not comprehensive. Nausea and vomiting are important side effects of these agents that can be adequately treated by current antiemetics alone or in combination. To tailor antiemetic therapy better to the emetic potential of the chemotherapy, a standard rating scale is used in these monographs. Several points to remember are that emetogenicity is dose dependent, combinations of chemotherapeutic agents result in greater emetogenic potential than the drug(s) used alone, and emetogenic potentials are best defined in adults and do not necessarily apply to children. The categories of emetogenicity used are as follows:[2]

EMETOGENICITY CATEGORY	PERCENTAGE OF PATIENTS AFFECTED
High	>90
Moderately high	60–90
Moderate	30–60
Moderately low	10–30
Low	<10

Class Instructions. Antineoplastics. This drug is very powerful, and some side effects can be expected to occur with its use. Be sure that you understand the possible benefits and dangers of the drug before you begin to take it.

Cytotoxic Agents. Because this drug can decrease your body's ability to fight infections, report any signs of infection such as fever, shaking chills, or sore throat immediately. Also report any unusual bruising or bleeding, shortness of breath, or painful or burning urination. Avoid the use of aspirin-containing products, and avoid alcohol or use it in moderation. Nausea, vomiting, or hair loss can sometimes occur with this drug. The severity of these effects depends on the individual, the dosage, and other drugs that might be given at the same time. This drug can cause temporary or sometimes permanent sterility in men and women. It also can cause birth defects if the father is taking the drug at the time of conception or if the mother is taking it any time during pregnancy. If you are breast feeding, this drug might appear in the milk and cause problems in your baby; therefore, use an alternate method of feeding your baby.

Missed Doses. This drug should be taken at regular intervals exactly as prescribed. If a dose is missed, it should be taken as soon as it is remembered. If it is almost time for the next dose, only that dose should be taken and the regular dosage schedule should be resumed. The dose should never be doubled or extra doses taken.

Alkylating Agents

ALTRETAMINE
Hexalen

Pharmacology. Altretamine (formerly hexamethylmelamine) acts primarily as an alkylating agent. It is used in combination chemotherapy of ovarian cancer and is active in cervical and lung cancers.[3–5]

Adult Dosage. PO as a single agent 260 mg/m^2/day in 4 divided doses for as long as 2–5 weeks. Lower dosages are required if altretamine is combined with other myelosuppressive agents.

Dosage Forms. Cap 50 mg.

Pharmacokinetics. Oral bioavailability is incomplete and erratic and may be dose dependent. Altretamine is *N*-demethylated to pentamethylmelamine by hepatic microsomal enzymes. The serum half-life is 4.7–10.2 hr, with >50% of a dose renally excreted in 24 hr and <1% excreted unchanged.

Adverse Reactions. Nausea, vomiting, and abdominal cramps can be dose limiting in some patients. Neurotoxicity is frequent, including agitation, hallucinations, and confusion; these are reversible and amenable to dosage reduction. Anemia, leukopenia, and thrombocytopenia are typically mild.

BUSULFAN
Busulfex, Myleran

CHLORAMBUCIL
Leukeran

MELPHALAN
Alkeran

Pharmacology. These drugs are water-soluble compounds that alkylate DNA, forming a variety of covalent cross-links. The drugs are polyfunctional and can form more than one covalent bond to susceptible cell constituents (typically the N^7 position of guanine). They are cell-cycle phase nonspecific and chemically stable enough for oral absorption before appreciable alkylator activation occurs.

Administration and Dosage.

	BUSULFAN	CHLORAMBUCIL	MELPHALAN
Administration	PO.	PO.	PO; IV.
Adult Dosage	Up to 8 mg/day (usually 1–3 mg/day).	0.1–0.2 mg/kg/day for 1 day; or 6–12 mg/day maintenance; or 0.4 mg/kg q 2–4 weeks.[6]	PO 7 mg/m² for 4 days; or 2–4 mg/day maintenance for multiple myeloma.[7] IV 16 mg/m² q 2 weeks for 4 doses, then q 4 weeks.
Pediatric Dosage	CML 0.06–0.12 mg/kg.	Non-Hodgkin's lymphoma, CLL, nephrotic syndrome, rheumatoid arthritis (initial) 0.1–0.2 mg/kg/day.	—
Geriatric Dosage	Same as adult dosage, but adjust for age-related reduction in renal function.		

Special Populations. *Other Conditions.* Elimination is significantly correlated with the GFR. Studies in nephrectomized animals demonstrate markedly increased myelotoxicity with unadjusted melphalan doses. Thus, one group currently recommends a 50% decrease in the melphalan dosage for BUN >30 mg/dL or Cr_s >1.5 mg/dL.[8] Reduce IV melphalan dosage to 75% of normal for WBC counts of 3000–4000/μL or platelet counts of 75,000–100,000/μL or to 50% for WBC counts of 2000–3000/μL or platelet counts of 50,000–75,000/μL, respectively; do not give it with WBC counts <2000/μL or platelet counts <50,000/μL.[9]

Dosage Forms. (Busulfan) **Tab** 2 mg; **Inj** 60 mg. (Chlorambucil) **Tab** 2 mg. (Melphalan) **Tab** 2 mg; **Inj** 50 mg.

Patient Instructions. (*See* Antineoplastics Class Instructions.)

Pharmacokinetics.

Fate.

	BUSULFAN	CHLORAMBUCIL	MELPHALAN
Absorption	Reported by manufacturer to be well absorbed orally.	Oral bioavailability is about 87 ± 20% by radiolabeled drug studies;[10,11] reduced by 10–20% if ingested with food.[12]	Oral bioavailability erratic and incomplete, (mean of 56%, range 25–89%); some patients have no levels after standard doses.[13,14]
Distribution	Homogeneous; good ascites penetration; V_d is 0.99 ±	V_d is 0.29 ± 0.21 L/kg; 99% plasma protein bound.[10]	V_d is 0.45 ± 0.15 L/kg; 90 ± 5% plasma protein bound.[10]

	BUSULFAN	CHLORAMBUCIL	MELPHALAN
	0.23 L/kg;[10] extensively bound to proteins.		
Metabolism	Extensively metabolized, major fraction as methanesulfonic acid. Cl is 0.27 ± 0.05 L/hr/kg.[10]	Rapid metabolism to a number of inactive metabolites. Cl is 0.16 ± 0.04 L/hr/kg.[10]	Not actively metabolized; spontaneous chemical degradation to mono- and dihydroxy products. Cl is 0.31 ± 0.17 L/hr/kg.[10]
Excretion	No unchanged drug found in urine; however, metabolites are renally excreted.	Less than 1% excreted unchanged in urine over 24 hr.	Unchanged drug 24-hr urinary excretion is 10–15% of a dose.
$t_{1/2}$	Rapid initial serum clearance: 90% of dose after 3 min. $t_{1/2\beta}$ is 2.6 ± 0.5 hr.[10]	1.3 ± 0.9 hr (unchanged drug); 2.5 hr (major metabolite, an aminophenylacetic acid derivative).[9,10]	IV: $t_{1/2\alpha}$ 8 min; $t_{1/2\beta}$ 1.4 ± 0.2 hr.[10,13,14]

Adverse Reactions. Emetic potential is low. Nausea and vomiting are rare with long-term administration, although large single doses can be strongly emetogenic. Dose-limiting toxicity for this group is typically myelosuppression, with nadirs of 14–21 days for leukopenia and thrombocytopenia after pulse dosage regimens; daily administration results in chronic low indices with cumulative effects. Blood counts commonly continue to drop after drug discontinuation; fatal pancytopenia has been reported. Therefore, hematologic assessments are important with long-term daily regimens. There might be some selectivity for different normal cell lines by these drugs; busulfan, and perhaps chlorambucil, selectively depresses granulocytes, relatively sparing platelets and lymphoid elements. The nadir for melphalan can be prolonged (4–6 weeks); continuous administration frequently leads to severe myelosuppression (especially platelets) that continues after the drug is discontinued. Pulmonary fibrosis can occasionally occur with all these drugs, especially busulfan; symptoms include cough, dyspnea, and fever; histopathologic changes include bilateral fibrosis. High-dose glucocorticoid therapy might help early evolving pulmonary disease caused by melphalan and chlorambucil, but "busulfan lung" is usually fatal within 6 months of diagnosis.[15–17] Busulfan frequently causes hyperpigmentation (especially of intertriginous areas) and broad suppression of testicular, ovarian, and adrenal functions (occasionally leading to Addisonian crisis). Long-term daily administration of these drugs predisposes patients to drug-induced carcinogenesis, often heralded by preleukemic pancytopenia and culminating in acute myelocytic leukemia. Allergic hypersensitivity reported, especially with melphalan. With prolonged use, sterility occurs with all alkylators; women seem more sensitive than men.

Contraindications. Documented hypersensitivity; inadequate marrow reserve.

Precautions. *See* Special Populations for melphalan use in renal impairment.

Drug Interactions. None known.

Parameters to Monitor. WBC and platelet counts at least monthly; reduce dosage at first sign of appreciable myelosuppression (ie, WBC <3000/μL or platelets <75,000/μL). Conversely, assess patients receiving oral melphalan for evidence of mild to moderate myelotoxicity to ensure that some absorption is occurring.

CARBOPLATIN   Paraplatin

Pharmacology. Carboplatin is a more stable cyclobutane carboxylato derivative of cisplatin that is slowly activated to expose two DNA binding sites on the platinum II coordinate complex. The drug binds to DNA by both inter- and intrastrand cross-links in a fashion similar to, but more delayed than, that with cisplatin.[18] It is more water soluble and commensurately less nephrotoxic than cisplatin. Action is cell-cycle phase nonspecific.

Administration and Adult Dosage. **IV for refractory ovarian cancer** 360 mg/m^2 q 4 weeks. Administration by continuous infusion has been reported but is not commonly used.[19–21]

Special Populations. *Pediatric Dosage.* Although not specifically labeled for pediatric use, carboplatin has been safely administered to children. **IV for recurrent brain tumors** 175 mg/m^2/week for 4 weeks.[22]

Geriatric Dosage. Same as adult dosage but adjust for age-related reduction in renal function.

Other Conditions. Reduce dosage in patients with reduced renal function, history of prior myelosuppressive therapy, and/or poor bone marrow reserve. Reduce dosage by about 25% if the prior nadir WBC count was <500/μL or the platelet count was <50,000/μL. When Cl_{cr} is 41–59 mL/min, a dose of 250 mg/m^2 is recommended; for Cl_{cr} of 16–40 mL/min, 200 mg/m^2 is recommended. Two prospectively validated formulas for dosage individualization are available. One formula seeks to achieve different target serum AUC values in untreated or pretreated patients: dose (mg) = AUC × (Cl_{cr} + 25), where "desired" AUC ranges are 6–8 mg/mL·min for untreated patients and 4–6 mg/mL·min for previously treated patients.[23] The second does not require Cl_{cr} estimates and uses a complex mathematical formula.[24]

Dosage Forms. **Inj** 50, 150, 450 mg.

Patient Instructions. (*See* Antineoplastics Class Instructions, particularly regarding infection risk.)

Pharmacokinetics. *Fate.* About 30% of carboplatin is irreversibly bound to plasma proteins; the half-life of this protein-bound fraction is >5 days.[25] V_d is 16–20 L for carboplatin. Carboplatin is slowly hydrolyzed in vivo to a form with two DNA binding sites; the rate of hydrolysis is much slower than the rate of chloride loss with cisplatin. The free (unbound) fraction of carboplatin and its hydrolyzed species are excreted in urine through glomerular filtration and tubular secretion. Urinary elimination accounts for over 65% of drug elimination in patients with normal renal function.

$t_{1/2}$. (Unbound) α phase 90 ± 50 min; β phase 180 ± 50 min.[25]

Adverse Reactions. The emetic potential is moderately high to high but is much less severe than with cisplatin and is easily controlled with antiemetics. Myelosuppression is the primary dose-limiting effect of carboplatin, and thrombocytopenia tends to be more severe than leukopenia; about 25% of previously untreated and 35% of previously treated ovarian cancer patients experience thrombocytopenia. The thrombocytopenic nadir for carboplatin as a single agent is approximately 21 days, and patients with pre-existing renal dysfunction or poor bone marrow reserve have an increased risk for severe thrombocytopenia. Anemia of a mild degree also can occur in up to 90% of patients; in some studies >40% of patients required transfusions and 5% of patients experienced hemorrhage. Diarrhea, abdominal pain, or constipation occur in 6–17% of patients. Nephrotoxicity occurs in 1–22% of patients. Unlike cisplatin, carboplatin does not cause cumulative damage to renal tubules. Transient decreases of 20–30% in some serum electrolytes occur, specifically magnesium, potassium, sodium, and calcium. Hepatic enzyme elevations occur in one-third of patients, but these elevations are not associated with serious or prolonged liver injury. Peripheral neuropathies occur in <10% of patients; however, the risk increases in patients >65 yr or if large dosages of cisplatin have been administered. CNS symptoms occur in ≤5% patients, and ototoxicity occurs in 1% of patients. Occasional reactions are allergic hypersensitivity, alopecia, and various cardiovascular events (eg, embolism, cerebrovascular accident, cardiac failure).

Contraindications. The manufacturer lists pre-existing renal impairment and myelosuppression as contraindications, but the drug has been given with appropriate dosage modification. (*See* Special Populations, Other Conditions.)

Precautions. Use with caution in patients with hearing impairment or reduced renal function, or if extensive prior chemotherapy has been administered. Patients with prior cisplatin therapy are at a higher risk for nephrotoxic and neurotoxic sequelae. Vigorous hydration and diuretics usually are not required with carboplatin.

Drug Interactions. Myelotoxicity of carboplatin is additive with other myelotoxic drugs. Concurrent use of other nephrotoxic drugs (eg, aminoglycosides) can delay carboplatin elimination and enhance toxicity. Although not well documented, cisplatin interactions also can occur with carboplatin, but at a lesser intensity.

Parameters to Monitor. Measure Cl_{cr} before dosage calculation. Monitor platelet and granulocyte counts and Cr_s during therapy.

CISPLATIN   Platinol, Various

Pharmacology. Cisplatin is a planar coordinate dichlorodiamino compound of platinum in the +II valence state. It is aquated in vivo to a positively charged species that can alkylate nucleophilic sites in DNA such as purine and pyrimidine bases. Its action is cell-cycle phase nonspecific.

Administration and Adult Dosage. **IV bolus or continuous infusion** (usually with aggressive hydration) single doses of up to 120 mg/m² have been used.[26] **IV**

in the Einhorn testicular cancer regimen 20 mg/m^2/day for 5 days.[27] (*See* Notes.)

Special Populations. *Pediatric Dosage.* IV 10–20 mg/m^2/day for 4–5 days, repeat q 3–4 weeks. IV maximum single dose is 100 mg/m^2 given q 2–3 weeks.[26]

Geriatric Dosage. Same as adult dosage but adjust for age-related reduction in renal function.

Other Conditions. Reduce dosage in renal impairment; specific dosage reduction guidelines have not been established.

Dosage Forms. Inj 50, 100 mg.

Patient Instructions. (*See* Antineoplastics Class Instructions.) Be prepared for severe nausea and vomiting after drug administration.

Pharmacokinetics. *Serum Levels.* In vitro cell culture data suggest cytotoxicity at levels of 50 mg/L for 1 hr or 5 mg/L for 8 hr.

Fate. Peak serum levels of free platinum after a 100 mg/m^2 bolus are about 3.4 mg/L when given with mannitol (12.5 g) and 2.7 mg/L without mannitol.[28] Over 90% of platinum is protein bound to RBCs, albumin, and prealbumin. It is freely distributed to most organs including kidneys, liver, skin, and lungs and has minimal accumulation in CSF only after repeated doses. Cumulative 24-hr urinary excretion of platinum is 20% with mannitol, 40% without.

t$_{1/2}$. (Free platinum) 59 min (with mannitol); 48 min (without mannitol). Terminal half-life is 58–73 hr, probably reflecting slow release of protein-bound drug.[28,29]

Adverse Reactions. Emetic potential is high. Nausea and vomiting are severe and often prolonged (days) and can be managed with aggressive prophylaxis using a serotonin 5HT$_3$-antagonist, butyrophenone (eg, droperidol), metoclopramide, a high-dose glucocorticoid, or a combination. Primary toxicity is dose-related nephrotoxicity, especially proximal tubular impairment. Ototoxicity and elevated hepatic enzymes occur frequently; total dose-related hypomagnesemia and severe cumulative peripheral neuropathy occur. Slight leukopenia, thrombocytopenia, and frequent anemia also occur. Epoetin alfa is useful in preventing severe anemia caused by cisplatin. Rare toxicities include transient cortical dysfunction (blindness) and hypersensitivity (including anaphylaxis).

Contraindications. Renal insufficiency (Cr$_s$ >1.5–2 mg/dL or Cl$_{cr}$ <60 mL/min); myelosuppression; hearing impairment; previous anaphylaxis. However, some patients with prior anaphylaxis have been successfully retreated with cisplatin and concomitant antihistamine, epinephrine, and glucocorticoid.

Precautions. Use with caution in renal impairment and with other nephrotoxic drugs, especially aminoglycosides.[30] Assure adequate hydration before administration. Both furosemide and mannitol are used to decrease platinum nephrotoxicity, although each apparently retards free platinum elimination.

Drug Interactions. Cisplatin can enhance nephrotoxicity and ototoxicity of the aminoglycosides. Use with ifosfamide can increase nephrotoxicity and potassium and magnesium loss, especially in children. Furosemide ototoxicity might be increased by cisplatin. Cisplatin can increase methotrexate serum levels and its toxicity. Cisplatin can decrease absorption and serum levels of valproic acid. Phenytoin serum levels can be decreased after cisplatin-containing combination regimens.

Parameters to Monitor. Assess renal function before each dose (eg, serial BUN or Cr_s) and serum magnesium levels periodically.

Notes. Reconstitute with sterile water; it may then be mixed in saline-containing solutions. It is stable for 24 hr in mannitol. Do not expose solution to metals (eg, metal drippers or cannulae) because platinum can rapidly plate onto these surfaces. Hydrate the patient with at least 1 L of a saline-containing solution with 20 mEq of KCl and 3 g of $MgSO_4/L.$[31]

CYCLOPHOSPHAMIDE
Cytoxan, Various

Pharmacology. Cyclophosphamide is inactive in vitro and must be enzymatically activated in the liver to yield active alkylating compounds and toxic metabolites.[32] Cell-cycle phase nonspecific.

Administration and Adult Dosage. **IV or PO alone or in combination regimens** 250–500 mg/m² q 3–4 weeks. **IV (usually) or PO in high-dose intermittent regimens (including bone marrow transplant)** maximum of 40–50 mg/kg given once or over 2–5 days, repeat q 2–4 weeks—these doses are not well tolerated orally. IV doses may be given in any convenient volume of all common IV solutions or by IV push. **Continuous daily administration PO** 1–5 mg/kg/day; during continuous therapy, dosage must be individualized based on patient bone marrow response.

Special Populations. *Pediatric Dosage.* **IV, PO for malignancies** same as adult dosage. **PO for nephrotic syndrome** 2.5–3 mg/kg/day for up to 8 weeks.

Geriatric Dosage. Same as adult dosage.

Other Conditions. No dosage alteration appears necessary in renal impairment because differences in toxicity between normals and patients with renal failure have not been reported.[33]

Dosage Forms. **Tab** 25, 50 mg; **Inj** 100, 200, 500 mg, 1, 2 g.

Patient Instructions. (*See* Antineoplastics Class Instructions.) Drink 2–3 quarts of fluids daily (1–2 quarts in smaller children) and urinate frequently; do *not* take oral doses at bedtime. Report any blood in the urine.

Pharmacokinetics. *Fate.* Oral absorption is 74 ± 22%.[10] Metabolized to active compounds (including the highly toxic nonalkylating aldehyde, acrolein, and the principal alkylator, phosphoramide mustard) primarily by hepatic microsomal mixed-function oxidases. Cyclophosphamide is 13% plasma protein bound; its alkylating metabolites are 50% bound. V_d is 0.78 ± 0.57 L/kg for parent drug; Cl is 0.078 ± 0.03 L/hr/kg.[10] Renal elimination accounts for 6.5 ± 4.3% of unchanged drug and 60% of metabolites,[34] with a mean renal clearance of 0.66 L/hr of unchanged drug.[33] Clearance may be reduced in obese patients. Elimination is linear over a wide range of doses.[32]

$t_{1/2}$. (Serum alkylating activity) 7.5 ± 4 hr, slightly longer in patients on allopurinol or those previously exposed to cyclophosphamide;[10,33,34] unchanged in renal dysfunction.[35]

Adverse Reactions. Emetic potential is moderate to high (>1 g). Nausea, vomiting, and alopecia are frequent and dose dependent. Dose-limiting toxicity is myelosuppression, with a WBC nadir of about 10 days; platelets also are suppressed, perhaps to a lesser extent. Transient, reversible blurred vision occurs frequently. The drug is locally nonirritating. Renally eliminated active metabolites occasionally cause sterile hemorrhagic cystitis, which can resolve slowly, often leading to a fibrotic, contracted bladder. Bladder epithelial changes range from minimal to frank neoplasia. An early sign of cystitis is microscopic hematuria, which can lead to hemorrhage. Prophylactic hydration is recommended. To prevent urotoxicity with high-dose regimens, administer **mesna.** (*See* Mesna.) **Acetylcysteine** (Mucomyst) bladder irrigations can have antidotal activity. Rarely, bladder dysplasia can lead to bladder cancer after very high doses or with concurrent or prior bladder radiation. Cross-allergenicity with other alkylators (eg, mechlorethamine) can occur. Ovarian and testicular function can be permanently lost after high-dose, long-term therapy. Rare reactions are a high-dose fatal cardiomyopathy, "allergic" interstitial pneumonitis, and a transient condition similar to SIADH that is preventable with vigorous isotonic hydration.

Contraindications. Previous life-threatening hypersensitivity to cyclophosphamide; marked leukopenia and thrombocytopenia; hemorrhagic cystitis; severe pulmonary toxicity caused by prior alkylator therapy.

Precautions. Pregnancy. Consider dosage reduction or discontinuation of drug in patients who develop infections.

Drug Interactions. Cyclophosphamide can prolong the action of neuromuscular blocking agents. Allopurinol and cimetidine can enhance cyclophosphamide myelotoxicity.

Parameters to Monitor. Before induction therapy, assess the patient for adequate numbers of WBCs (>3500/μL) and platelets (>120,000/μL). With long-term use, assess these counts at least monthly. Monitor closely for hematuria, especially if the patient has received a large cumulative dosage.

Notes. Do not dilute with benzyl alcohol-preserved solutions. Diluted solution is stable for 24 hr at room temperature and 6 days under refrigeration. Widely used in hematologic and solid malignancies and as an immunosuppressant in a variety of autoimmune disorders.

DACARBAZINE   DTIC-Dome, Various

Pharmacology. Dacarbazine is an imidazole analogue of a purine precursor that alkylates DNA via methyldiazonium in a cell-cycle phase nonspecific fashion. It is used in malignant melanoma with about a 10–20% objective response rate.[36,37]

Adult Dosage. IV as a single dose up to 850 mg/m^2, repeated in 3–4 weeks. Alternatively, it may be given in a dosage of up to 250 mg/m^2/day for 5 days, repeated in 3–4 weeks. Reduce the dosage in renal and/or hepatic impairment.

Dosage Forms. Inj 100, 200 mg.

Pharmacokinetics. Dacarbazine is extensively metabolized, some microsomally mediated (50% by *N*-demethylation); it is 5% plasma protein bound, with 30–45%

of a dose excreted unchanged in the urine. The drug has an α half-life of 35 min and a β half-life of about 5 hr; in one patient with renal and hepatic dysfunction, the terminal half-life increased to 7.2 hr.

Adverse Reactions. Nausea and vomiting, which occasionally are severe, occur almost invariably; these can decrease in severity with successive courses of therapy. Dose- and duration-dependent sterility, mutagenicity, and teratogenicity have been reported. Pain on injection also occurs. The dose-limiting toxicity is myelosuppression, with a leukopenic nadir at 21–25 days. Occasionally, a flu-like syndrome of myalgia, fever, and malaise occurs within 1 week of drug administration. Use dacarbazine with caution in patients with pre-existing bone marrow aplasia and avoid exposure to sunlight because of possible photosensitivity reactions. The drug is light sensitive so minimize exposure to light after reconstitution. The reconstituted solution is clear to pale yellow and is stable for 8 hr after reconstitution at room temperature; pink discoloration denotes drug decomposition.

IFOSFAMIDE   Ifex

Pharmacology. Ifosfamide is a structural analogue of the alkylating agent cyclophosphamide (CTX). The rate of hepatic conversion of ifosfamide to the active metabolite 4-hydroxyifosfamide is slightly slower than with CTX, although formation of the bladder toxin acrolein is not reduced. The ultimate metabolite ifosforamide mustard cross-links DNA to impair cell division. The drug is always given with mesna to prevent urotoxicity. Although labeled for use in refractory testicular cancer, ifosfamide also has useful activity against soft tissue sarcoma, malignant lymphoma, and small cell lung cancer.[38] Ifosfamide is cell-cycle phase nonspecific.

Administration and Adult Dosage. **IV for refractory testicular cancer** 1.2 g/m²/day over 30 min to 4 hr for 5 days, or 2 g/m²/day for 3 consecutive days. The recommended concurrent IV **mesna** dose is 20% of the ifosfamide dose, given 15 min before ifosfamide and again at 4 and 8 hr. It can be directly admixed with ifosfamide. The latter two mesna doses can be given orally at twice the dose (ie, each at 40% of the ifosfamide dose) if patient compliance and a lack of emesis can be assured.[39] **Alternatively, IV by continuous infusion** 5–8 g/m² over 24 hr with mesna added at the same concentration as ifosfamide.[40] However, more severe nephrotoxicity can occur with this regimen.[41]

Special Populations. *Pediatric Dosage.* **IV for sarcomas (Ewing's and osteosarcoma)** 1.2 g/m²/day over 30 min for 5 days, each with 3 IV mesna doses, as above.[42,43]

Geriatric Dosage. Same as adult dosage but adjust for age-related reduction in renal function.

Other Conditions. Dosage reduction is indicated in patients with reduced renal function, although specific guidelines are not available.

Dosage Forms. Inj 1, 3 g.

Patient Instructions. (*See* Antineoplastics Class Instructions.)

Pharmacokinetics. *Fate.* Ifosfamide, but not its metabolites, penetrates into the CNS; CSF levels are about 38–49% of simultaneous serum levels. Ifosfamide is metabolized to the active alkylating agent ifosforamide mustard by CYP2B6, which converts ifosfamide to 4-hydroxyifosfamide (which can act as the transport form of the molecule). The 4-hydroxy metabolite is then chemically or enzymatically broken down to active and inactive metabolites. Inactive metabolites include 4-carboxyifosfamide and several dechloroethylated species such as thiodiacetic acid. About 60–80% of a dose is excreted in the urine over 72 hr, including up to 50% of unchanged drug. In addition to 4-hydroxyifosfamide, the bladder irritant acrolein is excreted renally and can accumulate to high concentrations in the urinary bladder.[44,45]

$t_{\frac{1}{2}}$. 6.9 hr.[46]

Adverse Reactions. Emetic potential is moderate; nausea and vomiting can be readily managed with antiemetics. Alopecia occurs in most patients treated with ifosfamide. The major dose-limiting effect of ifosfamide is urotoxicity manifested as hematuria. The frequency of microscopic hematuria with ifosfamide and the chemoprotectant mesna are 5–18% of courses;[38] gross hematuria is less common (<5%). (*See* Mesna.) Renal tubular toxicity, manifested by elevations in BUN and Cr_s, occurs in <10% of patients. It is more frequent in patients who are poorly hydrated or have pre-existing abnormal renal function,[47] those with renal cell cancer,[48] those given high-dose 24-hr continuous ifosfamide infusions,[40] and those receiving concomitant treatment with other nephrotoxins.[47] Myelosuppression primarily involves leukopenia with a 7- to 14-day nadir. This effect is less severe than with cyclophosphamide and rarely affects platelets. However, in combination with other myelosuppressive drugs, additive leukopenia that is not reduced by mesna can occur. Leukopenia has been particularly severe in nephrectomized patients with renal cell cancer.[40] CNS toxicities occur in up to 50% of patients, but risk factors, including dosage, are unclear. The most common effect is slight sedation or somnolence, which rarely proceeds to coma and death. These signs appear within 2 hr and typically remit 1–3 days after drug administration. Other rare CNS neurotoxicities are cerebellar toxicity (ataxia), urinary incontinence, and seizures.[49] Some of these CNS effects might be caused by the minor metabolite chloracetaldehyde, which is excreted in the urine and accumulates in renal failure.[50] Transient elevation in LFTs is frequently reported but is rarely clinically important. Other occasional toxic effects are allergic reactions, diarrhea, peripheral neuropathy, and stomatitis.

Contraindications. Severe pre-existing myelosuppression.

Precautions. Because of more severe nephrotoxicity and CNS toxicities, patients with reduced renal function, and particularly nephrectomized renal cell cancer patients, are poor candidates for this agent. Withhold repeat therapy until there is resolution of microscopic hematuria (<10 RBCs per high-power field). An adequate state of hydration is critical to reducing urotoxicity.

Drug Interactions. Use with cisplatin can increase nephrotoxicity and potassium and magnesium loss, especially in children. Nephrotoxicity is also enhanced when ifosfamide is combined with other nephrotoxic drugs.

Parameters to Monitor. Ensure that renal function and peripheral WBC counts are normal before administration. During therapy, monitor hematuria daily because dosage reduction or higher mesna dosage can prevent more serious urotoxicity.

Notes. Ifosfamide is compatible with D5W, NS, Ringer's lactate injection, and sterile water. It also can be directly mixed with mesna. Exercise caution to reduce exposure during handling and disposal.

MECHLORETHAMINE HYDROCHLORIDE   Mustargen

Pharmacology. Mechlorethamine (nitrogen mustard; HN_2) is a prototype bis-chloroethylamine, polyfunctional alkylating agent. In solution, the compound readily ionizes to an active form, which can alkylate at a number of nucleophilic protein sites, principally the N^7 position of guanine in DNA and RNA. This action is cell-cycle phase nonspecific.

Administration and Adult Dosage. IV for Hodgkin's disease (in the classical MOPP regimen) 6 mg/m^2 by careful push on days 1 and 8 of a monthly treatment cycle.[51] Irritation, spasm, and sclerosis occur in exposed veins; therefore, it is common to begin venipunctures low on the limb and move up serially and administer mechlorethamine last in a combination drug sequence. **IV as a single agent** up to 0.4 mg/kg as a single monthly dose. **Top for mycosis fungoides and psoriasis** 10 mg/60 mL of water, applied to the affected body areas 1 or 2 times a day.[52]

Special Populations. *Pediatric Dosage.* **IV** same as adult dosage.

Geriatric Dosage. Same as adult dosage.

Dosage Forms. Inj 10 mg.

Patient Instructions. (*See* Antineoplastics Class Instructions.)

Pharmacokinetics. *Fate.* Chemical cyclization occurs in vivo to form positively charged carbonium ions, which rapidly react with various cellular components; unchanged drug cannot be detected in the blood within minutes of administration. Less than 0.01% of unchanged drug is recovered in the urine; however, up to 50% of radioactively labeled products can be found in urine within 24 hr.[1]

Adverse Reactions. Emetic potential is high; nausea and vomiting within the first 3 hr are severe and can last more than 1 day. The major dose-limiting toxicity is myelosuppression: leukopenic nadir occurs at 6–8 days, thrombocytopenic nadir at 10–16 days. Extravasation causes delayed and protracted (months) ulceration and necrosis; a 1/6 molar **sodium thiosulfate** solution (4 mL of 10% sodium thiosulfate plus 6 mL sterile water) and copious flushing with water may be used as topical antidotes to lessen serious tissue damage. Primary reproductive failure and alopecia are frequent in males and females. IV or topical use can cause maculopapular rashes and sometimes severe sensitivity reactions (anaphylaxis and occasional cross-reactivity with other alkylating agents).

Contraindications. Prior severe hypersensitivity reactions; pre-existing profound myelosuppression; infection.

Precautions. Give patients with lymphomas (especially "bulky" lymphomas) prophylactic allopurinol 2–3 days before and throughout therapy to prevent hyperuricemia and urate nephropathy after massive tumor lysis. Make every effort to avoid topical contact with this highly vesicant drug by health personnel.

Drug Interactions. None known.

Parameters to Monitor. Pretreatment and at least monthly assessment of bone marrow function, particularly WBC and platelet counts.

Notes. Mechlorethamine is a powerful vesicant and should be prepared with great caution. Use mask and rubber gloves during preparation and avoid inhalation of dust and vapors or contact with skin and mucous membranes, especially the eyes. Use the injection within 1 hr of preparation; topical solution and ointment are stable for 1 month under refrigeration.[53] Because of its extreme acute toxicity, use is limited primarily to malignant lymphomas[51] and topically in mycosis fungoides, a cutaneous non-Hodgkin's T-cell lymphoma.[54]

MITOMYCIN	Mutamycin

Pharmacology. Mitomycin (mitomycin C) is an antibiotic that contains quinone, urethane, and aziridine groups. It is activated chemically and metabolically to alkylating species; it is cell-cycle phase nonspecific, but maximum efficacy is in the G_1 and S phases. Mitomycin is used primarily in GI tract tumors intravenously and bladder cancer intravesically.[55-58]

Adult Dosage. **IV as a single agent** 10–15 mg/m² in a single dose and repeated q 6 weeks if hematologic toxicity has resolved. **IV in combination regimens** 5–10 mg/m² repeated in 4–6 weeks. **Intravesically in bladder cancer** up to 60 mg/week.

Dosage Forms. **Inj** 5, 20, 40 mg.

Pharmacokinetics. After IV doses of 15 mg/m², the peak serum level is about 1 mg/L (3 μmol/L). The drug is eliminated primarily by hepatic clearance, with about 20% hepatic extraction and 10–30% recovery of unchanged drug in the urine. Cl is 0.3–0.4 L/hr/kg. The drug has an α half-life of 5–10 min after IV injection and a β half-life of 46 min.

Adverse Reactions. Nausea, vomiting, diarrhea, alopecia, and nephrotoxicity occur frequently. The drug also produces sterility, mutagenicity, and teratogenicity. The dose-limiting toxicities are myelosuppression (with a long leukopenic nadir of 3–4 weeks), thrombocytopenia, and anemia, all of which can be cumulative. Monitor the patient carefully for delayed and prolonged myelosuppression. Severe ulceration can occur if the drug is extravasated (topical **DMSO** may be useful). Interstitial pneumonia, for which a **glucocorticoid** is helpful, occurs occasionally. Long-term therapy occasionally causes hemolytic-uremic syndrome. Mitomycin is contraindicated in patients with pre-existing severe myelosuppression or anemia.

NITROSOUREAS:	
CARMUSTINE	BiCNU, Gliadel
LOMUSTINE	CeeNU

Pharmacology. Carmustine (BCNU) and lomustine (CCNU) are highly lipid-soluble drugs that are metabolized to active alkylating and carbamoylating moieties. Several key cellular enzymatic steps are inhibited, including those involving

DNA polymerase and RNA and protein synthesis. There is typically only partial cross-resistance to classical alkylators. The nitrosoureas are cell-cycle phase non-specific and even have activity on G_0 (resting phase) cells.

Administration and Dosage. (*See also* Notes.)

	CARMUSTINE	LOMUSTINE
Administration	IV in 100–200 mL D5W in glass containers only over 15–45 min.	PO only.
Adult Dosage	75–100 mg/m²/day for 1–2 days or 200 mg/m² as a single dose, or 80 mg/m²/day for 3 days. Repeat at 6- to 8-week intervals.	100–130 mg/m² as a single dose, repeat at 6- to 8- week intervals.
Pediatric Dosage	Same as adult dosage.	Same as adult dosage.
Geriatric Dosage	Reduce dosage by 25–50% and/or increase treatment interval to at least 8 weeks.	Same as adult dosage.
Other Conditions	Treat patients with heavily pretreated bone marrow with 50–75% of the recommended dosage and/or at lengthened treatment intervals (8 weeks minimum).	

Dosage Forms. (Carmustine) **Inj** 100 mg with alcohol diluent (BiCNU); **Wafer** 7.7 mg (Gliadel). (Lomustine) **Cap** 10, 40, 100 mg—commercial packet contains two of each strength for a total of 300 mg. (*See* Notes.)

Patient Instructions. (*See* Antineoplastics Class Instructions.) Take lomustine on an empty stomach.

Pharmacokinetics. *Fate.*

	CARMUSTINE	LOMUSTINE
Absorption	—	Complete after 30 min.[59]
Distribution	Both drugs are diffusely distributed with decreasing relative concentrations in spleen, liver, and ovaries; both achieve substantial penetration into CNS with simultaneous CSF levels of >50% of serum for intact carmustine and its metabolites[60] and >30% for intact lomustine and its metabolites;[59] enterohepatic cycling of active metabolites is possible and may explain subsequent peaks in nitrosourea serum levels at 1 and 4 hr.	
Metabolism	Both drugs are rapidly and extensively metabolized (partly by liver microsomal enzymes) to a number of active products that have long serum half-lives compared with the parent compounds.	
Excretion	30% urinary drug recovery as metabolites after 24 hr, 65% after 96 hr.[60]	50% urinary drug recovery as metabolites after 12 hr, 60% after 48 hr; <5% fecal excretion.[59]
$t_{1/2}$	Intact drug 5 min; biologic effect 15–30 min; metabolites, slow decay over 3–4 days.[60]	Intact drug 15 min; cyclohexyl and carbonyl metabolites: α phase 4–5 hr, β phase 30–50 hr; chloroethyl metabolite 72 hr.[59]

Adverse Reactions. Emetic potential is moderately high to high; prophylactic antiemetics are recommended. Major dose-limiting toxicity is delayed and potentially cumulative myelosuppression; nadirs are unusually prolonged, with leukopenia at approximately 35 days and thrombocytopenia at about 30 days. Thus, doses are not repeated more often than q 6 weeks.[61] Carmustine frequently causes severe pain at injection site and venospasm, which can be reduced by slow, dilute infusions. Both drugs can transiently elevate liver enzymes. Pulmonary fibrosis can occur after cumulative dosages >1 g/m^2; nephrotoxicity consistently occurs after cumulative dosages of ≥ 1.5 g/m^2.[62] Variant carmustine-induced pulmonary fibrosis, highly responsive to early drug discontinuation and a glucocorticoid, has been reported.[63] Other occasional toxicities are CNS effects (eg, confusion, lethargy, ataxia), stomatitis, and alopecia. In animal models, the nitrosoureas are highly carcinogenic and several clinical cases of leukemia after nitrosourea therapy have been reported.

Contraindications. Demonstrated hypersensitivity; marked pre-existing myelosuppression.

Precautions. Pregnancy.

Drug Interactions. Experimentally in rats, carmustine, lomustine, and the investigational drug semustine are cleared much more rapidly (with reduced antitumor activity) by pretreatment with phenobarbital, which stimulates microsomal enzymes. Conversely, cimetidine can impair metabolism and increase nitrosourea myelotoxicity. Clinical resistance to carmustine and perhaps other nitrosoureas is reduced by concomitant amphotericin B. Digoxin and phenytoin serum levels might be decreased after carmustine-containing combination regimens.

Notes. Store carmustine under refrigeration; appearance of an oily film in the vial is evidence of decomposition, and such vials should be discarded. Carmustine is incompatible with sodium bicarbonate. Lomustine absorption is rapid; thus, vomiting 45 min or more after ingestion does not require readministration.

Carmustine implant wafers (Gliadel) are indicated for implantation in the resection cavity of patients undergoing surgery for recurrent glioblastoma multiforme. In a multicenter, placebo-controlled trial, 6-month survival in patients with glioblastoma was 50% greater with carmustine implants than with placebo. The typical adult dosage is 8 wafers (61.6 mg of carmustine) implanted at the time of surgery. In experimental systems, the polymer releases carmustine over 2 to 3 weeks in vivo. Intracranial infections occur at a higher rate (4% vs 1%), and seizures are more frequent in patients with carmustine wafers than in untreated patients. Mild to moderate healing abnormalities occur in 4% of treated patients compared with 1% of untreated patients. Other systemic and CNS side effects are equivalent in treated and untreated patients.[64,65]

PROCARBAZINE HYDROCHLORIDE   Matulane

Pharmacology. Procarbazine is an N-methylhydrazine derivative that undergoes auto-oxidation and microsomal activation to form several alkylating species, including the diazonium ion and several oxygen free radicals such as H_2O_2, $\cdot OH$, and $\cdot O_2$ (superoxide). It is cell-cycle phase nonspecific and used in brain tumors and Hodgkin's and non-Hodgkin's lymphomas.[66]

Adult Dosage. **PO** 50–200 mg/m^2/day for 10–25 days, repeated in 3–4 weeks. Calculate the dosage based on IBW and reduce dosage for a BUN >40 mg/dL, Cr$_s$ >2 mg/dL, or serum bilirubin >3 mg/dL.

Dosage Forms. **Cap** 50 mg.

Pharmacokinetics. The drug is rapidly and well absorbed after oral administration; CNS levels are equal to those in serum after 0.5–1.5 hr. Procarbazine is 70% recovered in the urine, primarily as an acid metabolite, with <5% excreted unchanged.

Adverse Reactions. Frequent CNS side effects include dizziness, headache, ataxia, nightmares, depression, and hallucinations (in up to 30% of patients). Paresthesias also can occur occasionally. Mild to moderate nausea and vomiting occur in 60–90% of patients, but tolerance usually develops rapidly. Dose- and duration-dependent sterility, mutagenicity, and teratogenicity are reported. The drug predisposes patients to secondary acute nonlymphocytic leukemias. The dose-limiting toxicity is myelosuppression with a pancytopenic nadir at 2–3 weeks. Occasional side effects include a flu-like syndrome, allergic pneumonitis, and rash. Procarbazine is contraindicated in patients with *severe* hypersensitivity to the drug or pre-existing bone marrow aplasia. Periodic evaluations of neurologic status and monthly CBCs may be useful.

Drug Interactions. Avoid concurrent use with MAO inhibitors, alcohol, heterocyclic antidepressants, sympathomimetics, or tyramine-containing foods. Microsomal enzyme-inducing drugs might augment procarbazine cytotoxicity. Procarbazine potentiates barbiturates, narcotics, and other hepatically metabolized drugs.

STREPTOZOCIN   Zanosar

Pharmacology. Streptozocin is a glucose-containing nitrosourea. It has some selective cytotoxic activity in insulinomas and malignant carcinoid and is active to a lesser extent in other adenocarcinomas of the GI tract. The drug inhibits DNA synthesis via inhibition of pyrimidine biosynthesis and blockade of key enzymatic reactions in gluconeogenesis pathways. It is cell-cycle phase nonspecific.[67]

Adult Dosage. **IV as a single agent** 1–1.5 g/m^2/week for 6 weeks, followed by a 4-week observation period; **IV in combination** 0.5–1 g/m^2/day for 5 days q 4–6 weeks.

Dosage Forms. **Inj** 1 g.

Pharmacokinetics. Streptozocin is highly lipophilic, achieving good CNS penetration. Streptozocin and metabolites have a short distribution phase ($t_{\frac{1}{2}\alpha}$ 6 min) followed by possibly two elimination phases representing active metabolites ($t_{\frac{1}{2}\beta}$ 3.5 hr; $t_{\frac{1}{2}\gamma}$ 40 hr). The drug is rapidly and extensively metabolized (unchanged drug half-life is 35 min), and only 10–20% is excreted unchanged in urine.

Adverse Reactions. Frequent acute toxicities include nausea, vomiting, and phlebitis; carefully avoid extravasation. The drug is moderately myelotoxic but extremely nephrotoxic. Signs of streptozocin nephrotoxicity include various renal tubular defects and proteinuria; adequate hydration can offer some protection. It also selectively destroys pancreatic β cells.

TEMOZOLOMIDE   Temodar

Pharmacology. Temozolomide is a synthetic oral alkylating agent structurally related to dacarbazine. Both are converted in vivo to 3-methyl-(triazen-1-yl)imidazole-4-carboxamide (MTIC). Dacarbazine requires metabolic activation through cytochrome P450 enzymes to form this intermediate, whereas temozolomide is spontaneously converted to MTIC under physiologic conditions.[68,69] Metabolites of MTIC methylate the O^6 position of guanine in DNA, with additional methylation at the N^7 position, resulting in cytotoxicity.[70]

Adult Dosage. **PO for refractory anaplastic astrocytoma** 150 mg/m^2 once daily for 5 days initially. Adjust subsequent dosages according to nadir neutrophil and platelet counts (see package insert for specific guidelines). The minimum recommended dose is 100 mg/m^2/day for 5 days q 4 weeks. The recommended maintenance dosage if tolerated is 200 mg/m^2/day for 5 days q 4 weeks. Treatment can be continued until disease progression. Temozolomide has not been studied in severe renal impairment (Cl_{cr} <36 mL/min/m^2) or in severe hepatic impairment.

Dosage Forms. **Cap** 5, 20, 100, 250 mg.

Pharmacokinetics. Temozolomide's oral bioavailability is 100%; food reduces the rate and extent of absorption. Peak plasma concentrations occur in 0.3–2 hr.[70] Temozolomide is 14% bound to plasma proteins[70] and penetrates the CNS in concentrations of about 30% of plasma levels.[71] V_d is 17–28 L/m^2.[72] At neutral or basic pH, temozolomide rapidly and spontaneously hydrolyzes to MTIC and temozolomide acid metabolite (AM). MTIC is further hydrolyzed to 5-aminoimidazole-4-carboxamide (AIC) and methylhydrazine, the active alkylating agent. Less than 1% of temozolomide is excreted in the feces. Five to 7% of temozolomide, 12% of AIC, 2.3% of AM, and 17% of unidentified polar compounds are excreted renally.[70] No accumulation of temozolomide or metabolites occurs.[73] Cl is 5.6–8.5 L/hr/m^2, with a half-life of 1.7–2.3 hr.[72]

Adverse Reactions. The dose-limiting toxicity of temozolomide, myelosuppression, is not cumulative. Thrombocytopenia and leukopenia are dose related and predictable with nadir platelet and leukocyte counts occurring around day 22 of treatment.[72] Anemia and lymphopenia also have been reported. The most frequent adverse effects are nausea, vomiting, constipation, and fatigue. Nausea and vomiting are usually moderate and can be controlled by taking the dose on an empty stomach and using prophylactic antiemetics. Occasional toxicities include headache, diarrhea, pain, fever, anorexia, and increased transaminase levels. Rare side effects include stomatitis, alopecia, flushing, dizziness, rash, and infection. Also reported are vomiting and elevation in liver enzymes.[74]

Contraindications. Hypersensitive to any components of temozolomide or dacarbazine.

Notes. If capsules are accidentally opened, inhalation or contact with skin or mucous membranes should be rigorously avoided. Temozolomide is equivalent to dacarbazine in melanoma and might have less CNS relapse than dacarbazine (which does not penetrate the CNS).[75,76]

THIOTEPA
Thioplex, Various

Pharmacology. Thiotepa (TESPA, TSPA) is a thiophosphoramide compound that is slowly hydrolyzed to release ethylenimine moieties that alkylate DNA. It is used systemically in the treatment of breast cancer, intracavitarily for bladder or pleural disease, and intrathecally for CNS disease. It is also given in high doses with autologous bone marrow transplantation.[77]

Adult Dosage. IV, IM, or SC 0.5 mg/kg monthly or 6 mg/m^2/day for 4 days. Reduce the dosage by all routes in patients with pre-existing bone marrow suppression. **Intracavitary** 60 mg; **IT** 1–10 mg/m^2.

Dosage Forms. Inj 15 mg.

Pharmacokinetics. Thiotepa is slowly metabolized, primarily to TEPA. Total body Cl is 8.5 L/hr/m^2, with 15% recovered in the urine as TEPA in 24 hr. Thiotepa has an α half-life of 7.5 min and a β half-life of 109 min.

Adverse Reactions. Mild nausea and vomiting occur frequently. The dose-limiting toxicity is myelosuppression (of granulocytes and platelets). Myelosuppression can occur after intravesicular or intrapleural administration. Anaphylaxis occurs rarely, and mutagenicity, teratogenicity, and sterility have been reported.

Antimetabolites

CLADRIBINE
Leustatin

Pharmacology. Cladribine (2CdA) is the 20-chloro analogue of deoxyadenosine. It is a purine nucleoside that is avidly phosphorylated to toxic metabolites that accumulate intracellularly. Lymphocytes, which lack inactivating deaminase activity, are selectively destroyed by inhibition of DNA synthesis and repair. Cladribine is highly active in hairy cell leukemia; other responsive tumors are malignant lymphoma and acute and chronic myelogenous leukemias. It is also promising in the treatment of chronic progressive multiple sclerosis.[78–81]

Adult Dosage. **IV for hairy cell leukemia** 0.09 mg/kg/day for 7 days by continuous infusion. New dosage regimens are exploring single daily SC injections because of the prolonged intracellular retention of active metabolites.

Dosage Forms. Inj 1 mg/mL.

Pharmacokinetics. Studies with oral administration indicate a bioavailability of 48%, implying that doubling the IV dose allows oral administration in hairy cell leukemia. The drug has a $V_{d\beta}$ of 9.2 ± 5.4 L/kg and biphasic elimination with half-lives of 35 min and 6.7 hr. About 40% of a dose is excreted renally as parent drug and metabolites.

Adverse Reactions. Frequent adverse reactions are severe neutropenia with fever and infection (70%), anemia (37%), and thrombocytopenia (12%). A flu-like syndrome is also common. Suppression of immune system function because of helper T-lymphocyte depletion can be quite long-lived and presents a risk of systemic opportunistic infections by fungi, bacteria, and/or parasites such as *Pneumocystis carinii*.

CYTARABINE	Cytosar-U, Tarabine PFS, Various
CYTARABNE, LIPOSOMAL	DepoCyt

Pharmacology. Cytarabine (cytosine arabinoside, ara-C) is an arabinose sugar analogue of the natural pyrimidine nucleoside deoxycytidine. Cytarabine is converted to the triphosphate derivative, ara-CTP, which interferes with one or more DNA polymerases and is incorporated into DNA strands, leading to DNA fragmentation and chain termination. Once a threshold level of ara-C–mediated DNA damage is exceeded, apoptosis occurs.[82] Cytarabine is cell-cycle S-phase specific, with activity markedly enhanced by continuous administration over several days.

Administration and Adult Dosage. (Conventional) **IV for remission induction** 100–150 mg/m^2/day as a continuous infusion for 5–10 days. Experimental therapy has successfully used induction doses of 2–3 g/m^2 q 12 hr as a 2-hr infusion for 4–12 doses in refractory AML.[83] **IV or SC for remission induction** 100 mg/m^2 q 12 hr for 5–10 days. **SC for remission maintenance** 70–100 mg/m^2/day for 5 days in 4 divided doses. (*See* Notes.) (Liposomal) **Intrathecal for lymphomatous meningitis** (induction and consolidation) 50 mg on weeks 1, 3, 5, 7, 9, and 13. (Maintenance) 50 mg on weeks 17, 21, 25, and 29. If neurotoxicity develops, reduce subsequent doses to 25 mg; if it persists, discontinue therapy. Administer each dose over 1–5 min directly into the CSF via an intraventricular reservoir or into the lumbar sac. Give dexamethasone 4 mg PO or IV bid for 5 days beginning on the day of each injection.

Special Populations. *Pediatric Dosage.* (Conventional) **IV or SC** same as adult dosage. (Liposomal) Safety and efficacy not established.

Geriatric Dosage. Same as adult dosage.

Dosage Forms. **Inj** (conventional) 100, 500 mg, 1, 2 g; (liposomal) 50 mg.

Patient Instructions. (Liposomal) Lie flat for 1 hour following administration via lumbar puncture. (*See also* Antineoplastics Class Instructions.)

Pharmacokinetics. *Serum Levels.* (Conventional) 50–100 mg/L (0.2–0.4 mmol/L) are required for cytotoxic effects.[84]

Fate. (Conventional) Not systemically available after oral absorption. After injection, there is a large interpatient variation in serum levels attained as measured by various assay techniques.[85] Serum levels of 100–400 mg/L (0.4–1.6 mmol/L) are produced by a 60-min continuous infusion of 300 mg/m^2.[86] Serum levels up to 240 mg/L (1 mmol/L) are achieved with high-dose regimens. It is widely distributed and deactivated by cytidine deaminase, primarily in the liver. The CSF-to-serum ratio is 0.1–0.14:1 with bolus doses and up to 0.4–0.5:1 with continuous infusion. There is slow elimination from the CSF caused by low CNS deaminating activity; however, to attain therapeutic CSF concentrations after standard IV doses, intrathecal administration is required. Tear fluid concentrations are detectable after high-dose therapy. The drug is about 13% plasma protein bound. V_d is 3 ± 1.9 L/kg; Cl is 0.78 ± 0.24 L/hr/kg.[10] The deamination product, uracil arabinoside (ara-U) is inactive and rapidly excreted in the urine; 24 hr after injection, 72% of the dose is recovered in the urine as ara-U, only 11 ± 8% as unchanged drug.[10,87]

t½. (Conventional) α phase 1.6–12 min; β phase 2.6 ± 0.6 hr.[10,86–88]

Adverse Reactions. (Conventional) Emetic potential is moderate (<250 mg) to moderately high (250 mg–1 g); prophylactic antiemetics are very effective. The principal side effect is dose-related myelosuppression with a leukopenic nadir of 3–11 days and a thrombocytopenic nadir of 12–14 days; megaloblastosis is typically noted in the recovering bone marrow and in the rare cases in which anemia develops. Ocular toxicity is frequent with high-dose therapy; typically, conjunctival injection and central punctate corneal opacities occur. Concurrent use of glucocorticoid eye drops is recommended with high-dose therapy.[89] Occasionally, mild oral ulceration and a flu-like syndrome, manifested by arthralgias, fever, and sometimes rash, occur. Irreversible cerebellar toxicity (ataxia, cognitive dysfunction) is a risk after cumulative doses of 30 g/m^2.[90] Hepatic enzyme elevation is rare, even with 3 g/m^2 doses; one instance of SIADH was reported with this large dose.[83] Cutaneous small vessel necrotizing vasculitis has occurred rarely after high-dose cytarabine, 3–5 days after initiation of therapy.[91](Liposomal) Arachnoiditis is frequent but sometimes can be related to disease progression or infection. Abnormal gait, confusion, headache, somnolence, asthenia, constipation, nausea, vomiting peripheral edema, neutropenia, and thrombocytopenia are frequent. Side effects are most likely during the 5 days after a dose.

Precautions. (Conventional) Myelosuppression is *not* a contraindication because marrow hypoplasia with complete suppression of the leukemic clone is the desired clinical endpoint; however, extensive supportive facilities must be available during therapy, including WBC and platelet transfusion capability. When IV (conventional) and intrathecal (liposomal) cytarabine are given within a few days of each other, spinal cord toxicity is more likely. Concurrent radiation might increase the rate of adverse reactions due to liposomal cytarabine.

Drug Interactions. Digoxin bioavailability from tablets may be decreased after cytarabine-containing combination regimens.

Parameters to Monitor. Routine WBC and platelet counts; RBC indices. (Liposomal) Monitor continuously for signs of neurotoxicity.

Notes. (Conventional) Patients can be taught sterile technique for self-administration of SC drug for leukemia remission maintenance. The use of small reconstitution volumes (1 mL/100 mg) and rotation of injection sites should be observed. Clinical activity is limited primarily to selected hematologic malignancies (eg, AML, ALL, DHL). The combination of cytarabine and **interferon** increases the rate of response and prolongs survival in patients with the chronic phase of chronic myelogenous leukemia compared with interferon alone.[92]

Conventional cytarabine is given by IT injection or intraventricular injection via an implanted Ommaya reservoir to prevent or treat malignant metastases from acute myeloid leukemia and other cancers. The usual adult dosage is 70 mg/m^2 (or a fixed 100 mg) per dose once or twice weekly. IT doses should not be repeated more often than q 3–5 days in adults. In children, the dose is reduced as follows: (<1 yr) reduce by one-half; (1–2 yr) reduce by one-third; (2–3 yr) reduce by one-sixth. The drug should be diluted only with nonpreserved, isotonic solutions such as NS or, preferably, Ringer's lactate (because of its buffering capacity). In these dilutions, conventional cytarabine is physically compatible with hydrocortisone sodium succinate and methotrexate if a neutral pH is maintained. The half-life in CSF is 2–11 hr (mean 3.5 hr). Typical toxicities include headache and vomiting, which are dose and frequency related. Patients with blocked or impaired CSF outflow might experience greater toxicity. With frequent, repeated administration, seizures and paraplegia can occur.[88,89]

(Liposomal) Use within 4 hr of withdrawal from vial and discard any unused drug. Do not dilute or mix with any other medications and do not use an in-line filter.

FLOXURIDINE   FUDR, Various

Pharmacology. Floxuridine is the deoxyribose metabolite of fluorouracil. The drug inhibits DNA synthesis by binding to thymidylate synthetase in S phase of cell division.

Administration and Adult Dosage. **Intra-arterially for colon cancer metastases to the liver** 0.1–0.6 mg/kg/day for 1–6 weeks by continuous hepatic artery perfusion.[93] Hospitalize patients for at least the first course of therapy.

Special Populations. *Pediatric Dosage.* Safety and efficacy not established.

Geriatric Dosage. Same as adult dosage.

Other Conditions. Reduce dosage when combined with other myelosuppressive drugs or in patients experiencing severe toxicity (usually mucositis or diarrhea) from previous doses.

Dosage Forms. **Inj** 500 mg.

Patient Instructions. (*See* Antineoplastics Class Instructions.)

Pharmacokinetics. *Fate.* Floxuridine has a high degree (69–92%) of hepatic extraction. A large fraction is converted to the active phosphorylated metabolite 5-fluorodeoxyuridylate monophosphate (FdUMP). Ultimately, the drug is almost completely metabolized to inactive compounds, which are eliminated by exhalation (60% of a dose) or by urinary excretion (about 10–30% of a dose).[94]

$t_{½}$. <15 min.

Adverse Reactions. Emetic potential with intra-arterial administration is low. Diarrhea and stomatitis occur frequently. Stomatitis can be life-threatening, as can an unusual dermatitis affecting the hands and feet; both toxicities are much more frequent with prolonged infusions. The primary dose-limiting toxicity of floxuridine is myelosuppression, principally leukopenia with some thrombocytopenia. Liver enzyme elevations occur frequently, but they rarely herald serious hepatic complications. Local complications involving the hepatic catheter are thrombosis, leakage, embolism, and infection. Some catheter placements also can result in gastric ulcers or biliary sclerosis if their respective arterioles are inadvertently perfused.[93]

Contraindications. Pregnancy; poor nutrition; pre-existing myelosuppression; serious infection.

Precautions. Biliary sclerosis can occur, requiring repositioning or removal of the catheter.

Drug Interactions. None known.

Parameters to Monitor. Monitor WBC count before and after each treatment. Observe for diarrhea (fluid and electrolyte status). Monitor for severe hepatic enzyme elevations, which might indicate biliary sclerosis.

Notes. Floxuridine can be administered in NS or D5W and it is compatible with heparin.

FLUDARABINE PHOSPHATE
Fludara

Pharmacology. Fludarabine is a fluorinated nucleotide analogue of vidarabine. It is rapidly converted to 2-fluoro-ara-A, which is then phosphorylated to 2-fluoro-ara-ATP, which inhibits DNA synthesis. Fludarabine has little cross-resistance with other agents used for chronic lymphocytic leukemia.

Adult Dosage. **IV for B-cell CLL that has not responded to at least one standard alkylating agent regimen** 25 mg/m^2/day for 5 days given over 30 min in 100–125 mL of D5W or NS. Refrigerate the drug before reconstitution and use within 8 hr after reconstitution.

Dosage Forms. **Inj** 50 mg.

Pharmacokinetics. The metabolite 2-fluoro-ara-A has a V_d of 98 L/m^2, a Cl of 8.9 L/hr/m^2, and a half-life of about 10 hr. About 23% of a dose is excreted in the urine as unchanged 2-fluoro-ara-A, and clearance is proportional to Cl_{cr}.

Adverse Reactions. The most frequent adverse effects are myelosuppression (neutropenia, thrombocytopenia, and anemia), fever and chills, infection, rash, myalgia, nausea, vomiting, and diarrhea. Frequent pulmonary symptoms include pneumonia, cough, and dyspnea. Fludarabine produced severe CNS toxicity (ie, blindness, coma, and death) in 36% of patients treated with a dosage of 4 times the currently recommended dosage. Similar CNS toxicity occurs occasionally (≤0.2% of patients) with recommended dosages. Other CNS effects are weakness, visual disturbances, paresthesias, agitation, confusion, and peripheral neuropathy.

FLUOROURACIL
Various

Pharmacology. Fluorouracil (5-fluorouracil, 5-FU) is a fluorinated antimetabolite of the DNA pyrimidine precursor uracil. It inhibits thymidine formation, thereby blocking DNA synthesis. Some fluorouracil might be incorporated into RNA, inhibiting subsequent protein synthesis. It is cell-cycle S-phase specific.

Administration and Adult Dosage. **Rapid IV** 15 mg/kg/week for 4 weeks followed by 20 mg/kg/week until severe toxicity develops. The drug is stopped until resolution is complete, then resumed at 5 mg/kg/week.[95] **IV "loading course"** 12 mg/kg (800 mg maximum) as a single daily dose for 4 days, then 12–15 mg/kg/week is recommended by manufacturer; however, this regimen has been associated with severe, life-threatening bone marrow toxicity.[96] **IV continuous infusion** 1–2 g/day for up to 5 days has been used by special treatment centers; continuous infusion does not consistently increase antitumor efficacy but does appear to lessen hematologic toxicity.[97] **IV for Dukes' stage C colon cancer after resection in combination with levamisole** 450 mg/m^2/day for 5 days initially, then 450 mg/m^2 once a week beginning in 28 days and continued for 1 yr. (*See* Notes.) **PO** doses are associated with low bioavailability and short clinical response. **Intra-arterial, intraperitoneal, and intracavitary** administration also have been used, although floxuridine is preferred. **Top for neoplastic keratoses** apply daily for 1–2 weeks as a thin layer with gloved hand or nonmetal applicator. Skin response progresses sequentially through erythema, vesiculation, erosion, ulceration, necrosis, and regranulation. Treatment is usually stopped once erosion is evident to allow healing to occur over the next 1–2 months. **Vag for condylomata acuminata** 1/3 applicatorful (1.5 g) of 5% cream once a week hs for 10 weeks.[98]

Special Populations. *Pediatric Dosage.* Generally indicated for adult malignancies, although theoretically; equivalent mg/kg doses could be used in children.

Geriatric Dosage. Same as adult dosage.

Other Conditions. Base dosage on ideal body weight in obesity or if the patient has excessive fluid retention.

Dosage Forms. **Inj** 50 mg/mL; **Top Crm** 1, 5%; **Top Soln** 1, 2, 5%.

Patient Instructions. (*See* Antineoplastics Class Instructions.) Avoid prolonged exposure to strong sunlight; report any severe sores in the mouth immediately.

Pharmacokinetics. *Fate.* Oral doses are erratically and incompletely absorbed, with bioavailability of 28%, and worsened by mixing with acidic fruit juices.[98] The drug is 8–12% plasma protein bound. The drug diffuses into effusions and CSF (peak CSF levels of 60–80 nmol/L after a 15 mg/kg IV bolus). V_d is about 25 ± 12 L/kg; Cl is 0.96 ± 0.42 L/hr/kg.[10] Extensively and rapidly metabolized, primarily in the liver, to a variety of inactive metabolites that are renally excreted. Up to 15% is renally excreted unchanged, 90% within 6 hr of administration. Fluoroacetate and citrate metabolites found in the CSF are believed to mediate rare CNS (cerebellar) toxicities.

$t_{\frac{1}{2}}$. α phase about 8 min; β phase 11 ± 4 min.[10,99]

Adverse Reactions. Emetic potential is moderately low (<1 g) to moderate (>1 g). Dose-limiting toxicity is myelosuppression (when given by bolus injection) with leukopenic and thrombocytopenic nadirs at 7–14 days. Severe stomatitis 5–8 days after therapy can herald severe impending myelosuppression; this occurs unpredictably with large bolus doses (>12 mg/kg). With continuous infusions, myelosuppression is reduced considerably, but mucositis and diarrhea can be dose limiting. Oral administration increases the severity of the frequent mild diarrhea. GI ulceration is occasionally severe. Cutaneous toxicities include mild to moderate alopecia, hyperpigmentation of skin and veins, and rashes that are often worsened by sunlight. Excessive lacrimation is frequent; occasionally tear duct fibrosis develops. Rare toxicities involve CNS dysfunction manifested by ataxia, confusion, visual disturbances, and headache. Cardiotoxicity occurs rarely.

Contraindications. Pregnancy. Pre-existing severe myelosuppression (WBCs <2000/μL, platelet count <100,000/μL); poor nutritional state; serious infections.

Precautions. Use with caution in patients with pre-existing coronary artery disease.

Drug Interactions. Concurrent allopurinol appears to block one activation pathway, thereby reducing fluorouracil hematologic toxicity. Fluorouracil can inhibit the antipurine effects of methotrexate. The clinical importance of these two interactions is unclear.

Parameters to Monitor. Pretreatment and monthly assessment of bone marrow function, particularly WBC and platelet counts. In the weeks after administration, observe for severe stomatitis, which can herald life-threatening myelosuppression.

Notes. If a precipitate is noted in the ampule, gently warm in a water bath and/or vigorously shake to redissolve. Fluorouracil is physically incompatible with diazepam, doxorubicin, cytarabine, and methotrexate injections. Mild to moderate activity in GI tract tumors and breast cancer; topical application of cream is often curative in superficial skin cancers. **Leucovorin** has been used with fluorouracil to increase fluorouracil binding to the target enzyme, thymidylate synthetase. **Levamisole** (Ergamisol) is an immunomodulator used to enhance fluorouracil efficacy in Dukes' C colon cancer. It is given orally in a dosage of 50 mg q 8 hr for 3 days, q 14 days for 1 yr.

GEMCITABINE Gemzar

Pharmacology. Gemcitabine is a difluorinated nucleoside analogue of cytarabine that is phosphorylated by intracellular deoxycytidine kinase to the active di- and triphosphate forms. These antimetabolites inhibit ribonucleotide reductase and reduce the normal pool of deoxycytidine triphosphate, respectively. This leads to an inhibition of DNA synthesis (of replication and repair). Compared with cytarabine, gemcitabine is preferentially phosphorylated and retained intracellularly. It is approved for palliative therapy in pancreatic cancer and is also active in breast cancer and non–small cell lung cancer.[100–102] (*See* Notes.)

Administration and Adult Dosage. IV 1 g/m^2/week infused over 30 min for 7 consecutive weeks, followed by 1 week rest, then once weekly for 3 weeks with 1 week rest thereafter.

Dosage Forms. **Inj** 200 mg, 1 g.

Patient Instructions. (*See* Antineoplastics Class Instructions.) Take acetaminophen before each dose to reduce flu-like symptoms.

Pharmacokinetics. *Fate.* A peak serum level of 14.7 mg/L (56 μmol/L) occurs after a 1 g/m^2 IV dose. The drug is metabolized to active di- and triphosphate forms and also deaminated to inactive difluorodeoxyuridine (dFdU) in liver and blood. Cl is 408 ± 121 L/hr/m^2 in men and 31% lower in women. Renal elimination of dFdU is 77% of a dose; 5% of a dose is recovered unchanged in urine.[100]

$t_{1/2}$. (Gemcitabine) 8–14 min (dose and infusion duration dependent); (dFdU) 10–14 hr.[100]

Adverse Reactions. Emetic potential is moderately low and well controlled by antiemetics. Thrombocytopenia is the dose-limiting toxicity; cumulative-dosage anemia is next most common. Neutropenia occurs but is rarely dose limiting. A transient, acute flu-like syndrome consisting of fever, fatigue, chills, headache, and arthralgias occurs in most patients. Fever responds to acetaminophen and usually does not recur. Erythematous pruritic maculopapular rashes on the neck and extremities are frequent but usually respond to a tropical glucocorticoid. Hepatic transaminases increase in two-thirds of patients but this is rarely serious. Diarrhea occurs rarely.

Contraindications. Severe pre-existing thrombocytopenia.

Precautions. Thrombocytopenia can lead to serious bleeding and anemia and may require transfusion therapy. Based on a similarity to cytarabine, CNS (cerebellar) toxicities might occur after high cumulative dosages, especially with impaired renal function.

Drug Interactions. None known.

Parameters to Monitor. Monitor platelet count, RBC count, and hemoglobin levels, and serum hepatic transaminase levels monthly.

Notes. Gemcitabine is clinically active in pancreatic cancer, breast cancer, and non-small cell lung cancer, although objective increases in tumor shrinkage and survival are minimal.[99–102] Gemcitabine produces primarily palliative responses such as reduced pain and enhanced quality of life with minimal serious toxicity compared with other cytotoxic agent therapies.

METHOTREXATE	Mexate, Various

Pharmacology. Methotrexate is a folic acid analogue that binds to dihydrofolate reductase, blocking formation of the DNA nucleotide thymidine; purine synthesis is also inhibited. It is most active in S phase.

Administration and Adult Dosage. *Single Agent Therapy.* **IM, IV, or PO for choriocarcinoma** 15–30 mg/day for 5 days, repeated q 1–2 weeks for 3–5 courses; **IM for mycosis fungoides** 50 mg once weekly or 25 mg twice weekly; **IM, IV, or PO for head and neck cancer** 25–50 mg/m^2 once weekly (watch for cumulative myelosuppression with continued administration of this regimen). **IT for meningeal leukemia** 12 mg/m^2 in a preservative-free, isotonic diluent (eg, Elliott's B solution, patient's own CSF, or D5LR); **IV high-dose therapy** (1–3 g/m^2) with leucovorin rescue should be used only by experts in major research centers; **IM or PO for psoriasis or arthritis** maintenance 5–10 mg initially, then **IM, IV, or PO** 10–25 mg/week, to a maximum of 50 mg/week, depending on clinical response; long-term daily administration results in increased hepatotoxicity compared with weekly oral or parenteral doses. **IM in glucocorticoid-dependent asthma** 7.5 mg, then 15 mg 1 week later, with subsequent weekly doses adjusted to 15–50 mg depending on 24-hr serum levels.[103] **PO for glucocorticoid-dependent asthma** 15 mg/week has been used.[104] **IM for ectopic pregnancy** 50 mg/m^2; some investigators repeat dose in 1 week if β-hCG levels do not drop.[105,106] **IM for induction of abortion** 50 mg/m^2, followed in 3–7 days by misoprostol 500–800 μg vaginally; exact timing of misoprostol dosage and oral administration of methotrexate are under investigation.[107–109]

Combined Modality Therapy. **For acute lymphocytic leukemia** various schedules are reported for remission-maintenance therapy: **IM or IV** 30 mg/m^2 twice weekly, or 7.5 mg/kg/day for 5 days, or **PO** 2.5 mg/kg/day for 2 weeks; repeat at monthly intervals. **IM, IV, or PO for Burkitt's lymphoma** 0.625–2.5 mg/kg/day for 1–2 weeks, then off drug for 7–10 days; **IM or IV for breast cancer** (combined with cyclophosphamide and fluorouracil) 40 mg/m^2 on days 1 and 8, then repeat monthly.[110]

Special Populations. *Pediatric Dosage.* **IM or IV for remission maintenance** same as adult dosage for acute lymphoblastic leukemia. **IT for meningeal cancer** use age-adjusted dosage rather than mg/m^2 dose:[111]

AGE (YR)	IT DOSE (MG)
>3	12
2–3	10
1–2	8
<1	6

Geriatric Dosage. Same as adult dosage but adjust for age-related reduction in renal function.

Other Conditions. Patients with any "third space" fluid (eg, ascites, pleural effusions) should have fluid removed before drug administration because of drug retention and slow release of drug from these compartments.[112] Reduce dosage in renal impairment as follows:[113]

CREATININE CLEARANCE (ML/MIN)	PERCENTAGE OF DOSAGE RECOMMENDED
>50	60–100 (0–40% reduction)
10–50	30–50 (50–70% reduction)
<10	15 (85% reduction)

Dosage Forms. **Tab** 2.5 mg; **Inj** (as sodium) 2.5, 25 mg/mL (preserved solution); 25 mg/mL (nonpreserved solution); 20, 50 mg, 1 g (nonpreserved powder).

Patient Instructions. (*See* Antineoplastics Class Instructions.) Inform your physician immediately if any of the following symptoms appear: dry cough, severe diarrhea, or mouth ulcers.

Pharmacokinetics. *Serum Levels.* After high-dose therapy, a threshold for bone marrow and mucosal toxicity is approximately 1 μmol/L 48 hr after administration. To prevent fatal bone marrow toxicity, keep serum levels below 10 μmol/L at 24 hr, 500 nmol/L at 48 hr, and 50 nmol/L at 72 hr.[114]

Fate. PO and IM absorption are rapid, peaking at 1–2 and 0.1–1 hr, respectively. Oral bioavailability is dose related but averages 30%.[113] After IT administration, the drug slowly diffuses into the bloodstream. About 34% is plasma protein bound; V_d is 0.55 ± 0.19 L/kg; Cl is 0.126 ± 0.048 L/hr/kg.[10] Over 90% of a dose is excreted in the urine, 90% unchanged after IV administration of high doses. Methotrexate solubility is markedly enhanced in slightly alkaline urine and reduced in acidic urine.

$t_{1/2}$. α phase 0.75 min; β phase 2 hr; γ phase 7.2 ± 2.1 hr.[10,115]

Adverse Reactions. Unless otherwise indicated, these reactions apply to high-dose chemotherapy of malignancies. Emetic potential is moderate. Nearly all reactions are dose and duration related. The primary toxicity is hematologic suppression, principally leukopenia, with the nadir at 7–14 days depending upon the administration schedule (more prolonged with daily administration). Thrombocytopenia and macrocytic anemia, dose-related nephrotoxicity, and ocular irritation occur frequently. Hepatotoxicity occurs frequently. Diarrhea and mucosal ulcerations of the mouth and tongue occasionally become severe within 1–3 weeks after administration, sometimes heralding severe myelotoxicity. Erythematous rashes have been reported. Leukoencephalopathy occurs rarely with IV or IT use. Other toxicities after IT use include nausea and vomiting, meningismus, paresthesias, and rarely convulsions. Long-term daily administration in psoriasis has led to hepatocellular damage including fibrotic liver changes and atrophy of the liver; the frequency may be lower with larger intermittent doses. Painful plaque erosion has occurred during psoriasis therapy. Pulmonary toxicity occurs rarely at any dosage and is not always reversible. A single low dose for use in medical abortion is generally well tolerated, with none of the severe reactions reported above.

Contraindications. Pregnancy; lactation; severe renal or hepatic dysfunction; psoriasis or rheumatoid arthritis patients with pre-existing immunodeficiency syndromes, blood dyscrasias or anemia.

Precautions. Renal function must be determined before administration. Alkalinize the urine before high doses to enhance methotrexate solubility. Concomitant use with radiotherapy can increase the risk of soft tissue and osteonecrosis.

Drug Interactions. Concomitant vinca alkaloids (vincristine or vinblastine) can impair methotrexate elimination from the CSF and enhance methotrexate toxicity. Cisplatin, NSAIDs, omeprazole, high-dose penicillins, probenecid, and sulfonamides can increase methotrexate serum levels and toxicity. Salicylate can decrease renal elimination of methotrexate and displace it from plasma protein binding sites. Alcohol can enhance hepatotoxicity of methotrexate. Asparaginase given 1 week before or 24 hr after methotrexate appears to reduce methotrexate hematologic toxicities. Cholesterol-binding resins can decrease oral methotrexate absorption. Broad-spectrum antibiotics can decrease methotrexate serum levels and efficacy after oral administration.

Parameters to Monitor. Monitor pretreatment and periodic hepatic, renal, and bone marrow functions (including WBCs, platelets, and RBCs). Follow high doses with 24-hr and/or 48-hr serum methotrexate levels and institution of appropriate leucovorin rescue. Observe for pulmonary symptoms, especially a dry, nonproductive cough and for diarrhea and ulcerative stomatitis.

Notes. Reconstitute lyophilized forms with NS, D5W, or Elliott's B solution (for intrathecal use). Reconstituted solutions are chemically stable for 7 days at room temperature. Methotrexate is physically incompatible with fluorouracil, prednisolone sodium phosphate, and cytarabine. It is clinically useful in a variety of hematologic and solid tumors as well as nonmalignant hyperplastic conditions such as psoriasis. If overdosage occurs, the antidote is **calcium leucovorin** (citrovorum factor), which can be given IV or IM in methotrexate-equivalent doses up to 75 mg q 6 hr for 4 doses. A delay of >36 hr lessens the chance of rescue.[114]

PENTOSTATIN   Nipent

Pharmacology. Pentostatin is an analogue of a normal purine intermediate involved in the conversion of adenosine to inosine. It is an irreversible inhibitor of the enzyme adenosine deaminase (ADA), which is found primarily in lymphoid cells. Pentostatin-induced inhibition of ADA leads to a build-up of deoxyadenosine and several phosphorylated derivatives that deplete cellular ATP. These metabolic products ultimately inhibit DNA synthesis in lymphatic tumor cells, including chronic lymphocytic leukemia, acute lymphoblastic leukemia, and especially hairy cell leukemia. Some data suggest that the cytotoxic effect is cell-cycle phase specific for G_1 phase.[116,117]

Adult Dosage. **IV for hairy cell leukemia refractory to interferon alfa** 4 mg/m^2 every other week.

Dosage Forms. **Inj** 10 mg.

Pharmacokinetics. Serum levels after doses of 2–10 mg/m^2 average 1.5–4.7 mmol/L. V_d is 20–23 L/m^2; Cl is 3.1 L/hr/kg. The terminal half-life of pentostatin averages 5–10 hr. Up to 90% of a dose is excreted in the urine in an active form, and dosage reduction is indicated in patients with reduced renal function.

Adverse Reactions. Renal tubular toxicity and myelosuppression are the major dose-limiting toxicities of pentostatin. Renal toxicity manifested by Cr_s elevation is much more frequent at doses over 5 mg/m^2/day. Adequate hydration and the avoidance of other nephrotoxins can reduce the frequency and severity of pentostatin-induced nephrotoxicity. Lymphocytopenia is frequent, with B- and T-lymphocytes depressed, possibly explaining the relatively frequent, severe systemic infections with organisms that include Gram-negative bacteria, *Candida albicans,* herpes zoster (varicella), and herpes simplex. Neurologic effects are frequent with pentostatin and include lethargy and fatigue; these rarely progress to coma and are more common and severe with high-dose regimens. Mild to moderate nausea and vomiting also occur frequently but are easily controlled with standard antiemetic regimens.

PURINE ANALOGUES:

MERCAPTOPURINE   Purinethol

THIOGUANINE

Pharmacology. Mercaptopurine (6-MP) and thioguanine (6-TG) are thiolated purines that act as antimetabolites after metabolic activation to the nucleotide forms (phosphorylated ribose sugar attachment). Subsequently, de novo purine biosynthesis is interrupted at a number of enzymatic sites, including the conversion of inosinic acid to adenine- or xanthine-based ribosides. DNA and RNA synthesis is halted in a cell-cycle S-phase–specific fashion.

Administration and Adult Dosage. (Mercaptopurine) **PO, IV** (investigational) 75–100 mg/m^2/day.[118] (*See* Drug Interactions.) (Thioguanine) **PO, IV** (investigational) 2–3 mg/kg/day.

Special Populations. *Pediatric Dosage.* Same as adult dosage.

Geriatric Dosage. Same as adult dosage.

Other Conditions. Purine antimetabolite toxicities are not consistently increased in patients with renal failure.[119,120] (*See* Precautions.)

Dosage Forms. (Mercaptopurine) **Tab** 50 mg; **Inj** (investigational) 500 mg. (Thioguanine) **Tab** 40 mg; **Inj** (investigational) 75 mg.

Patient Instructions. (*See* Antineoplastics Class Instructions.) To maximize absorption, do not take this drug with meals. Nausea and vomiting are uncommon with usual doses.

Pharmacokinetics. *Fate.* (Mercaptopurine) 12 ± 7% oral bioavailability, increasing to 60% with concurrent allopurinol.[121] The drug is approximately 20–30% plasma protein bound and freely distributed throughout the body including placental transfer; the CSF/serum ratio is 0.19–0.27. Mercaptopurine is metabolized extensively by xanthine oxidase, also methylated to active metabolite and sulfated to inactive thiouric acid. V_d is 0.56 ± 0.38 L/kg; Cl is 0.66 ± 0.24 L/hr/kg; 22% excreted unchanged in urine.[10] (Thioguanine) oral bioavailability is unknown. The drug is approximately 20–30% plasma protein bound and freely distributed throughout the body, including placental transfer; the CSF/serum ratio is 0.16. Thioguanine is metabolized predominantly to inactive metabolites.

$t_{1/2}$. (Mercaptopurine) 0.9 ± 0.37 hr;[10] (thioguanine) α phase 15 min, β phase 11 hr.

Adverse Reactions. Emetic potential is low to moderate. The dose-limiting toxicity is myelosuppression (leukopenia and thrombocytopenia). Mild to moderate mucositis occurs with large doses and low daily maintenance doses. Predominantly cholestatic liver toxicities occur frequently with long-term therapy. Marked crystalluria with hematuria has occurred with large IV mercaptopurine doses.[122] Various rashes also have been described with these drugs. Long-term immunosuppressive therapy with any of these agents predisposes patients to carcinogenesis; CNS lymphomas and acute myeloid leukemia are the most frequent malignancies.[123]

Contraindications. Pregnancy; pre-existing severe bone marrow depression.

Precautions. Investigational use of mercaptopurine for inflammatory bowel disease can predispose to pancreatitis.

Drug Interactions. Patients taking allopurinol *must* receive substantially reduced doses of oral mercaptopurine (25–33% of the normal dose) to avoid life-threatening myelosuppression caused by blocked inactivation. Thioguanine is inactivated primarily by methylation; thus, no dosage reduction is necessary with concomitant allopurinol. Enhanced bone marrow suppression can occur with the combination of trimethoprim/sulfamethoxazole and mercaptopurine.

Parameters to Monitor. WBC and platelet counts and total bilirubin at least monthly.

Notes. There is usually complete cross-resistance between mercaptopurine and thioguanine.

UFT (Investigational—Bristol-Myers Squibb)   Orzel

Pharmacology. UFT is a combination containing the fluorouracil prodrug **tegafur** (formerly ftorafur) and the ribonucleoside pyrimidine **uracil** in a fixed molar ratio of 1:4 (tegafur:uracil). Tegafur is gradually converted to the antimetabolite fluorouracil by metabolism in the liver. This approximates a continuous infusion of fluorouracil after oral ingestion of UFT. The uracil component slows the metabolism of fluorouracil and reduces production of the toxic metabolite, 2-fluoro-β-alanine, resulting in reduced GI and myelosuppressive toxicity with the combination.[124,125]

Administration and Adult Dosage. PO for colorectal cancer 800–900 mg/m^2 weekly or daily for 5 consecutive days, repeated q 28 days. Alternatively 360–400 mg/m^2/day for 28 consecutive days, repeated q 35–42 days. All daily dosages are given in 3 divided doses q 8 hr.[124]

Special Populations. *Pediatric Dosage.* Safety and efficacy not established.

Geriatric Dosage. Same as adult dosage.

Dosage Forms. Cap containing tegafur 100 mg and uracil 224 mg.

Patient Instructions. (*See* Antineoplastics Class Instructions.) Take this drug on an empty stomach with 4–8 fluid ounces of water.

Missed Doses. If you are taking this drug daily, take a missed dose as soon as possible if you remember within 12 hours. If it is within 2 hours of the next dose, skip the missed dose and do not double the next dose. If you miss 2 or more doses, contact your physician. If you are taking this drug weekly and miss a dose, contact your physician.

Pharmacokinetics. *Serum Levels.* No correlation has been found between the peak level or AUC of any component of UFT and myelotoxicity.

Fate. Tegafur and uracil are rapidly absorbed, but levels of tegafur are higher than those of uracil, despite the 4-fold higher uracil dosage. With a daily dosage of 800–900 mg/m^2, peak levels of tegafur, uracil, and 5-FU are 24.6, 13.6, and 1.4 mg/L, respectively. Tumor levels of 5-FU and its nucleotide metabolites are higher than in normal tissue. Uracil is quickly metabolized and excreted via nonbiliary pathways. Some tegafur metabolites are excreted in bile.[124]

Adverse Reactions. The dose-limiting toxicity in phase I trials using daily doses was GI, including nausea, vomiting, anorexia, and diarrhea. With daily schedules, the GI effects tend to be cumulative, resulting in moderate mucositis and diarrhea. Fatigue also occurs in over one-half of patients treated using the 28-day dosage schedule. With the shorter 5-day schedules, myelosuppression, principally neutropenia, is dose-limiting.

Notes. UFT also can be combined with oral **leucovorin** in the treatment of advanced colorectal cancer.[125]

Cytokines

ALDESLEUKIN
Proleukin

Pharmacology. Aldesleukin (interleukin-2, IL-2) is a cytokine produced by activated T-lymphocytes. It binds to T-cell receptors to induce a proliferative response and differentiation into lymphokine activated killer (LAK) cells in the blood and tumor-infiltrating lymphocytes (TIL cells) in specific tumors. The pharmaceutical product is a nonglycosylated molecule produced by recombinant DNA techniques in *Escherichia coli.*[126,127]

Administration and Adult Dosage. IV for metastatic renal cell carcinoma 600,000 IU/kg over 15 min q 8 hr for 14 doses; repeat after 9 days of rest for a total of 28 doses. **IV infusion** 3–6 million IU/m^2 infused over 6 hr is commonly used.

Special Populations. *Pediatric Dosage.* (<18 yr) safety and efficacy not established.

Geriatric Dosage. Same as adult dosage.

Other Conditions. Interpatient pharmacokinetic differences are not known; however, withholding dose(s) is required if severe cardiovascular collapse, pulmonary or renal insufficiency, coma, psychosis, or GI toxicity occurs.

Dosage Forms. Inj 22 million IU (1.3 mg protein). (*See* Notes.)

Patient Instructions. (*See* Antineoplastics Class Instructions.)

Pharmacokinetics. *Fate.* Limited human data indicate that the drug undergoes biphasic elimination after IV administration. The kidney is believed to be the major organ of elimination, and the drug undergoes intrarenal metabolism to inactive fragments.[128]

t$_{\frac{1}{2}}$. α phase 14 ± 7.7 min; β phase 80 ± 34 min.[128]

Adverse Reactions. Emetic potential is low. Severe cardiovascular toxicities include fluid retention (>10% of body weight) and pulmonary interstitial edema. Hypotension requiring treatment has occurred 2–4 hr after treatment with high-dose bolus or continuous infusion and low-dose SC regimens. Anemia occurs in up to 77% of high-dose bolus IV regimens. Frequently, nausea, vomiting, diarrhea, rash, pruritus, and nasal congestion occur. Abnormal laboratory findings include frequent increased Cr$_s$, oliguria, eosinophilia, and thrombocytopenia.[126] Increased serum transaminases and bilirubin occur occasionally; hepatic dysfunction occurs rarely. Myocardial ischemia also can occur and fatal MI has been reported. Capillary leak syndrome can occur and requires close monitoring of fluid balance.[126] When combined with adoptive cellular therapy (reinfused LAK cells), immediate fever and chills result; **indomethacin** 50 mg orally or **meperidine** 25–50 mg IM or IV can lessen these symptoms.

Precautions. Aldesleukin has produced severe cardiopulmonary toxicity and must be used cautiously in any patient with a history of cardiac insufficiency from any cause. Patients also must be in good general physical condition to tolerate the hypotension and pulmonary edema that can complicate high-dose aldesleukin therapy.

Drug Interactions. Glucocorticoids block some aldesleukin actions and usually are reserved for treating severe toxicity.

Parameters to Monitor. Monitor blood pressure, cardiac output, and fluid balance closely.

Notes. Some studies describe IL-2 activity in different units or by weight. Aldesleukin is labeled in IU (18 million IU = 1.1 mg protein), and doses for other IL-2 products should be converted to IU for proper dosage. Aldesleukin is active in metastatic renal cell carcinoma (MRCC) and metastatic malignant melanoma. In MRCC, response rates are 15% (with some complete remissions), lasting a median of 23 months. Response rates are higher in patients with good performance status and especially those with pulmonary metastases as the main site of disease.

INTERFERON ALFA:	
ALFA-2A	Pegasys, Roferon-A
ALFA-2B	Intron A, PEG-Intron
ALFA-N3	Alferon N

Pharmacology. Alpha interferons are single-chain proteins. The alfa-2 interferons are biosynthetic; alfa-2a has a lysine at position 23, alfa-2b an arginine. Alfa-n3 interferon is a multisubspecies form of natural interferons isolated from human leukocytes. Interferons bind to specific membrane receptors and are then taken up intracellularly to affect diverse cellular functions. These include cell membrane alterations (eg, enhanced antigen expression), cell-cycle blockade at the G_1–S portion, enhanced antiviral enzyme synthesis (eg, $2',5'$-oligo-adenylate synthetase with resultant products, which destroy double- and single-stranded viral RNA), and immunomodulatory activity (eg, increased activity of natural killer [NK] lymphocytes and phagocytic macrophages). General cellular protein synthesis also is decreased, including cytochrome P450 enzymes.[129] Linking the interferon to polyethylene glycol allows once weekly administration.

Administration and Adult Dosage. IM or SC for hairy cell leukemia (alfa-2a or 2b) 2 million IU/m^2 daily or 3 times a week. **IM or SC for AIDS-related Kaposi's sarcoma** (alfa-2b) slowly increase dose from 5 million IU/day up to 20–36 million IU/day.[130] **Intralesionally for condylomata acuminata** (alfa-2b) 1 million IU/wart 3 times weekly for 3 weeks, to a maximum 5 warts a day (use only the 10 million IU vial); (alfa-n3) 250,000 IU (0.05 mL)/wart twice weekly for up to 8 weeks, to a maximum 0.5 mL/day. **IM or SC for chronic hepatitis B** 5 million IU/day or 10 million IU 3 times a week for 16 weeks.[131] **IM or SC for chronic hepatitis C** (conventional) 3 million IU 3 times a week for 6 months or **SC for chronic hepatitis C** (PEGylated) 1μg/kg once weekly. (*See* Notes.) **IV and SC for malignant melanoma** (alfa-2b) 20 million IU/m^2 IV 5 times a week for 4 weeks, then 10 million IU/m^2 SC 3 times a week for 48 weeks. **IM or SC for chronic myeloid leukemia** (alfa-2a) 3–6 million IU/day.

Special Populations. *Pediatric Dosage.* (<18 yr) not recommended.

Geriatric Dosage. Same as adult dosage.

Dosage Forms. (Alfa-2a) **Inj** 3, 6, 10, 36 million IU/mL. (Alfa-2b) **Inj** (conventional) 3, 5, 10, 18, 25, 50 million IU; (PEGylated) 100, 160, 240, 300 μg/mL. (Alfa-n3) **Inj** 5 million IU/mL.

Patient Instructions. (Subcutaneous use) Instruct in proper method of aseptic preparation of vials and syringes, proper technique for subcutaneous administration, and proper disposal of syringes and needles. Rotate subcutaneous injection sites. Acetaminophen is recommended to reduce frequent flu-like symptoms, which usually decrease with continued therapy.

Missed Doses. Take this drug at regular intervals. If you miss a dose of this medicine, call your physician for instructions. Do not double the dose or take extra.

Pharmacokinetics. *Fate.* (Conventional) Alfa-2a and 2b are 100% bioavailable after IM or SC administration, with an absorption half-life of about 6 hr. IM or SC doses of 10 million IU produce peak serum levels of 100–200 IU/mL within 4 hr; the same dose IV produces peak serum levels of 500–600 IU/mL within 15–30 min. Alfa-n3 is not detectable in serum after intralesional administration, although a small amount is probably absorbed. Most of a dose is thought to be metabolized, with none filtered or secreted by the kidney.[132,133]

$t_{1/2}$. (Conventional) α phase 0.11 hr; β phase (IV or IM) 2 hr, (SC) 3 hr.[132,133]

Adverse Reactions. Emetic potential is negligible. The most frequent reactions are fevers of 38–39°C, chills, arthralgias, headache, malaise, and myalgias (flu-like syndrome). These reactions are more severe with initiation of therapy and ameliorated by acetaminophen or dosage reduction. Anorexia and nausea without vomiting also are frequent. With large doses (generally >1 million IU), hematologic suppression (eg, mild thrombocytopenia, leukopenia) occurs, as does slight elevation of hepatic enzymes (AST, LDH, alkaline phosphatase), and mild hypertension, occasionally associated with tachycardia. Very high doses (≥30 million IU) are associated with somnolence, dizziness, and confusion. Mild erythema and pruritus at the injection site also can occur. Interferons are not mutagenic or carcinogenic in standard animal or in vitro models. Alpha interferons can cause or aggravate life-threatening or fatal neuropsychiatric, autoimmune, ischemic and infectious disorders. These usually resolve with drug withdrawal.

Contraindications. Severe hypersensitivity; development of a neutralizing serum antibody (precludes the use of alternate recombinant product; switch to natural interferon alfa-n3). (*See* Notes.)

Precautions. Pregnancy. Use with caution in patients with cardiovascular disease, seizure disorder, or hepatic or renal impairment. Proper hydration during therapy may lessen hypotensive reactions. Neutralizing serum antibodies can form after prolonged interferon administration and has been associated with reduced toxicities and antitumor effects.[134]

Drug Interactions. Interferon can worsen the neutropenia of zidovudine in Kaposi's sarcoma. Interferon can increase theophylline serum levels. Combination with vidarabine can result in increased neurotoxicity.

Parameters to Monitor. Monitor periodically for clinical and laboratory signs of life-threatening adverse effects (*see* Adverse Reactions.)

Notes. A clear dose–response relationship is established for toxicity but not for antitumor effectiveness (except for Kaposi's sarcoma). Alpha interferons have activity in reducing the symptomatology of hairy cell leukemia; hematologic response rates of 80–90% are possible in this disease. Other cancers responsive to interferon alfa are renal cell cancer (10–30% partial response rate), acute leukemias (15–30% response rate), and the nonblastic phase of CML (40–60% response rate). Although not a labeled use, interferon alfa-n3 can be used systemically and is recommended specifically for antibody-positive patients receiving recombinant products. PEGylated forms appear to be more effective against hepatitis C than conventional forms. Patients who fail interferon treatment for hepatitis C can be given interferon alfa-2b plus oral **ribavirin** (Rebetol). It is available in a combination package (Rebetron).

DNA Intercalating Drugs

ANTHRACYCLINES:	
DAUNORUBICIN HYDROCHLORIDE	Cerubidine
DOXORUBICIN HYDROCHLORIDE	Adriamycin, Rubex
IDARUBICIN HYDROCHLORIDE	Idamycin

Pharmacology. Daunorubicin (daunomycin), doxorubicin (hydroxydaunomycin), and idarubicin (4-demethoxydaunorubicin) are tetracyclic amino sugar-linked antibiotics that are actively taken up by cells and concentrated in the nucleus; intercalation or fitting between DNA base pairs occurs, which impairs DNA synthesis. Other biochemical lesions produced include quinone moiety-generated production of oxygen and hydroxyl free radicals with lipid peroxidation of cellular membranes. The anthracyclines also interfere with the activity of the G_2-specific enzyme, topoisomerase-II, which leads to the formation of cleavable complexes between enzyme and DNA, resulting in DNA double-strand breaks. These agents are primarily cell-cycle phase nonspecific, but with slightly greater activity in late S- or G_2-phase cells.

Administration and Dosage.

	DAUNORUBICIN	DOXORUBICIN	IDARUBICIN
Administration	IV push, infusion.	IV push, infusion.	IV push, infusion.
	These compounds are extremely toxic (potent vesicants) if inadvertently extravasated; very careful IV technique is mandatory.		
Adult Dosage	IV 30–45 mg/m²/day for 1–3 days; generally not repeated more often than q 3 weeks.	IV 60–90 mg/m² for 1 dose or 20–30 mg/m²/day for 3 days; generally not repeated more often than q 3 weeks. Alternatively, 20 mg/m²/week.	IV 12 mg/m²/day for 3 days.[135]
Pediatric Dosage	Same as adult dosage.	Same as adult dosage.	Same as adult dosage.[136]
Cumulative Lifetime Dosage Limits[a]	550 mg/m², up to 850 mg/m².	550 mg/m². 400 mg/m² with prior chest irradiation or preexisting heart disease.[b]	Unknown.

[a]Attainment of maximal cumulative dosage generally precludes continued use, despite evidence of continuing drug response; however, some patients might continue to respond without development of cardiomyopathy.[137] Use of dexrazoxane can extend dosage limits in breast cancer. (*See* Dexrazoxane.)
[b]Low weekly doses or continuous 96-hr infusion[138] appear to be less toxic and might allow attainment of greater cumulative dosages (>550 mg/m²).[139,140]

Special Populations. *Other Conditions.* Cumulative dosages of all agents must be reduced in patients with prior irradiation of the cardiac chest region, pre-existing heart disease, or prior large cyclophosphamide dosage. Doxorubicin requires no dosage adjustment for severe renal impairment, whereas with daunorubicin 75% of the dosage is recommended in severe renal impairment. Doxorubicin dosages, however, must be substantially reduced with severe hepatic dysfunction.[141] Idarubicin dosage reductions are indicated for bilirubin of 2.6–5 mg/dL or Cr_s ≥2 mg/dL. For severe mucositis, administration is delayed until mucositis resolves, and then dosage is reduced by 25%.

SERUM BILIRUBIN (MG/DL)	PERCENTAGE OF DOSE RECOMMENDED	
	Doxorubicin	*Idarubicin*
≤1.2	100 (no reduction)	—
1.2–3	50 (50% reduction)	—
>3	25 (75% reduction)	50 (50% reduction)

Dosage Forms. (Daunorubicin) **Inj** 20, 50 mg. (Doxorubicin) **Inj** 10, 20, 50, 75, 100, 150, 200 mg. (Idarubicin) **Inj** 5, 10, 20 mg.

Patient Instructions. (*See* Antineoplastics Class Instructions.) Immediately report any change in sensation (eg, stinging) at the injection site during infusion (this might be an early sign of infiltration). Red-colored urine does not indicate toxicity.

	DAUNO-RUBICIN	DOXO-RUBICIN	IDARUBICIN	IDARUBICINOL
FATE				
Absorption	Extensively degraded to inactive aglycone in GI tract.		About 24% oral bioavailability.[142]	The primary active metabolite of idarubicin.
Distribution	Both drugs enter cells rapidly and concentrate in the nuclei. Tissue concentrations are highest in lung, kidney, small intestine, and liver; trivial amounts found in the CNS. Avid tissue binding is probably responsible for prolonged terminal half-lives and V_d of 500–600 L/m².		Peak serum level of 2 µg/L after a dose of 7–9 mg/m².[143] 94% plasma protein bound; V_d about 1700 L/m².	Peak serum level of 15 µg/L.[143] 94% plasma protein bound; V_d about 1700 L/m².
Metabolism	Both drugs are extensively metabolized, initially to less active alcohol metabolites; further metabolized by liver microsomes to inactive aglycones and demethylated glucuronide and sulfate conjugates.[144]		Both agents are partially metabolized and excreted as glucuronide conjugates. Idarubicin Cl is 60–77 L/hr/m².	
EXCRETION				
Biliary	20–30% of a dose.	40–60% of a dose.	Primary route of excretion.	Primary route of excretion.

	DAUNO-RUBICIN	DOXO-RUBICIN	IDARUBICIN	IDARUBICINOL
Urinary	14–23% as unchanged drug and metabolites (primarily daunorubicinol).	5–10% as metabolites over 5 days.[141]	8% of a dose over 24 hr.	8% of a dose over 24 hr.
$t_{1/2}$.	α 45 min β 18.5 hr (daunorubicinol 27 hr).	α 30 min β 3 hr γ 17 hr (metabolites 32 hr).[141]	α 14 min[145] β 19–34 hr.[143,145]	— 65.5 hr.[145]

Adverse Reactions. Emetic potential is moderate to moderately high with all three drugs. Stomatitis, nausea, and vomiting are dose dependent and frequent; prophylactic antiemetics are often helpful. Myelosuppression, affecting platelets and neutrophils, is the major acute dose-limiting side effect. Typical nadirs occur at 9–14 days, with recovery nearly complete within 3 weeks of administration. Hemorrhage occurs in up to 10% of induction courses with idarubicin. Excessive lacrimation is reported in about 25% of patients receiving doxorubicin. Alopecia usually occurs; during low-dose adjuvant chemotherapy administration, regional scalp hypothermia might decrease hair loss.[146] Severe, protracted ulceration and necrosis can occur with inadvertent perivenous infiltration; partially effective local treatments are limb elevation, ice packing, and topical **DMSO.** (*See* Notes.) Large evolving lesions necessitate early plastic surgery consultation. Long-term anthracycline use can lead to severe and often fatal cardiomyopathy. (*See* Cumulative Dosage Limits, Notes.) Symptoms such as shortness of breath, edema, and fatigue are nonspecific and indicative of advanced CHF. The frequency is low (overall 2.2%) when total dosage limits are observed and can be lower when monthly doses are given over several days or by continuous 96-hr infusion.[147] Late cardiotoxicity is reported in children receiving total dosages of doxorubicin <500 mg/m^2.[148] During drug infusion, various nonspecific ECG changes do not imply an increased risk of cardiotoxicity. Graded endomyocardial biopsy and graded radionuclide angiography have proved most effective for assessment of the emergence of severe cardiomyopathy. Other reactions are transient erythema and phlebitis during administration and a radiation–synergy phenomenon involving heightened tissue reactions in concurrently or previously irradiated tissues, especially the esophagus (avoid by spacing weeks apart). Urine remains red for 1–2 days after administration.

Contraindications. Pre-existing bone marrow suppression (WBCs <3000/μL; platelets <120,000/μL); MI in previous 6 months; history of CHF. Marrow suppression is not a contraindication in relapsed leukemia patients.

Precautions. Careful administration technique is mandatory to avoid extravasation and tissue necrosis. Hepatocellular disease or cirrhosis can slow production of alcohol metabolites.

Drug Interactions. A number of drugs might interact with the anthracyclines: vinca alkaloids (cross-resistance), amphotericin B (increased drug uptake), and cyclosporine and streptozocin (reduced drug clearance and increased toxicity).[149] Most of these drug interactions have been studied only in vitro and require clinical confirmation.

Parameters to Monitor. Obtain pretreatment and at least biweekly nadir WBC and platelet counts. Monitor general cardiac status and serial radionuclide scans of the heart in high-risk patients. Add up prior doses to estimate cardiotoxicity dosage limit.

Notes. These drugs are compatible with usual IV solutions but incompatible with heparin, sodium bicarbonate, and fluorouracil. IV push doses are best reconstituted with NS or D5W. These solutions are stable for prolonged periods and can withstand freezing and thawing.[150] Doxorubicin is widely effective in numerous solid tumors, such as ovarian, thyroid, and gastric carcinomas, sarcomas, and cancer of the breast, and hematologic malignancies, such as the lymphomas and leukemias. The iron-chelating agent dexrazoxane reduces doxorubicin-induced cardiotoxicity in patients with breast cancer.[151] (*See* Dexrazoxane.) The activity of idarubicin and daunorubicin is limited primarily to AML. Topical **DMSO** (1.5 mL of a 90% w/v solution q 6 hr for 2 weeks) has been effective at preventing extravasation ulceration in one trial.[152]

DAUNORUBICIN CITRATE, LIPOSOMAL   DaunoXome

Pharmacology. Daunorubicin is encapsulated in the lipid component of this red emulsion formulation, which consists of distearoylphosphatidylcholine and cholesterol in a fixed lipid:daunorubicin ratio of 1:18.6 (in mg/mL). These liposomes are taken up into tumor and reticuloendothelial system cells, which release prolonged but low serum levels of daunorubicin over time.[153] Murine studies suggest selective (enhanced) uptake of liposomal daunorubicin into tumor tissues compared with normal organs.[154] Liposomal daunorubicin is used to treat AIDS-related Kaposi's sarcoma.

Administration and Adult Dosage. **IV for Kaposi's sarcoma** 40 mg/m^2 q 2 weeks.

Special Populations. *Pediatric Dosage.* Safety and efficacy not established.

Geriatric Dosage. Same as adult dosage.

Other Conditions. Based on studies with daunorubicin, reduce dose by 25% for a serum bilirubin of 1.2–3 mg/dL and 50% for a serum bilirubin or Cr$_s$ >3 mg/dL. Do not administer if absolute granulocyte count is under 750/μL.

Dosage Forms. **Inj** 50 mg.

Patient Instructions. (*See* Antineoplastics Class Instructions.)

Pharmacokinetics. *Fate.* Mean peak serum levels (free plus liposomal) after doses of 20, 40, 60, and 80 mg/m^2 are 8.2, 18.2, 36.2, and 43.6 mg/L, respectively.[153] Compared with equivalent doses of the nonliposomal drug, the free drug levels are 100-fold lower and persist for up to 2.5 days after administration. In adults, V$_d$ is

2.9–4.1 L; Cl is 0.4–0.9 L/hr, about 5% of the Cl of the free drug.[153] Thus, the AUC is increased, Cl is slowed, but peak levels are low with the liposomal formulation.

$t_{1/2}$. 2.8–5.2 hr (total of liposomal plus free drug).

Adverse Reactions. Emetic potential is low to moderate. The most frequent symptoms are mild to moderate fatigue, which occurs in 56% of patients, and low-grade fever in 26% of patients. An acute triad of back pain, flushing, and chest tightness can occur in up to 14% of patients, usually with initial administration. This liposomal-component reaction subsides with interruption of the infusion and typically does not recur when restarting at a slower infusion rate. Neutropenia occurs in 17% of patients; mild anemia and thrombocytopenia occur in 7% and 4% of treatment courses, respectively. Diarrhea occurs in 10% of patients; mild liver enzyme elevation occurs in 4% of patients.[153] Cardiac toxicity appears to be less with this formulation than with aqueous daunorubicin.

Contraindications. Previous serious allergy to the drug or any component of the formulation. (*See* Anthracyclines, Daunorubicin.)

Precautions. Pregnancy; lactation. Do not administer if absolute granulocyte count is under 750/μL.

Drug Interactions. Not well studied with this formulation. (*See* Anthracyclines.)

Parameters to Monitor. Monitor the number of Kaposi's sarcoma lesions for response or evidence of disease progression (≥10 new lesions or an increase of 25%). Obtain WBC count before administration. Monitor left ventricular ejection fraction at cumulative dosages of 320 and 480 mg/m^2 and q 240 mg/m^2 thereafter.

Notes. Mix only in D5W; do not filter.

DOXORUBICIN HYDROCHLORIDE, LIPOSOMAL   Doxil

Pharmacology. Doxorubicin is encapsulated in the aqueous core of small (100-nm) liposomes composed of a phospholipid bilayer with an outer coating of polyethylene glycol (PEG). The small liposome size and PEG coating mask recognition by reticuloendothelial cells, thereby increasing the half-life of the liposomes in vivo. Once the liposomes accumulate in tissues, free doxorubicin is slowly released to exert its antitumor effect. Most toxicities are reduced by the liposomal formulation without compromising efficacy in solid tumors such as Kaposi's sarcoma. (*See* Anthracyclines.)

Administration and Adult Dosage. **IV for AIDS-related Kaposi's sarcoma** 20 mg/m^2 q 3 weeks.

Special Populations. *Pediatric Dosage.* Safety and efficacy not established.

Geriatric Dosage. Same as adult dosage.

Other Conditions. (Liver dysfunction) Reduce dosage 50% for serum bilirubin 1.2–3 mg/dL; reduce dosage by 75% for bilirubin >3 mg/dL. (Stomatitis) For patients who develop stomatitis, wait 1 week, re-evaluate, and readminister at 100% for grade II severity (painful ulcers but able to eat), 75% for grade III severity (painful ulcers and unable to eat), 50% for grade IV severity (extensive, disabling stomatitis requiring nutritional support). (Hematologic toxicity) Reduce dose and/or delay administration to allow for ANC and platelet count (PC) to return to at least 1000/μL and 50,000/μL, respectively. Then readminister at 100% of dosage if nadir ANC was 1000–1500/μL and/or PC was 50,000–150,000/μL; 75% of dosage if nadir ANC was 500/μL and/or PC was 25,000–50,000/μL; or 50% of dosage if nadir ANC was <500/μL and/or PC was <25,000/μL, respectively. (Erythrodysesthesia) For grade I erythrodysesthesia (mild swelling or erythema) present 4 weeks after the dose, administer 75% of standard dosage. For grade II erythrodysesthesia (erythema or desquamation not precluding physical activity) present 3 weeks after the dose, delay the dose for 1 week; if present 4 weeks after the dose, reduce the next dose by 50%. For grade III erythrodysesthesia (palmar–plantar [hand/foot] that is severe [diffuse blistering]) 3 weeks after drug administration, hold the next dose for 1 week; if it is still present at 4 weeks, discontinue the drug.

Dosage Forms. **Inj** 2 mg/mL.

Patient Instructions. (*See* Antineoplastics Class Instructions.)

Pharmacokinetics. *Fate.* Mean peak serum levels (±SE) after 10 and 20 mg/m^2 doses are 4.1 ± 0.2 and 8.3 ± 0.5 μg/mL, respectively. Most of this level is liposomally encapsulated drug; the assay does not differentiate. Liposomal doxorubicin has a smaller V_d (2.2–4.4 L/m^2) than free doxorubicin; Cl is 0.034–0.108 L/hr/m^2. The AUC for the 10 and 20 mg/m^2 doses are 277 ± 33 (±SE) and 590 ± 59 (±SE) mg·L/hr. A small amount (0.8–2.6 ng/mL) of the doxorubicinol metabolite is found in serum after a dose. Cl of parent drug is 24–35 L/hr/m^2. Tissue concentrations of drug can be 19 times higher in Kaposi's sarcoma lesions than in adjacent normal skin.[155]

$t_{1/2}$. (Liposomal and free drug) α phase 5.2 ± 1.4 hr; β phase 55 ± 4.8 hr.[155]

Adverse Reactions. Similar to free doxorubicin. Myelosuppression, principally neutropenia, occurs in 49% of patients and sepsis in 5%. Opportunistic infections also occur in AIDS patients, especially those with a high tumor burden, low CD4 count, or pre-existing infection. Palmar–plantar erythrodysesthesia is cumulative. It is manifested as painful red soles and palms, which can progress to ulceration and debilitating infection if doses are not reduced and/or delayed. Doxorubicin-induced cumulative dosage cardiomyopathy and inadvertent extravasation necrosis can be lessened, but not entirely eliminated, with the liposomal formulation. Radiation recall soft tissue toxicity has been reported.

Contraindications. (*See* Anthracyclines, Doxorubicin.)

Precautions. Sensitization of soft tissues to radiation damage can occur. To lessen frequency of irreversible cardiomyopathy, observe the cumulative anthracycline dosage limit of 500 mg/m^2. Avoid extravasation and do not give IM or SC.

Drug Interactions. (*See* Anthracyclines.)

Parameters to Monitor. Obtain absolute neutrophil count and platelet count, serum bilirubin level, and severity of stomatitis and palmar–plantar erythrodysesthesia before administration.

Notes. Do not filter. Overall response rates of 40–60% are reported for patients with AIDS-related Kaposi's sarcoma;[155,156] it also might be effective in other solid tumors in HIV-negative patients.

DACTINOMYCIN   Cosmegen

Pharmacology. Dactinomycin (actinomycin D) is a tricyclic, peptide-containing antibiotic that acts as an intercalator of DNA, resulting in decreased mRNA transcription in a phase-nonspecific fashion. It is used in the treatment of sarcomas and choriocarcinoma.[157,158]

Adult Dosage. IV 2 mg/week or 500 μg/day for up to 5 days, repeated at 3- to 4-week intervals. Reduce dosage in the presence of hepatobiliary dysfunction. Reconstitute dactinomycin with preservative-free diluents. It is bound by cellulose filters, so avoid in-line filtration.

Pediatric Dosage. IV 450 μg/m^2/day, to a maximum of 500 μg/day, for up to 5 days; the course is repeated in 3 weeks. (*See* Adult Dosage.)

Dosage Forms. Inj 0.5 mg.

Pharmacokinetics. About 30% of the drug is recovered from feces and urine after 1 week; there is no CNS penetration, and it is probably concentrated in the bile. The terminal half-life is >36 hr.

Adverse Reactions. Nausea, vomiting, mucositis, diarrhea, and reversible alopecia occur frequently. Dose- and duration-dependent hepatotoxicity and genotoxic effects have been reported. Severe ulceration occurs if the drug is extravasated. The dose-limiting toxicity is myelosuppression with a leukopenic nadir at 7–10 days. Rarely, radiation recall occurs.

MITOXANTRONE   Novantrone

Pharmacology. Mitoxantrone is a substituted salt of a planar anthracene. The drug binds to DNA by intercalation and inhibits topoisomerase-II, producing DNA strand breaks; DNA synthesis is impaired in a cell-cycle phase nonspecific fashion.[159]

Administration and Adult Dosage. IV for solid tumors 12 mg/m^2 q 4 weeks or 5 mg/m^2/week for 3 weeks. IV for leukemia 10–12 mg/m^2/day for 3 days. IV for multiple sclerosis 12 mg/m^2 q 3 months, to a usual lifetime maximum of 140 mg/m^2. Administer only through a freely flowing IV line.

Special Populations. *Pediatric Dosage.* IV for leukemia up to 8 mg/m^2/week for 3 weeks or up to 18 mg/m^2 q 4 weeks.[160]

Geriatric Dosage. Same as adult dosage.

Other Conditions. Reduce doses by approximately 30–50% in patients with abnormal hepatobiliary function and/or appreciable third-space fluid accumulations.[161] Reduced doses also are required in patients with poor bone marrow reserve. No dosage alteration is required with renal function impairment.

Dosage Forms. Inj 2 mg/mL.

Patient Instructions. (*See* Antineoplastics Class Instructions.) This drug might turn urine blue-green for 24 hr after administration because of its dark blue color. Discoloration of the whites of the eyes might occur.

Pharmacokinetics. *Fate.* The drug is >95% plasma protein bound and exhibits prolonged retention in tissues. Some liver metabolism to glucuronyl and glutathione conjugates occurs. Urinary recovery is <8% of a dose; the majority is eliminated in the bile; fecal recovery averages 18% of a dose over 5 days.[161]

$t_{1/2}$. α phase 14 min; β phase 1.1 hr; γ phase 38–43 hr.[161]

Adverse Reactions. Emetic potential is low. Myelosuppression, principally granulocytopenia (nadir at 10–14 days), occurs and is most severe in heavily pretreated or irradiated patients. Mucositis, which is dose limiting, occurs only with weekly regimens. CHF has been reported frequently, most often after prior anthracycline therapy. Cumulative cardiotoxicity limits are not well established but can approach 125 mg/m^2 with prior anthracyclines and 160 mg/m^2 without.[159] Alopecia and extravasation necrosis are minimal. Interstitial pneumonitis occurs rarely. Mitoxantrone is not usually a vesicant, although it causes necrosis rarely and usually tints the tissues a blue color.

Precautions. Reduce the dosage in patients with poor hepatobiliary function. Dosage reduction might be necessary in patients previously treated with marrow suppressant or cardiotoxic agents.

Drug Interactions. None known.

Parameters to Monitor. Obtain serum bilirubin before each dose. Assess cardiac function in patients with prior anthracycline therapy or severe pre-existing cardiovascular disease and in multiple sclerosis patients who reach a cumulative dosage of 100 mg/m^2. Monitor absolute granulocyte count before each dose; nadir counts 7–10 days after the dose are optimal.

PLICAMYCIN   Mithracin

Pharmacology. Plicamycin (mithramycin) is a complex, polycyclic, sugar-linked antibiotic that acts by DNA binding in a cell-cycle phase nonspecific fashion; it also has a separate calcium-lowering effect. It is used in testicular cancer and to control severe hypercalcemia caused by malignancy.[162,163]

Adult Dosage. **IV for testicular tumors** 25–30 μg/kg/day to a maximum of 3 mg for up to 5 days, repeat in 4 weeks if toxicity has resolved. **IV for hypercalcemia** 25 μg/kg/day to a maximum of 3 mg for 3–4 days. Reduce dosage by 25–50% in moderate to severe renal impairment. *Note:* Dosage is in μg/kg, with no single dose over 3 mg.

Dosage Forms. **Inj** 2.5 mg.

Pharmacokinetics. The metabolic fate of the drug is unknown, but the drug penetrates well into the CNS and 40% of radioactivity from a radiolabeled dose appears in the urine.

Adverse Reactions. Mild to moderate myelosuppression with a leukopenic nadir at 7–12 days, nausea, and vomiting occur frequently. Dose- and duration-dependent nephrotoxicity (increased Cr$_s$ and proteinuria) and hepatotoxicity (increased LDH and AST) occur frequently. Sterility, mutagenicity, and teratogenicity have been reported. The dose-limiting toxicity is a hemorrhagic tendency characterized by decreased platelet count and responsiveness and depressed clotting factor synthesis. Rarely, stomatitis, progressive skin thickening, and hyperpigmentation occur. The drug is an irritant, but not a vesicant if extravasated. The drug is contraindicated in patients with pre-existing bleeding diatheses, hypocalcemia, or severe renal or hepatic dysfunction. Use cautiously, if at all, with other drugs affecting platelet function (eg, aspirin).

Hormonal Drugs and Antagonists

ANTI-ANDROGENS:

BICALUTAMIDE	Casodex
FLUTAMIDE	Eulexin
NILUTAMIDE	Nilandron

Pharmacology. These drugs are nonsteroidal antiandrogens that competitively inhibit binding of testosterone at androgen receptors in the testes and prostate gland, reducing androgen-stimulated cell growth. They are used with a luteinizing hormone-releasing hormone (LHRH) analogue (eg, leuprolide or goserelin). Bicalutamide has a longer half-life and 4-fold higher affinity than flutamide for the androgen receptor, which allows once-daily administration.[164,165]

Administration and Adult Dosage. **PO for prostatic carcinoma** together with an LHRH analogue; (Bicalutamide) 50 mg once daily; (Flutamide) 250 mg q 8 hr; (Nilutamide) 300 mg/day for 30 days, then 150 mg/day.

Special Populations. *Geriatric Dosage.* Same as adult dosage.

Other Conditions. If PSA levels rise with clinical disease progression, consider discontinuing the antiandrogen temporarily and continuing the LHRH antagonist to re-establish androgen receptor sensitivity. Renal or hepatic impairment does not appear to alter elimination of either drug.

Dosage Forms. (Bicalutamide) **Tab** 50 mg. (Flutamide) **Cap** 125 mg. (Nilutamide) **Tab** 50 mg.

Patient Instructions. Take therapy continuously without interruption. Start bicalutamide at the same time as the luteinizing hormone-releasing hormone agonist. Hot flashes and some feminizing side effects (especially breast enlargement or tenderness) can occur during therapy.

Missed Doses. Take a missed dose as soon as possible. If you take the drug once daily and it is time for the next dose, take it at the regular time. Do not double the dose. If you take two or more doses daily, and it is about time for the next dose, skip the missed dose. Do not double the dose. If you miss two or more doses contact your physician.

Pharmacokinetics. *Fate.* These agents are well absorbed orally and absorption is unaffected by food, but absolute bioavailability is unknown. (Bicalutamide) With an oral dose of 50 mg/day, bicalutamide attains a peak serum level of 8.9 mg/L (21 μmol/L) 31 hr after a dose at steady state. Cl of (R)-bicalutamide is 0.32 L/hr. The active (R)-enantiomer of bicalutamide is oxidized to an inactive metabolite, which, like the inactive (S)-enantiomer, is glucuronidated and cleared rapidly by elimination in the urine and feces.[165] (Flutamide) Flutamide attains peak serum levels of 78 μg/L (283 nmol/L) 2–4 hr after a 250 mg dose at steady state, and its metabolite (α-hydroxyflutamide) achieves levels of 0.720–1.68 mg/L. Flutamide and its active metabolite α-hydroxyflutamide are bound to plasma proteins. Both drugs are extensively metabolized. The majority of a flutamide dose is excreted in the urine as 2-amino-5-nitro-4-(trifluoromethyl) phenol (inactive) with little parent and active metabolite (4.2% of a dose) excreted in the bile or feces.[166,167]

$t_{½}$. (Bicalutamide) 5.8 days; (flutamide) 7.8 hr; (nilutamide) 41–49 hr.[165–167]

Adverse Reactions. These agents are relatively well tolerated. When the drugs are combined with an LHRH agonist, the following side effects occur: hot flashes (50%), general pain (25%), back pain (16%), asthenia (16%), pelvic pain (12%), constipation (15%), diarrhea (10–24%, higher with flutamide, possibly because of lactose intolerance),[168] nausea (11%), nocturia (10%), liver enzyme elevation (6–10%), abdominal pain (8%), and chest pain (5%). Hepatic injury and jaundice occur rarely.

Contraindications. None known.

Precautions. Discontinue these drugs if LFTs are consistently over twice the upper limits of normal without hepatic metastases.

Drug Interactions. Dosage adjustment of warfarin, based on INR, might be necessary when bicalutamide is administered because it can displace warfarin from protein binding sites in vitro.

Parameters to Monitor. Monitor PSA levels q 3 months as an index of disease response. Obtain serum transaminases q 3–4 months to rule out drug-induced hepatic injury.

AROMATASE INHIBITORS:	
AMINOGLUTETHIMIDE	Cytadren
ANASTROZOLE	Arimidex
EXEMESTANE	Aromasin
LETROZOLE	Femara

Pharmacology. Aminoglutethimide, anastrozole, exemestane, and letrozole inhibit the metabolic conversion of androstenedione to estradiol, which is mediated by aromatase, primarily in peripheral adipose tissues. In postmenopausal women, this deprives hormonally sensitive breast cancers of estrogenic stimulation. Aminoglutethimide is less specific and blocks the cholesterol-based biosynthesis of all corticosteroid precursors (eg, hydrocortisone, aldosterone) in the adrenal gland and at peripheral sites.[169–171] Anastrozole, exemestane, and letrozole are much more specific inhibitors of estrogen synthesis that do not affect synthesis of other steroids. Exemestane's inhibition is irreversible and lasts for about 72 hr after a dose.

Administration and Adult Dosage. (Aminoglutethimide) **PO** 750 mg–1.5 g/day; (anastrozole) **PO** 1 mg/day; (exemestane) **PO** 25 mg/day after a meal; (letrozole) **PO** 2.5 mg/day. (*See* Notes.)

Special Populations. *Pediatric Dosage.* (Aminoglutethimide) safety and efficacy not established, but the following has been used: **PO for adrenal hyperplasia**

and adrenal tumors (>2.5 yr) 0.375–1.5 g/day. (Anastrozole, exemestane, letrozole) safety and efficacy not established.

Geriatric Dosage. Same as adult dosage.

Other Conditions. (Anastrozole, exemestane) No change required in hepatic or renal impairment. (Letrozole) No dosage adjustment is required with Cl_{cr} ≥10 mL/min.

Dosage Forms. (Aminoglutethimide) **Tab** 250 mg. (Anastrozole) **Tab** 1 mg. (Exemestane) **Tab** 25 mg. (Letrozole) **Tab** 2.5 mg.

Patient Instructions. (Aminoglutethimide) If severe stress or trauma occurs, increased hydrocortisone dosage might be needed. Marked drowsiness can occur during therapy. Skin rashes are common, especially at the start of therapy. (Exemestane) Take this drug after a meal. (Letrozole) This drug may be taken with food.

Missed Doses. This drug should be taken at regular intervals exactly as prescribed. If a dose is missed, it should be taken as soon as it is remembered. If it is almost time for the next dose, take only that dose and resume the regular dosage schedule. Do not double the dose.

Pharmacokinetics. *Fate.* (Aminoglutethimide) A 1 g oral dose yields serum levels of 9 μg/mL. Cl averages 5.5 L/hr in adults. About 50% is metabolized in liver to a less active *N*-acetyl derivative; this and other metabolites are excreted renally.[1,169] (Anastrozole) Extensively metabolized and excreted renally (10% as parent, 60% as metabolites).[170] (Exemestane) Absorption is increased by 40% when taken with a high-fat meal. Extensively metabolized by CYP3A4 and aldoketoreductases, with unchanged drug accounting for <10% of drug in plasma. Metabolites have less or no inhibitory activity against aromatase. Less than 1% excreted unchanged in urine. (Letrozole) Well absorbed. V_d is 1.9 L/kg. The drug is metabolized to a glucuronide metabolite, which is excreted in urine. Only 5% is excreted unchanged in urine.

$t_{½}$. (Aminoglutethimide) α phase 2.5 hr; β phase 13.3 hr. (Anastrozole) 50 hr. (Exemestane) 24 hr. (Letrozole) about 2 days.[1,169–171]

Adverse Reactions. (Aminoglutethimide) Lethargy and somnolence (80%), skin rashes (50%), visual blurring, dizziness (15–30%, especially in the elderly), nausea, vomiting, and hypotension (15%), hypothyroidism, hematologic suppression (eg, agranulocytosis, pancytopenia) (<1%). (Anastrozole) Asthenia, nausea, headache, hot flashes, back pain, emesis, dizziness, rash, constipation. (Exemestane) Hot flashes, nausea, fatigue, depression, insomnia, anxiety dizziness, headache, dyspnea, and GI disturbances occur frequently. About 4% of patients have androgenic side effects such as acne, hair loss, or hypertrichosis. (Letrozole) Musculoskeletal pain, nausea, hot flashes, headache, sweating, hair thinning, and edema are frequent.

Contraindications. These drugs should generally not be given to premenopausal women.

Precautions. (Aminoglutethimide) Supplemental **hydrocortisone** 50–100 mg/day and **fludrocortisone** 0.1 mg/day are required during therapy.

Drug Interactions. (Aminoglutethimide) Several drug interactions can occur because of the drug's enhancement of CYP3A metabolism; the effects of dexamethasone, digoxin, medroxyprogesterone, tamoxifen, theophylline, and warfarin might be reduced. Aminoglutethimide also induces its own metabolism, which decreases blood levels and half-lives during long-term therapy. (Exemestane) Although metabolized by CYP3A4, ketoconazole does not decease its metabolism, so CYP3A4 inhibitor interactions are unlikely. (Letrozole) Inhibits CYP2A6 and CYP2C9.

Parameters to Monitor. (Aminoglutethimide) Monitor thyroid function and blood pressure periodically during therapy.

Notes. Letrozole is approved for first-line treatment of breast cancer based on its superiority to tamoxifen. Anastrazole is also considered a first-line therapy for breast cancer.

ESTRAMUSTINE PHOSPHATE   Emcyt

Pharmacology. Estramustine is a conjugate of nor-nitrogen mustard linked by a carbamate bond to the 3 position of the steroidal nucleus of estradiol. Phosphorylation at position 17 adds water solubility. Estramustine originally was thought to act as a hormonally directed alkylating agent, but later studies suggest an alternate effect, impairment of mitotic spindle formation. Dephosphorylated estradiol and estrone metabolites produce typical estrogenic effects.[172]

Administration and Adult Dosage. **PO for prostatic carcinoma** 14 mg/kg/day in 3–4 divided doses.

Special Populations. *Geriatric Dosage.* Same as adult dosage.

Other Conditions. Diabetic and hypertensive patients might require increased doses of insulin or antihypertensives because of estrogenic effects.

Dosage Forms. **Cap** 140 mg.

Patient Instructions. Take this drug on an empty stomach; particularly avoid taking with milk, milk products, or calcium-containing foods or drugs.

Missed Doses. If you miss a dose, skip the missed dose and go back to your regular dosage regimen. Do not double the dose. If you miss two or more doses, contact your physician.

Pharmacokinetics. *Fate.* Milk and calcium salts reduce oral bioavailability by forming nonabsorbable calcium complexes. Dephosphorylated during absorption to estradiol and estrone congeners. (*See* Estradiol, Estrone.)

Adverse Reactions. Emetic potential is low. The major side effects are caused by estrogenic actions such as very frequent gynecomastia, cardiovascular effects (frequent edema, occasional leg cramps, or thrombophlebitis, and rare pulmonary embolism and infarction), and GI effects (frequent nausea without vomiting, diarrhea, and occasional anorexia). Laboratory abnormalities are minimal; there is no consistent hematologic suppression and only mild increases in AST or LDH in about 30% of patients.[172]

Contraindications. Thrombophlebitis or thromboembolic conditions (except when tumor is the cause).

Precautions. Use with caution in patients with severe underlying cardiovascular diseases. Poorly controlled CHF also can be exacerbated by estrogen-induced fluid retention. Type 1 diabetics and patients on antihypertensive medications can have increased medication requirements for these diseases.

Drug Interactions. Dairy products or calcium salts can reduce estramustine bioavailability.

Parameters to Monitor. Responses in prostate cancer are predominantly subjective, including reduced pain and less urinary retention. Objective responses can be followed with serial acid phosphatase determinations. Attention to cardiovascular or thromboembolic signs and symptoms is important.

Notes. Estramustine phosphate is principally used in the palliative treatment of advanced prostate cancer. Objective partial response rates of 20% are common. The drug can be safely combined with cytotoxic agents.[172]

GONADOTROPIN-RELEASING HORMONE ANALOGUES:	
GOSERELIN ACETATE	Zoladex
LEUPROLIDE ACETATE	Lupron, Viadur
TRIPTORELIN PAMOATE	Trelstar

Pharmacology. These drugs are synthetic peptide analogues of the natural hypothalamic hormone, gonadotropin-releasing hormone (GnRH). This hormone controls the release of pituitary luteinizing hormone (LH) and follicle-stimulating hormone (FSH) to stimulate sex hormone production in the testes (testosterone) and ovaries (estradiol, others). These synthetic agents have D-amino acid and other substitutions to increase stimulatory potency. FSH and LH are initially stimulated, followed by profound inhibition of circulating sex hormones to castration levels. This retards the growth of hormonally dependent organs including the prostate, breast, endometrium, and ovaries.[173,174]

Administration and Adult Dosage. SC for prostatic carcinoma (goserelin) insert 3.6 mg implant into upper abdominal wall q 28 days; (leuprolide aqueous) 1 mg/day; (leuprolide implant) insert 72 mg implant into inner aspect of upper arm. **IM for prostatic carcinoma** (leuprolide depot) 7.5 mg of 1-month formulation q 28–33 days or 22.5 mg of the 3-month formulation q 3 months; (triptorelin pamoate) 3.75 mg once monthly or 11.25 mg of the 3-month formulation q 3 months. **SC for endometriosis** (goserelin) insert 3.6 mg implant into upper abdominal wall q 28 days for 6 months; **IM for endometriosis** (leuprolide depot) 3.75 mg monthly for 6 months.

Special Populations. *Pediatric Dosage.* SC for central precocious puberty (CPP) (leuprolide aqueous) 50 μg/kg/day initially, increasing in 10 μg/kg/day increments until total down-regulation is achieved. **IM for CPP** initial dosage is (≤25 kg) 7.5 mg monthly; (25–37.5 kg) 11.25 mg monthly; (>37.5 kg) 15 mg monthly. Increase in 3.75 mg/month increments until total down-regulation is achieved.

Geriatric Dosage. (Prostatic carcinoma) same as adult dosage.

Dosage Forms. (Goserelin) **Implant** 3.6, 10.8 mg. (Leuprolide) **Inj (aqueous)** 5 mg/mL; **Inj (depot, 1-month)** 3.75, 7.5, 11.25, 15 mg; **(depot, 3-month)** 11.25, 22.5 mg with 1.5 mL diluent; **(depot, 4-month)** 30 mg with 1.5 mL diluent. (*Note:* Do not use a partial dose of the 3-month formulation in place of a 1-month formulation.) **Implant** 72 mg of leuprolide acetate equivalent to 65 mg of leuprolide. (Triptorelin) **Inj (depot, 1-month)** 3.75 mg; **(depot, 3-month)** 11.25 mg.

Patient Instructions. Instruct in proper method of aseptic preparation of vials and syringes, proper technique for subcutaenous administration, and proper disposal of syringes and needles. (Prostate cancer) Disease symptoms such as bone pain and urinary retention might become worse briefly with initiation of therapy. (Endometriosis) Do not become pregnant while on this drug; always use a barrier contraceptive. Notify your physician if regular menstruation continues. Because therapy can cause a loss of bone density, calcium supplementation is recommended. (Pediatric CPP) A slight increase in pubertal signs and symptoms might occur initially. Adherence to therapy is critical; symptoms such as menses or breast or testicular development might indicate inadequate therapy.

Pharmacokinetics. *Fate.* These drugs are inactive orally. The SC, IM, and IV routes provide comparable bioavailability. The metabolism of these compounds has not been described. (Goserelin) Goserelin is slowly absorbed over the first 8 days. Thereafter, absorption is steady for the remaining 28 days, with no evidence of dose-to-dose accumulation. Goserelin serum levels of about 2.5 µg/L occur on days 15–16 in males with prostate cancer. (Leuprolide) The absorption profile of leuprolide 3-month formulation is similar to the 7.5 mg 1-month formulation. Leuprolide serum levels after a 7.5 mg depot injection are 20 µg/L at 4 hr and 0.36 µg/L at 4 weeks. (Triptorelin) Triptorelin peak levels occur within 1 week and persist for 4 weeks.

$t_{1/2}$. (Goserelin) 4.2 hr with Cl_{cr} >70 mL/min; 12.1 hr with Cl_{cr} <20 mL/min. (Leuprolide) 2.9 hr. (Triptorelin) 0.5–3 hr.

Adverse Reactions. Emetic potential is low; nausea occurs in <5% of patients. Prostate cancer symptoms flare initially, causing bone pain or urinary retention. Sexual dysfunction and decreased erections are reported in about 20% of males. Hot flashes initially can occur in up to 80% of patients with endometriosis who also might experience calcium loss and estrogen-deficiency side effects (eg, decreased libido, vaginal discomfort, dizziness, general malaise, emotional lability, depression). Mild injection site reactions are rare, unless the patient is sensitive to benzyl alcohol (leuprolide aqueous only).

Contraindications. Pregnancy, because of an established teratogenic activity in animals. Do not initiate therapy for endometriosis until after negative pregnancy test.

Precautions. Monitor carefully initially in prostate cancer patients. Those with severe metastatic vertebral lesions are subject to spinal cord compression, and those with severe urinary retention might develop renal impairment.

Drug Interactions. None known.

Parameters to Monitor. (Prostate cancer) Monitor serum LH, FSH, estradiol, and testosterone; concentrations should fall to castrate levels with adequate GnRH analogue therapy. Close initial monitoring of disease symptom severity (bone pain, urinary retention) is required. Serum PSA levels should fall and remain low in patients who respond. (Endometriosis) Monitor pain and menstrual symptoms.

Notes. In prostate cancer, these drugs are often combined with an androgen receptor antagonist (eg, bicalutamide, flutamide) to provide complete hormonal blockade.

TAMOXIFEN CITRATE   Nolvadex, Various

Pharmacology. Tamoxifen is a synthetic, nonsteroidal antiestrogen that binds to cytosol or nuclear estrogen receptor (ER) proteins in hormonally sensitive organs including the breast, prostate, uterus, and ovary.[175] The tamoxifen–receptor complex binds to chromatin in the cell nucleus, thereby stopping estrogen-dependent growth-stimulatory mRNA synthesis.

Administration and Adult Dosage. **PO for breast cancer** usually 20 mg bid in premenopausal patients and 10 mg bid in postmenopausal patients. To rapidly achieve steady-state levels, an initial 2-week course of 40 mg/m^2 bid followed by the standard maintenance dosage has been recommended.[176] **PO for reduction of breast cancer risk in high-risk women** 20 mg/day for 5 yr.

Special Populations. *Geriatric Dosage.* Same as adult dosage.

Dosage Forms. **Tab** 10, 20 mg.

Patient Instructions. In premenopausal patients, the chance of becoming pregnant is increased and a barrier contraceptive should be used. You should have regular gynecologic examinations after taking this drug and report any menstrual irregularities, abnormal vaginal discharge or bleeding, or pelvic pain or pressure. Lactation can occur while you are on tamoxifen.

Missed Doses. If you miss a dose, skip the missed dose and go back to your regular dosage regimen. Do not double the dose. If you miss two or more doses, contact your physician.

Pharmacokinetics. *Onset and Duration.* Therapeutic levels are attained in ≥7 days with 10–20 mg/m^2/day but 3 hr after the loading dose regimen of ≥40 mg/m^2 bid.[176]

Serum Levels. There does not appear to be a direct relationship between serum levels and response or time to response, but all responders have tamoxifen levels >180 μg/L (0.48 μmol/L) at the time of remission.

Fate. Well absorbed orally, with a peak of 42 μg/L (0.11 μmol/L; 12 μg/L is *N*-desmethyl metabolite) achieved 3–4 hr after a 20 mg dose.[177] Initially, the *N*-desmethyl concentration is only 50% of the tamoxifen level, but after 21 days the metabolite level is higher because of its longer half-life. With low-dose continuous therapy, mean steady-state tamoxifen levels of ≥260 μg/L (0.7 μmol/L) are achieved after 16 weeks. Tamoxifen is slowly but extensively metabolized, mainly to *N*-desmethyltamoxifen, which is equally antiestrogenic to tamoxifen. Neither is readily conjugated, and both undergo hepatic hydroxylation and conjugation followed by elimination into the bile and feces; levels are measurable for up to 6 weeks after drug discontinuation.[176]

$t_{1/2}$. (Tamoxifen) 4 days; (N-desmethyltamoxifen) 9 days.[177] With long-term use, these half-lives increase slightly.[176]

Adverse Reactions. Emetic potential is moderately low. Well tolerated, producing rare minor myelosuppression (usually in heavily pretreated patients). Menopausal symptomatology, including hot flashes, nausea, and rarely vomiting, is produced in one-third of patients. Menstrual difficulties include irregularity, vaginal bleeding, and pruritus vulvae. A serious disease "flare" occurs occasionally during initial therapy, involving hypercalcemia and an increase in bone or soft tissue pain;[178] the flare often subsides even with continued therapy and might indicate early tumor response. Retinopathy has occurred, most commonly after very large dosages but also with usual dosages. The drug appears to produce estrogen-like effects in the bone; thus, skeletal demineralization is not a problem with long-term therapy. An increased risk of secondary uterine cancer has been reported.

Precautions. Pregnancy. Use with caution in patients with pre-existing leukopenia and thrombocytopenia.

Drug Interactions. Aminoglutethimide can decrease tamoxifen serum levels. Tamoxifen can attenuate the cytotoxic activities of fluorouracil and doxorubicin.[1]

Notes. The response rate in breast cancer is about 50–70% in ER-positive patients, whereas the rate in ER-negative patients is only about 5–10%.[179] Tamoxifen has been used in endometrial, stage D prostatic, and renal cell cancers and melanoma.[1] It has been used investigationally to decrease the size and pain of gynecomastia.

TOREMIFENE CITRATE
Fareston

Pharmacology. Toremifene is a chloro derivative of tamoxifen that binds to high-affinity estrogen receptors in hormonally dependent tissues. Like **tamoxifen,** it has antiestrogenic and estrogenic activities in different tissues. Effects on serum lipids are similar to those of tamoxifen (reduced total and LDL cholesterol), but toremifene slightly increases HDL levels. In ER-positive breast cancer, toremifene is comparable to tamoxifen but has minimal activity in tamoxifen-refractory patients. Unlike tamoxifen, toremifene does not produce DNA/genotoxic effects or hepatocellular carcinoma in animals, suggesting an improved long-term safety profile.[166,180,181]

Administration and Adult Dosage. **PO for breast cancer** 50 mg/day.

Special Populations. *Geriatric Dosage.* Same as adult dosage.

Dosage Forms. **Tab** 60 mg.

Patient Instructions. (*See* Tamoxifen.)

Pharmacokinetics. *Fate.* Peak serum levels occur 1.5–4.5 hr after a single dose, but the time to reach steady-state with long-term oral administration is 1–5 weeks. Steady-state levels with a dosage of 60 mg/day average 900 μg/L. The drug is metabolized extensively in the liver, primarily by CYP3A4. Major metabolites are N-desmethyl- and 4-hydroxytoremifene, both of which are active antiestrogens. However, only the N-desmethyl derivative is detectable in plasma with a dosage of 60 mg/day.[166,180]

$t_{1/2}$. (Toremifene) 5 days; (*N*-desmethyltoremifene) 6 days.[180]

Adverse Reactions. Toremifene is generally well tolerated; hot flashes (in 34%) are the most frequent side effect. Vaginal discharge or bleeding occurs in 13% of patients, dizziness in 9%, and edema in 5%. It causes minimal GI toxicity, consisting of nausea in 14% and vomiting in 4% of patients. Sweating, vaginal discharge or bleeding, dizziness, and edema also occur frequently. Acute tumor flare occurs in 16%, marked by transient increases in bone or musculoskeletal pain, cutaneous erythema, and/or hypercalcemia within 2 weeks of starting therapy. Worsening cataracts occur in 10%, which is similar to tamoxifen, and mild corneal keratopathies occur in 4%. All of these ocular effects are reversible with discontinuation. In a comparative trial, mild liver function abnormalities occurred in the toremifene group, although most were related to progressive metastatic breast cancer.

Drug Interactions. Drugs that induce CYP3A4 can decrease toremifene levels and those that inhibit CYP3A4 can increase levels. Toremifene can increase PT in patients taking warfarin.

Mitotic Inhibitors

DOCETAXEL   Taxotere

Pharmacology. Docetaxel is a semisynthetic derivative of a taxane extracted from the needles of the yew tree, *Taxus baccata*. It binds to microtubule tubulin sites distinct from paclitaxel, with the similar result of enhanced microtubule polymerization that causes clumps to form and halts cell division in metaphase. It is active in refractory breast cancer and non–small cell lung cancer.[182]

Administration and Adult Dosage. **IV for breast cancer** 60–100 mg/m^2 infused over 1 hr q 3 weeks. **IV for non–small cell lung cancer** 75 mg/m^2 over 1 hr q 3 weeks. Premedicate all patients with dexamethasone 16 mg/day for 5 days, starting 1 day before administering docetaxel.

Special Populations. *Pediatric Dosage.* (<16 yr) Safety and efficacy not established.

Geriatric Dosage. Same as adult dosage.

Other Conditions. Reduce dosage by 25–50% in patients with elevated hepatic enzymes (and probably elevated serum bilirubin).

Dosage Forms. **Inj** 40 mg/mL.

Patient Instructions. Immediately report fever or chills occurring 1–2 weeks after drug administration. This drug can cause swelling of the extremities and tingling sensations.

Pharmacokinetics. *Fate.* Peak serum levels average 3.6 μg/mL after a 1-hr IV infusion of 100 mg/m^2. Over 90% is plasma protein bound. Cl averages 40 L/hr in adults; Cl is reduced by ≥25% in patients with elevated LFTs (transaminases >1.5 times normal; alkaline phosphatase >2.5 times normal). Most of the drug is metabolized to less active hydroxylated forms and excreted by biliary secretion into the feces; <5% is excreted in urine.

$t_{1/2}$. α phase 5 min; β phase 38 min; γ phase 12 hr.

Adverse Reactions. Emetic potential is moderate. The dose-limiting toxicity is neutropenia, which is more severe with reduced liver function; the onset of febrile neutropenia can be as soon as 5 days after drug administration. Thrombocytopenia also occurs but is less severe. Anemia and alopecia also occur but are not dose limiting. Infusion-associated hypersensitivity symptoms (eg, facial flushing) occur in 50% of patients, whereas dyspnea, chest tightness, and low back pain are rare. A pruritic rash on the forearms, hands, and neck occurs in about 40% of patients. Mucositis, nausea, and vomiting occur in about one-third of patients. Peripheral nerve numbness and paresthesia, fluid retention, and edema are cumulative dose-related toxicities. Weight gain initially involves peripheral edema at cumulative dosages >500 mg/m^2; edema can become prominent after 6 cycles (600 mg/m^2 total dosage) and proceed to pulmonary edema. Pretreatment with oral dexamethasone (8 mg bid for 5 days, starting 24 hr before docetaxel) retards the development of serious fluid retention.

Contraindications. Severe hypersensitivity to drugs formulated with polysorbate 80; neutropenia <1500/μL; hepatic transaminase levels >1.5 times the upper limit of normal; hepatic alkaline phosphatase levels >2.5 times the upper limit of normal; severe pre-existing neutropenia, edema, or peripheral neuropathy.

Precautions. Febrile neutropenia is frequent, necessitating careful follow-up of infectious signs after administration.

Drug Interactions. In vitro, metabolism of docetaxel to its hydroxy metabolites is reduced by inhibitors of CYP3A such as cimetidine, erythromycin, ketoconazole, and troleandomycin. Barbiturates stimulate metabolism of docetaxel.[183] The clinical importance of these findings is not known.

Parameters to Monitor. WBC count, peripheral edema, LFTs (ALT, AST, alkaline phosphatase) and signs of infection.

ETOPOSIDE	VePesid, Various
ETOPOSIDE PHOSPHATE	Etopophos

Pharmacology. Etoposide (VP-16) is a substituted epipodophyllotoxin derivative from the May apple plant. The major cytotoxic activity is cell-cycle phase specific for G_2 and involves the induction of protein-linked DNA strand breaks by inhibiting DNA topoisomerase-II enzymes.

Administration and Adult Dosage. IV 200–250 mg/m^2 q 7 weeks, or 70 mg/m^2/day for 5 days. IV of etoposide should be administered over 30–60 min or longer; etoposide phosphate may be administered over 5–210 min. **IV continuous infusion** 125 mg/m^2/day for 5 days.[184] **PO for small cell lung cancer** 2 times the IV dose, rounded to the nearest 50 mg; alternatively, 50 mg/day for 30 days.

Special Populations. *Pediatric Dosage.* Safety and efficacy are not established. However, etoposide has been used in dosages similar to adult body surface area dosages.[185-187]

Geriatric Dosage. Same as adult dosage but adjust for age-related reduction in renal function.

Other Conditions. With $Cl_{cr} \leq 20$ mL/min, give 75% of standard dose; reduced dosage also is required with severe bone marrow compromise. Dosage reduction might be necessary with altered hepatobiliary function.

Dosage Forms. **Inj** (Etoposide) 20 mg/mL; (etoposide phosphate) 100 mg; **Cap** (etoposide) 50 mg.

Patient Instructions. (*See* Antineoplastics Class Instructions.)

Pharmacokinetics. *Fate.* Oral bioavailability is 52 ± 17% with inter- and intrapatient variabilities. CSF levels are <10% of serum levels. V_d is 0.36 ± 0.13 L/kg;[10] Cl is 1.1–1.7 L/hr/m^2 or 0.04 ± 0.014 L/hr/kg.[184,188] Inactive metabolites include the hydroxyacid and cis-lactones. Up to 16% of a dose can be eliminated in bile; 30 ± 5% is eliminated in urine, about 70% of this is unchanged drug.

$t_{1/2}$. 8.1 ± 4.3 hr, increased in uremia.[184,188]

Adverse Reactions. Emetic potential is low. Myelosuppression occurs, with a nadir at 7–10 days (longer with daily regimens), affecting principally the granulocytes but also platelets, with a nadir at 9–16 days. Myelosuppression might be less frequent with the phosphate form. Mild mucositis and alopecia can occur. Diarrhea is more frequent with oral administration. Hypotension occurs rarely with rapid IV bolus injections. There is one report of radiation recall skin injury in 13 of 23 patients with small cell lung cancer. Long-term administration can result in development of acute leukemia.

Precautions. Pregnancy; decrease dosage in severe renal dysfunction; avoid rapid IV bolus injection.

Drug Interactions. Anaphylaxis and possible synergistic neuropathy with vincristine and/or cardiomyopathy with anthracyclines have been reported. Cyclosporine can increase serum etoposide levels and toxicity. Phenytoin, phenobarbital, and possibly other CYP3A inducers can decrease etoposide serum levels.

Parameters to Monitor. Obtain peripheral granulocyte counts immediately before administration on repetitive courses. Nadir counts (1–2 weeks after dose) are optional.

Notes. Etoposide is indicated in the combination treatment of small cell carcinoma of the lung and refractory nonseminomatous testicular cancer. The drug is also active in lymphomas and acute leukemias (lymphoblastic and myeloblastic varieties). Etoposide is not a vesicant. Store capsules under refrigeration. Etoposide and cisplatin are compatible for 24 hr in the same container. Concentrated etoposide solutions (>1 mg/mL) can cause cracking of ABS plastic infusion system components and have short stability times of 2 hr. More dilute solutions in NS or D5W of 0.4–0.6 mg/mL have longer stability times of 8 hr and 48 hr, respectively.

IRINOTECAN
Camptosar

Pharmacology. Irinotecan is a water-soluble camptothecin derivative. It is a prodrug for the despiperidine metabolite SN-38, an inhibitor of topoisomerase-I enzymes. This causes single strand breaks in DNA. Irinotecan is approved for first-line treatment of colorectal cancer with 5-FU and leucovorin. The overall response rate in advanced fluorouracil-refractory colon cancer is about 15%, with a 5.2 month median duration of response.[189]

Adult Dosage. **IV as a single agent or in combination with fluorouracil and leucovorin** 125 mg/m^2 once weekly for 4 consecutive weeks administered in 500 mL of D5W over 90 min. Subsequent doses are increased by 25–50 mg/m^2 if no toxicity occurs; if severe toxicity occurs, dosage is decreased by 25–50 mg/m^2. **IV as a single agent** alternatively, 350 mg/m^2 q 3 weeks, with subsequent doses adjusted in 50 mg/m^2 increments.

Dosage Forms. Inj 40, 100 mg.

Pharmacokinetics. The half-lives of irinotecan and the active SN-38 metabolite are 5.7 and 9.8 hr, respectively, with peak SN-38 levels (2–5% of irinotecan) achieved 1 hr after administration. Renal excretion accounts for <10% of a dose as irinotecan and <1% as SN-38; hepatic elimination predominates.

Adverse Reactions. Diarrhea occurs in 90% of patients and can be severe, requiring aggressive prophylaxis with fluids and multiple doses of loperamide. Early diarrhea can be prevented or blunted with doses of 0.25-1 mg of atropine IV or SC. Leukopenia occurs in one-third of patients, although moderate to severe myelosuppression occurs in only 15% and 11% of patients, respectively. Other serious adverse reactions include anaphylactoid reactions, orthostatic hypotension, and rarely renal impairment.

PACLITAXEL Taxol, Various

Pharmacology. Paclitaxel is a naturally occurring diterpene taxane obtained from the bark of the Pacific yew tree, *Taxus brevifolia.* It binds to tubulin proteins, causing abnormal microtubule polymerization and cell-cycle arrest in metaphase.[190,191]

Administration and Adult Dosage. **IV** 135–175 mg/m^2 over 3 or 24 hr q 3 weeks. Doses up to 250 mg/m^2 have been used with hematopoietic colony stimulation factors. Use non-PVC infusion systems.

Special Populations. *Pediatric Dosage.* Safety and efficacy not established.

Geriatric Dosage. Same as adult dosage.

Dosage Forms. Inj 6 mg/mL.

Patient Instructions. (*See* Antineoplastics Class Instructions.)

Pharmacokinetics. *Fate.* Erratic oral bioavailability precludes oral administration. Cl is 18 L/hr/m^2. It is metabolized to a much less active hydroxylated species by CYP3A. Eliminated 30–40% by hepatobiliary excretion; only 1–5% excreted in urine.[192]

$t_{1/2}$. α phase 0.2 hr; β phase 1.9 hr (range 0.5–2.8); γ phase 20.7 hr (range 4–65).[192]

Adverse Reactions. Emetic potential is low. The usual dose-limiting toxicity is neutropenia, with an 8- to 11-day nadir; more severe with prolonged infusion. Dose-limiting toxicity in combination regimens with doxorubicin include neutropenia, inflammation of the cecum (typhlitis), and, with cisplatin, neuropathy.

Peripheral neuropathy (eg, numbness, paresthesias) is cumulative, dose related, and more severe with prior vinca alkaloid or concurrent cisplatin therapy. Alopecia can involve all body hair, with an abrupt onset of 2 weeks. Mucositis is dose dependent. Cardiotoxicity, primarily bradycardia, occurs in 10–30% of patients but rarely requires treatment. Myalgia and arthralgia are common but usually transient. Hypersensitivity reactions, thought to be caused by Cremophor, can occur within the first few minutes of infusion; symptoms include chest pain, hypotension, bronchospasm, urticaria, and flushing and can rapidly progress to anaphylaxis. (*See* Precautions.)

Contraindications. Hypersensitivity to Cremophor vehicle; neutropenia (<1500/μL).

Precautions. Recommended premedications are dexamethasone PO 20 mg at 12 and 6 hr before paclitaxel, and diphenhydramine IV 50 mg, plus cimetidine 300 mg, ranitidine 50 mg, or famotidine 20 mg 30 min before paclitaxel. Ensure that emergency resuscitation equipment is available at the start of infusion. Use cautiously in patients with heart rhythm disturbances.

Drug Interactions. Ketoconazole can decrease paclitaxel clearance and enhance toxicity. Although their effect is not well studied, use other CYP3A inhibitors with caution. (*See also* Adverse Reactions.)

Parameters to Monitor. Neutrophil count before administration.

Notes. Highly effective as a first-line or refractory treatment for ovarian cancer; typically used in platinum-containing regimens; also active in breast cancer, non–small cell lung cancer, lymphoma, and malignant melanoma.[191]

TENIPOSIDE   Vumon

Pharmacology. Teniposide is a semisynthetic podophyllum derivative that has cell-cycle S- and G_2-phase–specific cytotoxic activities similar to those of etoposide. Teniposide is active in acute leukemias and in children with relapsed acute leukemia or neuroblastoma.[188,193,194]

Pediatric Dosage. **IV for acute leukemias** 165–200 mg/m^2/week or 165 mg/m^2 twice weekly.

Dosage Forms. **Inj** 10 mg/mL.

Pharmacokinetics. Teniposide is >90% plasma protein bound and eliminated much more slowly than etoposide. Teniposide half-lives are α phase 45 min, β phase 4 hr, and γ phase 11–30 hr (average 20); 40% of a dose is eliminated in the feces; CSF drug levels are high (27% of serum levels).

Adverse Reactions. The dose-limiting side effect of teniposide is myelosuppression, with the leukopenic nadir at 10–14 days. Emetic potential is low; nausea and vomiting are typically mild (more severe after oral etoposide). Hypotension is reported with rapid drug infusions. Rarely severe hypersensitivity reactions (including anaphylaxis), alopecia, and chemical phlebitis during infusion occur.

TOPOTECAN	Hycamtin

Pharmacology. Topotecan is a topoisomerase-I inhibitor that causes single-strand breaks in DNA. It is a semisynthetic derivative of camptothecin, which is derived from the bark of the Chinese tree, *Camptotheca acuminata.* Topotecan is approved for metastatic ovarian carcinoma and small cell lung cancer after failure of a primary agent and being studied in colon and breast cancers.[1]

Adult Dosage. IV 1.5 mg/m^2/day administered over 30 min for 5 days, starting on day 1 of a 21-day course of therapy for at least 4 courses. With a Cl_{cr} of 20–39 mL/min, the dosage is reduced to 0.75 mg/m^2/day; no guidelines exist for Cl_{cr} <20 mL/min. If severe neutropenia occurs, reduce further doses by 0.25 mg/m^2/day or administer filgrastim with subsequent courses.

Dosage Forms. **Inj** 4 mg.

Pharmacokinetics. Topotecan is rapidly hydrolyzed in plasma. About 70% of the drug is excreted renally as metabolites.

Adverse Reactions. The primary dose-limiting side effect of topotecan is neutropenia, with a nadir at a mean of 11 days; severe neutropenia occurs in 80% of patients. Severe anemia in 40% of patients and severe thrombocytopenia in 26% also have been reported. Nausea and vomiting occur in most patients; other GI effects are frequent diarrhea, constipation, and abdominal pain. Alopecia occurs in about 60% of patients; fatigue and fever of ≥101°F also frequent. Topotecan is contraindicated in pregnancy, breastfeeding, or severe bone marrow depression.

VINCA ALKALOIDS:	
VINBLASTINE SULFATE	Velban, Various
VINCRISTINE SULFATE	Oncovin, Various
VINORELBINE TARTRATE	Navelbine

Pharmacology. The vinca alkaloids are *Vinca rosea* (periwinkle) plant-derived antimitotic agents; cytotoxic activity is related to specific binding to the microtubule protein tubulin, causing microtubule dissolution. This blocks formation of the mitotic spindle apparatus necessary for cell division. The vincas are lethal to cells at high concentrations; at lower concentrations, dividing cells are arrested in the metaphase portion of mitosis.

Administration and Dosage.

	VINBLASTINE	VINCRISTINE	VINORELBINE
Administration	IV push, infusion.	IV push.	IV short infusion.
Adult Dosage	IV push 4–12 mg/m^2 as a single agent at monthly intervals; or 1.5–1.7 mg/m^2/ day for 5 days as a continuous infusion.[195]	0.4–1.4 mg/m^2/ week (2.5 mg typical single dose limit).	30 mg/m^2/week.

	VINBLASTINE	VINCRISTINE	VINORELBINE
Pediatric Dosage	IV push 4–10 mg/m² q 1–2 weeks.	1.4–2 mg/m²/week (2 mg typical single dose limit).	Not used in children.
Geriatric Dosage	Same as adult dosage.	Same as adult dosage.	Same as adult dosage.

Special Populations. *Other Conditions.* Vinblastine and vinorelbine require substantial dosage reductions in heavily pretreated patients (ie, drug or radiation therapy). Reduce vinorelbine dosage by 50% in patients in whom >75% of the liver is replaced by tumor or for granulocyte counts on the day of treatment of 1000–1499/μL; do not administer at lower WBC counts.[196] Vinca alkaloids are eliminated extensively in the bile, and the dosages of vinblastine and vincristine must be reduced by approximately 50–75% with severe hepatobiliary dysfunction. Reduce vinorelbine dosages to 15 mg/m²/week for a serum total bilirubin of 2.1–3 mg/dL and 7.5 mg/m²/week for a bilirubin >3 mg/dL.

Dosage Forms. (Vinblastine) **Inj** 1 mg/mL, 10 mg vial. (Vincristine) **Inj** 1 mg/mL. (Vinorelbine) **Inj** 10 mg/mL.

Patient Instructions. (*See* Antineoplastics Class Instructions.)

Pharmacokinetics. *Fate.* Pharmacokinetics can be described by a two-compartment open model: an initial short phase with rapid tissue uptake (V_d approximating total body water) and a long terminal phase >1 day with a large V_d reflecting slow drug release from tissue binding sites—see below. Vincas do not effectively penetrate into the CNS or other fatty tissues and achieve their highest levels in the liver, gallbladder, and spleen. Approximately 50% of renally and fecally excreted products are closely related metabolites. An example is the formation of desacetyl vinblastine (which is more active on a weight basis than vinblastine) after vinblastine administration. Vinca alkaloids appear to be eliminated primarily in the bile and feces, some in the urine.

	VINBLASTINE	VINCRISTINE	VINORELBINE
***PHARMACOKINETIC PARAMETERS*[197–199]**			
V_c (L/kg)	0.7	0.33	—
V_d (L/kg)	27.3	8.4	40.1 (V_{dss})
Urinary Excretion	—	10% (24 hr)	—
(cumulative)	33% (72 hr)	13% (72 hr)	21% (21 days)
Fecal Excretion	—	33% (24 hr)	—
(cumulative)	21% (72 hr)	67% (72 hr)	34–58% (21 days)
$t_{1/2}$.			
$t_{1/2\alpha}$ (min)	<5	<5	<27
$t_{1/2\beta}$ (hr)	0.164	2.3	<1.9
$t_{1/2\gamma}$ (hr)	25	85	40

Adverse Reactions. Emetic potential is low (vincristine) to moderate (vinblastine and vinorelbine). Myelosuppression is the dose-limiting toxicity for vinblastine and vinorelbine, with the leukopenic nadir at 4–10 days; unless patients have been heavily pretreated with drugs or radiation, recovery from leukopenia is rather prompt, sometimes facilitating weekly or semimonthly drug administration. The major toxicity of vincristine is peripheral neuropathy manifested by paresthesias, constipation, jaw pain, decreased deep tendon reflexes, and rarely bladder atony or paralytic ileus; gut neurotoxicity occurs rarely with vinorelbine. All of these neurologic symptoms slowly resolve over 1 month and necessitate substantial dosage reduction if present at the time of drug administration. Seizures and ocular toxicity presenting as blurred vision or ptosis occur frequently. Mild laxatives or **metoclopramide** may be useful for constipation. The vincas are extremely toxic if inadvertently extravasated; **hyaluronidase** (150 units/mL) is sometimes effective as a local (subcutaneous) antidote. Vinorelbine also causes substantial phlebitis, which can be lessened by a short (6- to 10-min) infusion. Transiently severe pain in tumor masses occurs with vinblastine frequently. Alopecia is frequent with all agents.

Contraindications. Inadvertent intrathecal administration of any vinca alkaloid is fatal. (Vinblastine) Severe bone marrow compromise from prior therapy; uncontrolled infection. (Vincristine) Severe peripheral nervous system effects from prior doses, particularly paralytic ileus, tingling paresthesias, or decreased deep tendon reflexes; demyelinating form of Charcot-Marie-Tooth syndrome. (Vinorelbine) Pretreatment granulocyte count <1000/μL.

Precautions. Pregnancy. Use with caution in patients with neurologic deficiencies or hepatic disease.

Drug Interactions. Vinca administration (especially vincristine) has been associated with increased cellular retention of methotrexate (increased even in CNS tissues). Concurrent use of vincristine with zalcitabine can increase neuropathy.

Parameters to Monitor. (Vinblastine and vinorelbine) Obtain pretreatment and at least monthly WBC and hemoglobin/hematocrit assessments; (vincristine) obtain serial peripheral neurologic assessments; (all drugs) assess biliary function before making dosage adjustments for impaired hepatobiliary status and administering the drugs.

Notes. Protect these drugs from light and store under refrigeration. Place individual vincristine doses in an overwrap (eg, plastic bag) that is labeled, "Do not remove covering until the moment of injection. Fatal if given intrathecally. For intravenous use only." Useful in hematologic neoplasms (primarily vincristine) and solid tumors, including non–small cell lung cancer in combination with cisplatin (vinorelbine) and refractory breast cancer and Kaposi's sarcoma (vinblastine).[200]

Monoclonal Antibodies

IODINE I-131 TOSITUMOMAB
Bexxar

Pharmacology. This agent is a mouse-derived monoclonal antibody that binds to the CD-20 receptor of normal and malignant B-lymphocytes. The β-particle-emitting isotope ^{131}I is coupled to the antibody, forming a selective radioimmunoconjugate for patients with CD-20–positive non-Hodgkin's lymphoma refractory to chemotherapy.[201,202]

Adult Dosage. In clinical trials, a two-stage dosage schedule has been used. First, patients are administered unlabeled antibody IV to suppress nonspecific binding sites. Next, patients are given trace-labeled doses of ^{131}I-labeled antibody (15–20 mg containing 5 mCi IV) to assess antibody distribution. One week later, patients are given a 685 mg dose of unlabeled antibody IV, followed 1 day later by 2 individualized therapeutic (labeled) doses of 135 mg and 685 mg of antibody to deliver up to 75 cGy of whole-body radiation. A total body irradiation dosage of 55 cGy appears to be the maximum tolerated in patients who have undergone bone marrow transplantation. Give diphenhydramine 50 mg and acetaminophen 650 mg before each infusion.

Adverse Reactions. Nonhematologic toxicities after infusions are mild, with low-grade fever in 31% of patients and chills or rigors in 1%. Mild fatigue and nausea occur in 6–8% of radiolabeled infusions. The dose-limiting toxicity is hematologic suppression with grade 3 or 4 leukopenia and thrombocytopenia in 66% of patients who receive a whole-body radiation dose of 85 cGy. All patients develop complete or near-complete depletion of CD-19- and CD-20–positive B-cells from peripheral blood, recovering to normal levels in 3 months. Serum immunoglobulin levels are unchanged. Because of the short, single course of therapy, antimouse antibody (HAMA) reactions are uncommon. However, when they occur, they are usually marked by hypotension that can be treated with fluid hydration and vasopressors.

RITUXIMAB
Rituxan

Pharmacology. Rituximab is a chimeric murine/human monoclonal antibody that binds to the CD-20 antigen on the surface of normal and malignant B-lymphocytes. This blocks normal CD-20–dependent signaling of cell-cycle initiation and differentiation, leading to apoptosis. After binding to CD-20, the free Fc portion of the antibody can recruit immune effector functions to cause lysis of B-cells of B-lymphocytes.[203,204]

Administration and Adult Dosage. **IV infusion (not bolus) for relapsed or refractory low-grade B-cell non-Hodgkin's lymphoma** 375 mg/m^2 once weekly for 4 doses (days 1, 8, 15, and 22), diluted in NS or D5W. Premedicate the patient with diphenhydramine and acetaminophen and begin the first infusion at a rate of 50 mg/hr. Increase the rate by 50 mg/hr q 30 min to a maximum of 400 mg/hr if no hypotension or hypersensitivity develops. Subsequent infusions are started at a rate of 100 mg/hr and increased by 100 mg/hr q 30 min to the maximum rate of 400 mg/hr, if tolerated. If severe hypersensitivity reactions occur, stop the infusion and treat with diphenhydramine, acetaminophen, and a corticosteroid; for life-threatening reactions, add saline, epinephrine, and bronchodilators. If the reaction is not life-threatening, the infusion may be restarted at one-half of the earlier rate after symptoms subside.

Special Populations. *Pediatric Dosage.* Safety and efficacy not established.

Geriatric Dosage. Same as adult dosage.

Dosage Forms. Inj 10 mg/mL.

Patient Instructions. This drug might cause a flu-like syndrome including fever, chills, and weakness shortly after you receive it.

Pharmacokinetics. *Fate.* Peak serum levels are inversely correlated with the number of CD-20–positive B-cells. Levels average about 280 mg/L. Major sites of antibody distribution are to lymphoid cells of the thymus gland, white pulp of the spleen, and B-lymphocytes in peripheral blood and lymph nodes. Cl averages 0.054 L/hr; the antibody is still detectable in serum 3–6 months after the last dose.

$t_{1/2}$. Half-life is proportional to the dose (range 11–105 hr) with an average of 60 hr after a dosage of 375 mg/m^2.

Adverse Reactions. Most patients experience an infusion-related symptom complex with fever, chills, and rigors on the first infusion. Other frequent, acute infusion-related symptoms are nausea (18%), vomiting (10%), angioedema (13%), urticaria or pruritus (10%), and bronchospasm and rhinitis (8%). Hypotension and other acute effects are moderate or severe in 10% of the first doses. Overall, the frequency and severity of all reactions diminishes with subsequent injections. Most first-dose reactions occur within 30 min to 2 hr and resolve with slowing of the infusion rate for mild to moderate reactions or temporary halting the infusion and treating with supportive medications for severe reactions. Epinephrine is required only occasionally. Myelosuppression (neutropenia and thrombocytopenia) is typically mild and occurs in only 10% of patients, although long-term depletion of B-cells occurs in 70–80%; a minority also have decreased serum immunoglobulins. The frequency of grade 3 infections during the 4-week treatment period is 9% and grade 4 infections generally do not occur. Serious, sometimes fatal, skin reactions (bullous reactions, pemphigus) occur rarely.

Contraindications. Patients with a known type I hypersensitivity (or anaphylaxis) to mouse proteins.

Precautions. Pregnancy; lactation. Contraception is recommended in women of childbearing potential. The ability to respond immunologically to a vaccination is compromised after therapy; the safety of live virus vaccination is not known. Consider stopping antihypertensive medications on the day of treatment to reduce hypotensive reactions. Cardiac monitoring is recommended only in patients with pre-existing arrhythmias and angina that have worsened during the infusion.

Drug Interactions. Additive hypotension can occur in patients on antihypertensive therapy. There is no inhibition of cytotoxic activity in patients being treated for lymphoma with CHOP chemotherapy.

Parameters to Monitor. Monitor for allergic reactions and hypotension frequently during the infusion. Monitor CBC after therapy.

TRASTUZUMAB Herceptin

Pharmacology. Trastuzumab is a humanized monoclonal antibody that binds to the HER2 protein found on the surfaces of some normal cells and plays a role in regulating cell growth. It is used only to treat tumors with an overexpression of HER2 protein. It is used alone in the treatment of metastatic breast cancer in patients who have been treated with chemotherapy or with paclitaxel in patients who have not had chemotherapy for their metastatic diseases.

Adult Dosage. **IV for breast cancer in tumors with overexpression of HER2** 4 mg/kg over 90 min as a loading dose, then 2 mg/kg weekly. Subsequent doses can be infused over 30 min if the loading dose was well tolerated. Do not administer as an IV push or bolus.

Dosage Forms. Inj 440 mg.

Pharmacokinetics. With the recommended dosage regimen, steady-state peak and trough concentrations are 123 and 79 mg/L, respectively. Trough serum levels are 1.5 times higher when given with paclitaxel, possibly because of inhibition of metabolism. The drug is distributed primarily in serum, with a V_d of 0.44 L/kg. Pharmacokinetics appear to be dose related: Cl decreases and half-life increases with increasing dosages. Half-life averages 25 days (range 1–32 days) with the recommended regimen. Renal impairment appears not to affect pharmacokinetics.

Adverse Reactions. Side effects are frequent but usually not severe. Mild to moderate chills with or without fever occur in 40% of patients during the infusion and can usually be treated with acetaminophen, diphenhydramine, and/or meperidine. Other common side effects are diarrhea, pain, asthenia, nausea, vomiting, flu-like symptoms, cough, dyspnea, rash, edema, anemia, and leukopenia. Occasional serious reactions include anaphylaxis, thrombosis, pancytopenia, convulsions, apnea, hypoxia, and renal failure. Cardiac dysfunction and CHF have occurred. Use the drug with caution in pre-existing cardiac dysfunction; monitor cardiac function during therapy, and consider discontinuation if clinically important CHF develops. Serious infusion-related reactions including hypersensitivity (including anaphylaxis) and pulmonary events occur in about 0.25% of patients.

Precautions. Use with caution in patients with symptomatic intrinsic lung disease or extensive tumor involvement in the lungs. Interrupt infusion if the patient experiences dyspnea or clinically significant hypotension. Consider discontinuing therapy in patients who experience anaphylaxis, angioedema, or acute respiratory distress syndrome.

Miscellaneous Antineoplastics

| **ASPARAGINASE** | Elspar |
| **PEGASPARGASE** | Oncaspar |

Pharmacology. Asparaginase is the levo isomer of a macromolecular protein, isolated from *Escherichia coli* and other bacteria, that hydrolyzes the essential amino acid asparagine in the serum, thus depriving susceptible lymphocyte-derived malignancies of a necessary element for protein synthesis. Pegaspargase is a PEG-modified form of asparaginase that can be given to patients allergic to asparaginase. The drug is cell-cycle G-phase specific.

Administration and Adult Dosage. **IM (preferably) or IV for combination therapy of acute leukemia** (asparaginase) 200 IU/kg/day for 28 days,[205] or

1000–6000 IU/m^2/day for 5 days,[206] or 20,000 IU/m^2/week;[207] (pegaspargase) 2500 IU/m^2 q 14 days.

Special Populations. *Pediatric Dosage.* **IM (preferably) or IV for combination therapy of acute leukemia** (asparaginase) 1000–6000 IU/m^2/day for 5 days;[206,208] up to 20,000 IU/m^2/week; (pegaspargase) 2500 IU/m^2 q 14 days.

Geriatric Dosage. Same as adult dosage.

Dosage Forms. Inj (Asparaginase) 10,000 IU vial. (Pegaspargase) 750 IU/mL.

Patient Instructions. (*See* Antineoplastics Class Instructions.) Asparaginase often causes allergic reactions that can be life-threatening. This drug also can alter blood glucose levels and might worsen diabetes mellitus. Report any abdominal pain immediately because it might be a sign of pancreatitis.

Pharmacokinetics. *Fate.* (Asparaginase) IV and IM produce equivalent serum levels. There is negligible distribution out of the vascular compartment, with minimal urinary and biliary excretion. Clearance is probably immune mediated. Asparaginase remains detectable in serum 13–22 days after administration.[209] (Pegaspargase) asparaginase is slowly released from pegaspargase and distributed in the body similarly to native asparaginase.

$t_{½}$. (Asparaginase) α phase 4–9 hr; β phase 1.4–1.8 days.[209] (Pegaspargase) 3.2 ± 1.8 days in patients hypersensitive to asparaginase; 5.7 ± 3.3 days in nonsensitive patients.

Adverse Reactions. Emetic potential is low. Moderate to severe non–dose-related hypersensitivity reactions occur in about 20–35% of patients. (IM use might reduce and/or delay allergic complications);[205] a prophylactic antihistamine sometimes can be helpful. (*See* Precautions.) The drug is usually not myelotoxic. Transient blood glucose lowering followed by a pancreatitis-induced hyperglycemia can occur. Elevated serum cholesterol, severely elevated hepatic enzymes, steatosis, depressed clotting factors (especially profound for fibrinogen), and decreased albumin synthesis occur frequently. Lethargy and somnolence occur and might be more frequent in adults.[210] Fatal hyperthermia has been reported.

Contraindications. Anaphylactic reaction to commercial *E. coli* preparation; severe pancreatitis or history of pancreatitis.

Precautions. Onset of abdominal pain, serum amylase elevation, any changes in mental status, or severe elevation of prothrombin time require drug discontinuation. Some elevations of LFTs should be anticipated. Anaphylaxis can occur with any dose; ensure that emergency resuscitation equipment is available at the time of each dose. Intradermal scratch tests and desensitization procedures are not reliably predictive or preventive for anaphylaxis.[205,209]

Drug Interactions. None known.

Parameters to Monitor. Monitor serum hepatic enzymes, amylase, glucose, and prothrombin time routinely, and all vital signs during administration.

Notes. Reconstitute with NS or D5W (2 mL maximum for IM use); stable at least 24 hr; do not filter.

BLEOMYCIN SULFATE   Blenoxane

Pharmacology. Bleomycin is a mixture of 13 glycopeptide fractions produced by *Streptomyces verticillus.* Antineoplastic effects include single- and double-strand DNA scission, producing excision of thymine bases mediated through binding with ferric iron and subsequent production of highly reactive hydroxyl and superoxide radicals. It is cell-cycle phase specific, with maximal activity in the G_2 (premitotic) phase.[211]

Administration and Adult Dosage. **IM test dose** 1–2 units may be useful in malignant lymphoma patients to assess exaggerated hyperpyrexic response. If no reaction occurs in 2–4 hr, give regular dose. **SC, IM, or IV** 10–20 units/m^2 1–2 times/week.[211] **IV continuous infusion** 15–20 units/day for 4–5 days.[212] Experimental evidence in animals favors continuous administration to lessen pulmonary toxicity and maximize cell kill. A total lifetime dosage limit of 400 units is recommended to avoid pulmonary fibrosis. **Intracavitary for malignant effusion** 15–240 units (60 units for pleural effusion) in 50–100 mL or NS.[213]

Special Populations. *Pediatric Dosage.* **SC, IM, or IV** 10–20 units/m^2 1–2 times a week in combination regimens. **IV continuous infusion** 15–20 units/m^2/day for 4–5 days, usually as a single agent.

Geriatric Dosage. Same as adult dosage but use with caution in patients >70 yr and adjust dosage for age-related reduction in renal function.

Other Conditions. Dosage reduction has been recommended in renal impairment:[214]

SERUM CREATININE (MG/DL)	PERCENTAGE OF DOSE RECOMMENDED
2.5–4	25 (75% reduction)
4–6	20 (80% reduction)
6–10	5–10 (90–95% reduction)

Dosage Forms. **Inj** 15, 30 units.

Patient Instructions. (*See* Antineoplastics Class Instructions.) Report any coughing, shortness of breath, or wheezing. Skin rashes, shaking chills, or transient high fever can occur after administration. Hyperpigmentation of skin fold areas, scars, pressure areas, or sites of trauma can occur.

Pharmacokinetics. *Fate.* Poorly absorbed topically; roughly one-half of intracavitary-administered drug is systemically available (use this fraction to calculate lifetime exposure). After an IV dose of about 15 units/m^2, serum levels of 10–1000 milliunits/L are obtained.[212] Steady-state levels during continuous infusion of 20 units/day are 50–200 milliunits/L.[215] V_d is 0.27 ± 0.04 L/kg; Cl is 0.066 ± 0.018 L/hr/kg.[10] Tissue inactivation is mediated by specific bleomycin-hydrolase, which is low in skin and lung, the two main toxicity targets of the drug.[212,215] From 50% to 60% of a dose is recovered in the urine, 68% of this as unchanged drug.[10]

$t_{1/2}$. α phase 24 min; β phase 3.1 ± 1.7 hr.[10,212,215]

Adverse Reactions. Emetic potential is moderately low. Alopecia, acute fever, and generalized erythema with edema, eventually leading to hyperpigmentation and skin thickening, are frequent. The most serious long-term toxicity is pulmonary fibrosis manifested by dry cough, rales, dyspnea, and bilateral infiltrates. Pulmonary function studies show hypoxemia and reduced CO diffusing capacity. Pulmonary toxicity usually does not occur below 150 units/m^2, but the frequency increases to 55% at doses >283 units/m^2 and 66% at 360 units/m^2.[216] Life-threatening pulmonary fibrosis is rare if dosage limits are observed. Prior chest radiotherapy, age >70 yr, and hyperoxic ventilation predispose patients to toxicity. About 1% of high-dose bleomycin-treated patients die from pulmonary fibrosis. Low-dose hypersensitivity pneumonitis, which might be responsive to a glucocorticoid, also occurs.[217]

Precautions. Use with extreme caution in patients with renal or pulmonary disease, in those with lymphoma, and in those >70 yr.

Drug Interactions. Inspired oxygen concentrations >35% can cause acute respiratory failure in bleomycin-treated patients.

Parameters to Monitor. Calculate cumulative dosage before and after each treatment. Monitor temperature initially, especially in lymphoma patients. Assess renal function before administering. Pulmonary damage is best monitored with CO diffusing capacity and forced vital capacity; specific serial pulmonary function studies have been suggested before and during therapy. Characteristic x-ray findings include changes suggestive of progressive diffuse bilateral fibrosis.

Notes. One milligram of bleomycin equals 1 unit of activity. Reconstituted solution is stable for 1 month under refrigeration and 2 weeks at room temperature. Incompatible with divalent cations (especially copper), ascorbic acid, and compounds with sulfhydryl groups.

IMATINIB MESYLATE
Gleevec

Pharmacology. Imatinib inhibits the abnormal Bcr-Abl tyrosine kinase created by the Philadelphia chromosome abnormality of CML, inhibiting proliferation and inducing apoptosis in leukemic cells with this abnormality. It may also inhibit the tyrosine kinase of platelet-derived growth factor and stem cell factor. It is used in CML after failure of interferon alfa therapy and in chemotherapy-resistent GI stromal carcinoma.

Adult Dosage. PO for the chronic phase of CML 400 mg once daily, increasing to 600 mg once daily if conditions below are met; PO for the accelerated phase of CML or blast crisis 600 mg once daily, increasing to 400 mg bid if conditions below are met. All doses should be taken with a meal and a large glass of water. Dosages may be increased as indicated above in the absence of severe adverse reactions and severe non–leukemia-related neutropenia or thrombocytopenia for disease progression, failure to achieve a satisfactory hematologic response after ≥3 months of therapy, or with loss of a previous hematologic response.

Dosage Forms. Cap 100 mg.

Pharmacokinetics. Oral bioavailability is 98% with a peak at 2–4 hr. It is 95% plasma protein bound. Metabolism is primarily by CYP3A4 to the N-desmethyl metabolite that has activity similar to the parent drug. Imatinib Cl is 0.14–0.16 L/hr/kg. The drug is eliminated in feces, mostly as metabolites. Elimination half-lives are 18 and 40 hr for the drug and active metabolite, respectively.

Adverse Reactions. Most adverse reactions are mild to moderate and more frequent during the accelerated phase and especially during blast crisis. The most frequent are nausea, vomiting, and periorbital or lower limb edema. Edema is occasionally severe and can be managed by diuretics, supportive measures or imatinib dosage reduction. Muscle cramps and pain, hemorrhage, skin rash, headache, fatigue, abdominal pain, arthralgia and fever are also frequent. Dose-related neutropenia (duration 2–3 weeks) and thrombocytopenia (duration 3–4 weeks) also occur, and respond to dosage reduction or interruption of therapy. Elevated transaminases and bilirubin can occur, sometimes requiring dosage reduction or treatment interruption; one death from hepatotoxcity has been reported.

Drug Interactions. Inhibitors and inducers of CYP3A4 are expected to alter the metabolism of imatinib and should be used with caution. Imatinib decreases the metabolism of simvastatin, apparently through CYP3A4 inhibition. Use other drugs with caution that are metabolized by CYP3A4. Patients requiring anticoagulation should receive heparin or a LMWH rather than warfarin.

TRETINOIN   Vesanoid

Pharmacology. Tretinoin (all-trans-retinoic acid) is a modified form of vitamin A used in the treatment of acute promyelocytic leukemia. It causes immature promyeloblasts to differentiate into mature granulocytes, thereby halting cell division and inducing complete remissions in up to 90% of patients. Resistance rapidly develops during therapy because of accelerated drug catabolism to the 4-oxo metabolite, which is excreted in the urine, increased cellular retinoic acid binding protein (II), and tumors with high levels of a mutated α-retinoic acid receptor.[218–220]

Pediatric Dosage. PO 45 mg/m^2/day as a single dose until remission is obtained.

Dosage Forms. Cap 10 mg.

Pharmacokinetics. Peak serum levels of 294 μg/L occur 1–2 hr after a dose; the serum half-life is 0.8 hr.

Adverse Reactions. Hyperleukocytosis and effects typical of hypervitaminosis A (eg, headache, dry skin and mucosa, cheilitis, bone pain, hypertriglyceridemia) occur. Tolerance to these effects develops rapidly, and skin creams, lip balms, and eye and nasal drops are helpful. Liver and renal function test elevations occur occasionally.

Chemoprotectants

AMIFOSTINE   Ethyol

Pharmacology. Amifostine is a phosphorothiol compound metabolized by membrane-bound alkaline phosphatase to an active sulfhydryl form capable of binding electrophilic metabolites from DNA-binding anticancer agents or ionizing radiation. It is used prophylactically to block cisplatin-induced nephrotoxicity and neurotoxicity without altering antitumor efficacy in patients with advanced ovarian cancer.[221]

Administration and Adult Dosage. **IV to block cisplatin toxicity** 910 mg/m^2 in NS over ≤15 min, beginning 30 min before cisplatin.

Special Populations. *Pediatric Dosage.* Safety and efficacy not established.

Geriatric Dosage. Same as adult dosage, but limited experience exists in patients >70 yr.

Other Conditions. In patients who develop rare symptomatic acute hypocalcemia, reduce dose to 740 mg/m^2 and extend infusion time. Reduce dosage in patients who developed hypotension (drop of 15–20 mm Hg systolic) with prior courses. When used as a radioprotective agent, the maximally tolerated dosage is 340 mg/m^2 for 4 days/week.[222]

Dosage Forms. **Inj** 50 mg/mL.

Patient Instructions. The severity of chemotherapy-induced nausea and vomiting can increase with amifostine. Drink lots of fluids in the hours before receiving this medication to reduce its toxicity.

Pharmacokinetics. *Fate.* The mean peak serum level is 100 μmol/L after an IV dose of 740 mg/m^2. V_{dss} is 6.4 ± 1.5 L; Cl is 2.2 ± 0.4 L/min. Relatively little unchanged drug (1.1% of a dose), actifostine (1.4% of a dose), or disulfide metabolite (4.2% of a dose) is excreted renally.[223]

$t_{1/2}$. α phase 0.88 ± 0.12 min; β phase 8.8 ± 2 min.

Adverse Reactions. Toxic effects are all acute and include transient hypotension during or immediately after drug infusion; nausea; and vomiting.[224] Prophylactic antiemetics before administration can reduce nausea and vomiting. Rapid infusion (≤15 min) and aggressive hydration can lessen or eliminate hypotensive toxicity.[225] Stopping the infusion and placing the patient in the Trendelenberg position usually reverses the hypotension. Other less serious but common reactions are sneezing (27%), a flushed sensation (26%), somnolence (10–20%), a sensation of cold hands, or a metallic taste in the mouth (<5% each).

Contraindications. Allergy to aminothiol compounds or mannitol.

Precautions. Do not administer concurrently with or after cisplatin infusion. Use with caution in patients in whom hypotension or nausea might pose a serious risk. There is limited experience in patients with pre-existing cardiac or cardiovascular conditions such as CHF, angina pectoris, history of stroke, or TIAs.

Drug Interactions. Amifostine can reduce the systemic exposure to paclitaxel but not to docetaxel, cisplatin, carboplatin, or cyclophosphamide.[226]

Parameters to Monitor. Monitor blood pressure frequently during drug administration and immediately after infusion.

Notes. Amifostine has been safely combined with ionizing radiation, **carboplatin,** and **cyclophosphamide.** Amifostine markedly reduces mucositis when it is combined with carboplatin and radiotherapy in the treatment of head and neck cancer.[227] Amifostine allows dose escalation of **paclitaxel** and has hematopoietic activity in the investigational treatment of refractory myelodysplastic syndrome.

DEXRAZOXANE
Zinecard

Pharmacology. Dexrazoxane, a cardioprotectant for anthracyclines, is the water-soluble dextro isomer of razoxane. Dexrazoxane's two piperazinedione rings open to form sites that chelate intracellular ferrous ions, blocking the formation of doxorubicin-iron complexes capable of forming membrane-damaging oxygen free radicals. Dexrazoxane can extend **doxorubicin** cumulative dosage in patients with breast cancer. It also reduces the risk of short-term subclinical cardiotoxicity in pediatric sarcoma patients. It does not alter the pharmacokinetics of doxorubicin.[228-230]

Administration and Adult Dosage. IV as a cardioprotectant give in a 10:1 dexrazoxane:doxorubicin mg/m^2 ratio (eg, 500 mg/m^2 dexrazoxane:50 mg/m^2 doxorubicin). Infuse IV over 15 min, beginning not more than 30 min before an IV push dose of doxorubicin.

Special Populations. *Pediatric Dosage.* Safety and efficacy not established, but it has been used in a 20:1 dosage ratio (dexrazoxane:doxorubicin) in children with sarcomas.[230]

Geriatric Dosage. Same as adult dosage.

Dosage Forms. Inj 250, 500 mg.

Patient Instructions. (*See* Antineoplastics Class Instructions.)

Pharmacokinetics. *Fate.* The mean peak serum level after a dose of 500 mg/m^2 given over 15 min is 36.5 mg/L (136 μmol/L). The drug is not protein bound. V_d is 22 L/m^2 or approximately body water; Cl averages 7.9 L/hr/m^2. About 42% is renally eliminated as parent drug and mono- and diacid amide metabolites.[231]

$t_{1/2}$. α phase 0.2–0.3 hr; β phase 2.1–2.5 hr.[231]

Adverse Reactions. Dexrazoxane has little toxicity but slightly increases the myelosuppressive and emetogenic toxicities of doxorubicin-containing regimens. Pain on injection also occurs.

Contraindications. None known.

Precautions. Avoid use with bleomycin. Do not administer *after* doxorubicin.

Drug Interactions. None known.

Parameters to Monitor. WBC counts at nadir (7–11 days) after doxorubicin.

Notes. Dexrazoxane does not reduce the antitumor activity of fluorouracil, doxorubicin, and cyclophosphamide regimens in advanced breast cancer.[228] Effects on other antineoplastics are unknown.

MESNA
Mesnex

Pharmacology. Mesna (2-mercaptoethanesulfonate) is a sulfhydryl compound that minimizes urotoxicity from the alkylating agents cyclophosphamide (CTX) and ifosfamide (IFX) by binding to the irritant metabolite acrolein in the urinary bladder to prevent hemorrhagic cystitis.[35,232]

Administration and Adult Dosage. IV or PO (ampule contents dissolved in water or juice) in 3 doses as a percentage of the dose of ifosfamide or cyclophosphamide. Oral administration is not recommended for patients with poor compliance or those experiencing nausea or vomiting.

TIME BEFORE OR AFTER CTX OR IFX	PERCENTAGE OF CTX OR IFX DOSE[233]	
	IV MESNA ROUTE	PO MESNA ROUTE
15 min before	20	Not recommended
4 hr after	20	40
8 hr after	20	40

CTX = cyclophosphamide; IFX = ifosfamide.

Special Populations. *Pediatric Dosage.* Same as adult dosage.[42,234]

Geriatric Dosage. Same as adult dosage.

Dosage Forms. **Inj** 100 mg/mL.

Patient Instructions. This agent does not have antitumor activity but is essential to reduce or prevent permanent bladder damage from chemotherapy.

Pharmacokinetics. *Fate.* About 48% is orally absorbed.[235] V_d is 0.65 L/kg; Cl is 1.23 L/hr/kg. Mesna is oxidized to the inactive dimer, dimesna, which does not inactivate CTX or IFX metabolites in the serum. About 60% of the dimesna is converted back to mesna in the renal tubule and delivered to the bladder in the active sulfhydryl form. About two-thirds of a dose is excreted in the urine, one-half as mesna and one-half as dimesna.[236]

$t_{1/2}$. (Mesna) 22 min; (dimesna) 1.2 hr.[236]

Adverse Reactions. When administered alone, mesna produces little if any serious toxicity.[236] GI effects (eg, diarrhea, nausea, and, rarely, vomiting) of CTX or IFX might be slightly greater when mesna is administered. Other CTX or IFX toxicities such as myelosuppression or alopecia are not altered by mesna. With oral administration, a disagreeable sulfur odor might lessen palatability unless the drug is diluted with cola or juice.

Drug Interactions. Mesna inhibits the antitumor activity of cisplatin and carboplatin but not of other anticancer agents.

Notes. Mesna is compatible with solutions of CTX or IFX and has been administered concurrently as a continuous infusion of both agents at equal doses in the same infusion container.[237] It is stable in D5W or NS for at least 96 hr.

Immunosuppressants

General Precautions for Immunosuppressants. Immunosuppression increases the risk of infectious complications. Serious opportunistic infections can occur during immunosuppressive therapy. Long-term immunosuppression also increases the risk of malignancy or lymphoproliferative disease. Vaccinations might be less effective during immunosuppression. Live or live attenuated vaccines might proliferate excessively in immunosuppressed patients and should be avoided.

ANTILYMPHOCYTE IMMUNE GLOBULINS:

ANTITHYMOCYTE GLOBULIN (RABBIT)	Thymoglobulin
LYMPHOCYTE IMMUNE GLOBULIN (EQUINE)	Atgam

Pharmacology. Antilymphocyte immune globulins are polyclonal IgG purified from sera of horses or rabbits immunized with human thymus lymphocytes. These drugs are immunosuppressants that inhibit cell-mediated immunity. The immunosuppressive effects of antilymphocyte immune globulins may be secondary to clearance of alloreactive T-lymphocytes from the plasma. However, the exact pharmacologic mechanism of action has not been elucidated.

Administration and Adult Dosage. Antilymphocyte immune globulins are generally used in conjunction with other immunosuppressants. **Intradermal sensitivity testing** to identify patients at risk for anaphylaxis is *strongly* recommended before administration of equine lymphocyte immune globulin. Freshly diluted equine lymphocyte immune globulin (5 μg in 0.1 mL 0.9% NaCl) should be administered intradermally on the anterior aspect of one forearm, with intradermal administration of 0.9% NaCl 0.1 mL on the contralateral forearm as a control. During the hour after administration, the skin test should be observed q 15–20 min for swelling, urticaria, pruritus, and wheel or erythema. A positive skin test is defined as local wheel or erythema formation ≥10 mm in diameter. If the skin test is positive, the risk of serious hypersensitivity or anaphylaxis from drug administration should be weighed carefully against the anticipated benefits of drug administration. A systemic reaction to the skin test generally precludes further administration of equine lymphocyte immune globulin. Administration of equine lymphocyte immune globulin to patients after a positive skin test or systemic reaction to the skin test should be done only in a facility capable of supporting life-threatening allergic reactions. The skin test is not 100% predictive of subsequent hypersensitivity reactions. Allergic reactions and anaphylaxis to equine lymphocyte immune globulin have been reported after a negative skin test. The manufacturer does not recommend a test dose before administration of rabbit antithymocyte globulin.

IV for prevention of renal allograft rejection (equine lymphocyte immune globulin) 15 mg/kg/day for 14 doses, followed by the same dose every other day for an additional 14 days. This regimen administers up to 21 doses of equine lymphocyte immune globulin in 28 days. The first dose of equine lymphocyte immune globulin should be administered within 24 hr before or after surgery; (rabbit antithymocyte globulin) 1.5 mg/kg/day beginning on the day of surgery, for a total of at least 7 doses, has been used for prevention of renal allograft rejection.[238] **IV for treatment of renal allograft rejection** (equine lymphocyte immune globulin) same dosage regimen as above, with administration of the first dose at the diagnosis of the initial rejection episode; (rabbit antithymocyte globulin) 1.5 mg/kg/day for 7–14 days. **IV for prevention of rejection after heart transplantation** (rabbit antithymocyte globulin) 4 mg/kg/day administered as an IV infusion over 6 hr on postoperative days 1–5.[239] **IM for prevention of rejection after heart transplantation** (rabbit antithymocyte globulin) 1.5 mg/kg/day or 200 mg/day for

3–7 days has been administered.[240] **IV for treatment of aplastic anemia** (equine lymphocyte immune globulin) 10–30 mg/kg/day for 8-14 days, followed by the same dose every other day for 14 days, has been used. This regimen administers up to 21 doses of equine lymphocyte immune globulin in 28 days. An alternative regimen uses 40 mg/kg q 24–48 hr for 3–4 doses; (rabbit antithymocyte globulin) 3.5 mg/kg/day for 5 days has been administered with cyclosporine and filgrastim for treatment of severe aplastic anemia unresponsive to equine lymphocyte immune globulin.[241] **IV for prevention of acute graft-versus-host disease (GVHD) in allogeneic bone marrow transplant recipients** (equine lymphocyte immune globulin) 7–10 mg/kg every other day for 6 doses; (rabbit antithymocyte globulin) 2, 3.75, or 5 mg/kg/dose for 4–5 doses before unrelated bone marrow transplantation.[242] **IV for treatment of moderate-to-severe steroid-refractory acute GVHD** (equine lymphocyte immune globulin) 7–15 mg/kg for 6 doses or as indicated by the patient's clinical status. **IV for skin allograft survival in patients with full-thickness burns** (equine lymphocyte immune globulin) 10–15 mg/kg every other day is generally used; however, doses of 5 mg/kg every other day up to 40 mg/kg/day have been given. The duration of therapy is generally 40–60 days, ending when skin allografts cover <20% of the BSA. **The maximum tolerated cumulative dosage** of antilymphocyte polyclonal immune globulins has not been determined. A total of 50 doses of equine lymphocyte immune globulin has been administered over 4 months, and four 28-day courses of 28 equine lymphocyte immune globulin doses have been administered in renal allograft recipients without changing the frequency, severity, or character of adverse drug reactions. **Intravenous administration** (equine lymphocyte immune globulin) dilute in 0.45% or 0.9% NaCl to a final concentration ≤4 mg/mL and infuse slowly over 4–8 hr; (rabbit antithymocyte globulin) after reconstitution with the diluent provided, dilute to a final concentration of 0.5 mg/mL in 0.9% NaCl or 5% dextrose injection. Infuse the first dose at 0.25 mg/kg/hr (1.5 mg/kg/6 hr). In the absence of moderate-to-severe adverse effects, infuse subsequent doses over 4 hr. Antilymphocyte polyclonal immune globulins should be infused through an inline filter with pore sizes of 0.22–1 μ. Premedication and as-needed administration of a corticosteroid, acetaminophen, and an antihistamine are common practice intended to reduce infusion-related adverse effects.

Special Populations. *Pediatric Dosage.* Same as adult dosage.

Geriatric Dosing. Same as adult dosage.

Dosage Forms. Inj (equine lymphocyte immune globulin) 50 mg/mL; (rabbit antithymocyte globulin) 25 mg.

Patient Instructions. (Equine lymphocyte immune globulin) This medicine can cause serious allergic symptoms, especially in people allergic to horses and horse products. You will receive a skin test to check for allergy to this product. (Rabbit antithymocyte globulin, equine lymphocyte immune globulin) You might experience fever, shaking, and chills when this medication is being given. You may be given additional medications to reduce these side effects.

Pharmacokinetics. *Fate.* (Equine lymphocyte immune globulin) Peak concentrations of 727 μg/L occur with repeated doses of 10 mg/kg. Systemic distribution of equine immune globulin is not well defined. In vitro studies predict binding to circulating lymphocytes, granulocytes, and platelets. Binding to bone marrow cells, plus thymus and testis cell membranes, occurs in vitro. (Rabbit antithymocyte globulin) IV infusion of 1.25–1.5 mg/kg/day yields a peak concentration of 10–40 μg/L after the first dose and 23–170 μg/L after repeated doses. V_d is 0.12 L/kg.[243]

$t_{1/2}$. (Equine lymphocyte immune globulin) 3–9 days; (rabbit antithymocyte globulin) 14–45 days.[243]

Adverse Reactions. Anaphylaxis can occur anytime during therapy. If signs or symptoms of anaphylaxis occur, the infusion must be stopped immediately and appropriate management must be initiated. Serum sickness occurs frequently. The onset of serum sickness is typically 6–18 days after initiation of therapy with antilymphocyte immune globulins. A morbilliform rash generally starts as a truncal distribution of faint macules, with subsequent progression to the extremities. The macules can become confluent. Erythema can spread to involve palms of the hands and soles of the feet. Antihistamines are helpful for pruritus-associated serum sickness. Although not clearly shown to reduce serum sickness-related adverse effects, corticosteroids have been used. Antilymphocyte immune globulins might bind formed elements in the blood other than T-lymphocytes and promote splenic clearance of these blood constituents. Subsequently, patients might experience acute normochromic normocytic anemia, thrombocytopenia, or leukopenia during administration of antilymphocyte immune globulins that is reversible with drug discontinuation. Immunosuppression increases the risk of infectious complications from opportunistic and pathogenic microbes. Rare adverse effects reported with antilymphocyte immune globulins include Epstein-Barr virus infections, lymphoproliferative disorders and (equine lymphocyte immune globulin) periorbital edema, seizures, acute renal failure, headache, hypertension, edema, CHF, bradycardia, adult respiratory distress syndrome, myocarditis, pancytopenia, LFT abnormalities, hyperglycemia, and transient myopia; (rabbit antithymocyte globulin) tachycardia, dyspnea, and dizziness.[244–247]

Contraindications. (Equine lymphocyte immune globulin) allergy to equine lymphocyte immune globulin, horse serum, or horse products; (rabbit antithymocyte globulin) hypersensitivity or anaphylaxis to rabbit proteins; acute viral illness.

Precautions. Pregnancy; lactation.

Drug Interactions. None identified.

Parameters to Monitor. Observe for anaphylaxis during infusion and serum sickness 6–18 days after initiation of therapy. CBC and platelet count q 1–3 days during therapy.

Notes. Equine lymphocyte immune globulin is also known as ATG, antithymocyte globulin, antithymocyte gamma globulin, antithymocyte immunoglobulin, and horse antihuman thymocyte gamma globulin. Rabbit antithymocyte globulin is also known as r-ATG or RATG. Lot-to-lot variation of immunosuppressive potency and avidity for formed blood elements can occur with these products.

AZATHIOPRINE
Imuran

Pharmacology. Azathioprine is a thiopurine prodrug of 6-mercaptopurine (6-MP). Conversion to 6-MP with subsequent phosphoribosylation yields antimetabolites capable of inhibiting DNA and RNA synthesis. The metabolite 6-methylmercaptopurine ribotide is a potent inhibitor of de novo purine synthesis. T-lymphocytes are sensitive to inhibition of de novo purine synthesis because these cells lack efficient salvage pathways to maintain adequate intracellular stores.

Administration and Adult Dosage. **PO or IV for immunosuppression after solid organ transplantation** 3–5 mg/kg/day as a single daily dose beginning the day of, or 1–3 days preceding, transplantation. **Maintenance dosage** is 1–3 mg/kg/day as a single daily dose. **PO for rheumatoid arthritis** 1 mg/kg/day in 1 or 2 doses. The dosage may be increased after 6–8 weeks if indicated by disease response and patient tolerance. Increase the dosage in increments of 0.5 mg/kg/day q 4 weeks to a maximum of 2.5 mg/kg day. (*See* Drug Interactions.)

Special Populations. *Pediatric Dosage.* **PO or IV for immunosuppression after renal transplantation** same as adult dosage.

Geriatric Dosage. Same as adult dosage.

Dosage Forms. **Tab** 50 mg; **Inj** 100 mg.

Patient Instructions. This medication may be taken with food to reduce stomach upset. Notify your physician if any of the following symptoms occur: unusual bleeding or bruising, fever, sore throat, mouth sores, abdominal pain, yellowing of the eyes, pale stools, or dark urine, or if nausea, vomiting, diarrhea, skin rash, or joint pains become severe or persist.

Missed Doses. Take a missed dose as soon as possible. If you take the drug once daily and it is time for the next dose, take it at the regular time. Do not double the dose. If you take two or more doses daily, and it is time for the next dose, take both doses together. If two or more doses are missed, contact your physician.

Pharmacokinetics. *Onset and Duration.* Onset of immunosuppression occurs within days to weeks. Immunosuppression continues for days to weeks after drug discontinuation.

Serum Levels. No correlation between serum concentrations and efficacy or toxicity has been defined.

Fate. After oral absorption, conversion to 6-MP occurs rapidly.[1] (*See* Mercaptopurine.)

$t_{1/2}$. (Azathioprine) 9.6 ± 4.2 min; (6-MP) 0.9 ± 0.37 hr.[1,10]

Adverse Reactions. Dose-related bone marrow suppression, which can include leukopenia, thrombocytopenia, and anemia, occurs frequently. Macrocytic anemia, with megaloblastic features, or selective erythrocyte aplasia can occur with long-term azathioprine administration. Skin rash is a common adverse effect. Mouth sores can occur. Dose-related nausea and vomiting are frequent and can be reduced by administration in divided doses. Rare GI hypersensitivity characterized by severe nausea and vomiting, diarrhea, hyperpyrexia, malaise, myalgia, and

LFT abnormalities can occur early in the course of therapy. GI hypersensitivity is reversible with discontinuation of azathioprine and can recur with rechallenge. Hepatic veno-occlusive disease of the liver, secondary lymphomas, and other malignancies can occur with long-term administration. Azathioprine is teratogenic. Rare adverse effects include pancreatitis, constrictive lung disease, renal failure, alopecia, arthralgia, and retinopathy.

Contraindications. Pregnancy in patients treated for rheumatoid arthritis.

Precautions. Pregnancy; lactation. (*See also* General Precautions for Immunosuppressants.)

Drug Interactions. To reduce the risk of life-threatening myelosuppression, azathioprine dosage must be reduced to 25–33% of the normal dosage in patients receiving allopurinol. Enhanced bone marrow suppression can occur with concurrent use of drugs that inhibit hematopoiesis. Concurrent corticosteroids used for immunosuppression can mask fever.

Parameters to Monitor. Monitor CBC and platelet count weekly for 1 month after initiation of therapy or any dosage increase. Then, for patients with stable hemograms, the CBC and platelet count may be monitored twice monthly for 2 months and then monthly for the duration of therapy. Monitor serum transaminases, alkaline phosphatase, and total bilirubin periodically. Observe for signs of infection.

Notes. Azathioprine is used in combination with other immunosuppressants as an adjunct in the prevention of renal allograft rejection and for the prevention of solid organ rejection for cardiac and hepatic allografts. It is rarely used for the management of acute or chronic GVHD in allogeneic bone marrow transplant recipients because it markedly increases the risk for infections.[248]

CYCLOSPORINE   Gengraf, Neoral, Sandimmune, SangCya, Various

Pharmacology. Cyclosporine is a cyclic polypeptide immunosuppressant produced by the fungus *Tolypocladium inflatum Gams*. The intracellular drug-ligand complex formed by cyclosporine and cyclophilin indirectly blocks T-lymphocyte activation by inhibiting calcineurin-mediated dephosphorylation of transcription factors necessary for IL-2 transcription.

Administration and Adult Dosage. **PO for prophylaxis of organ rejection or GVHD** 8–12 mg/kg/day in 2 divided doses depending on the type of transplant and the other immunosuppressants being given. To hasten achievement of an immunosuppressant blood level, **an oral loading dose** of cyclosporine 15 mg/kg may be administered. Cyclosporine is usually started 4–12 hr before surgery. **Maintenance dosage** is based on cyclosporine blood levels, the risk of organ rejection or GVHD, and patient tolerance. **PO for rheumatoid arthritis** 2.5 mg/kg/day in divided doses bid. As patient tolerance allows, dosage may be increased by 0.5–0.75 mg/kg/day at 8 weeks and again at 12 weeks, to a maximum of 4 mg/kg/day. **PO for psoriasis** 2.5 mg/kg/day in divided doses bid. After 4 weeks of therapy, as patient tolerance allows, the dosage may be increased by 0.5–0.75 mg/kg/day q 2 weeks, to a maximum of 4 mg/kg/day. **An IV loading dose** of 3–4 mg/kg might be useful in patients with low cyclosporine levels during periods of mild-to-moderate diarrhea with oral maintenance therapy. **IV for patients unable to take oral medication** 2–6 mg/kg/day in 1–2 divided doses. **IV for prevention of GVHD** 3–4 mg/kg/day in 2 divided doses q 12 hr. Cyclosporine is generally started 1–2 days before bone marrow transplantation. Drug-induced mucositis or diarrhea usually necessitate use of IV cyclosporine in allogeneic bone marrow transplant recipients. Dilute IV cyclosporine in a glass container (it might leach plasticizers from PVC containers) with D5W or NS to a concentration of 50 mg/20–100 mL. Doses may be infused over 2–6 hr or given as a continuous infusion. **Conversion from IV to PO administration** the ratio of IV:PO dosage is typically 1:3 to 1:4 for Sandimmune capsules or 1:1 to 1:3 for microemulsion capsules or solution (Gengraf, Neoral, SangCya, various). **Conversion from PO Sandimmune to microemulsion capsules or solution** (Gengraf, Neoral, SangCya, various) give the same daily dosage or reduce microemulsion dose by 30% with prompt dosage adjustment based on subsequent blood levels. A cyclosporine blood level should be drawn 48 hr after dosage form conversion. Because of better bioavailability, maintenance dosages of the microemulsion formulation are usually lower than Sandimmune dosages. **Interchange of various microemulsion capsules or solutions** (Gengraf, Neoral, SangCya, various) give the same daily dosage with prompt dosage adjustment based on subsequent blood levels. A cyclosporine blood level should be drawn 48 hr after interchange. **Discontinuation** cyclosporine may eventually be discontinued in certain renal or allogeneic bone marrow transplant recipients. Cyclosporine dosage must be decreased gradually over time to reduce the risk of reactive immune stimulation and graft rejection or GVHD.

Special Populations. *Pediatric Dosage.* Initial dosage same as adult dose. Adjustment based on blood levels. Children may require higher weight-based maintenance dose.

Geriatric Dosage. Same as adult dosage. Age-related loss of renal function and co-morbid conditions can predispose geriatric patients to cyclosporine-induced nephrotoxicity or hypertension.

Other Conditions. Use IBW to calculate initial dosage in obese patients.

Dosage Forms. **Cap** (Neoral, various) 25, 100 mg; (Sandimmune) 25, 50, 100 mg; **Oral Soln** 100 mg/mL; **Inj** (Sandimmune) 50 mg/mL.

Patient Instructions. Take this medication on a regular schedule relative to the time of day and meals. Do not discontinue it unless directed to do so. Sandimmune cannot be interchanged with any other brands. The oral solution may taste better if mixed with another liquid. Sandimmune may be mixed with milk, chocolate milk, or orange juice. Neoral may be mixed with orange juice or apple juice. Using a glass container, mix the cyclosporine solution with the milk or juice, stir well, and drink immediately to ensure that the entire cyclosporine dose is swallowed. Do *not* refrigerate the oral solution. Use the oral solution within 2 months after opening. Grapefruit juice can interact with cyclosporine. Talk to the physician or coordinator who monitors your cyclosporine before drinking grapefruit juice and before starting, stopping, or changing the dose of any medication.

Missed Doses. Take a missed dose as soon as possible if you remember within 12 hours. If it is within 2 hours of the next dose, skip the missed dose and do not double the dose. If you miss 2 or more doses, contact the physician or coordinator who monitors your cyclosporine.

Pharmacokinetics. *Serum Levels.* The serum (blood) concentration–response relationship is not completely defined. Trough blood or serum levels are monitored for toxicity. Therapeutic and toxic concentrations vary with assay, biologic fluid, and time post-transplant. Therapeutic serum concentrations are: polyclonal radioimmunoassay (RIA) 100–250 μg/L; monoclonal RIA 50–125 μg/L; high-performance liquid chromatography (HPLC) 50–125 μg/L. Therapeutic whole blood concentrations are: polyclonal RIA 200–800 μg/L; monoclonal RIA 150–400 μg/L; HPLC 150–400 μg/L.[249] In routine clinical practice, spurious serum drug levels can result from in vitro drug redistribution. Artifactual serum or whole blood levels can occur when blood is drawn through the same central venous line used for IV cyclosporine administration.[250]

Fate. Oral absorption is formulation dependent (*See* Notes). Sandimmune absorption is incomplete and variable. The mean bioavailability of Sandimmune is 34%; however, the reported range is 5–90%. Absorption of Sandimmune is improved after a high-fat meal. Peak concentrations occur 2–6 hr after ingestion of Sandimmune capsules or oral solution. Absorption of cyclosporine microemulsion formulations is independent of food intake; peak concentrations occur 1.5–2 hr after ingestion of microemulsion capsules or solution. Factors that can decrease cyclosporine absorption are diarrhea, gastroenteritis, and short small bowel. Absorption may be reduced in allogeneic bone marrow transplant patients because of residual gut damage from intensive chemotherapy, radiation, or GVHD. Bioavailability of AB therapeutic equivalent cyclosporine capsules and liquid can vary by 20–30% for a particular patient or when mixed with various juices. Systemic cyclosporine distributes to erythrocytes (45%), leukocytes (15%), and plasma lipoproteins (35%). Marked elevations of plasma lipoproteins can increase measured cyclosporine levels without proportional changes in therapeutic or toxic effects. V_{dss} (whole blood, HPLC) is 4 ± 0.8 L/kg in renal transplant patients and 5.3 ± 2.9 L/kg in bone marrow transplant patients. Cl (whole blood, HPLC) is 0.4 ± 0.2 L/kg/hr in renal or liver transplant patients and 0.6 ± 0.4 L/kg/hr in allogeneic bone marrow transplant recipients. Cyclosporine is extensively metabolized by CYP3A. At least 25 metabolites, some with immunosuppressant activity, have been identified. Cyclosporine and its metabolites are cleared primarily in the bile. About 3% is excreted in the urine as cyclosporine and metabolites. Less than 1% is excreted in the urine as unchanged cyclosporine.[249]

$t_{1/2}$. (Whole blood, HPLC) 10 ± 3.5 hr, possibly prolonged in hepatic failure.

Adverse Reactions. Acute nephrotoxicity, which generally occurs during the first month of treatment, is characterized by Cr_s increasing by ≥ 0.3 mg/dL/24 hr or $\geq 30\%/24$ hr and usually abates with interruption of drug therapy. Dosage reduction may be required for continuation of therapy. Chronic progressive renal toxicity is characterized by a slow continual increase in Cr_s and BUN, mild proteinuria, and tubular dysfunction. $Cr_s > 2$ mg/dL in adult patients or doubling of Cr_s is an indication for interruption of therapy or dosage reduction. Electrolyte abnormalities, including hypomagnesemia, hypokalemia, hyperkalemia, and renal tubular acidosis, are consequences of cyclosporine-induced nephrotoxicity. Concurrent administration of nephrotoxic drugs increases the likelihood of renal dysfunction. Hypertension occurs frequently. **Calcium channel blockers** and **clonidine** are suitable agents for cyclosporine-induced hypertension because they do not have deleterious effects on renal blood flow. Fine tremors occur frequently and can persist and worsen after drug discontinuation. Neurotoxicity can also present as seizures, cortical blindness, paresthesias, hyperesthesia, headache, or expressive aphasia. Patients with low serum cholesterol may be at increased risk of neurotoxicity. Anaphylactic reactions to cyclosporine or the solubilizing agent, polyoxyethylated castor oil, can occur. Ethanol is a minor constituent in the intravenous and oral formulations. Cyclosporine-induced cholestasis is dose related and transient. Elevated serum transaminases and hypertriglyceridemia can occur. Additional side effects are hemolytic uremic syndrome, pancreatitis, hirsutism, gingival hyperplasia, nausea, vomiting, acne, and gynecomastia. Leukopenia, anemia, and thrombocytopenia occur rarely.

Contraindications. Allergy to cyclosporine or polyoxyethylated castor oil.

Precautions. Pregnancy; lactation. Use cautiously in patients with aldehyde dehydrogenase 2 (ALDH2) deficiency. (*See also* General Precautions for Immunosuppressants.)

Drug Interactions. Numerous important drug interactions have been identified. Additive or synergistic renal toxicity can occur with concomitant administration of nephrotoxic drugs. Sirolimus can potentiate cyclosporine nephrotoxicity. Potassium-sparing diuretics can exacerbate hyperkalemia. Concurrent use of the following drugs frequently increases cyclosporine blood levels: corticosteroids, erythromycin and macrolide antibiotics, itraconazole, and ketoconazole. Other drugs that can increase cyclosporine blood levels are acetazolamide, alcohol, allopurinol, calcium-channel blockers, cimetidine, colchicine, oral contraceptives, fluconazole, imipenem/cilastatin, metoclopramide, norfloxacin, and sulindac. Enzyme-inducing drugs such as carbamazepine, phenobarbital, phenytoin and rifampin reduce cyclosporine blood levels. Octreotide can decrease cyclosporine oral absorption. Additional drugs that can reduce cyclosporine blood levels are cotrimoxazole, nafcillin, and sulfonamides. Cyclosporine reduces the clearance of HMG-CoA reductase inhibitors, such as lovastatin and atorvastatin, and increases the risk of drug-induced rhabdomyolysis.

Parameters to Monitor. Observe for anaphylaxis with IV administration. Monitor Cr_s q 2–7 days and daily in patients at risk of acute renal dysfunction. Monitor blood pressure regularly. Monitor LFTs weekly, triglycerides and amylase monthly. Monitor blood or serum cyclosporine concentrations q 2–3 days when starting therapy. As the patient's clinical condition and renal function allow, reduce frequency to once or twice weekly and then monthly during the first year of therapy. After the first year of therapy, blood or serum concentration monitoring may be reduced to q 1–2 months in stable patients. Monitor for signs and symptoms of graft rejection or GVHD, especially after dosage reduction.

Notes. Assignment of AB therapeutic equivalency by the FDA requires bioequivalence testing in normal healthy volunteers. Absorption of bioequivalent products can vary in bone marrow or solid organ transplant patients with compromised gut function. Bioequivalence to Neoral in transplant patients has been established for microemulsion Gengraf capsules and SangCya solution.

Cyclosporine is generally used in combination with other immunosuppressant drugs for prevention of graft rejection or GVHD. Cyclosporine is used in the management of various immunologic diseases such as aplastic anemia, psoriasis, atopic dermatitis, acute ocular Behçet's syndrome, endogenous uveitis, primary biliary cirrhosis, and acute Crohn's disease. High-dose cyclosporine is administered with certain chemotherapy regimens as a modulator of P-glycoprotein-mediated drug resistance.[251] Optimmune (cyclosporine) ophthalmic (University of Georgia College of Veterinary Medicine) has orphan drug status for treatment of severe keratoconjunctivitis sicca with Sjögren's syndrome. Sandimmune 2% ophthalmic ointment (Allergan) has orphan drug status for patients at high risk for graft rejection after penetrating keratoplasty and for treatment of corneal melting syndrome.

Comparative trials found greater nephrotoxicity and neurotoxicity with tacrolimus than with cyclosporine.[252] Case reports describe resolution of certain drug-induced toxicities after replacement of cyclosporine with **tacrolimus** and resolution of cyclosporine-refractory GVHD with initiation of tacrolimus.[253,254]

INTERLEUKIN-2 RECEPTOR ANTAGONISTS:

BASILIXIMAB	Simulect
DACLIZUMAB	Zenapax

Pharmacology. Basiliximab and daclizumab (formerly dacliximab) are immunosuppressive, humanized, recombinant IgG1 monoclonal antibodies that bind specifically to the alpha subunit (p55 alpha, CD25, or Tac subunit) of the human high-affinity IL-2 receptor present on the surface of activated lymphocytes. They act as IL-2 receptor antagonists by preventing IL-2 from binding to lymphocytes, subsequently reducing IL-2–mediated immune activation. Both drugs are indicated for prevention of renal allograft rejection in a regimen that includes cyclosporine and a corticosteroid.

Administration and Adult Dosage. IV for prevention of renal allograft rejection (basiliximab) 20 mg infused over 30 min for 2 doses. The initial dose should be given about 2 hr before transplantation, the second dose is given 4 days after the transplant. Withhold the second dose if severe hypersensitivity or graft loss occurs. (Daclizumab) 1 mg/kg for 5 doses at 14-day intervals. The initial dose should be infused within 24 hr preceding surgery. The remaining 4 doses should be administered at 14-day intervals after surgery. Dilute each dose in 50 mL NS and infuse over 15 min through a peripheral or central venous line. **IV for treatment of steroid-refractory GVHD** (daclizumab) 1 mg/kg on days 1, 4, 8, 15, and 22, with day 1 representing the 1st day of daclizumab therapy; or 1.5 mg/kg, with repeated administration in 11–48 days for patients with transient improvement.[255,256]

Special Populations. *Pediatric Dosage.* (Basiliximab) 12 mg/m^2 to a maximum of 20 mg/dose, given as adult dosage above. (Daclizumab) same as adult dosage. Information about use in pediatric patients is limited.

Geriatric Dosage. Same as adult dosage. Information about use in patients >65 yr is limited.

Other Conditions. No dosage adjustment is necessary for patients with severe renal dysfunction.

Dosage Forms. **Inj** (basiliximab) 20 mg; (daclizumab) 5 mg/mL.

Patient Instructions. This drug is being used as part of combination therapy to prevent rejection of your transplanted kidney.

Pharmacokinetics. *Onset and Duration.* (Basiliximab) receptor saturation is maintained for 36 ± 14 days with the recommended regimen. (Daclizumab) receptor saturation is maintained for about 120 days with the recommended regimen.

Serum Levels. (Basiliximab) >200 µg/L maintains complete binding to IL-2 receptor and maintains effective T-lymphocyte suppression. (Daclizumab) 5–10 mg/L inhibits activated T-lymphocytes.

Fate. (Basiliximab) peak serum levels of 9.3 ± 4.5 mg/L are attained with the recommended dosage regimen. (Daclizumab) after the first dose of 1 mg/kg, a peak of 21 ± 14 mg/L occurs, and after the 5th dose, a peak of 32 ± 22 mg/L results. The trough is 7.6 ± 4 mg/L after repeated doses of 1 mg/kg in adult renal transplant recipients.

t½. (Basiliximab) about 14 days; (daclizumab) 11–38 days.

Adverse Reactions. Both drugs usually are well tolerated. The frequency and type of adverse events were similar between renal transplant patients receiving these drugs or placebo, along with a corticosteroid and cyclosporine.[257,258] Cases of severe acute hypersensitivity reactions have occurred with basiliximab, usually within 24 hr of a dose. Discontinue the drug permanently if this occurs. Hypertension and dehydration with daclizumab might be more frequent in children than in adults.

Precautions. Pregnancy; lactation. Use basiliximab with extreme caution in patients who have had previous courses of therapy. (*See also* General Precautions for Immunosuppressants.)

Drug Interactions. None known.

Parameters to Monitor. Monitor signs and symptoms of infection and graft rejection periodically.

Notes. After preparation, these drugs should be used within 4 hr if stored at room temperature or 24 hr if refrigerated. Although basiliximab and daclizumab have not been directly compared, their efficacies seem to be similar.

MUROMONAB-CD3	Orthoclone OKT3

Pharmacology. Muromonab-CD3 is a murine monoclonal antibody that recognizes the zeta chain of the CD3 protein complex associated with the T-cell receptor (TCR). CD3 protein complex is an integral component of TCR signal transduction. Muromonab-CD3 binding to CD3 blocks allograft rejection by inhibition of T-lymphocyte function. Muromonab-CD3 is used to treat acute renal allograft rejection or steroid-resistant heart or liver allograft rejection.

Administration and Adult Dosage. **IV for the treatment of allograft rejection** 5 mg/day as an IV push for 10–14 days. Administration of methylprednisolone 8 mg/kg IV 1–4 hr before muromonab is strongly recommended by the manufacturer to reduce the frequency and severity of reactions with the first dose. Acetaminophen and diphenhydramine also are often used to control symptoms. The manufacturer recommends that the patient's temperature be <37.8°C (<100°F) before infusion of muromonab-CD3.

Special Populations. *Pediatric Dosage.* Safety and efficacy are not established, but children have received dosages of ≤5 mg/day.

Geriatric Dosage. Same as adult dosage.

Dosage Forms. **Inj** 1 mg/mL.

Patient Instructions. This medication can cause shortness of breath, fever, and chills during the initial days of treatment.

Pharmacokinetics. *Serum Levels.* Levels ≥0.8 mg/L block cytotoxic T-lymphocyte function in vitro and in vivo.

Adverse Reactions. Cytokine release syndrome (CRS) occurs frequently with the initial 2–3 doses; it is related to cytokine release from activated lymphocytes. CRS can present as mild flu-like symptoms or as a life-threatening, shock-like reaction. Onset of CRS is usually 30–60 min after drug administration but can be delayed for hours. CRS might last for hours. Pretreatment and symptomatic treatment (*see* Administration and Adult Dosage) can reduce the frequency and severity of reactions with the first dose. Common symptoms are fever, headache, rigors, chills, tremor, nausea, vomiting, abdominal pain, myalgia, arthralgia, and rash. CRS can include CNS and cardiovascular adverse effects. CNS side effects are headache, seizures, encephalopathy, and aseptic meningitis. Cardiovascular side effects are angina, acute MI, CHF, hypertension, hypotension, and arrhythmias. Arterial and venous thromboses of allograft and other vascular beds have occurred. Consider coadministration of prophylactic antithrombotic agents in patients with histories of thrombotic events or underlying vascular disease. Pulmonary edema occurs frequently. Additional respiratory side effects are dyspnea, bronchospasm, wheezing, tachypnea, adult respiratory distress syndrome, and respiratory arrest. Hypersensitivity, including anaphylaxis and Stevens-Johnson syndrome, has been reported. Leukopenia, thrombocytopenia, pancytopenia, and lymphopenia also have occurred. Transient elevations of Cr_s and serum transaminases can occur 1–3 days after initiation of treatment.

Contraindications. Human antimouse antibody titer ≥1:1000.

Precautions. Pregnancy; lactation. Use with caution in patients with volume overload or history of thrombotic events or vascular disease. (*See also* General Precautions for Immunosuppressants.)

Drug Interactions. Concurrent use of indomethacin has been associated with encephalopathy and other CNS side effects.

Parameters to Monitor. A chest x-ray obtained ≤24 hr before starting muromonab should be free of evidence of volume overload or heart failure. Obtain human antimouse antibody before initiating treatment. (*See* Contraindications.) Obtain Cr_s q 2 days, AST and ALT q 3 days, CBC including differential and platelet counts q 3 days. Monitor one of the following immunologic tests during therapy: serum muromonab concentrations or quantitative T-lymphocyte surface phenotyping (target: CD3+ T-lymphocytes <25 cells/μL blood).

Notes. Transfer muromonab into a syringe through a 0.2 μ low protein-binding filter. Do not dilute with IV fluids for administration. Flush IV line with NS before and after injection.

MYCOPHENOLATE MOFETIL CellCept

Pharmacology. Mycophenolate mofetil is an ester prodrug of mycophenolic acid. Mycophenolic acid, which was isolated from the mold *Penicillium glaucum,* inhibits de novo purine synthesis by potent inhibition of inosine monophosphate dehydrogenase. Lymphocyte proliferation and antibody formation are subsequently inhibited by purine deficiency because lymphocytes lack an efficient salvage pathway for biosynthesis of purine bases. Mycophenolate is used in combination with cyclosporine and corticosteroids to prevent renal allograft rejection. Mycophenolate mofetil also has been used in combination with other immunosuppressants for the prevention of heart and liver allograft rejection.[259]

Administration and Adult Dosage. **PO or IV for prophylaxis of kidney or liver transplant rejection** 1 g bid beginning within 72 hr of transplantation.[260,261] **PO or IV for prophylaxis of heart transplant rejection** 1–1.5 g bid beginning within 72 hr of transplantation. **PO or IV for treatment of acute or chronic GVHD after allogeneic bone marrow transplantation** 1 g bid as adjunctive therapy for corticosteroid-refractory GVHD or to facilitate use of reduced corticosteroid dosage.[262,263] A dosage of 3 g/day does not confer a therapeutic advantage for any condition and is associated with more adverse effects.

Special Populations. *Pediatric Dosage.* **PO for renal transplantation** 600 mg/m² bid, to a maximum of 2 g/day as the suspension. Alternatively, (1.25–1.5 m² BSA) 750 mg bid as capsules; (>1.5 m² BSA) 1 g bid as capsules or tablets.

Geriatric Dosage. Same as adult dosage.

Other Conditions. With a chronic Cl_{cr} <25 mL/min, the dosage should not exceed 1 g bid. This does not apply to the immediate post-transplant period for renal transplant patients.

Dosage Forms. **Cap** 250; **Susp** 200 mg/mL; **Tab** 500 mg; **Inj** 500 mg.

Patient Instructions. Do not stop this medication without consulting your physician.

Missed Doses. Take a missed dose as soon as possible if you remember within 12 hours. If it is within 2 hours of next dose, skip the missed dose and do not double the next dose. If you miss 2 or more doses, contact your physician.

Pharmacokinetics. *Serum Levels.* Not established; but one study found that dosage adjustment to a blood level of 2.5–4 mg/L decreased heart transplant rejection rate.[264]

Fate. Bioavailability is 94% in normal, healthy volunteers. Food decreases the peak serum concentration by 40%, but not bioavailability. Bioavailability is decreased immediately after renal transplantation. Peak serum concentrations after 1 g PO bid are 8.2 ± 4.5 mg/L during the first 40 days post-transplant and 24 ± 12 mg/L 3 months post-transplant (similar to normal volunteers). The mean time to peak is prolonged to 1.3 ± 0.8 hr during the first 40 days post-transplant compared with 0.9 ± 0.2 hr after 3 months. AUC also is reduced by 42% during the first 40 days post-transplant; AUC is increased approximately 1.5-fold in patients with severe renal impairment. Alcoholic cirrhosis appears not to affect AUC. Mycophenolic acid is 97% bound to albumin. V_d in normal healthy volunteers is 4 ± 1.2 L/kg; Cl is 0.17 ± 0.04 L/hr/kg. Mycophenolate mofetil is rapidly hydrolyzed to mycophenolic acid, which is subsequently glucuronidated to an inactive metabolite. Enterohepatic recirculation can contribute to the mycophenolic acid AUC. Less than 1% of the dose is excreted in the urine as mycophenolic acid.

$t_{1/2}$. 16.6 ± 5.8 hr.

Adverse Reactions. Hematologic adverse effects are leukopenia, anemia, thrombocytopenia, and pancytopenia. Adverse effects of mycophenolate rarely necessitate discontinuation of therapy, but the drug should be stopped temporarily if neutropenia (ANC <1300/μL) develops during therapy. GI effects, including nausea, vomiting, dyspepsia, abdominal pain, constipation, and diarrhea, occur frequently. GI side effects can be reduced by giving the drug in 3–4 divided doses.

Contraindications. Allergy to mycophenolate mofetil.

Precautions. Pregnancy; lactation. Use with caution in patients with renal dysfunction. (*See also* General Precautions for Immunosuppressants.)

Drug Interactions. Concurrent iron or aluminum- or magnesium-containing antacids reduce absorption. Cholestyramine reduces the serum concentration of mycophenolate mofetil. In vitro, salicylate increases the unbound fraction of mycophenolic acid.

Parameters to Monitor. Monitor CBC, including differential and platelet counts, weekly during the first 1–2 months of therapy, q 2 weeks during the 2–4 months of therapy, and monthly thereafter. Monitor for signs and symptoms of infection, graft rejection, and GVHD.

Notes. Mycophenolate mofetil has been used in the treatment of certain dermatologic and immunologic disorders such as atopic dermatitis, inflammatory bowel disease, lupus nephritis, myasthenia gravis, pemphigus, psoriasis, rheumatoid arthritis, Takayasu's arteritis, uveitis, and Wegener's granulomatosis.

SIROLIMUS   Rapamune

Pharmacology. Sirolimus is a macrocyclic lactone immunosuppressant isolated from *Streptmyces hygroscopicus* that is structurally related to tacrolimus. It binds FK binding protein-12 (FKBP-12) and inhibits the cytosolic enzyme target of rapamycin (TOR). Inhibition of TOR restricts differentiation and proliferation of T-lymphocytes and B-lymphocytes subsequent to cytokine stimulation.

Administration and Adult Dosage. **PO for prevention of renal allograft rejection** ($\geq$40 kg) 6 mg on first day of therapy, followed by 2 mg daily. Dilute in glass or plastic container with at least 60 mL of water or orange juice. Mix thoroughly and administer immediately. Then fill container with at least 120 mL of liquid, stir vigorously, and administer immediately. Administer with or without food and consistently with respect to meals, oral cyclosporine, and substrates of CYP3A4 or P-glycoprotein.

Special Populations. *Pediatric Dosage.* **PO for prevention of renal allograft rejection** 3 mg/m^2 on first day of therapy, followed by 1 mg/m^2 daily.

Geriatric Dosage. Same as adult dosage.

Other Conditions. For adults <40 kg, same as pediatric dosage. In hepatic failure, reduce maintenance dosage by approximately one-third. In renal dysfunction, no dosage adjustment is necessary.

Dosage Forms. **Soln** 1 mg/mL; **Tab** 1 mg.

Patient Instructions. Take this medication on a regular schedule relative to the time of day and meals. Do not discontinue it unless directed to do so. If your sirolimus is in a bottle, use the amber syringe provided by the manufacturer to measure and take each dose out of the container. If your sirolimus is in a packet, squeeze contents to the lower part of the pouch and cut it across the top. Dilute sirolimus in a glass or plastic container with at least 2 fluid ounces of water or orange juice. Mix thoroughly and swallow immediately. Then fill container with at least 4 fluid ounces of water or orange juice, stir vigorously, and swallow immediately. Take each dose with or without food but consistently with respect to meals and medications. Refrigerate. Discard bottle 1 month after opening.

Missed Doses. Take a missed dose as soon as possible if you remember within 16 hours. If it is within 8 hours of the next dose, skip the missed dose and do not double the missed dose. If you miss 2 or more doses, contact the physician or coordinator who monitors your sirolimus.

Pharmacokinetics. *Serum Levels.* Relationship between whole blood levels and therapeutic or toxic effects is not well defined. Whole blood levels are not monitored routinely, although they may be monitored in pediatric patients or patients with markedly impaired hepatic function. Approximate whole blood trough levels (immunoassay) are 9 μg/L and 17 μg/L in patients receiving sirolimus 2 mg/day and 5 mg/day, respectively. The 24 hr post-dose whole blood concentration correlates with AUC. Marked interpatient variability of whole blood levels occurs.

Fate. Oral bioavailability is 14%. Time-to-peak whole blood concentration is 1–2 hr; it is delayed and AUC is increased by 35% when sirolimus is taken after a high-fat meal. P-glycoprotein–mediated countertransport affects absorption. The drug is extensively protein bound in plasma, primarily to albumin, α_1-acid glycoprotein, and lipoproteins. There is extensive sequestration in erythrocytes, with a whole blood:plasma ratio of 36:1. V_{dss} is 12 ± 7.5 L/kg. Sirolimus is a CYP3A4 substrate. After administration of radiolabeled drug, 2% is recovered in the urine and 91% is recovered in the bile.

$t_{1/2}$. 62 ± 16 hr.

Adverse Reactions. Phase I studies of sirolimus included concurrent administration of other immunosuppressants, including corticosteroids, and cyclosporine or tacrolimus. Subsequently, many reported side effects may not be directly attributable to sirolimus. Adverse effects related to use of sirolimus include hypercholesterolemia, hypertriglyceridemia, hypertension, anemia, thrombocytopenia, leukopenia, diarrhea, hypokalemia, arthralgia, rash, and acne. Thrombocytopenia and lipid abnormalities are dose related. Thrombocytopenia generally resolves after drug discontinuation. Additional adverse effects reported in patients taking sirolimus in combination with other immunosuppressants are nausea, emesis, dyspepsia, abdominal pain, diarrhea, constipation; renal and metabolic abnormalities such as increased Cr_s, hypophosphatemia, hyperkalemia, peripheral edema, and weight gain; respiratory system effects are dyspnea, pharyngitis and upper respiratory tract infection. Fever, headache, asthenia, body pain, arthralgia, insomnia, tremor, and posttransplant lymphoproliferative disorder also have been reported.

Contraindications. Hypersensitivity to sirolimus, derivatives of sirolimus, or any component of the formulation.

Precautions. Pregnancy; lactation. (*See also* General Precautions for Immunosuppressants.)

Drug Interactions. Concurrent administration of oral cyclosporine microemulsion capsules (Neoral) increases AUC, peak and trough, but administration of oral cyclosporine 4 hr after sirolimus has no effect on sirolimus whole blood levels. Sirolimus can potentiate cyclosporine nephrotoxicity. Diltiazem and ketoconazole increase sirolimus levels. Rifampin decreases sirolimus levels. AUC is unchanged with concurrent administration of acyclovir, glyburide, digoxin, nifedipine, norgestrel, or ethinyl estradiol. AUC can be affected by substrates, inhibitors, or inducers of CYP3A4 or P-glycoprotein.

Parameters to Monitor. Monitor WBC, erythrocyte, and platelet counts weekly during the first 2–3 months of therapy and monthly thereafter in stable patients. Monitor serum lipids monthly. Monitor for signs and symptoms of graft rejection, especially after dosage reduction.

Notes. Sirolimus has been used in the treatment of psoriasis.

TACROLIMUS   Prograf

Pharmacology. Tacrolimus (formerly FK506) is a macrolide antibiotic produced by *Streptomyces tsukubaensis*. The intracellular drug–ligand complex of tacrolimus and FK506 binding protein (FKBP-12) indirectly blocks T-lymphocyte activation. It inhibits calcineurin-mediated dephosphorylation of factors necessary for IL-2 transcription.

Administration and Adult Dosage. **PO for prophylaxis of organ rejection or GVHD** 0.15–0.3 mg/kg initially, depending on the type of transplant and coadministration of other immunosuppressants. Tacrolimus is usually started 4–12 hr before surgery and administered on a bid schedule. **Maintenance dosage** is based on tacrolimus blood concentrations, the magnitude of risk for organ rejection or GVHD, and patient tolerance. **IV for patients unable to take medication orally** 0.03–0.1 mg/kg/day as a continuous infusion diluted in D5W or NS in a glass container (it can leach plasticizers from PVC containers) to a concentration of 2 mg/100–500 mL (final concentration 4–20 mg/L).[265] Mucositis generally necessitates initial use of IV tacrolimus for allogeneic bone marrow transplant recipients. Tacrolimus is generally started 1 or 2 days before bone marrow transplantation. **Conversion from cyclosporine** the manufacturer recommends at least 24 hr between the last **cyclosporine** dose and the first tacrolimus dose. **To convert from IV to PO tacrolimus** the IV:PO dosage ratio is typically 1:3. A tacrolimus blood level should be drawn 48 hr after dosage form conversion. Absorption of oral medications may be reduced in allogeneic bone marrow transplant patients due to residual gut damage from intensive chemotherapy or radiation or GVHD. **Discontinuation** tacrolimus may be eventually discontinued in certain renal or allogeneic bone marrow transplant recipients. However, it must be decreased gradually to reduce the risk of reactive immune stimulation and consequent graft rejection or GVHD.

Special Populations. *Pediatric Dosage.* Same as adult dosage.

Geriatric Dosage. Same as adult dosage. Age-related reduction in renal function and comorbid conditions may predispose elderly patients to tacrolimus-induced nephrotoxicity and hypertension.

Special Populations. Use IBW to calculate initial dosage in obese patients.

Dosage Forms. Cap 0.5, 1, 5 mg; **Soln** 100 mg/mL; **Inj** 5 mg/mL.

Patient Instructions. Take this medication on a regular schedule in relation to the time of day and meals. Do not discontinue it unless directed to do so. Grapefruit juice can interact with cyclosporine. Talk to your physician before drinking grapefruit juice and before starting, stopping, or changing the dose of any medication.

Missed Doses. Take a missed dose as soon as possible if you remember within 12 hours. If it is within 2 hours of next dose, skip the missed dose and do not double the next dose. If you miss 2 or more doses, contact your physician.

Pharmacokinetics. *Serum Levels.* The serum (blood) concentration–response relationship is not completely defined. Trough blood or serum concentrations are monitored to reduce the risk of toxicity. Therapeutic and toxic concentrations vary with assay, biologic fluid, and time post-transplant. Artifactually elevated serum concentrations can occur when blood is drawn through the same central venous line used for IV tacrolimus administration. Whole blood trough levels of 10–20 μg/L are often considered therapeutic.

Fate. The mean absorption of tacrolimus capsules in normal healthy volunteers is $17 \pm 7\%$. In liver transplant patients absorption is $22 \pm 6\%$. Factors that can decrease absorption are diarrhea, gastroenteritis, and short small bowel. Food does not affect bioavailability but decreases and delays peak serum levels. Whole blood peak concentrations in liver transplant patients after 0.15 mg/kg is 52.4 μg/L fasting and 27.5 μg/L with food. Tacrolimus is extensively bound to erythrocytes and plasma proteins, primarily albumin and α_1-acid glycoprotein. V_d (whole blood) is 0.85 ± 0.3 L/kg in liver transplant patients; Cl (whole blood) is 0.053 ± 0.017 L/hr/kg in liver transplant recipients. Tacrolimus is extensively metabolized by CYP3A. At least 10 metabolites, some with immunosuppressant activity, have been identified. Less than 1% is excreted unchanged in the urine.

$t_{\frac{1}{2}}$. (Whole blood) 21.2 ± 8.5 hr in normal healthy volunteers; 11.7 ± 3.9 hr in liver transplant patients.

Adverse Reactions. Acute nephrotoxicity, which usually occurs within 1 month post-transplant and is characterized by Cr_s increasing ≥ 0.3 mg/mL/24 hr, frequently abates with interruption of drug therapy. Dosage reduction might be required for continued administration. Chronic progressive renal toxicity is characterized by a slow, continual increase in Cr_s and BUN, mild proteinuria, and tubular dysfunction. $Cr_s > 2$ mg/dL in adult patients, or doubling of Cr_s, is an indication for interruption of therapy or dosage reduction. Electrolyte abnormalities, including hypomagnesemia, hypokalemia or hyperkalemia, and renal tubular acidosis, are consequences of tacrolimus-induced nephrotoxicity. Concurrent administration of nephrotoxic drugs increases the likelihood of renal dysfunction. Hypertension occurs frequently. **Calcium-channel blockers** and **clonidine** are suitable agents for the management of tacrolimus-induced hypertension because these agents do not have deleterious effects on renal blood flow. Fine tremors occur frequently and can persist and worsen after drug discontinuation. Neurotoxicity symptoms are headache, seizures, encephalopathy, confusion, insomnia, cortical blindness, expressive aphasia, paresthesia, hyperesthesia, and myoclonic reactions. Anaphylactoid reactions to tacrolimus or the solubilizing agent, polyoxyethylated castor oil, can occur. After an allergic reaction to IV tacrolimus, patients may receive a trial of oral tacrolimus capsules under close observation. Hyperbilirubinemia, increased γ-glutamyltranspeptidase, serum alkaline phosphatase, and serum transaminases occur frequently. Additional adverse effects are photophobia, rash, hirsutism, pleural effusion, gingival hyperplasia, diarrhea, nausea, vomiting, and hypertriglyceridemia.

Contraindications. Allergy to tacrolimus or polyoxyethylated castor oil.

Precautions. Pregnancy; lactation. Use with caution in patients at risk for renal dysfunction. (*See also* General Precautions for Immunosuppressants.)

Drug Interactions. Additive or synergistic renal toxicity can occur with concurrent administration of nephrotoxic drugs. Potassium-sparing diuretics can exacerbate hyperkalemia. Because tacrolimus is metabolized by CYP3A, numerous drug interactions are possible with concurrent administration of drugs that affect this enzyme system. The following drugs can increase tacrolimus blood levels: corticosteroids, itraconazole, ketoconazole, erythromycin and other macrolide antibiotics, oral contraceptives, fluconazole, calcium-channel blockers, cimetidine, danazol, and metoclopramide. Enzyme-inducing drugs such as carbamazepine, phenobarbital, phenytoin, rifabutin, and rifampin can decrease tacrolimus blood levels. Tacrolimus can decrease the clearance of HMG-CoA reductase inhibitors and increase the risk of drug-induced rhabdomyolysis.

Parameters to Monitor. Observe for anaphylaxis with IV administration. Monitor Cr_s q 2–7 days and daily in patients at risk for acute renal dysfunction. Monitor

LFTs weekly, triglycerides monthly, and blood pressure regularly. Monitor blood or serum concentrations q 2–3 days when starting therapy. As the patient's clinical condition and renal function allow, reduce frequency to 1–2 times weekly and then monthly during the first year of therapy. After the first year of therapy, blood or serum concentration monitoring may be reduced q 1–2 months in stable patients. Monitor for signs and symptoms of graft rejection or GVHD, especially after dosage reduction.

Notes. Comparative clinical trials found greater nephrotoxicity and neurotoxicity with tacrolimus than with cyclosporine.[252] Case reports describe resolution of drug-induced toxicity after replacement of cyclosporine with tacrolimus and resolution of cyclosporine-refractory acute GVHD or chronic GVHD with tacrolimus.[253,254]

REFERENCES

1. Dorr RT, Von Hoff DD, eds. *Cancer chemotherapy handbook*. 2nd ed. Norwalk CT: Appleton & Lange; 1994.
2. Lindley CM et al. Incidence and duration of chemotherapy-induced nausea and vomiting in the outpatient oncology population. *J Clin Oncol* 1989;7:1142–9.
3. Wharton JT et al. Hexamethylmelamine: an evaluation of its role in the treatment of ovarian cancer. *Am J Obstet Gynecol* 1979;133:833–44.
4. Manetta A et al. Hexamethylmelamine as a single second-line agent in ovarian cancer. *Gynecol Oncol* 1990;36:93–6.
5. Ames MM et al. Phase I and clinical pharmacological evaluation of a parenteral hexamethylmelamine formulation. *Cancer Res* 1990;50:206–10.
6. Sawitsky A et al. Comparison of daily versus intermittent chlorambucil and prednisone therapy in the treatment of patients with chronic lymphocytic leukemia. *Blood* 1977;50:1049–59.
7. Alexanian R, Dreicer R. Chemotherapy of multiple myeloma. *Cancer* 1984;53:583–8.
8. Adair CG et al. Renal function in the elimination of oral melphalan in patients with multiple myeloma. *Cancer Chemother Pharmacol* 1986;17:185–8.
9. Hoogstraten B et al. Intermittent melphalan therapy in multiple myeloma. *JAMA* 1969;209:251–3.
10. Benet LZ et al. Design and optimization of dosage regimens: pharmacokinetic data. In, Hardman JG et al., eds. *Goodman and Gilman's the pharmacological basis of therapeutics*. 9th ed. New York: McGraw-Hill; 1996:1707–92.
11. McLean A et al. Pharmacokinetics and metabolism of chlorambucil in patients with malignant disease. *Cancer Treat Rev* 1979;6(suppl):33–42.
12. Adair CG et al. Can food affect the bioavailability of chlorambucil in patients with hematological malignancies? *Cancer Chemother Pharmacol* 1986;17:99–102.
13. Alberts DS et al. Oral melphalan kinetics. *Clin Pharmacol Ther* 1979;26:737–45.
14. Alberts DS et al. Kinetics of intravenous melphalan. *Clin Pharmacol Ther* 1979;26:73–80.
15. Taetle R et al. Pulmonary histopathologic changes associated with melphalan therapy. *Cancer* 1978;42:1239–45.
16. Heard BE, Cooke RA. Busulfan lung. *Thorax* 1968;23:187–93.
17. Lane SD et al. Fatal interstitial pneumonitis following high-dose intermittent chlorambucil therapy for chronic lymphocytic leukemia. *Cancer* 1981;47:32–6.
18. Micetich KC et al. A comparative study of the cytotoxicity and DNA-damaging effects of cis-(diamino) (1,1-cyclobutanedicarboxylato)-platinum(II) and cis-diaminedichloroplatinum(II) on L1210 cells. *Cancer Res* 1985;45:4043–7.
19. Curt GA et al. A phase I and pharmacokinetic study of diaminecyclobutane-dicarboxylatoplatinum (NSC 241240). *Cancer Res* 1983;43:4470–3.
20. Meyers FJ et al. Infusion carboplatin treatment of relapsed and refractory acute leukemia: evidence of efficacy with minimal extramedullary toxicity at intermediate doses. *J Clin Oncol* 1989;7:173–8.
21. Smit E et al. Continuous infusion carboplatin on a 21-day schedule: a phase I and pharmacokinetic study. *J Clin Oncol* 1991;9:100–10.
22. Allen JC et al. Carboplatin and recurrent childhood brain tumors. *J Clin Oncol* 1987;5:459–63.
23. Calvert AH et al. Carboplatin dosage: prospective evaluation of a simple formula based on renal function. *J Clin Oncol* 1989;7:1748–56.

24. Chatelut E et al. Prediction of carboplatin clearance from standard morphological and biological patient characteristics. *J Natl Cancer Inst* 1995;87:573–80.

25. Newell DR et al. Plasma free platinum pharmacokinetics in patients treated with high dose carboplatin. *Eur J Cancer Clin Oncol* 1987;23:1399–405.

26. Calvert AH et al. Early clinical studies with cis-diammine-1,1-cyclobutane dicarboxylate platinum(II). *Cancer Chemother Pharmacol* 1982;9:140–7.

27. Einhorn LH, Donahue J. Cis-diamminedichloroplatinum, vinblastine, and bleomycin combination chemotherapy in disseminated testicular cancer. *Ann Intern Med* 1977;87:293–8.

28. Belt RJ et al. Pharmacokinetics of non-protein-bound platinum species following administration of cis-dichlorodiammineplatinum (II). *Cancer Treat Rep* 1979;63:1515–21.

29. DeConti RC et al. Clinical and pharmacological studies with cis-diamminedichloroplatinum (II). *Cancer Res* 1973;33:1310–5.

30. Gonzalez-Vitale JC et al. Acute renal failure after cis-dichlorodiammineplatinum (II) and gentamicin-cephalothin therapies. *Cancer Treat Rep* 1978;62:693–8.

31. Macaulay VM et al. Prophylaxis against hypomagnesemia induced by cisplatinum combination therapy. *Cancer Chemother Pharmacol* 1982;9:179–81.

32. Brock N et al. Activation of cyclophosphamide in man and animals. *Cancer* 1971;6:1512–29.

33. Grochow LB, Colvin M. Clinical pharmacokinetics of cyclophosphamide. *Clin Pharmacokinet* 1979;4:380–94.

34. Bagley CM et al. Clinical pharmacology of cyclophosphamide. *Cancer Res* 1973;33:226–33.

35. Scheef W et al. Controlled clinical studies with an antidote against the urotoxicity of oxazophosphorines: preliminary results. *Cancer Treat Rep* 1979;63:501–5.

36. Carter SK, Friedman MA. 5-(3,3-dimethyl-l-triazeno)-imidazole-4-carboxamide (DTIC, DIC, NSC-45388)—a new antitumor agent with activity against malignant melanoma. *Eur J Cancer* 1972;8:85–92.

37. Loo TL et al. Mechanism of action and pharmacology studies with DTIC (NSC-45388). *Cancer Treat Rep* 1976;60:149–52.

38. Zalupski M, Baker LH. Ifosfamide. *J Natl Cancer Inst* 1988;80:556–66.

39. Araujo C, Tessler J. Treatment of ifosfamide-induced urothelial toxicity by oral administration of sodium 2-mercaptoethane sulphonate (mesna) to patients with inoperable lung cancer. *Eur J Cancer Clin Oncol* 1983;19:195–201.

40. Stuart-Harris RC et al. High-dose alkylation therapy using ifosfamide infusion with mesna in the treatment of adult advanced soft tissue sarcoma. *Cancer Chemother Pharmacol* 1983;11:69–72.

41. Sangster G et al. Failure of 2-mercaptoethane sulphonate sodium (mesna) to protect against ifosfamide nephrotoxicity. *Eur J Cancer Clin Oncol* 1984;20:435–6.

42. Pratt CB et al. Phase II trial of ifosfamide in children with malignant solid tumors. *Cancer Treat Rep* 1987; 71:131–5.

43. Miser JS et al. Ifosfamide with uroprotection and etoposide: an effective regimen in the treatment of recurrent sarcomas and other tumors of children and young adults. *J Clin Oncol* 1987;5:1191–8.

44. Creaven PJ et al. Clinical pharmacology of ifosfamide. *Clin Pharmacol Ther* 1974;16:77–86.

45. Colvin M. The comparative pharmacology of cyclophosphamide and ifosfamide. *Semin Oncol* 1982;9(suppl 1):2–7.

46. Allen LM et al. Studies on the human pharmacokinetics of ifosfamide (NSC-109724). *Cancer Treat Rep* 1976;60:451–8.

47. Wheeler BM et al. Ifosfamide in refractory male germ cell tumors. *J Clin Oncol* 1986;4:28–34.

48. Fossa SK, Talle K. Treatment of metastatic renal cancer with ifosfamide and mesnum with and without irradiation. *Cancer Treat Rep* 1980;64:1103–8.

49. Meanwell CA et al. Phase II study of ifosfamide in cervical cancer. *Cancer Treat Rep* 1986;70:727–30.

50. Goren MP et al. Dechlorethylation of ifosfamide and neurotoxicity. *Lancet* 1986;2:1219–20.

51. DeVita VT et al. Combination chemotherapy in the treatment of advanced Hodgkin's disease. *Ann Intern Med* 1970;73:881–95.

52. Taylor JR, Halprin KM. Topical use of mechlorethamine in the treatment of psoriasis. *Arch Dermatol* 1972; 106:362–4.

53. Taylor JR et al. Mechlorethamine hydrochloride solutions and ointment. *Arch Dermatol* 1980;116:783–5.

54. Van Scott EJ, Kalmanson JD. Complete remissions of mycosis fungoides lymphoma induced by topical nitrogen mustard (HN₂). *Cancer* 1973;32:18–30.

55. Crooke ST, Bradner WT. Mitomycin C: a review. *Cancer Treat Rev* 1976;3:121–39.

56. Buice RG et al. Pharmacokinetics of mitomycin C in non–oat cell carcinoma of the lung. *Cancer Chemother Pharmacol* 1984;13:1–4.

57. Dorr RT et al. Mitomycin C skin toxicity studies in mice. *J Clin Oncol* 1986;4:1399–1404.

58. DeFuria MD et al. Phase I-II study of mitomycin C topical therapy for low-grade, low-stage transitional cell carcinoma of the bladder: an interim report. *Cancer Treat Rep* 1980;64:225–30.

59. Sponzo RW et al. Physiologic disposition of 1-(2-chloroethyl)-3-cyclohexyl-1-nitrosourea (CCNU) and 1-(2-chloroethyl)-3-(4-methyl cyclohexyl)-1-nitrosourea (MeCCNU) in man. *Cancer* 1973;31:1154–9.

60. De Vita VT et al. Clinical trials with 1,3-bis(2-chloroethyl)-3-cyclohexyl-1-nitrosourea, NSC-409962. *Cancer Res* 1965;25:1876–81.

61. Oliverio VT. Toxicology and pharmacology of the nitrosoureas. *Cancer Chemother Pharmacol* 1973;4(part 3):13–20.

62. Aronin PA et al. Prediction of BCNU pulmonary toxicity in patients with malignant gliomas. *N Engl J Med* 1980;303:183–8.

63. Durant JR et al. Pulmonary toxicity associated with bischloroethylnitrosourea (BCNU). *Ann Intern Med* 1979;90:191–4.

64. Brem H et al. Placebo-controlled trial of safety and efficacy of intraoperative controlled delivery by biodegradable polymers of chemotherapy for recurrent gliomas. *Lancet* 1995;345:1008–12.

65. Tamargo RJ et al. Interstitial chemotherapy of the 9L gliosarcoma: controlled release polymers for drug delivery in the brain. *Cancer Res* 1993;53:329–33.

66. Spivack SD. Procarbazine. *Ann Intern Med* 1974;81:795–800.

67. Schein PS et al. Clinical antitumor activity and toxicity of streptozotocin (NSC-85998). *Cancer* 1974; 34:993–1000.

68. Hammond LA et al. Phase I and pharmacokinetic study of temozolomide on a daily-for-5-days schedule in patients with advanced solid malignancies. *J Clin Oncol* 1999;17:2604–13.

69. Dhodapkar M et al. Phase I trial of temozolomide (NSC 362856) in patients with advanced cancer. *Clin Cancer Res* 1997;3:1093–100.

70. Baker SD et al. Absorption, metabolism, and excretion of 14C-temozolomide following oral administration to patients with advanced cancer. *Clin Cancer Res* 1999;5:309–17.

71. Agarwala SS et al. Pharmacokinetic study of temozolomide penetration into CSF in a patient with dural melanoma. *Ann Oncol* 1998;9(suppl 4):659. Abstract.

72. Britten CD et al. A phase I and pharmacokinetic study of temozolomide and cisplatin in patients with advanced solid malignancies. *Clin Cancer Res* 1999;5:1629–37.

73. Reid JM et al. Pharmacokinetics of 3-methyl-(triazen-1-yl) imidazole-4-carboximide following administration of temozolomide to patients with advanced cancer. *Clin Cancer Res* 1997;3:2393–8.

74. Nicholson HS et al. Phase I study of temozolomide in children and adolescents with recurrent solid tumors: a report from the Children's Cancer Group. *J Clin Oncol* 1998;16:3037–43.

75. Middleton MR et al. Randomized phase III study of temozolomide versus dacarbazine in the treatment of patients with advanced metastatic malignant melanoma. *J Clin Oncol* 2000;18:158–66.

76. Summers Y et al. Effect of temozolomide (TMZ) on central nervous system (CNS) relapse in patients with advanced melanoma. *Am Soc Clin Oncol* 1999;2048. Abstract.

77. Cohen BE et al. Human plasma pharmacokinetics and urinary excretion of thiotepa and its metabolites. *Cancer Treat Rep* 1986;70:859–64.

78. Beutler E. Cladribine (2-chlorodeoxyadenosine). *Lancet* 1992;340:952–6.

79. Saven A et al. Treatment of hairy cell leukemia. *Blood* 1992;79:1111–20.

80. Sipe JC et al. Cladribine in treatment of chronic progressive multiple sclerosis. *Lancet* 1994;344:9–13.

81. Liliemark J et al. On the bioavailability of oral and subcutaneous 2-chloro-2′-deoxyadenosine in humans: alternative routes of administration. *J Clin Oncol* 1992;10:1514–8.

82. Grant S. Ara-C: cellular and molecular pharmacology. *Adv Cancer Res* 1998;72:197–233.

83. Rudnick SA et al. High dose cytosine arabinoside (HDARAC) in refractory acute leukemia. *Cancer* 1979;44:1189–93.

84. Wan SH et al. Pharmacokinetics of 1-β-D-arabinofuranosylcytosine in humans. *Cancer Res* 1974;34: 392–7.

85. Harris AL et al. Pharmacokinetics of cytosine arabinoside in patients with acute myeloid leukaemia. *Br J Clin Pharmacol* 1979;8:219–27.

86. van Prooijen R et al. Pharmacokinetics of cytosine arabinoside in acute myeloid leukemia. *Clin Pharmacol Ther* 1977;21:744–50.

87. Ho DHW, Frei E. Clinical pharmacology of 1-β-D-arabinofuranosylcytosine. *Clin Pharmacol Ther* 1971; 12: 944–54.

88. Chabner BA et al. Clinical pharmacology of anticancer drugs. *Semin Oncol* 1977;4:165–91.

89. Ritch PS et al. Ocular toxicity from high-dose cytosine arabinoside. *Cancer* 1983;51:430–2.

90. Lazarus HM et al. Central nervous system toxicity of high-dose systemic cytosine arabinoside. *Cancer* 1981;48:2577–82.

91. Ahmed I et al. Cytosine arabinoside-induced vasculitis. *Mayo Clin Proc* 1998;73:239–42.

92. Guilhot F et al. Interferon alfa-2b combined with cytarabine versus interferon alone in chronic myelogenous leukemia. French Chronic Myeloid Leukemia Study Group. *N Engl J Med* 1997;337:223–9.

93. Kemeny N et al. Intrahepatic or systemic infusion of fluorodeoxyuridine in patients with liver metastases from colorectal carcinoma. *Ann Intern Med* 1987;107:459–65.

94. Ensminger WD et al. A clinical pharmacological evaluation of hepatic arterial infusions of 5-fluoro-2'-deoxyuridine and 5-fluorouracil. *Cancer Res* 1978;38:3784–92.

95. Jacobs EM et al. Treatment of cancer with weekly 5-fluorouracil; study by the Western Cooperative Cancer Chemotherapy Group (WCCCG). *Cancer* 1971;27:1302–5.

96. Horton J et al. 5-Fluorouracil in cancer: an improved regimen. *Ann Intern Med* 1970;73:897–900.

97. Seifert P et al. Comparison of continuously infused 5-fluorouracil with bolus injection in treatment of patients with colorectal adenocarcinoma. *Cancer* 1975;36:123–8.

98. Cohen JL et al. Clinical pharmacology of oral and intravenous 5-fluorouracil (NSC-19893). *Cancer Chemother Rep* 1974;58(part 1):723–31.

99. Kirkwood JM et al. Comparison of pharmacokinetics of 5-fluorouracil and 5-fluorouracil with concurrent thymidine infusions in a phase I trial. *Cancer Res* 1980;40:107–13.

100. Abbruzzese JL et al. A phase I clinical, plasma, and cellular pharmacology study of gemcitabine. *J Clin Oncol* 1991;9:491–8.

101. Kaye SB. Gemcitabine: current status of phase I and II trials. *J Clin Oncol* 1994;12:1527–31.

102. Rothenberg ML et al. Gemcitabine: effective palliative therapy for pancreas cancer patients failing 5-FU. *Proc Am Soc Clin Oncol* 1995;14:198.

103. Mullarkey MF et al. Long-term methotrexate treatment in corticosteroid-dependent asthma. *Ann Intern Med* 1990;112:577–81.

104. Hedman J et al. Controlled trial of methotrexate in patients with severe chronic asthma. *Eur J Clin Pharmacol* 1996;49:347–9.

105. Henry MA, Gentry WL. Single injection of methotrexate for treatment of ectopic pregnancies. *Am J Obstet Gynecol* 1994;171:1584–7.

106. Corsan GH et al. Identification of hormonal parameters for successful systemic single-dose methotrexate therapy in ectopic pregnancy. *Hum Reprod* 1995;10:2719–22.

107. Wiebe ER. Abortion induced with methotrexate and misoprostol. *Can Med Assoc J* 1996;154:165–70.

108. Creinin MD. A randomized trial comparing misoprostol three and seven days after methotrexate for early abortion. *Am J Obstet Gynecol* 1995;173:1578–84.

109. Weibe ER. Abortion induced with methotrexate and misoprostol: a comparison of various protocols. *Contraception* 1997;55:159–63.

110. Bonadonna G et al. Combination chemotherapy as an adjuvant treatment in operable breast cancer. *N Engl J Med* 1976;294:405–10.

111. Bleyer WA. Clinical pharmacology of intrathecal methotrexate II. An improved dosage regimen derived from age-related pharmacokinetics. *Cancer Treat Rep* 1977;61:1419–25.

112. Evans WE, Pratt CB. Effect of pleural effusion on high-dose methotrexate kinetics. *Clin Pharmacol Ther* 1978;24:68–72.

113. Campbell MA et al. Methotrexate: bioavailability and pharmacokinetics. *Cancer Treat Rep* 1985;69:833–8. Dosages in the table were derived using the nomogram of Rowland M, Tozer TN. *Clinical pharmacokinetics: concepts and applications.* Philadelphia: Lea & Febiger; 1980:233.

114. Isacoff WH et al. Pharmacokinetics of high-dose methotrexate with citrovorum factor rescue. *Cancer Treat Rep* 1977;61:1665–74.

115. Shen DD, Azarnoff DL. Clinical pharmacokinetics of methotrexate. *Clin Pharmacokinet* 1978;3:1–13.

116. O'Dwyer PJ et al. 2'-deoxycoformycin (pentostatin) for lymphoid malignancies. *Ann Intern Med* 1988;108:733–43.

117. Malspeis L et al. Clinical pharmacokinetics of 2'-deoxycoformycin. *Cancer Treat Symp* 1984;2:7–15.

118. Wiernik PH, Serpick AA. A randomized clinical trial of daunorubicin and a combination of prednisone, vincristine, 6-mercaptopurine, and methotrexate in adult acute nonlymphocytic leukemia. *Cancer Res* 1967;32:2023–6.

119. Lin S-N et al. Quantitation of plasma azathioprine and 6-mercaptopurine levels in renal transplant patients. *Transplantation* 1980;29:290–4.

120. Bach JF, Dardenne M. The metabolism of azathioprine in renal failure. *Transplantation* 1971;12:253–9.

121. Zimm S et al. Variable bioavailability of oral mercaptopurine. *N Engl J Med* 1983;308:1005–9.

122. Duttera MJ et al. Hematuria and crystalluria after high-dose 6-mercaptopurine administration. *N Engl J Med* 1972;287:292–4.

123. Penn I, Starzl TE. A summary of the status of de novo cancer in transplant recipients. *Transplant Proc* 1972;4:719–32.

124. Ho DH et al. Clinical pharmacology of combined oral uracil and ftorafur. *Drug Metab Disp* 1992;20:936–40.

125. Salz LB et al. A fixed-ratio combination of uracil and ftorafur (UFT) with low dose leucovorin. *Cancer* 1995;75:782–5.

126. Rosenberg SA et al. Observations on the systemic administration of autologous lymphokine-activated killer cells and recombinant interleukin-2 to patients with metastatic cancer. *N Engl J Med* 1985;313:1485–92.
127. Winkelhake JL, Gauny SS. Human recombinant interleukin-2 as an experimental therapeutic. *Pharmacol Rev* 1990;42:1–28.
128. Konrad MW et al. Pharmacokinetics of recombinant interleukin-2 in humans. *Cancer Res* 1990;50:2009–17.
129. Goldstein D, Laszlo J. Interferon therapy in cancer: from imaginon to interferon. *Cancer Res* 1986;46:4315–29.
130. Krown SE. The role of interferon in the therapy of epidemic Kaposi's sarcoma. *Semin Oncol* 1987;14:27–33.
131. Perrillo RP et al. A randomized controlled trial of interferon alfa-2b alone and after prednisone withdrawal for the treatment of chronic hepatitis B. *N Engl J Med* 1990;323:295–301.
132. Spiegel RJ. Intron A (interferon alfa-2b): clinical overview. *Cancer Treat Rev* 1985;12(suppl B):5–16.
133. Wills RJ et al. Interferon kinetics and adverse reactions after intravenous, intramuscular, and subcutaneous injection. *Clin Pharmacol Ther* 1984;35:722–7.
134. Quesada JR et al. Antitumor activity of recombinant-derived interferon alpha in metastatic renal cell carcinoma. *J Clin Oncol* 1985;3:1522–8.
135. Berman E et al. Idarubicin in acute leukemia: results of studies at Memorial Sloan-Kettering Cancer Center. *Semin Oncol* 1989;16:30–4.
136. Lambertenghi-Deliliers G et al. Idarubicin plus cytarabine as first-line treatment of acute nonlymphoblastic leukemia. *Semin Oncol* 1989;16:16–20.
137. Blum RH, Carter SK. Adriamycin: a new anticancer drug with significant clinical activity. *Ann Intern Med* 1974;80:249–59.
138. Legha SS et al. Reduction of doxorubicin cardiotoxicity by prolonged continuous intravenous infusion. *Ann Intern Med* 1982;96:133–9.
139. Weiss AJ et al. Studies on adriamycin using a weekly regimen demonstrating its clinical effectiveness and lack of cardiac toxicity. *Cancer Treat Rep* 1976;60:813–22.
140. Von Hoff DD et al. Daunomycin-induced cardiotoxicity in children and adults: a review of 110 cases. *Am J Med* 1977;62:200–8.
141. Benjamin RS et al. Adriamycin chemotherapy—efficacy, safety, and pharmacologic basis of an intermittent single high-dosage schedule. *Cancer* 1974;33:19–27.
142. Smith DB et al. Clinical pharmacology of oral and intravenous 4-demethoxydaunorubicin. *Cancer Chemother Pharmacol* 1987;19:138–42.
143. Robert J et al. Pharmacokinetics of idarubicin after daily intravenous administration in leukemic patients. *Leuk Res* 1987;11:961–4.
144. Huffman DH et al. Daunorubicin metabolism in acute nonlymphocytic leukemia. *Clin Pharmacol Ther* 1972;13:895–905.
145. Lu K et al. Clinical pharmacology of 4-demethoxydaunorubicin (DMDR). *Cancer Chemother Pharmacol* 1986;17:143–8.
146. Dean JC et al. Scalp hypothermia: a comparison of ice packs and the Kold Kap in the prevention of doxorubicin-induced alopecia. *J Clin Oncol* 1983;1:33–7.
147. Von Hoff DD et al. Risk factors for doxorubicin-induced congestive heart failure. *Ann Intern Med* 1979;91:710–7.
148. Lipshultz SE et al. Late effects of doxorubicin therapy for acute lymphoblastic leukemia in childhood. *N Engl J Med* 1991;324:808–15.
149. Bartlett NL et al. Phase I trial of doxorubicin with cyclosporine as a modulator of multidrug resistance. *J Clin Oncol* 1994;12:835–42.
150. Dorr RT. Anthracycline update: stability and compatibility of adriamycin in solution. *Highlights Antineoplast Drugs* 1985;3:6–7.
151. Speyer JL et al. Protective effect of the bispiperazinedione ICRF-187 against doxorubicin-induced cardiac toxicity in women with advanced breast cancer. *N Engl J Med* 1988;319:745–52.
152. Olver IN et al. A prospective study of topical dimethylsulfoxide for treating anthracycline extravasation. *J Clin Oncol* 1988;6:1732–5.
153. Gill PS et al. Phase I/II clinical and pharmacokinetic evaluation of liposomal daunorubicin. *J Clin Oncol* 1995;13:996–1003.
154. Forssen EA et al. Selective in vivo localization of daunorubicin small unilamellar vesicles in solid tumors. *Cancer Res* 1992;52:3255–61.
155. Northfelt DW et al. Doxorubicin encapsulated in liposomes containing surface-bound polyethylene glycol: pharmacokinetics, tumor localization, and safety in patients with AIDS-related Kaposi's sarcoma. *J Clin Pharmacol* 1996;36:55–63.
156. Harrison M et al. Liposomal-entrapped doxorubicin: an active agent in AIDS-related Kaposi's sarcoma. *J Clin Oncol* 1995;13:914–20.

157. Frei E. The clinical use of actinomycin. *Cancer Chemother Rep* 1974;58:49–54.

158. Tattersall MHN et al. Pharmacokinetics of actinomycin D in patients with malignant melanoma. *Clin Pharmacol Ther* 1975;17:701–8.

159. Shenkenberg TD, Von Hoff DD. Mitoxantrone: a new anticancer drug with significant clinical activity. *Ann Intern Med* 1986;105:67–81.

160. Vietti TJ et al. Mitoxantrone in children with advanced malignant disease. In, Rozencweig M et al., eds. *New anticancer drugs: mitoxantrone and bisantrene*. New York: Raven Press; 1983:93–102.

161. Savaraj N et al. Pharmacology of mitoxantrone in cancer patients. *Cancer Chemother Pharmacol* 1982;8:113–7.

162. Slayton RE et al. New approach to the treatment of hypercalcemia: the effect of short-term treatment with mithramycin. *Clin Pharmacol Ther* 1971;12:833–7.

163. Kennedy BJ. Metabolic and toxic effects of mithramycin during tumor therapy. *Am J Med* 1970;49:494–503.

164. Newling DWW et al. The response of advanced prostatic cancer to a new non-steroidal antiandrogen: results of a multicenter open phase II study of Casodex. *Eur Urol* 1990;18:18–21.

165. Cockshott ID et al. The pharmacokinetics of Casodex in prostate cancer patients after single and during multiple dosing. *Eur Urol* 1990;18:10–7.

166. Katchen B, Buxbaum S. Disposition of a new nonsteroid antiandrogen, alpha, alpha, alpha-trifluoro-2-methyl-4'-nitro-m-propionotoluidide (flutamide) in men following a single oral 200 mg dose. *J Clin Endocrinol Metab* 1975;41:373–9.

167. Radwanski E et al. Single and multiple dose pharmacokinetic evaluation of flutamide in normal geriatric volunteers. *J Clin Pharmacol* 1989;29:554–8.

168. Yagoda A. Flutamide-induced diarrhea secondary to lactose intolerance. *J Natl Cancer Inst* 1989;81:1839–40. Letter.

169. Asbury RF et al. Treatment of metastatic breast cancer with aminoglutethimide. *Cancer* 1981;47:1954–8.

170. Plourde PV. Arimidex: a potent and selective fourth-generation aromatase inhibitor. *Breast Cancer Res Treat* 1994;30:103–11.

171. Anon. Toremifene and letrozole for advanced breast cancer. *Med Lett Drugs Ther* 1998;40:43–5.

172. Hauser AR, Marryman R. Estramustine phosphate sodium. *Drug Intell Clin Pharm* 1984;18:368–74.

173. Ahmann FR et al. Zoladex: a sustained-release, monthly luteinizing hormone-releasing hormone analogue for the treatment of advanced prostate cancer. *J Clin Oncol* 1987;5:912–7.

174. Leuprolide Study Group. Leuprolide versus diethylstilbestrol for metastatic prostate cancer. *N Engl J Med* 1984;311:1281–6.

175. Patterson JS, Battersby LA. Tamoxifen: an overview of recent studies in the field of oncology. *Cancer Treat Rep* 1980;64:775–8.

176. Fabian C et al. Clinical pharmacology of tamoxifen in patients with breast cancer: comparison of traditional and loading dose schedules. *Cancer Treat Rep* 1980;64:765–73.

177. Adam HK et al. Studies on the metabolism and pharmacokinetics of tamoxifen in normal volunteers. *Cancer Treat Rep* 1980;64:761–4.

178. Plotkin D et al. Tamoxifen flare in advanced breast cancer. *JAMA* 1978;240:2644–6.

179. Lippman ME, Allegra JC. Receptors in breast cancer: estrogen receptor and endocrine therapy of breast cancer. *N Engl J Med* 1978;299:930–3.

180. Wiebe VJ et al. Pharmacokinetics of toremifene and its metabolites with advanced breast cancer. *Cancer Chemother Pharmacol* 1990;25:247–51.

181. Saarto T et al. Antiatherogenic effects of adjuvant antiestrogens: a randomized trial comparing the effects of tamoxifen and toremifene on plasma lipid levels in postmenopausal women with node-positive breast cancer. *J Clin Oncol* 1996;14:429–33.

182. Cortes JE et al. Docetaxel. *J Clin Oncol* 1995;13:2643–55.

183. Royer I. Metabolism of docetaxel by human cytochromes P450: interactions with paclitaxel and other antineoplastic drugs. *Cancer Res* 1996;56:58–65.

184. O'Dwyer PJ et al. Etoposide (VP-16–213): current status of an active anticancer drug. *N Engl J Med* 1985;312:692–700.

185. Rivera GK et al. Epipodophyllotoxins in the treatment of childhood cancer. *Cancer Chemother Pharmacol* 1994;34(suppl):S89–95.

186. Chamberlain MC, Grafe MR. Recurrent chiasmatic-hypothalamic glioma treated with oral etoposide. *J Clin Oncol* 1995;13:2072–6.

187. Snyder DS et al. Fractionated total-body irradiation and high-dose etoposide as a preparatory regimen for bone marrow transplantation for 94 patients with chronic myelogenous leukemia in chronic phase. *Blood* 1994;84:1672–9.

188. Allen LM, Creaven PJ. Comparison of the human pharmacokinetics of VM-26 and VP-16, two antineoplastic epipodophyllotoxin glucopyranoside derivatives. *Eur J Cancer* 1975;11:697–707.

189. Wiseman LR, Markham A. Irinotecan. A review of its pharmacological properties and clinical efficacy in the management of advanced colorectal cancer. *Drugs* 1996;52:606–23.
190. Holmes FA et al. Phase II trial of taxol, an active drug in the treatment of metastatic breast cancer. *J Nat Cancer Inst* 1991;83:1797–805.
191. McGuire WP et al. Taxol: a unique antineoplastic agent with significant activity in advanced ovarian epithelial neoplasms. *Ann Intern Med* 1989;111:273–9.
192. Huizing MT et al. Pharmacokinetics of paclitaxel and metabolites in a randomized comparative study in platinum-pretreated ovarian cancer patients. *J Clin Oncol* 1993;11:2127–35.
193. Rozencweig M et al. VM-26 and VP 16-213: a comparative analysis. *Cancer* 1977;40:334–42.
194. Grem JL et al. Teniposide in the treatment of leukemia: a case study of conflicting priorities in the development of drugs for fatal diseases. *J Clin Oncol* 1988;6:351–79.
195. Yap H-Y et al. Vinblastine given as a continuous 5-day infusion in the treatment of refractory advanced breast cancer. *Cancer Treat Rep* 1980;64:279–83.
196. Robieux I et al. Pharmacokinetics of vinorelbine in patients with liver metastases. *Clin Pharmacol Ther* 1996;59:32–40.
197. Owellen RJ et al. Pharmacokinetics of vindesine and vincristine in humans. *Cancer Res* 1977;37:2603–7.
198. Nelson RL et al. Comparative pharmacokinetics of vindesine, vincristine and vinblastine in patients with cancer. *Cancer Treat Rev* 1980;7(suppl):17–24.
199. Wargin WA, Lucas VS. The clinical pharmacokinetics of vinorelbine (Navelbine). *Semin Oncol* 1994;21(suppl 10):21–7.
200. Le Chevalier T et al. Randomized study of vinorelbine and cisplatin versus vindesine and cisplatin versus vinorelbine alone in advanced non-small-cell lung cancer: results of a European multicenter trial including 612 patients. *J Clin Oncol* 1994;12:360–7.
201. Kaminski MS et al. Radioimmunotherapy of B-cell lymphoma with [¹³¹I]-anti-B1(anti-CD-20) antibody. *N Engl J Med* 1993;329:459–65.
202. Kaminski MS et al. Iodine-131-anti-B1 radioimmunotherapy for B-cell lymphoma. *J Clin Oncol* 1996; 14: 1974–81.
203. Maloney DG et al. IDEC-C2B8: results of a phase I multiple-dose trial in patients with relapsed non-Hodgkin's lymphoma. *J Clin Oncol* 1997;15:3266–74.
204. Maloney DG et al. Phase I clinical trial using escalating single-dose infusion of chimeric anti-CD20 monoclonal antibody (IDEC-C2B8) in patients with recurrent B-cell lymphoma. *Blood* 1994;84:2457–66.
205. Clarkson B et al. Clinical results of treatment with *E. coli* l-asparaginase in adults with leukemia, lymphoma and solid tumors. *Cancer* 1970;25:279–305.
206. Sutow WW et al. Evaluation of dose and schedule of l-asparaginase in multidrug therapy of childhood leukemia. *Med Pediatr Oncol* 1976;2:387–95.
207. Pratt CB et al. Comparison of daily versus weekly l-asparaginase for the treatment of childhood acute leukemia. *J Pediatr* 1970;77:474–83.
208. Nesbit M et al. Evaluation of intramuscular versus intravenous administration of l-asparaginase in childhood leukemia. *Am J Pediatr Hematol Oncol* 1979;1:9–13.
209. Ohnuma T et al. Biochemical and pharmacological studies with asparaginase in man. *Cancer Res* 1970;30:2297–305.
210. Haskell CM et al. L-asparaginase: therapeutic and toxic effects in patients with neoplastic disease. *N Engl J Med* 1969;281:1028–35.
211. Bennett JM, Reich SD. Bleomycin. *Ann Intern Med* 1979;90:945–8.
212. Alberts DS et al. Bleomycin pharmacokinetics in man. *Cancer Chemother Pharmacol* 1978;1:177–81.
213. Paladine W et al. Intracavitary bleomycin in the management of malignant effusions. *Cancer* 1976;38:1903–8.
214. Crooke ST et al. Effects of variations in renal function on the clinical pharmacology of bleomycin administered as an IV bolus. *Cancer Treat Rep* 1977;61:1631–6.
215. Kramer WG et al. The pharmacokinetics of bleomycin in man. *J Clin Pharmacol* 1978;18:346–52.
216. Sostman HD et al. Cytotoxic drug-induced lung disease. *Am J Med* 1977;62:608–15.
217. Yagoda A et al. Bleomycin, an antitumor antibiotic: clinical experience in 274 patients. *Ann Intern Med* 1972;77:861–70.
218. Muindi JRF et al. Clinical pharmacology of oral all-trans retinoic acid in patients with acute promyelocytic luekemia. *Cancer Res* 1992;52:2138–42.
219. Warrell RP et al. Differentiation therapy of acute promyelocytic leukemia with tretinoin (all-trans-retinoic acid). *N Engl J Med* 1991;324:1385–90.
220. Fenaux P et al. Effect of all transretinoic acid in newly diagnosed acute promyelocytic leukemia. Results of a multicenter randomized trial. European APL 91 Group. *Blood* 1993;82:3241–9.

221. Glick J et al. A randomized trial of cyclophosphamide and cisplatin ± amifostine in the treatment of advanced epithelial ovarian cancer. *Proc Am Soc Clin Oncol* 1994;13:432.

222. Kligerman MM et al. Final report on phase I trial of WR-2721 before protracted fractionated radiation. *Int J Radiat Oncol Biol Phys* 1988;14:1119–22.

223. Shaw LM et al. Pharmacokinetics of WR-2721. *Pharmacol Ther* 1988;39:195–201.

224. Kligerman MM et al. Phase I clinical studies with WR-2721. *Cancer Clin Trials* 1980;3:217–21.

225. Turrisi AT et al. Final report of the phase I trial of single-dose WR-2721 [S-2-(3-aminopropylamono)-ethylphosphorothiolic acid]. *Cancer Treat Rep* 1986;70:1389–93.

226. Korst AE et al. Pharmacokinetics of carboplatin with and without amifostine in patients with solid tumors. *Clin Cancer Res* 1997;3:697–703.

227. Büntzel J et al. Selective cytoprotection with amifostine in concurrent radiochemotherapy for head and neck cancer. *Ann Oncol* 1998;9:505–9.

228. Speyer JL et al. ICRF-187 permits longer treatment with doxorubicin in women with breast cancer. *J Clin Oncol* 1992;10:117–27.

229. Swain SM et al. Cardioprotection with dexrazoxane for doxorubicin-containing therapy in advanced breast cancer. *J Clin Oncol* 1997;15:1318–32.

230. Wexler LH et al. Randomized trial of the cardioprotective agent ICRF-187 in pediatric sarcoma patients treated with doxorubicin. *J Clin Oncol* 1996;14:362–72.

231. Hochster H et al. Pharmacokinetics of the cardioprotector ADR-529 (ICRF-187) in escalating doses combined with fixed-dose doxorubicin. *J Natl Cancer Inst* 1992;84:1725–30.

232. Burkert H. Clinical overview of mesna. *Cancer Treat Rev* 1983;10:175–81.

233. Antman KH et al. Phase II trial of ifosfamide with mesna in previously treated metastatic sarcoma. *Cancer Treat Rep* 1985;69:499–504.

234. Pratt CB et al. Phase II trial of ifosfamide in children with malignant solid tumors. *Cancer Treat Rep* 1987; 71:131–5.

235. Burkert H et al. Bioavailability of orally administered mesna. *Arzneimittelforschung* 1984;34:1597–600.

236. Pohl J et al. Toxicology, pharmacology and interactions of sodium 2-mercaptoethanesulfonate (mesna). *Curr Chemother* 1981;2:1387–9.

237. Stuart-Harris RC et al. High-dose alkylation therapy using ifosfamide infusion with mesna in the treatment of adults advanced soft-tissue sarcoma. *Cancer Chemother Pharmacol* 1983;11:69–72.

238. Brennan DC et al. A randomized, double-blinded comparison of Thymoglobulin versus Atgam for induction immunosuppression therapy in adult renal transplant recipients. *Transplantation* 1999;67:1011–8.

239. Laske A et al. Prophylactic cytolytic therapy in heart transplantation: monoclonal versus polyclonal antibody therapy. *J Heart Lung Transplant* 1992;11:557–63.

240. Copeland JG et al. Rabbit antithymocyte globulin. A 10-year experience in cardiac transplantation. *J Thorac Cardiovasc Surg* 1990;99:852–60.

241. Di Bona E et al. Rabbit antithymocyte globulin (r-ATG) plus cyclosporine and granulocyte colony stimulating factor is an effective treatment for aplastic anaemia patients unresponsive to a first course of intensive immunosuppressive therapy. *Br J Haematol* 1999;107:330–4.

242. Ringden O et al. Low incidence of acute graft-versus-host disease using unrelated HLA-A-, HLA-B-, and HLA-DR-compatible donors and conditioning, including anti-T-cell antibodies. *Transplantation* 1998;66: 620–5.

243. Bunn D et al. The pharmacokinetics of anti-thymocyte globulin (ATG) following intravenous infusion in man. *Clin Nephrol* 1996;45:29–32.

244. Levine JM, Lien YH. Antithymocyte globulin-induced acute renal failure. *Am J Kid Dis* 1999;34:1155. Letter.

245. Morishita Y et al. Antithymocyte globulin for a patient with systemic lupus erythematosus complicated by severe pancytopenia. *J Int Med Res* 1997;25:219–23.

246. Toren A et al. Impaired liver function tests in patients with antithymocyte globulin: implication for liver transplantation. *Med Oncol* 1997;14:125–9.

247. Milea D et al. Transient acute myopia induced by antilymphocyte globulins. *Ophthalmolgica* 1999;213: 133–4.

248. Sullivan KM et al. Prednisone and azathioprine compared with prednisone and placebo for treatment of chronic graft-v-host disease: prognostic influence of prolonged thrombocytopenia after allogenic marrow transplantation. *Blood* 1988;72:546–54.

249. Yee GC, Salomon DR. Cyclosporine. In, Evans WE et al., eds. *Applied pharmacokinetics. Principles of therapeutic drug monitoring.* 3rd ed. Vancouver, WA: Applied Therapeutics; 1992:28:1–40.

250. Brinch L. Fooled by cyclosporin levels. *Bone Marrow Transplant* 1992;9:77–8.

251. List AF et al. Phase I/II trial of cyclosporine as a chemotherapy-resistance modifier in acute leukemia. *J Clin Oncol* 1993;11:1652–60.

252. US Multicenter FK506 Liver Study Group. A comparison of tacrolimus (FK506) and cyclosporine for immunosuppression in liver transplantation. *N Engl J Med* 1994;331:1110–5.

253. Pratschke J et al. Treatment of cyclosporine-related adverse effects by conversion to tacrolimus after liver transplantation. *Transplantation* 1997;64:938–40.

254. Ohashi Y et al. Successful treatment of steroid-resistant severe acute GVHD with 24-h continuous infusion of FK506. *Bone Marrow Transplant* 1997;19:625–7.

255. Przepiorka D et al. Daclizumab, a humanized anti-interleukin-2 receptor alpha chain antibody, for treatment of acute graft-versus-host disease. *Blood* 2000;95:83–9.

256. Anasetti C et al. Treatment of acute graft-versus-host disease with humanized anti-Tac: an antibody that binds to the interleukin-2 receptor. *Blood* 1994;84:1320–7.

257. Vincenti F et al. Interleukin-2 receptor blockade with daclizumab to prevent acute rejection in renal transplantation. Daclizumab Triple Therapy Study Group. *N Engl J Med* 1998;338:161–5.

258. Nashan B et al. Randomised trial of basiliximab versus placebo for control of acute cellular rejection in renal allograft recipients. *Lancet* 1997;350:1193–8.

259. Sievers TM et al. Mycophenolate mofetil. *Pharmacotherapy* 1997;17:1178–97.

260. Jain AB et al. A prospective randomized trial of tacrolimus and prednisone versus tacrolimus, prednisone, and mycophenolate mofetil in primary adult liver transplant recipients: an interim report. *Transplantation* 1998;66:1395–8.

261. Papatheodoridis GV et al. Mycophenolate mofetil monotherapy in stable liver transplant patients with cyclosporine-induced renal impairment: a preliminary report. *Liver Transplant* 1999;68:155–7.

262. Basara N et al. Mycophenolate mofetil for the treatment of acute and chronic GVHD in bone marrow transplant patients. *Bone Marrow Transplant* 1998;22:61–5.

263. Mookerjee B et al. Salvage therapy for refractory chronic graft-versus-host disease with mycophenolate mofetil and tacrolimus. *Bone Marrow Transplant* 1999;24:517–20.

264. Meiser BM et al. Combination therapy with tacrolimus and mycophenolate mofetil following cardiac transplantation: importance of mycophenolic acid therapeutic drug monitoring. *J Heart Lung Transplant* 1999;18:143–9.

265. Przepiorka D et al. Tacrolimus and minidose methotrexate for prevention of acute graft-versus-host disease after matched unrelated donor marrow transplantation. *Blood* 1996;88:4383–9.

Cardiovascular Drugs

Antiarrhythmic Drugs

ADENOSINE
Adenocard

Pharmacology. Adenosine is a purinergic agonist that acts on the purine P_1 and P_2 receptors (although P_1 receptors are more sensitive to adenosine). Pharmacologic effects include coronary and peripheral vasodilation, negative inotropic actions, and depression of sinus node and AV nodal conduction. It is used most frequently for supraventricular tachycardia caused by re-entry (ie, AV nodal re-entry or AV re-entry associated with an extranodal pathway). In these instances, restoration of sinus rhythm occurs in 85–95% of patients. The drug also can be helpful in diagnosing wide-QRS tachycardias believed to be supraventricular in origin.[1–3]

Adult Dosage. IV for supraventricular tachycardia administer over 1–2 sec through an IV line with minimal dead space, followed by a saline flush; **initial dose** is 6 mg (3 mg if administered through a central line); if this is ineffective, 12 mg can be given 2 min later and repeated if necessary. An average effective dose of 1 mg has been reported in patients receiving concurrent dipyridamole.

Pediatric Dosage. IV 0.1–0.2 mg/kg increased in increments of 0.05 mg/kg q 2 min prn, to a maximum of 0.25 mg/kg.[4]

Dosage Forms. Inj 3 mg/mL.

Pharmacokinetics. Adenosine is rapidly metabolized in blood to inactive adenosine monophosphate and inosine; elimination half-life is about 1–10 sec.

Adverse Reactions. Frequent, but short-lived, subjective complaints include chest discomfort, dyspnea, flushing, and headache. Postconversion arrhythmias also are frequent but transient and include ventricular ectopy, sinus bradycardia, AV block, atrial fibrillation, and rapid reinitiation of supraventricular tachycardia. Adenosine is contraindicated in patients with pre-existing sinus node dysfunction or second- or third-degree heart block without a functioning pacemaker because of the risk of prolonged sinus arrest or AV block. Also use adenosine with caution in asthmatics because it can precipitate bronchospasm, and in patients with atrial fibrillation with an accessory AV pathway because it can accelerate ventricular response.

Drug Interactions. Dipyridamole blocks the cellular uptake of adenosine, enhancing the pharmacologic effect; theophylline, a purine antagonist, inhibits the therapeutic actions of adenosine.

AMIODARONE HYDROCHLORIDE
Cordarone, Pacerone

Pharmacology. Amiodarone is a type III antiarrhythmic that prolongs the effective refractory period of atrial and ventricular tissue by blocking potassium conductance. It decreases sinus rate and slows conduction through the AV node by β-adrenergic blockade. Amiodarone also blocks sodium and calcium channels. The antiarrhythmic actions can be caused by interruption of re-entrant substrate or abolition of premature beats that trigger re-entry.

Administration and Adult Dosage. **PO loading dosage** 800–1600 mg/day in divided doses for 1–2 weeks. Loading dosages are usually toward the lower end of this range for atrial arrhythmias and toward the upper end of the range for ventricular arrhythmias. **PO maintenance dosage** 100–600 mg/day (usually 300–400 mg/day for recurrent ventricular tachycardia and 100–200 mg/day for supraventricular tachycardias such as atrial fibrillation). Some suggest a 600–800 mg/day priming dosage for 1–2 months after the initial loading period and before maintenance therapy.[5] **IV for treatment or prevention of refractory ventricular tachycardia or fibrillation** 150 mg over 10 min 360 mg over the next 6 hr, and 540 mg over the next 18 hr. In one study, amiodarone was administered as a 300 mg IV bolus for cardiac arrest.[6] Initiate amiodarone only during hospitalization for the first several days of the loading phase.

Special Populations. *Pediatric Dosage.* Safety and efficacy not established. **PO** 10–15 mg/kg/day for 10 days and then 5 mg/kg/day maintenance therapy has been used.[7] **IV** 5 mg/kg in 1 mg/kg increments over 5–10 min each; an additional 1 to 5 mg/kg may be given in 30 min if needed.

Geriatric Dosage. Same as adult dosage.

Dosage Forms. **Tab** 200 mg; **Inj** 50 mg/mL.

Patient Instructions. Report any shortness of breath, tiredness, abdominal discomfort, or visual abnormalities. Avoid intense sunlight; use sunscreen. Divided doses during loading or maintenance dosage phases can reduce intestinal upset.

Missed Doses. Take this drug at regular intervals. If you miss a dose, do *not* take it. If it is about time for the next dose, take that dose only. Do not double the dose or take extra.

Pharmacokinetics. *Onset and Duration.* Onset is variable, from several days to a month; full effect might not occur for several months.[8]

Serum Levels. 1–2.5 mg/L (1.6–4 μmol/L) proposed but not well established.[9] Desethylamiodarone accumulates to serum levels similar to or greater than the parent drug.

Fate. Oral absorption is erratic and incomplete; bioavailability is 46 ± 22%. Peak serum concentrations occur in 3–7 hr. The drug is 99.9% plasma protein bound;[8,10] V_d is 66 ± 44 L/kg; Cl is 0.11 ± 0.024 L/hr/kg.[8,10,11] Amiodarone is primarily hepatically eliminated with at least one active metabolite, desethylamiodarone. No unchanged amiodarone or desethylamiodarone is found in urine.[8]

$t_{1/2}$. α phase 4–12 hr; β phase changes with duration of therapy and study sampling. Reported variously as 25 ± 12 days and 53 ± 23 days.[8,10,11] Similar for desethylamiodarone.[8,11]

Adverse Reactions. Corneal microdeposits occur in virtually all patients and are no reason for stopping treatment; however, visual disturbances are reported in about 5%.[11] Neurologic effects occur frequently and include tremor, ataxia, paresthesias, and nightmares, which can be more common during the loading phase.[11] Anorexia, nausea, vomiting, and/or constipation occur frequently. Transient elevations in hepatic enzymes occur in more than 50% of patients, but clinical hepatitis occurs only occasionally.[12] Photosensitivity occurs frequently, and a blue-gray skin pigmentation (sometimes irreversible) develops in 2–4% of patients.[11] Hypothyroidism (low-T_3 syndrome) or hyperthyroidism occurs frequently.[13] Occasional proximal muscle weakness and myopathy have been reported. Symptomatic pulmonary fibrosis has been reported in 1–6% of patients; it is probably not immunologic in etiology and seems to occur more often in patients with underlying lung disease.[11,14] Pulmonary symptoms usually improve with drug discontinuation, but up to 10% of cases result in death.[11,14] Aggravation of ventricular tachycardia and drug-induced torsades de pointes can occur.[11,15] Occasional severe sinus bradycardia (requiring a pacemaker) or AV block has been reported.

Contraindications. Sick sinus syndrome or second- or third-degree heart block in the absence of a ventricular pacemaker; patients in whom bradycardia has caused syncope; long-QT syndrome.

Precautions. Electrophysiologic studies may not predict the long-term efficacy of amiodarone.[16] The benzyl alcohol preservative can be hazardous in infants.

Drug Interactions. Amiodarone inhibits a wide array of cytochrome P450 enzymes including CYP1A2, 2C9, 2D6, and 3A4; it also inhibits *p*-glycoprotein.[17] Amiodarone increases serum levels of cyclosporine, digoxin, flecainide, phenytoin, procainamide, and quinidine. It potentiates the anticoagulant effects of warfarin; reduce the initial dosage of warfarin by one-third to one-half.

Parameters to Monitor. Monitor ECG daily during loading phase for heart rate, PR, QRS, and QT duration. Baseline and periodic thyroid function tests and liver enzymes (especially if symptoms present). Obtain baseline pulmonary function tests; repeat chest x-ray and clinical examination q 3–6 months.[11,14]

Notes. Because of the results of the Cardiac Arrhythmia Suppression Trial (CAST),[18] many clinicians use type III antiarrhythmics (eg, amiodarone, sotalol) as first-line therapy for supraventricular and ventricular arrhythmias. A noniodinated analogue of amiodarone under clinical investigation is **dronedarone**.

BRETYLIUM TOSYLATE   Bretylol, Various

Pharmacology. Bretylium is a type III antiarrhythmic with actions thought to be caused by an initial catecholamine release and subsequent catecholamine depletion and/or direct effect independent of the adrenergic nervous system. Direct actions can be mediated by blockade of potassium channels. Bretylium causes an initial increase in blood pressure, heart rate, and myocardial contractility (from catecholamine release), followed by hypotension (from neuronal blockade). Its greatest usefulness is in severe ventricular tachyarrhythmias resistant to other antiarrhythmics. Bretylium can be effective for ventricular fibrillation but is usually ineffective against ventricular tachycardia.

Administration and Adult Dosage. **IV loading dose** 5 mg/kg push with an additional dose of 10 mg/kg if no response. **Maintenance dosage** IM or IV (over 8 min or more) 5–10 mg/kg q 6 hr or as an IV infusion of 1–2 mg/min.

Special Populations. *Pediatric Dosage.* Not well established, although the following has been suggested: **IV loading dosage for ventricular fibrillation** 5 mg/kg, followed by 10 mg/kg at 15- to 30-min intervals, to a maximum total dosage of 30 mg/kg; **IV maintenance dosage** 5 mg/kg q 6–8 hr.[4]

Geriatric Dosage. Same as adult dosage.

Other Conditions. In renal impairment, lower dosages might be required.[19] A nomogram for dosage in renal insufficiency has been described.[20]

Dosage Forms. **Inj** 50 mg/mL.

Pharmacokinetics. *Onset and Duration.* IV onset usually 5–10 min but can be delayed to 20–60 min; myocardial levels increase gradually over 6–12 hr.[19,21] Duration is usually 6–12 hr after a single dose. Because of persistent myocardial levels, duration after multiple doses can be much longer.[21]

Fate. 23 ± 9% is orally absorbed.[10,19] The drug is not bound to plasma proteins.[19,22] V_d is 5.9 ± 0.8 L/kg;[23] Cl is 0.61 ± 0.11 L/hr/kg.[10] After IV administration, bretylium is primarily cleared renally, with 77 ± 15% excreted in the urine unchanged.[23] Disposition is probably route and concentration dependent.[19,24]

$t_{1/2}$. α phase about 25 min; β phase 8.9 ± 1.8 hr,[19,23] mean of 33.4 hr in renal insufficiency.[20]

Adverse Reactions. Hypotension (usually orthostatic) via adrenergic blockade occurs in up to 50% of patients. The drop in mean arterial pressure is usually not more than 20 mm Hg, but the drop can be severe, necessitating drug discontinuation. Nausea and vomiting occur frequently after rapid IV administration.

Contraindications. Suspected digitalis-induced ventricular tachycardia (can increase the rate of ventricular tachycardia or the likelihood of ventricular fibrillation).

Precautions. Use with caution if hypotension exists before administration. Keep patient supine until tolerance to hypotension develops. Prolonged effects can occur, and dosage reduction in patients with impaired renal function may be required.

Drug Interactions. Bretylium enhances pressor effects of catecholamines.

Parameters to Monitor. Closely monitor blood pressure and constantly monitor ECG.

DIGOXIN   Lanoxin, Various

Pharmacology. Digitalis glycosides exert positive inotropic effects through improved availability of calcium to myocardial contractile elements, thereby increasing cardiac output in CHF. In CHF, digoxin improves the symptoms of CHF but does not alter long-term mortality.[25] Antiarrhythmic actions of digoxin are caused primarily by an increase in AV nodal refractory period via increased vagal tone, sympathetic withdrawal, and direct mechanisms. Digoxin also exerts a moderate, direct vasoconstrictor action on arterial venous smooth muscle.

Administration and Adult Dosage. **IV loading dosage** 10–15 μg/kg in divided doses over 12–24 hr at intervals of 6–8 hr.[26] **PO loading dosage** adjust dosage for percent oral absorption. (*See* Fate.) Usually, 0.5–0.75 mg is given and then 0.125–0.375 mg q 6–8 hr until the desired effect or total digitalizing dosage is achieved. **Maintenance dosage** = (total body stores) × (% lost/day), where total body stores is the original calculated loading dosage and % lost/day is 14 + (Cl_{cr}/5). Usual maintenance dosage ranges from 0.125–0.5 mg/day.[26] A dosage nomogram has also been described.[27] **IM** not recommended.

Special Populations. *Pediatric Dosage.* Base all dosages on ideal body weight. **Total digitalizing dosage (TDD) PO** (premature newborn) 20 μg/kg; (full-term newborn) 30 μg/kg; (1–24 months) 40–50 μg/kg; (2–10 yr) 30–40 μg/kg; (>10 yr) 10–15 μg/kg. Give ½ TDD initially and then ¼ TDD q 8–18 hr twice. **PO maintenance dosage** (premature newborn) 5 μg/kg/day; (full-term newborn) 8–10 μg/kg/day; (1–24 months) 10–12 μg/kg/day; (2–10 yr) 8–10 μg/kg/day; (>10 yr) 2.5–5 μg/kg/day. In children <10 yr, give in 2 divided doses per day. **IV** (all ages) 75% of PO dosage.[4]

Geriatric Dosage. Maintenance dosage can be lower because of age-related decrease in renal function.[28]

Other Conditions. Decrease loading and maintenance dosages with renal impairment. Base dosage on ideal body weight in obese individuals.

Dosage Forms. **Cap** 0.05, 0.1, 0.2 mg; **Elxr** 50 μg/mL; **Tab** 0.125, 0.25 mg; **Inj** 0.1, 0.25 mg/mL.

Patient Instructions. Report feelings of tiredness, appetite loss, nausea, abdominal discomfort, or visual disturbances such as hazy vision, light sensitivity, spots, halos, or red–green blindness.

Missed Doses. Take this drug at regular intervals. If you miss a dose and it has been less than 12 hours since your dose was due, take it as soon as you remember. If it is about time for the next dose, take that dose only. Do not double the dose or take extra.

Pharmacokinetics. *Onset and Duration.* IV onset 14–30 min; peak 1.5–5 hr; somewhat slower after oral administration.

Serum Levels. Therapeutic 0.5–2 μg/L (0.6–2.5 nmol/L); toxic >3 μg/L (3.8 nmol/L). Considerable overlap exists between therapeutic and toxic ranges.[29] Signs or symptoms of toxicity can be evident below 3 μg/L, especially if other risk factors are present.[29] In CHF there does not seem to be an advantage in maintaining the digoxin level above 1 μg/L.[30] Obtain blood samples for digoxin levels at least 4 hr after an IV dose and 6–8 hr after an oral dose to allow central and tissue compartment equilibration. Digoxin concentrations (digitalis-like immunoreactive substance) have been detected in patients with renal failure, neonates, pregnant women, and those with severe liver disease not receiving a digitalis glycoside.[31]

Fate. Oral absorption is 70 ± 13% from tablets; 85% from elixir; 95% from capsules.[32] Enterohepatic recycling of digoxin can be as high as 30%.[33] Protein binding to albumin is 25 ± 5%; V_d is 7–8 L/kg; Cl is 0.16 ± 0.036 L/hr/kg; both depend on renal function.[32] The drug is excreted 60 ± 11% unchanged in the urine in patients with normal renal function.[32] Active metabolites include digitoxigenin, bisdigitoxoside, digoxigenin monodigitoxoside, and dihydrodigoxin.[32]

$t_{1/2}$. α phase 0.5–1 hr; β phase 39 ± 13 hr;[10,32] β phase 3.5–4.5 days in anephric patients.[26]

Adverse Reactions. Arrhythmias, listed by decreasing prevalence, are premature ventricular beats, second- and third-degree heart blocks, AV junctional tachycardia, atrial tachycardia with block, ventricular tachycardia, and SA nodal block.[34] Visual disturbances are related to serum level and occur in up to 25% of patients with digoxin intoxication. They include blurred vision, yellow or green tinting, flickering lights or halos, or red–green color blindness. GI symptoms occur frequently and include abdominal discomfort, anorexia, nausea, and vomiting. CNS side effects occur frequently but are nonspecific, such as weakness, lethargy, disorientation, agitation, and nervousness. Hallucinations and psychosis have been reported. Rare reactions include gynecomastia, hypersensitivity, and thrombocytopenia.

Contraindications. Hypertrophic obstructive cardiomyopathy; suspected digitalis intoxication; second- or third-degree heart block in the absence of mechanical pacing; atrial fibrillation with accessory AV pathway; ventricular fibrillation.

Precautions. Electrolyte abnormalities predisposing to digoxin toxicity include hypokalemia, hypomagnesemia, and hypercalcemia. Hypothyroidism can reduce digoxin requirements because of lower V_d and clearance.[32] Direct current cardioversion carries little risk in the absence of digoxin toxicity.[35] Use with caution in patients with pulmonary disease because hypoxia can sensitize the myocardium to arrhythmias and increase the risk of toxicity.[36] Serious bradyarrhythmias can occur with sick sinus syndrome, but controversy exists concerning the clinical importance of its effects on the SA node. Digoxin can increase infarct size in the nonfailing heart.

Drug Interactions. β-Blockers can worsen CHF or digoxin-induced bradycardia. Potassium loss caused by amphotericin B or diuretics can contribute to digoxin toxicity. Spironolactone can decrease digoxin renal elimination. ACE inhibitors, amiodarone, bepridil, diltiazem, nitrendipine, quinidine, and verapamil can increase digoxin levels. Oral antacids, kaolin-pectin, oral neomycin, and sulfasalazine can reduce digoxin absorption. Penicillamine can decrease serum digoxin levels.

Parameters to Monitor. Obtain serum levels only when compliance, effectiveness, or systemic availability is questioned or toxicity is suspected.[37] (*See* Serum Levels.) Monitor heart rate, ECG for digoxin-induced arrhythmias, subjective complaints of toxicity, and renal function. Monitor serum electrolytes (especially potassium) frequently initially and then q 1–2 months when stabilized.

Notes. Treatment of severe or life-threatening digoxin toxicity should include IV **digoxin immune Fab** (Digibind). About 40 mg (one vial) of digoxin-specific Fab fragments binds 0.6 mg of the glycoside. Exact dosage can be calculated based on estimated total body stores.

DISOPYRAMIDE PHOSPHATE   Norpace, Various

Pharmacology. Disopyramide has qualitatively the same electrophysiologic actions as procainamide and quinidine and is effective for ventricular and (unlabeled) supraventricular tachycardia. It increases systemic vascular resistance through vasoconstriction; it also can exert a profound negative inotropic effect and has marked anticholinergic properties systemically and on the heart. The isomers of disopyramide have stereospecific pharmacologic actions.[38,39]

Administration and Adult Dosage. **PO loading dosage** 300–400 mg. **PO maintenance dosage** 400–800 mg/day, to a maximum of 1.6 g/day. Give daily dosage in 4 equally divided doses q 6 hr with non-SR Cap or in 2 equally divided doses q 12 hr with SR Cap. Initiate disopyramide during hospitalization.

Special Populations. *Pediatric Dosage.* **PO** <1 yr, 10–30 mg/kg/day; 1–4 yr, 10–20 mg/kg/day; 4–12 yr, 10–15 mg/kg/day; 12–18 yr, 6–15 mg/kg/day. Daily dosage is divided into 4 equal doses q 6 hr.[4] (*See* Notes.)

Geriatric Dosage. Decreased dosage is probably necessary because the elderly might not tolerate anticholinergic side effects.

Other Conditions. In patients who weigh less than 50 kg or have hepatic disease or moderate renal insufficiency (Cl_{cr} >40 mL/min), load with 150–200 mg and then give 400 mg/day in 2 or 4 divided doses, depending on the dosage form used. Initial daily dosage in patients with hepatic disease is about 4.4 mg/kg/day.[40,41] In patients with severe renal insufficiency, give maintenance dosages as follows (non-SR Cap):

CREATNINE CLEARANCE	DAILY MAINTENANCE DOSAGE
30–40 mL/min	300 mg
15–30 mL/min	200 mg
<15 mL/min	100 mg

Dosage Forms. **Cap** 100, 150 mg; **SR Cap** 100, 150 mg. (*See* Notes.)

Patient Instructions. Report any symptoms such as difficulty in urination, constipation, blurred vision, or dry mouth. Also report shortness of breath, weight gain, or edema. Do not crush or chew sustained-release capsules. A sustained-release capsule core in the stool does not indicate lack of absorption.

Missed Doses. Take this drug at regular intervals. If you miss a dose, take it as soon as you remember. If it is about time for the next dose, take that dose only. Leave at least 4 hours between regular capsule doses and 6–8 hours between sustained-release capsule doses. Do not double the dose or take extra.

Pharmacokinetics. *Onset and Duration.* PO onset is within 1 hr. Duration differs with individual differences in drug disposition but is usually 6–12 hr.

Serum Levels. Usual range is 2–5 mg/L (6–15 μmol/L),[41,42] with toxicity more likely over 4 mg/L. Therapeutic range of unbound drug is 0.5–2 mg/L (1.5–6 μmol/L).[40] Monitoring unbound concentrations eliminates variability caused by concentration-dependent disposition.[41,43]

Fate. Oral absorption is rapid; systemic availability is 83 ± 11%.[41,42] Unbound drug in serum varies from 19–46% over a serum concentration range of 2–8 mg/L and is also age dependent.[44] V_d (unbound) is 1.4–1.7 L/kg in normal individuals;[10,41] Cl (unbound) is about 0.25 L/hr/kg;[41] Cl is stereospecific.[45] The major metabolite is a mono-*N*-dealkylated form that has weak antiarrhythmic but potent anticholinergic activity; 55 ± 6% is excreted unchanged in urine.[10]

$t_{1/2}$. α phase 2–4 min (IV);[42] β phase is concentration dependent, usually 6 ± 1 hr,[10] 11–17 hr in renal impairment, depending on severity.[44]

Adverse Reactions. Nausea or anorexia occur frequently. Dry mouth, urinary retention, blurred vision, and constipation are dose-related anticholinergic effects that can occur in up to 70% of patients and result in drug discontinuation in about 20%.[46] Through its vagolytic action, disopyramide can cause sinus tachycardia. Severe bradycardia, AV nodal block, or asystole also can occur, especially in patients with SA or AV nodal disease. Exacerbation of CHF is most prevalent (20–40%) in patients with left ventricular systolic dysfunction.[38] Torsades de pointes, similar to quinidine syncope, has been reported. Rarely, rash, hepatic cholestasis, psychosis, or peripheral neuropathy occur. Hypoglycemia also has been reported.

Contraindications. History of disopyramide-induced heart block or serious ventricular arrhythmias; second- or third-degree heart block without a ventricular pacemaker; long-QT syndrome; cardiogenic shock or severe CHF.

Precautions. In atrial fibrillation or flutter, give digoxin or drugs that slow AV nodal conduction before giving disopyramide. Use very cautiously, if at all, in patients with CHF because of negative inotropic and vasoconstrictive actions.[38] The drug can worsen sick sinus syndrome or aggravate underlying ventricular arrhythmias. If possible, use other antiarrhythmics in patients with prostatic hypertrophy or pre-existing urinary retention. Disopyramide can exacerbate glaucoma or myasthenia gravis.

Drug Interactions. Erythromycin inhibits disopyramide metabolism. Phenytoin can decrease disopyramide serum levels and increase its anticholinergic effects. Rifampin, barbiturates, and other enzyme inducers can decrease disopyramide serum levels. Concurrent use of disopyramide and quinidine can increase disopyramide serum levels or decrease quinidine serum levels.

Parameters to Monitor. Because of concentration-dependent protein binding, total drug levels unreliably reflect active drug concentration, and monitoring unbound drug concentrations is preferable. Monitor serum levels and symptoms or signs of toxicity closely in patients with altered states of drug disposition such as renal dysfunction. When initiating therapy, observe ECG daily for 3–4 days for QT, QRS, or PR prolongation. Frequently obtain vital signs initially for evidence of adverse hemodynamic effects (eg, CHF) and less frequently when a maintenance dosage is attained. Question the patient about anticholinergic manifestations such as urinary and visual abnormalities.

Notes. A 1–10 mg/mL suspension, prepared from capsules, in cherry syrup is stable for 1 month with refrigeration in an amber bottle.

DOFETILIDE
Tikosyn

Pharmacology. Dofetilide is a class III antiarrhythmic drug that selectively prolongs atrial and ventricular repolarization by blocking the delayed rectifier (rapid component) potassium current. It is indicated for the termination and prevention of atrial fibrillation and flutter.

Administration and Adult Dosage. PO 125–500 μg bid, adjusted based on response and QT interval prolongation. Initiate therapy during hospitalization.

Special Populations. *Pediatric Dosage.* Safety and efficacy not established.

Geriatric Dosage. Same as adult dosage.

Other Conditions. Reduce maintenance dosages patients with renal dysfunction: 250 μg bid for Cl_{cr} 40–60 mL/min and 125 μg bid for Cl_{cr} 20–40 mL/min.[47,48] Avoid the drug in patients with Cl_{cr} <20 mL/min.

Dosage Forms. Cap 125, 250, 500 μg.

Pharmacokinetics. Oral bioavailability is 96% and peak concentrations occur 2.5 hr after oral administration.[47] V_d is 3.9 ± 1.3 L/kg.[49] About 20% of dofetilide is metabolized hepatically and 80% is eliminated renally as unchanged drug.[47] Elimination half-life is 9.7 ± 2.7 hr with normal renal function.[49]

Adverse Reactions. The major side effect is drug-induced torsades de pointes, which occurs in 1–10% of patients; risk increases with higher dosages.[47] Other risk factors include female sex and underlying CHF.

Contraindications. Severe renal insufficiency; QT prolongation; hypokalemia; previous history of torsades de pointes; Cl_{cr} <20 mL/min.

Drug Interactions. Avoid using dofetilide with drugs that interfere with its renal elimination (eg, cimetidine, ketoconazole, trimethoprim and sulfamethoxazole, prochlorperazine, megestrol).[47,48] Use caution with concurrent use of agents that block CYP3A4 (eg, verapamil, erythromycin). Do not use with other drugs that can prolong the QT interval.

Parameters to Monitor. Initiate dofetilide during hospitalization with continuous ECG monitoring. Decrease dosage if QT prolongation occurs; discontinue if excessive. Monitor renal function q 3 months.

Notes. When administered properly and monitored closely, dofetilide does not seem to increase mortality in patients with CHF.[50] **Azimilide** is another agent currently under investigation that blocks potassium channels (both the rapid and slow components of the delayed rectifier).[51]

FLECAINIDE ACETATE
Tambocor

Pharmacology. Flecainide is a type Ic antiarrhythmic that predominantly slows conduction velocity, with minimal effect on refractoriness. (*See* Electrophysiologic Actions of Antiarrhythmics Comparison Chart.) Compared with type Ia or Ib antiarrhythmics, it binds to and dissociates from the sodium channel very slowly. It can decrease cardiac output by a negative inotropic action.

Administration and Adult Dosage. PO 50 mg q 12 hr initially, increasing in 50 mg increments q 12 hr q 4–7 days until desired response. **Usual maintenance dosage** is 100 mg PO q 12 hr to a maximum of 300 mg/day. Initiate flecainide during hospitalization.

Special Populations. *Pediatric Dosage.* Safety and efficacy not established. PO 100–200 mg/m^2/day (average 140 mg/m^2/day) in 2 divided doses has been used.[52]

Geriatric Dosage. Same as adult dosage.

Other Conditions. Lower maintenance dosage requirements are expected in patients with CHF, liver disease, or renal insufficiency. Start these patients with 50–100 mg q 12–24 hr and cautiously increase dosage as required with the aid of serum levels.[41,53]

Dosage Forms. **Tab** 50, 100, 150 mg.

Patient Instructions. Report any symptoms of dizziness, extra or rapid heart beats, or visual disturbances. Report symptoms of worsening shortness of breath or exercise intolerance.

Missed Doses. Take this drug at regular intervals. If you miss a dose and it has been less than 4 hours since your dose was due, take it as soon as you remember. If it is about time for the next dose, take that dose only. Do not double the dose or take extra.

Pharmacokinetics. *Onset and Duration.* Onset 1–6 hr (average 3); duration 12–30 hr.[53]

Serum Levels. (Therapeutic trough) 0.2–1 mg/L (0.5-2.5 μmol/L).[53,54]

Fate. Oral bioavailability is 70 ± 11%.[10,54] From 37–55% is bound to plasma proteins, but the percentage can be higher (61%) post-MI because of increases in α_1-acid glycoprotein.[53] V_d is 8–10 L/kg;[53] Cl has been reported as 0.34 ± 0.1 L/hr/kg[10] and 0.61 ± 0.23 L/hr/kg;[41,53] Cl decreases with CHF, renal failure, and liver disease. Flecainide is about 60% stereoselectively metabolized by the liver through the CYP2D6 isozyme[55] and about 30% excreted unchanged in urine.

$t_{1/2}$. α phase 3–8 min; β phase 14 ± 5 hr. β phase is 20 ± 4 hr in patients with ventricular ectopy and 37.8 ± 39.7 hr in those with severe renal dysfunction.[56]

Adverse Reactions. Neurologic side effects, which include dizziness and visual abnormalities, occur frequently. Exacerbation of CHF in patients with underlying left ventricular dysfunction occurs frequently. Nausea, dyspnea, and headache also can occur frequently. Flecainide has proarrhythmic effects that can result in new sustained ventricular tachycardia or aggravation of underlying ventricular arrhythmias. These reactions occur more frequently in patients with left ventricular dysfunction, coronary disease, or ventricular arrhythmias.[18,57] Risk can be sustained over time and not limited to the several days after initiation of therapy. Flecainide-induced ventricular tachycardia may be unresponsive to cardioversion or pacing but responsive to lidocaine therapy or sodium bicarbonate. Aggravation of underlying conduction disturbances also can occur.

Contraindications. Second- or third-degree AV block or bifasicular block without a ventricular pacemaker; severe CHF; history of type Ic–induced arrhythmia.

Precautions. Use with caution in patients with sick sinus syndrome and in combination with other negative inotropic drugs such as calcium-channel blockers or β-blockers or after recent therapy with a type Ia antiarrhythmic. Flecainide can increase pacemaker capture threshold.[58] (*See* Notes.)

Drug Interactions. Amiodarone and cimetidine can increase flecainide serum concentrations; flecainide slightly elevates serum digoxin levels.

Parameters to Monitor. Frequent or continuous (preferred) ECG when therapy is initiated and then periodically on an ambulatory basis. Obtain a baseline evaluation of left ventricular function before starting flecainide. Obtain periodic trough serum levels (particularly in those with renal or liver disease and CHF) once an individual's effective level is determined. Observe closely for neurologic toxicities and CHF symptoms when initiating therapy.

Notes. Because the CAST results showed increased mortality in patients with asymptomatic ventricular arrhythmias post-MI who were given flecainide,[18] it should be reserved for individuals with life-threatening ventricular arrhythmias (eg, sustained ventricular tachycardia) refractory to other drugs.

IBUTILIDE FUMARATE   Corvert

Pharmacology. Ibutilide is a class III antiarrhythmic that selectively prolongs atrial and ventricular repolarizations by increasing sodium influx (the window current) and blocking the rapid component of the delayed rectifier potassium current. It is indicated for the acute termination of atrial fibrillation or atrial flutter of recent onset. In these arrhythmias, sinus rhythm is restored in about 50% of patients.[59,60]

Adult Dosage. IV for atrial flutter or fibrillation (≥60 kg) 1 mg over 10 min; (<60 kg) 0.01 mg/kg. If the tachycardia is not terminated 10 min after the end of the initial infusion, the dose can be repeated.

Dosage Forms. Inj 0.1 mg/mL.

Pharmacokinetics. Ibutilide is approximately 40% bound to plasma proteins and has a V_d of 11 ± 4 L/kg.[59,60] It is metabolized primarily by the liver. Although many metabolites have been identified, only a hydroxylated form has shown weak class III activity. Less than 10% is excreted unchanged in urine. Elimination half-life is about 6 hr (range 2–12 hr).[60]

Adverse Reactions. The major side effect is drug-induced proarrhythmia; torsades de pointes (sustained or nonsustained) occurs in 4–5% of patients. Risk factors are hypokalemia, underlying left ventricular dysfunction, and female sex.[61] Rapid IV bolus administration can increase the risk of torsades de pointes.[60] Prior administration of IV $MgSO_4$ can prevent torsades de pointes. Heart block and heart failure have occurred rarely.

Contraindications. Pre-existing hypokalemia or hypomagnesemia; pre-existing long-QT interval; congenital long-QT syndromes; concurrent therapy with other drugs known to delay repolarization.

Precautions. Patients with atrial fibrillation of more than 2 days' duration must be anticoagulated with warfarin for 3 weeks before the administration of ibutilide.

Parameters to Monitor. Give ibutilide with continuous ECG monitoring. Monitor QT interval and serum electrolytes before and after administration.

LIDOCAINE HYDROCHLORIDE
Xylocaine, Various

Pharmacology. Lidocaine's electrophysiologic actions differ in healthy and diseased cardiac tissues. (*See* Electrophysiologic Actions of Antiarrhythmics Comparison Chart.) Most of its antiarrhythmic activity is caused by frequency-dependent blockade of the fast sodium channel in Purkinje fibers. In comparison with other antiarrhythmics, lidocaine binds to and dissociates from the sodium channel very quickly. It is used in the acute treatment of ventricular arrhythmias often associated with MI. Effectiveness in the treatment of supraventricular arrhythmia is limited.

Administration and Adult Dosage. **IV loading dose for ventricular tachycardia or fibrillation** 100 mg (1–1.5 mg/kg) over 1 min; if ineffective, repeat with 50–100 mg q 5–10 min, to a maximum of 300 mg.[62] **IV maintenance** 2–4 mg/min infusion.[62] **IV for neuropathic pain** 5 mg/kg/hr for 60–90 min has been used.[63] (*See* Notes.)

Special Populations. *Pediatric Dosage.* **IV (or intratracheal) loading dose** 1 mg/kg; can repeat q 10–15 min to a maximum of 3–5 mg/kg. **IV maintenance dosage** 20–50 μg/kg/min infusion.[4]

Geriatric Dosage. Same as adult dosage. The elderly can be at increased risk for toxicity because of decreased clearance.

Other Conditions. In CHF, use one-half of IV loading dose. In liver disease or CHF, initial maintenance infusion is 1 mg/min, to a maximum of 2–3 mg/min.[62] In MI without CHF, maintenance infusion rate might need to be decreased by 30–50% in 24 hr;[62] however, empiric dosage alterations in MI are not recommended because of increases in α_1-acid glycoprotein and lidocaine binding.[64]

Dosage Forms. **Inj** 10, 20, 40, 100, 200 mg/mL. Also available premixed in D5W in concentrations of 2, 4, and 8 mg/mL.

Patient Instructions. Report side effects such as drowsiness, perioral numbness or tingling, dizziness, and nausea during maintenance infusion.

Pharmacokinetics. *Onset and Duration.* IV onset is immediate; duration after initial IV bolus is 10–20 min. IM onset is 10 min; duration is 3 hr.[65]

Serum Levels. Therapeutic (total), 1.5–6 mg/L (7–28 μmol/L);[42] unbound, 0.5–1.5 mg/L (2–7 μmol/L).[64] Toxic reactions are more likely at total concentrations >5 mg/L (22 μmol/L).[62] (*See* Adverse Reactions.)

Fate. The drug is well absorbed orally, but a large hepatic first-pass effect limits systemic availability to 35 ± 11%.[66] IM absorption half-life is 12–28 min.[62] The drug is 70 ± 5% bound to plasma proteins;[62] V_d is 1.3 ± 0.4 L/kg in normal individuals and 0.9 ± 0.2 L/kg in patients with CHF.[67] Cl is 0.55 ± 0.14 L/hr/kg, decreased in CHF, liver disease, and during long-term infusion.[62,67,68] Lidocaine is metabolized primarily in the liver, with $2 \pm 1\%$ excreted unchanged in the urine.[67] The major metabolites, monoethylglycinexylidide (MEGX) and glycinexylidide (GX), have neurotoxic[69] and antiarrhythmic[70] actions. Accumulation of these metabolites in renal impairment or during prolonged infusions can contribute to lidocaine toxicity.

$t_{1/2}$. α phase about 8 min;[65,67] β phase 98 ± 24 min.[62,67] The β phases in CHF and liver disease can be prolonged to 4.5 ± 2.4 hr and 6.6 ± 1.1 hr, respectively.[62,67] Elimination half-life of total lidocaine increases to an average of 3.2 ± 0.5 hr 24 hr after MI without CHF and up to 10.2 ± 2 hr after MI with CHF.[71] In MI, the rise in total lidocaine half-life is greater than that of unbound lidocaine.[72]

Adverse Reactions. Serum level–related neurologic side effects including dizziness, nausea, drowsiness, speech disturbances, perioral numbness, muscle twitching, confusion, vertigo, and tinnitus are frequent at total serum levels >5 mg/L. Serious toxicities including psychosis, seizures, and respiratory depression occur at serum levels >9 mg/L.[62] Sinus arrest or severe bradycardia is associated with sinus node disease, toxic drug levels, or concomitant therapy with other antiarrhythmics. Complete AV block can occur, especially in patients with pre-existing bifasicular bundle branch block, AV nodal block, or inferior wall MI.[73,74]

Contraindications. History of hypersensitivity to any amide-type local anesthetic (rare); second- or third-degree heart block unless the site of the block can be localized to the AV node itself[73] or ventricular pacemaker is functional; severe sinus node dysfunction; Stokes–Adams syndrome; atrial fibrillation in association with Wolff–Parkinson–White syndrome.

Precautions. Lidocaine administered to prevent ventricular fibrillation in acute MI is no longer recommended.[74] Toxicity during bronchoscopy caused by tracheal lidocaine absorption has been reported.

Drug Interactions. Propranolol decreases lidocaine clearance, so close monitoring is necessary with concomitant administration of these drugs. Cimetidine can decrease lidocaine clearance, but empiric dosage reduction with concomitant cimetidine is not recommended.[75] Phenytoin can decrease lidocaine serum levels and increase myocardial depression.

Parameters to Monitor. Closely monitor serum levels and signs or symptoms of toxicity in patients with altered drug dispositions such as CHF, hepatic disease, acute MI, or prolonged IV infusion (>24 hr). Monitoring unbound levels is preferable post-MI. Minor subjective and objective toxicities are extremely important because they are often subtle and can forecast more serious toxicities (eg, psychosis or seizures). Continuously observe ECG for therapeutic and/or toxic actions. Frequently monitor vital signs such as blood pressure, heart rate, and respiration.

Notes. IV lidocaine has been used to treat pain of peripheral origin such as neuropathies and burns.[63]

MEXILETINE HYDROCHLORIDE   Mexitil, Various

Pharmacology. Mexiletine has electrophysiologic actions similar to those of lidocaine and tocainide. Depression of conduction is accentuated in ischemic/hypoxic tissue. It also has a slight negative inotropic action. It is used in the treatment of ventricular arrhythmias; effectiveness in supraventricular tachycardias is limited.

Administration and Adult Dosage. **PO loading dose** 400 mg once, followed by maintenance dosage in 8 hr; **PO maintenance dosage** 200–300 mg q 8 hr, to a maximum of 400 mg q 8 hr. **PO for neuropathic pain** 450 mg/day;[76] dosages as high as 10 mg/kg/day have been used to treat the thalamic pain syndrome.[77] (*See* Notes.) Initiate mexiletine during hospitalization.

Special Populations. *Pediatric Dosage.* Safety and efficacy not established.

Geriatric Dosage. Same as adult dosage.

Other Conditions. Reduce maintenance dosage by 30–50% in patients with hepatic disease or severe CHF.[41] Dosage also might need to be decreased with Cl_{cr} <10 mL/min.[78]

Dosage Forms. **Cap** 150, 200, 250 mg.

Patient Instructions. Report numbness, drowsiness, dizziness, or tingling. Nausea or loss of appetite can occur and reduced by taking the drug with food. Report any abnormal bruising.

Missed Doses. Take this drug at regular intervals. If you miss a dose and it has been less than 4 hr since your dose was due, take it as soon as you remember. If it is about time for the next dose, take that dose only. Do not double the dose or take extra.

Pharmacokinetics. *Onset and Duration.* **PO onset** 1–4 hr (average 2); duration 8–16 hr.

Serum Levels. Between 0.5 and 2 mg/L (3–11 μmol/L), although not well correlated with therapeutic or toxic effects.[79]

Fate. Oral bioavailability is 87 ± 13%, and, unlike lidocaine, mexiletine undergoes less than 10% first-pass hepatic elimination.[79,80] Absorption can be incomplete in MI patients receiving narcotic analgesics.[79,80] The drug is 63 ± 3% bound to plasma proteins;[10] V_d is large and has been variably reported as 6.6 ± 0.9 L/kg and 10.8 ± 7.2 L/kg.[79,80] Cl is variable, 0.4–0.6 L/hr/kg[45] decreased in CHF and liver disease.[79] Mexiletine is metabolized predominantly in the liver, where it undergoes polymorphic metabolism, primarily by the CYP2D6 isozyme;[81] 10–20% is excreted unchanged in urine, depending on urinary pH.[79,80]

$t_{1/2}$. α phase 3–12 min. β phase 9.2 ± 2.1 hr[82] and 18.5 hr in poor metabolizers,[81] 15.7 ± 4.9 hr in severe renal dysfunction,[78] and 15 ± 0.6 hr in CHF with or without MI;[83,84] and can be prolonged in cirrhosis.

Adverse Reactions. Neurologic toxicities are frequent and include tremor, ataxia, drowsiness, confusion, paresthesias, and occasionally psychosis or seizures. Minor CNS side effects can occur in up to 40% of patients.[85] Nausea, vomiting, and anorexia are frequent. Mexiletine can aggravate underlying ventricular arrhythmias or conduction disturbances. Thrombocytopenia has been reported rarely.[85] Mexiletine is an ether analogue of lidocaine, so cross-sensitivity between mexiletine and tocainide or lidocaine is not expected.[86]

Contraindications. Second- or third-degree AV block without a ventricular pacemaker; cardiogenic shock.

Precautions. Sick sinus syndrome can worsen. Mexiletine can increase pacemaker capture threshold and alter the effectiveness of internal defibrillators.[57]

Drug Interactions. Mexiletine increases theophylline concentrations by 30–50% by decreasing theophylline metabolism.[87] Phenytoin and rifampin can increase mexiletine metabolism. Quinidine and theophylline occasionally increase serum mexiletine levels.

Parameters to Monitor. ECG for 3–5 days when therapy is initiated and then q 3–6 months on an ambulatory basis. Obtain periodic serum levels once an individual's effective level is determined. Observe closely for neurologic toxicities when initiating therapy.

Notes. The efficacy of mexiletine for ventricular tachycardia can be increased by adding a type Ia antiarrhythmic such as **quinidine.**[88] Mexiletine has been used to treat neuropathic pain such as diabetic neuropathy and for thalamic pain syndrome.[76,77]

MORICIZINE HYDROCHLORIDE   Ethmozine

Pharmacology. Moricizine is a phenothiazinelike type I (probably Ic)[89] antiarrhythmic that (in normal tissue) slows conduction velocity by blocking sodium channels in a frequency-dependent manner. Its effects appear to be accentuated by ischemia.

Administration and Adult Dosage. **PO** 200 q 8 hr initially, increasing daily dosage q 3 days by 150 mg until desired effect or toxicity occurs, to a usual maintenance dosage of 200–300 mg q 8 hr. Initiate moricizine during hospitalization.

Special Populations. *Pediatric Dosage.* Safety and efficacy not established. **PO** 200–600 mg/m^2/day has been used.[90]

Geriatric Dosage. Same as adult dosage.

Other Conditions. Not well studied; patients with hepatic disease might require lower dosages.

Dosage Forms. **Tab** 200, 250, 300 mg.

Patient Instructions. Report any dizziness, rapid heartbeat, or gastrointestinal upset.

Missed Doses. Take this drug at regular intervals. If you miss a dose and it has been less than 4 hours since your dose was due, take it as soon as you remember. If it is about time for the next dose, take that dose only. Do not double the dose or take extra.

Pharmacokinetics. *Onset and Duration.* Onset is variable at 2–20 hr after multiple doses; duration is 12–36 hr after long-term use.[91]

Serum Levels. Correlation between serum levels and therapeutic effect is not well established, but 0.2–3.6 mg/L (0.5–8.4 μmol/L) has been suggested.[92]

Fate. Moricizine is well absorbed after oral administration, but the large hepatic first-pass metabolism limits bioavailability to 34–38%. About 81–90% is bound to plasma proteins.[93] V_d is 5.9 ± 3.2 and 11.6 ± 6.7 L/kg after 1 and 13 days of therapy, respectively.[94] Cl is 3.8 ± 1.8 to 4.7 ± 2.3 L/hr/kg, depending on length of therapy.[95] Moricizine undergoes extensive hepatic metabolism and appears to induce its own metabolism. More than 40 metabolites appear systemically in small quantities.[95] At least two, including moricizine sulfoxide, are active and probably account for some of the drug's antiarrhythmic activity and for its long duration of action. Less than 1% appears in the urine unchanged.[94,95]

$t_{½}$. α phase 4–20 min; β phase 1.6 ± 0.2 hr.[94,95]

Adverse Reactions. Frequent noncardiac side effects include nausea, anorexia, and dizziness. Dizziness can be lessened by administering more frequent, smaller doses. Moricizine has proarrhythmic actions that result in new or worsened ventricular tachycardia in 2–5% of patients. Exacerbation of CHF occurs occasionally. Underlying conduction disturbances such as AV block, ventricular conduction defects, or sick sinus syndrome can worsen. Drug fever has been reported.

Contraindications. Second- or third-degree AV block or bifasicular block without a ventricular pacemaker; cardiogenic shock; hypersensitivity to phenothiazines.

Precautions. Use with caution in patients with sick sinus syndrome. Because of the final results of CAST II,[96] moricizine is indicated only for life-threatening ventricular arrhythmias such as sustained ventricular tachycardia, where there is a clear benefit to therapy.

Drug Interactions. Cimetidine can increase moricizine serum levels. Moricizine decreases theophylline levels.

Parameters to Monitor. Daily ECG for the first 2–4 days, when therapy is initiated, and then q 3–6 months on an ambulatory basis; watch for PR and QRS lengthening and for GI side effects and dizziness.

Notes. Limited data exist on the use of moricizine in supraventricular tachycardias.

PROCAINAMIDE HYDROCHLORIDE   Procanbid, Pronestyl, Various

Pharmacology. Procainamide is a class Ia antiarrhythmic that alters conduction in normal and ischemic tissues by sodium-channel blockade in a fashion similar to that of quinidine. It can decrease systemic blood pressure by causing peripheral ganglionic blockade;[97] it also has weak anticholinergic action and a slight negative inotropic action. The active metabolite *N*-acetylprocainamide (NAPA) has primarily type III antiarrhythmic activity that predominantly delays repolarization by blocking potassium conductance.

Administration and Adult Dosage. **PO loading dose** (Cap, Tab) 1 g over 2 hr in 2 divided doses. **PO maintenance dosage** (Cap, Tab) 1–6 g/day in 4–6 divided doses, to a maximum of 9 g/day;[98] (SR Tab) can be given q 6–8 hr (Pronestyl-SR) or q 12 hr (Procanbid), to a maximum of 50 mg/kg/day. **IV loading dose** 1–1.5 g at 20–50 mg/min[97] or 15–20 mg/kg. **IV maintenance dosage** 1.5–5 mg/min

(20–80 μg/kg/min) infusion.[97] **Intermittent IV or IM** 1–6 g/day in 4–6 divided doses, to a maximum of 9 g/day. Initiate procainamide during hospitalization.

Special Populations. *Pediatric Dosage.* Safety and efficacy not established. **PO** 15–50 mg/kg/day in 4–8 divided doses, to a maximum of 4 g/day; **IV loading dose** 2–6 mg/kg over 5 min (up to 100 mg/dose); can repeat q 5–10 min, to a maximum of 15 mg/kg. **IV maintenance dosage** 20–80 μg/kg/min infusion, to a maximum of 2 g/day. **IM maintenance dosage** 20–30 mg/kg/day in 4–6 divided doses, to a maximum of 4 g/day.[4]

Geriatric Dosage. Same as adult dosage but adjust for age-related decrease in renal function.

Other Conditions. Reduce maintenance dosage in liver disease. In renal insufficiency, procainamide and its active metabolite accumulate, necessitating a lower maintenance dosage.[41] Recent data imply no need for decreasing loading and maintenance dosages in CHF and MI.[99]

Dosage Forms. **Cap, Tab** 250, 375, 500 mg; **SR Tab** (6-hr; Pronestyl-SR, various) 250, 500, 750, 1000 mg; (12-hr; Procanbid) 500, 1000 mg; **Inj** 100, 500 mg/mL.

Patient Instructions. Report any symptoms such as nausea, vomiting, fever, sore throat, joint pain, rash, chest or abdominal pain, and shortness of breath. Do not chew, split, or crush SR tablets. A sustained-release tablet shell in the stool does not indicate lack of absorption.

Missed Doses. Take this drug at regular intervals. If you miss a dose, take it as soon as you remember. If it is about time for the next dose, take that dose only. Leave at least 2 hours between regular capsule or tablet doses and 4–6 hours between sustained-release tablet doses. Do not double the dose or take extra.

Pharmacokinetics. *Onset and Duration.* IV onset is immediate; PO and IM onsets occur within 1 hr; SR Tab preparations are somewhat slower. Duration is usually 3–6 hr.

Serum Levels. Therapeutic range is 4–10 mg/L (17–43 μmol/L);[42] toxicity is more likely at serum levels above 12 mg/L (51 μmol/L). In some arrhythmias (eg, recurrent ventricular tachycardia), levels of at least 20 mg/L (85 μmol/L) may be required to prevent arrhythmias, with average effective levels of 13 mg/L.[98] Effective serum levels of NAPA are 15–25 mg/L (53–88 μmol/L), with overlap between the toxic and therapeutic ranges.[100]

Fate. Oral bioavailability is $83 \pm 16\%$;[10] about $16 \pm 5\%$ is bound to plasma proteins; V_d is 1.9 ± 0.3 L/kg.[10] The drug is $67 \pm 8\%$ excreted in the urine as unchanged; the remainder is metabolized, mostly to active NAPA by the liver, with smaller amounts excreted as para-aminobenzoic acid. Cl is highly variable depending on acetylator status and renal function. The total quantity of NAPA produced depends on liver function and acetylator phenotype.[10,101]

$t_{1/2}$. (Procainamide) α phase about 6 min; β phase 3 ± 0.6 hr in normal individuals, 5.3–20.7 hr in patients with renal dysfunction, and 12.5 ± 1.4 hr in anephric patients. (NAPA) 7 ± 1 hr, 41.5 ± 7.8 hr in renal failure.[10,100,101]

Adverse Reactions. About 50–80% of patients develop a positive ANA, with 30–50% developing symptoms of SLE; genetically slow acetylators more rapidly develop positive ANA and SLE symptoms.[102] Common SLE symptoms or signs are rash, arthralgias, fever, pericarditis, and pleuritis. Although drug cessation usually reverses these symptoms in about 2 weeks, some patients have prolonged manifestations; for others, the SLE syndrome initially can be life threatening.[102] Hypotension frequently can occur after rapid IV administration. Severe bradycardia, AV nodal block, or asystole has been reported. Procainamide can aggravate underlying ventricular arrhythmias and cause torsades de pointes.[103] GI symptoms occur frequently and include nausea and vomiting; drug fever and dermatologic reactions occasionally occur.[103] Agranulocytosis has been reported occasionally and can be fatal. Whether the SR product carries a higher risk of neutropenia than the fast-release preparation is controversial.[104] Hepatitis has been reported rarely.

Contraindications. SLE (including that induced by drugs); second- or third-degree heart block without a ventricular pacemaker; long-QT syndrome; severe sinus node dysfunction or torsades de pointes caused by other type Ia antiarrhythmics.

Precautions. In atrial fibrillation or flutter, procainamide paradoxically can increase ventricular rate; administer digoxin or other drugs that slow AV nodal conduction before procainamide. Procainamide can worsen symptoms of sick sinus syndrome and exacerbate myasthenia gravis.

Drug Interactions. Amiodarone, trimethoprim, cimetidine, and, to a lesser extent, ranitidine can increase procainamide levels; alcohol can decrease levels.

Parameters to Monitor. Monitor serum levels and symptoms or signs of toxicity in patients with suspected altered drug dispositions such as hepatic disease or renal dysfunction. Monitor ECG continuously (with IV) or daily initially (with PO) for QRS, QT, and PR prolongation; monitor oral therapy less frequently once maintenance dosage has been established. Monitor blood pressure frequently when therapy is initiated (especially with IV) and less frequently once a maintenance dosage has been established. Periodically monitor WBC count and signs of infection for development of drug-induced agranulocytosis. Observe closely for symptoms of drug-induced SLE.

PROPAFENONE HYDROCHLORIDE	Rhythmol

Pharmacology. Propafenone is a sodium-channel blocker that slows predominantly atrial and ventricular conduction velocities without appreciably prolonging repolarization. It is therefore classified as a type Ic antiarrhythmic, similar to flecainide. Propafenone is administered as a racemate; the enantiomers and the 5-hydroxy metabolite are equipotent sodium-channel blockers. Propafenone, in particular the (S)-enantiomer, and its active 5-hydroxy metabolite also have variable, nonselective β-blocking actions.[105]

Administration and Adult Dosage. **PO** 150 mg q 8 hr initially, increasing q 3–4 days to desired effect or toxicity. **PO maintenance** 150–200 mg q 8 hr, to a maximum of 1.2 g/day.[106] Initiate propafenone during hospitalization.

Special Populations. *Pediatric Dosage.* Safety and efficacy not established. **PO** 10–20 mg/kg/day in 2–3 divided doses has been used.[107]

Geriatric Dosage. Same as adult dosage. Lower initial dosages have been suggested.[108]

Other Conditions. Bioavailability and half-life are increased in patients with hepatic disease, and a dosage reduction of 50% has been suggested[109] and questioned.[106] Lower initial dosages have been suggested for patients with renal dysfunction.[106]

Dosage Forms. **Tab** 150, 225, 300 mg.

Patient Instructions. Report any symptoms of dizziness, rapid heartbeat, blurred vision, or shortness of breath.

Missed Doses. Take this drug at regular intervals. If you miss a dose, take it as soon as you remember. If it is about time for the next dose, take that dose only. Leave at least 4 hours between doses. Do not double the dose or take extra.

Pharmacokinetics. *Onset and Duration.* Onset 2–4 hr; peak 2–6 hr; duration 4–22 hr.[106,108]

Serum Levels. No established therapeutic range. Levels of parent compound and metabolite are highly variable, depending on genetically determined variations in hepatic metabolisms. Mean minimal effective concentration was 0.2 mg/L (6 μmol/L) in one study.[110] Side effects are more frequent when the trough propafenone level exceeds 0.9 mg/L (26 μmol/L).[111]

Fate. Completely absorbed after oral administration, but large hepatic first-pass metabolism limits bioavailability to $12.1 \pm 11\%$. First-pass elimination appears saturable, so bioavailability is highly variable and increases with larger oral doses and long-term therapy.[106,108,111] About 85–95% is bound to plasma proteins, primarily α_1-acid glycoprotein.[106] V_d is 3.6 ± 2.6 L/kg.[112] The parent drug undergoes polymorphic hepatic metabolism via CYP2D6. Extensive metabolizers (EMs; about 90% of patients) form clinically important quantities of the active metabolite 5-hydroxypropafenone; poor metabolizers (PMs; about 10% of patients) form little of this compound.[108,111] Another active metabolite, N-desethylpropafenone, is not subject to genetic polymorphism.[106,111] Cl is 0.96 ± 1.08 L/hr/kg in EMs and 0.23 ± 0.042 L/hr/kg in PMs.[113] Cl is also stereospecific.

$t_{1/2}$. α phase 5 min; β phase (EMs) 5.5 ± 2 hr; (PMs) 17 ± 8 hr.[111]

Adverse Reactions. Frequent noncardiac side effects include metallic or bitter taste in 15–20% of patients, and nausea and CNS toxicity such as dizziness and headache in 10–15% of patients.[112] Because of the β-blocking activity of propafenone, worsening of asthma or obstructive lung disease can occur.[105,112] Propafenone has proarrhythmic actions (sometimes life-threatening) that can result in new or worsened ventricular tachycardia. This can occur in 5–15% of patients, particularly in those with poor left ventricular function caused by structural heart disease or with underlying ventricular tachycardia. Worsening of existing CHF or underlying conduction disturbances, such as AV block or sick sinus syndrome, can occur. Cholestatic jaundice occurs rarely.[114]

Contraindications. Second- or third-degree AV block or bifasicular block without a ventricular pacemaker; history of type Ic-induced arrhythmia; bronchospastic disorders; uncontrolled CHF; cardiogenic shock; marked hypotension; sick sinus syndrome; bradycardia; electrolyte imbalance.

Precautions. Propafenone can increase pacemaker capture threshold and affect the efficacy of internal defibrillators.[57] Because of the CAST results (although not studied in this trial), propafenone is indicated only for arrhythmias where there is a clear benefit to therapy.

Drug Interactions. Propafenone inhibits hepatic enzymes and reportedly increases serum concentrations of digoxin, theophylline, warfarin, and β-blockers.[108]

Parameters to Monitor. Daily or continuous (preferred) ECG for 3–4 days initially and then q 3–6 months on an ambulatory basis. Observe closely for CNS symptoms such as dizziness.

Notes. Although not a labeled indication, propafenone can be effective for some supraventricular arrhythmias.

QUINIDINE SULFATE	Various
QUINIDINE GLUCONATE	Duraquin, Quinaglute, Quinora, Various

Pharmacology. Quinidine is a class Ia antiarrhythmic that slows conduction velocity, prolongs effective refractory period, and decreases automaticity of normal and diseased fibers. (*See* Electrophysiologic Actions of Antiarrhythmics Comparison Chart.) The cellular mechanism appears to be frequency-dependent blockade of the fast sodium channel. Quinidine also blocks potassium conductance, particularly at low concentrations. AV nodal conduction can be increased reflexly through vasodilation, attributed to peripheral α-adrenergic blockade or vagolytic action. Slight negative inotropic action might be clinically important in patients with severe CHF.

Administration and Adult Dosage. **IM and PO loading doses** not recommended. **PO maintenance dosage** generally 200–400 mg q 6–8 hr; **SR products** (gluconate) can be given q 12 hr, (polygalacturonate) can be given q 8 hr. **IV loading dose** (gluconate) 5–8 mg/kg (3.75–6 mg/kg in CHF) at a rate of 0.3 mg/kg/min. (*See* Notes.) Initiate quinidine during hospitalization.

Special Populations. *Pediatric Dosage.* **PO** (gluconate salt) 15–60 mg/kg/day in 4 divided doses. **IV and IM** not recommended.

Geriatric Dosage. (>60 yr) use lower initial dosages and adjust maintenance dosage based on side effects, therapeutic response, and serum levels.

Other Conditions. In liver disease, CHF, or renal disease, use lower initial dosages and adjust maintenance dosages based on side effects, therapeutic response, and serum levels.[41,115]

Dosage Forms. **Tab** (sulfate) 200, 300 mg; (polygalacturonate) 275 mg; **SR Tab** (gluconate) 324, 330 mg; (sulfate) 300 mg; **Inj** (gluconate) 80 mg/mL. (*See* Notes.)

Patient Instructions. Report any symptoms such as blurred vision, dizziness, tinnitus, diarrhea, abnormal bleeding or bruising, rash, or fainting episodes. Do not crush or chew sustained-release tablets. A sustained-release tablet shell in the stool does not indicate lack of absorption.

Missed Doses. Take this drug at regular intervals. If you miss a dose and it has been less than 2 hours since your dose was due, take it as soon as you remember. If it is about time for the next dose, take that dose only. Do not double the dose or take extra.

Pharmacokinetics. *Onset and Duration.* PO onset of sulfate within 1 hr; SR gluconate and polygalacturonate salts 2–4 hr. IM onset within 1 hr; IV is immediate. Duration (sulfate) 6–8 hr;[116] SR (gluconate) 12 hr; (polygalacturonate) 8–12 hr.

Serum Levels. Therapeutic range about 2–6 mg/L (6–18 μmol/L), depending on assay. Toxicity is more likely with serum levels above 6 mg/L.[41,42]

Fate. Oral sulfate and gluconate are 80 ± 15% and 71 ± 17% bioavailable, respectively, with some first-pass elimination; bioavailability is increased in the elderly; IM absorption is incomplete.[10,116] The drug is 87 ± 3% bound to plasma proteins.[10] V_d is 2.7 ± 1.2 L/kg and 1.8 ± 0.5 L/kg in patients with CHF; Cl is 0.28 ± 0.11 L/hr/kg.[10,117] The elderly and patients with liver disease or CHF are likely to have decreased clearance.[10] Quinidine is metabolized primarily in the liver to two active metabolites, 3-hydroxyquinidine and 2′-quinidinone, and 18 ± 5% of a dose is excreted unchanged in urine.

$t_{\frac{1}{2}}$. α phase about 7 min; β phase in normal individuals, 6.2 ± 1.8 hr.[10] In CHF, Cl and V_d are decreased, so elimination half-life remains about the same.[117] Half-life in alcoholic cirrhosis is prolonged to 9 ± 1 hr.[118]

Adverse Reactions. Diarrhea occurs in up to 30% of patients receiving quinidine and can be treated with **aluminum hydroxide gel** or lessened by using the polygalacturonate salt. Nausea or vomiting occurs frequently. Cinchonism can occur with high levels of quinidine; symptom complex includes tinnitus, blurred vision, headache, and nausea; in severe cases it can progress to delirium and psychosis. Hypotension can occur, especially after IV administration. Quinidine can aggravate underlying ventricular arrhythmias or CHF. Non–dose-related syncope, attributed to drug-induced torsades de pointes, can occur in 1–8% of patients, usually during the first week of therapy; it can occur in association with hypokalemia and/or hypomagnesemia.[119] Asystole or AV nodal block has been reported. Rare or occasional idiosyncratic reactions include hepatitis, drug fever, anaphylactoid reactions, SLE, thrombocytopenia, and hemolytic anemia. IM use can cause pain and muscle damage.[116]

Contraindications. History of immunologic reaction to quinidine or quinine; previous occurrence of quinidine syncope; second- or third-degree heart block without a ventricular pacemaker; severe sinus node dysfunction or long-QT syndrome; digitalis intoxication; myasthenia gravis.

Precautions. In atrial fibrillation or flutter, administer digoxin or other drugs that decrease AV nodal conduction before administering quinidine. Chronic quinidine use in patients with atrial fibrillation is associated with increased mortality,[120] which can be caused by torsades de pointes that occurs late in therapy.[121]

Drug Interactions. Quinidine inhibits CYP2D6 and can alter the disposition of many drugs that undergo genetically determined polymorphic metabolism through this pathway. Use care with concurrent digoxin and quinidine therapy because quinidine increases digoxin serum levels approximately 2-fold by inhibiting P-glycoprotein.[122] Urinary alkalinization (eg, with acetazolamide or antacids) can decrease quinidine clearance. Phenytoin can increase quinidine metabolism. Amiodarone and cimetidine can reduce quinidine clearance. Quinidine occasionally increases warfarin response and serum levels of tricyclic antidepressant.

Parameters to Monitor. Monitor serum levels and signs or symptoms of toxicity in patients with altered drug dispositions such as CHF or liver disease. With ECG, monitor daily for QT, QRS, or PR prolongation for the first 2–4 days of therapy and then q 3–6 months on an ambulatory basis. Frequently monitor blood pressure (especially with IV) when therapy is initiated. Monitoring can decrease after a maintenance dosage has been determined. Monitor liver enzymes during the first 4–8 weeks of therapy. Monitor other parameters such as platelet count and hematocrit only if idiosyncratic reactions are suspected.

Notes. Adjust dosage when switching from one salt form to another; sulfate salt contains 83% quinidine, gluconate 62%, and polygalacturonate 60%. The gluconate and polygalacturonate forms are slowly dissociating salts of quinidine.

SOTALOL HYDROCHLORIDE   Betapace, Betapace AF, Various

Pharmacology. Sotalol is a type III antiarrhythmic that is commercially available as a racemate: the L-isomer has nonselective β-blocking actions, and the D- and L-isomers delay repolarization by blockade of potassium channels. (*See* Electrophysiologic Actions of Antiarrhythmics Comparison Chart.) Sotalol is effective for ventricular and (unlabeled) supraventricular arrhythmias.

Administration and Adult Dosage. **PO for ventricular arrhythmias** (Betapace) 80 mg bid initially, increasing at 2- to 3-day intervals, to a maximum of 640 mg/day in 2 or 3 divided doses. Reserve high dosages (480–640 mg/day) for drug-refractory ventricular arrhythmias. **PO for atrial fibrillation or flutter** (Betapace AF) 80 mg bid initially, increasing at 3-day intervals, to a maximum of 160 mg bid. Initiate sotalol during hospitalization.

Special Populations. *Pediatric Dosage.* Safety and efficacy not established. **PO** 2–8 mg/kg/day in 2 divided doses has been used.[123]

Geriatric Dosage. Same as adult dosage.

Other Conditions. Reduce frequency of administration in patients with renal insufficiency as follows. **Ventricular arrhythmias** (Betapace) Cl_{cr} 30–60 mL/min, q 24 hr; Cl_{cr} 10–30 mL/min, q 36–48 hr.[124] Use with caution, if at all, in patients with Cl_{cr} <10 mL/min. **Atrial arrhythmias** (Betapace AF) Cl_{cr} 40–60 mL/min, q 24 hr; Cl_{cr} <40 mL/min, contraindicated.

Dosage Forms. **Tab** (Betapace) 80, 120, 160, 240 mg; (Betapace AF) 80, 120, 160 mg.

Patient Instructions. Report any symptoms of fainting, dizziness, shortness of breath, or fatigue.

Missed Doses. Take this drug at regular intervals. If you miss a dose and your next dose is more than 8 hours away, take it as soon as you remember. If it is about time for the next dose, take that dose only. Do not double the dose or take extra.

Pharmacokinetics. *Onset and Duration.* PO onset 1–3 hr; duration 12–18 hr.

Serum Levels. 1–3 mg/L (3.7–11 μmol/L), although not well correlated with therapeutic effect. Concentrations required to achieve delay in repolarization might be greater than those for β-blockade.[123]

Fate. Bioavailability is 90–100% with negligible first-pass metabolism.[124] AUC is decreased 20% by food.[124] The drug is not bound to plasma proteins. V_d is 1.2–2.4 L/kg; Cl is 0.13 ± 0.04 L/hr/kg;[124–126] 80–90% is excreted unchanged in urine.[124] The disposition of the D-isomer is similar to that of the racemate.[125,126]

$t_{1/2}$. α phase 3–5 min; β phase variously reported as 7.5 ± 0.8 to 17.5 ± 9.7 hr.[126,127] Half-life is highly dependent on renal function: 22.7 ± 6.4 hr for Cl_{cr} 30–80 mL/hr; 64 ± 27 hr for Cl_{cr} 10–30 mL/hr; and 98 ± 57 hr for Cl_{cr} <10 mL/min.[127]

Adverse Reactions. Fatigue, dyspnea, and bradycardia occur frequently, probably caused by the β-blocking actions of sotalol.[128] Exacerbation of CHF (1.7%) and asthma also can occur. (*See* Propranolol.) Sotalol induces arrhythmias, usually torsades de pointes, in 4.6% of patients.[128] Risk factors for torsades de pointes are hypokalemia, hypomagnesemia, concurrent diuretic usage, and high sotalol dosages.[129]

Contraindications. (Betapace and Betapace AF) Asthma; second- and third-degree AV blocks without a ventricular pacemaker; sinus bradycardia; cardiogenic shock; long QT-syndrome; uncontrolled CHF; (Betapace AF, additional) sick sinus syndrome; baseline QT interval > 450 msec; hypokalemia (<4 mEq/L); Cl_{cr} <40 mL/min.

Precautions. Use with caution in sinus node dysfunction. Because of its β-blocking actions, use sotalol with caution in patients with diabetes, depressed left ventricular function, obstructive pulmonary disease, or peripheral vascular disease. Do not abruptly discontinue the drug in patients with coronary artery disease. Use with caution with electrolyte disorders, other drugs that prolong QT interval, or pre-existing QT prolongation. Escalate dosage only after achieving steady state (2–3 days).[130]

Drug Interactions. Because of its β-blocking actions, observe β-blocker interaction precautions. (*See* Propranolol.)

Parameters to Monitor. Baseline and daily ECG for the first 2–5 days, when therapy is initiated or dosage is adjusted, and then q 3–6 months on an ambulatory basis. QT prolongation to over 550 msec is an indication to discontinue sotalol because of the risk of torsades de pointes.

Notes. Based on the CAST results,[18] many clinicians use type III antiarrhythmics (eg, amiodarone, sotalol) as first-line therapy in supraventricular and ventricular arrhythmias.

TOCAINIDE
Tonocard

Pharmacology. Tocainide has electrophysiologic actions similar to those of lidocaine and mexiletine. Depression of conduction is accentuated in ischemic/hypoxic tissue. Antiarrhythmic actions are somewhat stereospecific. It also has a slight negative inotropic action. It is used in the treatment of ventricular arrhythmias, but it has limited effectiveness in supraventricular tachycardias. There appears to be a concordance of response (and nonresponse) between tocainide and lidocaine.[131]

Administration and Adult Dosage. PO 400 mg q 8 hr initially; **usual maintenance dosage** 1.2–1.8 g/day, to a maximum of 2.4 g/day in 2–3 divided doses. **PO during lidocaine to tocainide conversion** 600 mg q 6 hr for 3 doses, then 600 mg q 12 hr; discontinue lidocaine infusion at the time of the second oral dose of tocainide.[132] Initiate tocainide during hospitalization.

Special Populations. *Pediatric Dosage.* Safety and efficacy not established.

Geriatric Dosage. Same as adult dosage.

Other Conditions. Reduce initial maintenance dosage by 50% in severe liver disease, by 25% in patients with Cl_{cr} 10–30 mL/min, and by 50% in patients with Cl_{cr} <10 mL/min.[133] Dosages might have to be reduced slightly in CHF, but more data are needed.[134]

Dosage Forms. **Tab** 400, 600 mg.

Patient Instructions. Report any symptoms of numbness, drowsiness, dizziness, or tingling. Nausea or loss of appetite can occur and reduced by taking the drug with food. Report sore throat, mouth sores, fever, or abnormal bruising.

Missed Doses. Take this drug at regular intervals. If you miss a dose, take it as soon as you remember. If it is about time for the next dose, take that dose only. Leave at least 4–6 hr between doses. Do not double the dose or take extra.

Pharmacokinetics. *Onset and Duration.* PO onset 1–2 hr (delayed by food); duration 12–24 hr.

Serum Levels. 3–10 mg/L (16–52 μmol/L), although not well correlated with therapeutic or toxic effects.[42,135]

Fate. Oral bioavailability is 89 ± 5% with negligible first-pass metabolism.[133–135] The drug is 10 ± 15% bound to plasma proteins.[10,136] V_d is 3 ± 0.2 L/kg but slightly lower in CHF;[133,134] Cl is 0.16 ± 0.03 L/hr/kg;[10] 38 ± 7% of the drug is excreted unchanged in urine, and 50–60% is hepatically eliminated.[133,135] Renal clearance depends on urine pH; hepatic metabolism is stereospecific, with the (S)-enantiomer eliminated more quickly.[137]

$t_{1/2}$. α phase 5–10 min;[136] β phase 13.5 ± 2.3 hr, 14–19 hr with ventricular arrhythmia or CHF,[135] and 22 ± 3.1 hr in severe renal insufficiency.[138]

Adverse Reactions. Neurologic toxicities, which include dizziness, tremor, ataxia, drowsiness, confusion, and paresthesias, are frequent (30–50%); psychosis and seizures occur occasionally. The neurologic toxicities of lidocaine and tocainide can be additive.[139] Nausea, vomiting, and anorexia occur frequently. Tocainide can exacerbate underlying ventricular arrhythmias or conduction disturbances. Agranulocytosis and other forms of bone marrow depression have been reported in up to 0.18% of patients.[135] Pulmonary fibrosis or interstitial pneumonitis occurs in 0.03–0.11% of patients.[132] Rash and fever occur occasionally, and cross-sensitivity between lidocaine and tocainide is possible.[86]

Contraindications. Second- or third-degree AV block without a ventricular pacemaker.

Precautions. Sick sinus syndrome and CHF can worsen.

Drug Interactions. Cimetidine can decrease tocainide serum levels; rifampin can decrease levels.

Parameters to Monitor. Monitor ECG daily for 2–4 days when therapy is initiated and then q 3–6 months on an ambulatory basis. Obtain periodic serum levels once an individual's effective level is determined. Monitor closely for neurologic toxicities when initiating therapy. Monitor WBC counts frequently, particularly during the first 3 months of therapy.[135] Obtain baseline chest x-ray; repeat if pulmonary symptoms arise.

Notes. Because of reports of bone marrow toxicity, pulmonary fibrosis, and hypersensitivity reactions, the indications for tocainide are restricted to patients with life-threatening ventricular arrhythmias.

ELECTROPHYSIOLOGIC ACTIONS OF ANTIARRHYTHMICS COMPARISON CHART

CLASS AND DRUG[a,b]	CONDUCTION VELOCITY	REFRACTORY PERIOD	AUTOMATICITY	AV NODAL CONDUCTION
IA (INTERMEDIATE SODIUM-CHANNEL BLOCKERS)				
Disopyramide	↓↓	↑↑	↓↓	↑
Procainamide	↓↓	↑↑	↓↓	↑/↓
Quinidine	↓↓	↑↑	↓↓	↑/↓
IB (FAST ON-OFF SODIUM-CHANNEL BLOCKERS)				
Lidocaine				
Normal Tissue	0	→	→	0
Ischemic Tissue	↓↓	↓	→↓	0
Mexiletine	0	→	→	0
Phenytoin				
Normal Tissue	0	→	→	↓
Ischemic Tissue	↓↓	↓	→↓	↓
Tocainide	0	→	→	0
IC (SLOW ON-OFF SODIUM-CHANNEL BLOCKERS)				
Flecainide	↓↓↓	0	→	0
Moricizine[c]	↓↓↓	↓/0	→	0
Propafenone[d]	↓↓↓	0	→	0
II (β—BLOCKERS)				
Propranolol[e]	→	↓ (acute) ↑ (chronic)	→	↑↑

(continued)

322

ELECTROPHYSIOLOGIC ACTIONS OF ANTIARRHYTHMICS COMPARISON CHART (*continued*)

CLASS AND DRUG[a,b]	CONDUCTION VELOCITY	REFRACTORY PERIOD	AUTOMATICITY	AV NODAL CONDUCTION
III (POTASSIUM-CHANNEL BLOCKERS)				
Amiodarone[d,f]	$0/\downarrow$	$\uparrow\uparrow$	0	$\downarrow$
Bretylium	0	$\uparrow\uparrow$	$\uparrow/0$	$\uparrow/0$
Dofetilide	0	$\uparrow\uparrow$	0	0
Ibutilide	0	$\uparrow\uparrow$	0	0
Sotalol[d,g]	0	$\uparrow\uparrow$	0	$\downarrow$
IV (CALCIUM-CHANNEL BLOCKERS)				
Diltiazem	0	0	0	$\downarrow$
Verapamil	0	0	0	$\downarrow\downarrow$

$\uparrow$ = increase, $\downarrow$ = decrease, 0 = minimal or no effect, $\uparrow/\downarrow$ = variable.

[a]Classification system from references 140 and 141.

[b]Type 1 antiarrhythmics are subdivided into Ia, Ib, and Ic based on their actions on repolarization in normal ventricular tissue and their binding characteristics to the sodium channel: type Ia prolongs repolarization; type Ib shortens repolarization; type Ic causes no change in repolarization.

[c]Classification of moricizine is controversial; it also has type Ia characteristics.

[d]Amiodarone, propafenone, and sotalol also have type II or β-adrenergic-blocking activity.

[e]When caused by sympathetic stimulation.

[f]Amiodarone also has type Ib sodium-channel-blocking activity.

[g]Most investigational antiarrhythmics are potassium-channel blockers, many of which are analogues of sotalol.

323

Antihypertensive Drugs

Class Instructions. Antihypertensives. This medication can control but not cure hypertension. Long-term treatment is necessary to control hypertension and prevent damage to several body systems. Do not start or stop taking medications or change the dosage without medical supervision and avoid running out of medications. Some prescription and nonprescription medications can interact with medications for hypertension; make sure that your physician and pharmacist know the names of any other medications that you are taking.

Missed Doses. Take this drug at regular intervals. If you miss a dose, take it as soon as you remember. If it is about time for the next dose, take that dose only. Do not double the dose or take extra.

α_1-ADRENERGIC–BLOCKING DRUGS:

DOXAZOSIN MESYLATE	Cardura
PRAZOSIN HYDROCHLORIDE	Minipress, Various
TERAZOSIN HYDROCHLORIDE	Hytrin, Various

Pharmacology. Doxazosin, prazosin, and terazosin are closely related quinazoline derivatives that selectively block postsynaptic α_1-adrenergic receptors. Total peripheral resistance is reduced through arterial and venous dilatations. Reflex tachycardia that occurs with other vasodilators is infrequent because there is no presynaptic α_2-receptor blockade. The drugs also decrease total cholesterol, increase HDL-c, and may improve glucose tolerance and reduce left ventricular mass during long-term therapy. They increase urine flow in BPH by relaxing smooth muscle tone in the bladder neck and prostate.[142,143]

Administration and Adult Dosage. Give the initial dose and the first dose of all increased dosage regimens at bedtime and observe the patient closely for syncope. **PO for hypertension** (doxazosin) 1 mg/day initially and then double the dose at 1- to 2-week intervals to a maximum of 16 mg/day in a single dose, although dosages over 4 mg/day are more likely to cause postural side effects. (Prazosin) 1 mg bid or tid initially, increasing the dosage slowly, based on response, to the usual dosage of 6–15 mg/day; although the maximum effective dosage is usually 20 mg/day, dosages up to 40 mg/day can be effective in some patients who fail to respond to lower dosages. (Terazosin) 1 mg/day initially, increasing to 2, 5, or 10 mg/day in 1–2 doses to a maximum of 20 mg/day. **PO for benign prostatic hypertrophy** (doxazosin) 1 mg/day initially, doubling the dose at 1- to 2-week intervals to a maximum of 8 mg/day. (Terazosin) 1 mg/day initially increasing to 2, 5, and 10 mg once daily.

Special Populations. *Pediatric Dosage.* **PO for hypertension** (prazosin) 0.05–0.4 mg/kg/day in 2–3 divided doses. Do not exceed single doses of 7 mg and a total daily dosage of 15 mg.[144] (Doxazosin, terazosin) safety and efficacy not established.

Geriatric Dosage. Same as adult dosage.

Dosage Forms. (Doxazosin) **Tab** 1, 2, 4, 8 mg. (Prazosin) **Cap** 1, 2, 5 mg; **Cap** 1, 2, 5 mg with polythiazide 0.5 mg (Minizide). (Terazosin) **Cap** 1, 2, 5, 10 mg.

Patient Instructions. (*See* Antihypertensives Class Instructions.) Take the initial dose of this drug at bedtime. Dizziness or drowsiness can occur with this medication, especially after the first dose or when the dosage is being increased. Do not arise suddenly, stand for long periods, or exercise too vigorously, especially in hot weather. Alcohol can worsen these effects.

Pharmacokinetics. *Onset and Duration.* (Doxazosin) onset 1–2 hr, duration 24 hr for hypertension; full effect for BPH might not occur for 1–2 weeks. (Prazosin) onset 1–2 hr, duration about 6–12 hr, up to 4–6 weeks might be required for full antihypertensive effect. (Terazosin) onset 15 min, duration 24 hr, but up to 6–8 weeks might be required for full antihypertensive effect. In BPH, at least 4–6 weeks might be required to fully evaluate response to a 10 mg/day dosage. (*See* α_1-Adrenergic–Blocking Drugs Comparison Chart.)

Serum Levels. No correlation between serum levels and clinical effect has been established.[10,143]

Fate. (Doxazosin) oral bioavailability is 63 ± 14%; absorption is slowed, but bioavailability is not affected by food; 98–99% is bound to plasma proteins. V_d is 1.5 ± 0.3 L/kg; Cl is 0.1 ± 0.024 L/kg/hr. Extensively metabolized and excreted primarily in the feces, with only about 9% excreted in urine as unchanged drug and metabolites.[10,143] (Prazosin) bioavailability is 68 ± 17%, 48 ± 16% in the elderly; food can delay but not affect the extent of absorption. About 95% is bound to plasma proteins, decreased in cirrhosis and uremia. V_d is 0.63 ± 0.14 L/kg and Cl is 0.24 ± 0.04 L/hr/kg in young patients; V_d is 0.89 ± 0.26 L/kg and Cl is 0.21 ± 0.06 L/hr/kg in the elderly; Cl is lower in CHF and pregnancy. Prazosin is metabolized in the liver by demethylation and conjugation; metabolites have about 20% of the activity of the drug. It is excreted renally as metabolites and 3.4% or less as unchanged drug.[145] (Terazosin) pharmacokinetics do not appear to be affected by uremia, CHF, or aging. Oral bioavailability is about 90%; 90–94% is bound to plasma proteins. V_d is 0.8 ± 0.18 L/kg, and Cl is 0.066 ± 0.012 L/hr/kg.[10] It is extensively metabolized in the liver, with 18% excreted unchanged in feces, 10% unchanged in urine, and the remainder excreted as metabolites.[146]

$t_{1/2}$. (Doxazosin) 10.5 ± 2.4 hr in young adults, 11.9 ± 4.7 hr in the elderly. (Prazosin) 2.1 ± 0.3 hr in young adults, 3.2 ± 0.6 hr in the elderly; also prolonged in CHF and pregnancy. (Terazosin) 13.5 ± 3.5 hr in young adults, 16.2 ± 2.2 hr in the elderly.[147]

Adverse Reactions. The most important adverse effect is first-dose syncope, which is more likely in patients being treated with other antihypertensive drugs, especially diuretics. During long-term treatment, the most frequent reactions are dizziness, headache, drowsiness, lack of energy or weakness, palpitations, or nausea, all of which occur in 5–20% of patients. Occasionally reported are rash, vomiting, diarrhea, edema, orthostatic hypotension, syncope, dyspnea, blurred vision, nasal congestion, or urinary frequency. Rarely, allergic reactions, priapism, or impotence occur.[148]

Contraindications. Allergy to a quinazoline derivative.

Precautions. Syncope can occur after the first dose (doxazosin, 2–6 hr; prazosin, 30–90 min; terazosin, 1–2 hr) and during rapid upward dosage titration or when adding an additional antihypertensive drug. Hold doses of diuretics for 1 day before starting an α_1-blocker. Increase dosage gradually, reduce dosage when adding another antihypertensive, and then retitrate dosage. Use doxazosin with caution in patients with hepatic impairment.

Drug Interactions. β-Blockers and verapamil can enhance postural effects of prazosin; NSAIDs can decrease the hypotensive effect of prazosin. The α_1-blockers can decrease the hypotensive effect of clonidine.

Parameters to Monitor. Monitor blood pressure regularly.

Notes. α_1-Antagonists can be particularly useful for hypertension in men with BPH, in those with hyperlipidemia or renal disease, in diabetics, in physically active young patients (no decrease in cardiac output), and in the elderly.[142,147] However, drugs in this class have not been shown to decrease long-term mortality of hypertension.[143] The doxazosin arm of the ALLHAT study was terminated prematurely because of inferior efficacy in reducing cardiovascular events compared with chlorthalidone.[149] **Tamsulosin** (Flomax) is a selective α_{1a}-receptor blocker, specific for adrenoreceptors in the prostate. Tamsulosin is not indicated for hypertension but rather for signs and symptoms of BPH. The initial oral dosage is 0.4 mg/day, increasing as needed up to 0.8 mg/day.

CAPTOPRIL
Capoten, Various

Pharmacology. Captopril is an ACE inhibitor pharmacologically similar to enalapril. Captopril's rapid onset and short duration of action are advantageous initially to assess patient tolerance to ACE inhibitors but inconvenient during long-term use. (*See* ACE Inhibitors Comparison Chart.)

Adult Dosage. **PO for hypertension** 12.5–25 mg bid–tid initially, increasing after 1–2 weeks to 50 mg bid–tid, to a maximum of 450 mg/day. **PO for CHF** 6.25–25 mg tid initially, increasing over several days based on the patient's tolerance to a dosage of 50 mg tid. Delay further dosage increases, if possible, for at least 2 weeks to evaluate response. Most patients respond to 50–100 mg tid. **For hypertension or CHF** use initial dosages of 6.25–12.5 mg bid–tid and increase slowly in patients on diuretic therapy, with sodium restriction, or with renal impairment. **PO for left ventricular dysfunction post-MI** 6.25 mg once at 3 or more days post-MI and then 12.5 mg tid; increase to 25 mg tid over several days to a target of 50 mg tid over several weeks as tolerated. **PO for diabetic nephropathy** 25 mg tid.

Pediatric Dosage. **PO for hypertension** (neonates) 0.01 mg/kg bid–tid initially; (children) up to 0.3 mg/kg tid initially.[144]

Dosage Forms. **Tab** 12.5, 25, 50, and 100 mg, and 25 or 50 mg in combination with hydrochlorothiazide 15 or 25 mg (Capozide, various).

Pharmacokinetics. Oral bioavailability is about 65%; food decreases absorption, so the drug should be taken on an empty stomach. About 30% is bound to plasma proteins and its V_d is 0.8 ± 0.2 L/kg, higher in CHF; Cl is 0.72 ± 0.08 L/hr/kg decreased with renal dysfunction.[10] Approximately 50% of a dose is metabolized, primarily to captopril disulfide, which can be converted back to active captopril in vivo. Urinary excretion of unchanged captopril is 24–38% over 24 hr. Its half-life is 2.2 ± 0.05 hr in healthy subjects and is prolonged in renal dysfunction or CHF.[10]

Adverse Reactions. Adverse reactions are similar to those of enalapril, although skin rashes and taste impairment can be more prevalent and cough less prevalent.

CLONIDINE HYDROCHLORIDE   Catapres, Various

Pharmacology. Clonidine stimulates postsynaptic α_2-adrenergic receptors in the CNS by activating inhibitory neurons to decrease sympathetic outflow. Clonidine is not a complete agonist, so some of its effects might result from antagonist actions at presynaptic α-receptors.[150] These actions reduce peripheral vascular resistance, renal vascular resistance, heart rate, and blood pressure.

Administration and Adult Dosage. **PO for hypertension** 0.1 mg bid initially, increasing weekly in increments of 0.1 mg/day until the desired response is achieved. **Maintenance dosage for monotherapy** is usually 0.2–0.6 mg/day, to a maximum of 2.4 mg/day. If rapid lowering of blood pressure is desired (eg, hypertensive urgency), give 0.1–0.2 mg initially and then 0.1 mg q 1 hr until the desired response is achieved or a total of 0.8 mg has been given. **SR patch for hypertension** initially apply one #1 (0.1 mg/24 hr) patch weekly; dosage can be increased at 1- to 2-week intervals up to a #3 patch that delivers 0.3 mg/24 hr. Dosages in excess of two #3 patches/week do not add efficacy. **PO for opiate withdrawal** 1.25–1.5 mg/day in 3–4 divided doses and then decreasing over 14 days by 0.1–0.2 mg/day.[151] **PO for smoking cessation** 0.15–0.675 mg/day in divided doses. **SR patch for smoking cessation** apply one #1 (0.1 mg/24 hr) patch weekly.[152] (*See* Notes.)

Special Populations. *Pediatric Dosage.* **PO for hypertension** 0.05–0.4 mg bid.

Geriatric Dosage. Lower oral dosages might be required, but decreased skin permeability might require higher transdermal dosages.[153]

Other Conditions. In renal impairment, lower oral dosages might be required, but decreased skin permeability might require higher transdermal dosages.[153]

Dosage Forms. **Tab** 0.1, 0.2, 0.3 mg; **Tab** 0.1, 0.2, 0.3 mg with chlorthalidone 15 mg (Combipres, various); **SR Patch** 0.1, 0.2, 0.3 mg/24 hr.

Patient Instructions. (*See* Antihypertensives Class Instructions.) Do not abruptly discontinue this drug or interrupt therapy unless under medical supervision. Apply transdermal patches weekly to a clean, hairless area of the upper arm or torso that is free of irritation, abrasions, or scars. Do not touch the adhesive surface. Apply patch to a different location with each application. If the system loosens during the 7 days, apply the adhesive overlay directly over the system. If a generalized rash or moderate to severe redness or vesicles appear at the site of application, notify the prescriber. Dispose of the patch by folding the sides together and placing it in a disposal site inaccessible to children.

Missed Doses. Take this drug at regular intervals. If you miss a dose, take it as soon as you remember. If it is about time for your next dose, take that dose only. Do not double the dose or take extra. Contact your physician if you miss two or more doses or if you are late in changing the transdermal system by 3 or more days.

Pharmacokinetics. *Onset and Duration.* (Hypertension) PO onset 30–60 min; peak 2–5 hr; duration 6–8 hr but can increase to 12–24 hr with long-term use.[153] Transdermally, maximal reduction in blood pressure occurs in 2–3 days and persists throughout the 7-day application period. After removal, blood pressure rapidly increases toward baseline, followed by a slower rate of increase, and returns to pretreatment levels over several days.[150]

Serum Levels. (Hypotensive effect) 0.2–2 μg/L (0.9–9 nmol/L); (dry mouth, sedation) 1.5–2 μg/L.[153]

Fate. Oral bioavailability is 75–95%.[153] Transdermally, maximum serum levels are reached in 3–4 days and remain constant throughout the 7-day application period.[150] Rate of release is a zero-order process and primarily controlled by the delivery system. Serum concentrations remain constant when a patch is removed and another is immediately applied to a different site.[150] Clonidine is 20% bound to plasma proteins; V_d is 2.1 ± 0.4 L/kg; Cl is 0.186 ± 0.072 L/hr/kg.[10] It is metabolized in the liver, with drug and metabolites excreted primarily in urine; remaining drug may undergo enterohepatic recycling. About 62% is excreted unchanged in urine.[10]

$t_{1/2}$. (PO) α phase 10.8 ± 4.7 min; β phase 12 ± 7 hr.[10] (Transdermal) 14 hr but can be up to 26 hr, reflecting continued absorption from a skin depot.[150]

Adverse Reactions. Frequent adverse reactions include dry mouth (40%), drowsiness (33%), dizziness (16%), constipation (10%), weakness (10%), sedation (10%), nausea or vomiting (5%), nervousness and agitation (3%), orthostatic hypotension (3%), and sexual dysfunction (3%). Occasionally rash, weight gain, anorexia, transient abnormalities in liver function tests, insomnia or vivid dreams, palpitations, tachycardia or bradycardia, or urinary retention occur. Rarely hepatitis, thrombocytopenia, parotitis, elevations of blood glucose or CPK, or cardiac conduction disturbances occur. Allergic contact dermatitis occurs in up to 50% of patients treated with patches.[154] Abrupt withdrawal of oral therapy can result in a withdrawal reaction characterized by rapid reversal of the antihypertensive effect within 24–48 hr up to or above pretreatment levels, a rise of blood pressure above 40 mm Hg systolic or 25 mm Hg diastolic, or blood pressure above 225/125 mm Hg. Subjective symptoms of sweating, palpitations, anxiety, and insomnia also can occur, even without marked blood pressure changes. The frequency and severity of symptoms appear to be greater in patients treated with high dosages for more than 3 months and in those with more severe hypertension.[155]

Precautions. Use with caution in patients with severe coronary insufficiency, conduction disturbances, recent MI, cerebrovascular disease, or chronic renal failure. Patients who develop rashes from the transdermal system can develop generalized skin rashes if oral clonidine is substituted.[154] Inadvertent person-to-person transfer of the patches has been reported; check the application site frequently and dispose of the patch by folding adhesive sides together and placing it in a container inaccessible to children.[156]

Drug Interactions. Tricyclic antidepressants can decrease the hypotensive effect of clonidine. Clonidine can inhibit the antiparkinson effect of levodopa. Clonidine use with propranolol can cause *hyper*tension, especially if clonidine is abruptly discontinued. Direct-acting sympathomimetics can have an exaggerated effect during clonidine use. Prazosin can decrease the effects of clonidine. Synergistic hypotension and conduction disturbances can occur with verapamil.

Parameters to Monitor. Monitor blood pressure regularly; check patient compliance.

Notes. Clonidine has been used to suppress symptoms of withdrawal of opiates and to reduce craving and other symptoms in alcohol and tobacco withdrawal.[151,152,157] It also has been used in a variety of psychiatric applications including treatment of mania, anxiety, panic disorders, schizophrenia, and antipsychotic-induced tardive dyskinesia.[157] As an aid in the diagnosis of pheochromocytoma, a single 0.3 mg dose has been administered after determination of baseline catecholamine levels, followed by three subsequent determinations at hourly intervals.[158] Other conditions for which it can be effective include diabetic diarrhea (0.1–0.6 mg q 12 hr), menopausal flushing (0.05–0.15 mg/day in divided doses), and premenstrual syndrome.[159–161]

DIAZOXIDE
Hyperstat I.V., Proglycem

Pharmacology. Diazoxide is a nondiuretic thiazide that reduces total peripheral resistance by direct relaxation of arteriolar smooth muscle. It also increases heart rate, cardiac output, and renal blood flow. Diazoxide increases blood glucose by inhibiting insulin release and peripheral utilization.

Adult Dosage. **IV for severe hypertension** 1–3 mg/kg, to a maximum single dose of 150 mg administered undiluted over less than 30 sec q 5–15 min, until adequate blood pressure reduction is achieved. Repeat q 4–24 hr as needed to maintain blood pressure control to a maximum of 10 days. **PO for hypoglycemia** 3–8 mg/kg/day in 2–3 equal doses q 8–12 hr, titrated to response.

Pediatric Dosage. **IV for severe hypertension** same as adult dosage. **PO for hypoglycemia** (neonates and infants) 8–15 mg/kg/day in 2–3 divided doses q 8–12 hr, titrated to response; (children) same as adult dosage.

Dosage Forms. **Inj** 15 mg/mL (Hyperstat I.V.); **Cap** 50 mg (Proglycem); **Susp** 50 mg/mL (Proglycem).

Pharmacokinetics. Antihypertensive onset is 1–4 min; peak within 5 min; duration is 3–12 hr. Hyperglycemia onset within 1 hr; duration 8 hr. Oral bioavailability is 86–96%; 94 ± 14% is bound to plasma proteins at typical concentrations, decreased at higher concentrations and in uremia. V_d is 0.21 ± 0.02 L/kg with normal renal function; Cl is 0.0036 ± 0.0012 L/hr/kg. The drug is metabolized by oxidation and sulfate conjugation and excreted slowly in urine as unchanged drug (20–50%) and metabolites.[10,162] Half-life is 48 ± 12 hr, prolonged in renal failure in proportion to Cl_{cr}.[10,162]

Adverse Reactions. (Hypertension) hypotension, nausea and vomiting, dizziness, and weakness are the most frequent reactions. Sodium and water retention and hyperglycemia can occur, especially with repeated administration. (Hypoglycemia) frequent reactions include sodium and fluid retention; hyperglycemia or glycosuria, which might require dosage reduction; hirsutism; tachycardia; palpitations; increases in uric acid; thrombocytopenia with or without purpura, which requires discontinuation of the drug. Rarely, diabetic ketoacidosis or hyperosmolar, nonketotic coma can develop rapidly.

Contraindications. Hypersensitivity to thiazides or other sulfonamide derivatives; compensatory hypertension, such as that seen secondary to coarctation of the aorta or arteriovenous shunts; functional hypoglycemia; dissecting aortic aneurysm.

Precautions. Use with caution with impaired cerebral or cardiac circulation. Avoid extravasation of the IV drug. Recent or co-administration of other antihypertensive drugs can produce excessive blood pressure reduction with the IV route.

Drug Interactions. Diazoxide and hydantoins can be mutually antagonistic. Use with a thiazide diuretic can potentiate hyperuricemia and hypotensive effects. Phenothiazines can potentiate the effects of oral diazoxide. Diazoxide can antagonize the effects of sulfonylureas.

Parameters to Monitor. (Hypertension) Obtain blood pressure frequently until stable and then hourly; monitor blood glucose and uric acid with repeated doses. Monitor for signs of cerebral or myocardial ischemia. (Hypoglycemia) Obtain frequent blood glucose and urine glucose and ketones initially, when dosage adjustments or dosage form changes are made, and then regularly during stabilization.

ENALAPRIL MALEATE	Vasotec
ENALAPRILAT	Vasotec I.V.

Pharmacology. Enalapril is a prodrug that is rapidly converted to its active metabolite, enalaprilat, by ester hydrolysis in the liver. Enalaprilat is a competitive ACE inhibitor. It also reduces serum aldosterone, leading to decreased sodium retention, potentiates the vasodilator kallikrein–kinin system, and can alter prostanoid metabolism, inhibit the sympathetic nervous system, and inhibit the tissue renin–angiotensin system. The net effect is reduction in total peripheral resistance and blood pressure in hypertensive patients, especially those with high pretreatment plasma renin activity and increased renal plasma flow, and reduction of elevated afterload in patients with CHF.[163]

Administration and Adult Dosage. **PO for hypertension** 5 mg/day initially. **Usual maintenance dosage** is 10–40 mg/day in 1–2 doses. If the patient has recently been receiving a diuretic, discontinue the diuretic for 2–3 days or start with a lower initial enalapril dose of 2.5 mg; bid administration might be necessary in some individuals to achieve adequate 24-hr blood pressure control. A diuretic can be added if blood pressure control is inadequate with enalapril monotherapy. **PO for CHF** 2.5 mg daily or bid initially, using the lower dosage for patients taking a diuretic. **Usual maintenance dosage** is 5–20 mg/day, to a maximum of 40 mg; bid administration is preferred. **IV for hypertension** 1.25 mg (0.625 mg initially if patient is taking a diuretic) over 5 min q 6 hr. Dosages as high as 5 mg q 6 hr can be tolerated for up to 36 hr, but there is inadequate experience with dosages over 20 mg/day. For patients converting from PO to IV, 5 mg/day PO is about equivalent to 1.25 mg IV q 6 hr.

Special Populations. *Pediatric Dosage.* Safety and efficacy not established.

Geriatric Dosage. No change necessarily required but observe cautions for impaired renal function.

Other Conditions. For patients with $Cl_{cr} \leq 30$ mL/min, $Cr_s >3$ mg/dL, or CHF with serum sodium <130 mEq/L, use lower initial doses (2.5 mg PO; 0.625 mg IV). For patients on dialysis, the initial dose should be no greater than 0.625 mg IV q 6 hr or 2.5 mg PO on dialysis days.

Dosage Forms. **Tab** 2.5, 5, 10, 20 mg (Enalapril); **Tab** 5 mg with hydrochlorothiazide 12.5 mg, 10 mg with hydrochlorothiazide 25 mg (Vaseretic); **SR Tab** 5 mg with diltiazem 180 mg (Teczem), 5 mg with 2.5 or 5 mg felodipine (Lexxel); **Inj** 1.25 mg/mL (enalaprilat).

Patient Instructions. (*See* Antihypertensives Class Instructions.) Use potassium supplements or salt substitutes only under medical supervision. Report any signs or symptoms of the following: infection (eg, sore throat or fever), angioedema (eg, swelling of face, eyes, lips, tongue, larynx, extremities, or hoarseness or difficulty in swallowing), or excessive fluid loss (eg, vomiting, diarrhea, or excessive perspiration). Report any skin rash, taste disturbance, or persistent, dry cough. If you become pregnant while taking this drug, contact your prescriber immediately.

Pharmacokinetics. *Onset and Duration.* PO onset is 1 hr; peak in 4–6 hr; duration is up to 24 hr.[164] The onset of action and maximal hemodynamic response correspond to the appearance of enalaprilat in serum.[10] IV onset is 15–30 min; peak is within 1 hr; duration is usually 4–6 hr with recommended doses but can be as long as 12 hr in some patients.[165]

Serum Levels. (Enalaprilat) 5–20 μg/L (13–52 nmol/L) is the EC_{50} for ACE inhibition; 40 μg/L (104 nmol/L) produces a mean blood pressure reduction of 12 mm Hg.[10,166]

Fate. Oral bioavailability is 41 ± 15%; it is not altered by meals but is decreased in cirrhosis.[10] Peak enalapril and enalaprilat serum levels after a 10 mg oral dose occur at about 1 and 4 hr, with ranges of 40–50 μg/L (104–130 nmol/L) and 30–40 μg/L (78–104 nmol/L), respectively.[166] About 60% of a dose is converted to enalaprilat; conversion can be reduced in patients with cirrhosis.[166] Enalapril and enalaprilat levels are increased in renal dysfunction. Less than 50% of enalaprilat is bound to plasma protein.[166] $V_{d\beta}$ is 1.7 ± 0.7 L/kg; Cl is 0.294 ± 0.09 L/hr/kg.[167] Cl is decreased in uremia, CHF, the elderly, and neonates.[10] After IV administration, 88% is excreted unchanged in urine;[10] after oral administration, 33% of the dose is recovered in the feces (6% as enalapril, 27% as enalaprilat) and 61% in the urine (18% as enalapril, 43% as enalaprilat).[166,168] Enalapril can be actively secreted into the urine; fecal recovery can indicate unabsorbed drug or biliary excretion.[166]

$t_{1/2}$. (Enalapril) estimated to be 11 hr; (enalaprilat) about 30–35 hr in normals, increased in CHF, renal dysfunction, cirrhosis, and uremia.[10,166]

Adverse Reactions. ACE inhibitors have a common side effect profile. Most adverse effects are related to dosage and renal function. A dry, nonproductive cough occurs in 1–3% or more (up to 20% in some surveys) of treated patients, most frequently in women and nonsmokers.[169] The cough is caused by potentiation of tissue kinins or prostaglandins in the lung. It can be more frequent with longer-acting drugs but is usually not resolved by switching to another ACE inhibitor. Taste disturbances occur in 2–7% but can resolve despite continued therapy.[169,170] Skin rashes occur in 1–7%, usually within a few days to weeks after starting.[170] Rashes often resolve with continued therapy and do not appear to cross-react among ACE inhibitors.[169] Angioedema is an occasional, serious, potentially fatal reaction, possibly more frequent with longer-acting ACE inhibitors and possibly in blacks.[163,169] Hypotension can occur, especially with the first dose, in vigorously diuresed patients, those who are hyponatremic or hypovolemic, those with severe hypertension, and the elderly. In salt-restricted patients with CHF receiving ACE inhibitors and continuous diuretic therapy, up to one-third can experience worsening of renal function that can improve when sodium is replenished.[170] Hyperkalemia occurs in 1–4% of patients, most often in those with diabetes mellitus or renal dysfunction. Proteinuria occurs occasionally with normal renal function and frequently with pre-existing renal disease,[163] although patients with progressive renal insufficiency tolerate the drug well and many experience a reduction in proteinuria despite transient reductions in renal function.[171] Neutropenia can occur, usually in the first 3 months of therapy; it is rare in normal patients but more frequent with high doses or in renal impairment.[169] Cholestatic hepatotoxicity is reported rarely and it can cross-react among ACE inhibitors;[169] it is reversible with drug discontinuation, but fatalities have been reported. Serious fetal harm, including renal failure, face or skull abnormalities, and increased risk of miscarriage, occurs with ACE-inhibitor use during the second and third trimesters of pregnancy.[169]

Contraindications. Angioedema caused by any ACE inhibitor.

Precautions. Pregnancy. It is best to avoid ACE inhibitors in women of childbearing potential who are not actively avoiding pregnancy. Monitor patients on dietary salt restriction, diuretic therapy, or dialysis (salt or volume depletion) for hypotensive episodes after the initial dose. If possible, discontinue these therapies before treatment. Titrate dosage slowly to the minimal effective dosage in patients with impaired renal function or collagen vascular disorders or in patients receiving drugs altering WBC count or immune function.[171,172] Patients with aortic stenosis can develop decreased coronary perfusion when treated with afterload reducers such as ACE inhibitors. Elevations in Cr_s and BUN might require dosage reduction or drug discontinuation. Patients with unilateral or bilateral renal artery stenosis might be more prone to increases in Cr_s and BUN. Hypotension responsive to volume expansion can occur during surgical procedures.

Drug Interactions. Hyperkalemia can develop with concomitant use of potassium-sparing diuretics, potassium supplements, or potassium-containing salt substitutes, particularly with pre-existing renal impairment.[169] Sodium and volume depletion because of a loop diuretic can cause postural hypotension when an ACE inhibitor is begun. ACE inhibitors can increase lithium levels. ACE inhibitors can potentiate oral hypoglycemic drugs and increase neutropenia caused by azathioprine and hypotensive reactions when used with IV plasma protein solutions. NSAIDs can antagonize the hypotensive effect of ACE inhibitors. Phenothiazines can increase the effects of ACE inhibitors and rifampin can decrease the effects of enalapril. ACE inhibitors can increase serum digoxin concentrations.

Parameters to Monitor. Monitor blood pressure regularly. Obtain baseline Cr_s and BUN to assess the potential for adverse effects and titrate dosages accordingly; then monitor periodically. Obtain WBC count with differential q 2 weeks for the first 3 months and then periodically in renally impaired patients or if signs of infection occur. Obtain baseline serum potassium and then monitor periodically, especially in patients receiving potassium-sparing diuretics, potassium supplements, or salt substitutes. Obtain periodic urinary protein estimates (morning urines) by dipstick in patients with renal impairment.

Notes. ACE inhibitors are considered first-line drugs, along with diuretics, β-blockers, and calcium-channel blockers, for the treatment of hypertension.[173] They are also first-line treatments for CHF in combination with digoxin and a diuretic because their use is associated with prolonged survival.[163,174] Regression or attenuation of left ventricular hypertrophy occurs in patients with hypertension and in post-MI patients.[163] Additional advantages of ACE inhibitors are their renal protective effects and improved insulin sensitivity in type 1 diabetics, their lack of adverse effects on serum lipid profile, an improvement in quality of life in hypertensive patients (with one study favoring **captopril** over **enalapril**), and possibly prevention of structural changes in the heart, systemic vasculature, and kidneys.[163,164] ACE inhibitors with greater tissue ACE inhibition (eg, **benazepril, quinapril, ramipril**) might be more effective in this latter regard, but studies are lacking.[163] Ramipril reduces mortality and cardiovascular morbidity in patients without CHF who are at high risk for cardiovascular events.[175](*See* ACE Inhibitors Comparison Chart.)

FENOLDOPAM   Corlopam

Pharmacology. Fenoldopam is a dopamine D_1-receptor agonist that dilates renal and mesenteric vascular beds, thereby reducing total peripheral resistance and increasing renal blood flow and sodium excretion. Stimulation of postsynaptic D_1-receptors leads to smooth muscle relaxation through activation of adenylate cyclase and a subsequent increase in intracellular cyclic AMP. Unlike dopamine, fenoldopam has no α- or β-adrenergic receptor activity, stimulation of which causes increases in blood pressure or heart rate, respectively.[176]

Administration and Adult Dosage. **IV for the in-hospital, short-term (up to 48 hr) management of severe hypertension** 0.03–0.1 μg/kg/min initially, increasing in increments of 0.05–0.1 μg/kg/min at intervals of >20 min to a maximum of 1.7 μg/kg/min.[177] Do not use bolus injections. Lower initial infusion rates and slower titration result in less reflex tachycardia. When the desired effect is achieved, the infusion can be stopped gradually or abruptly because rebound elevation of blood pressure has not been observed.[177]

Special Populations. *Pediatric Dosage.* Safety and efficacy not established.

Geriatric Dosage. Same as adult dosage.

Other Conditions. Dosage adjustments are not necessary for renal or hepatic disease or continuous ambulatory peritoneal dialysis. The effects of hemodialysis have not been evaluated.

Dosage Forms. Inj 10 mg/mL.

Pharmacokinetics. *Onset and Duration.* Onset <15 min; peak 2–6 hr. Blood pressure returns to baseline 2 hr after infusion discontinuation.[178]

Serum Levels. Plasma fenoldopam concentrations of 3.5 μg/L are required for demonstrable reduction in blood pressure. Each 1 μg/L increase in plasma fenoldopam concentration causes a 0.8% decrease in diastolic blood pressure. A concentration of 18 μg/L is required for each 10 mm Hg reduction in diastolic blood pressure.[177]

Fate. Fenoldopam has nonlinear increases in V_d with increases in dosage. V_d is 0.23, 0.66, and 0.67 L/kg at infusion rates of 0.025, 0.25, and 0.5 μg/kg/min, respectively.[177] Cl is dose dependent, increasing from 1.49 L/hr/kg at an infusion rate of 0.025 μg/kg/min to 2.29 L/hr/kg at a rate of 0.5 μg/kg/min.[179] Fenoldopam is about 88% bound to plasma proteins. Elimination is due primarily to conjugation to inactive metabolites. About 90% is excreted in the urine (4% unchanged), 10% in feces.

$t_{1/2}$. 5–10 min.

Adverse Reactions. Fenoldopam causes dose-related reduction in blood pressure and reflex tachycardia; excessive decreases in blood pressure and vasodilation are responsible for most adverse effects. Frequent adverse effects are headache (11–36%), flushing (7–11%), nausea (about 20%), asymptomatic ST-segment abnormalities (6–33%), and hypotension (>5%).[178] Most adverse events occur during the first 24 hr of therapy. Hypokalemia, elevated BUN, serum glucose, transaminase, and LDH have been reported in 0.5–5% of patients. Fenoldopam can cause reversible, dose-related increases in intraocular pressure.[180]

Contraindications. None known.

Precautions. Use with caution in patients with glaucoma or intraocular hypertension. Fenoldopam causes hypotension and reflex tachycardia, which can lead to increased myocardial oxygen demand and possibly ischemia. Closely monitor patients with low serum potassium concentrations, especially during the first 6 hr of fenoldopam therapy.

Drug Interactions. IV allopurinol can attenuate fenoldopam-induced increases in renal blood flow. If possible, avoid concomitant use of β-blockers, which can cause excessive hypotension and inhibition of reflex responses to fenoldopam.

Parameters to Monitor. Monitor blood pressure and heart rate at least q 15 min because of the rapid onset and termination of effects. Monitor serum potassium frequently during fenoldopam therapy, especially during the first 24 hr.

Notes. Fenoldopam reduces blood pressure similar to **nitroprusside**.[181–183] Fenoldopam might be preferred to nitroprusside in patients with renal dysfunction or requiring prolonged therapy due to the accumulation of thiocyanate with nitroprusside.[183,184] Prepare the infusion solution with NS or D5W. It is stable for 24 hr under normal light and temperature conditions.

HYDRALAZINE HYDROCHLORIDE   Apresoline, Various

Pharmacology. Hydralazine is a vasodilator that reduces total peripheral resistance by direct action on vascular smooth muscle, with an effect greater on arterioles than on veins. (*See* Notes.)

Administration and Adult Dosage. PO for hypertension 10 mg qid for the first 2–4 days and increase to 25 mg qid for the remainder of the first week; after the first week, the dosage can be increased to 50 mg qid, to a maximum of 300 mg/day; bid administration can be as effective as qid. **PO for CHF** 50–75 mg bid–qid initially. **Usual maintenance dosage** 200–600 mg/day, but dosages as high as 3 g/day have been used.[185] **IM or IV for hypertension and CHF** 10–40 mg prn.

Special Populations. *Pediatric Dosage.* **PO for hypertension and CHF** 0.75 mg/kg/day or 25 mg/m^2/day initially in 4 divided doses; the initial dose should not exceed 25 mg. Increase gradually over 3–4 weeks, to a maximum of 5 (infants) to 7.5 (children) mg/kg/day or 200 mg/day. **IM or IV for hypertension and CHF** 0.1–0.2 mg/kg q 4–6 hr prn; initial parenteral dosage should not exceed 20 mg.

Geriatric Dosage. Lower dosage and slower titration are desirable because of longer half-life in the elderly.

Dosage Forms. Inj 20 mg/mL; **Tab** 10, 25, 50, 100 mg; **Cap** 25 mg with hydrochlorothiazide 25 mg, 50 mg with hydrochlorothiazide 50 mg, 100 mg with hydrochlorothiazide 50 mg (Apresazide).

Patient Instructions. (*See* Antihypertensives Class Instructions.) This drug can cause headache, dizziness, or palpitations; report if these symptoms are persistent. Report symptoms of drug-induced SLE such as fever, joint pains, dermatitis, pleuritic chest pain, and generalized malaise.

Pharmacokinetics. *Onset and Duration.* **PO** onset in 1 hr; after 300 mg/day, a minimum of 30 hr is required for MAP to return to 50% of baseline value.[186] **IV** onset is in 10–20 min, peak in 10–80 min; **IM** onset is in 10–30 min; duration for IV and IM is 3–8 hr.

Serum Levels. 100 μg/L reduces MAP by 10–20 mm Hg.[10]

Fate. Bioavailability is a function of acetylator phenotype and averages 35 ± 4% for slow acetylators and 16 ± 6% for rapid acetylators. Food can enhance the bioavailability; the first-pass effect might be saturable. Plasma protein binding is 87%. V_d is 1.5 ± 1 L/kg; Cl is 3.36 ± 0.78 L/hr/kg, reduced in CHF. The drug is metabolized extensively by acetylation to multiple metabolites, principally hydrazones, at a rate that is genetically determined; only 1–15% of unchanged drug, as well as metabolites, is excreted in the urine.[10]

$t_{\frac{1}{2}}$. β phase 0.96 ± 0.28 hr, longer in CHF.[10]

Adverse Reactions. Frequently, headache, anorexia, nausea, vomiting, diarrhea, palpitations, tachycardia, and angina occur. Occasionally, hypotension, edema, peripheral neuritis, dizziness, tremors, muscle cramps, urinary retention, nasal congestion, and flushing occur. A syndrome similar to SLE with joint pain and skin rash (only rarely with cerebritis and nephritis) has been reported at an overall frequency of 6.7% in 281 patients over 51 months; daily dosage affects the frequency, with none at 50 mg/day, 5.4% at 100 mg/day, and 10.4% at 200 mg/day. Women had a higher overall frequency than men (11.6 and 2.8%, respectively), and women taking 200 mg/day had a 19.4% rate; slow acetylator phenotype also can increase the risk; the syndrome is reversible with drug discontinuation, although residual effects can be detected years later.[187] An immune complex glomerulonephritis has been reported in patients with hydralazine-induced SLE.[188]

Contraindications. Coronary artery disease, mitral valvular rheumatic disease.

Precautions. Reflex tachycardia can precipitate anginal attacks or ECG evidence of myocardial ischemia.

Drug Interactions. NSAIDs can antagonize the hypotensive effect of hydralazine.

Parameters to Monitor. Blood pressure and heart rate regularly. Baseline and periodic CBC. ANA titers can become positive after several months of therapy; routine monitoring is generally not warranted because the symptoms of hydralazine-induced SLE are characteristic and reversible with drug discontinuation.

Notes. Reflex increases in heart rate, cardiac output, and stroke volume and increases in plasma renin activity and retention of sodium and water can attenuate the antihypertensive action of hydralazine; therefore, long-term regimens for hypertension should include a diuretic and a sympatholytic drug. When hydralazine is used as an afterload-reducing drug in the treatment of CHF in patients on maintenance diuretics, the increase in cardiac output usually prevents the development of reflex tachycardia; likewise, hypotension is usually prevented by the increased cardiac output but can occur if myocardial reserves are inadequate or if the heart cannot respond by increasing output (eg, severe cardiomyopathy or aortic stenosis).[185]

LABELADOL HYDROCHLORIDE   Normodyne, Trandate, Various

Pharmacology. Labetalol is an adrenergic receptor blocking drug that has selective α_1- and nonselective β-adrenergic receptor blocking actions. Although its pharmacologic profile resembles that of other β-blockers and the postsynaptic α_1-adrenergic blocking action of prazosin, its β-blocking activity is approximately 3 times greater than the α-blocking activity after oral administration and 7 times greater after IV administration. During long-term treatment, α-blocking activity is reduced even more.[189,190]

Administration and Adult Dosage. **PO for hypertension** 100 mg bid initially, increasing at 2- to 3-day intervals in 100 mg bid increments until blood pressure is controlled. Usual **maintenance dosage** is 200–400 mg bid, to a maximum of 1.2–2.4 g/day for severe hypertension. **IV for hypertension** 20 mg by slow (2 min) injection, followed by 40–80 mg at 10-min intervals until blood pressure is controlled or to a total of 300 mg. Alternatively, administer a dilute solution by continuous infusion at a rate of 2 mg/min, to a maximum total dosage of 300 mg; the usual effective cumulative dosage is 50–200 mg; the infusion can be repeated q 6–8 hr.[173,189,190]

Special Populations. *Pediatric Dosage.* Safety and efficacy not established, but the following has been used: **IV for hypertension** 0.2–1 (average 0.55) mg/kg initially, followed by a continuous infusion of 0.25–1.5 (average 0.8) mg/kg/hr.[191]

Geriatric Dosage. **PO** Initiate therapy with 50 mg bid.[189]

Other Conditions. Titrate dosage to blood pressure control. No dosage adjustment is required in renal impairment. Patients with hepatic dysfunction might require lower than usual dosages.

Dosage Forms. **Tab** 100, 200, 300 mg; **Inj** 5 mg/mL.

Patient Instructions. (*See* Antihypertensives Class Instructions.) Do not discontinue medication abruptly except under medical supervision. Do not sit up or stand for 3 hours after intravenous administration.

Pharmacokinetics. *Onset and Duration.* PO onset is within 2 hr, peak in 3 hr, and duration of 8–12 hr; can be longer with higher dosages. IV injection onset <10 min, peak in 5–15 min, duration 3–6 hr.[173,190]

Fate. Almost completely absorbed, but bioavailability is only 18 ± 5% because of extensive first-pass metabolism, with the higher values reported in the elderly and patients with cirrhosis.[10,192] Peak serum levels occur within 1–2 hr after oral administration; food delays the time to peak but can increase bioavailability. Plasma protein binding averages 50%. There is little distribution into the brain because of low lipid solubility. V_d is 9.4 ± 3.4 L/kg; Cl is 1.5 ± 0.6 L/hr/kg, lower in young hypertensive patients and the elderly and unchanged in cirrhosis. The drug is metabolized extensively primarily in the liver and possibly gut wall to inactive compounds. Unchanged drug (<5%) and metabolites are excreted in urine and feces.[10,189,190,192]

$t_{1/2}$. β phase 4.9 ± 2 hr, independent of route of administration; increased in the elderly.[10,189,192]

Adverse Reactions. These are generally related to α- and β-adrenergic blockade and usually occur during the first few weeks of therapy. Frequently, dizziness, fatigue, headache, scalp tingling, nausea, dyspepsia, and nasal congestion occur. Occasionally, postural hypotension, edema, taste disturbance, impotence, rash, and blurred vision occur. IV administration causes ventricular arrhythmias rarely.

Contraindications. Bronchial asthma; overt cardiac failure; greater than first-degree heart block; cardiogenic shock; bradycardia.

Precautions. Lower dosages might be required in patients with impaired hepatic function.

Drug Interactions. Cimetidine can increase the bioavailability of oral labetalol. Glutethimide can decrease the effect of labetalol by inducing hepatic enzymes. Concurrent use with halothane can produce myocardial depression. Labetalol decreases the reflex tachycardia induced by nitroglycerin and the bronchodilator effects of β_2-agonist bronchodilators.

Parameters to Monitor. Monitor blood pressure regularly and hepatic and renal function as indicated.

Notes. Labetalol injection is incompatible with 5% sodium bicarbonate, furosemide, or other alkaline products.

LOSARTAN POTASSIUM   Cozaar

Pharmacology. Losartan is a selective, reversible, nonpeptide, competitive antagonist of the angiotensin II receptor (AT_1), which is responsible for the physiologic effects of angiotensin II including vasoconstriction, aldosterone secretion, sympathetic outflow, and stimulation of renal sodium reabsorption. Losartan and other angiotensin II receptor antagonists are highly selective for the AT_1 receptor over the AT_2 receptor, whose physiologic function is unknown. Angiotensin II receptor antagonists have no inhibitory effects on ACE and therefore decrease blood pressure with no appreciable effect on kinin metabolism.[193]

Administration and Adult Dosage. **PO for hypertension** 50 mg/day initially; 25 mg/day in patients on diuretics or volume depleted. The usual dosage is 25–100 mg/day given without regard to meals once daily; may increase to bid in patients not adequately controlled with once-daily administrations. Most patients respond to 50 mg/day, although further reductions in blood pressure are possible with 100 mg/day.[194] Patients who do not respond to 50 mg/day might benefit more with the addition of hydrochlorothiazide than an increased dosage. Dosages above 100 mg/day offer little added benefit.[193]

Special Populations. *Pediatric Dosage.* Safety and efficacy not established.

Geriatric Dosage. Same as adult dosage.

Other Conditions. No dosage adjustment is necessary in patients with renal impairment or on dialysis. Patients with hepatic insufficiency might require lower doses (eg, starting dose of 25 mg/day) because of decreased losartan clearance.

Dosage Forms. **Tab** 25, 50, 100 mg (Cozaar); **Tab** 50 mg with 12.5 mg hydrochlorothiazide, 100 mg with 25 mg hydrochlorothiazide (Hyzaar).

Patient Instructions. (*See* Antihypertensives Class Instructions.) This medication can cause dizziness, especially with the first few doses; do not drive or operate dangerous machinery until you know how you will react to this medicine. Do not use this medicine if you are pregnant or planning to become pregnant. If you become pregnant while taking this medicine, contact your prescriber immediately. Report any skin rash or signs or symptoms of angioedema (eg, swelling of face, eyes, lips, tongue, larynx, extremities, or hoarseness or difficulty in swallowing) immediately to your prescriber.

Pharmacokinetics. *Onset and Duration.* PO onset <2 hr; peak 6 hr; duration >24 hr, can be less with doses ≤25 mg/day.[195] Maximum antihypertensive effect occurs after 1 week in most patients but can take 3–6 weeks.

Serum Levels. Large interindividual variability, with IC_{50} for AT_1 inhibition occurring at losartan concentrations of 1.4–200 nmol/L.[196]

Fate. Oral absorption is rapid, but extensive first-pass metabolism results in a bioavailability of 33%, which might be doubled in hepatic insufficiency. About 14% of an oral dose is converted to an active carboxylic acid metabolite. Peak concentrations of losartan occur in 1 hr and those of its metabolite in 3–4 hr. The metabolite is approximately 10–40 times more potent than the parent compound and is believed to be responsible for most of the antihypertensive effects of losartan.[197] Losartan and its metabolite are about 99% bound to proteins, mainly to albumin. V_ds of losartan and its active metabolite are 34 and 12 L, respectively. Metabolism of losartan occurs through CYP2C9 and CYP3A4 to the active carboxylic acid metabolite and several inactive metabolites. Cl is about 36 L/hr for losartan (12–15% renal Cl) and 3 L/hr for the active metabolite (50% renal Cl). Losartan Cl can be 50% less with hepatic insufficiency.[197] About 4% of an oral losartan dose is excreted unchanged in the urine and 6% of the dose as active metabolite. After oral administration, 60% of a losartan dose is excreted in the feces.

$t_{1/2}$. (Losartan) 2 hr; (metabolite) 6–9 hr.

Adverse Reactions. Angiotensin II receptor antagonists are generally well tolerated, with adverse reactions occurring at frequencies similar to those of placebo; adverse events are not related to dose. The most frequent reactions are headache (10–20%) and upper respiratory tract infection (1–12%).[198] Nasal congestion, cough, and fatigue occur in fewer than 6% of patients.[198,199] Unlike ACE inhibitors, angiotensin II receptor antagonists induce cough about as frequently as placebo, probably because bradykinin concentrations are not elevated as they are with ACE inhibitors. Angiotensin II receptor antagonists are effective alternatives in patients who experience cough with ACE inhibitors.[200,201] Like ACE inhibitors, angiotensin II receptor antagonists can induce reversible renal dysfunction as a consequence of affecting the renin–angiotensin–aldosterone system. Increases in Cr_s and BUN also can occur in patients with unilateral or bilateral renal artery stenosis. Hypersensitivity reactions (eg, angioedema, rash) have been reported in patients receiving losartan or **valsartan.** Angiotensin II receptor antagonists can decrease hemoglobin and hematocrit and increase serum bilirubin, but these changes are rarely of clinical importance. Neutropenia has been reported in 1.8% of patients taking valsartan (0.9% for placebo). Hyperkalemia has been reported in 1.5% of losartan-treated patients (1.3% for ACE inhibitor) and 4.4% of valsartan-treated patients (2.9% for placebo).[199]

Contraindications. Hypersensitivity to any product components.

Precautions. Use of drugs affecting the renin–angiotensin–aldosterone system can cause injury and even death to the developing fetus if used in the second or third trimester of pregnancy. Increase dosage slowly in patients with liver dysfunction because of reduced drug clearance (losartan, valsartan) in these patients. Patients taking angiotensin II receptor antagonists whose renal function is dependent on the renin–angiotensin–aldosterone system (eg, CHF patients) can experience oliguria, progressive azotemia, and (rarely) acute renal failure or death. Reversible increases in Cr_s and/or BUN can occur in patients with unilateral or bilateral renal artery stenosis.

Drug Interactions. Inhibitors of the CYP3A4 or 2C9 isoenzymes (eg, ketoconazole) can impair the conversion of losartan to the active metabolite. **Telmisartan** can increase digoxin serum concentrations. No important interactions have been reported with other drugs in this class.

Parameters to Monitor. Monitor for hypersensitivity reactions (eg, flushing, dyspnea, facial swelling, rash) at the start of therapy. Monitor blood pressure regularly. Monitor patients on dietary salt restriction, diuretic therapy, or dialysis (salt or volume depletion) for hypotensive episodes after the initial dose. Obtain baseline and periodic Cr_s and BUN to assess the potential for adverse effects. Obtain baseline serum potassium, WBC count, hemoglobin, and hematocrit. Monitor periodically for hyperkalemia, neutropenia, and anemia.

Notes. Although the guidelines of the sixth report by the Joint National Committee on Prevention, Detection, Evlauation, and Treatment do not promote this, many clinicians consider AT_1 antagonists first-line therapy for hypertension because of their efficacy, safety, and ease of administration.[173,198] Losartan is a uricosuric, which can lower plasma uric acid concentration and increase the risk of acute uric acid nephropathy or acute gout.[197] Losartan has been shown to improve cardiac output and reduce peripheral vascular resistance and pulmonary capillary wedge pressure in patients with CHF.[202] The ELITE II study found losartan to be comparable but not superior to captopril in improving survival in elderly patients with CHF, although this study was not designed to test equivalence.[203] (*See* Angiotensin II Receptor Antagonists Comparison Chart.)

METHYLDOPA	Aldomet, Various
METHYLDOPATE HYDROCHLORIDE	Aldomet, Various

Pharmacology. The action of methyldopa is thought to be mediated through stimulation of central α-adrenergic receptors in a manner similar to that of clonidine. Stimulation is caused primarily by the metabolite α-methylnorepinephrine.

Administration and Adult Dosage. PO for hypertension 250 mg bid–tid initially, increasing at intervals of no less than 48 hr to the usual daily dosage of 500 mg–2 g/day in 2–4 divided doses. **IV for hypertension** usual dosage is 250–500 mg over 30–60 min in 100 mL D5W q 6 hr, to a maximum of 1 g q 6 hr.

Special Populations. *Pediatric Dosage.* **PO** 10 mg/kg/day in 2–4 doses initially, to a maximum of 65 mg/kg/day or 3 g/day, whichever is less. **IV** 20–40 mg/kg/day in divided doses q 6 hr, to a maximum of 65 mg/kg/day or 3 g/day, whichever is less.

Geriatric Dosage. Use lower dosages to avoid causing syncope.

Other Conditions. Patients with renal failure might respond to smaller dosages of methyldopa.

Dosage Forms. Tab 125, 250, 500 mg; **Tab** 250 mg with chlorothiazide 150 or 250 mg (Aldoclor); **Tab** 250 mg with hydrochlorothiazide 15, 25 mg, 500 mg with hydrochlorothiazide 30, 50 mg (Aldoril, various); **Susp** 50 mg/mL; **IV** 50 mg/mL.

Patient Instructions. (*See* Antihypertensives Class Instructions.) Report changes in mood (depression), loss of appetite, yellowing of eyes or skin, abdominal pain, or unexplained fever or joint pains. This drug can cause your urine to darken if it is exposed to air after voiding.

Pharmacokinetics. *Onset and Duration.* PO onset 2 hr, peak within 4–6 hr, duration 12–24 hr. IV onset 4–6 hr, duration 10–16 hr.

Serum Levels. No correlation between serum levels and therapeutic effect.

Fate. Oral bioavailability is $42 \pm 16\%$.[10] Peak serum levels occur in 2–4 hr but correlate poorly with the hypotensive effect. IV bioavailability is similar to oral, apparently because a large portion of methyldopate ester is not hydrolyzed to methyldopa. From 10 to 15% is bound to plasma proteins. V_d is 0.46 ± 0.15 L/kg; Cl is 0.22 ± 0.06 L/hr/kg and is decreased in uremia. The drug is excreted in the urine as metabolites, sulfate conjugate, and unchanged drug. About 49% (IV) and 70% (PO) of a dose are excreted in urine as sulfate conjugate and unchanged drug.[10,204]

$t_{1/2}$. α phase 0.21 hr (range 0.16–0.26); β phase 1.8 ± 0.6 hr, increased in uremia and in neonates.[10,204]

Adverse Reactions. Frequently, drowsiness, headache, weight gain, nasal stuffiness, postural hypotension, or dry mouth occur. A positive Coombs' test develops in 10–20% of patients, usually between 6 and 12 months of therapy; hemolytic anemia is rare. Occasionally, depression, sexual dysfunction, diarrhea, or nightmares occur. Rarely, hepatitis, drug fever, lupus-like syndrome, leukopenia, thrombocytopenia, or granulocytopenia occur.

Contraindications. Active hepatic disease such as acute hepatitis and active cirrhosis or liver dysfunction associated with previous methyldopa therapy; concurrent MAOI therapy.

Precautions. Use with caution in patients with histories of liver disease. A previously positive Coombs' test does not preclude methyldopa use, but early recognition of hemolytic anemia can be more difficult in such patients.

Drug Interactions. Methyldopa can potentiate the effect of tolbutamide and lithium. It also can cause confusion or disorientation when used with haloperidol. An increase in the pressor response of norepinephrine can occur with concurrent use. Iron products reduce methyldopa absorption. Amphetamines and heterocyclic antidepressants can decrease the efficacy of methyldopa. Levodopa and methyldopa can enhance each other's effects.

Parameters to Monitor. Obtain direct Coombs' test initially and at 6 and 12 months. Obtain baseline and periodic CBC and liver function tests to monitor for hemolytic anemia, blood dyscrasias, and hepatic dysfunction.

Notes. Methyldopa is not a first-line drug because of its frequent side effects, but it can be useful in those with ischemic heart disease or diastolic dysfunction because it reduces left ventricular mass.[205]

MINOXIDIL   Loniten, Rogaine, Various

Pharmacology. Minoxidil is a potent vasodilator that acts by direct relaxation of arteriolar smooth muscle, thereby reducing total peripheral resistance. The vasodilation and associated reduction in blood pressure lead to reflex sympathetic activation, vagal inhibition, and altered renal homeostatic mechanisms manifested as increases in heart rate and cardiac output, increase in renin secretion, and salt and water retention. Because these responses can attenuate the hypotensive actions, give minoxidil with a sympatholytic drug and a diuretic. Topically, minoxidil stimulates vertex hair growth by an unknown mechanism.

Administration and Adult Dosage. **PO for hypertension** 5 mg/day initially as a single daily dose, increasing to 10, 20, and then 40 mg/day q 3 days in single or divided doses based on blood pressure response, to a maximum of 100 mg/day; usual dosage is 10–40 mg/day. If a single dose reduces supine diastolic blood pressure by more than 30 mmHg, divide the total daily dosage into 2 equal doses. **Top for male pattern baldness or female alopecia androgenetica** 1 mL to affected areas bid.

Special Populations. *Pediatric Dosage.* **PO for hypertension** 0.2 mg/kg as a single daily dose, increasing in 50–100% increments q 3 days until optimum blood pressure control or a total daily dosage of 50 mg is achieved; usual dosage is 0.25–1 mg/kg/day.

Geriatric Dosage. Same as adult dosage.

Other Conditions. In renal impairment, lower dosages might be required.

Dosage Forms. **Tab** 2.5, 10 mg (Loniten, various); **Top** 20, 50 mg/mL (2, 5%) (Rogaine, various).

Patient Instructions. (*See* Antihypertensives Class Instructions.) If a dose is missed, wait until the next regularly scheduled dose and continue with your regular dose; do not double the next dose. Report any of the following: increase in resting heart rate of greater than 20 beats per minute, rapid weight gain of more than 5 pounds, or the development of edema, increased difficulty in breathing, new or worsening angina, dizziness, lightheadedness, or fainting.

Pharmacokinetics. *Onset and Duration.* PO single dose onset 30 min; peak 2–3 hr; duration up to 75 hr with a gradual return to baseline at a rate of about 30% per day. Time to maximum effect with repeated administration is a function of dose and averages 7 days at 10 mg/day, 5 days at 20 mg/day, and 3 days at 40 mg/day. Top onset 4 or more months; relapse can occur 3–4 months after drug discontinuation.

Serum Levels. No correlation between serum levels and effects.

Fate. Oral absorption is at least 90%, but bioavailability is probably lower. Protein binding is negligible. V_d is 2.7 ± 0.7 L/kg; Cl is 1.4 ± 0.4 L/hr/kg. The drug is primarily metabolized and renally excreted, with about 20% unchanged drug in the urine. The major metabolite, a glucuronide conjugate, is active and might contribute to the drug's effect.[10,205,206]

$t_{\frac{1}{2}}$. 3.1 ± 0.6 hr.[10]

Adverse Reactions. Frequently, hypertrichosis (elongation, thickening, and enhanced pigmentation) (80%), transient ECG T-wave changes (60%), temporary edema (7%), or tachycardia occur. Occasionally, pericardial effusion with or without tamponade (3%), CHF, or angina occur. Rarely, breast tenderness and rashes (including Stevens–Johnson syndrome) occur. Minor dermatologic reactions occur occasionally after topical application.

Contraindications. (Oral) pheochromocytoma, caused by possible stimulation of catecholamine release from the tumor; acute MI; dissecting aortic aneurysm.

Precautions. For hypertension, minoxidil must usually be administered with a diuretic to prevent fluid retention; a loop diuretic is almost always required. Drugs or regimens that provide around-the-clock sympathetic suppression are usually required to prevent tachycardia, which can precipitate or worsen existing angina. Degenerative myocardial lesions reported in animal studies have yet to be confirmed in humans.

Drug Interactions. Concomitant therapy with guanethidine can result in profound orthostatic hypotension; discontinue guanethidine 1–3 weeks before initiation of oral minoxidil therapy or initiate therapy in the hospital.

Parameters to Monitor. Blood pressure, pulse rate, body weight, cardiac and pulmonary function regularly.

Notes. Minoxidil is reserved for use in severe hypertension in combination with other drugs, usually a diuretic and a sympatholytic drug (eg, β-blocker).[205]

NITROPRUSSIDE SODIUM

Nitropress, Various

Pharmacology. Nitroprusside is a potent vasodilator that has direct action on vascular smooth muscle to reduce arterial pressure and produce a slight increase in heart rate, a mild decrease in cardiac output, and a moderate reduction in total peripheral resistance. The decrease in total peripheral resistance suggests arteriolar dilation (afterload reduction), whereas the reduction in cardiac output might be caused by peripheral pooling of blood (preload reduction). Nitroprusside is somewhat more active on veins than on arteries. The active component of sodium nitroprusside is the free nitroso (NO^-) group.

Administration and Adult Dosage. IV 0.3 μg/kg/min by continuous infusion initially, increasing to an average rate of 3 μg/kg/min based on blood pressure response with a range of 0.5–10 μg/kg/min. Infusion at the maximum rate should never exceed 10 min. Patients receiving other antihypertensives can usually be controlled with smaller dosages. Control administration rates carefully with a microdrip regulator or an infusion pump; avoid too rapid reduction in blood pressure. Infusion rates greater than 2 μg/kg/min generate more cyanide ion (CN^-) than the body can metabolize or eliminate. Maintain infusions at the lowest possible dosage for the shortest possible duration to avoid toxicity.[207] (*See* Adverse Reactions.)

Special Populations. *Pediatric Dosage.* IV same as adult dosage.

Geriatric Dosage. Initiate therapy with low infusion rates and carefully titrate the rate and degree of lowering blood pressure to avoid coronary and cerebral hypoperfusion.

Other Conditions. Patients with CHF, stroke, or receiving other antihypertensive drugs might be particularly sensitive to the blood-pressure–lowering effects of nitroprusside sodium; initiate therapy with low infusion rates and carefully titrate the rate and degree of lowering blood pressure to avoid coronary and cerebral hypoperfusions. Limit the total dosage in renal failure to avoid accumulation of thiocyanate. Use caution in hepatic insufficiency.

Dosage Forms. **Inj** 50 mg.

Pharmacokinetics. *Onset and Duration.* Onset within 1 min; peak 1–2 min; blood pressure usually returns to pretreatment levels in 2–10 min.[173]

Serum Levels. Therapeutic and toxic levels are not established for nitroprusside because of rapid metabolism to cyanide and thiocyanate. Thiocyanate levels >60 mg/L (1 mmol/L) are associated with toxicity.

Fate. Nitroprusside is distributed in a volume that approximates the extravascular space, from which it is rapidly metabolized by a reaction with hemoglobin, yielding cyanmethemoglobin and an unstable intermediate that dissociates, releasing cyanide ion. Cyanide is converted to thiocyanate by the enzyme thiosulfate–cyanide sulfur transferase (rhodanese) in the liver and the kidney. The rate of conversion is determined principally by the availability of sulfur, usually as thiosulfate. Thiocyanate is excreted largely by the kidneys and can accumulate with high infusion rates for prolonged periods or renal dysfunction.

$t_{1/2}$. (Nitroprusside) 2 min; (thiocyanate) 2.7 days, up to 9 days in patients with renal dysfunction.[208]

Adverse Reactions. Most adverse reactions are related to excessive or too rapid reduction of blood pressure and include nausea, retching, diaphoresis, apprehension, restlessness, headache, retrosternal discomfort, palpitations, dizziness, and abdominal pain, all of which resolve when the infusion rate is reduced or the infusion is temporarily discontinued. Thiocyanate is not particularly toxic and usually accumulates to toxic levels only with prolonged (>48 hr) or high-dosage (>10 μg/kg/min) infusions, when cyanide elimination is increased by the administration of thiosulfate, or in the presence of renal dysfunction. To limit the risk of thiocyanate toxicity, infuse at <3 μg/kg/min. Manifestations of thiocyanate toxicity include fatigue, anorexia, nausea, disorientation, toxic psychosis, and hallucinations. Cyanide toxicity usually occurs only when large dosages (>10 μg/kg/min) are infused rapidly or for longer than 1 hr. An early manifestation of cyanide toxicity can be apparent nitroprusside resistance, so increasing dosage requirements to achieve the same level of blood pressure control is an indication to look for metabolic acidosis, an indicator of cyanide toxicity, that might not be evident for more than 1 hr after accumulation of dangerous cyanide levels. Other symptoms of cyanide toxicity include dyspnea, vomiting, dizziness, loss of consciousness, weak pulse, distant heart sounds, areflexia, dilated pupils, shallow breathing, convulsions, and the occasional smell of bitter almonds on the breath. **Hydroxocobalamin** (25 mg/hr by continuous infusion) can facilitate the conversion of cyanide to cyanocobalamin,[209] but an appropriate hydroxocobalamin dosage form is unavailable. Concurrent **sodium thiosulfate** administration also can prevent cyanide toxicity, but thiocyanate levels can increase.[210] Management of cyanide toxicity includes immediate discontinuation of nitroprusside and the administration of sodium nitrite (0.2 mL/kg of a 3% solution IV over 2–4 min), followed by 12.5 g of sodium thiosulfate infused over 10 min. Methemoglobinemia can develop in patients congenitally unable to convert nitroprusside-induced methemoglobin back to hemoglobin. Management consists of IV administration of **methylene blue** 1–2 mg/kg over several minutes.

Contraindications. Compensatory hypertension (eg, arteriovenous shunt or coarctation of the aorta); controlled hypotension during surgery in patients with inadequate cerebral circulation; congenital (Leber's) optic atrophy; use of sildenafil. (*See* Drug Interactions.)

Precautions. If an adequate hypotensive response is not achieved after the maximum recommended infusion rate of 10 μg/kg/min for a maximum of 10 min, stop the infusion because these dosages increase the risk of toxicity. Use with caution in renal, hepatic, or thyroid disease, and in vitamin B_{12} deficiency or elevated intracranial pressure.

Drug Interactions. Use during general anesthesia can impair the capacity to compensate for hypovolemia and anemia and cause abnormal perfusion:ventilation ratio. Use in patients taking sildenafil can result in profound hypotension with serious consequences, including death.

Parameters to Monitor. Monitor blood pressure frequently (ie, every few minutes) because of the rapid onset and offset of effects. Monitor thiocyanate levels after 24–48 hr in patients with normal renal function and daily in patients with impaired renal function or receiving large dosages. However, these levels are of no value in detecting cyanide toxicity. Monitoring of serum cyanide concentrations has been recommended, but the assay is technically difficult and not readily interpretable if fluids other than packed RBCs are analyzed. Frequent monitoring of acid–base balance, particularly in patients with hepatic dysfunction, is considered adequate by most clinicians.

Notes. Protect from light and discard solution after 24 hr or if the color changes from the usual faint brownish tint to blue, green, or dark red. Do not administer IV push medications through the same line or use the solution for the simultaneous administration of any other drug.

OMAPATRILAT (Investigational—Bristol-Myers Squibb)   Vanlev

Pharmacology. Omapatrilat is the first of a new class of drugs called vasopeptidase inhibitors. Omapatrilat inhibits ACE and neutral endopeptidase, leading to blockades of the formation of angiotensin II and the breakdown of vasodilatory hormones such as natriuretic peptides, bradykinin, and adrenomedullin. This results in vasodilation, natriuresis, and diuresis.[211]

Adult Dosage. Not established.

Pharmacokinetics. Oral absorption is rapid, with peak plasma concentrations occurring 0.5–2 hr postdose. Biotransformation of the thiol group produces inactive metabolites; half-life is 14–19 hr; dosage adjustments are not necessary in renal dysfunction.[211]

Adverse Reactions. Omapatrilat is well tolerated, with an adverse event profile similar to that of placebo. The most commonly reported adverse reactions are hypotension (11%) and cough (about 10%). Flushing and syncope (about 1%) also have been reported, and angioedema is rare.[211]

Notes. Omapatrilat produces greater blood pressure reductions than lisinopril in hypertensive patients and in one study reduced morbidity and mortality (not the primary endpoint) to a greater extent than lisinopril in patients with CHF.[212,213]

ACE INHIBITORS COMPARISON CHART

DRUG	DOSAGE FORMS	DAILY ADULT DOSAGE (MG)[a]	INDICATED FOR CHF	PEAK EFFECT (HR)	DURATION (HR)	HALF-LIFE (HR)	ELIMINATION ROUTES
Benazepril Lotensin	Tab 5, 10, 20, 40 mg.	20–40	No	2–4	24+	10–11[b]	Renal, Hepatic.
Captopril Capoten Various	Tab 12.5, 25, 50, 100 mg.	50–150	Yes	1	6–10	2.2	Renal
Enalapril Vasotec	Tab 2.5, 5, 10, 20 mg. Inj 1.25 mg/mL.	PO 10–40; IV 1.25 mg q 6 hr.	Yes	4–6 (PO) 1–4 (IV)	24 (PO) 6 (IV)	11[b]	Renal.
Fosinopril Monopril	Tab 10, 20, 40 mg.	20–40	Yes	3–6	24	12–15[b]	Hepatic, Renal
Lisinopril Prinivil Zestril	Tab 2.5, 5, 10, 20, 30, 40 mg.	10–40	Yes	6	24	12[b]	Renal.
Moexipril Univasc	Tab 7.5, 15 mg.	7.5–30	No	3–8	24	2–9[b]	Hepatic, Renal.
Perindopril Aceon	Tab 2, 4, 8 mg.	4–8	No	3–7	24+	3–10[b]	Renal.
Quinapril Accupril	Tab 5, 10, 20, 40 mg.	20–80	Yes	2–4	24+	2–3[b]	Renal.

(continued)

ACE INHIBITORS COMPARISON CHART (*continued*)

DRUG	DOSAGE FORMS	DAILY ADULT DOSAGE (MG)[a]	INDICATED FOR CHF	PEAK EFFECT (HR)	DURATION (HR)	HALF-LIFE (HR)	ELIMINATION ROUTES
Ramipril Altace	Cap 1.25, 2.5, 5, 10 mg.	2.5–20	Yes[c]	3–8	24+	13–17[b]	Renal, Hepatic.
Trandolapril Mavik	Tab 1, 2, 4 mg.	2–4	Yes[c]	6–8	24+	10[b]	Hepatic, Renal.

[a]Usual maintenance dosage range for hypertension. Initial dosage is often lower, and higher dosages are sometimes effective.
[b]Half-life of active drug.
[c]Indicated for CHF post-MI.
From references 214 and 215 and product information.

ANGIOTENSIN II RECEPTOR ANTAGONISTS COMPARISON CHART

DRUG	DOSAGE FORMS	USUAL DAILY ADULT DOSAGE (MG)	PEAK EFFECT (HR)	DURATION (HR)	HALF-LIFE (HR)	ELIMINATION ROUTES
Candesartan Atacand	Tab 4, 8, 16, 32 mg.	8–32[a]	3–4	24+	9	Hepatic, Renal.
Eprosartan Teveten	Tab 400, 600 mg.	400–800[a]	1–3	24+	5–9	Hepatic, Renal
Irbesartan Avapro	Tab 75, 150, 300 mg.	150–300	3–6	24+	11–15	Hepatic, Renal.
Losartan Cozaar	Tab 25, 50, 100 mg.	25–100[b]	6	24+	2 6–9[b]	Hepatic. Renal, Hepatic.[b]
Telmisartan Micardis	Tab 40, 80 mg.	40–80	>3	24+	24	Hepatic
Valsartan Diovan	Cap 80, 160 mg.	80–320	6	24+	6	Hepatic.

[a]Occasionally, the daily dosage can be given in 2 divided doses.
[b]For active metabolite, which is responsible for most or all pharmacologic effects.
From references 197, 216, and 217 and product information.

α_1-ADRENERGIC–BLOCKING DRUGS COMPARISON CHART

DRUG	DOSAGE FORMS	DAILY ADULT DOSAGE (MG)[a]	PEAK EFFECT (HR)	DURATION (HR)	HALF-LIFE (HR)	ELIMINATION ROUTES
Doxazosin Cardura	Tab 1, 2, 4, 8 mg.	1–16	2–3	24	10–22	Hepatic.
Prazosin Minipress Various	Cap 1, 2, 5 mg.	2–20	1–3	6–12	2–3	Hepatic.
Terazosin Hytrin Various	Tab 1, 2, 5, 10 mg.	1–20	1–2	24	9–16	Hepatic, Renal.
Tamsulosin Flomax	Cap 0.4 mg.	0.4–0.8[b]	—	—	14–15	Hepatic.

[a]Usual maintenance dosage range for hypertension; higher dosages are sometimes effective. Dosage is the same in the elderly.
[b]Not for hypertension; for symptoms of benign prostatic hypertrophy only.
From references 147, and 218 and product information.

SECOND-LINE ANTIHYPERTENSIVES COMPARISON CHART

DRUG	DOSAGE FORMS	ADULT DOSAGE	DURATION	ADVERSE EFFECTS	MECHANISM
Guanabenz Acetate Wytensin Various	Tab 4, 8 mg.	PO 4 mg bid, increasing q 1–2 weeks to a maximum of 32 mg bid.	12 hr	See clonidine monograph	See clonidine monograph.
Guanadrel Sulfate Hylorel	Tab 10, 25 mg.	PO 5 mg bid, increasing q 1–4 weeks to 20–75 mg/day. Usual maximum is 150 mg/day in 2 divided doses.	4–14 hr	Orthostatic hypotension, diarrhea, drowsiness, sexual dysfunction, peripheral edema, nasal stuffiness, palpitations, shortness of breath, leg cramps, aching limbs.	Postganglionic adrenergic blockade.
Guanethidine Sulfate Ismelin	Tab 10, 25 mg.	PO 10 mg/day, increasing q 5–7 days to 25–50 mg once daily.	1–3 weeks	Same as guanadrel, but more f requent.	Postganglionic adrenergic blockade.
Guanfacine Hydrochloride Tenex Various	Tab 1, 2 mg.	PO 1 mg/day, increasing q 3–4 weeks to maximum of 3 mg/day.	2–4 days	See clonidine monograph.	See clonidine monograph.
Reserpine Various	Tab 0.1, 0.25 mg.	PO 0.5 mg/day for 1–2 weeks, then 0.1–0.25 mg/day.	24 hr	Drowsiness, weakness, GI disturbances, nasal congestion, sexual dysfunction, bradycardia. Dose-related mental depression occurs.	Depletes norepinephrine from post-ganglionic adrenergic neurons.

DRUGS FOR HYPERTENSIVE URGENCIES AND EMERGENCIES COMPARISON CHART

DRUG	DOSAGE RANGE	ONSET (MIN)	DURATION	COMMENTS
ORAL DRUGS FOR HYPERTENSIVE URGENCIES				
Captopril Capoten Various	PO, SL, 12.5–25 mg.	10–30	2–6 hr	Hypotensive effect is particularly large in patients on a diuretic or in hypertensive crisis. Subsequent doses may be less effective unless given with a diuretic. Acute renal failure can occur.
Clonidine Catapres	PO 0.1–0.2 mg initially, then 0.1 mg/hr, to a maximum total dosage of 0.8 mg.	30–120	6–8 hr	Rate of onset is slower after a meal; drowsiness or dry mouth can occur. Rebound hypertension is possible.
Labetalol Normodyne Trandate Various	PO 200–400 mg, may repeat q 2–3 hr.	30–120	6–12 hr	Orthostatic hypotension, bronchoconstriction, and heart block can occur. Avoid in COPD and asthma.
Prazosin Minipress Various	PO 1–2 mg, may repeat q 1 hr.	30–90	1–10 hr	Useful in presence of increased circulating catecholamines. First-dose syncope, palpitations, tachycardia, and headache reported.

(continued)

DRUGS FOR HYPERTENSIVE URGENCIES AND EMERGENCIES COMPARISON CHART (*continued*)

DRUG	DOSAGE RANGE	ONSET (MIN)	DURATION	COMMENTS
INTRAVENOUS DRUGS FOR HYPERTENSIVE EMERGENCIES				
Diazoxide Hyperstat I.V.	IV 1–3 mg/kg (up to 150 mg) over 30 sec, may repeat q 5–15 min. Alternatively, IV infusion 10–30 mg/min. After 300 mg given, give furosemide IV 40 mg before sub-sequent doses.	2–4	3–12 hr	Now obsolete, but can be useful in hypertensive encephalopathy, malignant hypertension, and eclampsia. Increases cardiac output; requires blood pressure monitoring at hourly intervals. Avoid with ischemic heart disease or intracranial hemorrhage.
Enalaprilat Vasotec I.V.	IV 0.625–1.25 mg. (*See monograph.*)	15–30	4–6 hr	Useful in CHF and those at risk for cerebral hypotension. Avoid in acute MI or severe renal impairment. Blacks may respond poorly. Hypotension may occur.
Esmolol Brevibloc	IV 250–500 µg/kg/min for 1–2 min, Then 50–100 µg/kg/min for 4 min; may repeat sequence.	1–2	10–20 min	Useful in perioperative patients with aortic dissection. Does not cause tachycardia but does decrease heart rate.
Fenoldopam Corlopam	IV 0.1–0.3 µg/kg/min initially by continuous infusion.	<5	30 min	Useful in patients with renal insufficiency who risk cyanide toxicity with nitroprusside. Use with caution in glaucoma.
Hydralazine Apresoline	IM or IV 10–40 mg q 3–6 hr.	10–20 (IV) 20–30 (IM)	3–8 hr	Limited to treatment of severe pre-eclampsia and eclampsia. Increases cardiac output; many patients sensitive to parenteral doses, resulting in excessive hypotension.
Labetalol Normodyne Trandate	IV push 20 mg initially, then 40–80 mg q 10 min until desired response achieved or a total dose of 300 mg. Alternatively, IV infusion 0.5–2 mg/min.	<10	3–6 hr	Hypotensive effect is predictable; contraindicated in CHF, head trauma, and intracranial hemorrhage; often causes marked postural hypotension. Avoid use in patients with COPD, CHF, or bradycardia.

(*continued*)

DRUGS FOR HYPERTENSIVE URGENCIES AND EMERGENCIES COMPARISON CHART (*continued*)

DRUG	DOSAGE RANGE	ONSET (MIN)	DURATION	COMMENTS
Nicardipine Cardene	IV infusion 5–15 mg/hr.	<5–15	1–4 hr	Predictable effect. Useful in coronary, cerebral, or peripheral artery disease and in surgical patients. Tachycardia can occur. Use with caution in patients with coronary ischemia.
Nitroglycerin Various	IV 0.3–6 mg/hr by continuous infusion.	1–5	3–5 min	Useful in myocardial ischemia and hypertension associated with MI. Hypotension, headache, tachycardia, and tachyphylaxis occur. Avoid in constrictive pericarditis, pericardial tamponade, or intracranial hypertension.
Nitroprusside Sodium Nipride Various	IV 0.3–10 µg/kg/min by continuous infusion. Infuse at maximal dosage for no more than 10 min. Average dosage is 3 µg/kg/min.	0.5–1	1–2 min	Especially useful in ischemic heart disease. Continuous monitoring required; arterial pressure response adjusted by changing infusion rate; hypotensive effect enhanced by elevating head of patient's bed. Decreases cardiac output; cyanide toxicity with prolonged, high infusion rates

Adapted from references 173, 195, 219 and 220.

β-Adrenergic Blocking Drugs

ESMOLOL HYDROCHLORIDE
Brevibloc

Pharmacology. Esmolol is an ultrashort-acting, cardioselective, β_1-adrenergic blocking agent. It is effective in controlling ventricular response in patients with atrial fibrillation and other supraventricular tachycardias and in slowing heart rate in patients with sinus tachycardia associated with acute MI or cardiac surgery. Esmolol is useful for treating hypertensive emergencies, particularly in patients with tachycardia, because it has a rapid onset, short duration of action, and reduces heart rate. It also can be effective in perioperative hypertension.[173,195,221,222]

Adult Dosage. Dilute injection to a final concentration of 10 mg/mL. **IV** loading dose is 500 μg/kg/min for 1 min and then 50 μg/kg/min. The IV loading dose can be repeated as often as q 5 min, with a concomitant increase of infusion rate in 50 μg/kg/min increments, titrated to ventricular response, heart rate, and/or blood pressure. Most patients respond to infusions of 100–200 μg/kg/min. Once the desired endpoint is obtained, the infusion rate can be decreased in 25–50 μg/kg/min increments at 5- to 10-min intervals. Infusions up to 48 hr are well tolerated.

Pediatric Dosage. **IV** 500 μg/kg/min for 1 min and then 25–200 (average 120) μg/kg/min.[222] Weight-adjusted dosages can be higher than in adults because of its more rapid elimination in children; infusion rates as high as 1 mg/kg/min have been required to achieve complete β blockade.[223]

Dosage Forms. **Inj** 10, 250 mg/mL.

Pharmacokinetics. Effective plasma levels are about 1–1.5 mg/L (3.4–5.1 μmol/L). The α half-life is about 2 min; V_d averages 3.5 L/kg (range 2–5). Esmolol is rapidly hydrolyzed by plasma and blood esterases to a metabolite with weak, clinically unimportant β-blocking activity and small amounts of methanol. No unchanged esmolol appears in the urine. The elimination half-life is about 9 min in adults and 3 min in children.[221,222]

Adverse Reactions. The side effect profile is similar to that of other β_1-selective β-blockers. Dose-related hypotension is frequent; IV site phlebitis occurs occasionally. Concurrent IV morphine can increase serum levels by 46%.

PROPRANOLOL HYDROCHLORIDE
Inderal, Various

Pharmacology. Propranolol is a nonselective β-adrenergic blocker used in arrhythmias, hypertension, angina pectoris, and CHF. It is also effective in decreasing post-MI mortality. The antiarrhythmic mechanism is caused by decreased AV nodal conduction in supraventricular tachycardias and blockade of catecholamine-induced dysrhythmias. Propranolol and other β-blockers are effective in preventing postoperative atrial fibrillation. The antihypertensive mechanism is unknown, but contributing factors are a CNS mechanism, renin blockade, and decreases in myocardial contractility and cardiac output. Propranolol also lowers myocardial oxygen demand by decreasing contractility and heart rate, which symptomatically alleviates anginal pain and increases exercise tolerance in coronary artery disease. **Metoprolol** and **carvedilol** (and perhaps other β-blockers) are effective in reduc-

ing mortality and improving quality of life in patients with CHF by blocking deleterious neurohumoral compensatory factors. β-Blockers and diuretics are recommended as first-line drugs for hypertension because of demonstrated reductions in
morbidity and mortality.[173] (*See* β-Adrenergic Blocking Drugs Comparison
Chart.)

Administration and Adult Dosage. PO 10–20 mg q 6 hr initially, increasing gradually to desired effects. In hypertension, more than 1 g/day has been used; however, consider adding another drug if 480 mg/day is ineffective. In angina pectoris, the dosage is titrated to pain relief and exercise evidence of β-blockade
(bradycardia). The endpoint for dosage escalation in acute arrhythmias is the return to sinus rhythm or, in atrial fibrillation or flutter, to a ventricular rate below
100 beats/min with hemodynamic stability. Twice-daily administration is effective in angina pectoris and hypertension. Administer **SR Cap** in the same daily
dosage once or twice daily (not indicated post-MI). **PO for post-MI prophylaxis
(non-SR)** 180–240 mg/day in 2–3 divided doses. **IV slow push** 1 mg q 5 min, to a
maximum of 0.15 mg/kg; some investigators have recommended that the first
dose be given over 2–10 min.

Special Populations. *Pediatric Dosage.* **PO for hypertension** 0.5–1 mg/kg/day in
2–4 divided doses, increasing to a maximum of 8 mg/kg/day. **IV slow push**
0.01–0.1 mg/kg/dose over 10 min up to 1 mg (infants) or 3 mg (children); may repeat in 6–8 hr.[4]

Geriatric Dosage. Bioavailability is increased in the elderly, necessitating lower
initial doses.

Other Conditions. Therapeutic endpoints can be achieved with lower dosages in
hypothyroidism or liver disease. Begin with lower dosages and titrate to clinical
response. Patients with thyrotoxicosis require higher dosages to achieve the desired effect.[224]

Dosage Forms. **Soln** 4, 8, 80 mg/mL; **Tab** 10, 20, 40, 60, 80, 90 mg; **SR Cap** 60,
80, 120, 160 mg; **Inj** 1 mg/mL.

Patient Instructions. Report any symptoms such as shortness of breath, swelling,
wheezing, fatigue, depression, nightmares, or inability to concentrate. Do not stop
therapy abruptly. Do not crush or chew SR capsule. A sustained-release capsule
core in the stool does not indicate lack of absorption.

Missed Doses. Take this drug at regular intervals. If you miss a dose take it as
soon as you remember. If it is about time for the next dose, take that dose only.
Leave at least 4 hours between regular tablet doses and 6–8 hours between
extended-release capsule doses. Do not double the dose or take extra.

Pharmacokinetics. *Onset and Duration.* PO onset is variable; the duration varies
from 6 to longer than 12 hr.[224]

Serum Levels. No definite relation has been established between serum concentrations and therapeutic effect in the treatment of arrhythmias, angina pectoris, or
hypertension. β-Blockade is associated with serum concentrations >100 μg/L
(340 nmol/L).[225]

Fate. Propranolol is rapidly and completely absorbed after oral administration; however, a large hepatic first-pass effect occurs, limiting systemic availability to 26 ± 10%. First-pass elimination is saturable with an oral dose greater than about 30 mg.[225] The drug is 87 ± 6% bound to α_1-acid glycoprotein and other plasma proteins.[10,224] V_d is 4.3 ± 0.6 L/kg; Cl is 0.96 ± 0.3 L/hr/kg. Unlike most other drugs, displacement from plasma proteins increases elimination half-life and V_d because of high tissue affinity (nonrestrictive elimination). An active metabolite, 4-hydroxypropranolol, is formed after oral, but not IV, administration. Less than 0.5% of a dose is excreted unchanged in urine.[10]

$t_{1/2}$. α phase is about 10 min;[224] β phase after a single PO dose is 3.9 ± 0.4 hr.[10] With long-term oral therapy, β phase is 4–6 hr but can be as long as 10–20 hr in patients with liver disease.[226]

Adverse Reactions. Adverse effects often are not related to dose. Depression, nightmares, insomnia, fatigue, and lethargy occur frequently; less often, psychotic changes have been reported. CNS side effects probably occur more often with the lipophilic β-blockers (eg, propranolol). The drug can cause occasional life-threatening reactions when therapy (especially IV) is initiated, and acute CHF with pulmonary edema and hypotension or symptomatic bradycardia and heart block can occur. Acute drug cessation in patients with coronary artery disease can precipitate unstable angina pectoris or MI. The drug can precipitate hypoglycemia, but probably more important in diabetics is its ability to mask hypoglycemic symptoms (except for sweating). It can exacerbate symptoms of peripheral vascular disease or Raynaud's disease. β-Blockers can exacerbate previously stable asthma or chronic airway obstruction by causing bronchospasm or renal dysfunction by further depressing GFR.

Contraindications. Severe obstructive pulmonary disease, asthma or active allergic rhinitis; cardiogenic shock or severe CHF; second- or third-degree heart block; severe sinus node disease.

Precautions. In coronary artery disease, discontinue drug by tapering the dosage over 4–7 days. Use cautiously in patients with Prinzmetal's vasospastic angina to prevent worsening of chest pain. Use caution in peripheral vascular disease or CHF and in patients with brittle diabetes or history of hypoglycemic episodes. Can worsen atrial fibrillation associated with accessory AV pathway.

Drug Interactions. Concurrent digoxin therapy can lessen the β-blocker exacerbation of CHF. When taken with oral hypoglycemics, nonselective β-blockers such as propranolol prolong hypoglycemic episodes and inhibit tachycardia and tremors, which are signs of hypoglycemia (sweating is not inhibited); hypertension can occur during hypoglycemia. Epinephrine can produce hypertensive reactions in patients on propranolol (and probably other nonselective β-blockers); this can occur with other sympathomimetics such as phenylephrine and phenylpropanolamine. Barbiturates and rifampin can increase the metabolism of hepatically eliminated β-blockers such as propranolol. Cimetidine can increase propranolol effects. Combined use of clonidine and propranolol can result in *hyper*tensive reactions, especially if clonidine is abruptly discontinued. β-Blockers can increase the first-dose hypotensive effect of prazosin and similar drugs. NSAIDs can blunt the hypotensive response of β-blockers.

Parameters to Monitor. During IV administration, obtain blood pressure and pulse q 5 min with constant ECG monitoring for signs of AV nodal block (lengthened PR interval) or bradycardia. Evaluate vital signs routinely for hemodynamic endpoints (eg, blood pressure in hypertension and heart rate or pressure rate product in angina pectoris). Question the patient about subjective complaints such as nightmares or fatigue. When a patient at risk for adverse reactions is first given propranolol, evaluate signs and symptoms of toxicity (eg, CHF, shortness of breath or edema; bronchospasm, wheezing or shortness of breath; diabetes, blood glucose; peripheral vascular disease, painful or cold extremities).

Notes. Propranolol can be beneficial for treatment of symptomatic hypertrophic obstructive cardiomyopathy by increasing end-diastolic volume, producing ventricular relaxation, and relieving ventricular outflow obstruction. Other uses include migraine prophylaxis, prevention of GI bleeding in patients with esophageal varicies, prevention of sudden death in congenital long-QT syndromes, and as a cardiac protectant in patients with heart disease undergoing noncardiac surgery. If a β-blocker must be used in lung disease, $β_1$-selective drugs (eg, **acebutolol, atenolol,** or **metoprolol**) cause alterations in pulmonary function that are more easily reversed by bronchodilators; these drugs are probably a better choice than propranolol or other nonselective β-blockers. (*See* β-Adrenergic Blocking Drugs Comparison Chart.)

β-ADRENERGIC BLOCKING DRUGS COMPARISON CHART

DRUG	DOSAGE FORMS	CARDIO-SELECTIVITY	β HALF-LIFE (HR)	EXCRETED UNCHANGED IN URINE	PROTEIN BINDING	LABELED USES	STARTING DOSAGE	MAXIMUM DOSAGE
Acebutolol[a] Sectral Various	Cap 200, 400 mg.	+	3–4 (diacetolol) 8–13	30–40%	25%	Hypertension, arrhythmias.	PO 400 mg/day.	PO 1.2 g/day.
Atenolol Tenormin Various	Tab 25, 50, 100 mg Inj 0.5 mg/mL.	+ (up to 100 mg)	6–7	85%	10%	Hypertension. Post-MI prophylaxis.	PO 50 mg/day. IV 5 mg × 2, then PO 100 mg/day.	PO 200 mg/day.
Betaxolol Kerlone	Tab 10, 20 mg.	+	14–20	15%	50%	Hypertension.	PO 10 mg/day.	PO 40 mg/day.
Bevantolol Vantol (Investigational—Pfizer)	—	+	1–3	<10%	95%	—	PO 150 mg/day.	PO 400 mg/day.
Bisoprolol Zebeta	Tab 5, 10 mg.	+	9–12	50%	30%	Hypertension.	PO 2–5 mg/day.	PO 20 mg/day.

(continued)

β-ADRENERGIC BLOCKING DRUGS COMPARISON CHART (*continued*)

DRUG	DOSAGE FORMS	CARDIO-SELECTIVITY	β HALF-LIFE (HR)	EXCRETED UNCHANGED IN URINE	PROTEIN BINDING	LABELED USES	STARTING DOSAGE	MAXIMUM DOSAGE
Carteolol[a] Cartrol	Tab 2.5, 5 mg.	0	6–11	60%	15%	Hypertension.	PO 2.5 mg/day.	PO 10 mg/day.
Carvedilol[b] Coreg	Tab 3.125, 6.25, 12.5, 25 mg.	0	6–8	1%	95%	Hypertension, CHF.	PO 3.125 mg bid, increasing q 2 weeks.	PO (<85 kg) 50 mg/day; (>85 kg) 100 mg/day.
Esmolol Brevibloc	Inj 10, 250 mg/mL.	+	9 min	0%	55%	Supraventricular tachycardia.	IV 50 µg/kg/min.	IV 200 µg/kg/min.
Labetalol[b] Trandate Normodyne Various	Tab 100, 200, 300 mg Inj 5 mg/mL.	0	4–9	5%	50%	Hypertension.	PO 100 mg/day. IV 20 mg, then 40–80 mg q 10 min.	PO 2.4 g/day. IV 300 mg.
Metoprolol Lopressor Toprol-XL	Tab 50, 100 mg SR Tab 50, 100, 200 mg Inj 1 mg/mL.	+ (up to 100 mg)	3–7	39%	10%	Hypertension. Hypertension, angina pectoris. Acute MI. CHF (Toprol-XL).	PO 100 mg/day. PO SR 50–100 mg/day. IV 5 mg × 3, then PO 50 mg q 6 hr × 48 hr. PO SR 12.5–25 mg/day.	PO 450 mg/day. PO SR 400 mg/day. PO SR 200 mg/day.

(continued)

β-ADRENERGIC BLOCKING DRUGS COMPARISON CHART (continued)

DRUG	DOSAGE FORMS	CARDIO-SELECTIVITY	β HALF-LIFE (HR)	EXCRETED UNCHANGED IN URINE	PROTEIN BINDING	LABELED USES	STARTING DOSAGE	MAXIMUM DOSAGE
Nadolol Corgard Various	Tab 20, 40, 80, 120, 160 mg.	0	17–24	70%	25%	Hypertension, angina pectoris.	PO 40 mg/day.	PO 320 mg/day.
Penbutolol[a] Levatol	Tab 20 mg.	0	4–8	5%	80–90%	Hypertension.	PO 20 mg/day.	PO 80 mg/day.
Pindolol[a] Visken	Tab 5, 10 mg.	0	3–4	40%	57%	Hypertension.	PO 10 mg/day.	PO 60 mg/day.
Propranolol Inderal Various	(See monograph.)	0	4–6	<0.5%	87%	Hypertension, angina pectoris, arrhythmias. Post-MI prophylaxis.	PO 40–80 mg/day. PO 180 mg/day.	PO 480 mg/day. PO 240 mg/day.
Sotalol[c] Betapace	Tab 80, 120, 160, 240 mg.	0	7–15	80–90%	0%	Life-threatening ventricular arrhythmias.	PO 160 mg/day.	PO 640 mg/day.
Timolol[b] Blocadren	Tab 5, 10, 20 mg.	0	4–5	20%	<10%	Hypertension. Post-MI prophylaxis.	PO 20 mg/day. PO 20 mg/day.	PO 60 mg/day. PO 20 mg/day.

[a]Acebutolol, carteolol, penbutolol, and pindolol have intrinsic agonist (sympathomimetic) activity (ISA).
[b]Carvedilol has α_1-blocking actions. Labetalol has potent α_1-blocking actions (ratio of α- to β-blockade 1:3 and 1:7 with PO and IV, respectively).
[c]Sotalol also has type III antiarrhythmic properties.
From references 123, 221, 227–232 and product information.

Calcium-Channel Blocking Drugs

DILTIAZEM HYDROCHLORIDE
Cardizem, Dilacor XR, Tiazac, Various

Pharmacology. Diltiazem is a calcium-channel blocking drug that decreases heart rate, prolongs AV nodal conduction, and decreases arteriolar and coronary vascular tone. It also has negative inotropic properties. Diltiazem is effective in symptomatic angina pectoris, essential hypertension, and supraventricular tachycardias. It also can reduce early reinfarction rates in patients with non–Q-wave MI and normal left ventricular functions. (*See* Calcium-Channel Blocking Drugs Comparison Chart.)

Administration and Adult Dosage. IV loading dose 0.25 mg/kg (about 20 mg) over 2 min; can repeat in 15 min with 0.35 mg/kg (about 25 mg). **IV infusion** 5–15 mg/hr, titrated to ventricular response. **PO for angina** 30–60 mg q 6–8 hr initially; dosages up to 480 mg/day may be required for symptomatic relief of angina;[233,234] 180–300 mg once daily with Cardizem CD. **PO for hypertension** 120–240 mg/day initially in 2 divided doses using Cardizem SR, or 180–300 mg once daily using Cardizem CD or Dilacor XR, titrated to clinical response; **maintenance dosages** of 180–480 mg/day are usually necessary.

Special Populations. *Pediatric Dosage.* Safety and efficacy are not established. **PO** 1.5–2 mg/kg/day in 3–4 divided daily doses up to a maximum of 3.5 mg/kg/day.[4]

Geriatric Dosage. Same as adult dosage but titrate dosage slowly.

Other Conditions. Patients with liver disease may require lower dosages; titrate to clinical response.

Dosage Forms. Tab 30, 60, 90, 120 mg; **SR Cap** (12 hr; Cardizem SR, various) 60, 90, 120 mg; **SR Cap** (24 hr; Cardizem CD) 120, 180, 240, 300 mg; (24 hr; Dilacor XR) 120, 180, 240 mg; (24 hr; Tiazac) 120, 180, 240, 300, 360 mg; **SR Tab** 120, 180, 240 mg (Tiamate); **Inj** 5 mg/mL; **SR Tab** 180 mg with enalapril 5 mg (Teczem).

Patient Instructions. Report dizziness, leg swelling, or shortness of breath. (For angina) Maintain a diary to document the numbers of episodes of chest pain and sublingual nitroglycerin tablets used.

Missed Doses. Take this drug at regular intervals. If you miss a dose, take it as soon as you remember. If it is about time for the next dose, take that dose only. Do not double the dose or take extra.

Pharmacokinetics. *Onset and Duration.* PO onset 0.5–3 hr, duration 6–10 hr;[235] 12–24 hr with SR cap, depending on the product.

Serum Levels. Levels >95 μg/L (230 nmol/L) are necessary to cause hemodynamic changes, but their clinical usefulness is questionable.[236] Levels of desacetyldiltiazem are similar to those of diltiazem.[237]

Fate. Oral bioavailability is 38 ± 11% with the first dose and 90 ± 21% with long-term therapy.[237] The drug is 78 ± 3% bound to plasma proteins; V_d is 5.3 ± 1.7 L/kg;[237] Cl is 0.72 ± 0.3 L/hr/kg.[10] Enterohepatic recycling occurs. The drug is almost entirely metabolized by the liver, with only 1–3% excreted unchanged in urine. One metabolite, desacetyldiltiazem, has 40–50% the activity of diltiazem. Metabolites are excreted primarily in the feces.

$t_{1/2}$. α phase 2–5 min; β phase 4.9 ± 0.4 hr,[235,237] longer in the elderly.[234] β phase (desacetyldiltiazem) 6.1 ± 1.2 hr.[237]

Adverse Reactions. Frequency of side effects is dose related. Headache, flushing, dizziness, and edema occur frequently. Sinus bradycardia and AV block occur frequently, often in association with concomitant β-blockers.[234] CHF can worsen in patients with underlying left ventricular dysfunction. A variety of skin reactions have been occasionally reported.[234] Hepatitis occurs rarely.

Contraindications. Second- or third-degree block or sick sinus syndrome without a ventricular pacemaker; symptomatic hypotension or severe CHF, acute MI, or pulmonary congestion; atrial fibrillation with accessory AV pathway.

Precautions. Use caution with concomitant use of β-blockers in patients with underlying CHF, especially those with poor left ventricular function.[234]

Drug Interactions. Cimetidine and propranolol increase diltiazem serum levels.[234] Diltiazem inhibits CYP3A4 and the metabolism of many drugs, including carbamazepine, cyclosporine, and theophylline.[234] It also inhibits P-glycoprotein.[238]

Parameters to Monitor. Monitor blood pressure, heart rate, and ECG, especially when initiating therapy. Watch for symptoms of hypotension and CHF. Serial treadmill exercise tests can assess efficacy in angina. Monitor the number of episodes of chest pain and SL nitroglycerin used.

NIFEDIPINE
Adalat, Procardia

Pharmacology. Nifedipine is a dihydropyridine calcium-channel blocking drug with potent arterial and coronary vasodilating properties. A reflex increase in sympathetic tone (in response to vasodilation) counteracts the direct depressant effects on SA and AV nodal conduction. This renders nifedipine ineffective in the treatment of supraventricular tachycardias. It is used for vasospastic and chronic stable angina and in the treatment of hypertension. (*See* Calcium-Channel Blocking Drugs Comparison Chart.)

Administration and Adult Dosage. PO for angina (Cap) 10 mg tid initially, increasing to a usual maximum of 20–30 mg tid or qid; dosages above 180 mg/day are not recommended. **PO for hypertension** (SR Tab only) 30–60 mg/day initially, increasing up to 120 mg/day prn. **PO for severe hypertension** (non-SR) 10 mg, may repeat prn in 20 min. The capsule can be punctured or bitten and swallowed, usually resulting in a more rapid onset than SL administration.[239]

Special Populations. *Pediatric Dosage.* Safety and efficacy not established. **PO for hypertensive crisis** 0.25–0.5 mg/kg q 4–6 hr.[4]

Geriatric Dosage. Same as adult dosage.

Other Conditions. Patients with liver disease might require lower dosages;[240] titrate to clinical response.

Dosage Forms. Cap 10, 20 mg; **SR Tab** 30, 60, 90 mg.

Patient Instructions. Report flushing, edema, dizziness, or increased frequency of chest discomfort. Do not split, chew, or crush sustained-release tablets. A sustained-release tablet core in the stool does not indicate lack of absorption. Maintain a diary to document the number of episodes of chest pain and sublingual nitroglycerin tablets used.

Missed Doses. Take this drug at regular intervals. If you miss a dose, take it as soon as you remember. If it is about time for the next dose, take that dose only. Do not double the dose or take extra.

Pharmacokinetics. *Onset and Duration.* PO onset 0.5–2 hr; duration (Cap) 4–8 hr; (SR Tab) 12–24 hr. PO (punctured capsule) onset 10–20 min; duration 3–4 hr.

Serum Levels. (Therapeutic) >90 μg/L (260 nmol/L), although clinical utility is questionable.[241]

Fate. Bioavailability is 52 ± 37% in normals and 91 ± 26% in cirrhosis because of extensive and variable first-pass hepatic elimination.[240] It is 96 ± 1% bound to plasma proteins; V_d is 0.8 ± 0.2 L/kg;[241,242] Cl is 0.42 ± 0.12 L/hr/kg.[10] Nifedipine is almost entirely eliminated by hepatic metabolism via the CYP3A4 isozyme, which is present in variable amounts (but is not a true polymorphism).[243] Only traces of drug are excreted unchanged in urine.[241]

$t_{½}$. α phase 4–7 min; β phase 2 ± 0.4 hr.[241,242]

Adverse Reactions. Most side effects relate to vasodilatory actions and occur frequently; symptoms include dizziness (with or without hypotension), flushing, and headache. These types of side effects seem less frequent with SR dosage forms.[244] Avoid long-term treatment of hypertension with immediate-release products because they can increase mortality.[173,245] Edema occurs frequently and is related to venous pooling and usually not exacerbation of CHF. Nifedipine paradoxically can worsen anginal chest pain, possibly because of a reflex increase in sympathetic tone or redistribution of coronary blood flow away from ischemic areas. Acute, reversible renal failure can occur in patients with chronic renal insufficiency;[246] rare reactions include hepatitis and hyperglycemia.

Contraindications. Symptomatic hypotension.

Precautions. Use with caution in unstable angina pectoris when used alone (ie, without a β-blocker) and in patients with CHF caused by systolic dysfunction because mortality can be increased.[245,247] Do not use immediate-release products to treat hypertension. Nifedipine has an antiplatelet action and can increase bleeding time.[248] Nifedipine can worsen symptoms of obstructive cardiomyopathy.

Drug Interactions. Barbiturates increase nifedipine metabolism. Cimetidine can increase nifedipine serum levels. Nifedipine occasionally increases PT in patients on oral anticoagulants. Nifedipine and IV magnesium sulfate can cause neuromuscular blockade and hypotension.

Parameters to Monitor. Monitor blood pressure and heart rate, especially when initiating therapy. Observe for symptoms of hypotension and edema. Serial treadmill exercise tests can assess efficacy.

Notes. Other potential uses for nifedipine are migraine prophylaxis, achalasia, and Raynaud's phenomenon.

VERAPAMIL HYDROCHLORIDE   Calan, Covera-HS, Isoptin, Verelan, Various

Pharmacology. Verapamil is a calcium-channel blocking drug that prolongs AV nodal conduction. It is used to convert re-entrant supraventricular tachycardias and slow ventricular rate in atrial fibrillation or flutter. Because it decreases contractility and arteriolar resistance, it is used in angina caused by coronary obstruction or vasospasm. Verapamil also is effective in the treatments of hypertension, hypertrophic obstructive cardiomyopathy, and migraine prophylaxis. (*See* Calcium-Channel Blocking Drugs Comparison Chart.)

Administration and Adult Dosage. **PO for angina** 80–120 mg tid initially, increasing at daily (for unstable angina) or weekly intervals to a maximum of 480 mg/day. **PO for hypertension** usually 240 mg/day using SR tablet; SR dosages of 120 mg/day to 240 mg bid have been used. Covera HS is designed to be taken hs. **PO for migraine prophylaxis** 160–320 mg/day. **IV for supraventricular arrhythmias** 5–10 mg (0.075–0.15 mg/kg) over at least 2 min (3 min in elderly); can repeat with 10 mg (0.15 mg/kg) in 30 min if arrhythmia is not terminated or desired endpoint is not achieved. **IV constant infusion** 5–10 mg/hr.[249]

Special Populations. *Pediatric Dosage.* **PO** 4–8 mg/kg/day in 3 divided doses. **IV** (<1 yr) 0.1–0.2 mg/kg; (1–15 yr) 0.1–0.3 mg/kg, to a maximum of 5 mg over 2–3 min.[4]

Geriatric Dosage. Same as adult dosage but administer over 3 min.

Other Conditions. Dosage might need to be decreased in patients with liver disease; titrate to clinical response.

Dosage Forms. **Tab** 40, 80, 120 mg; **SR Tab** 120, 180, 240 mg; **SR Cap** 100, 120, 180, 200, 240, 300 mg; **Inj** 2.5 mg/mL; **SR Tab** 180 mg with trandolapril 2 mg, 240 mg with trandolapril 1, 4 mg (Tarka).

Patient Instructions. Report any dizziness, shortness of breath, or edema. Constipation occurs often. Maintain a diary to document the number of episodes of chest pain and sublingual nitroglycerin tablets used.

Missed Doses. Take this drug at regular intervals. If you miss a dose, take it as soon as you remember. If it is about time for the next dose, take that dose only. Do not double the dose or take extra.

Pharmacokinetics. *Onset and Duration.* IV onset immediate; duration 2–6 hr, up to 12 hr with long-term use.[250]

Serum Levels. 50–400 μg/L (100–800 nmol/L), although therapeutic range is not well established.

Fate. Although the drug is well absorbed orally, only 22 ± 8% is bioavailable because of extensive first-pass elimination; bioavailability increases in liver disease.[251] Covera-HS provides a 4- to 5-hr delay before releasing the drug. Verapamil has stereospecific pharmacology and pharmacokinetics; L-verapamil is a more potent AV nodal blocking drug, but it undergoes greater first-pass metabolism.[252] Norverapamil is an active metabolite. Verapamil is about 90 ± 2% bound to plasma proteins, with the more active L-isomer having a greater unbound fraction.[251,253] V_d is 5 ± 2 L/kg and increases in liver disease;[10,251] Cl is 0.9 ± 0.36 L/hr/kg. About 1% is excreted unchanged in urine.[10]

$t_{1/2}$. (Verapamil) α phase 5–30 min; β phase 4 ± 1.5 hr; can increase during long-term use; 13.6 ± 3.9 hr in severe liver disease; (norverapamil) 8 ± 1.9 hr.[10,251,253]

Adverse Reactions. Constipation occurs frequently (5–40%), particularly in elderly patients. CHF can occur in patients with left ventricular dysfunction. Serious hemodynamic side effects (eg, severe hypotension) and conduction abnormalities (eg, symptomatic bradycardia or asystole) have been reported; these reactions usually occur when the patient is concurrently receiving a β-blocker or has underlying conduction disease.[254] Infants appear to be particularly susceptible to arrhythmias. IV **calcium** (gluconate or chloride salts, 10–20 mL of a 10% solution) and/or **isoproterenol** can, in part, reverse these adverse effects.[254] The administration of IV calcium before verapamil can prevent hypotension without abolishing the antiarrhythmic actions.[255]

Contraindications. Shock or severely hypotensive states; second- or third-degree AV nodal block; sick sinus syndrome, unless functioning ventricular pacemaker is in place; hypotension or CHF unless caused by supraventricular tachyarrhythmias amenable to verapamil therapy; atrial fibrillation and an accessory AV pathway.

Precautions. Use caution with any wide-QRS tachycardia; severe hypotension and shock can ensue if the tachycardia is ventricular in origin. Use with caution in combination with oral β-blockers and poor left ventricular function.

Drug Interactions. Verapamil can increase serum levels of several drugs, including carbamazepine, cyclosporine, digoxin (probably by inhibiting P-glyco-protein[238]), and theophylline. Barbiturates and rifampin can increase verapamil metabolism.

Parameters to Monitor. Monitor blood pressure and ECG continuously during IV administration. Pay particular attention to signs and symptoms of CHF and hypotension. Also, monitor the ECG for PR prolongation and bradycardia.

CALCIUM-CHANNEL BLOCKING DRUGS COMPARISON CHART

DRUG	DOSAGE FORMS	ADULT DOSAGE	CONTRACTILITY	HEART RATE	AV NODAL CONDUCTION	VASCULAR RESISTANCE
Amlodipine[a] Norvasc	Tab 2.5, 5, 10 mg.	PO for hypertension or angina 5–10 mg/day.	0	0	0	→↓
Bepridil[b] Vasocor	Tab 200, 300, 400 mg.	PO for refractory angina 200–400 mg/day.	0/↓	0/↓	0/↓	→
Diltiazem[c] Cardizem Dilacor XR	(See monograph.)	(See monograph.)	→	→	→	→
Felodipine[d] Plendil	SR Tab 2.5, 5, 10 mg.	PO for hypertension 2.5–20 mg once daily.	0/↑	0/↑	0/↑	→↓
Isradipine[d] DynaCirc DynaCirc CR	Cap 2.5, 5 mg SR Tab 5, 10 mg.	PO for hypertension 2.5–10 mg bid or SR 5–10 mg once daily.	0/↑	0/↑	0/↑	→↓
Nicardipine[d] Cardene Various	Cap 20, 30 mg SR Cap 30, 45, 60 mg Inj 2.5 mg/mL.	PO for angina or hypertension 20–40 mg tid or SR 30–60 mg q 12 hr. IV for hypertension 5–15 mg/hr.	0/↑	0/↑	0/↑	→↓
Nifedipine[d] Adalat Procardia	Cap 10, 20 mg SR Tab 30, 60, 90 mg.	(See monograph.)	0/↑	0/↑	0/↑	→↓

(continued)

CALCIUM-CHANNEL BLOCKING DRUGS COMPARISON CHART (*continued*)

DRUG	DOSAGE FORMS	ADULT DOSAGE	CONTRACTILITY	HEART RATE	AV NODAL CONDUCTION	VASCULAR RESISTANCE
Nimodipine[d] Nimotop	Cap 30 mg.	PO postsubarachnoid hemorrhage 60 mg q 4 hr for 21 days.	0/↑	0/↑	0/↑	↓↓
Nisoldipine[d] Sular	SR Tab 10, 20, 30, 40 mg.	PO for hypertension SR 20–40 mg once daily.	0/↑	0/↑	0/↑	↓↓
Verapamil[c] Calan Isoptin Verelan	(*See* monograph.)	(*See* monograph.)	↓↓	↓	↓↑	↓

↑ = increase; ↓↓ = marked decrease, ↓ = decrease, 0 = no change.
[a]Selective vascular actions.
[b]Complex pharmacology with probable sodium- and potassium-channel blockade (quinidine-like).
[c]Vascular and eletrophysiologic actions.
[d]Predominantly vascular actions.
From reference 256 and product information.

Hypolipidemic Drugs

Class Instructions. **Hypolipidemics.** There is a strong relationship between elevated serum cholesterol and death caused by coronary heart disease (CHD). Lowering cholesterol decreased events related to CHD and can slow or even reverse atherosclerosis. These effects are associated with a decrease in CHD mortality. In general, each 1% decrease in serum cholesterol results in a 2% decrease in the risk of coronary events. Hypolipidemic drugs must be taken daily to achieve these results. Drug therapy does not eliminate the need for appropriate diet and other measures such as weight reduction (if appropriate), smoking cessation, and physical activity. Use of estrogen and progestin in postmenopausal women also has beneficial effects on lipoprotein levels, but the overall risk/benefit assessment of hormone-replacement therapy remains controversial. Depending on their overall state of health, elderly patients can benefit from secondary prevention with hypolipidemic therapy. Hypolipidemic drug therapy (with the exception of niacin) has been associated with an increase in cancer in animals, but it is not known if they have this effect in humans.

Missed Doses. Take this drug at regular intervals. If you miss a dose, take it as soon as you remember. If it is about time for the next dose, take that dose only. Do not double the dose or take extra.

CHOLESTYRAMINE RESIN   Questran, Various

Pharmacology. Cholestyramine is a bile acid sequestrant that acts as an anion exchange resin; it releases chloride ions and adsorbs bile acids in the intestine to form a nonabsorbable complex that is excreted in feces. The resulting increase in activity of hepatic low-density lipoprotein cholesterol (LDL-c) receptors leads to the oxidation of cholesterol to form new bile acids. Despite a compensatory increase in hepatic cholesterol synthesis, total serum cholesterol and LDL-c levels are reduced by 15–30%. The increase in cholesterol synthesis sometimes results in an increase in VLDL cholesterol levels, which can increase triglyceride levels by 10–50%.[257,258] Cardioprotective HDL-c levels can increase by 3–8%.[258]

Administration and Adult Dosage. PO for hyperlipidemia 4 g daily–bid initially, increasing slowly to a maintenance dosage of 8–16 g/day in 1–6 (usually 2) divided doses, to a maximum of 24 g/day. Compliance appears to be best in the range of 8–10 g/day in 1–2 divided doses. **PO for treatment of cholestatic pruritus** 4–8 g/day is usual. **PO for treatment of relapsing enterocolitis caused by** *Clostridium difficile* 4 g tid or qid (with or without vancomycin) has been used.

Special Populations. *Pediatric Dosage.* Limited data are available, especially concerning long-term use. Drug therapy is generally reserved for children at least 10 yr old, initiated at the lowest possible dosage, and gradually increased until the desired response is achieved. Base initial dosage on serum LDL-c level rather than body weight, and adjust dosage based on response: **PO for hyperlipidemia** (LDL-c <195 mg/dL) 4 g/day; (LDL-c 195–235 mg/dL) 8 g/day; (LDL-c 236–280 mg/dL) 12 g/day; (LDL-c >280 mg/dL) 16 g/day.[259,260] (*See* Precautions.)

Geriatric Dosage. Initiate therapy at lowest possible dosage and slowly titrate to desired effect. Maximum dosage might not be required or tolerated.

Other Conditions. In patients with histories of constipation, start at the low end of the dosage range. In patients with GI intolerance, reduce dosage and increase gradually. (*See* Adverse Reactions.)

Dosage Forms. **Pwdr** 4 g resin/9 g powder (Questran); 4 g resin/5, 5.5, 5.7 g powder (Questran Light, various); **Tab** 1 g.

Patient Instructions. (*See* Hypolipidemics Class Instructions.) It is preferable to take this drug before meals, but you can adjust the time of the dosages around the scheduling of other oral medications. Take other oral medications at least 1 hour before or 4–6 hours after taking cholestyramine. Do not take dry; mix each packet or level scoopful with at least 60–180 mL (2–6 fluid ounces) of water or noncarbonated beverage, highly fluid soup, or pulpy fruit such as applesauce or crushed pineapple. You can experiment with different products and vehicles to determine your preference based on taste, cost, and caloric restrictions. Mixtures can be refrigerated to improve palatability but do not cook because the drug can be inactivated. This drug frequently causes constipation. If this becomes a problem, contact your physician or pharmacist to discuss measures to minimize constipation. It can cause other gastrointestinal symptoms that usually decrease over time.

Pharmacokinetics. *Onset and Duration.* Reduction in cholesterol begins the first month.

Fate. It is not absorbed from the GI tract. Resin and complex are excreted in the feces.

Adverse Reactions. Almost 70% of patients experience at least one GI side effect.[261] Constipation frequently occurs, especially with higher dosages, in the elderly and patients with previous constipation; fecal impaction is rare. Nausea, heartburn, abdominal pain, bloating, steatorrhea, and belching also occur frequently but tend to decrease over time.[257] GI side effects tend to be milder in children than in adults. Hemorrhoids can be aggravated or develop. Rash can occur. Chloride absorption in place of bicarbonate can lead to hyperchloremic acidosis, especially in children, and calcium excretion can increase. Absorption of vitamins D and K can be impaired, leading to osteomalacia and bleeding, respectively. Absorption of folic acid also can be impaired, especially in children. Alimentary cancers in rats are somewhat more prevalent with cholestyramine treatment because of enhancement of other carcinogens, but the importance of this in humans is unknown.[262]

Contraindications. Complete biliary obstruction.

Precautions. Pregnancy and lactation because of possible malabsorption of fat-soluble vitamins. Avoid constipation in patients with symptomatic coronary artery disease. Constipation can be controlled by reducing dosage, slowly titrating dosage, increasing dietary fiber, or using stool softeners. Avoid use in the presence of diverticular disease and local intestinal tract lesions because constipation can be a problem.[263] Discontinue if a clinically important elevation in serum triglycerides occurs. Vitamin supplementation might be needed with high dosage or long-term therapy. Children in particular might need multivitamins with folate and iron.[260] Patients with osteoporosis might need to restrict dietary chloride to limit calcium excretion.[264] Phenylketonurics should avoid Questran Light because it contains aspartame.

Drug Interactions. Absorption of many drugs can be delayed or reduced, including acetaminophen, coumarin anticoagulants, digoxin, furosemide, gemfibrozil, hydrocortisone, oral hypoglycemic drugs,[265] iron, loperamide, methotrexate, naproxen, penicillin G, phenobarbital, oral phosphate supplements, pravastatin, propranolol, tetracyclines, thyroid hormones, thiazides, and vancomycin. Monitor for concurrent drug therapy effects when initiating and altering sequestrant therapy, particularly for drugs with a narrow therapeutic index.

Parameters to Monitor. Monitor LDL-c and triglycerides 4 weeks and 3 months after initiation of therapy. If therapy goals are achieved, monitor q 4 months unless adverse effects are suspected. Periodically monitor hemoglobin and serum folic acid during long-term therapy. Monitor efficacy of and appropriate tests for concurrent drug therapy that might be affected by cholestyramine. In children, monitor serum concentrations of vitamins A, D, and E and erythrocyte folate, liver function tests, and CBC annually.[260]

Notes. Bile acid sequestering resins are indicated as an adjunct to diet for primary hypercholesterolemia (types IIa and IIb) in patients for whom hypertriglyceridemia is not a primary concern (triglyceride levels <300 mg/dL).[264] Bile acid sequestrants moderately lower LDL-c compared with some of the other hypolipidemic drugs but are considered safer because they are not absorbed. These drugs can be particularly useful with moderately elevated LDL-c and when the risk of CHD is low and long-term safety is of concern (eg, primary prevention and in young men and premenopausal women).[257,266] They can be used in combination with other hypolipidemic drugs for additive effects when a larger decrease in LDL-c is required. Long-term use reduces cardiovascular morbidity and mortality, including the incidence of first heart attacks. Because over one-third of patients discontinue bile acid sequestrants in the first year, primarily because of adverse effects, conservative dosage titration, education, and support are needed to manage and avoid adverse effects.[261,267] Maximum dosage is rarely needed.[258] Low-dose therapy (8–10 g/day) appears to be best tolerated[257] and the most cost effective, alone or in combination therapy.[268] Increased dosage can increase adverse effects without meaningful decreases in cholesterol. Resins are not effective in patients with homozygous familial hypercholesterolemia.[258] (*See* Recommendations for Initiation of Drug Therapy in Hypercholesterolemia Chart.)

The resins also are used to reduce pruritus caused by dermal deposition of bile acids in patients with partial biliary obstruction, and cholestyramine has been used to treat relapsing *Clostridium difficile* colitis.[269,270] Interference with digoxin absorption suggests a possible role in the management of the mild intoxication caused by these drugs; however, do not rely on cholestyramine alone in cases of severe digoxin toxicity.[265] Questran contains 14 kcal/9 g packet or scoop; Questran Light is flavored with aspartame and contains 1.6 kcal and 16.8 mg of phenylalanine/5 g packet or scoop.

COLESEVELAM   Welchol

Pharmacology. Colesevelam is a nonabsorbed, polymeric, lipid-lowering agent that binds intestinal bile acids, resulting in the increased clearance of LDL-c and a reduction of total cholesterol. Unlike cholestyramine and colestipol, colesevelam is not an anion exchange resin but binds bile acids and impedes their reabsorption. Clinical trials have demonstrated a mean LDL-c reduction of 15–18% after 24 weeks of therapy. HDL-c was increased by approximately 3% and triglyceride levels were elevated 4–5% compared with placebo.

Administration and Adult Dosage. PO for hyperlipidemia 3 tablets bid with meals or 6 tablets once daily with a meal.[271] **PO combination therapy for hyperlipidemia** 4–6 tablets/day is safe and effective when coadministered with an HMG-CoA reductase inhibitor. The drugs can be administered together or separately.[271]

Special Populations. *Pediatric Dosage.* Safety and efficacy not established.

Geriatric Dosage. Same as adult dosage.

Dosage Forms. Tab 625 mg.

Patient Instructions. Take this drug with meals for maximum benefit.

Pharmacokinetics. *Onset and Duration.* Maximum effect occurs after 2 weeks.[271]

Fate. Colesevelam is not absorbed orally. It is excreted unchanged in the feces.

Adverse Reactions. Unlike cholestyramine and colestipol, colesevelam is generally well tolerated. GI effects, including flatulence, constipation, diarrhea, nausea, and dyspepsia, are the most common side effects, but the frequency is similar to that of placebo.[271,272]

Contraindications. Bowel obstruction.

Precautions. Caution in patients with elevated triglyceride levels or GI disorders (ie, GI motility disorders, dysphagia, swallowing disorders, or recent GI surgery).

Drug Interactions. Colesevelam does not affect the bioavailability of digoxin, lovastatin, metoprolol, quinidine, valproic acid, or warfarin. The bioavailability of SR verapamil can be reduced by colesevelam. Colesevelam does not interfere with the lipid-lowering activity of the HMG-CoA reductase inhibitors. Colesevelam did not appear to affect the bioavailability of vitamin A, D, E, or K during clinical trials of up to 1 yr.[271] The manufacturer states that caution should be exercised when treating patients with a susceptibility to vitamin K or fat-soluble vitamin deficiencies.

Parameters to Monitor. Monitor serum total cholesterol, LDL-c, and triglyceride levels initially and periodically during therapy.

Notes. The tolerability and the apparent lack of GI side effects can make colesevelam a good alternative to other bile acid binding agents and potentially the drug of choice in this class.[271] It is a good choice for use with an HMG-CoA reductase inhibitor in patients with inadequate responses to the maximal HMG-CoA dose.

COLESTIPOL HYDROCHLORIDE
Colestid

Pharmacology. Colestipol is a bile acid sequestrant similar to cholestyramine, with equivalent lipid-lowering effects in most patients. Selection of a bile acid sequestrant is generally based on patient preference and cost. The palatability of cholestyramine–vehicle combinations is often preferred over colestipol granules, although colestipol tablets are well tolerated. A 5 g dose of colestipol lowers cholesterol in an amount equivalent to 4 g of cholestyramine; a 4 g dose of colestipol tablets is about equivalent to 5 g of the granules.[273–279] (*See* Hypolipidemic Drugs Comparison Chart and Recommendations for Initiation of Drug Therapy in Hypercholesterolemia Chart.)

Adult Dosage. **PO for hypercholesterolemia** (Granules) 5 g bid initially, increasing in 5 g/day increments at 1- to 2-month intervals to a maximum of 30 g/day in 1–4 doses; (tablets) 2 g bid initially, increasing in 2 g/day increments at 1- to 2-month intervals to a maximum of 16 g/day. (*See* Adverse Effects.) **PO for relapsing enterocolitis caused by *Clostridium difficile*** 5 g q 12 hr has been used with oral vancomycin but avoid coadministration with vancomycin to prevent vancomycin binding.

Dosage Forms. **Granules** 5 g resin/7.5 g packets and bulk containers; **Tab** 1 g.

Adverse Effects. Adverse effects, precautions, monitoring instructions, and drug interactions are similar to those of cholestyramine. Patients with moderate hypercholesterolemia who cannot tolerate colestipol granules due to GI side effects can benefit from one-half the colestipol dose mixed with 2.5 g of **psyllium.**

FENOFIBRATE
TriCor

Pharmacology. Fenofibrate is a fibric acid derivative indicated for the treatment of type IV and V hyperlipidemias. It reduces serum LDL-c by 17–35% and triglycerides by 15–43% and increases HDL. It appears to act by enhancing lipoprotein lipase activity, inhibiting VLDL synthesis, and reducing cholesterol synthesis, possibly by inhibiting acyltransferase activity. It also can reduce platelet aggregation and decrease serum uric acid.[280–282]

Adult Dosage. **PO for type IV or V hyperlipidemia in those at risk of pancreatitis** 67 mg/day initially, increasing q 4–8 weeks to a maximum of 201 mg/day. Take doses with a meal.

Dosage Forms. **Cap** 67, 134 mg.

Pharmacokinetics. After absorption, fenofibrate is hydrolyzed to the active drug, fenofibric acid, which is more than 99% bound to plasma proteins. It is excreted predominantly unchanged in urine with a half-life of 20 hr, which is prolonged in renal dysfunction.

Adverse Reactions. Side effects include GI disturbances, skin rash, muscle pain, and headache. Elevations in serum transaminases and CPK have occurred. Cholelithiasis has been reported, but it is not clear if the frequency is as great as with clofibrate. Avoid fenofibrate in those with liver, gallbladder, or kidney disease.

GEMFIBROZIL
Lopid, Various

Pharmacology. Gemfibrozil is a fibric acid derivative that decreases triglyceride and VLDL-c concentrations and increases HDL-c concentrations. Effects on LDL-c are variable. LDL-c can increase in some patients, especially those with type IV hyperlipoproteinemia. Its exact mechanism is unclear, but it appears to act through many mechanisms. There is increased secretion of cholesterol into bile, increased affinity of LDL receptors for LDL particles, activation of lipoprotein lipase, inhibition of triglyceride synthesis, suppression of free fatty acid release from adipose tissue, and a change in LDL-c toward a potentially less atherosclerotic form.[258,282]

Administration and Adult Dosage. **PO as a hypolipidemic** 600 mg bid.

Special Populations. *Pediatric Dosage.* Safety and efficacy not established.

Geriatric Dosage. Initiate therapy at lowest possible dosage and slowly titrate to desired effect. Maximum dosage might not be required or tolerated.

Other Conditions. Some investigators advise decreasing dose by one-half with Cl_{cr} of 20–50 mL/min.

Dosage Forms. **Tab** 600 mg.

Patient Instructions. (*See* Hypolipidemics Class Instructions.) Take doses 30 minutes before morning and evening meals. Gemfibrozil can slightly increase the risk of cancer and is similar to another medication that increases the risk of cancer, gallstones, and pancreatitis. You and your physician might decide that the benefit of reducing the risk of coronary heart disease is worth these other risks. Promptly report any muscle pain, tenderness, or weakness, especially if you also are taking lovastatin or a similar drug.

Pharmacokinetics. *Onset and Duration.* The maximum decrease in serum triglyceride and total cholesterol occurs within 4–12 weeks; lipids return to pretreatment levels after drug discontinuation.

Fate. The drug is rapidly and completely absorbed after oral administration. Mean peak serum concentrations of 15–25 mg/L (60–100 μmol/L) occur 1–2 hr after administration of 600 mg bid. Serum concentrations are directly proportional to dose. The drug is 97–98.6% bound to albumin. Cl appears to be independent of renal function. Gemfibrozil is metabolized in the liver to a number of compounds. Approximately 70% of a dose is excreted in the urine, primarily as glucuronide conjugates of the drug and metabolites; less than 2% is excreted renally as unchanged drug.[283–285]

$t_{\frac{1}{2}}$. Reportedly 1.5–2 hr but might be longer.[283]

Adverse Reactions. Dyspepsia (20%), abdominal pain (10%), diarrhea (7%), fatigue (3%), and nausea and vomiting (3%) are frequent; acute appendicitis, dizziness, eczema, rash, vertigo, constipation, headache, paresthesia (all 1–2%) also occur. Occasional side effects include atrial fibrillation and elevations in liver function tests (AST, ALT, LDH, bilirubin, and alkaline phosphatase) that return to normal with drug discontinuation. Occasional mild decreases in WBC count, hematocrit, and hemoglobin occur but usually stabilize. However, there have been rare reports of severe blood dyscrasias. Serum glucose can be slightly elevated, as can LDL-c in some patients with high triglyceride levels. Gemfibrozil can increase biliary lipogenicity and possibly increase long-term risk of cholelithiasis.[258] Cholelithiasis requiring gallbladder surgery developed in 0.9% of gemfibrozil-treated patients, compared with 0.5% of patients in a placebo group. This excess was similar to that which occurred with clofibrate. (*See* Notes.) An acute infection-like syndrome characterized by arthralgias, myalgia, and myositis has occurred during therapy. Rhabdomyolysis with elevated CPK levels can precipitate acute renal failure, especially with the combination of gemfibrozil and lovastatin.[263] This has occurred as early as several weeks to months after initiating therapy. Routine monitoring of CPK might not detect rhabdomyolysis in a timely manner. Many have recommended avoiding the combination of gemfibrozil and any HMG-CoA reductase inhibitor.[265] Worsening of renal insufficiency has been reported with an initial Cr_s >2 mg/dL. Carcinogenesis, impairment of fertility, and development of cataracts occur in rats. (*See* Precautions and Notes.)

Contraindications. Hepatic or severe renal dysfunction; primary biliary cirrhosis; pre-existing gallbladder disease.

Precautions. Pregnancy, lactation. Evaluate any reports of muscle pain, tenderness, or weakness for myositis, including a determination of serum CPK. Discontinue if an adequate effect does not occur after 3 months, if cholelithiasis is suspected, or if liver function tests remain elevated.

Drug Interactions. Gemfibrozil can potentiate the effect of oral anticoagulants. Cholesterol-binding resins can decrease absorption of gemfibrozil. Insulin or an oral hypoglycemic might be required.[283,285] Displacement of glyburide from plasma protein binding sites, an action that produces hypoglycemia, has been reported.[286] Gemfibrozil and lovastatin (and possibly other HMG-CoA reductase inhibitors) together might increase the risk of myotoxicity. (*See* Adverse Reactions.)

Parameters to Monitor. Serum lipids, initially every few weeks, and then about q 3 months.[266] Liver function tests and CBC q 3–6 months. Monitor serum glucose if the patient is receiving insulin or an oral hypoglycemic and prothrombin time if patient is taking an oral anticoagulant.

Notes. Gemfibrozil is not considered a major treatment for hypercholesterolemia because of its effects on LDL-c, but it does increase HDL-c and decrease triglycerides, so it is useful in some patients.[257] Gemfibrozil is indicated for the treatment of type IV and V hyperlipidemias with very high serum triglycerides (usually >2000 mg/dL) in patients at risk for pancreatitis and not responding to diet. It is also indicated in type IIb patients (only those without history or symptoms of CHD) with low HDL-c and an inadequate response to weight loss, diet, exercise, and other drugs that raise HDL-c (eg, bile acid sequestrants, niacin), but is not indicated in type I or IIa hyperlipidemias or in those patients who have low HDL-c only. The Helsinki Heart Study showed a 34% reduction in the incidence of CHD in middle-aged men (initially without CHD symptoms) treated with gemfibrozil in a 5-yr study, although total death rate was no different between treated and placebo groups.[287,288] A substudy of the Helsinki Heart Study showed an increase in gallstone and gallbladder surgery in gemfibrozil-treated patients. After a 3.5-yr extension of this study, all-cause mortality was slightly higher in the original gemfibrozil group, primarily because of cancer deaths.[288] An ancillary study of the Helsinki Heart Study investigated the use of gemfibrozil in patients with signs or symptoms of CHD.[289] The rate of serious adverse cardiac advents and total mortality with gemfibrozil treatment did not significantly differ from that of placebo; however, information on key prognostic indicators and their distribution was not known.[289] Gemfibrozil is chemically and pharmacologically similar to **clofibrate**. A 44% relative increase in age-adjusted, all-cause mortality occurred in a study of long-term clofibrate use related to a 33% increase in noncardiovascular disease such as malignancy, gallbladder disease, and pancreatitis. Because of the smaller size of the gemfibrozil studies, the increase in mortality in the gemfibrozil group relative to placebo might not be statistically significantly different from the excess mortality associated with clofibrate use.

HMG-COA REDUCTASE INHIBITORS:	
ATORVASTATIN	Lipitor
CERIVASTATIN	Baycol
FLUVASTATIN	Lescol, Lescol XL
LOVASTATIN	Mevacor
PRAVASTATIN	Pravachol
SIMVASTATIN	Zocor

Pharmacology. Hydroxymethylglutaryl-CoA (HMG-CoA) reductase inhibitors competitively inhibit conversion of HMG-CoA to mevalonate, an early rate-limiting step in cholesterol synthesis. A compensatory increase in LDL receptors, which bind and remove circulating LDL-c, results. Production of LDL-c also can decrease because of decreased production of VLDL or increased VLDL removal by LDL receptors. These drugs produce dose-dependent, maximum reductions in LDL of 30–40% (up to 60% with atorvastatin) and triglycerides of 10–30% and increases in HDL levels of 2–15%. Drug effects are dose dependent until the following doses are reached: 80 mg for atorvastatin, 0.3 mg for cerivastatin, 20 mg for fluvastatin and simvastatin, and 40 mg for lovastatin and pravastatin. Fluvastatin is about 30% less effective in lowering lipids than the other drugs. These drugs stabilize arterial plaques, which might be an important factor in their reduction of MI risk. They also appear to reduce the risk of bone fracture by increasing bone density, the risk of DVT and the risk of becoming diabetic.[258,290-292]

Administration and Adult Dosage. Adjust dosage at no less than 4-week intervals. **PO for hyperlipidemia** (Atorvastatin) 10 mg/day initially, increasing to a maximum of 80 mg/day. (Cerivastatin) 0.2–0.8 mg/day in the evening. (Fluvastatin) 20 mg hs initially, increasing up to 80 mg/day; a slight increase in fluvastatin LDL-c lowering occurs with a bid schedule. (Lovastatin) 20 mg (40 mg with serum cholesterol >300 mg/dL) with the evening meal initially. Start with 10 mg/day in patients requiring <20% decrease in LDL-c or when concurrent use with cyclosporine is unavoidable. Increase to a maintenance dosage of 20–80 mg/day. Do not exceed a lovastatin dosage of 20 mg/day when used with cyclosporine. (Pravastatin) 10–20 mg hs initially, increasing to 10–40 mg/day hs. (Simvastatin) 5–10 mg/day in the evening initially, increasing to 5–40 mg/day in the evening.

Special Populations. *Pediatric Dosage.* Safety and efficacy not established.

Geriatric Dosage. **PO** (Pravastatin) 10 mg/day initially; (Simvastatin) 5 mg/day initially; the elderly can achieve maximal reductions in LDL-c at doses ≤20 mg/day. Maximum dosage might not be required or tolerated.

Other Conditions. (Atorvastatin) no dosage adjustment necessary in renal impairment. (Cerivastatin) start with 0.2 mg/day in moderate to severe renal impairment. (Lovastatin) start with 10 mg/day when concurrent use with cyclosporine is unavoidable; maximum dosage is 20 mg/day with concurrent immunosuppressant therapy. (Pravastatin) start with 10 mg/day with renal or hepatic impairment and in patients concurrently taking cyclosporine; do not exceed a dose of 20 mg/day in the latter case. (Simvastatin) start with 5 mg/day in patients requiring <20% reductions in LDL-c and with severe renal insufficiency. Use dosages >20 mg/day only with extreme caution in patients with Cl_{cr} <30 mL/min.

Dosage Forms. (*See* Hypolipidemic Drugs Comparison Chart.)

Patient Instructions. (*See* Hypolipidemics Class Instructions.) Atorvastatin can be taken any time of day without regard to meals. Take lovastatin with the evening meal to increase its absorption; other drugs can be taken without regard to meals. Take pravastatin 1 hour before or 4 hours after a dose of a cholesterol-binding resin. Promptly report any unexplained muscle pain or tenderness, especially if accompanied by malaise or fever. Avoid excessive concurrent use of alcohol, but abstinence is not required. Do not take these drugs during pregnancy because of possible harm to the fetus. Inform your physician if you become or intend to become pregnant.

Pharmacokinetics. *Onset and Duration.* Onset is within 2 weeks; peak effect is within 4–6 weeks; cholesterol levels return to baseline after drug discontinuation.

Fate. Absorption is rapid. Lovastatin and simvastatin are prodrugs that undergo extensive first-pass metabolism to active metabolites. Serum concentrations of the active lovastatin metabolite when taken under fasting conditions are two-thirds of that when taken with food. Absorption of other drugs is unaffected by food. Systemic bioavailability of all drugs is low because of extensive (>60%) first-pass extraction. Peak serum concentrations of active inhibitors are achieved in 1–4 hr for all drugs. Protein binding is 98% for atorvastatin, 99% for cerivastatin, 55–60% for pravastatin, 95% for simvastatin, >95% for lovastatin, and 98% for fluvastatin. Atorvastatin, lovastatin, and simvastatin are lipophilic and cross the blood–brain barrier; cerivastatin, fluvastatin, and pravastatin are hydrophilic and do not. All the drugs are primarily (>70%) hepatically metabolized to active and inactive metabolites, which then undergo extensive fecal elimination. Renal elimination accounts for <2% for atorvastatin, 5% for fluvastatin, 10% for lovastatin, 13% for simvastatin, 20% for pravastatin, and 26% for cerivastatin. Severe renal insufficiency (Cl_{cr} 10–30 mL/min) results in a 2-fold increase in serum concentrations of renally excreted drugs (ie, cerivastatin, pravastatin).[257,291–297]

$t_{1/2}$. (Fluvastatin, lovastatin, pravastatin, simvastatin) <2 hr; (cerivastatin) 2–3 hr; (atorvastatin) 14 hr.[292]

Adverse Reactions. The drugs are generally well tolerated, with discontinuation rates less than other hypolipidemic drugs.[267] The frequency of side effects appears to be similar for all drugs.[292–298] GI complaints such as diarrhea, constipation, flatulence, abdominal pain, and nausea occur in about 5% of patients. Headache (4–9%), rash (3–5%), dizziness (3–5%), and blurred vision (1–2%) are other frequent side effects. Myopathy and myositis occur rarely with single therapy and can be associated with mild elevations of CPK. Rhabdomyolysis leading to acute renal failure is a rare complication but occurs more frequently in combination with gemfibrozil, cyclosporine, or ≥1 g/day of niacin. Pravastatin can cause less myopathy than lovastatin with cyclosporine.[292] Increases in liver function tests greater than 3 times normal occur in up to 2% of patients, but most are asymptomatic and reverse with discontinuation.[258] There have been 62 cases of serious liver disease directly associated with statin use reported to the Food and Drug Administration.[299] Anomalies have been reported with intrauterine exposure. Carcinogenicity occurs in mice and rats at higher than human doses, but the clinical implications are unclear.[262,300]

Contraindications. Pregnancy; lactation; active liver disease; unexplained persistent elevations of serum transaminases.

Precautions. Administer to women of childbearing age only when possibility of becoming pregnant is unlikely. Use with caution in patients who consume substantial quantities of alcohol and/or have histories of liver disease. Discontinue therapy if liver function tests are >3 times normal. Consider withholding the drug in any patient with risk factors for renal failure secondary to rhabdomyolysis, such as severe acute infection; hypotension, major surgery, or trauma; severe electrolyte, endocrine, or metabolic abnormalities; or uncontrolled seizures.

Drug Interactions. Myositis and rhabdomyolysis can be more common in combination with cyclosporine (lovastatin levels are quadrupled), erythromycin, gemfibrozil, itraconazole, ketoconazole (and possibly other inhibitors of CYP3A4), or lipid-lowering dosages of niacin (>1 g/day).[292] HMG-CoA reductase inhibitors can increase the effect of warfarin. Bile acid sequestrants can markedly decrease pravastatin oral bioavailability when taken together; take pravastatin 1 hr before or 4 hr after resin doses.

Parameters to Monitor. Obtain serum lipid and liver function tests on initiation, 6 and 12 weeks after initiation, after dosage increases, and at least semiannually thereafter. Others have recommended more frequent monitoring.[257,258] Increase the frequency of monitoring if adverse effects are suspected. Routine monitoring of muscle enzymes might not adequately identify patients at risk for rhabdomyolysis but might be warranted in patients with skeletal muscle complaints and risk factors.

Notes. HMG-CoA reductase inhibitors are indicated for the treatment of type IIa and IIb hyperlipoproteinemias. They are the most effective in decreasing LDL-c, and their effect on decreasing coronary morbidity and mortality is proven.[292] The choice of drug depends on cost, amount of cholesterol lowering desired, and risk factors for CHD. Lovastatin, pravastatin, and simvastatin are more effective than fluvastatin and are therefore preferable when a >25% reduction in LDL-c is required.[292,301] They can have additive effects with the bile acid sequestrants and have been used in combination with niacin and gemfibrozil. (*See* Adverse Reactions and Drug Interactions.) Cholesterol reduction with these agents can reduce the risk of stroke and total mortality.[302] One large study found a reduced CHD risk with lovastatin in men and women with "average" serum cholesterol and no evidence of pre-existing heart disease.[303] Pravastatin appears to reduce inflammation in vessel walls based on its effective lowering of C-reactive protein levels in patients with coronary artery disease.[304] C-reactive protein concentrations can be a predictive and sensitive measure of vessel wall inflammation resulting from elevated cholesterol levels.[305]

NIACIN
Niaspan, Various

Pharmacology. Niacin (nicotinic acid), in dosages of 1 g/day or more, decreases serum total cholesterol, LDL-c and VLDL-c, and triglycerides, and increases HDL-c. Mean serum cholesterol and triglyceride levels are reduced by 10% and 26%, respectively. The mechanism for these effects is not entirely known but might involve inhibition of lipolysis, reduced LDL and VLDL synthesis, and increased lipoprotein lipase activity.[306,307] Niacin consistently decreases lipoprotein (a).[257] **Niacinamide** (nicotinamide) does not have hypolipidemic effects and cannot be substituted for niacin.

Administration and Adult Dosage. **PO as a hypolipidemic** 250 mg/day with evening meal initially, increasing at 4- to 7-day intervals to 1.5–2 g/day in 3 divided doses. Continue this dosage for 2 months. If necessary, the dosage can then be increased at 2- to 4-week intervals to 1 g tid; the dose can be increased again, if necessary, to reach the desired clinical effect or the maximum tolerated dosage to a usual maximum of 2 g tid. Use of >3–4 g/day does not appear to increase efficacy appreciably and is associated with increased side effects.[306] (Niaspan) 375 mg hs initially, increasing as tolerated to a maximum of 2 g hs. (*See* Notes.) If an **SR product** is substituted for an immediate-release form, reduce the dosage by one-half. Risk of hepatotoxicity increases at SR doses >1.5–3 g/day, and these are not recommended.[258]

Special Populations. *Pediatric Dosage.* Safety and efficacy not established. Although niacin is effective in reducing triglycerides and cholesterol in children and adolescents, adverse effects are common and can be severe. Some investigators have recommended niacin use be avoided in children or used only under close supervision by a lipid specialist if diet and bile acid sequestrants have failed.[259,308] In these cases, niacin should generally be used in combination with diet and a bile acid sequestrant, if tolerated.[259] Close monitoring is necessary. (*See* Adverse Reactions and Precautions.)

Geriatric Dosage. Initiate therapy at lowest possible dosage and slowly titrate to desired effect. Maximum dosage might not be required or tolerated.

Patient Instructions. Use only under medical supervision. Effects can differ with different preparations. Almost everyone experiences some flushing. Tolerance to flushing generally occurs with time. Taking 325 mg of aspirin or 200 mg of ibuprofen (or an equivalent dose of another NSAID) 30–60 minutes before each niacin dose might reduce flushing. Taking niacin with meals also might minimize flushing and reduce GI upset. Avoid hot liquids or alcohol after taking a dose. Avoid interruptions in therapy; tolerance can be lost if therapy is interrupted, so slow resumption of the usual dosage is recommended. Avoid sudden changes in posture if you are also taking medicine for high blood pressure. Report any persistent nausea.

Dosage Forms. **Tab** 50, 100, 250, 500 mg; **Elxr** 10 mg/mL; **SR Cap** 125, 250, 400, 500 mg; **SR Tab** 250, 500, 750, 1000 mg. (*See* Notes.)

Pharmacokinetics. *Onset and Duration.* The onset of triglyceride and cholesterol reductions usually occurs within several days, although some studies have demonstrated a response after a single dose.[306] Pretreatment lipid levels return 2–6 weeks after drug discontinuation.

Fate. The drug is almost completely absorbed from standard formulations; peak serum levels 30–60 min after 1 g standard formulations are 15–30 μg/L (120–240 nmol/L). Niacin is largely metabolized in the liver to niacinamide (nicotinamide) and its derivatives (eg, nicotinuric acid), which can contribute to the lipid-lowering activity, especially after long-term use. The majority is excreted as unchanged drug or metabolites in urine.[306]

$t_{½}$. 20–48 min.[306]

Adverse Reactions. Dose-related flushing of the neck and face (usually in "blush" areas) occurs in almost all patients and is related to the rate of rise of serum levels rather than the absolute serum concentrations. Tolerance can develop but disappear if therapy is interrupted. Administration with food, gradual upward dosage titration, use of a SR formulation, or premedication with 325 mg of aspirin or 200 mg of ibuprofen (or equivalent dose of another NSAID) 30–60 min before each dose can reduce flushing. Postural hypotension can occur, especially when niacin is used with antihypertensive drugs or when it is taken with alcohol or hot liquids. Vasodilatory effects can precipitate or aggravate angina. Rash, pruritus, and stomach discomfort also occur frequently; the latter can occur more commonly with SR preparations. Increases in AST, ALT , bilirubin, and LDH concentrations occur frequently and might be related to increasing the daily dosage by more than 2.5 g/month. Severe hepatotoxicity (hepatic necrosis) is rare and tends to occur with abrupt dosage increases, SR forms substituted for immediate-release products without dosage reduction, or brand interchange. Hepatotoxicity can occur at low dosages (≤3 g/day) of SR products and as soon as 2 days after initiation. Discontinue therapy if liver function tests remain over 3 times pretreatment values.[307]

Contraindications. Arterial hemorrhage; severe hypotension; hepatic dysfunction; unexplained elevations of transaminases, active peptic ulcer disease.

Precautions. Pregnancy; lactation. Use with caution in patients with gallbladder disease or histories of liver disease, unstable angina, gout, gouty arthritis, glaucoma, or diabetes.[258,309] Nausea can be a presenting sign of hepatotoxicity.[258] If the SR form is substituted for the immediate-release form, reduce dosage by about one-half. If use with an HMG-CoA reductase inhibitor is unavoidable, use with extreme caution. Some formulations contain tartrazine dye, which can cause allergic reactions in sensitive patients.

Drug Interactions. Concurrent use with HMG-CoA reductase inhibitors can increase the risk of rhabdomyolysis. Concurrent therapy with α-adrenergic blocking antihypertensives can result in hypotension. Diet and/or dosage of oral hypoglycemic drugs or insulin might require adjustment with concurrent niacin use. Hepatotoxic drugs can have additive effects.[257]

Parameters to Monitor. Monitor serum lipids q 2 weeks initially and then q 1–3 months. Periodic liver function tests, blood glucose, and serum uric acid levels are recommended, especially at dosages >1.5 g/day.[257] Obtain liver function tests at baseline and q 6–12 weeks for the first year and then semiannually unless hepatotoxicity is suspected.

Notes. Indicated for type IIa, IIb, III, IV, and V hyperlipoproteinemias. Reductions in sudden cardiac deaths and fatal and nonfatal MI and an 11% decrease in mortality (compared with placebo) occur in patients treated with niacin.[298] The cost of standard niacin formulations can be much lower than alternative drugs; the cost of SR products can be higher. SR products appear to have equal efficacy at lowering LDL-c at one-half the dosage of standard products, but the SR form might be less effective in lowering triglycerides or raising HDL at dosages equal to standard forms.[257,308,310] Some have advocated avoidance of SR preparations altogether for treatment of hyperlipidemia because of their potentially greater hepatotoxicity.[308,310]

Niaspan is an extended-release product that may be safer than other SR products because of its release rate. It is available as 500, 750 and 1000 mg tablets.[369]

HYPOLIPIDEMIC DRUGS COMPARISON CHART

DRUG	DOSAGE FORMS	ADULT ORAL DOSAGE[a] INITIAL (I) MAINTENANCE (M)	RELATIVE EFFECT ON LIPIDS[b] LDL	RELATIVE EFFECT ON LIPIDS[b] HDL	RELATIVE EFFECT ON LIPIDS[b] TG	INDICATIONS BY WHO CATEGORY TYPE[c]	COMMENTS
BILE ACID SEQUESTRANTS							
Cholestyramine Questran Questran Light Various	Pwdr 4 g resin/9 g drug packet or scoop Pwdr 4 g resin/5, 5.5, 5.7 g packet or scoop Tab 1g.	(I) 4 g daily–bid. (M) 8–16 g/day in 1–6 doses, to a maximum of 24 g/day.[d]	↓↓	↑	↑	IIa	Constipation frequent. Can be used in children. Numerous interactions. Decrease in mortality demonstrated. Take before meals.
Colesevelam Welchol	Tab 625 mg.	6 tablets/day in 1–2 doses.	↓↓	↑	↑	IIa	Better tolerated than cholestyramine or colestipol.
Colestipol HCl Colestid	Gran 5 g resin/7.5 g packet or scoop Tab 1 g.	(I) (gran) 5 g daily–bid. (M) (gran) 15–30 g/day in 1–4 doses.[e]	↓↓	↑	↑	IIa	Similar to cholestyramine. (See above.)
FIBRIC ACID DERIVATIVES							
Fenofibrate Tricor	Cap 67, 134 mg.	(I) 67 mg/day. (M) up to 201 mg/day.	↓↓↓	↑↑	↓↓↓	IV, V	Avoid in liver, gallbladder, or kidney disease. Take with food.
Gemfibrozil Lopid Various	Tab 600 mg.	(M) 600 mg bid.	↑↓	↑↑	↓↓↓	IIb, IV, V	Overall mortality rate with long-term therapy is increased. Take 30 min before AM and PM meals.
Clofibrate	Not recommended because of a large increase in overall mortality.						*(continued)*

381

HYPOLIPIDEMIC DRUGS COMPARISON CHART (continued)

DRUG	DOSAGE FORMS	ADULT ORAL DOSAGE[a] INITIAL (I) MAINTENANCE (M)	RELATIVE EFFECT ON LIPIDS[b] LDL	RELATIVE EFFECT ON LIPIDS[b] HDL	RELATIVE EFFECT ON LIPIDS[b] TG	INDICATIONS BY WHO CATEGORY TYPE[c]	COMMENTS
NICOTINIC ACID							
Niacin Various	Tab 50, 100, 250, 500 mg Elxr 10 mg/mL SR Cap 125, 250, 400, 500 mg[e] SR Tab 250, 500, 750, 1000 mg.[e] Inj 100 mg/mL.	(I) Titrate slowly. (See monograph.) (M) 1.5–3 g/day, to a maximum of 6 g/day.	↓↓	↑↑	↓↓↓	IIa, IIb, III, IV, V	Frequent flushing and GI side effects. Must titrate dosage slowly. Decrease in mortality demonstrated. Avoid SR products. Low cost. Take with food or milk.
HMG-COA REDUCTASE INHIBITORS							
Atorvastatin Lipitor	Tab 10, 20, 40, 80 mg.	(I) 10 mg/day. (M) 10–80 mg/day.	↓↓↓↓	↑	↓↓↓	IIa, IIb	Take at any time without regard to meals.
Cerivastatin Baycol	Tab 0.2, 0.3, 0.4, 0.8 mg.	0.2–0.8 mg/day.	↓↓↓	↑	↓↓	IIa, IIb	Take in evening without regard to meals.
Fluvastatin Lescol Lescol XL	Cap 20, 40 mg SR Tab 80 mg.	(I) 20 mg q hs. (M) 20–80 mg q hs.	↓↓	↑	↓	IIa, IIb	Take without regard to meals. Monitor for myositis and hepatic dysfunction. Important drug interactions.

(continued)

HYPOLIPIDEMIC DRUGS COMPARISON CHART (continued)

DRUG	DOSAGE FORMS	ADULT ORAL DOSAGE[a] INITIAL (I) MAINTENANCE (M)	RELATIVE EFFECT ON LIPIDS[b]			INDICATIONS BY WHO CATEGORY TYPE[c]	COMMENTS
			LDL	HDL	TG		
Lovastatin Mevacor	Tab 10, 20, 40 mg.	(I) 20 mg/day. (M) 20–80 mg/day in 1–2 divided doses.	↓↓↓	↑	↓↓	IIa, IIb	Take with evening meal. (*See* Fluvastatin.)
Pravastatin Pravachol	Tab 10, 20, 40 mg.	(I) 10–20 mg q hs. (M) 10–40 mg q hs.	↓↓↓	↑	↓↓	IIa, IIb	Take without regard to meals. (*See* Fluvastatin.)
Rosuvastatin Crestor (Investigational— AstraZeneca)	—	(I) 5–10 mg/day. (M) 10–80 mg/day.	↓↓↓↓↓↓	↑↑	↓↓	IIa, IIb	Take at anytime of day.
Simvastatin Zocor	Tab 5, 10, 20, 40, 80 mg.	(I) 5–10 mg q hs. (M) 5–80 mg/day.	↓↓↓	↑	↓↓	IIa, IIb	Take without regard to meals. (*See* Fluvastatin.)

LDL = serum low-density lipoprotein cholesterol, shown to have a graded, positive relationship with coronary heart disease (CHD); HDL = serum high-density lipoprotein, shown to have a cardioprotective effect against CHD; TG = serum triglycerides, which have a positive relationship to CHD.

[a] Clinical trials in the elderly are limited, but the drugs are considered effective. Base decision on drug treatment on life expectancy, concomitant disease, potential adverse effects, patient desire for treatment, quality of life, assessment of coronary heart disease risk, and cost. A conservative approach is recommended; generally initiating therapy at the lowest possible dosage and slowly titrating to desired effect while closely monitoring possible side effects. Maximum dosage might not be required or tolerated.

[b] Arrows represent approximate relative effects based on results achieved with usual dosage. Study results differ because of differences in patient groups, administration schedules, dosages, and degrees of hypercholesteremia.

[c] World Health Organization (WHO) classification by characteristics of dyslipidemia.

[d] All dosages are expressed in terms of anhydrous resin.

[e] Do not substitute SR niacin products for an equal dosage of immediate-release products; use one-half the dosage of immediate-release products.

From references 266, 285, 311, and 312 and product information.

RECOMMENDATIONS FROM THE THIRD REPORT OF THE NATIONAL CHOLESTEROL EDUCATION PROGRAM (NCEP) EXPERT PANEL ON DETECTION, EVALUATION, AND TREATMENT OF HIGH BLOOD CHOLESTEROL IN ADULTS (ADULT TREATMENT PANEL [ATP] III)

STEP 1. Classification of lipoprotein levels

ATP III CLASSIFICATION OF LDL, TOTAL, AND HDL CHOLESTEROL (MG/DL)

LDL CHOLESTEROL–PRIMARY TARGET OF THERAPY		TOTAL CHOLESTEROL		HDL CHOLESTEROL	
<100 mg/dL	Optimal	<200 mg/dL	Desirable	<40 mg/dL	Low
100–129 mg/dL	Near Optimal/Above Optimal	200–239 mg/dL	Borderline High	≥60 mg/dL	High
130–159 mg/dL	Borderline High	≥240 mg/dL	High		
160–189 mg/dL	High				
≥190 mg/dL	Very High				

STEP 2. Identify the presence or absence of clinical atherosclerotic disease that confers a high risk for coronary heart disease (CHD) events. These include clinical CHD, symptomatic carotid artery disease, peripheral arterial disease or abdominal aortic aneurysm.

STEP 3. Identify major risk factors other than LDL: cigarette smoking, hypertension (BP ≥140/90 mmHg or on antihypertensive medication, HDL cholesterol <40 mg/dL, family history of premature CHD, age (men ≥45 years; women ≥55 years). Diabetes is considered a risk equivalent.

STEP 4. If 2+ risk factors (other than LDL) are present without CHD or CHD risk equivalent, assess 10-year (short-term) CHD risk (refer to Framingham tables).

STEP 5. Determine Risk Category

RISK CATEGORY	LDL GOAL	LDL LEVEL AT WHICH TO INITIATE THERAPEUTIC LIFESTYLE CHANGES (TLC)	LDL LEVEL AT WHICH TO CONSIDER DRUG THERAPY
CHD or CHD risk equivalents (10-yr risk >20%)	<100 mg/dL	≥100 mg/dL	≥130 mg/dL (100–129 mg/dL: drug therapy optional)
2+ risk factors (10-yr risk ≤20%)	<130 mg/dL	≥130 mg/dL	10-yr risk 10–20%: ≥130 mg/dL; 10-yr risk < 10%: ≥160 mg/dL
0–1 risk factor	<160 mg/dL	≥160 mg/dL	≥190 mg/dL (160–189 mg/dL: LDL-lowering drug is optional)

STEP 6. Initiate therapeutic lifestyle changes (TLC): diet (refer to guidelines for precise recommendations), weight management, increased physical activity.

STEP 7. Consider adding drug therapy if LDL exceeds levels shown in Step 5 of table: consider drug simultaneously with TLC for CHD and CHD equivalents; consider adding drug to TLC after 3 months for other risk categories.

(continued)

RECOMMENDATIONS FROM THE THIRD REPORT OF THE NATIONAL CHOLESTEROL EDUCATION PROGRAM (NCEP) EXPERT PANEL ON DETECTION, EVALUATION, AND TREATMENT OF HIGH BLOOD CHOLESTEROL IN ADULTS (ADULT TREATMENT PANEL [ATP] III) *(continued)*

STEP 8. Identify metabolic syndrome and treat, if present, after 3 months of TLC.

CLINICAL IDENTIFICATION OF METABOLIC SYNDROME

Risk Factor	Defined Level
Abdominal obesity	For men: waist circumference >102 cm (40 in); For women: waist circumference >88 cm (35 in)
Triglycerides	≥150 mg/dL
HDL cholesterol	For men: <40 mg/dL; For women: <50 mg/dL
Blood pressure	≥130/≥85 mmHg
Fasting glucose	≥110 mg/dL

STEP 9. Treat elevated triglycerides

ATPIII—CLASSIFICATION OF SERUM TRIGLYCERIDES (TG) (MG/DL)

<150 mg/dL	Normal
150–199 mg/dL	Borderline High
200–499 mg/dL	High
≥500 mg/dL	Very High

- Primary aim of therapy is to reach LDL goal
- Intensify weight management
- Increase physical activity

If triglycerides are ≥200 mg/dL after LDL goal is reached, set secondary goal for non-HDL cholesterol (total HDL) 30 mg/dL higher than LDL goal.

COMPARISON OF LDL CHOLESTEROL AND NON-HDL CHOLESTEROL GOALS FOR THREE RISK CATEGORIES

Risk Category	LDL Goal	Non-HDL Goal	
CHD and CHD RE (10-yr risk for CHD >20%)	<100 mg/dL	<130 mg/dL	If TG ≥500 mg/dL: reduce to prevent pancreatitis (low fat diet, weight management, a fibrate or niacin).
Multiple (2+) risk factors and 10-yr risk ≤20%)	<130 mg/dL	<160 mg/dL	Treatment of low HDL: weight management; increased physical activity; if TG = 200–499 mg/dL, then achieve non-HDL goal; if TG <200 mg/dL in CHD or CHD risk equivalent, consider niacin or a fibrate.
0–1 risk factor	<160 mg/dL	<190 mg/dL	

From reference 266 and The National Heart Lung and Blood Institute (http://www.nhlbi.nih.gov/).

Inotropic Drugs

DOBUTAMINE HYDROCHLORIDE
Dobutrex, Various

Pharmacology. Dobutamine is a synthetic sympathomimetic amine that exists as the racemic mixture of an L-isomer with predominantly α-adrenergic agonist actions and a D-isomer that has β_1- and β_2-adrenergic agonist actions. The net clinical effect is typically that of a potent β_1-agonist with mild vasodilatory properties. At low dosages, it increases myocardial contractility without markedly increasing heart rate; this specificity is dose dependent and is lost at high dosages. Unlike dopamine, dobutamine does not release stored catecholamines and has no effect on dopaminergic receptors.[313,314]

Administration and Adult Dosage. IV for inotropic support, by infusion only (in any nonalkaline IV fluid) 2.5 μg/kg/min initially, increasing gradually in 2.5 μg/kg/min increments to 20 μg/kg/min, and adjusting dosage to desired response. Maintenance dosages are typically 2–10 μg/kg/min.[315] Although dosages up to 40 μg/kg/min have been used, use dosages above 20 μg/kg/min with caution because of increased risks of tachycardia, arrhythmias, and myocardial ischemia.[316]

Special Populations. *Pediatric Dosage.* Safety and efficacy not established. However, **IV infusion** 2 μg/kg/min initially, followed by adjustment to desired hemodynamic response, up to 20 μg/kg/min, has been used.[317]

Geriatric Dosage. Same as adult dosage.

Dosage Forms. Inj 12.5 mg/mL.

Pharmacokinetics. *Onset and Duration.* Onset <2 min; peak within 10 min; duration <10 min.[318]

Fate. Wide interpatient variability exists, especially between adult and pediatric patients. V_d in CHF is 0.2 ± 0.08 L/kg; Cl in CHF is 3.5 ± 1.3 L/hr/kg. The drug is eliminated primarily in the liver to inactive glucuronide conjugates and 3-O-methyldobutamine.[10,313]

$t_{½}$. 2.4 ± 0.7 min.[10]

Adverse Reactions. Precipitation or exacerbation of ventricular ectopy occurs frequently; ventricular arrhythmias can occur (although these are less likely than with other sympathomimetics).[313] Modest increases in heart rate or systolic blood pressure occur frequently; dosage reduction usually reverses these effects rapidly. Occasionally, nausea, headache, angina, nonspecific chest pain, palpitations, and shortness of breath are noted. Patients with atrial fibrillation might be at risk of developing rapid ventricular responses because dobutamine facilitates AV conduction.

Contraindications. Idiopathic hypertrophic subaortic stenosis.

Precautions. Correct hypovolemia before using in patients who are hypotensive. Although most cases of extravasation cause no signs of tissue damage, at least one case of dermal necrosis after extravasation of a 2.5 μg/kg/min infusion has been reported. Dobutamine contains a sulfite preservative that can be problematic in sensitive individuals, especially asthmatics.

Drug Interactions. Bretylium, guanethidine, and heterocyclic antidepressants can potentiate the pressor response to direct-acting vasopressors. Oxytocics used in obstetrics can cause severe, persistent hypertension when used with vasopressors. Halogenated hydrocarbon anesthetics can predispose patients to serious arrhythmias.

Parameters to Monitor. Monitor heart rate, arterial blood pressure, urine output, pulmonary capillary wedge pressure, cardiac index, ECG for ectopic activity, and infusion rate of solution continuously in the acute care setting and during periods of dosage titration or adjustment.

Notes. The drug is physically incompatible with sodium bicarbonate, furosemide, and other alkaline solutions. Use the reconstituted solution within 24 hr. (*See* Sympathomimetic Drugs for Hemodynamic Support Comparison Chart.)

DOBUTAMINE DILUTION GUIDE

| AMOUNT ADDED | | VOLUME OF | FINAL |
mg	*Volume*	DILUENT	CONCENTRATION[a]
250	1 vial (20 mL)	1000 mL	250 mg/L
250	1 vial (20 mL)	500 mL	500 mg/L
250	1 vial (20 mL)	250 mL	1 g/L

[a]Recommended concentrations, but concentrations up to 5 g/L have been used.

DOPAMINE HYDROCHLORIDE
Dopastat, Intropin, Various

Pharmacology. Dopamine is a catecholamine that acts directly, in a dose-dependent fashion, on postsynaptic dopaminergic (DA_1) receptors to produce renal and mesenteric vasodilation and on postsynaptic α_1-, α_2-, and β_1-adrenergic receptors. It also acts indirectly by releasing norepinephrine from sympathetic nerve storage sites. Clinical response depends on the patient's clinical condition and baseline sympathetic nervous system activity.[319] Approximate ranges: dopaminergic 0.5–2 μg/kg/min; β_1 5–10 μg/kg/min; mixed α and β 10–20 μg/kg/min; predominantly α >20 μg/kg/min.[313]

Administration and Adult Dosage. IV for shock, by infusion only (in any *non*alkaline IV fluid) 2.5 μg/kg/min initially, increasing gradually in 5–10 μg/kg/min increments up to 20–50 μg/kg/min, and adjusting dosage to desired response. If a dosage over 20 μg/kg/min is required, consider other pressors.[316] Use dosages over 50 μg/kg/min only with careful monitoring of hemodynamic parameters and urine output. **IV for chronic refractory CHF** 2–3 μg/kg/min initially and then increasing gradually until desired increases in urine flow, diastolic blood pressure, or heart rate are observed.[320] Dosages over 20 μg/kg/min are rarely used in CHF.[315,319,320] (*See* Notes.)

Special Populations. *Pediatric Dosage.* Safety and efficacy not established. However, **IV for shock** (recommendations for pediatric advance life support by the

American College of Cardiology and the American Heart Association) 2–5 μg/kg/min initially, increasing to 10–20 μg/kg/min to improve blood pressure, perfusion, and urine output.[317]

Geriatric Dosage. Same as adult dosage.

Dosage Forms. **Inj** 40, 80, 160 mg/mL. Also available prediluted, 0.8, 1.6, 3.2 mg/mL.

Pharmacokinetics. *Onset and Duration.* Onset within 5 min, duration <10 min.

Fate. There is large interpatient variability.[313] One evaluation in adult surgery patients derived a V_d of 0.89 ± 0.25 L/kg.[321] Cl is usually 3–4.2 L/hr/kg and 4.48 ± 0.94 L/hr/kg in adult surgery patients.[313,316] The drug is metabolized primarily to homovanillic acid (HVA) and related metabolites; the remainder is metabolized to norepinephrine and excreted in urine as HVA and metabolites of both HVA and norepinephrine; very little is excreted as unchanged dopamine.

$t_{1/2}$. α phase 1–2 min, β phase 6–9 min.[313,318]

Adverse Reactions. Increases in ventricular ectopy and ventricular arrhythmias can occur, particularly at high dosages (although this is less likely than with other sympathomimetics); reduce dosage if the number of ventricular ectopic beats increases. Hypertension can occur at high infusion rates. Nausea, vomiting, headache, anxiety, and angina pectoris also have been observed. Gangrene of the extremities has occurred in patients given large dosages of dopamine for long periods and in patients with occlusive vascular disease given low dosages.[313,322]

Contraindications. Pheochromocytoma; presence of uncorrected tachyarrhythmias or ventricular fibrillation.

Precautions. Correct hypovolemia before using in patients with shock. If increased diastolic pressure, decreased pulse pressure, or decreased urine flow occurs, decrease infusion rate and monitor patient for signs of excessive vasoconstriction. Use with caution in patients with occlusive vascular disease and extreme caution in patients receiving halogenated hydrocarbon anesthesia. Avoid extravasation of solution; however, if it occurs, the area can be infiltrated with 5–10 mg of phentolamine diluted in 10–15 mL of NS. Dopamine contains a sulfite preservative that can be problematic in sensitive individuals, especially asthmatics.

Drug Interactions. MAOIs (including furazolidone and linezolid) can increase the pressor response to dopamine by up to 20-fold; avoid these combinations. Bretylium, guanethidine, and heterocyclic antidepressants can potentiate the pressor response to direct-acting vasopressors. Oxytocics used in obstetrics can cause severe, persistent hypertension when used with vasopressors. IV phenytoin can produce hypotension in severely ill patients receiving IV dopamine. Halogenated hydrocarbon anesthetics can predispose patients to serious arrhythmias.

Parameters to Monitor. In shock, closely monitor heart rate, ECG, pulmonary capillary wedge pressure, cardiac index, arterial blood pressure, arterial blood gases, acid–base balance, toe temperature, urine output, and infusion rate of solution and watch for signs of vasoconstriction or extravasation (eg, blanching). With low dosages for dopaminergic effects, monitor urine output and ECG.

Notes. The drug is physically incompatible with sodium bicarbonate, furosemide, and other alkaline solutions. (*See* Sympathomimetic Drugs for Hemodynamic Support Comparison Chart.) Low-dose dopamine is ineffective in preventing renal failure in critically ill patients with signs of early renal dysfunction.[323]

DOPAMINE DILUTION GUIDE

AMOUNT ADDED		VOLUME OF	FINAL
mg	*Volume*	DILUENT	CONCENTRATION[a]
200	5 mL (1 amp, 40 mg/mL)	250 mL	800 mg/L
200	5 mL (1 amp, 40 mg/mL)	500 mL	400 mg/L
400	5 mL (1 amp, 80 mg/mL)	500 mL	800 mg/L
800	5 mL (1 amp, 160 mg/mL)	500 mL	1.6 g/L

[a]Recommended concentrations, but concentrations up to 3.2 g/L have been used.

EPINEPHRINE AND SALTS   Adrenalin, Sus-Phrine, Various

Pharmacology. Epinephrine stimulates α_1-, α_2- (vasoconstriction, pressor effects), β_1- (increased myocardial contractility and conduction), and β_2-adrenergic (bronchodilation and vasodilation) receptors. It is used for reversible bronchospasm, anaphylactic reactions, laryngeal edema (croup), open-angle glaucoma, and cardiac arrest. (*See* Medical Emergencies.)

Administration and Adult Dosage. **SC for anaphylaxis** 0.2–0.5 mg (0.2–0.5 mL of 1:1000 aqueous soln), may repeat q 10–15 min prn; if SC is ineffective, then **IV** 0.1–0.25 mg (1–2.5 mL of 1:10,000) q 5–15 min may be given and followed by an IV infusion, if necessary. **SC for asthma** same dosage as SC for anaphylaxis; may repeat q 20 min to 4 hr as needed.[144] **SC aqueous suspension for asthma** 0.5–1.5 mg (0.1–0.3 mL of 1:200), may repeat with 0.5–1.5 mg no sooner than q 6 hr. **IV infusion for hemodynamic support** 1 μg/min (1 mg in 500 mL NS or D5W) initially, adjust to hemodynamic response (usually 2–10 μg/min).[316] **Inhal (metered dose) not recommended** because of low efficacy and ultrashort duration of action.

Special Populations. *Pediatric Dosage.* **SC for anaphylaxis or asthma** 0.01 mL/kg/dose of 1:1000 aqueous solution, to a maximum of 0.5 mL; may repeat q 15–20 min for 2 doses, then q 4 hr prn. **SC aqueous suspension for asthma** (1 month–12 yr) 0.005 mL/kg/dose of 1:200, to a maximum of 0.15 mL/dose for children ≤30 kg; repeat no sooner than q 6 hr.[144] **Inhal for croup** 0.25–0.5 mL of 2.25% racemic aqueous solution diluted in 1.5–4.5 mL of NS q 1–2 hr prn by nebulizer.[324,325] Alternatively, 5 mL of prediluted L-epinephrine in NS (1:1000) has been used.[325] **IV for hemodynamic support** 0.05–0.3 μg/kg/min initially, adjusted to desired hemodynamic response; avoid dosages >0.3 μg/kg/min, if possible, because they are associated with marked vasoconstrictor effects.[317,326]

Geriatric Dosage. Same as adult dosage. (*See* Precautions.)

Dosage Forms. **Inhal Pwdr** 200 μg/spray; **Inhal Pwdr** (bitartrate) 160 μg/spray; **Inhal Soln** (HCl) 1% (1:100); **Inhal Soln** (racepinephrine) 2.25%; **Inj** (aqueous solution as HCl) 0.01 mg/mL (1:100,000), 0.1 mg/mL (1:10,000), 0.5 mg/mL (1:2000), 1 mg/mL (1:1000); **Inj** (aqueous suspension as free base) 5 mg/mL (1:200).

Patient Instructions. (Autoinjectors) Periodically familiarize yourself with instructions for use so you maintain an adequate comfort level. Obtain new kit by expiration date or sooner if precipitate or color change is noted in solution.

Pharmacokinetics. *Onset and Duration.* Onset SC (aqueous soln or susp) 3–10 min; inhal peak 3–5 min. Duration SC (aqueous soln) 0.5–2 hr, (aqueous susp) up to 6–10 hr; inhal 15–60 min.[323,327]

Fate. Parenteral action is terminated by uptake into adrenergic neurons. Metabolism is by MAO and COMT.[313,323] Cl is 2.1–5.3 L/hr/kg.[313]

t½. About 1 min.[144]

Adverse Reactions. Dose-related restlessness, anxiety, tremor, cardiac arrhythmias, palpitations, hypertension, weakness, dizziness, and headache occur. Cerebral hemorrhage can be caused by a sharp rise in blood pressure from overdosage. Angina can be precipitated when coronary insufficiency is present, and elevation of blood glucose has been reported. Local necrosis from repeated injections and tolerance with prolonged use also can occur.[313,323]

Contraindications. Intra-arterial administration is not recommended because of marked vasoconstriction. Do not use with local anesthetics in fingers or toes or during general anesthesia with halogenated hydrocarbons. Other contraindications include α-adrenergic blocker-induced (including phenothiazines) hypotension; cerebral arteriosclerosis; organic heart disease; narrow-angle glaucoma; shock; labor.

Precautions. Use with caution in patients with cardiovascular disease, hypertension, diabetes, or hyperthyroidism and in psychoneurotic patients. Caution is usually recommended in the elderly because of a higher frequency of cardiovascular intolerance. However, one evaluation of patients with acute asthma attacks found no difference in hemodynamic alterations or arrhythmias between those older and younger than 40 yr in response to SC epinephrine.[328] IM injection can produce local tissue necrosis. Epinephrine infusions are administered preferably through a central venous line. Extravasation can cause necrosis; if extravasation occurs, infiltrate the area with **phentolamine** 5–10 mg diluted in 10–15 mL of NS.

Drug Interactions. Bretylium, guanethidine, and heterocyclic antidepressants can potentiate the pressor response to epinephrine. Oxytocics used in obstetrics can cause severe, persistent hypertension when used with vasopressors. Halogenated hydrocarbon anesthetics can predispose patients to serious arrhythmias. A hypertensive reaction can occur when epinephrine is given with nonselective β-adrenergic blockers (eg, propranolol, nadolol).

Parameters to Monitor. (IV infusion) ECG, infusion rate and site; (in the elderly) ECG; (asthma or allergy) blood pressure, heart rate, relief of symptoms.

Notes. Do not use solution if it is brown or contains a precipitate. Protect solution from light. The solution is incompatible with sodium bicarbonate, furosemide, and other alkaline solutions. Suspension provides a sustained effect; shake suspension well before use. Nonprescription inhalers have only a transient effect because of their low dosage[327] and should be used only by patients who have infrequent symptoms (less than once a week) and obtain total relief of symptoms from administration of two inhalations. Parenteral administration offers no advantage over inhalation for the treatment of acute bronchospasm.[329] (*See* Sympathomimetic Drugs for Hemodynamic Support Comparison Chart.)

INAMRINONE LACTATE   Inocor, Various

Pharmacology. Inamrinone (formerly amrinone) increases cyclic AMP and calcium availability through the inhibition of phosphodiesterase III, which improves cardiac output through vasodilatory and positive inotropic actions.[330]

Administration and Adult Dosage. **IV loading dose** 0.5–1 mg/kg (usually 0.75 mg/kg) over 2–3 min; can repeat in 30 min based on response. **IV maintenance dosage by continuous infusion** 5–10 μg/kg/min.

Special Populations. *Pediatric Dosage.* Safety and efficacy not established,[331] but the following dosages have been suggested:[144] **IV loading dosage** (neonates and infants) 3–4.5 mg/kg, then **IV maintenance dosage by continuous infusion** (neonates) 3–5 μg/kg/min; (infants) 10 μg/kg/min.

Geriatric Dosage. Same as adult dosage.

Dosage Forms. **Inj** 5 mg/mL.

Pharmacokinetics. *Onset and Duration.* IV onset 2–5 min after bolus, peak 10 min, duration 60–90 min.[330]

Serum Levels. A level of 1.5–4 mg/L (8–21.3 μmol/L) is associated with therapeutic response. Although a correlation exists between inamrinone levels and increased cardiac output, the clinical usefulness of serum level monitoring is not established.[332,333]

Fate. Bioavailability is 93 ± 12%. The drug is 20–50% bound to plasma proteins; V_d is 1.8 ± 0.9 L/kg; Cl is 0.28 ± 0.1 L/hr/kg. The drug is eliminated primarily by hepatic metabolism, with 30 ± 20% excreted unchanged in urine.[332]

$t_{1/2}$. α phase 1–5 min; β phase 4.3 ± 1.3 hr in normals, 7.3 ± 4.6 hr in CHF.[332,333]

Adverse Reactions. Dose-dependent, asymptomatic thrombocytopenia occurs frequently. Platelet counts return to normal within 2–4 days of discontinuing therapy; in some cases, this side effect is be reversible when dosage is maintained or reduced. Thrombocytopenia might be caused primarily by the metabolite *N*-acetylinamrinone.[334] Nausea and vomiting are unusual with IV use.[330] Occasional side effects include nephrogenic diabetes insipidus, liver enzyme elevation, fever, taste disturbances, flu-like syndrome, rash, and aggravation of underlying arrhythmias.[335,336]

Precautions. Caution in hypertrophic obstructive cardiomyopathy. One study found decreased survival rates in patients on long-term inamrinone therapy.[336] Use concomitant antiplatelet drugs with caution.

Drug Interactions. None known.

Parameters to Monitor. Continuous ECG and frequent vital signs. Invasive hemodynamic monitoring is necessary in seriously ill patients for adequate dosage titration.

Notes. Do not dilute with dextrose-containing solutions but can infuse through dextrose-containing IV lines. Do not administer furosemide through IV lines containing inamrinone.

MILRINONE LACTATE   Primacor

Pharmacology. Milrinone is a phosphodiesterase inhibitor, positive inotropic agent, and a vasodilator similar to inamrinone, but 10–15 times more potent on a weight basis. Milrinone is labeled for temporary use in patients with severe left ventricular dysfunction and CHF. It is also used for postoperative hemodynamic support and those awaiting cardiac transplantation.[337,338]

Adult Dosage. IV loading dose 50 μg/kg over 10 min and then **IV continuous infusion** 0.375–0.5 μg/kg/min; adjust dosage depending on the patient's response and hemodynamic variables to a maximum of 0.75 μg/kg/min. In renal impairment, reduce dosage as follows: Cl_{cr} 50 mL/min, 0.43 μg/kg/min; 40 mL/min, 0.38 μg/kg/min; 30 mL/min, 0.33 μg/kg/min; 20 mL/min, 0.28 μg/kg/min; 10 mL/min, 0.23 μg/kg/min; 5 mL/min, 0.2 μg/kg/min.

Pediatric Dosage. Safety and efficacy not established, but weight-based dosages similar to adult dosages have been used.

Dosage Forms. Inj 200 μg/mL (100 mL), 1 mg/mL.

Pharmacokinetics. Although well absorbed orally, milrinone is available only for IV use; 70% bound to plasma proteins; V_d is 0.47 ± 0.3 L/kg. It is 88–90% eliminated as unchanged drug by renal excretion. Elimination half-life in patients with CHF is 2.3 ± 0.1 hr, longer than in normal volunteers.

Adverse Reactions. Thrombocytopenia is less frequent (0.4%) with milrinone than with inamrinone. Milrinone can cause or worsen existing ventricular and supraventricular arrhythmias. Hypotension and headaches occur frequently.

Precautions. Long-term milrinone therapy can lead to increased mortality in patients with CHF. Use with caution in patients with severe obstructive aortic or pulmonary disease (eg, hypertrophic subaortic stenosis).

Parameters to Monitor. Continuous ECG and frequent vital signs. Invasive hemodynamic monitoring is necessary in seriously ill patients for adequate dosage titration.

Notes. Physically incompatible with IV furosemide.

NOREPINEPHRINE BITARTRATE
Levophed

Pharmacology. Norepinephrine is a catecholamine that directly stimulates β_1-, α_1-, and α_2-adrenergic receptors. It has little action on β_2-receptors.[314]

Administration and Adult Dosage. **IV for shock, by infusion only** (in any *non*alkaline IV fluid) 8–12 μg of base/min initially; adjust rate to maintain a systolic blood pressure of about 80–100 mm Hg or to a specific hemodynamic response; average maintenance dosage range is 2–4 μg of base/min. Very large dosages (up to 1.5 μg/kg/min) have been used in patients with septic shock.[313,339]

Special Populations. *Pediatric Dosage.* Safety and efficacy not established. **IV for shock, by infusion only** 0.05–0.1 μg/kg/min of base initially, adjust dosage to blood pressure response, to a maximum of 1.5 μg/kg/min.[313]

Geriatric Dosage. Same as adult dosage. (*See* Precautions.)

Dosage Forms. **Inj** 1 mg (of base)/mL.

Pharmacokinetics. *Onset and Duration.* Onset 1–2 min; duration 1–2 min after discontinuing infusion.[323]

Fate. Action is terminated primarily by uptake into adrenergic neurons. Free drug is metabolized primarily by COMT and, to a lesser extent, MAO to inactive metabolites and their conjugates.

$t_{1/2}$. 2–2.5 min.[313]

Adverse Reactions. Dose-related hypertension (sometimes indicated by headache), reflex bradycardia, increased peripheral vascular resistance, and decreased cardiac output occur. Volume depletion can occur if fluid is not replaced. Arrhythmias can occur in extreme hypoxia or hypercarbia.

Contraindications. Hypotension secondary to uncorrected blood volume deficit; severe visceral or peripheral vasoconstriction; mesenteric or peripheral vascular thrombosis, unless drug is life-saving; halogenated hydrocarbon anesthesia.

Precautions. Use with caution in patients receiving MAOIs or heterocyclic antidepressants. Administer into a large vein (antecubital preferred) to avoid necrosis secondary to vasoconstriction; avoid the leg veins whenever possible, especially in the elderly or in those with occlusive vascular diseases. Avoid extravasation of solution; however, if it occurs, the area can be infiltrated with 5–10 mg of **phentolamine** diluted in 10–15 mL of NS.

Drug Interactions. Bretylium, guanethidine, MAOIs, methyldopa, and heterocyclic antidepressants can potentiate the pressor response to direct-acting vasopressors. Oxytocics used in obstetrics can cause severe, persistent hypertension when used with vasopressors. Halogenated hydrocarbon anesthetics can predispose patients to serious arrhythmias.

Parameters to Monitor. In shock, closely monitor heart rate, pulmonary capillary wedge pressure, cardiac index, arterial blood pressure, arterial blood gases, acid–base balance, urine output, and infusion rate of solution and watch for signs of vasoconstriction or extravasation (eg, blanching).

Notes. Do not use solution if it is brown or contains precipitate; 2 mg of norepinephrine bitartrate = 1 mg norepinephrine base. (*See* Sympathomimetic Drugs for Hemodynamic Support Comparison Chart.)

NOREPINEPHRINE DILUTION GUIDE

AMOUNT ADDED		VOLUME OF 5% DEXTROSE	FINAL CONCENTRATION
mg (base)	*Volume*		
2 mg	2 mL	500 mL	4 mg/L[a]
4 mg	4 mL	500 mL	8 mg/L
8 mg	8 mL	500 mL	16 mg/L

[a]Recommended pediatric concentration.[340]

SYMPATHOMIMETIC DRUGS FOR HEMODYNAMIC SUPPORT COMPARISON CHART[a]

DRUG	ADRENERGIC RECEPTOR SELECTIVITY					TOTAL PERIPHERAL RESISTANCE	CARDIAC OUTPUT
	Inotropic Activity (β_1)	Chronotropic Activity (β_1)	Vasodilation (β_2)	Vasoconstriction (α)	Renal/ Mesenteric Vasodilation (DA_1)		
Dobutamine Dobutrex Various	++	0/+[b]	+	0/+[b]	0	↓	↑
Dopamine Inotropin Various	++	+/++[b,c]	++	+/++	+++	↓/↑[b]	↑
Epinephrine Adrenalin Various	+++	+++	++	++++	0	↓	↑
Isoproterenol Isuprel Various	++++	++++	+++++	0	0	↓	↑
Norepinephrine[d] Levophed	++	++[e]	0	++++	0	↑	0/↓/↑
Phentolamine[f] Regitine	0	g	0	0	0	↓	↑

(continued)

SYMPATHOMIMETIC DRUGS FOR HEMODYNAMIC SUPPORT COMPARISON CHART[a] (continued)

DRUG	ADRENERGIC RECEPTOR SELECTIVITY					TOTAL PERIPHERAL RESISTANCE	CARDIAC OUTPUT
	Inotropic Activity (β_1)	Chronotropic Activity (β_1)	Vasodilation (β_2)	Vasoconstriction (α)	Renal/ Mesenteric Vasodilation (DA_1)		
Phenylephrine[h] Neo-Synephrine	0	0[e]	0	+++++	0	↑	↓

+++++ = Pronounced effect; + = Minimal effect; 0 = No effect; ↓ = Decreased; ↑ = Increased.

[a] This table compares only a few of the many factors important in the treatment of shock. Consult references 313, 315 and 341–343 for clinical use. Cross-table comparisons of the adrenergic selectivity properties between this table and the Sympathomimetic Bronchodilators Comparison Chart cannot be made because: (1) the rating scale of this table reflects a finer degree of differentiation of effects (hence 0–5+ vs 0–4+); (2) the routes of administration are different; and (3) vascular β_2-receptors appear to respond slightly differently from bronchiolar β_2-receptors.

[b] Dose dependent.

[c] Releases stored norepinephrine via tyramine-like mechanism.

[d] Used primarily to increase peripheral vascular resistance in volume-repleted hypotensive patients.

[e] Decrease in heart rate can result from reflex mechanisms.

[f] α-Adrenergic blocking drug; useful in severe vasoconstriction (eg, extravasation of norepinephrine or dopamine).

[g] Increase in heart rate can result from reflex and direct mechanisms.

[h] Primary use is to increase blood pressure to reflexly increase vagal tone in paroxysmal supraventricular tachycardias. Other pressors are preferred in most shock states because they also have positive inotropic activity. Phenylephrine has no inotropic activity and with its strong α-agonist properties functions as a pure vasopressor (afterload increaser).

Nitrates

Class Instructions. **Nitrates.** This drug can cause headache, dizziness, and/or flushing; alcohol can worsen these side effects. Tolerance to side effects of long-acting nitrates such as headache can occur with continued therapy. If necessary, a mild analgesic can be used until tolerance to side effects occurs. During an acute angina attack, discontinue activity, assume a sitting position, and dissolve one sublingual tablet under the tongue. If chest discomfort does not improve after use of the tablets, seek medical attention. Keep tablets in the tightly closed original container. If you have been taking this medication for a long time, do not discontinue it abruptly.

ISOSORBIDE DINITRATE
Isordil, Sorbitrate, Various

Pharmacology. (*See* Nitroglycerin.)

Administration and Adult Dosage. **SL tab for acute anginal attack** 2.5–10 mg q 2–3 hr prn;[344,345] **Chew Tab for acute anginal attack** 5 mg initially and then 5–10 mg q 2–3 hr prn.[345] **PO for prophylaxis of angina and for CHF** 10–60 mg q 4–6 hr; individual doses up to 120 mg have been used.[344,346] (*See* Vasodilators in Heart Failure Comparison Chart.) **SR products for prophylaxis of angina** 40–80 mg q 8–12 hr (once daily–bid at 8 AM and 2 PM preferred). Start the dosage low and adjust upward slowly over several days to weeks to patient tolerance or to the desired therapeutic effect. A daily nitrate-free period of at least 12 hr is desirable to minimize tolerance.[346]

Special Populations. *Pediatric Dosage.* Safety and efficacy not established.

Geriatric Dosage. Same as adult dosage. However, some clinicians have recommended lower doses and that initial SL doses be given under medical observation because of increased likelihood of postural hypotension.[347]

Dosage Forms. **Chew Tab** 5, 10 mg; **SL Tab** 2.5, 5, 10 mg; **SR Cap** 40 mg; **SR Tab** 40 mg; **Tab** 5, 10, 20, 30, 40 mg.

Patient Instructions. (*See* Nitrates Class Instructions.) Do not crush or chew sustained-release preparations.

Missed Doses. Take this drug at regular intervals. If you miss a dose, take it as soon as you remember. If it is about time for the next dose, take that dose only. Leave a minimum of 2 hours between regular tablet doses and 6 hours between sustained-release tablet or capsule doses. Do not double the dose or take extra.

Pharmacokinetics. *Onset and Duration.* Onset is 5–20 min after SL and Chew Tab administration, 15–45 min after PO tab administration, up to 4 hr in rare cases or with SR products; peak occurs 15–60 min after SL administration and 45–120 min after PO tab administration.[344,345] Duration is 1–3 hr after SL or Chew Tab, 2–6 hr after PO tab, up to 8 hr after SR.[344,348] Although PO administration can improve exercise tolerance for 4–8 hr after the first dose, with long-term, around-the-clock administration, the duration of action declines to 2–3 hr, probably because of nitrate tolerance.[348]

Fate. Oral bioavailability is 22 ± 14%. There is extensive first-pass metabolism by the liver after oral administration to less active isosorbide mononitrate metabolites (2-ISMN, 5-ISMN). Larger doses and long-term administration saturate metabolic processes, with appreciable increases in serum concentrations of the parent compound and metabolites.[349] The drug is 28 ± 12% bound to plasma proteins; V_d is 1.5 ± 0.8 L/kg; Cl is 2.7 ± 1.2 L/hr/kg.[10] (*See* Isosorbide Mononitrate *Fate*.)

$t_{1/2}$. (Isosorbide dinitrate) 50 ± 20 min; (2-ISMN) 1.9 ± 0.5 hr; (5-ISMN) 4.6 ± 0.7 hr.[10,350]

Adverse Reactions. (*See* Nitroglycerin.)

Contraindications. (*See* Nitroglycerin.)

Precautions. (*See* Nitroglycerin.)

Drug Interactions. (*See* Nitroglycerin.)

Parameters to Monitor. Monitor for headache, orthostatic hypotension, and dizziness. In angina, monitor frequency of angina. In CHF, monitor hemodynamic and functional measurements.

Notes. Because of their slower onset of action, reserve SL and chewable isosorbide dinitrate (ISDN) for acute anginal attacks only in patients intolerant of or unresponsive to nitroglycerin. ISDN is a mainstay of antianginal and CHF therapy because of its long record of efficacy in these disorders. It is also less expensive than other long-term nitrate preparations. However, patients must take multiple doses daily on an eccentric schedule to achieve and maintain efficacy.

ISOSORBIDE MONONITRATE
Imdur, ISMO, Monoket

Pharmacology. Isosorbide mononitrate (ISMN) is the active 5-mononitrate metabolite of isosorbide dinitrate. (*See* Nitroglycerin.)

Administration and Adult Dosage. PO for prophylaxis of angina (ISMO, Monoket) 20 mg bid, doses 7 hr apart. **SR for prophylaxis of angina** (Imdur) 30–60 mg once daily in the morning, can increase to 120 mg once daily, to a maximum (rarely) of 240 mg once daily. There can be some attenuation of antianginal efficacy after 6 weeks of therapy with the 30 and 60 mg doses, but not with the 120 mg dose.[348,351]

Special Populations. *Pediatric Dosage.* Safety and efficacy not established.

Geriatric Dosage. Same as adult dosage.

Other Conditions. For persons of particularly small stature, the manufacturer of Monoket recommends an alternative initial dosage of 5 mg bid, but to increase it to at least 10 mg bid by the second or third day of therapy.

Dosage Forms. SR Tab (Imdur) 30, 60, 120 mg; **Tab** (ISMO, Monoket) 10, 20 mg.

Patient Instructions. (*See* Nitrates Class Instructions.) Follow the prescribed administration schedule closely. Do not crush the sustained-release product.

Missed Doses. Take this drug at regular intervals. If you miss a dose, take it as soon as you remember. If it is about time for the next dose, take that dose only. Leave a minimum of 6 hours between regular tablet doses and 12 hours between sustained-release tablet doses. Do not double the dose or take extra.

Pharmacokinetics. *Onset and Duration.* Non-SR tablet onset 30–60 min,[351] peak 1–2 hr, duration 12–14 hr with bid administration.[348] SR Tab onset within 4 hr, peak 4 hr, duration about 12 hr.[348,351]

Fate. The tablet is rapidly absorbed and essentially 100% bioavailable; SR Tab bioavailability is 78–86%.[351] The drug is distributed into total body water with negligible plasma protein binding and a V_d of 0.62 ± 0.05 L/kg.[350,352] Cl is 0.094 ± 0.005 L/hr/kg.[350] It is primarily hepatically metabolized by denitration and glucuronidation to inactive products that are renally eliminated; less than 2% of a dose is excreted unchanged in urine.[352]

$t_{1/2}$. 4.6 ± 0.7 hr.[350]

Adverse Reactions. (*See* Nitroglycerin.)

Contraindications. (*See* Nitroglycerin.)

Precautions. (*See* Nitroglycerin.)

Drug Interactions. (*See* Nitroglycerin.)

Parameters to Monitor. Monitor for headache, orthostatic hypotension, and dizziness; antianginal efficacy; and compliance with 7-hr dosage regimen for non-SR tablet.

Notes. ISMN is an effective nitrate with dosage schedules proven to avoid tolerance. Patient compliance is favored with the use of ISMN because the products are administered once (Imdur) or twice (ISMO, Monoket) daily. Although the available preparations are comparable to each other in cost, at relatively low dosages (ie, 20 mg bid for the immediate-release products and 60 mg/day or less of the SR products) they are much more expensive than generic ISDN, which is also effective when taken properly. Compliance and cost factors must be assessed carefully in the individual patient when choosing an oral nitrate product.

NITROGLYCERIN   Various

Pharmacology. Nitroglycerin and other organic nitrates are believed to be converted to nitric oxide (NO) by vascular endothelium. NO activates guanylate cyclase, increasing cyclic GMP that in turn decreases intracellular calcium, resulting in direct relaxation of vascular smooth muscle.[344,346,353] The venous (capacitance) system is affected to a greater degree than the arterial (resistance) system. Venous pooling, decreased venous return to the heart (preload), and decreased arterial resistance (afterload) reduce intracardiac pressures and left ventricular size, thereby decreasing myocardial oxygen consumption and ischemia. In myocardial ischemia, nitrates dilate large epicardial vessels, enhance collateral size and flow, and reduce coronary vasoconstriction.[344] The various organic nitrate preparations have the same pharmacologic effects and differ only in bioavailability and pharmacokinetics.[320]

Administration and Adult Dosage. **SL Tab for acute anginal attack** 150–600 μg prn, up to 3 doses in 15 min; **SL aerosol for acute anginal attack** 400–800 μg prn, up to 1200 μg/15 min; **Buccal for acute anginal attack and/or prophylaxis and treatment of angina pectoris or CHF** 1–3 mg q 4–6 hr; **PO SR for prophylaxis of angina or CHF** 2.5–19.5 mg bid or tid;[344,348] **Top ointment for prophylaxis and treatment of angina pectoris or CHF** 1.3–5 cm (0.5–2 inches) q 6–8 hr.[344,348] Start the dosage low and adjust slowly upward over a several days to weeks to patient tolerance or to the desired therapeutic effect. **SR Patch for prophylaxis and treatment of angina pectoris** 0.2–0.8 mg/hr, patch applied once daily, dosage adjusted to patient response.[344] Greater antianginal efficacy has been noted with patches delivering at least 0.4 mg/hr.[344,354] A daily nitrate-free period of 12 hr is desirable to minimize nitrate tolerance.[346,348] **IV for CHF, post-MI, angina pectoris, perioperative blood pressure control, or hypotensive anesthesia** 5 μg/min initially by constant infusion using an infusion pump. Dosage must be adjusted to the individual patient's response. Increase dosage initially in 5 μg/min increments q 3–5 min until response is noted. If no response occurs at 20 μg/min, increments of 10 μg/min and then perhaps 20 μg/min can be used. Once partial blood pressure response occurs, decrease incremental increases and increase intervals. (*See* Notes.)

Special Populations. *Pediatric Dosage.* Safety and efficacy not established. **IV** 0.5–20 μg/kg/min has been suggested.[355]

Geriatric Dosage. Same as adult dosage but some clinicians have recommended lower doses and that initial SL doses be given under medical observation because of increased likelihood of postural hypotension.[347]

Dosage Forms. **Buccal SR Tab** 1, 2, 3 mg; **Oint** 2%; **SL Aerosol** 400 μg/spray; **SL Tab** 300, 400, 600 μg; **SR Cap** 2.5, 6.5, 9, 13 mg; **SR Tab** 2.6, 6.5, 9 mg; **SR Patch** 0.1, 0.2, 0.3, 0.4, 0.6, 0.8 mg/hr; **Inj** 0.5, 5 mg/mL.

Patient Instructions. (*See* Nitrates Class Instructions.)

Pharmacokinetics. *Onset and Duration.* Onset immediate after IV, 2–5 min after SL or buccal, 20–45 min after SR Cap or Tab, 15–60 min after topical ointment, and 30–60 min after transdermal administration.[344] Peak 4–8 min after SL, 4–10 min after buccal, 45–120 min after SR Cap or Tab, 30–120 min after topical ointment, and 1–3 hr after transdermal administration.[344] Duration 10–30 min after IV and SL, 0.5–5 hr after buccal, 2–6 hr after oral, 4–8 hr after SR, and 3–8 hr after topical administration.[344,348] Although the SR patch can act longer after the first application, long-term continuous therapy limits the duration of action to 4 hr or less, probably because of tolerance.[356] With sustained intermittent therapy (removal of patch after 12 hr), duration is 8–12 hr.[348]

Fate. Bioavailability of SL and Top are 38 ± 26% and 72 ± 20%, respectively.[10,357] Extensive first-pass metabolism occurs after oral administration. The drug is 87 ± 1% bound to plasma proteins. V_d is 3.3 ± 1.2 L/kg; Cl is 13.8 ± 5.4 L/hr/kg.[10,357] It is metabolized in the liver to 1ess active dinitro and inactive mononitro metabolites. Larger doses and long-term administration can saturate metabolism and result in increased serum concentrations of drug and metabolites.[357]

$t_{1/2}$. β phase estimated to be 2.3 ± 0.6 min.[10]

Adverse Reactions. Headache occurs very frequently; dizziness occurs frequently, especially with oral or topical administration. Occasionally, flushing, weakness, nausea, vomiting, palpitations, tachycardia, and postural hypotension occur. Many of these effects are dose related and can be minimized by slowly increasing the dosage. Tolerance and dependence can occur with prolonged use. Contact dermatitis occurs in up to 40% of patients using transdermal patches.[358]

Contraindications. Severe anemia; severe hypotension or uncompensated hypovolemia; increased intracranial pressure; purported hypersensitivity or idiosyncrasy to nitroglycerin, nitrates, or nitrites; use of sildenafil. (*See* Drug Interactions.) Constrictive pericarditis, pericardial tamponade, and inadequate cerebral circulation are also considered contraindications by some clinicians.[348]

Precautions. Some tolerance and cross-tolerance with other nitrates can occur with long-term or excessive use.[348] Use with caution in patients with severe renal or hepatic disease, those with low or normal pulmonary capillary wedge pressure, and those receiving drugs that lower blood pressure. With intermittent therapy, anginal episodes can increase during the nitrate-free interval.[359]

Drug Interactions. Nitrates can produce additive vasodilation and severe postural hypotension when combined with alcohol or hypotensive drugs. Use in patients taking sildenafil can result in profound hypotension with serious consequences, including death.

Parameters to Monitor. Observe for headache, dizziness, and other side effects. Monitor for orthostatic hypotension, especially with first SL dose in elderly. (Angina) monitor frequency of angina. (CHF) obtain hemodynamic and functional measurements. (IV use) monitor blood pressure and heart rate constantly in all patients; monitoring pulmonary capillary wedge pressure in some patients also can be useful.

Notes. Large and unpredictable amounts of nitroglycerin are lost through polyvinylchloride (PVC) containers, most IV administration sets and tubing, and certain IV filters.[360,361] The manufacturers recommend that IV nitroglycerin infusions be prepared and stored in glass bottles and infused through special non-PVC tubing to avoid the use of in-line filters. However, because nitroglycerin infusion rate is usually adjusted to response rather than by a microgram/kilogram dosage, the need for special tubing has been questioned.[344] Some institutions have discontinued use of nitroglycerin tubing to reduce costs and achieved good results clinically when using PVC tubing to infuse nitroglycerin.[362,363] However, because substantial amounts of nitroglycerin are adsorbed onto PVC tubing, special attention to patient response is advisable at the time of IV tubing changes. Stored in glass containers, the diluted injection is stable for 48 hr at room temperature and 7 days under refrigeration. When administration sets with large dead spaces are used, flush the line whenever the concentration of solution is changed. (*See* Vasodilators in Heart Failure Comparison Chart.)

APPROXIMATE EQUIVALENT DOSAGES OF NITRATES

PRODUCT	LOW DOSAGE	HIGH DOSAGE
Nitroglycerin Ointment	≤1 inch q 6 hr	1–2 inches q 6 hr
Nitroglycerin Patch	0.4 mg/hr	0.4–0.6 mg/hr
Isosorbide Dinitrate	20 mg tid	20–40 mg tid
Isosorbide Mononitrate		
Immediate-Release	10–20 mg bid	20 mg bid
Sustained-Release	30–60 mg/day	60–120 mg/day

VASODILATORS IN HEART FAILURE COMPARISON CHART

DRUG	DOSAGE[a]	DURATION	SITE OF ACTION[b]	HR	MAP	PCWP	CI	SVR
ACE INHIBITORS								
Captopril	PO 25–100 mg tid.	hours	A, V	0/↓	↓	↓	↑	↓
Capoten								
Enalapril	PO 2.5–10 mg bid;							
Vasotec	IV 0.625–5 mg q 6–12 hr.							
Lisinopril	PO 5–20 mg/day.							
Prinivil								
Zestril								
Quinapril	PO 5–20 mg q 12 hr.							
Accupril								
HYDRALAZINE								
Hydralazine	PO 50–75 mg	hours	A	0/↑	sl↓	sl↓	↑	↓
Apresoline	q 6–8 hr; usual							
Various	maintenance 200–600 mg/day.							
NITRATES								
Isosorbide	PO 10–60 mg	hours	V,(A)	sl↑/↓	↓	↓	↑/↓	sl↓
Dinitrate	q 4–6 hr.							
Isordil								
Sorbitrate								
Various								

(continued)

VASODILATORS IN HEART FAILURE COMPARISON CHART (*continued*)

DRUG	DOSAGE[a]	DURATION	SITE OF ACTION[b]	HR	MAP	PCWP	CI	SVR
Nitroglycerin Various	(*See* monograph.)	minutes	V,(A)	sl↑/↓	↓	↓	↑/↓	sl↓
NITROPRUSSIDE								
Nitroprusside Sodium Various	IV 0.1–3 μg/kg/min.	minutes	A,V	0	sl↓	↓	↑	↓

A = arterial; V = venous; HR = heart rate; MAP = mean arterial pressure; PCWP = pulmonary capillary wedge pressure; CI = cardiac index; SVR = systemic vascular resistance; ↑ = increase; ↓ = decrease; sl = slight; 0 = no change

[a]Start with low dosages of these drugs and increase gradually with continuous hemodynamic monitoring. To avoid adverse rebound effects, carefully taper the dosages of these drugs if they are to be discontinued. (*See* Nitroglycerin Notes.)

[b]Predominant site of action. Parentheses denote lesser activity.

From references 320, 364–368 and product information.

REFERENCES

1. Parker RB, McCollam PL. Adenosine in the episodic treatment of paroxysmal supraventricular tachycardia. *Clin Pharm* 1990;9:261–71.
2. DiMarco JP et al. Adenosine for paroxysmal supraventricular tachycardia: dose ranging and comparison with verapamil. *Ann Intern Med* 1990;113:104–10.
3. McIntosh-Vellin NL et al. Safety and efficacy of central intravenous bolus administration of adenosine for termination of supraventricular tachycardia. *J Am Coll Cardiol* 1993;22:741–5.
4. Siberry GK, Iannone R, eds. *The Harriet Lane handbook*. 15th ed. St. Louis: Mosby; 2000.
5. Podrid PJ. Amiodarone: reevaluation of an old drug. *Ann Intern Med* 1995;122:689–700.
6. Kudenchuck PJ et al. Amiodarone for resuscitation after out-of-hospital cardiac arrest due to ventricular fibrillation. *N Engl J Med* 1999;341:871–8.
7. Gilette PC et al. Amiodarone for children. *Clin Prog Electrophysiol Pacing* 1986;4:328–30.
8. Roden DM. Pharmacokinetics of amiodarone: implications for drug therapy. *Am J Cardiol* 1993;72:45F–50.
9. Rotmensch HH et al. Steady-mate serum amiodarone concentrations: relationship with antiarrhythmic efficacy and toxicity. *Ann Intern Med* 1984;101:462–9.
10. Benet LZ et al. Design and optimization of dosage regimens; pharmacokinetic data. In, Hardman JG et al., eds. *Goodman and Gilman's the pharmacological basis of therapeutics*. 9th ed. New York: McGraw-Hill; 1996:1707–92.
11. Gill J et al. Amiodarone. An overview of its pharmacologic properties, and review of its therapeutic use in cardiac arrhythmias. *Drugs* 1992;43:69–110.
12. Rigas B et al. Amiodarone hepatotoxicity. A clinicopathologic study of five patients. *Ann Intern Med* 1986;104:348–51.
13. Figge HL, Figge J. The effects of amiodarone on thyroid hormone function: a review of the physiology and clinical manifestations. *J Clin Pharmacol* 1990;30:588–95.
14. Dusman RE et al. Clinical features of amiodarone-induced pulmonary toxicity. *Circulation* 1990;82:51–9.
15. Hohnloser SH et al. Amiodarone-associated proarrhythmic effects. A review with special reference to torsade de pointes tachycardia. *Ann Intern Med* 1994;121:529–35.
16. Roberts SA et al. Invasive and noninvasive methods to predict the long-term efficacy of amiodarone: a compilation of clinical observations using meta-analysis. *PACE Pacing Clin Electrophysiol* 1994;17:1590–602.
17. Bauman JL et al. Pharmacokinetic and pharmacodynamic drug interactions with antiarrhythmic agents. *Cardiol Rev* 1997;5:292–304.
18. Echt DS et al. Mortality and morbidity in patients receiving encainide, flecainide, or placebo. The Cardiac Arrhythmia Suppression Trial. *N Engl J Med* 1991;324:781–8.
19. Rapeport WG. Clinical pharmacokinetics of bretylium. *Clin Pharmacokinet* 1985;10:248–56.
20. Adir J et al. Nomogram for bretylium dosing in renal impairment. *Ther Drug Monit* 1985;7:265–8.
21. Anderson JL et al. Kinetics of antifibrillatory effects of bretylium: correlation with myocardial drug concentrations. *Am J Cardiol* 1980;46:583–92.
22. Anderson JL et al. Oral and intravenous bretylium disposition. *Clin Pharmacol Ther* 1980;28:468–78.
23. Narang PK et al. Pharmacokinetics of bretylium in man after intravenous administration. *J Pharmacokinet Biopharm* 1980;8:363–73.
24. Anderson JL et al. Clinical pharmacokinetics of intravenous and oral bretylium tosylate in survivors of ventricular tachycardia or fibrillation: clinical application of a new assay for bretylium. *J Cardiovasc Pharmacol* 1981;3:485–99.
25. The Digitalis Investigation Group. The effect of digoxin on mortality and morbidity in patients with heart failure. *N Engl J Med* 1997;336:525–33.
26. Jelliffe RW. An improved method of digoxin therapy. *Ann Intern Med* 1968;69:703–17.
27. Jelliffe RW, Brooker G. A nomogram for digoxin therapy. *Am J Med* 1974;57:63–8.
28. Mooradian AD, Wynn EM. Pharmacokinetic prediction of serum digoxin concentration in the elderly. *Arch Intern Med* 1987;147:650–3.
29. Doherty JE et al. Clinical pharmacokinetics of digitalis glycosides. *Prog Cardiovasc Dis* 1978;21:141–58.
30. Slatton ML et al. Does digoxin provide additional hemodynamic and autonomic benefit at higher doses in patients with mild to moderate heart failure and normal sinus rhythm? *J Am Coll Cardiol* 1997;29:1206–13.
31. Soldin SJ. Digoxin—issues and controversies. *Clin Chem* 1986;32:5–12.
32. Iisalo E. Clinical pharmacokinetics of digoxin. *Clin Pharmacokinet* 1977;2:1–16.
33. Caldwell JH, Cline CT. Biliary excretion of digoxin in man. *Clin Pharmacol Ther* 1976;19:410–5.
34. Ewy GA et al. Digitalis intoxication—diagnosis, management and prevention. *Cardiol Clin* 1974;6:153–74.
35. Mann DL et al. Absence of cardioversion-induced ventricular arrhythmias in patients with therapeutic digoxin levels. *J Am Coll Cardiol* 1985;5:882–8.

36. Green LH, Smith TW. The use of digitalis in patients with pulmonary disease. *Ann Intern Med* 1977;87:459–65.
37. Slaughter RL et al. Appropriateness of the use of serum digoxin and digitoxin assays. *Am J Hosp Pharm* 1978;35:1376–9.
38. Podrid PJ et al. Congestive heart failure caused by oral disopyramide. *N Engl J Med* 1980;302:614–7.
39. Lima JJ et al. Antiarrhythmic activity and unbound concentrations of disopyramide enantiomers in patients. *Ther Drug Monit* 1990;12:23–8.
40. Lima JJ. Disopyramide. In, Taylor WJ, Caviness MHD, eds. *A textbook for the clinical application of therapeutic drug monitoring*. Irving, TX: Abbott Diagnostics; 1986:97–108.
41. Bauman JL et al. Practical optimisation of antiarrhythmic drug therapy using pharmacokinetic principles. *Clin Pharmacokinet* 1991;20:151–66.
42. Latini R et al. Therapeutic drug monitoring of antiarrhythmic drugs: rationale and current status. *Clin Pharmacokinet* 1990;18:91–103.
43. Piscitelli DA et al. Bioavailability of total and unbound disopyramide: implications for clinical use of the immediate and controlled-release forms. *J Clin Pharmacol* 1994;34:823–8.
44. Siddoway LA, Woosley RL. Clinical pharmacokinetics of disopyramide. *Clin Pharmacokinet* 1986;11:214–22.
45. Hasselstrom J et al. Enantioselective steady-state kinetics of unbound disopyramide and its dealkylated metabolite in man. *Eur J Clin Pharmacol* 1991;41:481–4.
46. Bauman JL et al. Long-term therapy with disopyramide phosphate: side effects and effectiveness. *Am Heart J* 1986;111:654–60.
47. Lenz TL, Hilleman DE. Dofetilide: a new class III antiarrhythmic agent. *Pharmacotherapy* 2000;20: 776–86.
48. Kalus JS, Mauro VF. Dofetilide: a class III–specific antiarrhythmic agent. *Ann Pharmacother* 2000;34:44–56.
49. Rasmussen HS et al. Dofetilide, a novel class III antiarrhythmic agent. *J Cardiovasc Pharmacol* 1992;20(suppl 2):S96–105.
50. Torp-Pedersen C et al. Dofetilide in patients with congestive heart failure and left ventricular dysfunction. *N Engl J Med* 1999;341:857–65.
51. Karam R et al. Azimilide dihydrochloride, a novel antiarrhythmic agent. *Am J Cardiol* 1998;81:40D–6.
52. Perry JC, Garson A. Flecainide acetate for treatment of tachyarrhythmias in children: review of world literature on efficacy, safety and dosing. *Am Heart J* 1992;124:1614–21.
53. Holmes B, Heel RC. Flecainide. A preliminary review of its pharmacodynamic properties and therapeutic efficacy. *Drugs* 1985;29:1–33.
54. Conrad GJ, Ober RE. Metabolism of flecainide. *Am J Cardiol* 1984;53:41B–51B.
55. Gross AS et al. Polymorphic flecainide disposition under conditions of uncontrolled urine flow and pH. *Eur J Clin Pharmacol* 1991;40:155–62.
56. Forland SC et al, Flecainide pharmacokinetics after multiple dosing in patients with impaired renal function. *J Clin Pharmacol* 1988;28:727–35.
57. McCollam P et al. Proarrhythmia: a paradoxical response to antiarrhythmic drugs. *Pharmacotherapy* 1989;9:144–53.
58. Tworek DA et al. Interference by antiarrhythmic agents with function of electrical cardiac devices. *Clin Pharm* 1992;11:48–56.
59. Anon. Ibutilide. *Med Lett Drugs Ther* 1996;38:38.
60. Howard PA. Ibutilide: an antiarrhythmic agent for the treatment of atrial fibrillation or flutter. *Ann Pharmacother* 1999;33:38–47.
61. Kowey PR et al. Safety and risk/benefit analysis of ibutilide for acute conversion of atrial fibrillation/flutter. *Am J Cardiol* 1996;78(suppl 8A):46–52.
62. Benowitz NL, Meister W. Clinical pharmacokinetics of lignocaine. *Clin Pharmacokinet* 1978;3:177–201.
63. Galer BS et al. Response to intravenous lidocaine infusion differs based on clinical diagnosis and site of nervous system injury. *Neurology* 1993;43:1233–5.
64. Routledge PA et al. Control of lidocaine therapy: new perspectives. *Ther Drug Monit* 1982;4:265–70.
65. Rowland M et al. Disposition kinetics of lidocaine in normal subjects. *Ann N Y Acad Sci* 1971;179:383–98.
66. Boyes RN et al. Pharmacokinetics of lidocaine in man. *Clin Pharmacol Ther* 1971;12:105–16.
67. Thomson PD et al. Lidocaine pharmacokinetics in advanced heart failure, liver disease, and renal failure in humans. *Ann Intern Med* 1973;78:499–508.
68. Bauer LA et al. Influence of long-term infusions on lidocaine kinetics. *Clin Pharmacol Ther* 1982;31:433–7.
69. Blumer J et al. The convulsant potency of lidocaine and its N-dealkylated metabolites. *J Pharmacol Exp Ther* 1973;186:31–6.
70. Burney RG et al. Anti-arrhythmic effects of lidocaine metabolites. *Am Heart J* 1974;88:765–9.

71. LeLorier J et al. Pharmacokinetics of lidocaine after prolonged intravenous infusions in uncomplicated myocardial infarction. *Ann Intern Med* 1977;87:700–2.

72. Routledge PA et al. Increased alpha-l-acid glycoprotein and lidocaine disposition in myocardial infarction. *Ann Intern Med* 1980;93:701–4.

73. Gupta PK et al. Lidocaine-induced heart block in patients with bundle branch block. *Am J Cardiol* 1974;33:187–92.

74. Singh BN. Routine prophylactic lidocaine administration in acute myocardial infarction, an idea whose time is all but gone? *Circulation* 1992;86:1033–5. Editorial.

75. Berk SI et al. The effect of oral cimetidine on total and unbound serum lidocaine concentrations in patients with suspected myocardial infarction. *Int J Cardiol* 1987;14:91–4.

76. Stracke H et al. Mexiletine in the treatment of diabetic neuropathy. *Diabetes Care* 1992;15:1550–5.

77. Awerbuch GI, Sandyk R. Mexiletine for thalamic pain syndrome. *Int J Neurosci* 1990;55:129–33.

78. Allaf et al. Pharmacokinetics of mexiletine in renal insufficiency. *Br J Clin Pharmacol* 1982;14:431–5.

79. Schrader BJ, Bauman IL. Mexiletine: a new type I antiarrhythmic agent. *Drug Intell Clin Pharm* 1986;20: 255–60.

80. Woosley RL et al. Pharmacology, electrophysiology, and pharmacokinetics of mexiletine. *Am Heart J* 1984; 107:1058–65.

81. Lledo P et al. Influence of debrisoquine hydroxylation phenotype on the pharmacokinetics of mexiletine. *Eur J Clin Pharmacol* 1993;44:63–7.

82. Campbell NPS et al. The clinical pharmacology of mexiletine. *Br J Clin Pharmacol* 1978;6:103–8.

83. Leahey EB et al. Effect of ventricular failure on steady state kinetics of mexiletine. *Clin Res* 1982;31:239A. Abstract.

84. Pentikainen PJ et al. Pharmacokinetics of oral mexiletine in patients with acute myocardial infarction. *Eur J Clin Pharmacol* 1983;25:773–7.

85. Campbell NPS et al. Long-term oral antiarrhythmic therapy with mexiletine. *Br Heart J* 1978;40:796–801.

86. Duff HJ et al. Molecular basis for the antigenicity of lidocaine analogs: tocainide and mexiletine. *Am Heart J* 1984;107:585–9.

87. Hurwitz A et al. Mexiletine effects on theophylline disposition. *Clin Pharmacol Ther* 1991;50:299–307.

88. Duff HJ et al. Mexiletine in the treatment of resistant ventricular arrhythmias: enhancement of efficacy and reduction of dose-related side effects by combination with quinidine. *Circulation* 1983;67:1124–8.

89. Vaughan Williams EM. Classification of the antiarrhythmic action of moricizine. *J Clin Pharmacol* 1991;31:216–21.

90. Moak JP et al. Newer antiarrhythmic drugs in children. *Am Heart J* 1987;61:179–85.

91. Morganroth J. Dose effect of moricizine on suppression of ventricular arrhythmias. *Am J Cardiol* 1990;65:26D–31.

92. Giardina EG et al. Moricizine concentration to guide arrhythmia treatment with attention to elderly patients. *J Clin Pharmacol* 1994;34:725–33.

93. Yang JM et al. Distribution of moricizine in human blood: binding to plasma proteins and erythrocytes. *Ther Drug Monit* 1990;12:59–64.

94. Siddoway LA et al. Clinical pharmacokinetics of moricizine. *Am J Cardiol* 1990;65:21D–5D.

95. Carnes CA, Coyle JD. Moricizine: a novel antiarrhythmic agent. *DICP* 1990;24:745–53.

96. The Cardiac Arrhythmia Suppression Trial II Investigators. Effect of the antiarrhythmic agent moricizine on survival after myocardial infarction. *N Engl J Med* 1992;327:227–33.

97. Hoffman BF et al. Electrophysiology and pharmacology of cardiac arrhythmias. VII. Cardiac effects of quinidine and procain amide. *Am Heart J* 1975;89:804–8.

98. Greenspan AM et al. Large dose procain amide therapy for ventricular tachyarrhythmia. *Am J Cardiol* 1980;46:453–62.

99. Kessler KM et al. Procainamide pharmacokinetics in patients with acute myocardial infarction or congestive heart failure. *J Am Coll Cardiol* 1986;7:1131–9.

100. Connolly SJ, Kates RE. Clinical pharmacokinetics of N-acetylprocain amide. *Clin Pharmacokinet* 1982;7: 206–20.

101. Karlsson E. Clinical pharmacokinetics of procainamide. *Clin Pharmacokinet* 1978;3:97–107.

102. Henningsen NC et al. Effects of long-term treatment with procainamide. A prospective study with special regard to ANF and SLE in fast and slow acetylators. *Acta Med Scand* 1975;198:475–82.

103. Strasberg B et al. Procainamide-induced polymorphous ventricular tachycardia. *Am J Cardiol* 1981;47: 1309–14.

104. Meyers DG et al. Severe neutropenia associated with procainamide: comparison of sustained release and conventional preparations. *Am Heart J* 1985;109:1393–5.

105. Lee JT et al. The role of genetically determined polymorphic drug metabolism in the beta-blockade produced by propafenone. *N Engl J Med* 1990;322:1764–8.

106. Funck-Brentano C et al. Propafenone. *N Engl J Med* 1990;322:518–25.

107. Musto et al. Electrophysiological effects and clinical efficacy of propafenone in children with recurrent paroxysmal supraventricular tachycardia. *Circulation* 1988;78:863–9.

108. Hii JTY et al. Clinical pharmacokinetics of propafenone. *Clin Pharmacokinet* 1991;21:1–10.

109. Lee JT et al. Influence of hepatic dysfunction on the pharmacokinetics of propafenone. *J Clin Pharmacol* 1987;27:384–9.

110. Capucci A et al. Minimal effective concentration values of propafenone and 5-hydroxy-propafenone in acute and chronic therapy. *Cardiovasc Drugs Ther* 1990;4:281–7.

111. Siddoway LA et al. Polymorphism of propafenone metabolism and disposition in man: clinical and pharmacokinetic consequences. *Circulation* 1987;75:785–91.

112. Parker RB et al. Propafenone: a novel type Ic antiarrhythmic agent. *DICP* 1989;23:196–202.

113. Bryson HM et al. Propafenone. A reappraisal of its pharmacology, pharmacokinetics and therapeutic use in cardiac arrhythmias. *Drugs* 1993;45:85–130.

114. Mondardini A et al. Propafenone-induced liver injury: report of a case and review of the literature. *Gastroenterology* 1993;104:1524–6.

115. Verme CN et al. Pharmacokinetics of quinidine in male patients. A population analysis. *Clin Pharmacokinet* 1992;22:468–80.

116. Greenblatt DJ et al. Pharmacokinetics of quinidine in humans after intravenous, intramuscular and oral administration. *J Pharmacol Exp Ther* 1977;202:365–78.

117. Ueda CT, Dzindzio BS. Quinidine kinetics in congestive heart failure. *Clin Pharmacol Ther* 1978;23:158–64.

118. Kessler KM et al. Quinidine pharmacokinetics in patients with cirrhosis or receiving propranolol. *Am Heart J* 1978;96:627–35.

119. Bauman JL et al. Torsade de pointes due to quinidine: observations in 31 patients. *Am Heart J* 1984; 107:425–30.

120. Coplen SE et al. Efficacy and safety of quinidine therapy for maintenance of sinus rhythm after cardioversion. *Circulation* 1990;82:1106–16.

121. Oberg KC et al. "Late" proarrhythmia due to quinidine. *Am J Cardiol* 1994;74:192–4.

122. Fromm MF et al. Inhibition of P-glycoprotein–mediated drug transport. A unifying mechanism to explain the interaction between digoxin and quinidine. *Circulation* 1999;99:552–7.

123. Nappi JM, McCollam PL. Sotalol: a breakthrough antiarrhythmic? *Ann Pharmacother* 1993;27:1359–68.

124. Hanyok JJ. Clinical pharmacokinetics of sotalol. *Am J Cardiol* 1993;72:19A–26A.

125. Fiset C et al. Stereoselective disposition of (±)-sotalol at steady-state conditions. *Br J Clin Pharmacol* 1993;36:75–7.

126. Poirer M et al. The pharmacokinetics of d-sotalol and d,l-sotalol in healthy volunteers. *Br J Clin Pharmacol* 1990;38:579–82.

127. Dumas M et al. Variations of sotalol kinetics in renal insufficiency. *Int J Clin Pharmacol Ther Toxicol* 1989;27:486–9.

128. MacNeil DJ et al. Clinical safety profile of sotalol in the treatment of arrhythmias. *Am J Cardiol* 1993; 72:44A–50.

129. Campbell RW, Furniss SS. Practical considerations in the use of sotalol for ventricular tachycardia and ventricular fibrillation. *Am J Cardiol* 1993;72:80A–5.

130. Kehoe RF et al. Safety and efficacy of oral sotalol for sustained ventricular tachyarrhythmias refractory to other antiarrhythmic agents. *Am J Cardiol* 1993;72:56A–66.

131. Winkle RA et al. Tocainide for drug-resistant ventricular arrhythmias: efficacy, side effects, and lidocaine responsiveness for predicting tocainide success. *Am Heart J* 1980;100:1031–6.

132. Kutalek SP et al. Tocainide: a new oral antiarrhythmic agent. *Ann Intern Med* 1985;103:387–91.

133. Routledge PA. Tocainide. In, Taylor WJ, Caviness MHD, eds. *A textbook for the clinical application of therapeutic drug monitoring.* Irving, TX: Abbott Diagnostics; 1986:175–80.

134. Mohiuddin SM et al. Tocainide kinetics in congestive heart failure. *Clin Pharmacol Ther* 1983;34:596–603.

135. Roden DM, Woosley RL. Tocainide. *N Engl J Med* 1986;315:41–5.

136. Holmes B et al. Tocainide. A review of its pharmacological properties and therapeutic efficacy. *Drugs* 1983;26:93–123.

137. Hoffmann K-J et al. Analysis and stereoselective metabolism after separate oral doses of tocainide enantiomers to healthy volunteers. *Biopharm Drug Dispos* 1990;11:351–63.

138. Braun J et al. Pharmacokinetics of tocainide in patients with severe renal failure. *Eur J Clin Pharmacol* 1985;28:665–70.

139. Forrence E et al. A seizure induced by concurrent lidocaine-tocainide therapy—is it just a case of additive toxicity? *Drug Intell Clin Pharm* 1986;20:56–9.

140. Vaughan Williams ED. A classification of antiarrhythmic actions reassessed after a decade of new drugs. *J Clin Pharmacol* 1984;24:129–47.

141. Task Force of the Working Group on Arrhythmias of the European Society of Cardiology. The Sicilian gambit. A new approach to the classification of antiarrhythmic drugs based on their actions on arrhythmogenic mechanisms. *Circulation* 1991;84:1831–51.

142. Cauffield JS et al. Alpha blockers: a reassessment of their role in therapy. *Am Fam Physician* 1996; 54:263–70.

143. Fulton B et al. Doxazosin. An update of its clinical pharmacology and therapeutic applications in hypertension and benign prostatic hypertrophy. *Drugs* 1995;49:295–320.

144. Drug information for the health professional, Vol I. In, *USP DI*, 20th ed. Englewood, CO: Micromedex; 2000.

145. Vincent J et al. Clinical pharmacokinetics of prazosin—1985. *Clin Pharmacokinet* 1985;10:144–54.

146. Titmarsh S, Monk JP. Terazosin. A review of its pharmacodynamic and pharmacokinetic properties, and therapeutic efficacy in essential hypertension. *Drugs* 1987;33:461–77.

147. Studer JA, Piepho RW. Antihypertensive therapy in the geriatric patient: II. A review of the alpha$_1$-adrenergic blocking agents. *J Clin Pharmacol* 1993;33:2–13.

148. Carruthers SG. Adverse effects of α_1-adrenergic blocking drugs. *Drug Saf* 1994;11:12–20.

149. ALLHAT Officers and Coordinators. Major cardiovascular events in hypertensive patients randomized to doxazosin vs chlorthalidone. *JAMA* 2000;283:1967–75.

150. Langely MS, Heel RC. Transdermal clonidine: a preliminary review of its pharmacodynamic properties and therapeutic efficacy. *Drugs* 1988;35:123–42.

151. Guthrie SK. Pharmacologic interventions for the treatment of opioid dependence and withdrawal. *DICP* 1990;24:721–34.

152. Nunn-Thompson CL, Simon PA. Pharmacotherapy for smoking cessation. *Clin Pharm* 1989;8:710–20.

153. Lowenthal DT el al. Clinical pharmacokinetics of clonidine. *Clin Pharmacokinet* 1988;14:287–310.

154. Holdiness MR. A review of contact dermatitis associated with transdermal therapeutic systems. *Contact Dermatitis* 1989;20:3–9.

155. Reid JL et al. Withdrawal reactions following cessation of central α-adrenergic receptor agonist. *Hypertension* 1984;6(suppl II):71II–5II.

156. Harris JM. Clonidine patch toxicity. *DICP* 1990;24:1191–4.

157. Bond WS. Psychiatric indications for clonidine: the neuropharmacologic and clinical basis. *J Clin Psychopharmacol* 1986;6:81–7.

158. Bravo EL et al. Clonidine-suppression test: a useful aid in the diagnosis of pheochromocytoma. *N Engl J Med* 1981;305:623–6.

159. Fedorak RN. Treatment of diabetic diarrhea with clonidine. *Ann Intern Med* 1985;102:197–9.

160. Hammer M, Berg G. Clonidine in the treatment of menopausal flushing. *Acta Obstet Gynecol Scand Suppl* 1985;132:29–31.

161. Nilsson LC et al. Clonidine for the relief of premenstrual syndrome. *Lancet* 1985;2:549–50.

162. Ogilvie RI et al. Diazoxide concentration-response relation in hypertension. *Hypertension* 1982;4:167–73.

163. Burris JF. The expanding role of angiotensin converting enzyme inhibitors in the management of hypertension. *J Clin Pharmacol* 1995;35:337–42.

164. Leonetti G, Cuspidi C. Choosing the right ACE inhibitors. A guide to selection. *Drugs* 1995;49:516–35.

165. DiPette DJ et al. Enalaprilat, an intravenous angiotensin-converting enzyme inhibitor, in hypertensive crisis. *Clin Pharmacol Ther* 1985;38:199–204.

166. Todd PA, Heel RC. Enalapril: a review of its pharmacodynamic and pharmacokinetic properties and therapeutic use in hypertension and congestive heart failure. *Drugs* 1986;31:198–248.

167. Till AE et al. Pharmacokinetics of repeated oral doses of enalapril maleate (MK-421) in normal volunteers. *Biopharm Drug Dispos* 1984;5:273–80.

168. Ulm EH et al. Enalapril maleate and a lysine analogue (MK-521): disposition in man. *Br J Clin Pharmacol* 1982;14:357–62.

169. Alderman CP. Adverse effects of the angiotensin-converting enzyme inhibitors. *Ann Pharmacother* 1996; 30:55–61.

170. Brogden RN et al. Captopril. An update of its pharmacodynamic and pharmacokinetic properties, and therapeutic use in hypertension and congestive heart failure. *Drugs* 1988;36:540–600.

171. Keane WF et al. Angiotensin converting enzyme inhibitors and progressive renal insufficiency; current experience and future directions. *Ann Intern Med* 1989;111:503–16.

172. Cooper RA. Captopril-associated neutropenia: who is at risk? *Arch Intern Med* 1983;143:659–60.

173. Joint National Committee on Prevention, Detection, Evaluation, and Treatment of High Blood Pressure. The sixth report of the Joint National Committee on Prevention, Detection, Evaluation, and Treatment of High Blood Pressure. *Arch Intern Med* 1997;157:2413–46.

174. CONSENSUS Trial Study Group. Effects of enalapril on mortality in severe congestive heart failure. *N Engl J Med* 1987;316:1430–5.

175. The Heart Outcomes Prevention Evaluation Study Investigators. Effects of an angiotensin-converting enzyme inhibitor, ramipril, on cardiovascular events in high-risk patients. *N Engl J Med* 2000;342:145–53.

176. Murphy MB, Elliott WJ. Dopamine and dopamine receptor agonists in cardiovascular therapy. *Crit Care Med* 1990;18:S14–8.

177. Brogden RN, Markham A. Fenoldopam. *Drugs* 1997;54:634–50.

178. White WB, Halley SE. Comparative renal effects of intravenous administration of fenoldopam mesylate and sodium nitroprusside in patients with severe hypertension. *Arch Intern Med* 1989;149:870–4.

179. Allison NL et al. The effect of fenoldopam, a dopaminergic agonist, on renal hemodynamics. *Clin Pharmacol Ther* 1987;41:282–8.

180. Everitt DE et al. Effect of intravenous fenoldopam on intraocular pressure in ocular hypertension. *J Clin Pharmacol* 1997;37:312–20.

181. Pilmer BL et al. Fenoldopam mesylate versus sodium nitroprusside in the acute management of severe systemic hypertension. *J Clin Pharmacol* 1993;33:549–53.

182. Panacek EA et al. Randomized, prospective trial of fenoldopam vs sodium nitroprusside in the treatment of acute severe hypertension. *Acad Emerg Med* 1995;2:959–65.

183. Bednarczyk EM et al. Comparative acute blood pressure reduction from intravenous fenoldopam mesylate versus sodium nitroprusside in severe systemic hypertension. *Am J Cardiol* 1989;63:993–6.

184. Reisin E et al. Intravenous fenoldopam versus sodium nitroprusside in patients with severe hypertension. *Hypertension* 1990;15(suppl I):I-59–I-62.

185. Mulrow JP, Crawford MH. Clinical pharmacokinetics and therapeutic use of hydralazine in congestive heart failure. *Clin Pharmacokinet* 1989;16:86–99.

186. O'Malley K et al. Duration of hydralazine action in hypertension. *Clin Pharmacol Ther* 1975;18:581–6.

187. Cameron HA, Ramsay LE. The lupus syndrome induced by hydralazine: a common complication with low-dose treatment. *Br Med J* 1984;289:410–2.

188. Shapiro KS et al. Immune complex glomerulonephritis in hydralazine-induced SLE. *Am J Kidney Dis* 1984;3:270–4.

189. Goa KL et al. Labetalol: a reappraisal of its pharmacology, pharmacokinetics and therapeutic use in hypertension and ischaemic heart disease. *Drugs* 1989;37:583–627.

190. MacCarthy EP, Bloomfield SS. Labetalol: a review of its pharmacology, pharmacokinetics, clinical uses and adverse effects. *Pharmacotherapy* 1983;3:193–219.

191. Bunchman TE et al. Intravenously administered labetalol for treatment of hypertension in children. *J Pediatr* 1992;120:140–4.

192. McNeil JJ, Louis WJ. Clinical pharmacokinetics of labetalol. *Clin Pharmacokinet* 1984;9:157–67.

193. Oliverio MI, Coffman TM. Angiotensin-II receptors: new targets for antihypertensive therapy. *Clin Cardiol* 1997;20:3–6.

194. Weber MA et al. Blood pressure effects of the angiotensin II receptor blocker, losartan. *Arch Intern Med* 1995;115:405–11.

195. Abdelwahab W et al. Management of hypertensive urgencies and emergencies. *J Clin Pharmacol* 1995; 35:747–62.

196. Timmermans PBMWM et al. Angiotensin II receptors and angiotensin II receptor antagonists. *Pharmacol Rev* 1993;45:205–51.

197. Csajka C et al. Pharmacokinetic–pharmacodynamic profile of angiotensin II receptor antagonists. *Clin Pharmacokinet* 1997;32:1–29.

198. Gavras HP, Salerno CM. The angiotensin II type I receptor blocker losartan in clinical practice: a review. *Clin Ther* 1996;18:1058–67.

199. Ellis ML, Patterson JH. A new class of antihypertensive therapy: angiotensin II receptor antagonists. *Pharmacotherapy* 1996:16:849–60.

200. Benz J et al. Valsartan, a new angiotensin II receptor antagonist: a double-blind study comparing the incidence of cough with lisinopril and hydrochlorothiazide. *J Clin Pharmacol* 1997;37:101–7.

201. Lacourcière Y et al. Effects of modulators of the renin–angiotensin–aldosterone system on cough. *J Hypertens* 1994;12:1387–93.

202. Crozier I et al. Losartan in heart failure. Hemodynamic effects and tolerability. *Circulation* 1995;91:691–7.

203. Pitt B et al. Effect of losartan compared with captopril on mortality in patients with symptomatic heart failure—the Losartan Heart Failure Survival Study ELITE II. *Lancet* 2000;355:1582–7.

204. Myhre E et al. Clinical pharmacokinetics of methyldopa. *Clin Pharmacokinet* 1982;7:221–33.

205. Oates JA. Antihypertensive agents and drug therapy of hypertension. In, Hardman JG et al., eds. *Goodman and Gilman's the pharmacological basis of therapeutics.* 9th ed. New York: McGraw-Hill; 1996:-780–808.

206. Fleishaker JC et al. The pharmacokinetics of 2.5 to 10 mg oral doses of minoxidil in healthy volunteers. *J Clin Pharmacol* 1989;29:162–7.

207. Vesey CJ, Cole PV. Blood cyanide and thiocyanate concentrations produced by long-term therapy with sodium nitroprusside. *Br J Anaesth* 1985;57:148–55.

208. Schultz V et al. Kinetics of elimination of thiocyanate in 7 healthy subjects and in 8 subjects with renal failure. *Klin Wochenschr* 1979;57:243–7.

209. Cottrell JE et al. Prevention of nitroprusside induced cyanide toxicity with hydroxocobalamin. *N Engl J Med* 1978;298:809–11.

210. Pasch TH et al. Nitroprusside-induced formation of cyanide and its detoxification with thiosulphate during deliberate hypotension. *J Cardiovasc Pharmacol* 1983;5:77–82.

211. Nawarskas JJ, Anderson JR. Omapatrilat. A unique new agent for the treatment of cardiovascular disease. *Heart Dis* 2000;2:266–74.

212. Neutel J et al. Antihypertensive efficacy of omapatrilat, a vasopeptidase inhibitor, compared with lisinopril. *J Hypertens* 1999;17(suppl 3):S67. Abstract.

213. Rouleau JL et al. Vasopeptidase inhibitor or angiotensin converting enzyme inhibitor in heart failure? Results of the IMPRESS Trial. *Circulation* 1999;99(suppl):1847. Abstract.

214. McAreavey D, Robertson JI. Angiotensin-converting enzyme inhibitors and moderate hypertension. *Drugs* 1990;40:326–45.

215. Salvetti A. Newer ACE inhibitors: a look at the future. *Drugs* 1990;40:800–28.

216. Tenero D et al. Effect of hepatic disease on the pharmacokinetics and plasma protein binding of eprosartan. *Pharmacotherapy* 1998;18:42–50.

217. McClellan KJ, Balfour JA. Eprosartan. *Drugs* 1998;55:713–8.

218. Frishman WH et al. Terazosin: a new long-acting α_1-adrenergic antagonist for hypertension. *Med Clin North Am* 1988;72:441–8.

219. Stumpf JL. Drug therapy of hypertensive crises. *Clin Pharm* 1988;7:582–91.

220. Hirschl MM. Guidelines for the drug treatment of hypertensive crisis. *Drugs* 1995;50:991–1000.

221. Angaran DM et al. Esmolol hydrochloride: an ultrashort-acting β-adrenergic blocking agent. *Clin Pharm* 1986;5:288–303.

222. Cuneo BF et al. Pharmacodynamics and pharmacokinetics of esmolol, a short-acting β-blocking agent, in children. *Pediatr Cardiol* 1994;15:296–301.

223. Trippel DL et al. Cardiovascular and antiarrhythmic effects of esmolol in children. *J Pediatr* 1991;119 (1, pt 1):142–7.

224. Routledge PA, Shand DG. Clinical pharmacokinetics of propranolol. *Clin Pharmacokinet* 1979;4:73–90.

225. Nies AS, Shand DG. Clinical pharmacology of propranolol. *Circulation* 1975;52:6–15.

226. Johnsson G, Regardh CG. Clinical pharmacokinetics of β-adrenoreceptor blocking drugs. *Clin Pharmacokinet* 1976;1:233–63.

227. McTavish D et al. Carvedilol. A review of its pharmacodynamic and pharmacokinetic properties, and therapeutic efficacy. *Drugs* 1993;45:232–58.

228. MacCarthy EP, Bloomfield SS. Labetalol. A review of its pharmacology, pharmacokinetics, clinical uses and adverse effects. *Pharmacotherapy* 1983;3:193–219.

229. Ryan JR. Clinical pharmacology of acebutolol. *Am Heart J* 1985;109:1131–6.

230. Frishman WH, Covey S. Penbutolol and carteolol: two new beta-adrenergic blockers with partial agonism. *J Clin Pharmacol* 1990;30:412–21.

231. Frishman WH et al. Bevantolol. A preliminary review of its pharmacodynamic and pharmacokinetic properties, and therapeutic efficacy in hypertension and angina pectoris. *Drugs* 1988;35:1–21.

232. Lancaster SG, Sorkin EM. Bisoprolol. A preliminary review of its pharmacodynamic and pharmacokinetic properties, therapeutic efficacy in hypertension and angina pectoris. *Drugs* 1988;36:256–85.

233. Petru MA et al. Long-term efficacy of high-dose diltiazem for chronic stable angina pectoris: 16-month serial studies with placebo controls. *Am Heart J* 1985;109:99–103.

234. Markham A, Brogden RN. Diltiazem. A review of its pharmacology and therapeutic use in older patients. *Drugs Aging* 1993;3:363–90.

235. Zelis RF, Kinney EL. The pharmacokinetics of diltiazem in healthy American men. *Am J Cardiol* 1982;49:529–32.

236. Joyal M et al. Pharmacodynamic aspects of intravenous diltiazem administration. *Am Heart J* 1986;111:54–60.

237. Smith MS et al. Pharmacokinetic and pharmacodynamic effects of diltiazem. *Am J Cardiol* 1983;51:1369–74.

238. Rodriguez I et al. P-glycoprotein in clinical cardiology. *Circulation* 1999;99:472–4.

239. McAllister RG. Kinetics and dynamics of nifedipine after oral sublingual doses. *Am J Med* 1986;81(suppl 6A):2–5.

240. Kleinbloesem CH et al. Nifedipine: kinetics and hemodynamic effects in patients with liver cirrhosis after intravenous and oral administration. *Clin Pharmacol Ther* 1986;40:21–8.

241. Sorkin EM et al. Nifedipine. A review of its pharmacodynamic and pharmacokinetic properties, and therapeutic efficacy, in ischemic heart disease, hypertension and related cardiovascular disorders. *Drugs* 1985;30:182–274.

242. Kleinbloesem CH et al. Nifedipine: kinetics and dynamics in healthy subjects. *Clin Pharmacol Ther* 1984;36:742–9.

243. Breimer DD et al. Nifedipine: variability in its kinetics and metabolism in man. *Pharmacol Ther* 1989;44:445–54.

244. Vetrovec GW et al. Comparative dosing and efficacy of continuous release nifedipine versus standard nifedipine for angina pectoris: clinical response, exercise performance and plasma nifedipine levels. *Am Heart J* 1988;115:793–8.

245. Opie LH. Calcium channel blockers for hypertension: dissecting the evidence for adverse effects. *Am J Hypertens* 1997;10(5, pt 1):565–77.

246. Diamond JR et al. Nifedipine-induced renal dysfunction. Alterations in renal hemodynamics. *Am J Med* 1984;77:905–9.

247. Elkayam U et al. A prospective, randomized, double-blind, crossover study to compare the efficacy and safety of chronic nifedipine therapy with that of isosorbide dinitrate and their combination in the treatment of chronic congestive heart failure. *Circulation* 1990;82:1954–61.

248. Dale J et al. The effects of nifedipine, a calcium antagonist, on platelet function. *Am Heart J* 1983;105:103–5.

249. Barbarash RA et al. Verapamil infusions in the treatment of atrial tachyarrhythmias. *Crit Care Med* 1986;14:886–8.

250. Schwartz JB et al. Prolongation of verapamil elimination kinetics during chronic oral administration. *Am Heart J* 1982;104:198–203.

251. Hamann SR et al. Clinical pharmacokinetics of verapamil. *Clin Pharmacokinet* 1984;9:26–41.

252. Hoon TJ et al. The pharmacodynamic and pharmacokinetic differences of the D- and L-isomers of verapamil: implications in the treatment of paroxysmal supraventricular tachycardia. *Am Heart J* 1986;112:396–403.

253. McTavish D, Sorkin EM. Verapamil. An updated review of its pharmacodynamic and pharmacokinetic properties, and therapeutic use in hypertension. *Drugs* 1989;38:19–76.

254. Singh BN et al. New perspectives in the pharmacologic therapy of cardiac arrhythmias. *Prog Cardiovasc Dis* 1980;22:243–301.

255. Schoen MD et al. Evaluation of the pharmacokinetics and electrocardiographic effects of intravenous verapamil with intravenous calcium chloride pretreatment in normal subjects. *Am J Cardiol* 1991;67:300–4.

256. Singh BN et al. Second generation calcium antagonists: search for greater selectivity and versatility. *Am J Cardiol* 1985;55:214B–21.

257. Bays HE, Dujovne CA. Drugs for treatment of patients with high cholesterol blood levels and other dyslipidemias. *Prog Drug Res* 1994;43:9–41.

258. Larsen ML, Illingworth DR. Drug treatment of dyslipoproteinemia. *Med Clin North Am* 1994;78:225–45.

259. National Cholesterol Education Program. Report of the Expert Panel on Blood Cholesterol Levels in Children and Adolescents. *Pediatrics* 1992;89:S525–70.

260. Kwiterovich PO. Diagnosis and management of familial dyslipoproteinemia in children and adolescents. *Pediatr Clin North Am* 1990;37:1489–521.

261. Lipid Research Clinics Program. Lipid research clinics coronary primary prevention trial results. I. Reduction in incidence of coronary heart disease. *JAMA* 1984;251:351–64.

262. Newman TB, Hulley SB. Carcinogenicity of lipid-lowering drugs. *JAMA* 1996;275:55–60.

263. Smellie WAS, Lorimer AR. Adverse effects of the lipid-lowering drugs. *Adverse Drug React Toxicol Rev* 1992;11:71–92.

264. Ast M, Frishman WH. Bile acid sequestrants. *J Clin Pharmacol* 1990;30:99–106.

265. Farmer JA, Gotto AM Jr. Antihyperlipidaemic agents. Drug interactions of clinical significance. *Drug Saf* 1994;11:301–9.

266. Expert Panel on Detection, Evaluation and Treatment of High Blood Cholesterol in Adults. Executive summary of the third report of the National Cholesterol Education Program (NCEP) Expert Panel on Detection, Evaluation, and Treatment of High Blood Cholesterol in Adults (Adult Treatment Panel III). *JAMA* 2001;285:2486–97.

267. Andrade SE et al. Discontinuation rates of antihyperlipidemic drugs—do rates reported in clinical trials reflect rates in primary care settings? *N Engl J Med* 1995;332:1125–31.

268. Hilleman DE et al. Comparative cost-effectiveness of bile acid sequestering resins, HMG Co-A reductase inhibitors, and their combination in patients with hypercholesterolemia. *J Managed Care Pharm* 1995;1:188–92.

269. Bartlett JG. Antibiotic-associated diarrhea. *Clin Infect Dis* 1992;15:573–81.

270. Kelly CP et al. *Clostridium difficile* colitis. *N Engl J Med* 1994;330:257–62.

271. Anon. Colesevelam (Welchol) for hypercholesterolemia. *Med Lett Drugs Ther* 2000;42:102–4.

272. Davidson MH et al. Colesevelam hydrochloride (Cholestagel): a new, potent bile acid sequestrant associated with a low incidence of gastrointestinal side effects. *Arch Intern Med* 1999;159:1893–900.

273. Jungnickel PW et al. Blind comparison of patient preference for flavored Colestid granules and Questran Light. *Ann Pharmacother* 1993;27:700–3.
274. Shaefer MS et al. Acceptability of cholestyramine or colestipol combinations with six vehicles. *Clin Pharm* 1987;6:51–4.
275. Shaefer MS et al. Sensory/mixability preference evaluation of cholestyramine powder formulations. *DICP* 1990;24:472–4.
276. Ito MK, Morreale AP. Acceptability of cholestyramine and colestipol formulations in three common vehicles. *Clin Pharm* 1991;10:138–40.
277. Insull W Jr et al. The effects of colestipol tablets compared with colestipol granules on plasma cholesterol and other lipids in moderately hypercholesterolemic patients. *Atherosclerosis* 1995;112:223–35.
278. Spence JD et al. Combination therapy with colestipol and psyllium mucilloid in patients with hyperlipidemia. *Ann Intern Med* 1995;123:493–9.
279. Superko HR et al. Effectiveness of low-dose colestipol therapy in patients with moderate hypercholesterolemia. *Am J Cardiol* 1992;70:135–40.
280. Balfour JA et al. Fenofibrate. *Drugs* 1990;40:260–90.
281. Adkins JC, Faulds D. Micronized fenofibrate. *Drugs* 1997;54:615–33.
282. Sheperd J. Mechanism of action of fibrates. *Postgrad Med J* 1993;69:S34–41.
283. Todd PA, Ward A. Gemfibrozil. A review of its pharmacodynamic and pharmacokinetic properties, and therapeutic use in dyslipidemia. *Drugs* 1988;36:314–39.
284. Evans JR et al. Effect of renal function on the pharmacokinetics of gemfibrozil. *J Clin Pharmacol* 1987;27:994–1000.
285. Shen D et al. Effect of gemfibrozil treatment in sulfonylurea-treated patients with noninsulin-dependent diabetes mellitus. *J Clin Endocrinol Metab* 1991;73:503–10.
286. Lozada A, Dujovne CA. Drug interactions with fibric acids. *Pharmacol Ther* 1994;63:163–76.
287. Frick MH et al. Helsinki heart study: primary prevention trial with gemfibrozil in middle-aged men with dyslipidemia. *N Engl J Med* 1987;317:1237–45.
288. Heinonen OP et al. Helsinki heart study: coronary heart disease incidence during an extended follow-up. *J Intern Med* 1994;235:41–9.
289. Frick MH et al. Efficacy of gemfibrozil in dyslipidaemic subjects with suspected heart disease. An ancillary study in the Helsinki heart study frame population. *Ann Med* 1993;25:41–5.
290. Furberg CD et al. Effect of lovastatin on early carotid atherosclerosis and cardiovascular events. *Circulation* 1994;90:1679–87.
291. Freeman DJ et al. Pravastatin and the development of diabetes mellitus. *Circulation* 2001;103:357-62.
292. Hsu I et al. Comparative evaluation of the safety and efficacy of HMG-CoA reductase inhibitor monotherapy in the treatment of primary hypercholesterolemia. *Ann Pharmacother* 1995;29:743–59.
293. Henwood JM, Heel RC. Lovastatin. A preliminary review of its pharmacodynamic properties and therapeutic use in hyperlipidaemia. *Drugs* 1988;429–54.
294. McTavish D, Sorkin EM. Pravastatin. A review of its pharmacological properties and therapeutic potential in hypercholesterolemia. *Drugs* 1991;65–89.
295. Todd PA, Goa KL. Simvastatin. A review of its pharmacological properties and therapeutic potential in hypercholesterolemia. *Drugs* 1990;40:583–607.
296. Mauro VF, MacDonald JL. Simvastatin: a review of its pharmacology and clinical use. *DICP* 1991;25:257–64.
297. Jungnickel PW et al. Pravastatin: a new drug for the treatment of hypercholesterolemia. *Clin Pharm* 1992;11:677–89.
298. Canner PL et al. Fifteen year mortality in coronary drug project patients: long-term benefit with niacin. *J Am Coll Cardiol* 1986;8:1245–55.
299. Anon. Statin class labeling should include liver failure as adverse event—OPDRA. *FDC Rep* 2000;July 24:26–8.
300. Dalen JE, Dalton WS. Does lowering cholesterol cause cancer? *JAMA* 1996;275:67–9. Commentary.
301. Scandinavian Simvastatin Survival Study Group. Randomised trial of cholesterol lowering in 4444 patients with coronary artery disease: the Scandinavian Simvastatin Survival Study (4S). *Lancet* 1994;344:1383–9.
302. Blauw GJ et al. Stroke, statins, and cholesterol. A meta-analysis of randomized, placebo-controlled, double-blind trials with HMG-CoA reductase inhibitors. *Stroke* 1997;28:946–50.
303. Downs JR et al. Primary prevention of acute coronary events with lovastatin in men and women with average cholesterol levels. *JAMA* 1998;279:1615–22.
304. Ridker PM et al. Long-term effects of pravastatin on plasma concentrations of C-reactive protein. *Circulation* 1999;100:230–5.
305. Ridker PM et al. C-reactive protein and other markers of inflammation in prediction of cardiovascular disease in women. *N Engl J Med* 2000;342:836–43.

306. Figge HL et al. Nicotinic acid: a review of its clinical use in the treatment of lipid disorders. *Pharmacotherapy* 1988;8:287–94.

307. ASHP Therapeutic Position Statement on the safe use of niacin in the management of dyslipidemias. *Am J Health-Syst Pharm* 1997;54:2815–9.

308. Colletti RB et al. Niacin treatment of hypercholesterolemia in children. *Pediatrics* 1993;92:78–82.

309. Hunninghake DB. Diagnosis and treatment of lipid disorders. *Med Clin North Am* 1994;78:247–57.

310. McKenney JM et al. A comparison of the efficacy and toxic effects of sustained- vs immediate-release niacin in hypercholesterolemic patients. *JAMA* 1994;271:672–7.

311. Chong PH, Seeger JD. Atorvastatin calcium: an addition to HMG-CoA reductase inhibitors. *Pharmacotherapy* 1997;17:1157–77.

312. Anon. Cerivastatin for hypercholesterolemia. *Med Lett Drugs Ther* 1998;40:13–4.

313. Zaritsky AL. Catecholamines, inotropic medications, and vasopressor agents. In, Chernow B et al., eds. *The pharmacologic approach to the critically ill patient.* 3rd ed. Baltimore: Williams & Wilkins; 1994: 387–404.

314. Kulka PJ, Tryba M. Inotropic support of the critically ill patient. A review of the agents. *Drugs* 1993; 45:654–67.

315. Trujillo MH, Bellorin-Font E. Drugs commonly administered by intravenous infusion in intensive care units: a practical guide. *Crit Care Med* 1990;18:232–8.

316. American College of Cardiology, American Heart Association Task Force. Adult advanced cardiac life support. *JAMA* 1992;268:2199–241.

317. American College of Cardiology, American Heart Association Task Force. Pediatric advanced life support. *JAMA* 1992;268:2262–75.

318. Bhatt-Mehta V, Nahata MC. Dopamine and dobutamine in pediatric therapy. *Pharmacotherapy* 1989;9:303–14.

319. Murphy MB, Elliott WJ. Dopamine and dopamine receptor agonists in cardiovascular therapy. *Crit Care Med* 1990;18:S14–8.

320. Geraci SA. Pharmacologic approach in patients with heart failure. In, Chernow B et al., eds. *The pharmacologic approach to the critically ill patient.* 3rd ed. Baltimore: Williams & Wilkins; 1994:80–94.

321. Jarnberg P-O et al. Dopamine infusion in man. Plasma catecholamine levels and pharmacokinetics. *Acta Anaesthesiol Scand* 1981;25:328–31.

322. Hoffman BB, Lefkowitz RJ. Catecholamines and sympathomimetic drugs. In, Gilman AG et al., eds. *Goodman and Gilman's the pharmacological basis of therapeutics.* 8th ed. New York: Pergamon Press; 1990:187–220.

323. Australian and New Zealand Intensive Care Society Clinical Trials Group. Low-dose dopamine in patients with early renal dysfunction: a placebo-controlled randomised trial. *Lancet* 2000;356:39-43.324. Skolnik NS. Treatment of croup. A critical review. *Am J Dis Child* 1989;143:1045–9.

325. Waisman Y et al. Prospective randomized double-blind study comparing L-epinephrine and racemic epinephrine aerosols in the treatment of laryngotracheitis (croup). *Pediatrics* 1992;89:302–6.

326. Zaritsky A, Chernow B. Use of catecholamines in pediatrics. *J Pediatr* 1984;105:341–50.

327. Tashkin DP, Jenne JW. Alpha and beta adrenergic agonists. In, Weiss EB et al., eds. *Bronchial asthma: mechanisms and therapeutics.* 2nd ed. Boston: Little, Brown; 1985:604–39.

328. Cydulka R et al. The use of epinephrine in the treatment of older adult asthmatics. *Ann Emerg Med* 1988;17:322–6.

329. Kelly HW. New β_2-adrenergic agonist aerosols. *Clin Pharm* 1985;4:393–403.

330. Wynne J, Braunwald E. New treatment for congestive heart failure: amrinone and milrinone. *J Cardiovasc Med* 1984;9:393–405.

331. Lawless ST et al. The acute pharmacokinetics and pharmacodynamics of amrinone in pediatric patients. *J Clin Pharmacol* 1991;31:800–3.

332. Rocci ML, Wilson H. The pharmacokinetics and pharmacodynamics of newer inotropic agents. *Clin Pharmacokinet* 1987;13:91–109.

333. Edelson J et al. Relationship between amrinone plasma concentration and cardiac index. *Clin Pharmacol Ther* 1981;29:723–8.

334. Ross MP et al. Amrinone-associated thrombocytopenia: pharmacokinetic analysis. *Clin Pharmacol Ther* 1993;53:661–7.

335. Dunkman WB et al. Adverse effects of long-term amrinone administration in congestive heart failure. *Am Heart J* 1983;105:861–3.

336. Packer M et al. Hemodynamic and clinical limitations of long-term inotropic therapy with amrinone in patients with severe chronic heart failure. *Circulation* 1984;70:1038–47.

337. Edelson J et al. Pharmacokinetics of the bipyridines amrinone and milrinone. *Circulation* 1986;73(suppl III):145-III–52-III.

338. Young RA, Ward A. Milrinone. A preliminary review of its pharmacological properties and therapeutic use. *Drugs* 1988;36:158–92.

339. Martin C et al. Norepinephrine or dopamine for the treatment of hyperdynamic septic shock? *Chest* 1993;103:1826–31.

340. Notterman DA. Pediatric pharmacotherapy. In, Chernow B et al., eds. *The pharmacologic approach to the critically ill patient.* 3rd ed. Baltimore: Williams & Wilkins; 1994:139–55.

341. Neugebauer E et al. Pharmacotherapy of shock. In, Chernow B et al., eds. *The pharmacologic approach to the critically ill patient.* 3rd ed. Baltimore: Williams & Wilkins; 1994:1104–21.

342. Rackow EC, Astiz ME. Mechanisms and management of septic shock. *Crit Care Clin* 1993;9:219–37.

343. Zaloga GP et al. Pharmacologic cardiovascular support. *Crit Care Clin* 1993;9:335–62.

344. Abrams J. Nitroglycerin and long-acting nitrates. *P&T* 1992;59–64,67–9.

345. Parker JO. Nitrate therapy in stable angina pectoris. *N Engl J Med* 1987;316:1635–42.

346. Elkayam U. Tolerance to organic nitrates: evidence, mechanisms, clinical relevance, and strategies for prevention. *Ann Intern Med* 1991;114:667–77.

347. Cannon LA, Marshall JM. Cardiac disease in the elderly population. *Clin Geriatr Med* 1993;9:499–525.

348. Thadani U, Opie LH. Nitrates. In, Opie LH, ed. *Drugs for the heart.* 4th ed. Philadelphia: WB Saunders; 1995:31–48.

349. Sporl-Radun S et al. Effects and pharmacokinetics of isosorbide dinitrate in normal man. *Eur J Clin Pharmacol* 1980;18:237–44.

350. Abshagen WWP et al. Pharmacokinetics of intravenous and oral isosorbide-5-mononitrate. *Eur J Clin Pharmacol* 1981;20:269–75.

351. Frishman WH et al. Mononitrates: defining the ideal long-acting nitrate. *Clin Ther* 1994;16:130–9.

352. Abshagen WWP. Pharmacokinetics of isosorbide mononitrate. *Am J Cardiol* 1992;70:61G–6G.

353. Fung H-L. Clinical pharmacology of organic nitrates. *Am J Cardiol* 1993;72:9C–15C.

354. Fletcher A. Transdermal nitroglycerin. Does it really work in the treatment of angina? *Drugs Aging* 1991;1:6–16.

355. Friedman WF, George BL. New concepts and drugs in the treatment of congestive heart failure. *Pediatr Clin North Am* 1984;31:1197–226.

356. Anon. Nitroglycerin patches—do they work? *Med Lett Drugs Ther* 1989;31:65–6.

357. Abrams J. Pharmacology of nitroglycerin and long-acting nitrates and their usefulness in the treatment of chronic congestive heart failure. In, Gould L, Reddy CVR, eds. *Vasodilator therapy for cardiac disorders.* Mount Kisco, NY: Futura Publishing; 1979:129–67.

358. Schrader BJ et al. Acceptance of transcutaneous nitroglycerin patches by patients with angina pectoris. *Pharmacotherapy* 1986;6:83–6.

359. DeMots H, Glasser SPP. Intermittent transdermal nitroglycerin therapy in the treatment of chronic stable angina. *J Am Coll Cardiol* 1989;13:786–93.

360. Baaske DM et al. Nitroglycerin compatibility with intravenous fluid filters, containers, and administration sets. *Am J Hosp Pharm* 1980;37:201–5.

361. Amann AH et al. Plastic I.V. container for nitroglycerin. *Am J Hosp Pharm* 1980;37:618. Letter.

362. Haas CE et al. Effect of using a standard polyvinyl chloride intravenous infusion set on patient response to nitroglycerin. *Am J Hosp Pharm* 1992;49:1135–7.

363. Altavela JL et al. Clinical response to intravenous nitroglycerin infused through polyethylene or polyvinyl chloride tubing. *Am J Hosp Pharm* 1994;51:490–4.

364. Mulrow CD et al. Relative efficacy of vasodilator therapy in chronic congestive heart failure. Implications of randomized trials. *JAMA* 1988;259:3422–6.

365. Chaterjee K et al. Vasodilator therapy in chronic congestive heart failure. *Am J Cardiol* 1988;62:46A–54A.

366. Cohn JN et al. A comparison of enalapril with hydralazine-isosorbide dinitrate in the treatment of chronic congestive heart failure. *N Engl J Med* 1991;325:303–10.

367. Parillo JE. Vasodilator therapy. In, Chernow B et al., eds. *The pharmacological approach to the critically ill patient.* 3rd ed. Baltimore: Williams & Wilkins; 1994:470–83.

368. Johnson JA, Lalonde RL. Congestive heart failure. In, DiPiro JT et al., eds. *Pharmacotherapy: a pathophysiologic approach.* 2nd ed. East Norwalk, CT: Appleton & Lange; 1993:160–93.

369. Guyton JR et al. Effectiveness of once-nightly dosing of extended-release niacin alone and in combination for hypercholesterolemia. *Am J Cardiol* 1998;82:737–43.

Central Nervous System Drugs

Anticonvulsants

Class Instructions. Anticonvulsants. It is important to take this medication as prescribed to control seizures; stopping it suddenly can increase seizures. This medication can cause drowsiness. Until the extent of this effect is known, use caution when driving, operating machinery, or performing other tasks requiring mental alertness. Avoid concurrent use of alcohol or other drugs that cause drowsiness. Report unusual or bothersome side effects. Always use an effective contraceptive; contact your physician if you plan to become or become pregnant.

CARBAMAZEPINE
Carbatrol, Tegretol, Various

Pharmacology. Carbamazepine is an iminostilbene compound related structurally to the tricyclic antidepressants. In animals, carbamazepine acts presynaptically to block firing of action potentials, which decreases the release of excitatory neurotransmitters, and postsynaptically by blocking high-frequency repetitive discharge initiated at cell bodies.

Administration and Adult Dosage. **PO for epilepsy** 100–200 mg bid with meals initially, increasing in increments of up to 200 mg/day at weekly intervals to effective dosage. **Usual maintenance dosage** is 10–30 mg/kg/day or 600–1600 mg/day in 2–4 divided doses;[1,2] tid or qid administration is recommended when enzyme-inducing antiepileptic drugs are administered concurrently. **SR** product can be given bid. **PO for trigeminal neuralgia** 100 mg bid initially, increasing in 200 mg/day increments until relief of pain, to a maximum of 1.2 g/day. **Usual maintenance dosage** is 400–800 mg/day in 2–3 divided doses. **PO loading dose** 8 mg/kg in a single dose achieves therapeutic levels in 2 hr (with suspension) or 5 hr (with tablets) and is well tolerated. **Rectal administration** has been reported. (*See* Fate.)

Special Populations. *Pediatric Dosage.* **PO for epilepsy** (<6 yr) 10–20 mg/kg/day in 3–4 divided doses with the chewable tablets or in 4 divided doses with the suspension; (6–12 yr) 10–20 mg/kg/day with meals initially, increasing weekly in 100 mg/day increments as needed to achieve optimal clinical response. **Usual maintenance dosage** is 15–35 mg/kg/day or 400–800 mg/day in 3–4 divided doses. (>12 yr) same as adult dosage.[2]

Geriatric Dosage. Clearance of carbamazepine is reduced in some elderly patients, so a lower maintenance dosage might be required.[3]

Other Conditions. During pregnancy, increases in carbamazepine clearance can occur; dosage increases guided by serum levels and patient status might be necessary.[2]

Dosage Forms. **Chew Tab** 100 mg; **Susp** 20 mg/mL; **Tab** 200 mg; **SR Cap** 200, 300 mg (Carbatrol); **SR Tab** 100, 200, 400 mg (Tegretol XR).

Patient Instructions. (*See* Anticonvulsants Class Instructions.) Immediately report sore throat, fever, mouth ulcers, or easy bruising, which can be an early sign of a severe, but rare, blood disorder. The Tegretol XR shell might appear in the stool, but does not indicate a lack of absorption.

Missed Doses. Take this drug at regular intervals. If you miss a dose, take it as soon as you remember. If it is about time for the next dose, take that dose only. Do not double the dose or take extra. If you miss more than one dose in a day, call your physician.

Pharmacokinetics. *Onset and Duration.* Steady-state serum levels are attained within 2–4 days and subsequently can decline because of autoinduction of metabolism.[2] (*See* Fate.)

Serum Levels. (Anticonvulsant) 4–12 mg/L (17–50 μmol/L). Variability exists in the relationship between serum levels and CNS side effects. (*See* Notes.)

Fate. Absorption from tablets is slow and erratic, with a bioavailability of 75–85%; peak serum levels occur 4–8 hr after a dose of immediate-release product and 19 ± 7 hr after a dose of SR product.[2] Absorption is rapid with the suspension, with a peak serum level of 7.9 ± 1.9 mg/L at 1.6 ± 1.3 hr in the fasting state or 3.4 ± 3.4 hr with concomitant enteral tube feeding after a 500 mg oral dose.[4] A peak serum level of 5.1 ± 1.6 mg/L occurs 6.3 ± 1.5 hr after rectal administration of 6 mg/kg oral suspension (100 mg/5 mL) diluted with an equal volume of water.[5] The drug is 75–78% bound to plasma proteins.[2,6] V_d is 0.88 ± 0.06 L/kg in adults[4] and 1.2 ± 0.2 L/kg in children.[7] Large differences in Cl occur because of autoinduction of liver enzymes; autoinduction is completed within 1–2 weeks of monotherapy; Cl is 0.052 ± 0.04 L/hr/kg at end of week 1, 0.04 ± 0.02 L/hr/kg at week 2, and 0.054 ± 0.04 L/hr/kg at week 4.[8] Carbamazepine is metabolized to pharmacologically active carbamazepine-10,11-epoxide; the epoxide metabolite (CBZ-E) serum level ratios at steady state are 0.19 ± 0.06 at a carbamazepine level of 6.9 ± 1.5 mg/L and 0.28 ± 1.4 at a carbamazepine level of 10.5 ± 2.6 mg/L.[9] (*See* Notes.) Only about 2% of drug is excreted unchanged in the urine.[2,6]

$t_{1/2}$. There are large interindividual differences because of autoinduction of liver enzymes. (Adults) 31.3 ± 5.9 hr after a single dose,[4] 14.5 ± 5.3 hr after 2 months;[9] (children) 29.4 ± 3.6 hr after a single dose, 15.2 ± 5.2 hr after 5 months.[7]

Adverse Reactions. Dizziness, drowsiness, headache, diplopia, nausea, and vomiting occur frequently with initiation of therapy and are minimized by slow titration of dosage. Mild, transient, morbilliform rash and thrombocytopenia also occur frequently. Occasionally, confusion, stomatitis, or rash occur. Hyponatremia and water intoxication occur, and risk factors include carbamazepine monotherapy, elevated serum levels, patient age >25 yr, diuretic use, vomiting, or diarrhea.[2] Transient leukopenia has been observed in 10–20% of patients; persistent leukopenia occurs in 2% of patients.[2] Discontinue drug if leukopenia (ANC <1500/μL) persists or any evidence of bone marrow depression develops. Rare effects include aplastic anemia, agranulocytosis, hepatitis, lenticular opacities, and arrhythmias.

Contraindications. History of bone marrow depression; hypersensitivity to tricyclic antidepressants.

Precautions. Pregnancy; history of liver disease. Abrupt withdrawal of the drug in patients with epilepsy can precipitate status epilepticus. Exacerbation of atypical absence seizures can occur in children receiving carbamazepine for mixed seizure disorders.[2] Use carbamazepine cautiously in patients with histories of severe hypersensitivity reactions to phenytoin or phenobarbital.

Drug Interactions. Because of structural similarities to tricyclic antidepressants, discontinue MAOIs for a minimum of 14 days before starting carbamazepine. Carbamazepine can stimulate the metabolism of many drugs metabolized by CYP3A4, including oral anticoagulants, oral contraceptives, corticosteroids, cyclosporine, doxycycline, haloperidol, heterocyclic antidepressants, protease inhibitors, and theophylline. Many drugs inhibit carbamazepine metabolism, including cimetidine, clarithromycin, danazol, erythromycin, fluoxetine, isoniazid, ketoconazole, propoxyphene, quinine, troleandomycin, verapamil, and diltiazem.

Parameters to Monitor. Baseline CBC and platelet counts; monitor more frequently if WBC or platelet counts decrease. Monitor liver function tests periodically during long-term therapy. Monitor serum levels at least weekly during the first month of therapy because of autoinduction. Periodic serum level monitoring is useful in evaluating therapeutic efficacy or potential for adverse effects.[2]

Notes. The contribution of CBZ-E to the therapeutic or adverse effects of carbamazepine is uncertain. One study found no significant correlation between toxicity score or seizure frequency and serum levels of carbamazepine, CBZ-E, or their sum in patients receiving carbamazepine monotherapy, or combination therapy with phenytoin or valproic acid.[9] (*See* Anticonvulsants Comparison Chart.)

CLONAZEPAM   Klonopin

Pharmacology. Clonazepam is a benzodiazepine anticonvulsant that limits the spread of seizure activity, possibly by enhancing the postsynaptic effect of the inhibitory neurotransmitter, γ-aminobutyric acid (GABA).

Administration and Adult Dosage. **PO for epilepsy** no more than 0.5 mg tid initially; increase in 0.5–1 mg/day increments q 3 days to effective dosage or to a maximum of 20 mg/day. **Usual maintenance dosage** is 4–8 mg/day.[1] **PO for panic disorder** 0.25 mg bid initially, increasing to 1 mg/day after 3 days. **Usual maintenance dosage** is 1 mg/day; some patients require up to 4 mg/day. (*See* Notes.) **Rectal administration** has been reported. (*See* Fate.)

Special Populations. *Pediatric Dosage.* **PO for epilepsy** ($\leq$10 yr or $\leq$30 kg) 0.01–0.03 mg/kg/day initially in 2–3 divided doses, increase in 0.25–0.5 mg/day increments q 3 days to effective dosage, to a maximum of 0.2 mg/kg/day in 3 divided doses. Rectal administration has been reported. (*See* Fate.)

Geriatric Dosage. **PO for epilepsy and as an antipanic agent** same as adult dosage initially. **Maintenance dosage** requirements might be lower in elderly patients because of reduced drug clearance and enhanced pharmacodynamic response.[10]

Dosage Forms. Tab 0.5, 1, 2 mg.

Patient Instructions. (*See* Anticonvulsants Class Instructions.)

Missed Doses. Take this drug at regular intervals. If you miss a dose, take it as soon as you remember. If it is about time for the next dose, take that dose only. Do not double the dose or take extra.

Pharmacokinetics. *Onset and Duration.* Steady-state serum levels are attained in 4–8 days.[2] (*See* Notes.)

Serum Levels. 13–72 μg/L (40–230 nmol/L); however, some patients controlled with clonazepam can have levels below this range. There is a poor correlation between serum levels and efficacy or adverse effects.[2]

Fate. Rapidly absorbed orally; peak serum levels occur 1–3 hr after a dose. Serum levels of 18–40 μg/L occur 20–120 min after rectal administration of a 0.1 mg/kg dose of clonazepam suspension.[11] The drug is $86 \pm 0.5\%$ bound to plasma proteins;[2] V_d is 3.1 ± 1.2 L/kg; Cl is 0.059 ± 0.011 L/hr/kg.[12] The principal metabolite, 7-aminoclonazepam, is inactive. Less than 0.5% of clonazepam is excreted unchanged in urine.[2]

$t_{1/2}$. 34.1 ± 7.5 hr.[12]

Adverse Reactions. Drowsiness, ataxia, behavior disturbances, and personality changes (hyperactivity, restlessness, and irritability, especially in children) occur frequently and require dosage reduction.[2] Occasionally, hypersalivation and bronchial hypersecretion occur and can cause respiratory difficulties. Rarely, anemia, leukopenia, thrombocytopenia, and respiratory depression occur. Nearly 50% of patients receiving long-term clonazepam can experience transient exacerbations of seizures, dysphoria, restlessness, or autonomic signs during clonazepam withdrawal.[13] An increased seizure frequency and status epilepticus occur rarely, possibly associated with supratherapeutic serum levels.[2]

Contraindications. Severe liver disease; acute narrow-angle glaucoma.

Precautions. Pregnancy; lactation; patients with chronic respiratory disease. Clonazepam can increase frequency of generalized tonic-clonic seizures in patients with mixed seizure types. Abrupt withdrawal of the drug in patients with epilepsy can precipitate status epilepticus. Absence status has been reported in patients receiving valproic acid concurrently.

Drug Interactions. Concurrent use with other CNS depressants can potentiate the sedation caused by clonazepam.

Parameters to Monitor. Periodic serum level monitoring is of limited value. Close attention to changes in patient's seizure frequency is necessary to monitor for the development of tolerance to the therapeutic effect. (*See* Notes.)

Notes. Tolerance to the anticonvulsant effect of clonazepam occurs in approximately one-third of patients within 3–6 months of starting the drug. Taper and discontinue clonazepam if therapeutic benefit cannot be demonstrated. Because of prominent CNS adverse effects and the development of tolerance, it is considered an alternative to **valproic acid** for myoclonic seizures and an alternative to **ethosuximide** or valproic acid for absence seizures.[16] (*See* Anticonvulsants Comparison Chart.) Clonazepam also has become an alternative to **alprazolam** for treatment of panic disorder. For patients who experience interdose symptom recurrence or morning rebound with alprazolam, clonazepam offers an equally effective alternative with the benefit of a longer duration of effect. When switching a patient from alprazolam to clonazepam, an equivalent dosage of clonazepam is one-half that of alprazolam.[14–16]

ETHOSUXIMIDE   Zarontin

Pharmacology. Ethosuximide is a succinimide that produces an anticonvulsant effect by blockade of T-type calcium currents in the thalamus. In humans, it suppresses 3 cycle per second spike and wave activity. (*See* Notes.)

Administration and Adult Dosage. PO for epilepsy 250 mg bid initially; increase in 250 mg/day increments at 4- to 7-day intervals to an effective dosage, to a maximum of 1.5 g/day. **Usual maintenance dosage** 750–1250 mg/day in 1–2 doses.[1,2]

Special Populations. *Pediatric Dosage.* PO for epilepsy (3–6 yr) 250 mg/day initially; increase in 250 mg/day increments q 4–7 days to effective dosage, to a maximum of 1 g/day. **Usual maintenance dosage** 20–40 mg/kg/day in 1–2 doses.[1,2] (>6 yr) same as adult dosage.

Geriatric Doses. Same as adult dosage.

Dosage Forms. **Cap** 250 mg; **Syrup** 50 mg/mL.

Patient Instructions. (*See* Anticonvulsants Class Instructions.) This drug can be taken with food or milk to minimize stomach upset.

Missed Doses. Take this drug at regular intervals. If you miss a dose, take it as soon as you remember. If it is about time for the next dose, take that dose only. Do not double the dose or take extra.

Pharmacokinetics. *Onset and Duration.* Steady-state serum levels are attained in 7–12 days.[2]

Serum Levels. 40–100 mg/L (280–710 μmol/L).[2]

Fate. The drug is well absorbed orally, with peak serum level in 3–7 hr in adults and children. Plasma protein binding is less than 10%. V_d is 0.69 L/kg;[17] Cl is 0.01 ± 0.04 L/hr/kg, greater in children.[2] Ethosuximide is metabolized to three inactive metabolites. About 20% of the drug is excreted unchanged in urine.[2,6]

$t_{1/2}$. (Adults) 52.6 hr;[18] (children) 31.6 ± 5.4 hr.[17]

Adverse Reactions. Nausea, vomiting, drowsiness, headache, hiccups, and dizziness occur frequently during initiation of therapy and usually are dose related. Occasionally, behavior changes or rashes occur. Rarely, SLE, leukopenia, aplastic anemia, or Stevens–Johnson syndrome occur.

Precautions. Pregnancy; patients with known liver or renal disease. Generalized tonic-clonic seizures can occur in patients with mixed seizure types who are treated with ethosuximide alone. Abrupt withdrawal of the drug can precipitate absence status epilepticus.

Contraindications. None known.

Drug Interactions. Ethosuximide can increase phenytoin serum levels and decrease levels of primidone (and its phenobarbital metabolite).

Parameters to Monitor. Periodic serum level monitoring, after attaining steady state (7–12 days), is useful in evaluating therapeutic efficacy or potential adverse effects.[2] Periodically monitor CBC, urinalysis, and liver function tests.

Notes. Ethosuximide is indicated only for treatment of absence seizures. Because of the drug's low potential for serious or long-term toxicity and its proven efficacy, it is considered the drug of choice for absence seizures. (*See* Anticonvulsants Comparison Chart.)

FELBAMATE   Felbatol

Pharmacology. Felbamate is a dicarbamate that is structurally related to meprobamate; its mechanism of action is not known but might involve inhibition of N-methyl-D-aspartate responses and potentiation of $GABA_a$ receptor chloride currents.[19]

Administration and Adult Dosage. PO for epilepsy 1.2 g/day initially in 3–4 divided doses while reducing the dosage of concomitant antiepileptic drugs (phenytoin, carbamazepine, valproic acid, or phenobarbital) by 20–30%. Increase in 1200 mg/day increments at weekly intervals to a maximum of 3.6 g/day. Further reduction in the dosage of concomitant antiepileptic drugs might be required during felbamate titration.

Special Populations. *Pediatric Dosage.* PO for epilepsy 15 mg/kg/day initially in 3–4 divided doses while reducing the dosage of concomitant antiepileptic drugs (phenytoin, carbamazepine, valproic acid, or phenobarbital) by 20–30%. Increase in 15 mg/kg/day increments at weekly intervals to a maximum of 45 mg/kg/day. Further reduction in the dosage of concomitant antiepileptic drugs may be required during felbamate titration.

Geriatric Dosage. Dosage reduction might be required in patients with reduced hepatic or renal function and should be guided by clinical response.

Dosage Forms. **Tab** 400, 600 mg; **Susp** 120 mg/mL.

Patient Instructions. (*See* Anticonvulsants Class Instructions.) Felbamate has been associated with severe blood and liver disorders that can be fatal. Report signs of infection, bleeding, easy bruising, or signs of anemia (fatigue, weakness) immediately; also report abdominal pain or yellowing of the skin immediately. Give the patient the information/consent section of the Felbatol prescribing information and obtain informed consent at the time of initial prescribing.

Missed Doses. Take this drug at regular intervals. If you miss a dose, take it as soon as you remember. If it is about time for the next dose, take that dose only. Do not double the dose or take extra.

Pharmacokinetics. *Onset and Duration.* Steady-state serum levels are attained in 2–3 days.[2]

Serum Levels. A therapeutic range has not been established. Serum concentrations reported in clinical studies are 20–137 mg/L.[20,21]

Fate. Rapidly absorbed with over 90% bioavailability; peak serum levels occur 1–4 hr after an oral dose.[22] Food and antacids have no appreciable effect on absorption.[2] The drug is 22–25% bound to plasma proteins, primarily to albumin. V_d is 0.76 ± 0.08 L/kg; Cl is 0.030 ± 0.008 L/hr/kg in adults. From 40% to 50% is excreted unchanged in urine; 5% is excreted unchanged in feces; the remainder is excreted as inactive metabolites.[2]

$t_{\frac{1}{2}}$. 20.2 hr in normal volunteers;[22] 14.7 ± 2.8 hr in epileptic patients on concomitant enzyme-inducing antiepileptic drugs.[23]

Adverse Reactions. Anorexia, vomiting, insomnia, nausea, headache, weight loss, dizziness, and somnolence occur frequently. Adverse reaction frequency is lower when felbamate is used as monotherapy, and reactions often resolve during long-term therapy. Adverse reactions during adjunctive therapy can be the result of drug interactions. Felbamate is occasionally associated with aplastic anemia and hepatic failure (*see* Precautions), with fatality rates of 20–30%. It is not known whether the risks of aplastic anemia and hepatic failure are related to the duration of felbamate exposure.[24]

Contraindications. History of any blood dyscrasia or hepatic dysfunction.

Precautions. Do not use felbamate as a first-line antiepileptic drug. Because of the risk of aplastic anemia and hepatic failure, use felbamate only in patients whose seizures cannot be controlled with other antiepileptic drugs or whose epilepsy is so severe that the risks are deemed acceptable. Fully inform patients of the risks of felbamate therapy. (*See* Patient Instructions.)

Drug Interactions. Felbamate increases serum concentrations of phenytoin, CBZ-E (the active metabolite of carbamazepine), and valproate; therefore, reduce the dosage of these antiepileptics by 20–30% when felbamate is initiated.

Parameters to Monitor. Close monitoring of CBC, platelets, liver function tests, and clinical signs or symptoms of infection, bruising, bleeding, or hepatitis is essential. Monitor liver function tests (ie, AST, ALT, bilirubin) q 1–2 weeks while treatment continues. The acceptable frequency of hematologic monitoring is not established. Routine monitoring of serum levels is of limited value because of the lack of a well-defined therapeutic range.

Notes. Felbamate is effective for the treatment of partial and secondarily generalized seizures in adults and for partial and generalized seizures associated with the Lennox–Gastaut syndrome in children.

FOSPHENYTOIN   Cerebyx

Pharmacology. Fosphenytoin is a phosphate ester prodrug that is rapidly and completely converted to phenytoin in vivo by phosphatases after parenteral administration. Fosphenytoin has no pharmacologic activity before its conversion to phenytoin. (*See* Phenytoin.)

Administration and Adult Dosage. IV loading dose 15–20 mg phenytoin equivalents (PE)/kg at a maximum rate of 150 mg PE/min. **IM loading dose** 10–20 mg

PE/kg in 1 or more injection sites. **IV or IM maintenance dosage** 4–6 mg PE/kg/day in 1 or 2 divided doses. Safety and effectiveness have not been established for therapy lasting more than 5 days. **IV or IM substitution for oral phenytoin therapy** use same total daily dosage in PEs.

Special Populations. *Pediatric Dosage.* Safety and efficacy not established.

Geriatric Dosage. Advanced age has no effect on fosphenytoin pharmacokinetics, but phenytoin clearance and protein binding might be reduced. (*See* Phenytoin.)

Other Conditions. In patients with renal or hepatic disease, fosphenytoin conversion to phenytoin might be increased because of protein binding changes.[25] Because of an increased fraction of unbound phenytoin in patients with renal or hepatic diseases or hypoalbuminemia, dosage adjustments should be guided by patient status and measurement of unbound phenytoin concentrations.

Dosage Forms. **Inj** 50 mg PE/mL.

Patient Instructions. Itching or tingling can occur during intravenous infusion, particularly in the facial and groin areas. These sensations are usually mild and disappear within minutes of stopping the infusion. These symptoms do not indicate an allergic reaction to fosphenytoin or phenytoin.

Pharmacokinetics. *Onset and Duration.* Therapeutic concentrations of unbound phenytoin (≥ 1 μg/mL) are attained within 8–10 min after the start of an IV infusion of fosphenytoin (administered at a rate of 100–150 mg PE/min) and are similar to those attained after an equivalent dose of phenytoin administered at 50 mg/min. Therapeutic concentrations of unbound phenytoin are attained within 30 min after IM injection of fosphenytoin.

Serum Levels. Monitoring fosphenytoin serum concentration is not clinically useful. Phenytoin serum concentrations correlate with efficacy and toxicity. (*See* Phenytoin.)

Fate. Fosphenytoin is completely converted to phenytoin by phosphatases. Peak-free phenytoin concentrations occur 30 min after completion of fosphenytoin infusion administered at rates of 100–150 mg PE/min and occur 3 hr after an IM dose of fosphenytoin. (*See* Onset and Duration.) Fosphenytoin is 95–99% bound to plasma proteins, primarily albumin. Fosphenytoin binding is saturable and the V_d of fosphenytoin is 4.3–10.8 L depending on plasma concentration. Fosphenytoin displaces phenytoin from protein binding sites. The free (unbound) fraction of phenytoin ranges from 0.30 (in the presence of fosphenytoin) to 0.12 (after complete conversion of fosphenytoin to phenytoin).[26,27] (*See* Phenytoin.)

$t_{\frac{1}{2}}$. (Conversion to phenytoin) 15 min.

Adverse Reactions. Fosphenytoin commonly causes burning, itching, or paresthesias during IV infusion, particularly in the groin and facial areas. These symptoms usually disappear within minutes and can be minimized by slowing or stopping the infusion. The frequency and severity of these symptoms increase with fosphenytoin dose and infusion rate and might be related to the phosphate load. Venous irritation including pain, erythema, swelling, tenderness, and cording (hardening of the vessel) occurs less often than with phenytoin.[28] IM fosphenytoin injections are well tolerated and no significant differences in local symptoms were reported when compared with IM saline injections.[29] No significant differences between fosphenytoin and phenytoin have been reported with regard to adverse cardiovascular effects with IV infusion. CNS adverse effects are common and likely represent reactions to phenytoin. (*See* Phenytoin.)

Contraindications. Sinus bradycardia; sinoatrial block; second- or third-degree AV block; Adams–Stokes syndrome.

Precautions. Consider the phosphate load of fosphenytoin (0.0037 mmol phosphate/mg PE fosphenytoin) in patients with renal insufficiency and those requiring phosphate restriction. (*See* Phenytoin.)

Drug Interactions. No drugs are known to affect the conversion of fosphenytoin to phenytoin. (*See* Phenytoin.)

Parameters to Monitor. Common immunoassays (eg, TDx, TDx/FLx) overestimate phenytoin concentrations when fosphenytoin is present. Determine serum phenytoin concentrations no earlier than 2 hr after an IV infusion or 4 hr after an IM dose of fosphenytoin. Obtain samples in tubes containing ethylenediaminetetraacetic acid to minimize the ex vivo conversion of fosphenytoin to phenytoin. Monitor blood pressure and ECG during and 1–2 hr after IV fosphenytoin infusion.

Notes. Unlike parenteral phenytoin, fosphenytoin is not formulated with propylene glycol and is compatible with most common IV solutions (including those containing dextrose). Fosphenytoin, undiluted or admixed in NS or D5W, is stable for 30 days at room temperature.[30]

GABAPENTIN   Neurontin

Pharmacology. Gabapentin is a cyclohexane compound that is structurally related to GABA; its mechanism of action is not known. Gabapentin does not interact with GABA receptors or alter the formation, release, degradation, or reuptake of GABA.

Administration and Adult Dosage. **PO for epilepsy** 300 mg hs on day 1; 300 mg bid on day 2; 300 mg tid on day 3. However, many patients tolerate initiation with 300 mg bid or tid. Dosage can be increased according to clinical response. **Usual maintenance dosage** 900–2400 mg/day in 3 divided doses.[1] Dosages of 3.6–4.8 g/day have been well tolerated in some patients.[31] Give dosages ≥3.6 g/day in 4 divided doses qid. (*See* Notes.)

Special Populations. *Pediatric Dosage.* (<12 yr) safety and efficacy not established.

Geriatric Dosage. Lower dosages might be required because of normal age-related decreases in renal function.

Other Conditions. Reduce dosage in patients with compromised renal function as indicated on the following page:

CL$_{CR}$ (ML/MIN)	DOSAGE REGIMEN
>60	400 mg tid
30–60	300 mg bid
15–30	300 mg daily
<15	300 mg every other day
Hemodialysis	200–300 mg after dialysis

Dosage Forms. Cap 100, 300, 400 mg.

Patient Instructions. (*See* Anticonvulsants Class Instructions.) Do not take this drug with antacids.

Missed Doses. Take this drug at regular intervals. If you miss a dose, take it as soon as you remember. If it is about time for the next dose, take that dose only. Do not double the dose or take extra.

Pharmacokinetics. *Onset and Duration.* Steady-state serum levels are attained in 1–2 days in patients with normal renal function.[32]

Serum Levels. A therapeutic range has not been established. One study found that therapeutic effect correlated with serum concentrations greater than 2 mg/L.[33]

Fate. Rapidly absorbed and food has no effect on absorption. Absorption occurs via a saturable transport mechanism, so bioavailability decreases with dosages greater than 1.8 g/day; at this dosage it is 60%. At a dosage of 4.8 g/day, bioavailability is 35%.[32] The drug is not bound to plasma proteins. V_d is 58 ± 6 L in adults; Cl is 0.17 ± 0.05 L/kg/hr in adults with normal renal function; Cl is linearly related to Cl$_{cr}$. Gabapentin is not appreciably metabolized but is eliminated unchanged in urine and normal renal function.[34]

t$_{1/2}$. 4.8 ± 1.4 hr in adults with epilepsy and normal renal function.[34]

Adverse Reactions. Somnolence, dizziness, ataxia, nystagmus, and headache occur frequently. Symptoms are of mild to moderate severity and resolve within 2 weeks with continued treatment.[35] Weight gain (mean 4.9% of body weight) and peripheral edema also occur frequently.[36] Occasionally, rash occurs. Rarely, behavioral changes in children occur.[37]

Contraindications. None known.

Precautions. Abrupt withdrawal of gabapentin in patients with epilepsy can precipitate status epilepticus. In vivo carcinogenicity studies have demonstrated a high incidence of pancreatic acinar cell tumors in male rats; the relevance of this observation to humans is not known.

Drug Interactions. Gabapentin does not induce or inhibit hepatic microsomal enzymes and does not affect the metabolism of other antiepileptic drugs or oral contraceptives. Antacids decrease the oral bioavailability of gabapentin by about 20%.

Parameters to Monitor. Serum level monitoring is of limited value because of the lack of a well-defined therapeutic range. Routine monitoring of clinical laboratory parameters during gabapentin therapy is not indicated.

Notes. Gabapentin is indicated as adjunctive treatment for partial and secondarily generalized seizures in adults. Preliminary studies have indicated that the drug can be efficacious as an adjunct in children with refractory partial seizures.[38] Gabapentin might not be effective as monotherapy.[39] Gabapentin is effective for the treatment of postherpetic neuralgia and painful diabetic peripheral neuropathy.[40,41] Preliminary evidence has suggested efficacy in other painful conditions (eg, reflex sympathetic dystrophy), bipolar disorder, and other psychiatric conditions.[42,43]

LAMOTRIGINE   Lamictal

Pharmacology. Lamotrigine is a phenyltriazine derivative unrelated to other marketed antiepileptic drugs. Lamotrigine inhibits voltage-dependent sodium channels, thereby stabilizing neuronal membranes and reducing the release of excitatory neurotransmitters such as glutamate and aspartate. (*See* Notes.)

Administration and Adult Dosage. Adjust starting dosages, titration schedules, and maintenance dosage based on concomitant therapy. **PO for epilepsy in patients receiving enzyme-inducing antiepileptic drugs** (eg, carbamazepine, phenytoin, phenobarbital, and primidone) 50 mg/day for 2 weeks and then increase to 50 mg bid for 2 more weeks. Thereafter, increase dosage in 100 mg/day increments at weekly intervals to a maintenance dosage of 300–500 mg/day in 2 divided doses. **PO for epilepsy in patients receiving enzyme-inducing antiepileptic drugs with valproic acid** 25 mg every other day for 2 weeks and then increase to 25 mg/day for 2 more weeks. Thereafter, increase dosage in 25–50 mg/day increments at 1- to 2-week intervals to a **maintenance dosage** of 100–200 mg/day in 2 divided doses. Dosage recommendations are not available for patients receiving valproic acid alone, but dosages are expected to be lower due to prolonged half-life.

Special Populations. *Pediatric Dosage.* **PO for Lennox–Gastaut syndrome in patients receiving enzyme-inducing antiepileptic drugs with valproic acid** 0.15 mg/kg/day in 1–2 divided doses for 2 weeks and then increase to 0.3 mg/kg/day in 1–2 divided doses. Increase by 0.3 mg/kg/day at weekly intervals if needed. **PO for epilepsy (Lennox–Gastaut syndrome only) in patients receiving enzyme-inducing antiepileptic drugs** 0.6 mg/kg/day in 1–2 divided doses for 2 weeks and then increase to 1.2 mg/kg/day in 1–2 divided doses. Increase in increments of 1.2 mg/kg/day at weekly intervals, if needed.

Geriatric Dosage. Dosage reduction might be required in patients with reduced hepatic or renal function and should be guided by clinical response.

Other Conditions. Patients with chronic renal failure or liver disease might require lower dosages of lamotrigine; specific dosage guidelines are not available.

Dosage Forms. **Chew Tab** 5, 25 mg; **Tab** 25, 100, 150, 200 mg.

Patient Instructions. (*See* Anticonvulsants Class Instructions.) Inform your physician immediately if a skin rash develops.

Missed Doses. Take this drug at regular intervals. If you miss a dose, take it as soon as you remember. If it is about time for the next dose, take that dose only. Do not double the dose or take extra.

Pharmacokinetics. *Onset and Duration.* Steady-state serum levels are attained in 2–3 days.[2]

Serum Levels. A therapeutic range has not been established. In most clinical trials, trough serum concentrations of lamotrigine were 1–3 mg/L.[44]

Fate. The drug is rapidly absorbed, with a bioavailability of 98 ± 5%; peak serum levels occur 2.8 ± 1.3 hr after an oral dose. Food does not affect absorption. Lamotrigine is 56% bound to plasma proteins. V_d is 1.2 ± 0.12 L/kg;[45] Cl is 0.049 ± 0.028 L/hr/kg in adults.[46] From 7% to 30% is excreted unchanged in urine; 80–90% is excreted as the inactive glucuronide conjugate.[45]

$t_{1/2}$. 24.1 ± 5.7 hr in normal volunteers taking no other medications;[45] 14.3 ± 6.9 hr in patients taking enzyme-inducing antiepileptic drugs; 29.6 ± 10 hr in patients taking enzyme-inducing antiepileptic drugs with valproic acid;[46] 59 hr in patients taking valproic acid alone.[45]

Adverse Reactions. Dose-related dizziness, ataxia, somnolence, headache, diplopia, nausea, vomiting, and rash occur frequently. Rash occurs in about 10% of patients, usually within 4–6 weeks of treatment initiation. The rash is usually maculopapular and erythematous. Potentially life-threatening rashes (including Stevens–Johnson syndrome and toxic epidermal necrolysis) are reported in 1:1000 adults and as many as 1:100 children. Risk factors for rash include concomitant valproic acid therapy, high initial dosage of lamotrigine, and rapid escalation of lamotrigine dosage. Discontinue lamotrigine at the first sign of rash.

Contraindications. None known.

Precautions. Initiate lamotrigine cautiously in patients taking valproic acid because of a higher risk of rash. (*See* Administration and Adult Dosage.)

Drug Interactions. Dizziness, diplopia, and ataxia are more common in patients taking carbamazepine concomitantly and appear to be the result of a pharmacodynamic interaction.[47] Lamotrigine has no important effect on blood levels of phenytoin, carbamazepine, or its metabolite CBZ-E. Lamotrigine reduces steady-state valproic acid levels by 25%. Valproic acid increases lamotrigine levels by about 2-fold, and carbamazepine, phenobarbital, primidone, and phenytoin each decrease lamotrigine serum levels.

Parameters to Monitor. Serum level monitoring is of limited value because of the lack of a well-defined therapeutic range. Routine monitoring of clinical laboratory parameters during lamotrigine therapy is not necessary.

Notes. Lamotrigine is indicated as adjunctive treatment for partial and secondarily generalized seizures in adults and for the treatment of the Lennox–Gastaut syndrome in adults and children.[48] Lamotrigine can be effective as monotherapy and appears to be better tolerated than carbamazepine monotherapy at dosages that are equally effective for the treatment of partial epilepsy.[49] (*See* Anticonvulsants Comparison Chart.)

LEVETIRACETAM
Keppra

Pharmacology. Levetiracetam is a pyrollidine derivative that is structurally unrelated to other antiepileptic drugs. Its mechanism of action is unclear and does not relate to any known mechanisms of neuronal excitation or inhibition. The action of levetiracetam in animal models of seizures and epilepsy is unique from other antiepileptic drugs.[50]

Administration and Adult Dosage. **PO for epilepsy** 500 mg bid initially, increasing in increments of 1 g/day at 2-week intervals as needed. **Usual maintenance dosage** 2–3 g/day in 2 divided doses. Higher dosages have been used, but there is little evidence of increased effectiveness above 3 g/day.

Special Populations. *Pediatric Dosage.* Safety and efficacy not established.

Geriatric Dosage. Lower dosages might be required because of age-related decreases in renal function.[51]

Other Conditions. Dosage reduction is not necessary for patients with hepatic impairment. Reduce dosage in patients with compromised renal function, as indicated below:

CL$_{CR}$ (ML/MIN)	DOSAGE REGIMEN
>80	0.5–1.5 g bid
50–80	0.5–1 g bid
30–50	0.25–0.75 g bid
<30	0.25–0.5 g bid
ESRD with hemodialysis	0.5–1 g/day*

*Supplemental doses of 250–500 mg recommended after dialysis.

Dosage Forms. **Tab** 250, 500, 750 mg.

Patient Instructions. (*See* Anticonvulsants Class Instructions.)

Missed Doses. Take this drug at regular intervals. If you miss a dose, take it as soon as you remember. If it is about time for the next dose, take that dose only. Do not double the dose or take extra.

Pharmacokinetics. *Onset and Duration.* Steady-state serum levels are attained in 2 days.[51]

Serum Levels. Not established.

Fate. Rapidly and completely absorbed within 1–1.5 hr; food has no effect on bioavailability. The drug is largely unbound to plasma proteins (<10% bound). V_d is 0.5–0.7 L/kg in adults; Cl is 0.96 mL/kg/min in adults with normal renal function; reduced by 38% in elderly patients with Cl$_{cr}$ of 30–74 mL/min. Levetiracetam is eliminated primarily as unchanged drug in urine (66% of an administered dose). Metabolism is a minor route of elimination; three inactive metabolites have been identified. CYP pathways are not involved.[51]

$t_{\frac{1}{2}}$. (Adults with normal renal function) 7 ± 1 hr.

Adverse Reactions. Somnolence, asthenia (lack of energy), infection, and dizziness occur frequently. Symptoms are of mild to moderate severity and usually occur within the first 4 weeks of treatment. Skin rash is rare.

Contraindications. None known.

Precautions. Minor decreases in RBC and WBC counts, hemoglobin, and hematocrit have been seen. The clinical importance of these findings appears to be minimal.

Drug Interactions. Levetiracetam does not induce or inhibit hepatic microsomal (CYP) enzymes and does not affect the metabolism of other antiepileptic drugs, oral contraceptives, warfarin, or digoxin. Antacids have no effect on levetiracetam bioavailability.

Parameters to Monitor. Serum level monitoring is not of value because of the lack of a defined therapeutic range. Routine monitoring of clinical laboratory parameters during levetiracetam therapy is not required.

Notes. Levetiracetam is indicated as adjunctive treatment for partial and secondarily generalized tonic-clonic seizures in adults. Seizures are reduced in frequency by $\geq 50\%$ in 20–40% of patients taking 1–3 g/day.

OXCARBAZEPINE   Trileptal

Pharmacology. Oxcarbazepine is a 10-keto analogue of carbamazepine that exerts its anticonvulsant effect through an active 10-monohydroxy metabolite (MHD). Its mechanism of action is not known but likely involves blockade of voltage-dependent sodium channels and inhibition of repetitive neuronal firing.

Administration and Adult Dosage. **PO for epilepsy** 300 mg bid initially, increasing in increments of 300 mg/day at weekly intervals to effective dosage. **Usual maintenance dosage** is 1200–2400 mg/day in 2 divided doses.[52]

Special Populations. *Pediatric Dosage.* **PO for epilepsy** 8–10 mg/kg/day in 2 divided doses initially, increasing at weekly intervals as needed. **Usual maintenance dosage** in 2 divided doses: (20–29 kg) 900 mg/day; (29.1–39 kg) 1200 mg/day; (>39 kg) 1800 mg/day.

Geriatric Dosage. Clearance of the active MHD is reduced in some elderly patients, so lower maintenance dosages might be required.[52]

Other Conditions. No dosage adjustment is required in patients with mild to moderate hepatic impairment. Begin oxcarbazepine at one-half the usual starting dosage in patients with Cl_{cr} <30 mL/min and reduce the rate of titration.

Dosage Forms. **Tab** 150, 300, 600 mg.

Patient Instructions. (*See* Anticonvulsants Class Instructions.) Report symptoms of nausea, malaise, headache, lethargy, or confusion.

Missed Doses. Take this drug at regular intervals. If you miss a dose, take it as soon as you remember. If it is about time for the next dose, take that dose only. Do not double the dose or take extra.

Pharmacokinetics. *Onset and Duration.* Steady-state serum levels of MHD are attained in 2 days.[53]

Serum Levels. A therapeutic range has not been established.

Fate. Completely absorbed; food has no effect. Oxcarbazepine is converted into MHD, which is primarily responsible for the anticonvulsant activity of oxcarbazepine. MHD is 40% bound to plasma proteins, primarily albumin. V_d (MHD) is 0.7–0.8 L/kg in adults; Cl (MHD) is 2.5 ± 0.1 L/kg/hr after a single dose in epilepsy patients taking other antiepileptic drugs.[54] MHD is eliminated primarily by glucuronidation to inactive products (47%) and renal excretion of unchanged MHD (27%).

$t_{1/2}$. (Oxcarbazepine) 2.4 ± 1.1 hr; (MHD) 9.3 ± 1.8 hr in healthy adult volunteers.

Adverse Reactions. Dizziness, somnolence, diplopia, fatigue, and nausea occur frequently. Symptoms are more common with rapid dosage titration. Rash occurs in 2.8% of patients.[52] Among patients with histories of hypersensitivity to carbamazepine, 25–30% experience hypersensitivity to oxcarbazepine. Hyponatremia (Na <125 mEq/L) occurs in 2.5% of patients.

Contraindications. None known.

Precautions. Patients with histories of severe hypersensitivity reactions to carbamazepine (eg, exfoliative dermatitis) appear to be at high risk for similar reactions to oxcarbazepine.[55] Patients should report symptoms of nausea, malaise, headache, lethargy, or confusion, which might indicate hyponatremia.

Drug Interactions. Oxcarbazepine does not induce its own metabolism but does reduce estrogen and progestin levels by 50%. Thus, the efficacy of oral contraceptives might be reduced. Oxcarbamazepine can increase phenytoin levels by up to 40% in adults; no effects on the metabolism of other antiepileptic drugs are reported. Carbamazepine, phenytoin, and phenobarbital increase the metabolism of MHD. Cimetidine, erythromycin, and propoxyphene do not affect MHD levels. Verapamil reduces MHD concentrations by 20%.

Parameters to Monitor. Consider measuring serum sodium levels during oxcarbazepine therapy, particularly in patients taking other drugs known to reduce sodium concentrations or those who develop signs or symptoms of hyponatremia. (*See* Precautions.)

Notes. Oxcarbazepine is indicated as monotherapy and adjunctive therapy for the treatment of partial and secondarily generalized seizures in adults and as adjunctive therapy for the treatment of partial-onset seizures in children (4–16 yr).

PHENOBARBITAL   Various

Pharmacology. Phenobarbital is a barbiturate that exerts an anticonvulsant effect by depressing excitatory postsynaptic seizure discharge and increasing the convulsive threshold for electric and chemical stimulation.

Administration and Adult Dosage. **PO or IM for epilepsy** 60–90 mg/day initially, increasing in 30–60 mg/day increments q 7–14 days to an effective dosage. **Usual maintenance dosage** 90–240 mg/day or 1–3 mg/kg/day hs.[1] **IV for status epilepticus** 20 mg/kg at a rate of 100 mg/min.[56] **Rectal administration** has been reported. (*See* Fate.) (*See also* Adverse Reactions and Notes.)

Special Populations. *Pediatric Dosage.* **PO or IM for epilepsy** 0.5 mg/kg/day initially, increasing q 7–14 days to minimize sedation. **Usual maintenance dosage** is 2–5 mg/kg/day or 125 mg/m²/day given at bedtime.[2] **IV for status epilepticus** 20 mg/kg at a rate of 50–100 mg/min.[57] (*See* Adverse Reactions and Notes.)

Geriatric Dosage. Clearance of phenobarbital is reduced in the elderly, so lower maintenance dosages might be required.[3]

Other Conditions. During pregnancy, phenobarbital clearance can increase. Dosage increases might be necessary and should be guided by serum levels and patient status.[2]

Dosage Forms. **Cap** 16 mg; **Tab** 15, 16, 30, 60, 90, 100 mg; **Elxr** 3, 4 mg/mL; **Inj** 30, 60, 65, 130 mg/mL.

Patient Instructions. (*See* Anticonvulsants Class Instructions.)

Missed Doses. Take this drug at regular intervals. If you miss a dose, take it as soon as you remember. If it is about time for the next dose, take that dose only. Do not double the dose or take extra.

Pharmacokinetics. *Onset and Duration.* Steady-state serum levels are attained in about 21 days.[2]

Serum Levels. (Anticonvulsant) 15–35 mg/L (65–150 μmol/L); dysarthria, ataxia, and nystagmus appear as serum level approaches 40 mg/L (172 μmol/L).[1,2,58]

Fate. The drug is slowly absorbed orally with 95–100% bioavailability; peak serum level occurs 2–4 hr after a PO or IM dose.[2] Rectal bioavailability is 90%, with a peak of 7.2 ± 0.8 mg/L (31 ± 3.4 μmol/L) 4.4 ± 0.6 hr after rectal administration of a 5 mg/kg dose of parenteral phenobarbital sodium solution.[59] The drug is 45–60% bound to plasma proteins. V_d is 0.61 ± 0.05 L/kg; Cl is 0.004 ± 0.0008 L/hr/kg in adults,[60] with 50–80% metabolized in the liver to *p*-hydroxyphenobarbital (inactive). The drug is 20–50% excreted unchanged in urine; alkalinization of urine increases renal phenobarbital clearance.[2,6]

$t_{1/2}$. (Adults) 100 ± 17 hr;[61] (cirrhosis) 130 ± 15 hr;[60] (children 1–5 yr) 69 ± 3.2 hr.[62]

Adverse Reactions. (*See* Serum Levels.) Sedation is frequent and dose related; tolerance usually develops with long-term administration. In adults, phenobarbital can impair cognition, reaction time, and motor performance.[63] Loss of concentration, mental dulling, depression of affect, insomnia, and hyperkinetic activity occur frequently with long-term therapy in children and the elderly.[58] Connective tissue disorders associated with barbiturates occur in 6% of patients, usually within the first year of treatment.[64] Occasionally, skin rashes or folate deficiency occur. Rarely, megaloblastic anemia, hepatitis, exfoliative dermatitis, or Stevens–Johnson syndrome is reported. Patients can be at risk for similar hypersensitivity reactions if rechallenged with phenytoin or carbamazepine.[65] Neonatal hemorrhage has been reported in newborns whose mothers were taking phenobarbital. SC or intra-arterial injection can produce tissue necrosis. IV administration, especially when given after IV benzodiazepines, can produce severe respiratory depression and provision for respiratory support should be made.

Contraindications. History of porphyria or severe respiratory disease where dyspnea or obstruction is present.

Precautions. Pregnancy; lactation. Use with caution in patients with marked liver or renal disease because drug clearance is slowed. Abrupt withdrawal of the drug in patients with epilepsy can precipitate status epilepticus.

Drug Interactions. Concurrent use with other CNS depressants can potentiate the sedation caused by phenobarbital. Numerous drugs can increase phenobarbital serum levels, possibly requiring phenobarbital dosage reduction; phenobarbital can stimulate CYP2D6 and CYP3A and increase the metabolism of many drugs.

Parameters to Monitor. Periodic serum level monitoring, after attaining steady state (about 21 days), is useful in guiding dosage changes or evaluating adverse effects.[2] Monitor CBC and liver function tests periodically during long-term therapy.

Notes. In tonic-clonic status epilepticus, phenobarbital is usually considered a third agent after IV phenytoin plus IV diazepam or lorazepam have failed to control seizures.[56] Considering clinical efficacy and patient tolerance, phenobarbital is a third- or fourth-line choice for single-drug therapy of partial or generalized tonic-clonic seizures compared with the drugs of first choice: carbamazepine, phenytoin, or valproic acid.[2] (*See* Anticonvulsants Comparison Chart.)

PHENYTOIN
Dilantin, Various

Pharmacology. Phenytoin is a hydantoin that suppresses the spread of seizure activity mainly by inhibiting synaptic post-tetanic potentiation and blocking the propagation of electric discharge. Phenytoin might decrease sodium transport and block calcium channels at the cellular level to produce these actions.

Administration and Adult Dosage. PO maintenance dosage 300 mg/day in 1–3 doses initially. Using serum levels as a guide, increase in 30–100 mg/day increments q 10–21 days to effective dosage.[2] Because of dose-dependent saturable metabolism, small increases in dosage can produce disproportionate increases in serum levels. **Usual maintenance dosage** 300–400 mg/day or 4–8 mg/kg/day in 1 or 2 doses.[1] Only extended-release phenytoin sodium capsules are approved for once-daily administration. **PO loading dosage** 15 mg/kg in 3 divided doses, administered at 2-hr intervals. Using serum levels as a guide, a maintenance dosage can be initiated within 24 hr of starting the loading dosage. **IV loading dose** 15–20 mg/kg by direct IV injection, at a rate not greater than 50 mg/min or 0.75 mg/kg/min in adults.[58] Therapeutic serum levels persist for 12–24 hr in most patients.[66] Alternatively, dilute the loading dose in 50–150 mL of 0.45% or 0.9% NaCl and infuse through an IV volume control set with an in-line filter at a rate not greater than 50 mg/min.[2,67] In nonemergency situations, an IV dose of 5 mg/kg q 2 hr for 3 doses at a rate of 50 mg/min results in phenytoin serum levels of 10–20 mg/L 12 hr after the third dose.[68] (*See* Adverse Reactions and Notes.) **IM administration** is painful and results in slow, but complete, absorption because of deposition of phenytoin crystals in muscle.[2] The IM route is not recommended. The IV route is preferred in patients unable to take phenytoin by mouth. (*See* Fosphenytoin.)

Special Populations. *Pediatric Dosage.* **PO maintenance dosage** 5 mg/kg/day initially in 2–3 divided doses. Increase initial dosage in small increments q 7–10 days to effective dosage.[2] Because of dose-dependent metabolism, small increases in dosage can produce disproportionate increases in serum levels. **Usual maintenance dosage** 4–8 mg/kg/day in 2–3 divided doses.[1] **IV loading dose** (neonates)

15–20 mg/kg given at a rate of 0.5 mg/kg/min; (older infants and children) same as adult dosage.

Geriatric Dosage. **PO maintenance dosage** 200–300 mg/day in 1–3 doses. Advanced age can be associated with a decrease in phenytoin clearance and a reduction in albumin concentration.[69] Dosage adjustment should be guided by phenytoin levels and patient status. (*See* Serum Levels.)

Other Conditions. During pregnancy or febrile illness or after acute traumatic injury, phenytoin clearance can increase; dosage adjustment might be necessary and should be guided by serum levels and patient status.[70–72] Renal disease and hypoalbuminemia can alter phenytoin binding to plasma proteins, resulting in a change in the usual ratio of free to total phenytoin levels; renal disease alters phenytoin protein binding because of decreased affinity of plasma proteins. Increases in fraction unbound are most pronounced in patients with Cl_{cr} <25 mL/min. Ideally, adjust dosage guided by patient status and actual measurement of unbound and total phenytoin levels. (*See* Serum Levels.)

Dosage Forms. (Phenytoin) **Chew Tab** 50 mg; **Susp** 25 mg/mL. (Phenytoin sodium) **Cap** (extended or prompt) 30, 100 mg; **Inj** 50 mg/mL. Phenytoin sodium is 92% phenytoin.

Patient Instructions. (*See* Anticonvulsants Class Instructions.) Good dental hygiene and regular dental visits can minimize gum tenderness, bleeding, or enlargement (especially in children). Shake oral suspension well before each dose and use a calibrated measuring device. (*See* Notes.) Call physician if skin rash develops.

Missed Doses. Take this drug at regular intervals. If you miss a dose, take it as soon as you remember. If it is about time for the next dose, take that dose only. When taking multiple daily doses, leave a minimum of 4–6 hours between doses. If you are taking the drug only once daily and you do not remember until the next day, skip the missed dose and return to your normal schedule. Do not double the dose or take extra. If doses are missed for 2 or more days in a row, consult your physician.

Pharmacokinetics. *Onset and Duration.* Time to steady state increases with increasing dosage and serum level. Steady state is usually attained within 7–14 days but can take as long as 28 days.[2]

Serum Levels. 10–20 mg/L (40–80 μmol/L) in patients with normal renal function and serum albumin concentration. Nystagmus, slurred speech, ataxia, or dizziness appear in most patients as serum levels approach 20 mg/L; drowsiness, diplopia, behavioral changes, and cognitive impairment occur with serum levels above 30 mg/L (120 μmol/L).[2] The equation $C_{normal} = C_{observed}/([0.2 \times albumin] + 0.1)$ estimates the concentration of phenytoin that would be expected if the albumin concentration were normal (C_{normal}) from the measured total phenytoin concentration in a hypoalbuminemia patient ($C_{observed}$) and the patient's albumin concentration in g/dL (albumin). In patients with end-stage renal disease (Cl_{cr} <10 mL/min), the equation $C_{normal} = C_{observed}/([0.1 \times albumin] + 0.1)$ is used.[73] (*See also* Special Populations, Other Conditions.)

Fate. Oral phenytoin absorption is very slow and incomplete in infants <3 months of age.[2] Bioavailability of the suspension is decreased in patients receiving concomitant enteral feedings. (*See* Precautions.) IM injection is slowly absorbed over several days because of deposition of phenytoin crystals in muscle. Peak serum levels occur 4–8 hr after a single dose of an extended-release capsule;[2] after oral loading given in divided doses, the times to reach a serum level of 10 mg/L are 4.5 ± 2.1 hr for prompt-release capsules and 9.6 ± 2.5 hr for extended-release capsules.[74] Time to peak serum level increases with increasing oral dosages.[75] About 90% is bound to plasma proteins.[2] Hypoalbuminemia, chronic liver or renal disease, nephrotic syndrome, AIDS, or acute traumatic injury alter protein binding and increase the fraction of unbound phenytoin.[2,70] V_d is 0.83 ± 0.2 L/kg in adults with acute seizures[67] and 0.79 ± 0.25 L/kg in critically ill adults after trauma.[70] Hepatic metabolism is capacity limited, exhibiting Michaelis–Menden pharmacokinetics; therefore, Cl decreases as serum level increases. Mean apparent V_{max} is 0.45 mg/L/hr; mean apparent K_m is 6.2 mg/L in adults.[2] About 70% of phenytoin is excreted in urine as the inactive metabolite, 5-(*p*-hydroxyphenyl)-5-phenyl hydantoin. Less than 5% of the parent drug is excreted unchanged in urine.[2,6]

$t_{1/2}$. Phenytoin has no true half-life, but its apparent half-life increases as serum level increases; at phenytoin serum levels of 1, 10, 20, and 40 mg/L, the predicted mean phenytoin half-lives are 13, 26, 40, and 69 hr, respectively.[2,76]

Adverse Reactions. (*See* Serum Levels.) Erythematous morbilliform rash occurs frequently. Do not resume phenytoin if rash is exfoliative, purpuric, bullous, or accompanied by fever. With long-term administration, hirsutism, gingival hypertrophy (especially in children and adolescents), coarsening of facial features, acneiform eruption, osteomalacia, and folate deficiency with mild macrocytosis occur frequently.[2,58] Bradycardia or hypotension caused by rapid IV administration are reported occasionally; slowing the rate of administration can minimize these complications.[56,66] Severe soft tissue injury after IV phenytoin is more likely in elderly (>70 yr) women who receive 2 or more infusions through small (<20 gauge) IV devices.[77] Hepatotoxicity occurs occasionally, usually within the first 6 weeks, and presents with fever, rash, lymphadenopathy, and hepatomegaly.[78] Other idiosyncratic reactions are rare, can occur together within the first 2 months, and include fever, lymphoid hyperplasia, eosinophilia, erythema multiforme, exfoliative dermatitis, Stevens–Johnson syndrome, leukopenia, anemia, thrombocytopenia, serum sickness, and SLE.[2] These patients are at risk for similar hypersensitivity reactions if rechallenged with phenobarbital or carbamazepine.[65] Concurrent cranial irradiation predisposes patients to the development of erythema multiforme.[79] A syndrome of anomalies in infants of phenytoin-exposed mothers has been described (fetal hydantoin syndrome).

Contraindications. (Parenteral phenytoin) sinus bradycardia; sinoatrial block; second- and third-degree AV blocks; Adams–Stokes syndrome.

Precautions. Pregnancy; lactation. Use with caution in patients with severe liver disease or diabetes or with histories of severe hypersensitivity reactions to carbamazepine or phenobarbital. Abrupt withdrawal of the drug in patients with epilepsy can precipitate status epilepticus. If the patient's nutritional status allows, interrupt tube feeding 2 hr before and after the dose and irrigate the feeding tube to improve absorption; nevertheless, the patient might require an increase in phenytoin dosage. If the feedings are discontinued after the phenytoin dosage is increased, the dosage must be adjusted to prevent toxic serum levels from occurring.[80]

Drug Interactions. Chronic alcohol use, barbiturates, rifampin, and some other drugs can stimulate phenytoin metabolism and increase phenytoin dosage requirements. Numerous drugs can increase phenytoin serum levels, possibly requiring phenytoin dosage reduction; phenytoin can stimulate CYP2D6 and CYP3A and increase the metabolism of many drugs. IV phenytoin can produce hypotension in severely ill patients receiving IV dopamine. The antiparkinson effect of levodopa can be inhibited by phenytoin.

Parameters to Monitor. Serum level monitoring, after attaining steady state (10–21 days), is useful in evaluating therapeutic efficacy or potential for adverse effects.[2] Patient and serum level monitoring are recommended when changing phenytoin dosage form or brand; monitor serum levels q 5–7 days to assess trend in concentrations. Monitor CBC and liver function tests periodically with long-term therapy.

Notes. Agitation or shaking is needed to resuspend phenytoin suspension; settling occurs 5 weeks after resuspension.[81] In tonic-clonic status epilepticus, the anticonvulsant effect of phenytoin appears 20–30 min after start of the infusion. Thus, in this situation, concurrent use of phenytoin with a rapidly acting injectable benzodiazepine (**diazepam** or **lorazepam**) is recommended.[56] Phenytoin is recommended, as is **carbamazepine,** as a drug of first choice for single-drug therapy of partial or generalized tonic-clonic seizures.[82] (*See* Anticonvulsants Comparison Chart.)

PRIMIDONE   Mysoline, Various

Pharmacology. Primidone (desoxyphenobarbital) is structurally related to the barbiturates. Primidone and its metabolites, phenylethylmalonamide (PEMA) and phenobarbital, exert anticonvulsant activity. (*See* Phenobarbital.)

Administration and Adult Dosage. PO for epilepsy 50–100 mg hs initially; increase in 100–125 mg/day increments q 2–3 days to effective dosage, to a maximum of 2 g/day. **Usual maintenance dosage** 250–500 mg tid.[1]

Special Populations. *Pediatric Dosage.* **PO for epilepsy** (<8 yr) 50 mg hs initially, increasing by 50 mg in 3 days and thereafter in 100–125 mg/day increments q 3 days to effective dosage; **usual maintenance dosage** is 125–250 mg tid or 10–20 mg/kg/day in 3 divided doses; (≥8 yr) same as adult dosage.

Geriatric Dosage. Clearance of primidone is unchanged in elderly patients, but phenobarbital clearance is reduced. Lower maintenance dosages might be required.

Dosage Forms. **Susp** 50 mg/mL; **Tab** 50, 250 mg.

Patient Instructions. (*See* Anticonvulsants Class Instructions.)

Missed Doses. Take this drug at regular intervals. If you miss a dose, take it as soon as you remember. If it is about time for the next dose, take that dose only. Do not double the dose or take extra.

Pharmacokinetics. *Onset and Duration.* Steady-state serum levels are attained in about 3 days.[2]

Serum Levels. (Primidone) 6–12 mg/L (28–55 μmol/L).[1,2,58] (*See also* Phenobarbital.) During monotherapy, the serum level ratio of phenobarbital to primidone is about 1:1.[2] During polytherapy with enzyme-inducing agents, this ratio increases to 4:1.[2] During monotherapy, the serum level ratio of PEMA to primidone at steady state is 0.74 ± 0.38 for samples drawn before the first morning dose.[2]

Fate. The drug is rapidly absorbed with 90–100% bioavailability; peak serum levels occur 2–6 hr after an oral dose. The drug is 0–20% bound to plasma proteins; V_d is 0.86 ± 0.22 L/kg;[83] Cl with monotherapy is 0.035 ± 0.02 L/hr/kg; with concomitant anticonvulsants, it is 0.052 ± 0.02 L/hr/kg;[2] in monotherapy with concomitant acute viral hepatitis, it is 0.042 ± 0.14 L/hr/kg.[83] Primidone is metabolized in the liver to PEMA and phenobarbital; 76% of the drug is excreted into the urine within 5 days after a single dose as 64% primidone, 7% PEMA, 2% phenobarbital, and 3% unidentified products.[2]

$t_{1/2}$. (Primidone) 15.2 ± 4.8 hr (monotherapy); 8.3 ± 2.9 hr (with concomitant enzyme-inducing anticonvulsants); 18 ± 3.1 hr (with acute viral hepatitis).[83] (PEMA) 21 ± 3 hr (primidone monotherapy); 17 ± 4.3 hr (with concomitant anticonvulsants).[84] (*See also* Phenobarbital.)

Adverse Reactions. Drowsiness, ataxia, nausea, weakness, and dizziness occur frequently during the first month of therapy and might become tolerable with time. Behavioral disturbances, depression of affect, and cognitive impairment occur frequently with long-term therapy in children and the elderly.[2] Occasionally, skin rashes and, rarely, impotence, leukopenia, thrombocytopenia, megaloblastic anemia, or lymphadenopathy occur.[2,58]

Contraindications. History of porphyria; hypersensitivity to phenobarbital.

Precautions. Pregnancy; lactation. Use with caution in patients with severe liver or renal disease. Abrupt withdrawal of the drug can precipitate status epilepticus. (*See* Phenobarbital Notes.)

Drug Interactions. Concurrent use with other CNS depressants can potentiate the sedation caused by phenobarbital. Primidone levels can be decreased by concurrent acetazolamide, carbamazepine, or succinimides. Primidone levels can be increased by concurrent hydantoins, isoniazid, or niacinamide.

Parameters to Monitor. Periodic serum level monitoring of primidone and phenobarbital, after attaining steady state (primidone, 3 days; phenobarbital, 21 days), is useful in guiding dosage changes, detecting noncompliance, or evaluating adverse effects.[2] Monitor CBC, electrolytes, and liver function tests periodically during long-term therapy.

Notes. Considering comparative efficacy and good patient tolerance of **carbamazepine, phenytoin,** and **valproic acid,** primidone is a fourth- or fifth-line choice for single-drug therapy of generalized tonic-clonic seizures. In a large, multicenter trial comparing carbamazepine, phenytoin, phenobarbital, and primidone, primidone was least successful in controlling seizures with acceptable adverse effects.[82]

TIAGABINE
Gabitril

Pharmacology. Tiagabine is a nipecotic acid derivative unrelated to other marketed antiepileptic drugs. It interacts with the GABA uptake carrier and is thought to enhance the inhibitory effect of GABA by preventing its reuptake into neurons. Tiagabine is indicated in adults and adolescents (>12 yr) as adjunctive therapy for patients with partial-onset seizures.[85,86]

Administration and Adult Dosage. **PO for epilepsy** in patients taking enzyme-inducing antiepileptic drugs (eg, carbamazepine, phenytoin, phenobarbital, primidone), initiate at 4 mg/day for 1 week, increasing in increments of 4–8 mg/day at weekly intervals according to clinical response. **Usual maintenance dosage** is 32–56 mg/day. The daily dosage is given in 2–4 divided doses; with dosages >32 mg/day, tid or qid administration might be required. Patients taking only non–enzyme-inducing antiepileptic drugs (eg, gabapentin, lamotrigine, valproate) might require lower doses or a slower titration schedule.

Special Populations. *Pediatric Dosage.* (≤12 yr) safety and efficacy not established; (>12 yr) same as adult dose.

Geriatric Dosage. Same as adult dosage.

Other Conditions. No apparent need to adjust tiagabine dosage in renal impairment. Patients with liver disease might require lower dosages of tiagabine; however, specific dosage guidelines are not available.

Dosage Forms. **Tab** 2, 4, 12, 16, 20 mg.

Patient Instructions. (*See* Anticonvulsants Class Instructions) Take this medication with food.

Missed Doses. Take this drug at regular intervals. If you miss a dose, take it as soon as you remember. If it is about time for the next dose, take that dose only. Do not double the dose or take extra.

Pharmacokinetics. *Onset and Duration.* Steady-state serum levels are attained within 2 days.

Serum Levels. A therapeutic range has not been established.

Fate. Rapidly absorbed with a bioavailability of 89.9 ± 9.7%.[87,88] Food slows the rate, but not the extent, of tiagabine absorption. Peak serum concentrations of 241 ± 79 μg/L occurred 1.3 ± 1 hr after a single 12 mg dose in healthy volunteers.[89] Tiagabine is 96% bound to plasma proteins, primarily albumin and α_1-acid glycoprotein. V_d is 1.07 ± 0.22 L/kg[89] and Cl is 6.5 ± 1.5 L/hr in healthy volunteers.[88] Cl is increased in patients taking enzyme-inducing antiepileptic drugs. Tiagabine is metabolized by oxidation (primarily CYP3A) and glucuronidation; about 2% is excreted unchanged in urine.

$t_{1/2}$. 7–9 hr in healthy subjects taking no other medications; reduced by 50–65% in patients with epilepsy taking enzyme-inducing antiepileptic drugs.[88,89]

Adverse Reactions. Dizziness, asthenia/lack of energy, somnolence, nausea, nervousness, tremor, abdominal pain, and difficulty with concentration occur frequently. Tremor, difficulty with concentration, and asthenia appear to be dose related. The most common reasons for discontinuation are dizziness, somnolence, depression, confusion, and asthenia. Moderate to severe generalized weakness occurs occasionally. Tiagabine rarely induces absence status.

Contraindications. None known.

Precautions. Dosage reduction might be required in hepatic impairment.

Drug Interactions. Carbamazepine, phenytoin, and phenobarbital reduce tiagabine levels by 60% compared with noninduced patients. Valproate has no important effect on tiagabine levels. Tiagabine has no effect on serum concentrations of phenytoin, carbamazepine, phenobarbital, or primidone. Valproate concentrations decrease approximately 10% during tiagabine therapy. Tiagabine has no effect on the pharmacokinetics of warfarin, theophylline, digoxin, or oral contraceptives.

Parameters to Monitor. Serum level monitoring is of limited value because of the lack of a well-defined therapeutic range. No routine laboratory test monitoring is required during therapy.

TOPIRAMATE Topamax

Pharmacology. Topiramate, a derivative of the naturally occurring monosaccharide D-fructose, reduces the frequency of action potentials elicited by depolarizing currents in a manner suggestive of sodium-channel blocking action. Topiramate also increases GABA-induced chloride flux, although the drug has no direct effect on GABA binding sites. It also inhibits kainate activation of a subtype of the excitatory glutamate receptor. Topiramate inhibits carbonic anhydrase, but this action might not contribute to the drug's anticonvulsant effect. (*See* Notes.)

Administration and Adult Dosage. PO for epilepsy 25–50 mg/day initially, increasing in 25–50 mg/day increments at weekly intervals to 200–400 mg/day in 2 divided doses. **Usual maintenance dosage** 400 mg/day. Higher dosages have not been shown to be more effective; however, individual patients might require ≥1 g/day.[90] (*See* Notes.)

Special Populations. *Pediatric Dosage.* **PO for epilepsy** (<2 yr) Safety and efficacy not established; (2–16 yr) 5–9 mg/kg in 2 divided doses. Increase in increments of 1–3 mg/kg/day at weekly intervals, if needed.

Geriatric Dosage. Same as adult dosage.

Other Conditions. With Cl_{cr} <70 mL/min/1.73 m^2, reduce dosage by 50%. Topiramate clearance increases during hemodialysis to a rate 4–6 times greater than in a normal person. Additional doses of topiramate might be required depending on dialysis method and duration.

Dosage Forms. **Cap** 15, 25, 50 mg; **Tab** 25, 100, 200 mg. (*See* Notes.)

Patient Instructions. (*See* Anticonvulsants Class Instructions.) Maintain adequate fluid intake (6 to 8 glasses of water daily) to minimize the formation of kidney stones. If you are taking oral contraceptives, report any change in menstrual bleeding patterns to your health care provider.

Missed Doses. Take this drug at regular intervals. If you miss a dose, take it as soon as you remember. If it is about time for the next dose, take that dose only. Do not double the dose or take extra.

Pharmacokinetics. *Onset and Duration.* Steady-state serum concentrations are attained in 4 days in patients with normal renal function.

Serum Levels. A therapeutic range has not been established.[91]

Fate. The bioavailability of oral tablets is 80% compared with oral solution and peak concentrations occur 3.5 ± 0.6 hr after 400 mg.[2] Administration with food delays absorption (by approximately 2 hr) but does not affect extent of absorption.[2] Topiramate is 13–17% bound to plasma proteins and binds to a saturable, low-capacity binding site on or in erythrocytes.[85] V_d is 0.6–0.8 L/kg in healthy volunteers.[2] Cl is 0.021 ± 0.004 L/kg/hr in adults on topiramate monotherapy after tapering of valproic acid.[91] Approximately 70% is eliminated unchanged in urine. Six metabolites (each <5% of the administered dose) have been identified.

$t_{1/2}$. 23 hr after a single 400 mg dose in healthy adults.[2]

Adverse Reactions. Somnolence, dizziness, ataxia, speech problems, psychomotor slowing, nystagmus, and paresthesias occur commonly and are not dose related. Common dose-related adverse effects include fatigue, nervousness, difficulty with concentration or attention, confusion, depression, weight loss, and tremor. These adverse effects are minimized by slow dose titration. Psychomotor slowing and difficulty with concentration are the most common reasons for topiramate discontinuation. Kidney stones occur in 1.5% of patients and might be related to carbonic anhydrase inhibition.

Contraindications. None known.

Precautions. Avoid concomitant use of other carbonic anhydrase inhibitors (eg, acetazolamide) because of the potential increased risk of kidney stones.

Drug Interactions. Concomitant phenytoin and carbamazepine reduce topiramate concentrations by 48% and 40%, respectively. Concomitant valproate reduces topiramate concentrations by 17%.[91] Topiramate variably affects phenytoin concentrations (0–25% decrease) and has no important effect on other anticonvulsants. Topiramate can reduce the effectiveness of oral contraceptives; consider using products containing ≥35 µg of ethinyl estradiol.[92]

Parameters to Monitor. Serum level monitoring is of limited value because of the lack of a well-defined therapeutic range. Routine monitoring of clinical laboratory parameters during topiramate therapy is not indicated.

Notes. Topiramate is indicated for adult and pediatric patients as adjunctive treatment for partial-onset and primary generalized tonic-clonic seizures. Preliminary evidence suggests that topiramate also might be effective as monotherapy for partial-onset seizures[93] and as adjunctive treatment of Lennox–Gastaut syndrome.[94] Capsules can be opened and sprinkled on food.

VALPROIC ACID	Depakene, Depacon, Various
DIVALPROEX SODIUM	Depakote

Pharmacology. Valproic acid is a carboxylic acid compound whose anticonvulsant activity might be mediated by an inhibitory neurotransmitter, GABA. Valproic acid might increase GABA levels by inhibiting GABA metabolism or enhancing postsynaptic GABA activity. Valproic acid also limits repetitive neuronal firing through voltage- and usage-dependent sodium channels. Divalproex is comprised of sodium valproate and valproic acid. (*See* Notes.)

Administration and Adult Dosage. **PO for epilepsy** (valproic acid) 15 mg/kg/day in 2–3 divided doses initially, increasing in 5–10 mg/kg/day increments at weekly intervals to an effective dosage, to a maximum of 60 mg/kg/day. **Usual maintenance dosage** 15–40 mg/kg/day in 3 divided doses.[95] In patients receiving valproic acid, divalproex can be substituted at the same daily dosage; in selected patients, it can be given bid. **PO for migraine prophylaxis** (divalproex) 250 mg bid, to a maximum of 1 g/day. **PO for mania** (divalproex) 750 mg/day in divided doses, increasing as rapidly as possible to the lowest dosage that produces the desired effect, to a maximum of 60 mg/kg/day. (*See* Serum Levels.) Long-term experience with this use is minimal and characterized by a high drop-out rate. **IV for epilepsy** (valproic acid) same as oral dosage. Administer infusion over 60 min or at a rate of ≤20 mg/min. **Rectal administration** has been reported. (*See* Fate.)

Special Populations. *Pediatric Dosage.* Same as adult dosage.

Geriatric Dosage. Reduce the starting dosage in the elderly. Protein binding and unbound clearance of valproic acid are reduced in the elderly, and the desired clinical response can be achieved with lower dosages than in younger adults. Adjust dosage guided by valproic acid levels (preferably free levels in patients with low serum albumin) and patient status.[3]

Dosage Forms. (Valproic acid) **Cap** 250 mg; **Syrup** 50 mg/mL; **Inj** 100 mg/mL; (divalproex) **EC Tab** 125, 250, 500 mg; **Cap** (EC granules) 125 mg; **SR Tab** 500 mg.

Patient Instructions. (*See* Anticonvulsants Class Instructions). This drug can be taken with food or milk to minimize stomach upset. Do not chew, break, or crush the tablet or capsule because this may irritate your mouth or throat. Sprinkle capsule can be swallowed whole or administered by sprinkling the entire contents on small amount (1 teaspoonful) of soft food such as pudding or applesauce; swallow the drug/food mixture immediately (avoid chewing). Polymer from the sprinkles might appear in the stools, but does not indicate a lack of absorption. Immediately report weakness, tiredness, repeated vomiting, or loss of seizure control, which might be early signs of severe, but rare, liver disorder.

Missed Doses. Take this drug at regular intervals. If you miss a dose, take it as soon as you remember. If it is about time for the next dose, take that dose only. Leave a minimum of 6 hours between doses. Do not double the dose or take extra.

Pharmacokinetics. *Onset and Duration.* Steady-state serum levels are attained in 2–4 days.[2] Several weeks might be required to attain maximal therapeutic effect.[95] For mania, levels should be above 45 mg/L for efficacy and below 125 mg/L to minimize adverse effects.

Serum Levels. 50–120 mg/L (350–830 μmol/L) for epilepsy and mania. Some patients require and can tolerate serum levels up to 150 mg/L.[95] Tremor, irritability, confusion, and restlessness might be observed with levels >100–150 mg/L.[2]

Fate. The bioavailability of the oral capsule is 93 ± 13%, with peak levels occurring 1–2 hr after the dose. The bioavailability of the EC divalproex tablet is

$90 \pm 14\%$, with peak levels in 4 hr.[2,96] The peak time of both is delayed by food: (Cap) 5.2 ± 1.7 hr; (EC divalproex tab) 8.1 ± 3.6 hr.[97] Bioavailability of the SR tab is 80–90% of the EC product. Bioavailability is $80 \pm 7\%$ after a 250 mg suppository.[98] Peak serum levels of 40–50 mg/L (280–350 μmol/L) occur 2–4 hr after a 15–20 mg/kg dose of syrup diluted 1:1 with water as a retention enema.[11] V_d is 0.19 ± 0.05 L/kg in adults and 0.26 ± 0.09 L/kg in children.[2] Plasma protein binding is about 90%.[96] Increasing serum concentrations, hypoalbuminemia, severe liver disease, renal disease, or pregnancy reportedly increases the unbound fraction and might alter clearance. Cl is (healthy adults) 0.0066 ± 0.0005 L/hr/kg; (epileptic adults) 0.018 ± 0.011 L/hr/kg; (children) 0.027 ± 0.015 L/hr/kg.[2] Over 96% is metabolized to at least 10 metabolites. Only 1.8–3.2% of drug is excreted unchanged in urine.[2]

$t_{1/2}$. (Healthy adults) 13.9 ± 3.4 hr; (epileptic adults) 8.5 ± 3.3 hr; (children) 7.2 ± 2.3 hr.[2]

Adverse Reactions. (*See* Serum Levels.) Nausea, vomiting, diarrhea, and abdominal cramps occur frequently during initiation of therapy and are minimized by slow titration of valproic acid or substitution of EC divalproex for valproic acid. Transient elevations in liver function tests occur frequently. The risk of valproate-exposed women having children with spina bifida is approximately 1–2%. Drowsiness, ataxia, tremor, behavioral disturbances, transient hair loss, asymptomatic hyperammonemia, or weight gain occurs occasionally. Drowsiness and ataxia are more prominent in patients taking valproic acid with other anticonvulsants.[2] Rarely, thrombocytopenia, acute pancreatitis, abnormal coagulation parameters, or hyperglycinemia occurs. Liver failure occurs rarely; the greatest risk is during the first 6 months of therapy and in children <2 yr who receive multiple anticonvulsants.[99]

Contraindications. Hepatic dysfunction or disease.

Precautions. Pregnancy; lactation. The drug can alter results of urine ketone tests.

Drug Interactions. Valproate levels can be decreased by concurrent carbamazepine, lamotrigine, phenytoin, or rifampin. Valproate levels can be increased by concurrent aspirin, chlorpromazine, cimetidine, or felbamate. Lamotrigine and phenobarbital levels can be increased by valproate.

Parameters to Monitor. Baseline liver function tests and platelets; repeat liver function tests frequently, especially during the first 6 months. Monitor platelet count and coagulation tests before surgery. Periodic serum level monitoring is useful for guiding dosage changes and evaluating potential adverse effects. Serum levels fluctuate considerably over 24 hr, making a single random measurement of limited value. Predose blood sampling at standard times is recommended.[2,96]

Notes. Valproic acid and ethosuximide are equally effective for treating absence seizures, although **ethosuximide** is sometimes preferred as a first-line agent because of its lower risk of serious toxicity. Valproic acid is preferred for patients with absence and generalized tonic-clonic seizures. Many clinicians in the United States use valproic acid as a second-line agent (after **phenytoin** or **carbamazepine**) for the treatment of partial seizures. Valproic acid is as effective as phenytoin and carbamazepine for tonic-clonic seizures and is a drug of choice for atonic and myoclonic seizures.[2,95,100] (*See* Anticonvulsants Comparison Chart.)

Divalproex is equivalent to **lithium** in bipolar disorder and is more effective than lithium for rapid-cycling bipolar patients (four or more episodes in 1 yr) and comorbid substance abuse. Carbamazepine is more effective as an adjunctive treatment with lithium to enhance partial efficacy than with lithium alone.[101-103]

For migraine prophylaxis, divalproex is effective and well tolerated. It might be more effective in those having frequent migraines than in those characterized as having tension headaches.[104,105] The sustained-release formulation is approved for migraine prophylaxis only.

ZONISAMIDE Zonegran

Pharmacology. Zonisamide is a 1,2-benzisoxazole sulfonamide derivative that is chemically unrelated to other antiepileptic drugs. It blocks seizure spread and inhibits epileptic foci in animals. The anticonvulsant effect is likely related to blockade of voltage-sensitive sodium and T-type calcium channels. It is also a weak carbonic anhydrase inhibitor.[106]

Administration and Adult Dosage. PO as adjunctive therapy for partial seizures 100 mg/day initially, increasing in 100 mg/day increments at intervals of 2 weeks as needed. **Usual maintenance dosage** is 200–400 mg/day in 1–2 divided doses. Some patients might require dosages of 600 mg/day; there is little evidence of increased effectiveness above 400 mg/day.

Special Populations. *Pediatric Dosage.* Safety and efficacy not established. Zonisamide is used in Japan for the treatment of epilepsy in children. The recommended dosage is 2–4 mg/kg/day initially, increasing at 2-week intervals to 4–12 mg/kg/day as needed.

Geriatric Dosage. Advanced age has no effect on zonisamide pharmacokinetics. No dosage adjustment is necessary.

Other Conditions. Zonisamide clearance is reduced in patients with renal disease. These patients might require slower titration because of the prolonged half-life of the drug. The effect of liver disease on zonisamide pharmacokinetics is unknown.

Dosage Forms. Cap 100 mg.

Patient Instructions. (*See* Anticonvulsants Class Instructions). Drink 6–8 glasses of water daily to lessen the likelihood of kidney stone formation.

Missed Doses. Take this drug at regular intervals. If you miss a dose, take it as soon as you remember. If it is about time for the next dose, take that dose only. Do not double the dose or take extra.

Pharmacokinetics. *Onset and Duration.* Steady-state serum levels are attained in 14 days in patients with normal renal function.

Serum Levels. Therapeutic range not established.

Fate. Rapidly absorbed after oral administration with peak serum concentrations occurring 2.8 ± 1.4 hr after a dose in healthy volunteers. Food delays the rate but has no effect on the extent of zonisamide absorption. Zonisamide is 40% bound to plasma proteins, mainly albumin. In healthy volunteers, V_d/F is 1.47 ± 0.39 L/kg;

Cl/F is 0.019 ± 0.004 L/kg/hr. Cl is increased 30–40% during concomitant therapy with enzyme-induced antiepileptic drugs. Elimination is mainly by urinary excretion of unchanged drug and glucuronide metabolite. Other metabolic pathways include acetylation and reduction of an acetylated metabolite (via CYP3A4).

$t_{1/2}$. (Adults with normal renal function) 63 hr.

Adverse Reactions. Frequent adverse effects include somnolence, ataxia, anorexia, confusion, abnormal thinking, and nervousness. Kidney stones occur in 2.6% of patients.[2]

Contraindications. Allergy to sulfonamides.

Drug Interactions. Enzyme-inducing antiepileptic drugs (carbamazepine, phenytoin, barbiturates) enhance zonisamide's metabolism and reduce its half-life to 27–36 hr. Zonisamide has no apparent effect on the pharmacokinetics of other antiepileptic drugs.[88]

Notes. Zonisamide is indicated as adjunctive treatment for partial and secondarily generalized tonic-clonic seizures in adults. It reduces the frequency of seizures by ≥50% in 30–40% of patients as adjunctive therapy. The drug also appears to be effective for generalized and progressive myoclonic epilepsies.[2]

ANTICONVULSANTS COMPARISON CHART

DRUG	CHOICE OF ANTICONVULSANT FOR CLINICAL SEIZURE TYPE[a]					ANTICONVULSANT DOSAGE RANGE AND SERUM LEVELS			
	Generalized Seizures				Partial Seizures[b]	Dosage Range (mg/kg/day)		Therapeutic Serum Levels	
	Tonic-Clonic	Absence	Myoclonic	Atonic		Adult	Pediatric	(mg/L)	(μmol/L)
Carbamazepine	1	W	—	—	1	10–30	15–35	4–12	17–50
Clonazepam	W	3	2	1	—	0.01–0.2	0.01–0.2	13–72 µg/L	40–230 nmol/L
Ethosuximide	—	1	—	—	—	10–30	20–40	40–100	280–710
Gabapentin	—	—	—	—	4	15–35	—	—	—
Lamotrigine	—	—	—	—	4	1.5–7	—	—	—
Levetiracetam	—	—	—	—	4	30–45	—	—	—
Oxcarbazepine	—	—	—	—	4	20–40	30–45	—	—
Phenytoin	1	W	—	—	1	4–8	4–8	10–20	40–80
Tiagabine	—	—	—	—	4	0.5–0.8	—	—	—
Topiramate	—	—	—	—	4	4–8	—	—	—
Valproic Acid[c]	1	2	1	1	2	15–60	15–60	50–120	350–830
Zonisamide	—	—	—	—	4	3–6	4–12	—	—

1 = Drug of first choice; initial agent; given as monotherapy.

2 = Drug of second choice; alternative to first choice; given as monotherapy or in combination with agent of first choice;

3 = Drug of third choice; alternative to first or second choice; given as monotherapy or in combination with another agent;

4 = Useful as adjunctive therapy after failure of monotherapy with preferred agents;

W = May worsen clinical seizure type.

[a]Choice of anticonvulsant based on relative and comparative efficacy and potential for adverse effects. Choice of agent should consider individual patient factors. (See references 1, 82, 95, and 100.)

[b]Includes simple-partial, complex-partial, and secondarily generalized tonic-clonic seizures.

[c]Drug of first choice when both generalized tonic-clonic and absence seizures are present.

Antidepressants

Class Instructions. Antidepressants. This drug can cause drowsiness. Until the extent of this effect is known, use caution when driving, operating machinery, or performing other tasks requiring mental alertness. Avoid excessive concurrent use of alcohol or other drugs that cause drowsiness.

BUPROPION
Wellbutrin, Zyban

Pharmacology. Bupropion is a monocyclic antidepressant, unique as a mild dopamine and norepinephrine uptake inhibitor with no direct effect on serotonin receptors or MAO. It is essentially devoid of anticholinergic, antihistaminic, and peripheral adrenergic effects. In contrast with heterocyclic antidepressants, bupropion produces no clinically important effect on cardiac conduction, no orthostatic hypotension, minimal anticholinergic effects, and it is not associated with weight gain. Compared with SSRIs, bupropion offers a similar side effect profile without sexual dysfunction. Its lack of sedation and its activating effect can be advantageous for patients with decreased psychomotor activity and lethargy. Disadvantages of bupropion include seizures and the necessity of multiple daily doses.[107–109] (*See* Antidepressants Comparison Chart.)

Administration and Adult Dosage. Small initial doses and gradual dosage escalation is necessary to minimize the risk of seizures. **PO for depression** (immediate-release) 100 mg bid initially, increasing to 100 mg tid no sooner than 3 days after the start of therapy. The maximum daily dosage is 450 mg, with a maximum single dose of 150 mg; (sustained-release) 150 mg given in the morning initially, increasing to 150 mg bid no sooner than 4 days after the start of therapy, to a maximum of 200 mg bid. **PO as an aid to smoking cessation** (sustained-release) Zyban is identical to Wellbutrin SR and is given in the same dosage regimen as Wellbutrin SR for depression for 7–12 weeks.[110]

Dosage Forms. Tab 75, 100 mg (Wellbutrin); **SR Tab** 100, 150 mg (Wellbutrin SR, Zyban).

Pharmacokinetics. Elimination half-life is 11–14 hr, but an active hydroxy metabolite has a half-life longer than 24 hr.

Adverse Reactions. Frequent adverse effects include insomnia, agitation, headache, and nausea. With dosages of ≤450 mg/day, seizures occur in 0.4% of patients, with a 1-yr cumulative incidence of 0.5%. Bupropion is contraindicated in patients with psychotic disorders (its dopamine agonist effect can increase psychotic symptoms), seizure disorders, anorexia, or bulimia, and in those receiving MAOIs. Bupropion seems to offer better safety in overdose than heterocyclic antidepressants.

Drug Interactions. Bupropion can increase levodopa side effects. Phenelzine can increase bupropion's acute adverse reactions.

CLOMIPRAMINE
Anafranil, Various

Pharmacology. Clomipramine is a 3-chloro analogue of imipramine that is a potent inhibitor of serotonin reuptake and, unlike other tricyclic antidepressants, antagonizes dopaminergic neurotransmission. It has a specific indication for treatment of obsessive-compulsive disorder (OCD). Few patients experience complete OCD symptom relief; typically, about 40–50% of patients have marked symptom improvement. Although it is an effective antidepressant, its adverse effect profile makes other antidepressants preferred for this indication.[111–113] (*See* Antidepressants Comparison Chart.)

Adult Dosage. **PO for OCD** 25 mg/day initially, increasing to 100 mg/day during the first 2 weeks, and then gradually increasing over several weeks to a maximum of 250 mg/day. **PO as an antidepressant** 100–150 mg/day. Clomipramine can be given safely once daily at bedtime.

Dosage Forms. **Cap** 25, 50, 75 mg.

Pharmacokinetics. Antiobsessional effects are first seen at week 4, with maximum effects between weeks 10 and 18. Clomipramine is a highly lipophilic drug with a large first-pass effect and oral bioavailability of 36–62%. The major route of elimination is metabolism by demethylation and then hydroxylation and conjugation, with an elimination half-life of 20–24 hr.

Adverse Reactions. Clomipramine's adverse effect profile is similar to that of amitriptyline (ie, frequent sedation, anticholinergic effects, orthostatic hypotension, tremor, nausea, and sweating), but it has a much higher prevalence of sexual dysfunction and seizures. In controlled studies, 42% of patients experienced ejaculatory failure and 20% were impotent. Frequency of sexual dysfunction increases to >90% of patients when asked directly rather than relying on self-reporting.[114] Seizures occur in 0.5% of patients receiving 250 mg/day or less, and 2% of patients experience seizures with dosages above 250 mg/day. Clomipramine is contraindicated in patients who have received MAOIs within the past 14 days. Use with caution in patients with cardiovascular disease (eg, arrhythmias, angina, MI).

Drug Interactions. Drug interactions are the same as other tricyclic antidepressants (TCAs). (*See* Heterocyclic Antidepressants.)

FLUOXETINE Prozac, Sarafem

Pharmacology. Fluoxetine is a bicyclic antidepressant that is a selective and potent inhibitor of presynaptic reuptake of serotonin (an SSRI). It does not affect reuptake of norepinephrine or dopamine and has a relative lack of affinity for muscarinic, histamine, α_1- and α_2-adrenergic, and serotonin receptors.[115]

Administration and Adult Dosage. (*See* Antidepressants Comparison Chart.) **PO for depression or OCD** 20 mg/day initially, administered in the morning. Increase dosage no more frequently than q 3–5 weeks. Divide higher dosages, with the last dose given in early afternoon. Although the maximum labeled dosage is 80 mg/day, 20 mg is equal in efficacy for major depression to higher dosages with the benefit of fewer adverse effects.[115,116] For depression maintenance, Prozac Weekly 90 mg once/week can be started one week after the last 20 mg/day dose. **PO for bulimia** 60 mg/day in the morning. **PO for premenstrual dysphoric disorder** 20 mg/day; higher dosages appear to have no increased efficacy. Administration for the 14 days before menses can be as effective as continuous use.[117]

Special Populations. *Pediatric Dosage.* (<18 yr) safety and efficacy not established.

Geriatric Dosage. Reduce initial dosage and rate of dosage increase in the elderly. Single-dose studies suggest no difference in maintenance dosage in the elderly, but data from multiple-dose studies are needed. (*See* Notes.)

Other Conditions. Reduce initial dosage and rate of dosage increase in patients with hepatic impairment. Dosage adjustment in renal impairment is unnecessary.[115]

Dosage Forms. **Cap** 10, 20, 40 mg; **SR cap** 90 mg (Prozac Weekly); **Soln** 4 mg/mL; **Tab** 10 mg.

Patient Instructions. This drug requires at least 2 weeks for a noticeable response in mood and up to 4 weeks for full therapeutic benefit. Take fluoxetine in the morning or early afternoon. Inform your physician of any other medications you are taking.

Pharmacokinetics. *Onset and Duration.* Onset is delayed 2–4 weeks, which is similar to other antidepressants.

Serum Levels. Not established.

Fate. Oral bioavailability is 95% with all dosage forms. It is 94% bound to plasma proteins, with a V_d of 35 ± 21 L/kg; Cl is 0.58 ± 0.41 L/hr/kg, decreasing with repeated administration. The primary active metabolite is norfluoxetine; the metabolic rate is possibly under polygenic control.

$t_{1/2}$. (Fluoxetine) 1–3 days after a single oral dose, increasing with multiple doses to 4–5 days; (norfluoxetine) 7–15 days. Half-lives do not appear to be altered in the elderly or in patients with renal impairment. Patients with alcohol-induced cirrhosis have fluoxetine half-life increased by 100% and norfluoxetine half-life increased by 60% compared with controls.[115,118]

Adverse Reactions. Nausea, anxiety, insomnia, nervousness, diarrhea, anorexia, dry mouth, headache, and tremor occur with a frequency greater than 10%. Delayed ejaculation and anorgasmia occurs with fluoxetine and all SSRIs in at least 30–55% of patients.[119,120] Unlike TCAs, which typically cause weight gain, fluoxetine dosages over 40 mg/day cause a weight loss of 1–2 kg within the first 6 weeks of treatment.[121] Fluoxetine rarely causes sedation except at dosages over 40 mg/day and has no adverse cardiovascular or anticholinergic effects.[122] Initial case reports of patients developing new and intense suicidal preoccupation, agitation, and impulsiveness after several weeks of fluoxetine therapy have been adequately evaluated and found not to be directly related to the drug.[123]

Contraindications. Pregnancy. Concurrent use of an MAOI; 5 weeks must elapse between discontinuation of fluoxetine and starting an MAOI.[124]

Precautions. Use cautiously in the elderly and in patients with hepatic impairment. Use fluoxetine with caution in depressed patients with psychomotor agitation and anxiety or with anorexia and weight loss.

Drug Interactions. Fluoxetine is a potent inhibitor of CYP2D6, causing decreased metabolism and increased serum levels and adverse effects of many drugs, including most other antidepressants, antipsychotics, β-blockers, and type Ic antiarrhythmics. Fluoxetine's effect on other P450 isoenzymes has not been well defined.

Parameters to Monitor. Monitor liver function tests periodically during long-term therapy.

Notes. Fluoxetine is a useful alternative to TCAs because of its greater safety in overdose and relative lack of anticholinergic and cardiovascular effects. For severely depressed elderly patients, fluoxetine is less effective than **nortriptyline.**[125] Fluoxetine and other SSRIs have demonstrated efficacy for OCD and panic disorder. (*See* Antidepressants Comparison Chart.)

FLUVOXAMINE   LUVOX

Pharmacology. Fluvoxamine has a selective and potent inhibitory effect on serotonergic presynaptic reuptake, similar to fluoxetine. Although it is also an effective antidepressant, fluvoxamine has been marketed for use in OCD. Fluvoxamine is equal in efficacy to **clomipramine** in OCD and causes fewer anticholinergic effects and sexual dysfunction but more headache and insomnia.[126–128] (*See* Antidepressants Comparison Chart.)

Adult Dosage. PO for OCD 50 mg/day initially, with a **maintenance dosage** of 100–300 mg/day. Give dosages over 100 mg/day in 2 divided doses. The elderly and those with hepatic impairment might require a lower starting dosage and slower dosage titration.

Pediatric Dosage. PO for OCD (<8 yr) safety and efficacy not established; (8–17 yr) 25 mg hs initially, increasing in 25 mg/day increments q 4–7 days to a **usual maintenance dosage** of 50–200 mg/day. Divide dosages >50 mg/day into 2 doses, either equal or with a greater portion given hs.

Dosage Forms. **Tab** 25, 50, 100 mg.

Pharmacokinetics. Bioavailability is about 50% and not affected by food. Fluvoxamine is the least protein bound of the SSRIs (77%). On the same dosage, elderly patients have 40% higher serum concentrations than younger patients. Fluvoxamine is metabolized to inactive metabolites. Elimination half-life is about 16 hr in adults and 26 hr in the elderly.

Adverse Reactions. Frequent adverse effects include nausea, somnolence or insomnia, dry mouth, and sexual dysfunction.

Drug Interactions. Unlike other SSRIs, fluvoxamine is a potent inhibitor of CYP1A2, so increased levels and adverse effects are possible with warfarin, propranolol, metoprolol, caffeine, and theophylline. As with all SSRIs, do not administer fluvoxamine with MAOIs.

HETEROCYCLIC ANTIDEPRESSANTS

Pharmacology. Heterocyclic antidepressants (**tricyclic antidepressants, amoxapine,** and **maprotiline**) have specific effects on neurotransmitters and receptor sensitivity. The primary pharmacologic effect of heterocyclic antidepressants is blockade of presynaptic reuptake of norepinephrine, with subsequent downregulation of adrenergic receptors. Amoxapine, a metabolite of **loxapine**, retains some postsynaptic dopamine reuptake inhibition. Heterocyclic antidepressants have less effect on serotonergic activity than on other neurotransmitters.[129,130]

Administration and Adult Dosage. (*See* Antidepressants Comparison Chart for dosage ranges.) **PO for depression** initiate dosage at lower limit of range. Administer in divided doses to assess tolerance to side effects and then once-daily hs can be used.[129,131] **Maintenance dosage** should be the same as the dosage necessary to treat the acute depressive episode.[132] **IM** rarely used (eg, surgical patient NPO for 1–2 days). **PO for chronic pain (amitriptyline** or **imipramine)** 10–25 mg/day initially; most patients respond to a dosage of 25–75 mg/day, although dosages up to 200 mg/day have been used.[133,134] (*See* Notes.)

Special Populations. *Pediatric Dosage.* Not recommended <12 yr except for childhood enuresis. **PO for enuresis (imipramine)** (<12 yr) 25–50 mg/day; (≥12 yr) up to 75 mg/day.[135] Imipramine maximum dosage in children is 2.5 mg/kg/day; however, use in prepubertal major depression disorder often requires up to 5 mg/kg/day with serum levels over 150 μg/L.[136]

Geriatric Dosage. (>65 yr) reduce initial dosage by at least 50% of adult dosage and increase the dosage slowly.[137]

Other Conditions. Reduce initial dosage and rate of titration in patients with cardiovascular or hepatic disease.[138] During the last trimester of pregnancy, the mean dosage of TCAs required is 1.6 times that of nonpregnant women.[139]

Dosage Forms. (*See* Antidepressants Comparison Chart.)

Patient Instructions. (*See* Antidepressants Class Instructions.) These drugs usually take 2 weeks for a noticeable response in mood and up to 4 weeks for full therapeutic benefit. If you have small children, be sure to keep this medication in a secure place.

Pharmacokinetics. *Onset and Duration.* Physiologic symptoms of depression (eg, sleep and appetite disturbance, decreased energy) should improve after 1 week, but mood (pessimism, hopelessness, anhedonia) often requires 2–4 weeks for response.

Serum Levels. **Nortriptyline** has a well-established therapeutic range and a curvilinear relationship of serum levels and response ("therapeutic window"). Other antidepressants show a linear response relationship.[140] (*See* Antidepressants Comparison Chart.)

Fate. Bioavailability is variable (30–70%) because of first-pass metabolism. Major metabolites for TCAs are desmethyl (for tertiary amines) and hydroxy compounds; rate is possibly genetically determined and can result in 30-fold variation in steady-state levels in patients given the same dosage.[141]

$t_{½}$. (Tertiary amine TCAs) 10–25 hr; (secondary amine TCAs) 12–44 hr.[140]

Adverse Reactions. Sedation, postural hypotension, anticholinergic effects (dry mouth, blurred near vision, constipation, urinary retention, aggravation of narrow-angle glaucoma, and prostatic hypertrophy), weight gain, and cardiac effects (ECG changes and slowed AV conduction) are frequent. **Nortriptyline** is least likely of the TCAs to cause postural hypotension. (*See* Antidepressants Comparison Chart for relative differences in frequency of common adverse reactions.) Fine hand tremors, seizures, cardiac arrhythmia, or cholestasis can occur, as can hypomanic or manic episodes in bipolar patients. Seizures and blood dyscrasias are rare.[142,143]

Contraindications. Cardiac arrhythmias, especially bundle-branch block.

Precautions. Use with caution in the elderly, in pregnancy, or in patients with CHF and angina pectoris, epilepsy, glaucoma, prostatic hypertrophy, or renal or liver disease. When discontinuing therapy, taper the heterocyclic antidepressant dosage to prevent cholinergic rebound. Cases of sudden cardiac death have been reported in children with attention deficit disorder who received **desipramine** in therapeutic or subtherapeutic dosages.[144] Ingestion of ≥1 g of a heterocyclic antidepressant constitutes a life-threatening medical emergency. Limit the quantities dispensed to depressed patients with suicidal ideation. **Maprotiline** has an increased frequency of seizures at dosages above 225 mg/day. **Amoxapine** has a metabolite with dopamine-blocking activity, resulting in possible extrapyramidal effects, tardive dyskinesia, endocrine effects, and neuroleptic malignant syndrome. Neither amoxapine nor maprotiline offers greater efficacy or safety in overdose than TCAs.

Drug Interactions. Many drug interactions occur. Use with caution with MAOIs. The antihypertensive effects of guanethidine, clonidine, and closely related drugs might be reduced.

Parameters to Monitor. Monitor hepatic and renal function tests periodically during long-term therapy. Obtain ECG in the elderly, children, and those with pre-existing heart disease. With **amoxapine**, monitor carefully for signs of tardive dyskinesia.

Notes. TCAs are commonly used in treating pain associated with diabetic neuropathy and postherpetic neuralgia; **amitriptyline, desipramine,** and **nortriptyline** have proven efficacy, but **SSRIs** are less effective.[133,134] (*See* Antidepressants Comparison Chart.)

MIRTAZAPINE   Remeron

Pharmacology. Mirtazapine is an antidepressant that antagonizes presynaptic α_2-adrenergic auto- and heteroreceptors that are responsible for controlling the release of norepinephrine and serotonin (5-HT). It is also a potent antagonist of postsynaptic 5-HT_2 and 5-HT_3 receptors. The net outcome of these effects is increased noradrenergic activity and enhanced 5-HT activity, especially at 5-HT_{1A} receptors. This unique mechanism of action preserves antidepressant efficacy but minimizes many of the adverse effects common to heterocyclic antidepressants and SSRIs. Mirtazapine is effective in moderate and severe major depression.[145,146] (*See* Antidepressants Comparison Chart.)

Administration and Adult Dosage. **PO for depression** 15 mg/day at bedtime initially, increasing at 1–2-week intervals to a maximum of 45 mg/day.

Dosage Forms. **Tab** (conventional and rapidly dissolving) 15, 30, 45 mg.

Pharmacokinetics. Mirtazapine has an onset of clinical effect in 2–4 weeks, similar to other antidepressants. It has an elimination half-life of 20–40 hr, allowing once-daily administration at bedtime.

Adverse Reactions. Sedation, increased appetite, and weight gain are the most frequent side effects. Sedation is most frequent at lower doses (15 mg) and decreases in frequency with increasing dosage. Although two cases of agranulocytosis occurred in clinical trials, no specific or additional blood count monitoring is required. Mirtazapine has minimal cardiovascular and anticholinergic effects and essentially lacks adverse GI effects, insomnia, and sexual dysfunction. Do not use mirtazapine within 14 days of an MAOI. Overdose up to 975 mg in combination with a benzodiazepine has caused marked sedation but no difficulty with cardiovascular or respiratory effects.

MONOAMINE OXIDASE INHIBITORS

Pharmacology. MAOIs are thought to exert their antidepressant action because of alterations in adrenergic and serotonergic receptor sensitivity. The most consistent findings during long-term MAOI therapy include downregulation of β-adrenergic and adenyl cyclase activities. **Isocarboxazid** and **phenelzine** are hydrazine derivatives; **tranylcypromine** is a nonhydrazine.

Administration and Adult Dosage. PO for depression (isocarboxazid) 20–30 mg/day; (phenelzine) 45–90 mg/day; (tranylcypromine) 30–60 mg/day. Initiate dosage at the lower limit and titrate upward depending on tolerance to side effects. Dosage schedule should remain divided, usually bid or tid. Avoid bedtime administration because MAOIs can delay onset of sleep.

Special Populations. *Pediatric Dosage.* (<16 yr) not recommended.

Geriatric Dosage. Limited information, but decrease initial dosage by 50% because of orthostatic hypotension. Contraindicated in patients older than 60 yr.

Other Conditions. Reduce the initial dosage and rate of upward titration if the patient has taken a heterocyclic antidepressant within 7–10 days.

Dosage Forms. (Isocarboxazid) **Tab** 10 mg; (phenelzine) **Tab** 15 mg; (tranylcypromine) **Tab** 10 mg.

Patient Instructions. (*See* Antidepressants Class Instructions.) This drug usually takes 2 weeks for noticeable response in mood and up to 4 weeks for full therapeutic benefit to occur. This drug can cause faintness or dizziness, especially after rising suddenly or standing for prolonged periods, or after exertion or alcohol intake. Immediately report nausea, vomiting, sweating, severe occipital headache, and stiff neck, which might be signs of a serious adverse effect. Avoid concurrent use of diet pills and cough and cold remedies and restrict consumption of aged foods high in tyramine. (*See* Foods That Interact with MAO Inhibitors Chart.)

Pharmacokinetics. *Onset and Duration.* Onset 2 weeks; maximum improvement occurs after 3–4 weeks.[147]

Serum Levels. Not used clinically.

Fate. Termination of drug action is dependent on MAO regeneration because the drugs or their active metabolites chemically combine with the MAO enzyme.

Adverse Reactions. Autonomic effects are frequent and not necessarily dose dependent; these include postural hypotension, dry mouth, and constipation. Drowsiness is more frequent with phenelzine, whereas overstimulation and agitation are more likely with tranylcypromine; isocarboxazid is mildly stimulating. Occasionally, delayed ejaculation, edema, skin rash, urinary retention, and blurred vision occur. MAOIs are much less likely than TCAs to cause weight gain, with tranyl-cypromine the least likely.[148]

Contraindications. Patients older than 60 yr; patients with confirmed or suspected cerebrovascular defect; cardiovascular disease; pheochromocytoma; history of liver disease or abnormal liver function tests.

Precautions. Always consider the possibility of suicide in depressed patients and take adequate precautions. Like other antidepressant drugs, MAOIs can switch bipolar patients to a hypomanic or manic state.

Drug Interactions. Postural hypotension can increase with co-administration of antipsychotic, heterocyclic antidepressant, or antihypertensive drugs, and in patients with CHF. Avoid concurrent use with buspirone, heterocyclic antidepressants, meperidine, sympathomimetic drugs, SSRIs, and other MAOIs. A 1–2-week drug-free interval is necessary when switching from an MAOI to a TCA, but a drug-free interval is not necessary when switching from a TCA to an MAOI.[149] Although uncommon, hypertensive crisis can result from concurrent use of sympathomimetic amines or ingestion of food and drinks high in tyramine.[150,151] Avoid diets high in tyramine content. (*See* Foods That Interact with MAO Inhibitors Chart.)

Parameters to Monitor. Monitor blood pressure frequently.

Notes. MAOIs are excellent alternatives to heterocyclic antidepressants in major depressive disorder, are very effective in panic disorder, and are drugs of choice for atypical depression.[150,152]

FOODS THAT INTERACT WITH MAO INHIBITORS

Many fermented foods contain tyramine as a byproduct formed by the bacterial breakdown of the amino acid tyrosine; it also can be formed by parahydroxylation of phenylethylamine or dehydroxylation of dihydroxyphenylalanine (DOPA) and dopamine. Tyramine and some other amines found in food can cause hypertensive reactions in patients taking MAO inhibitors. MAO found in the GI tract inactivates tyramine; when drugs prevent this, exogenous tyramine and other monoamines are absorbed and release norepinephrine from sympathetic nerve endings and epinephrine from the adrenal gland. If sufficient quantities of these pressor compounds are released, palpitations, severe headache, and hypertensive crisis can result.

FOODS THAT CONTAIN TYRAMINE

Avocados	Particularly if overripe.
Bananas	Reactions can occur if eaten in large amounts; tyramine levels are high in peel.
Bean curd	Fermented bean curd, fermented soya bean, soya bean pastes, soy sauces, and miso soup, prepared from fermented bean curd, contain tyramine in large amounts; miso soup has caused reactions.
Beer and ale	Major domestic brands do not contain appreciable amounts; some imported brands have had high levels. Nonalcoholic beer might contain tyramine and should be avoided.
Caviar	Safe if vacuum-packed and eaten fresh or refrigerated only briefly.

FOODS THAT CONTAIN TYRAMINE

Cheese	Reactions possible with most, except unfermented varieties such as cottage cheese. In others, tyramine concentration is higher near the rind and close to fermentation holes.
Figs	Particularly if overripe.
Fish	Safe if fresh; avoid dried products. Caution required in restaurants. Vacuum-packed products are safe if eaten promptly or refrigerated only briefly.
Liver	Safe if very fresh, but rapidly accumulates tyramine; caution required in restaurants.
Meat	Safe if known to be fresh; caution required in restaurants.
Milk products	Milk and yogurt appear to be safe.
Protein extracts	See also soups; avoid liquid and powdered protein dietary supplements.
Sausage	Fermented varieties such as bologna, pepperoni, and salami have a high tyramine content.
Shrimp paste	Contains large amounts of tyramine.
Soups	Might contain protein extracts and should be avoided.
Soy sauce	Contains large amounts of tyramine; reactions have occurred with teriyaki.
Wines	Generally do not contain tyramine, but many reactions have been reported with Chianti, champagne, and other wines.
Yeast extracts	Dietary supplements (eg, Marmite) contain large amounts; yeast in baked goods, is safe.

FOODS THAT DO NOT CONTAIN TYRAMINE

Caffeine	A weak pressor agent; large amounts can cause reactions.
Chocolate	Contains phenylethylamine, a pressor agent that can cause reactions in large amounts.
Fava beans	(Broad beans, "Italian" green beans) Contain dopamine, a pressor amine, particularly when overripe.
Ginseng	Some preparations have caused headache, tremulousness, and manic-like symptoms.
Liqueurs	Reactions reported with some (eg, Chartreuse, Drambuie); cause unknown.
New Zealand prickly spinach	Single case report; patient ate large amounts.
Whiskey	Reactions have occurred; cause unknown.

For more information, consult Lippman SB, Nash K. Monoamine oxidase inhibitor update. Potential adverse food and drug interactions. *Drug Saf* 1990;5:195–204; and, Shulman KI, Walker SE. Redefining the MAOI diet: tyramine content of pizzas and soy products. *J Clin Psychiatry* 1999;60: 191-13.

From Anon. Foods interacting with MAO inhibitors. Med Lett Drugs Ther 1989;31:11–2, reproduced with permission.

NEFAZODONE   Serzone

Pharmacology. Nefazodone is a postsynaptic serotonin 5-HT$_{2A}$ antagonist and presynaptic serotonin reuptake inhibitor. These two serotonergic effects make it different from SSRIs and TCAs.[153–156] (*See* Antidepressants Comparison Chart.)

Administration and Adult Dosage. **PO for depression** 100 mg bid initially (50 mg bid in the elderly), increasing q 4–7 days to the effective dosage range of 150–300 mg bid. After initial dosage titration, once-daily bedtime administration is preferred to minimize daytime sedation.[157]

Dosage Forms. **Tab** 50, 100, 150, 200, 250 mg.

Pharmacokinetics. Nefazodone has an oral bioavailability of about 20%. Single-dose studies in the elderly have shown a 100% larger AUC; with multiple doses, the AUC differences decreased to 10–20% above those in younger populations. It is >99% protein bound and extensively metabolized, with a dose-dependent elimination half-life of about 1–2.3 hr in young patients, modestly prolonged in the elderly, and 2–3 times longer in hepatic disease. The major active metabolite, hydroxynefazodone, has a half-life of 1.2–1.6 hr in young and elderly patients, increasing to 2–4 hr with hepatic disease. Renal impairment does not markedly affect nefazodone pharmacokinetics.

Adverse Reactions. Although chemically similar to trazodone, it causes less sedation and orthostatic hypotension, and its lower α-adrenergic blockade makes priapism much less likely (no cases reported). Frequent adverse effects include sedation, dry mouth, nausea, and dizziness. Unlike SSRIs, nefazodone's effects on sexual function, agitation, tremor, insomnia, and weight are no different from placebo.

Drug Interactions. Nefazodone is a potent inhibitor of the CYP3A4 isoenzyme and a weak inhibitor of the CYP2D6 isoenzyme. Drug interactions of particular concern include the triazolobenzodiazepines (ie, alprazolam, triazolam, midazolam). A 1- to 2-week washout period is recommended when converting a patient to or from a MAOI and nefazodone.

PAROXETINE   Paxil

Pharmacology. Paroxetine is a highly selective and potent inhibitor of serotonin reuptake (an SSRI) similar to fluoxetine.[126,158–164] (*See* Antidepressants Comparison Chart.)

Administration and Adult Dosage. **PO for depression** 20 mg/day; a few patients require 30–50 mg/day for full efficacy. **PO for social anxiety disorder and panic disorder** 10 mg/day initially; usual maintenance dosage is 20–60 mg/day. **PO for OCD** 20 mg/day initially; maintenance dosage is 40 mg/day to a maximum of 60 mg/day, preferably as a single dose in the morning or evening. The starting dosage for all uses in elderly patients and those with marked renal or hepatic impairment is 10 mg/day. For the elderly or those with severe renal or hepatic impairment, the maximum dosage is 40 mg/day.

Dosage Forms. **Tab** 10, 20, 30, 40 mg; **SR Tab** 12.5, 25 mg; **Susp** 2 mg/mL.

Pharmacokinetics. Paroxetine is completely orally bioavailable; protein binding is 93–95%. Unlike fluoxetine, paroxetine is metabolized to inactive metabolites and has an elimination half-life of 24 hr.

Adverse Reactions. Paroxetine causes the typical SSRI adverse effects of nausea, sexual dysfunction, and headache but is more likely to cause sedation than insomnia and can cause more delay of orgasm or ejaculation and more impotence than other SSRIs.[165] Like the other SSRIs, it is much safer in overdose than TCAs.

Drug Interactions. Paroxetine is a potent inhibitor of CYP2D6, so most other antidepressants, antipsychotics, β-blockers, and type Ic antiarrhythmics can have increased serum levels and adverse effects when paroxetine is combined with these drugs. Do not use paroxetine within 14 days of using an MAOI.

REBOXETINE (Investigational—Pharmacia)   Vestra

Pharmacology. Reboxetine is the first in a new class of selective norepinephrine reuptake inhibitors with no affinity for serotonin or dopamine reuptake sites. It has negligible affinity for muscarinic, histaminic, or adrenergic receptors. This noradrenergic mechanism for antidepressant efficacy is similar to TCAs such as desipramine without the potential for appreciable adverse anticholinergic, cardiovascular, and sedative effects. It has efficacy for major depression equal to fluoxetine and desipramine.[166,167] (*See* Antidepressants Comparison Chart.)

Administration and Adult Dosage. PO for depression 8–10 mg/day given bid, 4–6 mg/day given bid in the elderly.

Dosage Forms. **Tab** 4 mg (investigational).

Pharmacokinetics. Reboxetine is rapidly absorbed. Metabolism occurs through three oxidative pathways: hydroxylation, dealkylation, and oxidation. The CYP450 isoenzymes responsible for metabolism have not been identified, and the degree of activity of the metabolites is unknown. Reboxetine has no inhibitory effect on CYP450 isoenzymes. Elimination half-life is 13 hr.[166]

Adverse Reactions. The most common adverse effects include dry mouth, constipation, increased sweating, insomnia, and urinary hesitancy, which are greater than placebo, but less frequent than imipramine. These "anticholinergic-like" effects are believed to result from increased norepinephrine levels. Side effects commonly associated with serotonin reuptake inhibitors such as nausea, anxiety or agitation, and daytime somnolence were no more common with reboxetine than with placebo.[167] No information is available regarding reboxetine overdose in humans.

SERTRALINE   Zoloft

Pharmacology. Sertraline is an SSRI similar to fluoxetine, which indirectly results in a downregulation of β-adrenergic receptors. It has no clinically important effect on noradrenergic or histamine receptors and no effect on MAO. It lacks stimulant, cardiovascular, anticholinergic, and convulsant effects. Sertraline has antidepressant effects equal to TCAs and fluoxetine and might have anorectic effects and efficacy in OCD.[130,168–170] (*See* Antidepressants Comparison Chart.)

Administration and Adult Dosage. **PO for depression, panic disorder, OCD, and posttraumatic stress disorder** 50 mg/day initially, increasing if necessary at weekly intervals to a maximum of 200 mg/day in a single dose in the morning or evening.

Dosage Forms. **Tab** 25, 50, 100 mg; **Soln** 20 mg/mL.

Pharmacokinetics. Sertraline has an oral bioavailability of 36%, and, when it is taken with food, peak serum concentrations and bioavailability increase by 30–40%. Peak serum concentrations are reached in 6–8 hr. Sertraline concentrations in breast milk are the lowest of the SSRIs and produce minimal serum levels in the breast-fed infant.[171] Its primary metabolite is *N*-desmethylsertraline, which has 5–10 times less activity than sertraline as an SSRI and has no demonstrated antidepressant activity. Cl is decreased by up to 40% in the elderly. Steady-state half-life is 27 hr.

Adverse Reactions. Frequent adverse effects include nausea, diarrhea, ejaculatory delay, tremor, and increased sweating. It causes less agitation, anxiety, and insomnia than fluoxetine and is a less potent inhibitor of the CYP2D6 isoenzyme at a dosage of 50 mg/day. Use with caution in patients with renal or hepatic impairment and do not use it within 14 days of using an MAOI. SIADH has been reported.[172]

VENLAFAXINE   Effexor

Pharmacology. Venlafaxine is a potent reuptake inhibitor of serotonin and norepinephrine, like many TCAs, but lacks effects on muscarinic, α-adrenergic, or histamine receptors.[173–176] (*See* Antidepressants Comparison Chart.)

Administration and Adult Dosage. **PO for depression** (immediate-release) 75 mg bid or tid initially, increasing q 4–7 days to an effective antidepressant dosage of 225–375 mg/day in 2 or 3 divided doses; (sustained-release) 75 mg once daily initially, increasing in increments of up to 75 mg/day at intervals of 4 or more days to a maximum of 225 mg/day. The sustained-release preparation does not reduce side effects but allows once-daily administration. **PO for generalized anxiety disorder** 75–225 mg/day in 2–3 divided doses. Patients with renal impairment or on hemodialysis require a 25–50% dosage reduction.

Dosage Forms. **Tab** 25, 37.5, 50, 75, 100 mg; **SR Cap** 37.5, 75, 150 mg (Effexor XR).

Pharmacokinetics. Venlafaxine is well absorbed orally; food has no effect on absorption. Serum concentrations in elderly patients are no different from those in younger patients. Unlike SSRIs, venlafaxine has minimal protein binding (27–30%). It undergoes extensive hepatic metabolism. Venlafaxine has an elimination half-life of 5 hr, and one major active metabolite has an 11-hr half-life. Venlafaxine exhibits linear pharmacokinetics over the recommended dosage range, and steady state is reached in 3 days.

Adverse Reactions. Frequent adverse effects include expected serotonin-related effects (eg, nausea, headache, insomnia or somnolence, and sexual dysfunction). At higher dosages (375 mg/day), venlafaxine is unique in causing a consistent but mild elevation in diastolic blood pressure (6 mm Hg). Regular blood pressure monitoring is required for all patients.

Drug Interactions. Venlafaxine is not a potent inhibitor of the cytochrome P450 enzyme system, making it different from most of the SSRIs. Avoid it in patients who have received an MAOI within the past 14 days.

ANTIDEPRESSANTS COMPARISON CHART[a]

CLASS AND DRUG	DOSAGE FORMS	USUAL DAILY ADULT DOSAGE RANGE (MG)	THERAPEUTIC SERUM LEVELS (μG/L)	RELATIVE FREQUENCY OF SIDE EFFECTS		
				Sedation	Anticholinergic	Orthostatic Hypotension
α₂-ADRENERGIC BLOCKERS						
Mirtazapine Remeron	Tab (conventional and rapidly dissolving) 15, 30, 45 mg.	15–45	b	Moderate	None	None
CHLOROPROPIOPHENONES						
Bupropion Wellbutrin Zyban	Tab 75, 100 mg SR Tab 100, 150 mg.	300–450	b	None	None	None
DIBENZOXAZEPINES[c]						
Amoxapine Asendin Various	Tab 25, 50, 100, 150 mg.	300–600	b	Low	Low	Low
MONOAMINE OXIDASE INHIBITORS (MAOIs)						
Phenelzine Nardil	Tab 15 mg.	45–90	b	Moderate	Low	Very High
Tranylcypromine Parnate	Tab 10 mg.	30–60	b	Low	Low	Very High
MORPHOLINES						
Reboxetine Vestra		8–10	b	Very Low	Low	Very Low

(continued)

ANTIDEPRESSANTS COMPARISON CHART[a] (*continued*)

| CLASS AND DRUG | DOSAGE FORMS | USUAL DAILY ADULT DOSAGE RANGE (MG) | THERAPEUTIC SERUM LEVELS (µG/L) | RELATIVE FREQUENCY OF SIDE EFFECTS | | |
				Sedation	Anticholinergic	Orthostatic Hypotension
SELECTIVE SEROTONIN REUPTAKE INHIBITORS (SSRIs)						
Citalopram Celexa	Tab 20, 40 mg Soln 2 mg/mL.	20–60	b	Very Low	Very Low	None
Fluoxetine Prozac	Cap, Tab 10, 20, 40 mg SR Cap 90 mg Soln 4 mg/mL Tab 10 mg.	10–80	b	None	Very Low	None
Fluvoxamine Luvox	Tab 25, 50, 100 mg.	100–300[d]	b	None	None	None
Paroxetine Paxil	Tab 10, 20, 30, 40 mg SR Tab 12.5, 25 mg Susp 2 mg/mL.	20–50	b	Low	Low	Very Low
Sertraline Zoloft	Tab 25, 50, 100 mg Soln 20 mg/mL.	50–200	b	None	None	None
SEROTONIN NOREPINEPHRINE REUPTAKE INHIBITORS (SNRIs)						
Venlafaxine Effexor Effexor XR	Tab 25, 37.5, 50, 75, 100 mg SR Cap 37.5, 75, 150 mg.	225–375	b	Very Low	Very Low	Very Low
TETRACYCLICS[c]						
Maprotiline Ludiomil Various	Tab 25, 50, 75 mg.	150–225	200–300[b]	Moderate	Moderate	Moderate

(continued)

457

ANTIDEPRESSANTS COMPARISON CHART[a] (*continued*)

CLASS AND DRUG	DOSAGE FORMS	USUAL DAILY ADULT DOSAGE RANGE (MG)	THERAPEUTIC SERUM LEVELS (μG/L)	RELATIVE FREQUENCY OF SIDE EFFECTS		
				Sedation	Anticholinergic	Orthostatic Hypotension
TRIAZOLOPYRIDINES						
Trazodone Desyrel Various	Tab 50, 100, 150, 300 mg.	50–100 (hypnotic) 200–400 (antidepressant)	b	High	Very Low	High
Nefazodone Serzone	Tab 50, 100, 150, 200, 250 mg.	300–600	b	Moderate	Very low	Moderate
TRICYCLICS (TCAs)[d]						
Amitriptyline Elavil Various	Tab 10, 25, 50, 75, 100, 150 mg Inj 10 mg/mL.	150–300	75–175[e]	High	High	High
Clomipramine Anafranil Various	Cap 25, 50, 75 mg.	100–250[d] 100–150[f]	b	High	High	High
Desipramine Norpramin Various	Tab 10, 25, 50, 75, 100, 150 mg.	150–300	100–160	Low	Low	Moderate
Doxepin Adapin Sinequan Various	Cap 10, 25, 50, 75, 100, 150 mg Soln 10 mg/mL.	150–300	110–250[e]	High	Moderate	High

(continued)

ANTIDEPRESSANTS COMPARISON CHART[a] (continued)

CLASS AND DRUG	DOSAGE FORMS	USUAL DAILY ADULT DOSAGE RANGE (MG)	THERAPEUTIC SERUM LEVELS (MG/L)	RELATIVE FREQUENCY OF SIDE EFFECTS		
				Sedation	Anticholinergic	Orthostatic Hypotension
Imipramine Tofranil Janimine Various	Tab 10, 25, 50 mg Cap (as pamoate) 75, 100, 125, 150 mg.	150–300	>200[e]	Moderate	Moderate	High
Nortriptyline Aventyl Pamelor Various	Cap 10, 25, 50, 75 mg Soln 2 mg/mL.	100–200	50–150	Moderate	Moderate	Low
Protriptyline Vivactil Various	Tab 5, 10 mg.	30–60	70–260[b]	Very Low	Moderate	Moderate
Trimipramine Surmontil	Cap 25, 50, 100 mg.	150–300	b	Moderate	Moderate	High

[a]Antidepressants with serotonergic activity (SSRIs, nefazodone, venlafaxine, and mirtazapine) have established efficacy for many indications other than depression. Some have received approval from the Food and Drug Administration for generalized anxiety disorder, bulimia nervosa, obsessive-compulsive disorder, social phobia, panic disorder, posttraumatic stress disorder, and premenstrual dysphoric disorder. Effective doses for major depression for most patients are in the low to moderate ranges listed, which is also true for generalized anxiety disorder, social phobia, panic disorder, and premenstrual dysphoric disorder. The middle to high end of the listed dosage ranges is usually necessary for efficacy when treating bulimia nervosa, obsessive-compulsive disorder, and posttraumatic stress disorder.[180]

[b]Not well established.

[c]Amoxapine, maprotiline, and the tricyclic antidepressants are categorized together as heterocyclic antidepressants because their therapeutic and side effect profiles are similar.

[d]For obsessive-compulsive disorder.

[e]Includes active metabolites.

[f]Major depression.

From references 106, 112, 122, 126, 127, 140, 141, 145, 146, 148, 153, 159, 160, 175, and 177–179.

Antipsychotic Drugs

Class Instructions. **Antipsychotics.** This drug can cause drowsiness. Until the extent of this effect is known, use caution when driving, operating machinery, or performing other tasks requiring mental alertness. Avoid excessive concurrent use of alcohol or other drugs that cause drowsiness.

Missed Doses. If you miss a dose, take it as soon as you remember. If it is almost time for your next dose, skip it and resume your normal schedule. Do not double doses.

ANTIPSYCHOTIC DRUGS

Pharmacology. Antipsychotic efficacy is most likely related to blockade of post-synaptic dopaminergic receptors in the mesolimbic and prefrontal cortexes of the brain, although other neurotransmitter systems also are involved.[181]

Administration and Adult Dosage. (*See* Antipsychotic Drugs Comparison Chart for oral dosage ranges.) Initiate therapy with divided doses until therapeutic dosage is found; then, for most patients, once-daily hs administration is preferred. For maintenance, decrease acute dosage by 25% q 3 months, with a target maintenance dosage being 50–67% of the acute treatment dosage.[182] Recent concern has focused on the need to establish a minimum effective dosage for antipsychotic drugs, and treatment regimens at the low end of the dosage range are preferred. Oral dosages of high-potency antipsychotics (eg, **fluphenazine, haloperidol**) in the range of 5–20 mg/day are better tolerated and equal in efficacy to dosages >20 mg/day.[183] Most patients can be given a maintenance dosage of 50% the acute dosage by the end of 1 yr, although 10–15% of chronically ill patients require a maintenance dosage >15 mg/day of **haloperidol** or its equivalent.[184,185] For manic episodes, no additional benefit is achieved with dosages >10 mg/day of haloperidol.[186] **Mesoridazine** and **thioridazine** are indicated only in patients who fail with other drugs because of inefficacy or intolerable side effects.

Special Populations. *Pediatric Dosage.* As with adults, dosage is determined primarily by titration to individual response. No precise dosage range exists, but in general the initial dosage is lower and increased more gradually in children.

Geriatric Dosage. Initial dosage is 20–25% of the dosage used in younger adults. Typical starting dosages in the elderly are **haloperidol** 0.5–2 mg/day. Dosage adjustments also must be done more slowly than in younger adults.[187]

Other Conditions. Dosages in the lower range are sufficient for most elderly patients, and the rate of dosage titration is slower.

Dosage Forms. (*See* Antipsychotic Drugs Comparison Chart.)

Patient Instructions. (*See* Antipsychotics Class Instructions.) These drugs usually take several weeks for clinical response and up to 8 weeks for full therapeutic response.

Pharmacokinetics. *Onset and Duration.* Onset of antipsychotic activity is variable, with noticeable response requiring days to weeks.

Serum Levels. Correlation of serum levels with clinical response is not consistently established. The best evidence exists for **haloperidol,** with serum concentrations of 5–15 μg/L (13–40 nmol/L) correlating well with therapeutic effects in adult psychotic patients, and an increasing risk of adverse effects and decreased efficacy when steady-state concentrations exceed 15 μg/L.[188,189]

Fate. **Haloperidol** is well absorbed; peak serum levels are achieved 2–6 hr after liquid or tablets and within 30 min after IM. Oral bioavailability of haloperidol is 60–70%. Haloperidol is extensively metabolized, with one active hydroxy metabolite. **Chlorpromazine** and other phenothiazines are well absorbed but undergo extensive and variable presystemic metabolism in the gut wall and liver; more than 20 chlorpromazine metabolites with different activities have been identified in human plasma. SR formulations result in a greater first-pass effect.

$t_{\frac{1}{2}}$. Serum half-lives have no clinical correlation with biologic half-lives for antipsychotic drugs. **Chlorpromazine** serum half-life is 30 hr, **thioridazine** 4–10 hr, **thiothixene** 34 hr, and **haloperidol** 12–24 hr. Of more clinical importance is that steady-state CNS levels and tissue saturation allow once-daily administration of all antipsychotic drugs.[141]

Adverse Reactions. (*See* Antipsychotic Drugs Comparison Chart for relative frequency of common adverse reactions.) Frequently, sedation, extrapyramidal effects (eg, parkinsonism, dystonic reactions, akathisia), tardive dyskinesia, anticholinergic effects (eg, dry mouth, blurred vision, constipation, urinary retention), photosensitivity, and postural hypotension occur. Occasionally, weight gain, amenorrhea, galactorrhea, ejaculatory disturbance, neuroleptic malignant syndrome, agranulocytosis, skin rash, cholestatic jaundice, and skin or eye pigmentation occur. Rarely, seizures, thermoregulatory impairment, and slowed AV conduction occur. **Mesoridazine** and **thioridazine** can prolong QT_c interval, leading to torsades de pointes and sudden death. Low-potency drugs are more likely to cause sedation, anticholinergic effects, and orthostatic hypotension, whereas high-potency drugs cause more extrapyramidal effects. Tardive dyskinesia is a long-term adverse effect, untreatable, and sometimes irreversible. Tardive dyskinesia occurs at a 4% yearly incidence for at least the first 5–6 yr of treatment. Neuroleptic malignant syndrome (ie, fever, extrapyramidal rigidity, autonomic instability, alterations in consciousness) occurs more frequently with high-potency antipsychotics, with a prevalence of 1.4% and a fatality rate of 4%.[183,190,191]

Contraindications. Coma; circulatory collapse or severe hypotension; bone marrow depression; history of blood dyscrasia. (Mesoridazine and thioridazine) concurrent use with drugs that prolong QT_c interval; baseline QT_c >450 msec.

Precautions. Use cautiously in patients with myasthenia gravis, Parkinson's disease, seizure disorders, or hepatic disease.

Drug Interactions. Barbiturates can enhance phenothiazine metabolism; carbamazepine can enhance haloperidol metabolism. Phenothiazines can decrease efficacy of guanethidine or guanadrel or have additive hypotensive effects with hypotensive drugs. Phenothiazines can inhibit the antiparkinson activity of levodopa. Haloperidol can increase the CNS toxicity of lithium. Combined use of haloperidol and methyldopa can result in dementia.

Parameters to Monitor. (Mesoridazine and thioridazine) obtain baseline and periodic ECGs and serum potassium.

Notes. (*See also* Prochlorperazine Salts in the Antiemetics section for antiemetic uses.)

CLOZAPINE
Clozaril

Pharmacology. Clozapine is an atypical antipsychotic drug that is chemically similar to loxapine and has unique pharmacologic effects and indications, as well as very serious adverse effects. Whereas typical antipsychotic drugs exert their effects primarily with a blockade of dopamine-D_2 receptors, clozapine affects several dopamine and serotonin receptors. Its high serotonin-$5HT_2$ to dopamine-D_2 ratio is the likely explanation for its unique efficacy. Compared with traditional antipsychotic drugs, clozapine is more effective for negative symptoms of schizophrenia, is more effective in treatment-resistant patients, and rarely causes extrapyramidal effects.[192-195]

Adult Dosage. PO 100–200 mg tid is effective for most patients, but some might require up to 900 mg/day. A therapeutic trial of 12–24 weeks is required for the full therapeutic effect to become apparent.

Dosage Forms. **Tab** 25, 100 mg.

Pharmacokinetics. Clozapine is nearly completely absorbed after oral administration, with about 30% oral bioavailability because of extensive first-pass metabolism. Clozapine is 95% bound to plasma proteins; with multiple doses, its elimination half-life is 12 hr.[196]

Adverse Reactions. Frequent adverse effects include sedation, orthostatic hypotension, anticholinergic effects, fever, and excessive salivation. Seizures are dose related, with a frequency up to 5% in the therapeutic dosage range and a 1-yr cumulative incidence of 10%. Agranulocytosis is the major adverse effect of concern, occurring in 0.8% of patients after 1 yr.[197] Most cases of agranulocytosis occur within the first 3 months of therapy. Substantial weight gain has been reported in most patients receiving clozapine.[198] (*See* Antipsychotic Drugs Comparison Chart.)

Paramaters to Monitor. Patients must have a baseline WBC count and differential before initiating therapy, mandatory weekly WBC monitoring for the first 6 months, and then q 2 weeks throughout treatment and for 4 weeks after discontinuation.

HALOPERIDOL DECANOATE
Haldol Decanoate, Various

Pharmacology. Haloperidol decanoate (HD) is the preferred long-acting depot antipsychotic drug. Depot antipsychotics are indicated only for patients who demonstrate good response but are consistently drug-noncompliant with resultant frequent psychotic relapses. Depot antipsychotics provide fewer relapses and hospitalizations, stable serum drug levels, and side effects equal to oral antipsychotic drugs. HD can be given q 4 weeks; **fluphenazine decanoate** (FD) is similar in efficacy and adverse effects, but it must be administered q 2 weeks. Do not use HD or FD to treat acute psychotic symptoms; rather, use the drug only after a patient has been stabilized on an oral antipsychotic drug.[199-203]

Adult Dosage. IM do not exceed an initial HD dosage of 100 mg, with a target monthly dosage 20 times the oral haloperidol daily dosage. An IM loading dose technique has been described that gives 20 times the daily oral dosage, using 100–200 mg of depot q 3–7 days to reach the calculated amount, with a maximum of 450 mg. In geriatric or hepatically impaired patients, use a monthly HD dose of 15 times the oral haloperidol dosage. Experience with HD doses greater than 500 mg is limited; divide injections >5 mL into 2 equal portions given at 2 sites. Oral haloperidol supplementation might be necessary between monthly injections to treat re-emergence of psychotic symptoms until steady-state concentrations are reached.

Dosage Forms. Inj 50, 100 mg/mL.

Pharmacokinetics. After IM administration of HD, esterases cleave the decanoate chain to release the active drug. Peak serum concentrations of haloperidol occur in 3–9 days, with an apparent half-life of 3 weeks; steady-state levels are reached after 12–16 weeks.

Adverse Reactions. There is no evidence that HD causes adverse effects with a frequency different from that of oral haloperidol.

OLANZAPINE   Zyprexa

Pharmacology. Olanzapine is an atypical antipsychotic agent that is a potent serotonin-5HT$_2$ and dopamine-D$_2$ antagonist. It also has anticholinergic and histamine H$_1$-receptor antagonistic effects that might account for some of its side effects.[204,205] (*See* Antipsychotic Drugs Comparison Chart.)

Adult Dosage. **PO for psychotic disorders** 5–10 mg/day initially (5 mg/day in patients >65 yr, debilitated patients, or those with a predisposition to hypotensive reactions). Increase in 5 mg/day increments at ≥7-day intervals. **Usual maintenance dosage** 10–15 mg/day, to a maximum of 20 mg/day, although dosages >10 mg/day are generally no more effective than 10 mg/day. **IM for acute psychosis** 2.5–10 mg/dose has been used investigationally.

Dosage Forms. **Tab** (conventional) 2.5, 5, 7.5, 10, 15 mg; (rapidly dissolving) 5, 10, 15, 20 mg (Zyprexa Zydis); **Inj** (investigational).

Pharmacokinetics. Olanzapine is well absorbed orally; food has no effect, but bioavailability is about 60% because of a first-pass effect. It is 93% bound to plasma proteins and has a V$_d$ of about 1000 L. The drug is hepatically metabolized, probably by CYP1A2 and CYP2D6. Only 7% is excreted unchanged in urine. Its half-life is 30 hr.

Adverse Reactions. Frequent adverse effects include drowsiness, agitation, nervousness, orthostatic hypotension, dizziness, tachycardia, headache, rhinitis, constipation, akathisia, and weight gain. As with other atypical antipsychotic drugs, weight gain is the most troublesome long-term adverse effect, often affecting compliance.

Drug Interactions. Inducers of CYP2D6 may decrease olanzapine serum levels. Olanzapine does not appear to affect cytochrome P450 enzymes.

PIMOZIDE Orap

Pharmacology. Pimozide is indicated for the treatment of Tourette's disorder. Although structurally different from other antipsychotic drugs, pimozide shares their ability to block dopaminergic receptors. Its lack of effect on norepinephrine receptors led to the hope that pimozide would have a more favorable adverse effect profile than other antipsychotic drugs. **Haloperidol** is the drug of choice for Tourette's disorder.[206,207]

Adult Dosage. **PO** 1–2 mg/day in divided doses initially, with dosage increased every other day up to a maximum of 20 mg/day. Most patients who respond require ≤10 mg/day. Periodically decrease the dosage and attempt to withdraw treatment.

Pediatric Dosage. **PO** 0.05 mg/kg/day initially (preferably hs), increasing q 3 days to a maximum of 0.2 mg/kg or 10 mg daily.

Dosage Forms. **Tab** 2 mg.

Pharmacokinetics. Pimozide is about 50% absorbed orally. It undergoes extensive first-pass metabolism in the liver to two metabolites with unknown activity. The elimination half-life averages 55 hr.

Adverse Reactions. The relative frequencies of adverse effects of pimozide and haloperidol are similar, and pimozide remains an alternative to haloperidol for treating Tourette's disorder.

RISPERIDONE Risperdal

Pharmacology. Risperidone is a potent serotonin-5-HT_2 antagonist with dopamine-D_2 antagonism. Whereas typical antipsychotics are dopamine antagonists, the additional serotonin antagonism increases efficacy for negative symptoms of schizophrenia and reduces the likelihood of extrapyramidal symptoms. Initial evidence also suggests that risperidone is more effective than traditional antipsychotic drugs for treatment-resistant schizophrenic patients.[208–211] (*See* Antipsychotic Drugs Comparison Chart.)

Adult Dosage. **PO** 1 mg bid initially (0.5 mg bid in the elderly or patients with severe renal or hepatic impairment), increasing q 2–4 days to the usual effective dosage of 4–6 mg/day in 1 or 2 doses. Occasionally, dosages above 6 mg/day might be necessary, but adverse effects increase and efficacy can be less. The solution can be mixed with water, coffee, orange juice, or low-fat milk; do not mix with cola or tea.

Dosage Forms. **Tab** 0.25, 0.5, 1, 2, 3, 4 mg; **Soln** 1 mg/mL.

Pharmacokinetics. Risperidone is well absorbed orally. The free fraction of risperidone in serum increases in hepatic disease, necessitating lower dosages. It is metabolized by CYP2D6 to an active metabolite. Risperidone's elimination half-life is 3 hr; its active metabolite has a half-life of 24 hr. The half-lives of one or both are prolonged in patients with renal disease.[212]

Adverse Reactions. Frequent dose-related adverse effects are extrapyramidal effects, orthostatic hypotension, headache, rhinitis, and insomnia.

Drug Interactions. Inhibitors of CYP2D6 can increase risperidone levels and have adverse effects.

ZIPRASIDONE HYDROCHLORIDE   Geodon

Pharmacology. Ziprasidone is an atypical antipsychotic drug with a very high ratio of 5-HT_{2A} to dopamine-2 blockade, suggesting a very low risk of extrapyramidal effects. In addition, it is a 5-HT_{1A} agonist like buspirone, and inhibits reuptake of both serotonin and norepinephrine like antidepressants. The clinical value of the latter two effects are not established.[213]

Adult Dosage. **PO as an antipsychotic** 20 mg bid with food initially, increasing as necessary at intervals of at least 2 days to a maximum of 80 mg bid. Maintenance dosage may be as low as 40 mg/day. **IM ziprasidone for acute agitation in a psychotic patient** 10–20 mg, may repeat in 2–4 hr.[213]

Dosage Forms. **Cap** 20, 40, 60, 80 mg; **Inj** investigational.

Patient Instructions. (*See* Antipsychotics Class Instructions.) Take this medication with food.

Pharmacokinetics. Oral bioavailability is 60% when taken with food. With oral twice daily administration, peak blood levels occur at 6–8 hr. Ziprasidone is metabolized by aldehyde oxidase and to a lesser extent by CYP3A4 to inactive metabolites. The elimination half-life is 5–10 hr (range 3–18) for oral ziprasidone and 3 hr for IM ziprasidone. The pharmacokinetics are unaffected by sex, age, or moderate renal or hepatic disease.

Adverse Reactions. Extrapyramidal effects are minimal, but comparative data with other atypical antipsychotic drugs are not available. A major potential advantage of ziprasidone is that it is the least likely atypical antipsychotic drug to cause weight gain.[214] Compared to placebo, the only side effect greater with ziprasidone is sedation. Ziprasidone increases the QT_c interval by up to 14 msec. Ziprasidone should be avoided in patients with pre-existing QT_c prolongation, after acute MI, in severe CHF, and in patients taking other drugs that prolong the QT_c interval. The drug should be discontinued if the QT_c interval is persistently >500 msec.

ANTIPSYCHOTIC DRUGS COMPARISON CHART

DRUG AND CLASS	DOSAGE FORMS	ADULT ORAL DOSAGE RANGE (MG/DAY)	ORAL EQUIVALENT ANTIPSYCHOTIC DOSE (MG)	USUAL SINGLE IM DOSE (MG)	RELATIVE FREQUENCY OF SIDE EFFECTS			
					Sedation	Anticholinergic	Extrapyramidal	Orthostatic Hypotension
LOW POTENCY								
Chlorpromazine Thorazine Various	Soln 30, 100 mg/mL Syrup 2 mg/mL Tab 10, 25, 50, 100, 200 mg Inj 25 mg/mL Supp 25, 100 mg SR Cap not recommended.	50–1200	100	25–50	High	Moderate	Moderate	High
Thioridazine Mellaril Various	Soln 30, 100 mg/mL Susp 5, 20 mg/mL Tab 10, 15, 25, 50, 100, 150 200 mg.	50–800	100	—	High	High	Low	High
INTERMEDIATE POTENCY								
Loxapine Loxitane Various	Cap 5, 10, 25, 50 mg Soln 25 mg/mL Inj 50 mg/mL.	20–250	10	12.5–50	Low	Low	Moderate	Low

(continued)

ANTIPSYCHOTIC DRUGS COMPARISON CHART (*continued*)

DRUG AND CLASS	DOSAGE FORMS	ADULT ORAL DOSAGE RANGE (MG/DAY)	ORAL EQUIVALENT ANTIPSYCHOTIC DOSE (MG)	USUAL SINGLE IM DOSE (MG)	RELATIVE FREQUENCY OF SIDE EFFECTS			
					Sedation	Anticholinergic	Extrapyramidal	Orthostatic Hypotension
Molindone Moban	Tab 5, 10, 25, 50, 100 mg Soln 20 mg/mL.	25–225	10	—	Very Low	Low	Moderate	Low
ATYPICAL								
Clozapine Clozaril	Tab 25, 100 mg.	300–900	50	—	High	High	Very Low	High
Olanzapine Zyprexa	Tab 2.5, 5, 7.5, 10, 15 mg. Inj (Investigational)	10–15	—	2.5–10	Low	Low	Very Low	Low
Quetiapine Seroquel	Tab 25, 100, 200 mg.	150–500	—	—	Moderate	Low	Very Low	Low
Risperidone Risperdal	Tab 0.25, 0.5, 1, 2, 3, 4 mg Soln 1 mg/mL.	4–6[a]	—	—	Very Low	Very Low	Low[a]	Moderate
Ziprasidone Geodon	Cap 20, 40, 60, 80 mg. Inj (Investigational)	40–160	—	10	Moderate	Very Low	Very Low	Low

(continued)

ANTIPSYCHOTIC DRUGS COMPARISON CHART (*continued*)

DRUG AND CLASS	DOSAGE FORMS	ADULT ORAL DOSAGE RANGE (MG/DAY)	ORAL EQUIVALENT ANTIPSYCHOTIC DOSE (MG)	USUAL SINGLE IM DOSE (MG)	RELATIVE FREQUENCY OF SIDE EFFECTS			
					Sedation	Anticholinergic	Extrapyramidal	Orthostatic Hypotension
HIGH POTENCY								
Fluphenazine Permitil Prolixin Various	Elxr 0.5 mg/mL Soln 5 mg/mL Tab 1, 2.5, 5, 10 mg Inj 2.5 mg/mL	2–40	2	2–5	Low	Low	Very High	Low
Fluphenazine Decanoate Prolixin Various	Inj 25 mg/mL	—	—	12.5–75 q 2 weeks	Low	Low	Very High	Low
Haloperidol Haldol Various	Soln 2 mg/mL Tab 0.5, 1, 2, 5, 10, 20 mg Inj 5 mg/mL	2–100	2	2–5	Very Low	Very Low	Very High	Very Low
Haloperidol Decanoate Haldol Decanoate	Inj 50, 100 mg/mL	—	—	50–450 monthly	Very Low	Very Low	Very High	Very Low

(continued)

ANTIPSYCHOTIC DRUGS COMPARISON CHART (*continued*)

DRUG AND CLASS	DOSAGE FORMS	ADULT ORAL DOSAGE RANGE (MG/DAY)	ORAL EQUIVALENT ANTIPSYCHOTIC DOSE (MG)	USUAL SINGLE IM DOSE (MG)	RELATIVE FREQUENCY OF SIDE EFFECTS			
					Sedation	Anticholinergic	Extrapyramidal	Orthostatic Hypotension
Perphenazine Trilafon Various	Soln 3.2 mg/mL Tab 2, 4, 8, 16 mg Inj 5 mg/mL	12–64	8	5–10	Low	Low	High	Low
Trifluoperazine Stelazine Various	Soln 10 mg/mL Tab 1, 2, 5, 10 mg Inj 2 mg/mL	5–40	5	1–2	Low	Low	High	Low
Thiothixene Navane Various	Cap 1, 2, 5, 10, 20 mg Soln 5 mg/mL Inj 5 mg/mL	5–60	4	2–4	Low	Low	High	Low

[a]At dosages over 6 mg/day, nausea and insomnia are limiting side effects; extrapyramidal symptoms markedly increase at dosages over 6 mg/day.
From references 181–183, 192, 196, 200, 201, 209, and 215–219.

469

Anxiolytics, Sedatives, and Hypnotics

Class Instructions. **Sedatives and Hypnotics.** This drug causes drowsiness and can produce sleep. Do not exceed the prescribed dosage and use caution when driving, operating machinery, or performing other tasks requiring mental alertness. Avoid concurrent use of alcohol or other drugs that cause drowsiness or sleep. Do not abruptly stop taking this medication; the dosage must be decreased slowly.

Missed Doses. If you miss a dose, take it as soon as you remember. If it is almost time for your next dose, skip it and resume your normal schedule. Do not double doses.

ALPRAZOLAM
Xanax, Various

Pharmacology. Alprazolam is a triazolobenzodiazepine that is equal in efficacy to other benzodiazepines for generalized anxiety disorder but more effective in the treatment of panic disorder. Although alprazolam has some efficacy in major depression, it is less effective than heterocyclic antidepressants.[220,221] (*See also* Clonazepam, and the Benzodiazepines and Related Drugs Comparison Chart.)

Adult Dosage. **PO for generalized anxiety disorder** 0.25 mg tid initially, increasing gradually to 4 mg/day. **PO for panic disorder** 0.5 mg tid is recommended initially; most panic patients require 5–6 mg/day, and occasionally 10 mg/day can be needed for full response. **SL** alprazolam tablets can be administered SL with no difference from oral administration in onset, peak, or pharmacokinetics.[222] **Discontinuation** decrease the daily dosage by no more than 0.5 mg/day q 3 days until the daily dosage reaches 2 mg and then decrease dosage in 0.25 mg/day increments q 3 days.

Dosage Forms. **Tab** 0.25, 0.5, 1, 2 mg; **Soln** 0.1, 1 mg/mL.

Pharmacokinetics. Like diazepam, alprazolam has a rapid onset of effect after oral administration, but its shorter half-life requires tid administration. The half-life is 11 hr in adults; the elderly might have decreased clearance and an increased half-life of 21 hr.[221–223]

Adverse Reactions. (*See* Benzodiazepines.) Patients do not show complete cross-tolerance between triazolobenzodiazepines and other benzodiazepines, but **clonazepam** has been shown to be an effective long–half-life substitute drug for use in alprazolam withdrawal.[224]

BENZODIAZEPINES

Pharmacology. Benzodiazepines have a more specific anxiolytic effect than other sedatives. Benzodiazepines facilitate the inhibitory effect of GABA on neuronal excitability by increasing membrane permeability to chloride ions.[225]

Administration and Adult Dosage. (*See* Benzodiazepines and Related Drugs Comparison Chart.) Optimal oral use requires individual dosage titration to clinical response. The long-acting drugs can be administered once daily hs; the short-acting drugs require multiple daily doses. (*See* Benzodiazepines and Related Drugs Comparison Chart.) Determine the dosage schedule by the individual patient's relative degree of dysfunction from daytime anxiety compared with insomnia. Despite physiologic dependence, benzodiazepines might need to be used for months and sometimes years for treatment of panic disorder and generalized anxiety disorder; situational anxiety, adjustment disorders, and anxiety secondary to other causes require only days to weeks of drug treatment.[226] **PO for alcohol withdrawal** evidence suggests no superiority of any benzodiazepine in alcohol withdrawal, although **chlordiazepoxide** has been most adequately studied; **(chlordiazepoxide)** 25–100 mg for agitation, anxiety, and tremor; on the first day, up to 400 mg can be given in divided doses, with gradual dosage reductions over 4 days; **(diazepam)** 5–20 mg for agitation, anxiety, and tremor; alternatively, it can be given in 20 mg doses q 2 hr until complete suppression of signs and symptoms is achieved. After this loading dose, further administration is unnecessary;[227] **(oxazepam)** 15–60 mg q 4–6 hr for agitation, anxiety, and tremor. Oxazepam is preferred in patients with severe liver disease. **IM chlordiazepoxide** is not recommended because of slow, erratic absorption; however, **lorazepam** is suitable for IM administration.[141,227] Diazepam injectable solution (Valium, various) can be administered **IM or IV;** the injectable emulsion (Dizac) is for **IV use only** (do not administer IM or SC); neither the solution nor the emulsion should be administered faster than 5 mg/min into a peripheral vein, and small veins should be avoided; neither product is recommended to be added to other drugs or solutions. (*See* Fate.) **PR diazepam for seizures** 0.2 mg/kg of Diastat rectal gel, rounded up to the next dosage size (2.5, 5, 10, 15, 20 mg); an additional dose can be given 4–12 hr after the first dose. Treat no more than 1 episode q 5 days or 5 episodes/month with Diastat.

Special Populations. *Pediatric Dosage.* **PO** (diazepam, >6 months) 1–2.5 mg tid or qid. Most benzodiazepines are not recommended in children because of insufficient clinical experience and concern about the stimulating and paradoxical effects that occur because of disinhibition. **Midazolam** is commonly used in children for preanesthetic sedation. (*See* Midazolam.) **PR diazepam for seizures** (2–5 yr) 0.5 mg/kg of Diastat rectal gel, rounded up to the next dosage size (2.5, 5, 10, 15, 20 mg); (6–11 yr) 0.3 mg/kg of Diastat rectal gel, rounded up to the next dosage size. An additional dose may be given 4–12 hr after the first dose. Treat no more than 1 episode q 5 days or 5 episodes/month with Diastat.

Geriatric Dosage. The elderly might have reduced clearance and enhanced CNS sensitivity, which requires initial dosage to be reduced by 33–50%.[228]

Other Conditions. Higher dosages might be needed in heavy smokers. Patients with liver disease might have reduced clearance and/or enhanced CNS sensitivity, which requires reduction of initial and subsequent doses. Alcoholic patients with reduced plasma proteins might require a lower dosage because of decreased protein binding.

Dosage Forms. (*See* Benzodiazepines and Related Drugs Comparison Chart.)

Patient Instructions. (*See* Sedatives and Hypnotics Class Instructions.)

Pharmacokinetics. *Serum Levels.* Not used clinically.

Fate. Diazepam and chlordiazepoxide are absorbed faster and more completely orally than intramuscularly. Lorazepam and midazolam have rapid and reliable IM absorption.[141,229] (*See* Benzodiazepines and Related Drugs Comparison Chart.)

Adverse Reactions. Frequent effects include drowsiness, dizziness, ataxia, and disorientation; these effects rarely require drug discontinuation and are easily managed by dosage reduction. Anterograde amnesia is frequent.[141] Occasionally, agitation and excitement occur.[230] With parenteral therapy, hypotension and respiratory depression occur occasionally. Rarely, hepatotoxicity or blood dyscrasias occur. Diazepam emulsion is associated with less venous thrombosis and phlebitis than the solution, which can be very irritating to veins.

Contraindications. Acute narrow-angle glaucoma; (diazepam emulsion injection) hypersensitivity to soy protein.

Precautions. Pregnancy; impaired hepatic function. Abrupt drug withdrawal can result in rebound insomnia, abstinence syndrome similar to barbiturate withdrawal, seizures, or, rarely, psychosis. Patients do not show complete cross-tolerance between triazolobenzodiazepines and other benzodiazepines. History of substance abuse can indicate increased likelihood of benzodiazepine misuse.[225]

Drug Interactions. Concurrent use with other CNS depressants can potentiate the sedation caused by benzodiazepines. Nefazodone inhibits alprazolam and triazolam metabolism; fluoxetine and fluvoxamine increase levels of alprazolam and diazepam; omeprazole increases serum diazepam levels.

Parameters to Monitor. Periodically reassess the need for therapy during long-term use.

BUSPIRONE HYDROCHLORIDE BuSpar, Various

Pharmacology. Buspirone is the first of a class of selective serotonin-5-HT$_{1A}$ receptor partial agonists. It also has some effect on dopamine-D$_2$ autoreceptors and, like antidepressants, can downregulate β-adrenergic receptors. Unlike benzodiazepines, it lacks amnestic, anticonvulsant, muscle relaxant, and hypnotic effects. Its exact anxiolytic mechanism of action is complex and not clearly defined.[231,232]

Administration and Adult Dosage. PO for anxiety 5 mg tid or 7.5 mg bid for 1 week, increasing in 5 mg/day increments q 2–3 days to a maximum of 60 mg/day in 2 or 3 divided doses. Most patients require 20–30 mg/day in divided doses.

Special Populations. *Pediatric Dosage.* Safety and efficacy not established.

Geriatric Dosage. Same as adult dosage.

Other Conditions. Decrease the initial dose to 5 mg bid in patients with hepatic or renal impairment.[231,233]

Dosage Forms. **Tab** 5, 7.5, 10, 15 mg.

Patient Instructions. This drug requires several weeks of continuous use for therapeutic effect and is not effective when used intermittently.

Pharmacokinetics. *Onset and Duration.* Onset of anxiolytic effect can take several weeks.

Fate. The drug is well absorbed; oral bioavailability is 3.9 ± 4.3%. Administration after meals increases bioavailability by 80%. It is extensively metabolized by oxidative dealkylation pathways.[234]

$t_{1/2}$. 2.1 ± 1.2 hr.[234]

Adverse Reactions. Dosages >60 mg/day can cause dysphoria.[225] Frequent nausea, dizziness, headache, and insomnia occur. Unlike benzodiazepines, buspirone does not cause dependence or withdrawal effects.[231,235]

Contraindications. None known.

Precautions. Buspirone has no cross-tolerance with benzodiazepines, so patients being switched from a benzodiazepine should have their dosages of the benzodiazepine decreased slowly.

Drug Interactions. Unlike benzodiazepines, buspirone does not interact with alcohol.[231,235] Buspirone can increase haloperidol serum levels. Avoid concurrent buspirone and an MAOI because the combination can cause hypertension.

Parameters to Monitor. Monitor renal and hepatic function initially and periodically during long-term therapy.

Notes. Buspirone is indicated only for the treatment of generalized anxiety disorder and is not effective as a prn medication or hypnotic. Buspirone's anxiolytic effect without sedation or respiratory depression has led to its use in agitation and anxiety, dementia, mental retardation, and spinal cord injury. Its unique effect on the 5-HT$_{1A}$ receptor has led to uncontrolled studies and clinical use for premenstrual tension syndrome and to decrease craving in smoking cessation.[236]

FLUMAZENIL   Romazicon

Pharmacology. Flumazenil is a selective inhibitor of the CNS effects of benzodiazepine sedatives. It competitively blocks the effect of benzodiazepines and zolpidem on GABA-mediated inhibitory pathways within the CNS. Flumazenil finds its greatest use in the reversal of benzodiazepine sedation after medical and surgical procedures and occasionally in the management of benzodiazepine overdose.[237-239]

Adult Dosage. **IV for reversal of conscious sedation** 0.2 mg over 15 sec; this dose can be repeated after 45 sec and every minute thereafter prn, to a total dosage of 1 mg. **IV for benzodiazepine overdose** 0.2 mg over 30 sec, followed, if necessary, by 0.3 mg after 30 sec. Further doses of 0.5 mg over 30 sec can be given at 1-min intervals to a cumulative dosage of 3 mg. Rarely, patients who respond partially to 3 mg respond more completely to a dosage of 5 mg. If resedation occurs after either use, additional doses of up to 1 mg can be given at 20-min intervals to a maximum of 3 mg/hr. Flumazenil does not consistently reverse benzodiazepine amnesia, so give patients written instructions to avoid operation of motor vehicles or hazardous equipment, or ingestion of alcohol or nonprescription medications for 18–24 hr, or longer if benzodiazepine effects persist.

Dosage Forms. **Inj** 0.1 mg/mL.

Pharmacokinetics. Reversal of benzodiazepine coma can occur within 1–2 min and last 1–5 hr, depending on the dosages of the benzodiazepine and flumazenil.

First-pass hepatic metabolism limits the bioavailability of oral flumazenil, so the drug is administered by IV injection. It is rapidly hydroxylated in the liver to inactive metabolites. V_d is 0.6–1.6 L/kg; its elimination half-life is 0.7–1.3 hr.

Adverse Reactions. Frequent side effects have been minimal and are usually limited to nausea and vomiting, anxiety, and agitation. However, seizures have occurred, most often in patients on long-term benzodiazepine therapy or after overdose with heterocyclic antidepressants or other potentially convulsant drugs (eg, bupropion, cocaine, cyclosporine, isoniazid, lithium, methylxanthines, MAOIs, propoxyphene). Be prepared to manage seizures before giving flumazenil.[240]

MIDAZOLAM HYDROCHLORIDE   Versed

Pharmacology. Midazolam is a short-acting triazolobenzodiazepine for use in anesthesia. It is unique in its physicochemical properties; at a pH under 4 the drug exists as a highly water-soluble, stable compound, but at physiologic pH, it becomes lipophilic. This allows IV administration of a water-soluble, rapidly acting drug with a very low frequency of venous irritation. Midazolam is given IM for preoperative sedation and IV for induction of anesthesia or for conscious sedation for endoscopy and other procedures.[241-243]

Adult Dosage. **IM for preoperative sedation** 0.07–0.08 mg/kg (about 5 mg) 1 hr before surgery. **IV for endoscopy and other conscious sedation procedures** dosage must be individualized and not administered by rapid bolus. Titrate slowly to desired effect; some patients might respond to as little as 1 mg. Give no more than 2.5 mg over at least 2 min as the 1 mg/mL (or more dilute) solution; in elderly, debilitated, or chronically ill patients, limit the initial dose to 1.5 mg. Further small doses can be given after waiting at least 2 min. Do not give the drug IV without oxygen and resuscitation equipment immediately available.

Pediatric Dosage. **PO for sedation** (6 mo–16 yr) 0.25–1 mg/kg (usually 0.5 mg/kg) to a maximum of 20 mg. **PR for preanesthetic sedation** 0.3 mg/kg as a solution diluted in 5 mL of saline is a safe and effective alternative to IM administration.[244]

Dosage Forms. **Inj** 1, 5 mg/mL; **Syrup** 2 mg/mL.

Pharmacokinetics. Midazolam is >90% absorbed after IM injection; peak serum levels occur within 30 min. Peak levels after IM administration are about 50% of IV levels. PO onset is 10–20 min; IM onset is about 15 min. The drug is 97% bound to plasma proteins and has a V_d of 1–3 L/kg; Cl is 0.25–0.54 L/hr/kg. Midazolam is hepatically metabolized via CYP3A4 to the 1-hydroxy- and 4-hydroxy-metabolites; the 1-hydroxy-metabolite is at least as active as midazolam. Midazolam's half-life is 1.8–6.4 hr.

Adverse Reactions. Respiratory depression and respiratory arrest occur frequently. Impairment of psychomotor skills continues after acute sedation has passed, so patients should not drive or operate machinery until it is clear that they have recovered fully.

TRIAZOLAM
Halcion, Various

Pharmacology. Triazolam is a triazolobenzodiazepine hypnotic whose effect is likely related to its facilitation of GABA-mediated neurotransmission, but its exact mechanism is unknown.

Administration and Adult Dosage. (*See* Benzodiazepines and Related Drugs Comparison Chart.) **PO as a hypnotic** 0.25 mg hs initially; do not exceed 0.5 mg.

Special Populations. *Pediatric Dosage.* (<18 yr) safety and efficacy not established.

Geriatric Dosage. **PO** decrease initial dose to 0.125 mg, increase if necessary to 0.25 mg hs.[245,246]

Other Conditions. **PO** 0.125 mg initially in debilitated patients and those with low body weights or with hepatic impairment.

Dosage Forms. **Tab** 0.125, 0.25 mg.

Patient Instructions. (*See* Sedatives and Hypnotics Class Instructions.)

Pharmacokinetics. *Onset and Duration.* Onset of hypnotic effect is 0.5–1 hr, with peak serum levels achieved within 2 hr.

Fate. Oral bioavailability 44%, SL 53%, because of nonhepatic presystemic metabolism. V_d is 1.2 ± 0.5 L/kg; Cl is 0.34 ± 0.2 L/hr/kg. Cl decreases with advancing age (attributed to reduced hepatic oxidizing capacity in the elderly). Triazolam undergoes hydroxylation and rapid conjugation. Smoking does not affect elimination.[118,247] Accumulation does not occur with multiple doses.

$t_{1/2}$. 2.6 ± 1 hr. Half-life is not affected by end-stage renal disease or liver disease.[118,247,248]

Adverse Reactions. Frequently, anterograde amnesia,[249] daytime anxiety, and ataxia occur. Occasionally, agitation, confusion, or mood disturbance occur. Rarely, respiratory depression, depersonalization, and derealization, or psychosis occur. Unlike other benzodiazepines, several fatalities have been reported in elderly patients who overdosed on triazolam.[250,251]

Contraindications. Pregnancy.

Precautions. Pregnancy; impaired hepatic function. Abrupt drug withdrawal can result in rebound insomnia, abstinence syndrome similar to barbiturate withdrawal, seizures, or, rarely, psychosis. Patients do not show complete cross-tolerance between triazolam and other benzodiazepines. History of substance abuse can indicate an increased likelihood of triazolam misuse.[225] Do not prescribe the drug for more than 7–10 days of consecutive therapy or in quantities larger than a 30-day supply.

Drug Interactions. Concurrent use with other CNS depressants can potentiate the sedation caused by benzodiazepines. Nefazodone inhibits triazolam metabolism.

Notes. Compared with other benzodiazepine hypnotics, triazolam is equally effective in reducing sleep latency and less likely to cause daytime sedation; however, it is less likely to prevent early morning awakening and more likely to cause rebound insomnia. Hypnotic drugs are most effective when used to treat transient situational insomnia (1–3 days) and short-term insomnia (1–3 weeks maximum).[251,252]

ZALEPLON
Sonata

Pharmacology. Zaleplon is a nonbenzodiazepine hypnotic that, like zolpidem, selectively binds only to the ω_1 receptor. This selectivity suggests a sedative effect with less potential for memory impairment, interaction with alcohol, and psychomotor effects than with benzodiazepines.[253]

Administration and Adult Dosage. **PO as a hypnotic** 10 mg hs initially (5 mg in the elderly). Because of its very rapid onset and offset, zaleplon can be given during the night after the patient experiences difficulty falling asleep rather than being given before bedtime in anticipation of sleep difficulty. Zaleplon can be given during the night without morning hangover as long as there are 4 hr remaining in bed after administration.

Dosage Forms. **Cap** 5, 10 mg.

Pharmacokinetics. After oral administration, zaleplon reaches peak serum concentrations in 1.1 hr. Zaleplon is metabolized by CYP3A4 but has no active metabolites. Its half-life is 0.8–1.4 hr (average 1).[254]

Adverse Reactions. Dose-related side effects include dizziness, headache, and somnolence. Symptoms begin to appear approximately 30 min after a dose, peak at 1–2 hr, and are no longer evident at 4 hr. After a 10-mg dose, zaleplon has no residual effects on performance and memory tests after 2 hr; in contrast, residual effects persist for up to 5 hr with zolpidem.[255]

ZOLPIDEM TARTRATE
Ambien

Pharmacology. Zolpidem is a short-acting nonbenzodiazepine hypnotic indicated for the short-term treatment of insomnia. Most benzodiazepines bind to all GABA-benzodiazepine (ω) receptor complexes, but zolpidem selectively binds only to the ω_1 receptor. This difference suggests a more selective sedative–hypnotic effect without anxiolytic, anticonvulsant, or muscle relaxant effects.[256–258] (*See* Benzodiazepines and Related Drugs Comparison Chart.)

Adult Dosage. **PO as a hypnotic** 10 mg immediately before bedtime. In the elderly, patients with hepatic impairment, or patients taking other CNS depressants, the dose is 5 mg.

Dosage Forms. **Tab** 5, 10 mg.

Pharmacokinetics. After oral administration, zolpidem reaches peak serum concentrations in 1.6 hr, is 93% bound to plasma proteins, has no active metabolites, and has an elimination half-life of 1.5–4 hr (average 2.5). Half-life is increased by one-third in the elderly and greatly increased in patients with hepatic impairment (9.9 hr).

Adverse Reactions. Dose-related side effects include daytime drowsiness, dizziness, and diarrhea. Clinical trials with 20 mg doses have reported headache, nausea, memory problems, and CNS stimulation. Tolerance has not been reported, nor has rebound insomnia after therapeutic doses. Psychomotor performance is impaired when zolpidem is combined with alcohol. Efficacy has been demonstrated for 35 nights at doses of 10 mg without affecting sleep stages or psychomotor performance.

BENZODIAZEPINES AND RELATED DRUGS COMPARISON CHART

DRUG AND SCHEDULE[a]	DOSAGE FORMS	ADULT ORAL DOSAGE RANGE	PEAK ORAL SERUM LEVELS (HR)	HALF-LIFE (HR)[b]
SHORT-ACTING ANXIOLYTICS				
Alprazolam (C-IV) Xanax Various	Tab 0.25, 0.5, 1, 2 mg Soln 0.1, 1 mg/mL.	0.75–4 mg/day[c] 5–10 mg/day[d]	0.7–1.6	11–21
Lorazepam[e] (C-IV) Ativan Various	Tab 0.5, 1, 2 mg Soln 2 mg/mL Inj 2, 4 mg/mL.	2–10 mg/day	2	10–20
Oxazepam (C-IV) Serax Various	Cap 10, 15, 30 mg Tab 15 mg.	30–120 mg/day	1–2	5–15
LONG-ACTING ANXIOLYTICS				
Chlordiazepoxide (C-IV) Librium Libritabs Various	Cap 5, 10, 25 mg Tab 10, 25 mg Inj 100 mg.	15–100 mg/day	2–4	>24
Clorazepate (C-IV) Tranxene Various	Cap 3.75, 7.5, 15 mg Tab 3.75, 7.5, 15 mg SR Tab 11.25, 22.5 mg.	15–60 mg/day	1–2[f]	>24
Diazepam (C-IV) Dizac Valium Various	Tab 2, 5, 10 mg Soln 1, 5 mg/mL Inj 5 mg/mL.	6–40 mg/day	1–2	>24
Halazepam (C-IV) Paxipam	Tab 20, 40 mg.	60–160 mg/day	1–3	>24
SHORT-ACTING HYPNOTICS				
Midazolam[e] (C-IV) Versed	Inj 1, 5 mg/mL Syrup 2 mg/mL.	—	—	1.5–3
Triazolam (C-IV) Halcion Various	Tab 0.125, 0.25 mg.	0.125–0.25 mg	0.5–2	1.5–3.6
Zaleplon[g] (C-IV) Sonata	Cap 5, 10 mg.	10 mg	1.1	0.8–1.4
Zolpidem[g] (C-IV) Ambien	Tab 5, 10 mg.	5–20 mg	2	1.5–4

(continued)

BENZODIAZEPINES AND RELATED DRUGS COMPARISON CHART (*continued*)

DRUG AND SCHEDULE[a]	DOSAGE FORMS	ADULT ORAL DOSAGE RANGE	PEAK ORAL SERUM LEVELS (HR)	HALF-LIFE (HR)[b]
INTERMEDIATE-ACTING HYPNOTICS				
Estazolam (C-IV) Pro-Som Various	Tab 1, 2 mg.	1–2 mg	1–2	12–15
Temazepam (C-IV) Restoril Various	Cap 7.5, 15, 30 mg.	7.5–30 mg	2–3	10–15
LONG-ACTING HYPNOTICS				
Flurazepam (C-IV) Dalmane Various	Cap 15, 30 mg.	15–30 mg	h	>24[b]
Quazepam (C-IV) Doral	Tab 7.5, 15 mg.	7.5–15 mg	1–2	>24[b]

[a]Controlled substance schedule designated after each drug (in parentheses).
[b]Parent drug plus active metabolites.
[c]For generalized anxiety disorder.
[d]For panic disorder.
[e]Also used as an IV anesthetic; well absorbed IM.
[f]Hydrolyzed to nordazepam (desmethyldiazepam) before absorption.
[g]Not a benzodiazepine chemically, but an imidazopyridine, which is a selective benzodiazepine-1 receptor agonist.
[h]Rapidly and completely metabolized to desalkylflurazepam.
From references 221, 222, 225, 229, 241, 247, 249, and 258–262.

SEDATIVES AND HYPNOTICS COMPARISON CHART

DRUG AND SCHEDULE[a]	DOSAGE FORMS	ADULT ORAL DOSAGE	HALF-LIFE (HR)
SEDATIVES			
Meprobamate (C-IV) Equanil Miltown Various	Tab 200, 400, 600 mg SR Cap 200, 400 mg.	400 mg tid or qid or 600 mg bid	6–16
Phenobarbital (C-IV) Various	Cap 16 mg Elxr 3, 4 mg/mL Tab 8, 15, 16, 30, 60, 90, 100 mg Inj 30, 60, 65, 130 mg/mL.	15–30 mg bid–qid	48–120
HYPNOTICS			
Chloral Hydrate (C-IV) Noctec Various	Cap 500 mg Supp 325, 500, 650 mg Syrup 50, 100 mg/mL.	500 mg–1.5 g	8 (Trichloro-ethanol)
Ethchlorvynol (C-IV) Placidyl Various	Cap 200, 500, 750 mg.	500 mg–1 g	6
Glutethimide (C-II) Various	Tab 250 mg.	250–500 mg	5–22
Pentobarbital (C-II) Nembutal Various	Cap 50, 100 mg Elxr 4 mg/mL Supp 30, 60, 120, 200 mg (C-III) Inj 50 mg/mL.	100–200 mg	21–42
Secobarbital (C-II) Seconal Various	Cap 100 mg	100–200 mg	19–34

[a]Controlled substance schedule designated after each drug (in parentheses).
From references 251, 252, 262, and 263.

Lithium

| **LITHIUM CARBONATE** | Various |
| **LITHIUM CITRATE** | Cibalith-S, Lithonate-S |

Pharmacology. Lithium's mechanism of antimanic effect is unknown; it alters the actions of several second-messenger systems (eg, adenylate cyclase and phosphoinositol).[264,265]

Administration and Adult Dosage. Individualize dosage according to serum levels and clinical response. Acute manic episodes typically require **PO** 1.2–2.4 g/day; **maintenance therapy** requires 900 mg–1.5 g/day. A **loading dose** of 30 mg/kg, in 3 divided doses, can be given to achieve the desired serum level within 12 hr.[266] A number of predictive dosage techniques have been developed based on estimated steady state after one serum level.[267,268]

Special Populations. *Pediatric Dosage.* **PO** (<12 yr) 15–20 mg (0.4–0.5 mEq)/kg/day in 2–3 divided doses; (12–18 yr) same as adult dosage.[269]

Geriatric Dosage. (>65 yr) decrease adult dosage by 33–50%.[270]

Other Conditions. Adjust the dosage more carefully in patients with decreased renal function and in patients receiving thiazide diuretics or NSAIDs.

Dosage Forms. **Cap** 150, 300, 600 mg; **Tab** 300 mg; **SR Tab** 300, 450 mg; **Syrup** 1.6 mEq/mL (as citrate).

Patient Instructions. This drug can be taken with food, milk, or antacid to minimize stomach upset. Report immediately if signs of toxicity occur, such as persistent diarrhea, vomiting, coarse hand tremor, drowsiness, or slurred speech, or before beginning any diet. In hot weather, ensure adequate water and salt intake.

Pharmacokinetics. *Onset and Duration.* Onset 7–10 days for therapeutic effect.[141]

Serum Levels. (Acute mania or hypomania) 0.8–1.5 mEq/L; (prophylaxis) 0.6–1.2 mEq/L, although concern about long-term renal effects suggests most patients should be maintained <0.9 mEq/L. Levels >1.5 mEq/L are regularly associated with some signs of toxicity, and levels >2 mEq/L result in serious toxicity.[271] (*See* Adverse Reactions.)

Fate. Absorption is virtually complete within 8 hr after oral administration, with peak levels occurring in 2–4 hr. Distribution is throughout total body water, but tissue uptake is not uniform. The drug is not protein bound or metabolized, but freely filtered through the glomerulus, with about 80% being reabsorbed.

$t_{1/2}$. 18–20 hr; up to 36 hr in the elderly.[141]

Adverse Reactions. Frequent, dose-related effects with therapeutic serum levels include nausea, diarrhea, polyuria, polydipsia, fine hand tremor, and muscle weakness. Signs of toxicity include coarse hand tremor, persistent GI effects, muscle hyperirritability, slurred speech, confusion, stupor, seizures, increased deep tendon reflexes, irregular pulse, and coma. Frequent, non–dose-related effects include nontoxic goiter, hypothyroidism, nephrogenic diabetes insipidus-like syndrome, folliculitis, aggravation of acne or psoriasis, leukocytosis, hypercalcemia, and weight gain.[272,273]

Contraindications. Pregnancy; fluctuating renal function; severe renal or cardiovascular disease.

Precautions. Use with caution in patients with cardiac disease, dehydration, sodium depletion, diuretic therapy, or dementia, in nursing mothers, and in the elderly. (*See* Special Populations.)

Drug Interactions. ACE inhibitors can increase serum lithium concentrations. Theophylline or excess sodium enhance renal lithium clearance; sodium deficiency can promote lithium retention and increase risk of toxicity. Long-term diuretic or NSAID use can result in decreased lithium elimination. Haloperidol can increase the CNS toxicity of lithium; with methyldopa or phenytoin, signs of lithium toxicity can occur without increased serum lithium.

Parameters to Monitor. Prelithium workup should include thyroid function tests, Cr_s, BUN, CBC (for baseline WBC count), urinalysis (for baseline specific gravity), electrolytes, and ECG (if patient is older than 40 yr). During therapy, obtain serum lithium levels (drawn 12 hr after last dose) weekly during initiation and monthly during maintenance.[274,275]

Notes. Divalproex sodium is equivalent in efficacy to lithium for bipolar disorder and more effective than lithium for rapid-cycling bipolar illness.[276–278]

Neurodegenerative Disease Drugs

AMANTADINE
Symmetrel, Various

Pharmacology. Amantadine is an antiviral compound that prevents the release of viral nucleic acid into the host cell. In Parkinson's disease, the drug increases presynaptic dopamine release, blocks the reuptake of dopamine into the presynaptic neurons, and exerts anticholinergic effects. Amantadine also can reduce levodopa-induced dyskinesias in patients with Parkinson's disease, possibly by acting as an *N*-methyl-*D*-aspartate receptor antagonist.[279,280]

Administration and Adult Dosage. PO for Parkinson's disease, give 100 mg/day initially, increasing in 100 mg/day increments q 7–14 days to effective dosage, or to a maximum of 300 mg/day in divided doses. **Usual maintenance dosage** 100 mg bid. **PO for extrapyramidal reactions** 100 mg bid, to a maximum of 300 mg/day in 3 divided doses. **PO for prophylaxis of influenza A** 200 mg/day in 1–2 divided doses continuing for at least 10 days after exposure, for 2–3 weeks after giving influenza A vaccine, or for up to 90 days when vaccine is unavailable or contraindicated. **PO for treatment of influenza A** 200 mg/day in 1–2 divided doses starting within 24–48 hr after onset of illness and continuing for 24–48 hr after symptoms disappear.

Special Populations. *Pediatric Dosage.* **PO for prophylaxis or treatment of influenza A** (<1 yr) safety and efficacy not established; (1–9 yr) 4.4–8.8 mg/kg/day in 2 divided doses, to a maximum of 150 mg/day; (9–12 yr) 100 mg bid. For prophylaxis, continue therapy for at least 10 days after exposure, for 2–3 days after giving influenza A vaccine, or for up to 90 days when vaccine is unavailable or contraindicated. For treatment, continue for 24–48 hr after symptoms disappear.

Geriatric Dosage. **PO for influenza prophylaxis or treatment** (>65 yr) 100 mg/day. **PO for Parkinson's disease** same as adult dosage, adjusting for renal impairment.

Other Conditions. Reduce dosage in renal impairment as follows: with Cl_{cr} of 30–50 mL/min, give 200 mg first day and then 100 mg/day; with Cl_{cr} of 15–29 mL/min, give 200 mg first day and then 100 mg every other day; with Cl_{cr} <15 mL/min or for patients on hemodialysis, give 200 mg q 7 days.

Dosage Forms. **Cap** 100 mg; **Syrup** 10 mg/mL.

Patient Instructions. This medication can cause dizziness, confusion, or difficulty in concentrating. Until the extent of these effects is known, use caution when driving, operating machinery, or performing other tasks requiring mental alertness. Avoid excessive concurrent use of alcohol. **Parkinson's disease** Stopping this medication suddenly can cause your Parkinson's disease to worsen.

Missed Doses. Take this drug at regular intervals. If you miss a dose, take it as soon as you remember. If it is about time for the next dose, take that dose only. Do not double the dose or take extra.

Pharmacokinetics. *Onset and Duration.* Antiparkinson effects disappear in most patients after 6–12 weeks of therapy.[281]

Serum Levels. (Therapeutic trough, antiviral) 300 μg/L (2 μmol/L).

Fate. Peak serum levels occur in 1–4 hr in young adults, 4.5–7 hr in older adults. Steady-state serum levels occur in healthy volunteers and Parkinson's patients within 4–7 days;[282] V_d is 6.6 ± 1.5 L/kg; Cl is 0.39 ± 0.13 L/hr/kg with normal renal function. From 78% to 88% is excreted unchanged in urine.[283]

$t_{1/2}$. (Healthy young adults) 11.8 ± 2.1 hr,[284] (elderly adults) 31 ± 7.2 hr,[285] (during chronic hemodialysis) 8.3 ± 1.5 days.[284]

Adverse Reactions. Nausea, dizziness, insomnia, confusion, hallucinations, anxiety, restlessness, depression, irritability, peripheral edema, orthostatic hypotension, or livedo reticularis occur frequently. Occasionally, CHF, psychosis, urinary retention, or reversible elevation of liver enzymes can occur. Seizures, corneal opacities, or leukopenia rarely occur.

Drug Interactions. Amantadine can potentiate the CNS effects of anticholinergic agents.

Precautions. Pregnancy; lactation. Use with caution in patients with CHF, seizures, renal or hepatic disease, peripheral edema, orthostatic hypotension, psychosis, or history of eczematoid rash or in those receiving CNS stimulants. Abrupt drug discontinuation in patients with Parkinson's disease can result in rapid clinical deterioration. Observe patients carefully when dosages of amantadine are reduced abruptly or discontinued, especially if patients are receiving neuroleptics. Sporadic cases of neuroleptic malignant syndrome have been reported in association with amantadine withdrawal or dosage reduction. Suicide attempts have been reported in patients treated with amantadine, including short influenza treatment, and in patients with and without psychiatric histories. Amantadine can exacerbate mental problems in patients with psychiatric disorders.

Parameters to Monitor. Monitor renal function and disease symptoms periodically in parkinsonian patients.

Notes. In Parkinson's disease, amantadine is indicated as initial treatment alone or in combination with **levodopa**. Amantadine produces clinical improvements in akinesia and rigidity, but to a lesser degree than levodopa.[281,282] Amantadine also can be beneficial in Parkinson's disease patients with nighttime monoclonus, freezing, or dystonia. There is no evidence that amantadine alters the course of Parkinson's disease. **Anticholinergics** appear to reduce tremor to a greater degree than amantadine.

    Rimantadine (Flumadine) is an antiviral compound with efficacy similar to amantadine against influenza A. It appears to be slightly better tolerated than amantadine. Dosage is 100 mg bid in adults. In elderly nursing home patients or those with severe hepatic dysfunction or renal failure ($Cl_{cr} \leq 10$ mL/min), reduce dosage to 100 mg/day. In children younger than 10 yr (prophylaxis only), give 5 mg/kg once daily, not to exceed 150 mg. For children 10 yr and older, use the adult dose. Available as 100 mg tablets and 10 mg/mL syrup.

BENZTROPINE MESYLATE
Cogentin

Pharmacology. Benztropine is a synthetic competitive antagonist of acetylcholine. In Parkinson's disease, the drug reduces the relative excess of cholinergic activity in the basal ganglia that develops because of absolute dopamine deficiency in this area.

Administration and Adult Dosage. PO, IM, or IV for Parkinson's disease 0.5–1 mg/day initially, increasing in 0.5 mg/day increments q 5–6 days to effective dosage, to a maximum of 6 mg/day. **Usual maintenance dosage** 1–2 mg/day in 2–3 divided doses. When used concurrently with levodopa, the dosages of both drugs might require reduction. **PO, IM, or IV for drug-induced extrapyramidal disorders** 1–4 mg/day in 1–2 doses.

Special Populations. *Pediatric Dosage.* (<3 yr) contraindicated; (>3 yr) 0.02–0.05 mg/kg/dose once or twice daily.

Geriatric Dosage. Same as adult dosage, although older patients often can be controlled with 1–2 mg/day. Some consider it best to avoid this drug in the elderly.[286]

Dosage Forms. Tab 0.5, 1, 2 mg; **Inj** 1 mg/mL.

Patient Instructions. This drug can cause constipation, difficult or painful urination, dry mouth, blurred vision, or drowsiness. Use caution when driving, operating machinery, or performing other tasks requiring mental alertness. Avoid excessive concurrent use of alcohol and other drugs that cause drowsiness.

Missed Doses. Take this drug at regular intervals. If you miss a dose, take it as soon as you remember. If it is about time for the next dose, take that dose only. Do not double the dose or take extra.

Pharmacokinetics. *Onset and Duration.* Onset of resolution of drug-induced extrapyramidal symptoms is within 15 min after IV or IM administration and 1–2 hr after oral administration. Duration is 24 hr.[269]

Fate. Benztropine pharmacokinetics are not well studied, but the drug apparently is hepatically metabolized to conjugates and might undergo enterohepatic recycling.[287]

Adverse Reactions. Frequent adverse effects are dose related and include dry mouth, blurred vision, nausea, dizziness, constipation, nervousness, and urinary retention. Confusional states, impairment of recent memory, and hallucinations occur with use of high doses and in patients with advanced age and underlying dementia. Rarely, paralytic ileus, parotitis, hyperthermia, or skin rash occurs.

Contraindications. Children <3 yr; narrow-angle glaucoma; pyloric or duodenal obstruction; stenosing peptic ulcers; achalasia; bladder-neck obstructions; myasthenia gravis; cognitive disturbances.[286]

Precautions. Pregnancy; elderly patients. Use with caution in hot weather or during exercise and in patients with tachycardia, prostatic hypertrophy, open-angle glaucoma, or obstructive diseases of the GI tract.

Drug Interactions. Carefully observe patients given concomitant phenothiazines and/or heterocyclic antidepressants because intensification of mental symptoms, paralytic ileus, or hyperthermia can occur. Anticholinergics can decrease the effectiveness of phenothiazines. Use with amantadine can result in increased CNS anticholinergic effects. Anticholinergics can decrease digoxin absorption from digoxin tablets.

Parameters to Monitor. Intraocular pressure monitoring and gonioscope evaluation periodically. Monitor for Parkinson's disease symptoms periodically.

Notes. Anticholinergic agents are considered useful for the initial treatment of parkinsonism in patients ≤60 yr with a rest tremor and without akinesia or rigidity.[281,282] The drug does not alleviate the symptoms of tardive dyskinesia.

CARBIDOPA AND LEVODOPA   Sinemet

Pharmacology. Levodopa is centrally converted to dopamine by DOPA decarboxylase and replenishes dopamine, which is deficient in the basal ganglia of patients with Parkinson's disease. Carbidopa, which does not cross the blood–brain barrier, inhibits peripheral DOPA decarboxylase, thereby increasing the amount of levodopa available to the brain for conversion to dopamine and limiting peripheral side effects. Addition of carbidopa decreases levodopa-induced nausea and vomiting but does not decrease adverse reactions caused by the central effects of levodopa.[288]

Administration and Adult Dosage. **PO for Parkinson's disease in patients not receiving levodopa (standard formulation)** 25 mg carbidopa/100 mg levodopa tid initially, increasing in 1 tablet/day increments q 1–2 days to effective dosage, to a maximum of 8 tablets/day. Alternatively, 10 mg carbidopa/100 mg levodopa tid or qid initially, to a maximum of 8 tablets/day. Initial use of 10 mg carbidopa/100 mg levodopa can result in more nausea and vomiting because 70–100 mg/day of carbidopa is needed to saturate peripheral DOPA decarboxylase. If initial dosage maximum is reached with 10/100 tablets and further titration is necessary, substitute 25 mg carbidopa/250 mg levodopa tid or qid, increasing in 0.5–1 tablet/day increments q 1–2 days to effective dosage, to a maximum of

8 tablets/day. Some long-term users with advanced disease might need >2 g/day.[286] **SR Tab** (patients already taking non-SR tablets) start with a dosage that provides 10% more levodopa daily. Initially, divide dosage bid or tid with an interval of 4–8 hr between doses while awake. Ultimately, dosages up to 30% greater might be needed, depending on patient response; (patients not receiving carbidopa/levodopa) 1 tablet bid initially, at least 6 hr apart, and allow 3 days between dosage adjustments. **Usual dosage** 2–8 tablets/day. If given in combination with a dopamine agonist or selegiline, lower dosages can be effective.

Special Populations. *Pediatric Dosage.* (<18 yr) safety and efficacy not established.

Geriatric Dosage. Same as adult dosage.

Dosage Forms. **Tab** 10 mg carbidopa/100 mg levodopa, 25 mg carbidopa/100 mg levodopa, 25 mg carbidopa/250 mg levodopa; **SR Tab** 25 mg carbidopa/100 mg levodopa, 50 mg carbidopa/200 mg levodopa. (*See* Notes.)

Patient Instructions. Stopping this medication suddenly can cause Parkinson's disease to worsen quickly. Report bothersome or unexpected side effects. Unless prescribed, do not take levodopa in addition to this drug. Avoid pyridoxine (vitamin B_6) if you are taking levodopa alone, although it can be taken with carbidopa/levodopa. Avoid high-protein meals for maximum absorption. If you are taking the sustained-release tablet, swallow a whole or one-half tablet without chewing or crushing it. Onset of effect of the first morning dose of the sustained-release product could be delayed up to 1 hour compared with the quick-release product. A dark color (red, brown, or black) might appear in saliva, urine, or sweat and can stain clothing.

Missed Doses. Take this drug at regular intervals. If you miss a dose, take it as soon as you remember. If it is about time for the next dose, take that dose only. Do not double the dose or take extra.

Pharmacokinetics. *Onset and Duration.* Up to 50% of patients experience a reduction in efficacy after 5 yr.[289] (*See* Notes.)

Fate. Carbidopa's inhibition of peripheral levodopa decarboxylation doubles the oral bioavailability of levodopa and decreases its clearance by one-half.[289–291] Dietary proteins compete with levodopa for intestinal absorption and decrease its effectiveness. (Rapid-release 50 mg carbidopa/200 mg levodopa) levodopa bioavailability is 99 ± 21%. A peak of 3.2 ± 1.1 mg/L occurs in 0.7 ± 0.3 hr.[292] (SR 50 mg carbidopa/200 mg levodopa) levodopa bioavailability is 71 ± 24% and increases with food. A peak of 1.14 ± 0.42 mg/L occurs in 2.4 ± 1.2 hr.[292] Levodopa V_d is 1.09 ± 0.59 L/kg; Cl is 0.28 ± 0.06 L/hr/kg; 90% of clearance is nonrenal.[293]

$t_{1/2}$. (Carbidopa) 2.1 ± 0.6 hr;[292] (levodopa alone) 1.4 ± 0.3 hr; (levodopa with carbidopa) 2 ± 1.3 hr.[293]

Adverse Reactions. Anorexia, nausea, vomiting, and involuntary muscle movements (dyskinesias) occur frequently and are generally reversible with dosage reduction. Occasionally, mental changes, depression, dementia, palpitations, or orthostatic hypotensive episodes, increased libido, and bullous lesions occur. Rarely, psychosis, hemolytic anemia, leukopenia, or agranulocytosis is reported.

Compared with levodopa alone, carbidopa/levodopa has markedly reduced GI and cardiovascular side effects. However, mental disturbances are not eliminated and dyskinesias can appear earlier in therapy. These dyskinesias might require a decrease in dosage or dosage interval.[289,291] Side effects can be more pronounced in patients receiving **selegiline** or a dopamine agonist as adjunctive therapy.

Contraindications. Lactation; nonselective MAO inhibitors concurrently or 2 weeks before carbidopa/levodopa; narrow-angle glaucoma; undiagnosed skin lesions; history of melanoma.

Precautions. Pregnancy. Use with caution in patients with histories of MI complicated by arrhythmias; peptic ulcer disease; severe cardiovascular, pulmonary, renal, hepatic, or endocrine disease; open-angle glaucoma; bronchial asthma; urinary retention; or psychosis. Also, use caution in patients receiving antihypertensives. Symptoms resembling neuroleptic malignant syndrome can occur when carbidopa/levodopa in combination with other antiparkinson agents is reduced abruptly or discontinued.

Drug Interactions. Iron salts, including low doses in multivitamins, can decrease levodopa absorption. Other agents for Parkinson's disease, such as dopamine agonists, COMT inhibitors, and selegiline, can increase levodopa side effects when added to carbidopa/levodopa. Dosage of the levodopa product might need to be reduced by 10–30%. Metoclopramide and older neuroleptics (eg, chlorpromazine, haloperidol) have antidopaminergic effects and oppose the action of levodopa. Atypical neuroleptics have less antidopaminergic effect (clozapine has the least) but still can reduce the effectiveness of Parkinson's disease therapy. Cholinergic agents such as tacrine, donepezil, and rivastigmine can worsen Parkinson's symptoms by changing the dopamine–acetylcholine balance in the brain. Bupropion elicits a higher frequency of side effects in patients taking levodopa. Administer bupropion with caution, using small initial doses and small, gradual increases. There are rare reports of adverse reactions, including hypertension and dyskinesias, resulting from the concomitant use of TCAs and levodopa. Isoniazid, phenytoin, and papaverine can decrease the therapeutic effects of levodopa.

Parameters to Monitor. Monitor CBC, renal, cardiovascular, and liver functions periodically during long-term therapy. Monitor symptoms of Parkinson's disease periodically. In patients with open-angle glaucoma, monitor intraocular pressure.

Notes. Levodopa produces sustained improvement in rigidity and bradykinesia in 50–60% of patients.[289] Tremor is variably affected, and postural stability is unresponsive.[281,282] Loss of therapeutic effect is manifested by fluctuations in motor performance. Patients can experience periods of lack of drug effect ("off" periods) alternating with periods of therapeutic efficacy ("on" periods). Response can be predictable, where the effect fades before the next dose ("wearing-off" or "end-of-dose"), or unpredictable ("yo-yo"), where there is no relation to the time of dose.[288] SR carbidopa/levodopa reduces "off" time an average of 30–40 min/day and allows a mean 33% reduction in the frequency of administration; the lower bioavailability of the SR product necessitates a 25% median increase in the daily dosage of levodopa compared with non-SR carbidopa/levodopa.[294] With disease progression, adjunctive therapy with an MAO-B inhibitor, a dopamine agonist, or a COMT inhibitor (eg, tolcapone, entacapone) might be required to decrease the frequency of fluctuations caused by dyskinesia or dystonia.

DONEPEZIL   Aricept

Pharmacology. Donepezil enhances the action of acetylcholine by reversibly inhibiting acetylcholinesterase (AChE), the enzyme responsible for its hydrolysis. It has a high degree of selectivity for AChE in the CNS, which might explain the relative lack of peripheral side effects. Donepezil is indicated for the treatment of mild to moderate dementia of the Alzheimer's type. No evidence suggests that donepezil alters the course of the disease.

Administration and Adult Dosage. **PO for Alzheimer's disease** 5 mg once daily at bedtime, with or without food. The 10 mg dose is associated with a higher frequency of side effects but can provide extra benefit in some individuals. If a 10 mg dose is desired, first allow 4–6 weeks at 5 mg/day.

Special Populations. *Geriatric Dosage.* Same as adult dosage.

Other Conditions. No dosage adjustment is necessary in patients with renal or hepatic disease.

Dosage Forms. **Tab** 5, 10 mg.

Patient Instructions. This drug can be taken with or without food. Side effects can occur when you first start taking donepezil, but these frequently subside after 1 to 2 weeks. The maximum benefits of the drug might not occur until 4 to 8 weeks after starting the drug. Because there is variability in the way patients respond to donepezil, decide with your doctor how long to take donepezil. Do not abruptly discontinue donepezil on your own.

Missed Doses. Take this drug at regular intervals. If you miss a dose, take it as soon as you remember. If it is about time for the next dose, take that dose only. Do not double the dose or take extra.

Pharmacokinetics. *Onset and Duration.* Onset is in about 3 weeks, with maximum benefits occurring in 4–8 weeks.[295] The manufacturer recommends waiting 3 months before evaluating the full effects of the drug.[296]

Fate. Donepezil is completely absorbed and is 96% protein bound. V_{dss} is 12 L/kg; Cl is 0.13 L/hr/kg. About 60% is eliminated as hepatic metabolites including products of CYP2D6 and CYP3A4 and glucuronides. About 17% is excreted unchanged in urine.[297,298]

$t_{1/2}$, >70 hr.

Adverse Reactions. Occasionally, nausea, vomiting, muscle cramps, fatigue, anorexia, and headache occur.

Contraindications. Hypersensitivity to donepezil or piperidine derivatives (eg, biperiden, bupivacaine, methylphenidate, paroxetine, rifabutin, trihexyphenidyl).

Precautions. Use with caution in peptic ulcer disease, syncope, sick sinus syndrome, bradycardia, altered supraventricular cardiac conduction, asthma, seizures, or COPD.

Drug Interactions. There are few in vivo studies. In vitro, ketoconazole and quinidine decrease donepezil metabolism; enzyme inducers might increase its metabolism. Although extensively bound to plasma proteins, donepezil does not interact with warfarin or furosemide or with cimetidine or digoxin. Donepezil can increase the risk of GI side effects from NSAIDs because of the possible increase in stomach acid production.

Parameters to Monitor. Monitor mental status and improvements in activities of daily living initially and then periodically during therapy.

Notes. Because Alzheimer's disease is a neurodegenerative disorder, patients might improve or show no change in their cognitive functions.

DOPAMINE AGONISTS:	
BROMOCRIPTINE	Parlodel
PERGOLIDE	Permax
PRAMIPEXOLE	Mirapex
ROPINIROLE	Requip

Pharmacology. Bromocriptine and pergolide are ergot-derived dopamine agonists that stimulate dopamine-D_2 receptors; in addition, pergolide stimulates and bromocriptine partly antagonizes D_1 receptors. Pramipexole and ropinirole are non–ergot-derived dopamine subtype selective agonists that exert activity in the CNS at D_2 and D_3 receptors but have no activity at the D_1 receptor.[299–301] D_2 receptors are thought to play an important role in improving the akinesia, bradykinesia, rigidity, and gait disturbances of Parkinson's disease. Pramipexole, unlike other dopamine agonists, binds with 7-fold greater affinity to D_3 receptors than to D_2 receptors and can affect mood. Although bromocriptine also can inhibit prolactin secretion, it is no longer indicated for the prevention of postpartum lactation. Other uses of bromocriptine are the treatment of acromegaly, prolactin-secreting pituitary adenomas, and amenorrhea/galactorrhea secondary to hyperprolactinemia without a primary tumor. (*See* Dopamine Agonists Comparison Chart.)

Administration and Adult Dosage. (Bromocriptine) **PO for acromegaly** 1.25 mg/day or bid with food initially and then increasing in 1.25–2.5 mg/day increments q 3–7 days to a **usual maintenance dosage** of 2.5 mg bid–tid. **Maximum dosage** is 100 mg/day. **PO for hyperprolactinemia** 2.5 mg tid. **PO for Parkinson's disease** (*see* Dopamine Agonists Comparison Chart).

Special Populations. *Pediatric Dosage.* Safety and efficacy not established. **PO for treatment of prolactin-secreting pituitary adenomas** (≥11 yr) 1.25–2.5 mg daily; increase in 2.5 mg/day increments q 2–7 days as tolerated until therapeutic response is achieved.

Geriatric Dosage. Same as adult dosage.

Other Conditions. (Pramipexole) adjust for renal impairment as follows: Cl_{cr} 35–59 mL/min, give 1.5 mg bid initially, to a maximum of 1.5 mg bid; Cl_{cr} 15–34 mL/min, give 0.125 mg/day initially, to a maximum of 1.5 mg/day.

Dosage Forms. (*See* Dopamine Agonists Comparison Chart.)

Patient Instructions. This medication might improve the symptoms of Parkinson's disease but will not cure it. Take this drug with food to minimize stomach upset. This drug can cause dizziness, drowsiness, or fainting, especially after the first dose. Until the extent of these effects is known, use caution when driving, operating machinery, or performing tasks requiring mental alertness. Mental disturbances, including vivid dreams, confusion, and paranoid delusions, can occur even with low doses, especially when added to levodopa therapy. Avoid concurrent use of alcohol. Inform your physician and pharmacist of any other prescription or over-the-counter medications you might be taking because these can interact with your antiparkinsonian medications. Do not abruptly stop taking this medication or change your dosage without medical supervision. (Bromocriptine) women taking this drug to induce ovulation should use a barrier contraceptive. (Pramipexole and ropinirole) some patients have reported sudden excessive drowsiness, causing them to fall asleep during activities of daily living, including driving. Notify your doctor immediately if you notice significant daytime drowsiness. Avoid use of other sedating medications.

Missed Doses. Take this drug at regular intervals. If you miss a dose, take it as soon as you remember. If it is about time for the next dose, take that dose only. Do not double the dose or take extra.

Pharmacokinetics. *Onset and Duration.* Onset (bromocriptine) 0.5–1 hr;[302,303] (pergolide and pramipexole) 1–2 hr; (ropinirole) 1–2 hr on an empty stomach, 3–4 hr with food.[304] Duration (bromocriptine, ropinirole) 3–6 hr; (pergolide, pramipexole) 8–12 hr.[305] (Bromocriptine in amenorrhea) normal menstrual function usually returns within 6–8 weeks.

Fate. (Bromocriptine) bioavailability is about 28%; it is 90% bound to plasma proteins. Peak serum concentrations occur in 1.2 ± 0.4 hr, and detectable concentrations are found for up to 12 hr after discontinuation of drug;[302] Cl is 4.4 ± 2.6 L/hr/kg.[303] The majority (98%) is excreted in the feces via bile.[302] (Pergolide) bioavailability is about 60%; it is 90% bound to plasma proteins. Approximately 40–50% of a dose is excreted in feces over 7 days as at least 10 metabolites.[306] (Pramipexole) bioavailability is about 90%; it is 15% bound to plasma proteins. V_d is 7 L/kg; renal Cl is about 0.4 L/hr/kg and markedly exceeds the GFR. About 90% of a dose is excreted unchanged in urine. (Ropinirole) although completely absorbed, bioavailability is 55% because of first-pass metabolism. It is 36% bound to plasma proteins and undergoes extensive metabolism in the liver to inactive metabolites. The *N*-despropyl metabolite is the major metabolite; the drug also is hydroxylated and glucuronidated.

$t_{1/2}$. (*See* Dopamine Agonists Comparison Chart.)

Adverse Reactions. Nausea, headache, hallucinations, dyskinesias, somnolence, vomiting, symptomatic hypotension, dizziness, fatigue, constipation, and light-headedness occur frequently. Occasionally, abdominal cramps and diarrhea occur. (Bromocriptine, pergolide) rarely, hypertension, stroke, seizures, rhinorrhea, or erythromelalgia are reported. Pleuropulmonary disease is rare and usually occurs in men, especially in smokers receiving 20–100 mg/day of bromocriptine for 3–6 months; it presents with dyspnea and improves with drug discontinuation.[307]

Contraindications. (Bromocriptine, pergolide) pregnancy; lactation; uncontrolled hypertension; pre-eclampsia; concurrent use of other ergot alkaloids; hypersensitivity to ergot alkaloids.

Precautions. (Bromocriptine, pergolide) use with caution in patients with symptoms of peptic ulcer disease, history of pulmonary disease, MI, liver disease, severe angina, or psychiatric disease. (Bromocriptine) use a barrier contraceptive during treatment for amenorrhea, galactorrhea, or infertility. If pregnancy is detected, discontinue the drug. (Pramipexole, ropinirole) several patients have reported "sleep attacks," or falling asleep during activities of daily living. These sudden occasions of sleepiness have resulted in motor vehicle accidents. Advise patients of this possibility and assess them regularly for symptoms of drowsiness. Instruct patients to avoid other sedating medications and drugs that can increase blood levels of these agents (eg, cimetidine with pramipexole, ciprofloxacin with ropinirole). Sudden episodes of falling asleep might necessitate discontinuation of the dopamine agonist. If pramipexole or ropinirole is continued after such an incident, instruct the patient not to drive or use dangerous machinery.

Drug Interactions. When used with carbidopa/levodopa, it might be necessary to reduce the dosage of levodopa by as much as 30% to reduce the potential for developing dyskinesias. Drugs that antagonize dopamine (eg, phenothiazines, butyrophenones, metoclopramide) can reduce the effectiveness of these drugs. (Bromocriptine) erythromycin can increase bromocriptine serum levels. (Bromocriptine, pergolide) other ergot alkaloids can exacerbate cardiotoxic effects. (Pramipexole) pramipexole can result in an earlier and higher peak serum level of levodopa. Drugs that interfere with renal tubular secretion of cations (eg, cimetidine, ranitidine, verapamil, quinidine) can decrease pramipexole renal elimination. (Ropinirole) ropinirole is metabolized by CYP1A2; therefore, it might interact with inhibitors or inducers of this isozyme; ciprofloxacin markedly increases AUC and peak serum concentrations. Ropinirole might require dosage reduction with co-administration of estrogen.

Parameters to Monitor. Monitor blood pressure frequently during the first few days of therapy and periodically thereafter. Periodically evaluate hepatic, hematopoietic, cardiovascular, and renal function during long-term therapy. Monitor symptoms of Parkinson's disease periodically.

Notes. These drugs can be used as single agents for the treatment of early Parkinson's disease and as adjunctive agents in moderate- to late-stage disease.[305,308–312] As first-line agents, dopamine agonists can offer neuroprotection by regulating dopamine turnover and delaying the introduction of levodopa. However, as single agents, they are less effective than **levodopa.**

ENTACAPONE Comtan

Pharmacology. Entacapone is a peripheral acting, selective, and reversible inhibitor of COMT, similar in mechanism to tolcapone. Entacapone is indicated as an adjunct to levodopa/carbidopa to treat patients with Parkinson's disease who experience end-of-dose "wearing-off."[313]

Administration and Adult Dosage. **PO for Parkinson's disease** 200 mg, taken with each levodopa/carbidopa dose, to a maximum of 8 times daily (1600 mg/day).

The 200 mg dose is optimal and is more efficacious than higher doses, possibly because of interference with carbidopa absorption at doses ≥400 mg.[313]

Special Populations. *Geriatric Dosage.* Same as adult dosage.

Dosage Forms. **Tab** 200 mg.

Patient Instructions. Take one tablet of entacapone with each dose of levodopa/carbidopa. Be aware of the possibility of developing dizziness and hypotension when rising from a sitting or supine position. This effect is more likely to occur when the drug is first started. Nausea is another potential side effect in early therapy. Entacapone can cause a brownish-orange discoloration of the urine that is harmless. Dyskinesias and hallucinations can occur with entacapone, which can necessitate the reduction of the carbidopa/levodopa dose. Do not drive a car or operate machinery until you know how entacapone will affect your mental alertness or motor abilities.

Missed Doses. Take this drug at regular intervals. If you miss a dose, take it as soon as you remember. If it is close to the time of the next dose, take that dose only. Do not double the dose or take extra.

Pharmacokinetics. *Onset and Duration.* Onset is rapid and occurs with first dose. Peak effect is 0.7–1.3 hr after oral administration. Entacapone can prolong the effects of a carbidopa/levodopa dose by about 30 min.[313]

Fate. Oral bioavailability 35%. Food does not affect entacapone pharmacokinetics, but bioavailability is doubled with liver cirrhosis. Peak after a single 200 mg dose is approximately 1.2 μg/mL. Plasma binding is 98%, mainly to serum albumin. Entacapone does not distribute into tissues or CNS; V_{dss} is 0.4 ± 0.16 L/kg. Cl is 0.6 ± 0.1 L/kg/hr. Entacapone is metabolized almost completely before elimination, mainly by isomerization followed by glucuronidation. Metabolites are eliminated primarily by biliary excretion, with 90% of the metabolized dose found in the feces and 10% in urine. Only about 0.2% of the dose is eliminated unchanged in urine.[314]

$t_{½}$. β phase 0.4-0.7 hr; γ phase 2.4 hr, which accounts for about 10% of the total AUC.

Adverse Reactions. Orthostatic hypotension, diarrhea, dyskinesias, and hallucinations can occur with entacapone therapy, especially during the initial days of therapy. Dopaminergic side effects, including dyskinesias, nausea, dizziness, hallucinations, and insomnia, can occur. Dyskinesias are the most common side effect, usually early in therapy. Their frequency is reduced with lowering of the levodopa/carbidopa dose. Diarrhea is a frequent side effect that is mild to moderate in 4–10% of patients but severe in 1.3%. Orthostatic hypotension, urine discoloration, abdominal pain, and constipation occur occasionally. Elevation of liver enzymes was the same as that with placebo (0.8%). Rarely, rhabdomyolysis, hyperpyrexia and confusion, resembling neuroleptic malignant syndrome, occur.

Contraindications. Concurrent use with nonselective MAOIs but it can be taken with a selective MAO-B inhibitor (eg, selegiline).

Precautions. Because 90% of drug elimination is by biliary excretion, use caution in patients with biliary obstruction.

Drug Interactions. Entacapone does not inhibit cytochrome P450 enzymes at doses used for Parkinson's disease. Despite its extensive protein binding, in vitro studies have not shown binding displacement between entacapone and other highly bound drugs such as warfarin, salicylic acid, and diazepam. Drugs that interfere with biliary excretion, glucuronidation, and intestinal β-glucuronidase, such as probenecid, cholestyramine, erythromycin, ampicillin, rifampin, and chloraphenicol, have the potential to interfere with entacapone elimination. Drugs that are metabolized by COMT, such as methyldopa, dobutamine, isoproterenol, and epinephrine, can have enhanced effects when given with entacapone.

Parameters to Monitor. Monitor symptoms of Parkinson's disease and excessive dopaminergic activity. The dose of carbidopa/levodopa might need to be reduced if side effects such as dyskinesias and hallucinations are excessive or intolerable.

GALANTAMINE HYDROBROMIDE   Reminyl

Pharmacology. Galantamine is a competitive, reversible acetylcholinesterase inhibitor similar to donepezil and rivastigmine.[315,316]

Administration and Adult Dosage. **PO for Alzheimer's disease** 4 mg bid initially with a meal, increasing in 4 mg bid increments at 4-week intervals to a maximum of 12 mg bid. In moderate hepatic or renal dysfunction the maximum dosage is 8 mg bid. Avoid in severe hepatic (Child-Pugh 10–15) or renal (Cl_{cr} <9 mL/min) impairment. If more than a few days of therapy are missed, resume therapy at 4 mg bid.

Dosage Forms. **Tab** 4, 8, 12 mg.

Pharmacokinetics. Oral bioavailability is ≥90%; food decreases peak concentration and rate, but not extent of absorption. Peak cholinesterase inhibition occurs 1 hr after a dose. It is 18% plasma protein bound and distributed extensively into RBCs. V_{dss} is 2.6 L/kg; Cl is 0.34 L/hr/kg. Metabolism is primarily by CYP2D6 and 3A4. About 20–25% is excreted unchanged in urine in 24 hr. Half-life is 5–7 hr.[315]

Adverse Reactions. GI side effects (eg, nausea, vomiting, diarrhea, anorexia, weight loss), are most prominent during dosage escalation. Dizziness, headache, chest pain, tremor, depression, rhinitis, urinary incontinence, flatulence and bradycardia also occur frequently. Various cardiac arrhythmias, increased alkaline phosphatase, thrombocytopenia, GI bleeding, hyperglycemia, and psychiatric symptoms occur occasionally. Esophageal perforation has been reported.

RILUZOLE   Rilutek

Pharmacology. In the treatment of amyotrophic lateral sclerosis, riluzole is hypothesized to protect motor neurons from degeneration and death. Although the exact mechanism of action is unknown, there are three pharmacologic properties of the drug that are thought to be relevant: inhibition of glutamate release, inactivation of voltage-dependent sodium channels, and interference with intracellular events that follow activation of excitatory amino acid receptors.

Administration and Adult Dosage. **PO for amyotrophic lateral sclerosis** 50 mg bid.

Special Populations. *Geriatric Dosage.* Same as adult dosage.

Dosage Forms. **Tab** 50 mg.

Patient Instructions. Take this medication at the same time each day on an empty stomach. It can cause dizziness, drowsiness, or vertigo. Until the extent of these effects is known, use caution when driving, operating machinery, or performing tasks requiring mental alertness. Do not drink alcohol while taking this medication. Contact your doctor if fever or flulike symptoms occur. Protect the drug from exposure to light.

Missed Doses. Take this drug at regular intervals. If you miss a dose, take it as soon as you remember. If it is about time for the next dose, take that dose only. Do not double the dose or take extra.

Pharmacokinetics. *Fate.* Riluzole is rapidly absorbed, with about 90% absorbed, but absolute bioavailability is 60 ± 9% because of a first-pass effect. Peak serum concentrations occur within 60–90 min.[317] A high-fat meal decreases the AUC by about 20%. About 96% is bound to serum proteins, mainly albumin and lipoproteins; it is distributed extensively throughout the body, with a V_d of about 3.4 L/kg; Cl is 0.7 L/hr/kg in white males. Riluzole is metabolized extensively in the liver to at least six major metabolites, mainly by CYP1A2 (hydroxylated derivatives) and P450-dependent glucuronidation.[318] Its metabolism is slower by 32% in women and by 50% in Japanese subjects native to Japan than in white males. Glucuronides account for about 85% of urine metabolites.[317-319]

$t_{½}$. 12 ± 1.8 hr.

Adverse Reactions. Nausea, constipation, vomiting, abdominal pain, elevations in AST and ALT, asthenia, dizziness, diarrhea, vertigo, and circumoral paresthesia occur frequently. Decreased lung function, pneumonia, somnolence and neutropenia occur occasionally (3 cases of neutropenia in 4000 during clinical trials).

Precautions. Use with caution in patients with renal or hepatic disease, especially the elderly.

Drug Interactions. Riluzole might interact with other drugs that also are metabolized by CYP1A2, including theophylline, caffeine, fluoroquinolones, and amitriptyline. Enzyme inducers and cigarette smoking increase the metabolism of riluzole.[319]

Parameters to Monitor. Monitor liver function tests and CBC periodically as well as response to therapy.

Notes. In amyotrophic lateral sclerosis, riluzole prolongs the time to tracheostomy or death (a 21% risk reduction) compared with placebo.[320,321] The difference in rates of muscle deterioration between riluzole and placebo was significant in some studies but not in others.

RIVASTIGMINE   Exelon

Pharmacology. Rivastigmine is an intermediate-acting (pseudo-irreversible) AChE inhibitor that binds to AChE, resulting in a carbamated form of AChE that cannot hydrolyze acetylcholine. This action increases CNS acetylcholine activity. It is indicated for treatment of mild to moderate symptoms of dementia of the Alzheimer's type.[322]

Administration and Adult Dosage. **PO for Alzheimer's disease** 1.5 mg bid initially. After at least 2 weeks, increase in 1.5 mg bid increments q 2 weeks as tolerated, to a maximum of 6 mg bid. If more than a few days of therapy are missed, resume therapy at the initial dose of 1.5 mg bid.

Special Populations. *Geriatric Dosage.* No specific dosage adjustment is needed because the dose is adjusted to patient tolerance.

Dosage Forms. **Cap** 1.5, 3, 4.5, 6 mg; **Soln** 2 mg/mL.

Patient Instructions. Take this drug with food in the morning and evening. Dosage will be increased about every 2 weeks until the maximum tolerable dose is reached. If you experience adverse effects, such as loss of appetite, nausea, vomiting or abdominal pain, stop treatment for several doses and then resume at the same or next lower dose level. Inform your physician if these symptoms occur.

Missed Doses. Take this drug at regular intervals. If you miss a dose, take it as soon as you remember. If it is within a few hours of the next dose, take that dose only. Do not double the dose or take extra. If you miss more than a few doses, do not resume the same dosage. Inform your physician.

Pharmacokinetics. *Onset and Duration.* After 6 mg, anticholinesterase activity is present in the CSF for about 10 hr, with a maximum inhibition of about 60% 5 hr after a dose.

Fate. Rivastigmine is rapidly and completely absorbed with bioavailability of about 36% after a 3 mg dose. Peak plasma concentrations occur within 1 hr, with peak CSF concentrations achieved in 1.4–2.6 hr. Food delays plasma peak time by 90 min, lowers the peak by 30%, and increases bioavailability by 30%. Rivastigmine is 40% bound to plasma proteins; V_d is 1.8–2.7 L/kg.[323] Cl is 108 ± 36 L/hr after 6 mg bid. Pharmacokinetics are nonlinear at doses above 3 mg bid. Metabolism is mainly by cholinesterase-mediated hydrolysis. It is then eliminated renally, with 97% of the dose detected in the urine as metabolites, most commonly as the sulfate conjugate of the decarbamylated metabolite (40%). Cl is reduced in the elderly (by 30%) and in patients with renal (by 64%) or hepatic (by 60%) disease. Only 0.4% is eliminated in the feces.

$t_{½}$. 1.5 hr.[324]

Adverse Reactions. Nausea (47%) and vomiting (31%) are frequent occurrences in patients, especially women, treated with 6–12 mg/day and are more likely during the titration phase rather than the maintenance phase. Anorexia and weight loss also occur more frequently in women. Other side effects are dizziness, headache, tremor, abdominal pain, dyspepsia, hypotension, orthostatic hypotension, insomnia, tinnitus, palpitations, confusion, anemia, and rash.[322-324] Resumption of a high dose after a few days without taking the drug can result in severe vomiting and esophageal perforation.

Contraindications. Sensitivity to carbamate derivatives.

Precautions. *See* Donepezil.

Drug Interactions. Excessive cholinergic effect can occur if rivastigmine is given with cholinergic drugs (eg, succinylcholine, bethanecol). Rivastigmine can antagonize the effects of anticholinergic drugs and antiparkinson's drugs. Based on in vitro studies, rivastigmine does not interact with digoxin, warfarin, diazepam, or fluoxetine. Rivastigmine pharmacokinetics are not altered by antacids, antihypertensives, calcium channel blockers, antidiabetics, NSAIDs, salicylates, antianginals, antihistamines, estrogens, or β-blockers. Rivastigmine can increase the risk of GI side effects from NSAIDs due to the possible increase in stomach acid production.

Parameters to Monitor. Because of the high frequency of nausea, vomiting, and anorexia, monitor patients for these reactions and for possible weight loss.

Notes. Metrifonate (ProMem—Bayer) is an organophosphate being studied for Alzheimer's disease.

SELEGILINE HYDROCHLORIDE   Eldepryl

Pharmacology. Selegiline (formerly L-deprenyl) is a selective, irreversible MAO-B inhibitor that is used as adjunctive therapy in the management of Parkinson's disease. MAO-B is found in the brain and plays a role in the catabolism of dopamine.[325,326] By preventing the breakdown of dopamine by MAO-B, selegiline increases the net amount of dopamine available in the brain. Selegiline also can exert a protective effect by preventing the accumulation of neurotoxic free radicals generated by dopamine metabolism.[327–331] However, the exact mechanism of the beneficial effects of selegiline is unclear and might be symptomatic, neuroprotective, or both.

Administration and Adult Dosage. **PO for Parkinson's disease** 5 mg bid taken at breakfast and lunch. Alternatively, give an initial dosage of 2.5 mg/day and slowly increase to 10 mg/day over several weeks to minimize side effects.[325] There is no evidence that dosages >10 mg/day increase efficacy, and they can lead to nonspecific inhibition of MAO-A.

Special Populations. *Pediatric Dosage.* Safety and efficacy not established.

Geriatric Dosage. Same as adult dosage.

Dosage Forms. **Cap** 5 mg; **Tab** 5 mg.

Patient Instructions. Take this medication with morning and midday meals to minimize nausea and night-time insomnia. At a dosage of 10 mg/day or less, tyramine-containing foods and medications containing amines are safe to consume. Initiation of selegiline might require a reduction of carbidopa/levodopa dosage. Report immediately any severe headache or other unusual or unexpected symptoms.

Missed Doses. Take this drug at regular intervals. If you miss a dose, take it as soon as you remember. If it is about time for the next dose, take that dose only. Do not double the dose or take extra.

Pharmacokinetics. *Onset and Duration.* Recovery of platelet MAO-B activity after a single oral dose is 2–4 days; after long-term treatment, >90% of platelet MAO-B remains inhibited after 5 days.[332] With continual use, clinical efficacy lasts 6–12 months in most patients, to a maximum of 12–24 months.[327–330]

Fate. Selegiline is readily absorbed from the GI tract, with a peak at 0.5–2 hr; 94% is bound to plasma proteins.[332] It is metabolized by the liver to N-desmethylselegiline, L-amphetamine, and L-methamphetamine; these isomers, however, are only 10% as potent as the D-isomers. After long-term therapy with 10 mg/day in 2 divided doses, mean trough serum levels of selegiline and N-desmethylselegiline are undetectable; L-amphetamine is 5.9 ± 2.7 µg/L (22 ± 10 nmol/L), and L-methamphetamine is 14.9 ± 6.8 µg/L (100 ± 45 nmol/L). The concentrations of these metabolites are probably too low to contribute to the drug's clinical efficacy but can contribute to adverse effects. About 86% is excreted in urine as inactive metabolites.[325,326]

$t_{\frac{1}{2}}$. (N-desmethylselegiline) 2 ± 1.2 hr; (L-amphetamine) 17.7 ± 16.3 hr; (L-methamphetamine) 20.5 ± 11.4 hr.[325,326]

Adverse Reactions. Nausea, abdominal pain, dry mouth, confusion, hallucinations, dizziness, insomnia, lightheadedness, and/or fainting occur frequently. Vivid dreams, dyskinesias, and headache occur occasionally. In decreasing order of frequency—nausea, hallucinations, confusion, depression, loss of balance, and insomnia—can lead to discontinuation of the drug. Mild, asymptomatic elevations in liver function tests can occur.

Precautions. Pregnancy; lactation. Concurrent use with meperidine. Do not use at dosages exceeding 10 mg/day.

Drug Interactions. Concurrent administration of selegiline and serotonin reuptake inhibitors (eg, SSRIs, nefazondone, venlafaxine) can cause serotonin syndrome; do not give them within 1–2 weeks of each other (5 weeks after stopping fluoxetine).

Parameters to Monitor. Evaluate cardiovascular status and monitor liver function tests periodically. Monitor Parkinson's disease symptoms periodically.

Notes. Selegiline is indicated as adjunctive treatment with **carbidopa/levodopa** in Parkinson's disease. Although the efficacy of selegiline is not superior to that of other adjunctive drugs such as dopamine agonists, it appears to be better tolerated.[299,300] Approximately 60% of patients who receive selegiline experience a modest (<10%) reduction in "off" periods and can reduce their levodopa dosage by 20%.[329] A role for the drug as an initial agent in patients with mild disease is supported by results of a study comparing selegiline 10 mg/day with placebo in patients with early (<5 yr) untreated Parkinson's disease; selegiline delayed the onset of disease-related disability by nearly 1 yr.[327] **Zelepar** (Athena) is a rapidly dissolving form of selegiline in phase III clinical trials.

TOLCAPONE   Tasmar

Pharmacology. Tolcapone reversibly inhibits at least 80% of the activity of COMT. This action prevents the metabolism of levodopa to 3-O-methyldopa and thus prolongs its duration of action, especially with co-administration of carbidopa.[333,334] Tolcapone increases plasma levodopa bioavailability by about 2-fold and variably prolongs the terminal half-life of levodopa (given with carbidopa) in the elderly from 2 hr to as long as 3.5 hr, but has no effect on the peak serum levels of levodopa or the time at which they occur. (*See* Notes.)

Administration and Adult Dosage. PO for Parkinson's disease 100 mg tid initially, always as an adjunct to levodopa/carbidopa therapy, increasing to a maximum of 200 mg tid. If the patient shows no substantial clinical benefit after 3 weeks of therapy, discontinue tolcapone. (*See* Parameters to Monitor.)

Special Populations. *Geriatric Dosage.* Same as adult dosage.

Dosage Forms. **Tab** 100, 200 mg.

Patient Instructions. This drug can lower blood pressure and cause unsteadiness, nausea, or sweating initially. Do not rise rapidly after sitting or lying down. It also can cause drowsiness. Until the extent of these effects is known, use caution when driving, operating machinery, or performing tasks that require mental alertness. This drug also can worsen dyskinesias or dystonia when it is first started and might require adjustment of the amount of carbidopa/levodopa you are taking. Because of the risk of liver damage with this drug, you will require regular liver enzyme tests. Notify your physician immediately if signs of liver toxicity develop.

Missed Doses. Take this drug at regular intervals. If you miss a dose, take it as soon as you remember. If it is about time for the next dose, take that dose only. Do not double the dose or take extra.

Pharmacokinetics. *Onset and Duration.* Onset 1–2 hr; duration 12–24 hr.

Fate. About 65% is orally absorbed. A peak serum concentration of 6.3 ± 2.9 mg/L occurs 1.8 ± 1.3 hr after a 200 mg dose. Food increases the peak time and decreases the peak and AUC of tolcapone. About 99.9% is bound to plasma proteins, mainly albumin. The predominant metabolic pathway is glucuronidation. Major metabolites that are a product of oxidative processes include 3-*O*-methyltolcapone and carboxylic acid derivatives metabolized by CYP2A6 and CYP3A4. Those that are a product of reductive processes include amines and *N*-acetyl derivatives. Cl is about 0.1 L/kg/hr. About 40% of an orally administered dose is excreted in the urine and feces in 24 hr and >95% in 7–9 days. Less than 0.5% of tolcapone is excreted unchanged in urine.[333,334]

$t_{1/2}$. (Tolcapone) 2 ± 0.8 hr; (3-*O*-methyltolcapone) 32 ± 7 hr.[333,334]

Adverse Reactions. Tolcapone has caused several cases of severe, fulminant liver failure that were sometimes fatal. Monitor liver function carefully. Adverse reactions consistent with increased levodopa exposure include worsening dyskinesia, nausea, sleep disorders, dystonia, somnolence, anorexia, hallucinations, and postural hypotension. They might be lessened by reducing levodopa dosage. Urine discoloration also occurs and is attributable to the yellow color of tolcapone and its metabolites. Other tolcapone-related side effects include headache, abdominal pain, and diarrhea. The most common reason for drug discontinuation from clinical studies was severe diarrhea in 3% of patients. The onset is often delayed and usually occurs within 0.5–3 months after initiation of therapy.

Contraindications. Liver disease or in patients who have discontinued tolcapone therapy because of liver toxicity; history of rhabdomyolysis caused by any medication; history of hyperpyrexia and confusion related to medication use or to medication discontinuation.

Precautions. Orthostatic hypotension, hallucinations, diarrhea, or dyskinesias can occur at the initiation of therapy. Use with caution in patients with renal impairment. Follow recommended plan for monitoring liver enzymes. Discontinue tolcapone if ALT or AST exceeds the upper limit of normal or if the patient develops signs and symptoms of liver failure (jaundice, anorexia, dark urine, pruritus, nausea, and right upper quadrant tenderness). The patient should sign a consent form before therapy is initiated.

Drug Interactions. Tolcapone can inhibit the metabolism of other drugs also metabolized by COMT (eg, dobutamine, isoproterenol) and exacerbate the dopaminergic side effects of other antiparkinsonian agents. It does not interact with ephedrine or desipramine (a substrate for CYP2D6) but has in vivo affinity for CYP2C9 (although the clinical relevance is undetermined).

Parameters to Monitor. Before starting treatment, conduct tests to exclude the presence of liver disease. Obtain ALT and AST levels at baseline and then q 2 weeks for the first year of therapy, q 4 weeks for the next 6 months, and q 8 weeks thereafter. If the dose is increased, begin liver enzyme monitoring again as when the drug was initiated.

Notes. Tolcapone can be administered on a schedule (3 times daily) and does not need to be administered with each dose of levodopa. The increase in "on time" in nonfluctuating and fluctuating patients was 1.7–2.9 hr over baseline (vs 0.7–1 hr for placebo).[335–337] In clinical trials, the average decrease in daily levodopa dosage was about 30% in about 70% of patients.

TRIHEXYPHENIDYL HYDROCHLORIDE   Artane, Various

Pharmacology. Trihexyphenidyl is a competitive antagonist of acetylcholine at central muscarinic receptors. In Parkinson's disease, it is an adjunctive treatment that balances cholinergic and dopaminergic activities in cerebral synapses.

Administration and Adult Dosage. PO for Parkinson's disease 1 mg/day initially, increasing in 2 mg/day increments q 3–5 days, to a maximum of 12–15 mg/day. **Usual maintenance dosage** 6–10 mg/day in 3 divided doses or 3–6 mg/day in 3 divided doses concurrent with levodopa. SR caps can be given bid once the maintenance dosage has been determined. **PO for drug-induced extrapyramidal disorders** 1 mg initially, increasing in 1 mg increments every few hours until symptoms are controlled, usually 5–15 mg/day in 3–4 divided doses.

Dosage Forms. Elxr 0.4 mg/mL; **Tab** 2, 5 mg; **SR Cap** 5 mg.

Pharmacokinetics. The onset of action is within 1 hr, and the peak effect lasts 2–3 hr; the duration of action is 6–12 hr. The majority of the drug is excreted in the urine probably unchanged, and the elimination half-life is 10.2 ± 4.7 hr.

Adverse Reactions. Adverse reactions, precautions, contraindications, and drug interactions are the same as those for benztropine. When trihexyphenidyl is used concurrently with levodopa, the dosages of both drugs might require reduction.

Precautions. Use with great caution in patients older than 65 yr because they are more sensitive to the effects of anticholinergic agents.

DOPAMINE AGONISTS COMPARISON CHART

DRUG	DOSAGE FORMS	ADULT DOSAGE	DOPAMINE RECEPTOR SELECTIVITY			EFFECT ON CYTOCHROME P450 ISOZYMES	HALF-LIFE (HR)
			D_1	D_2	D_3		
Bromocriptine[a] Parlodel	Cap 5 mg Tab 2.5 mg.	PO 1.25 mg bid initially, increasing in 2.5 mg/day increments q 2 weeks to a usual dosage of 10–40 mg/day.	0/+	++	+	*Inhibits* CYP3A4	4
Pergolide[a] Permax	Tab 0.05, 0.25, 1 mg.	PO 0.05 mg/day for 2 days initially, increasing in 0.1–0.15 mg/day increments q 3 days for 12 days, then in 0.25 mg/day increments q 3 days to a usual dosage of 1–4 mg/day.	0/+	++	++	*Inhibits* CYP2D6	27

(continued)

DOPAMINE AGONISTS COMPARISON CHART (*continued*)

DRUG	DOSAGE FORMS	ADULT DOSAGE	DOPAMINE RECEPTOR SELECTIVITY D_1	D_2	D_3	EFFECT ON CYTOCHROME P450 ISOZYMES	HALF-LIFE (HR)
Pramipexole Mirapex	Tab 0.125, 0.25, 1, 1.5 mg.	PO 0.125 mg tid initially, increasing in increments of 0.75 mg/day at weekly intervals to a usual dosage of 1.5–4.5 mg/day in 3 divided doses.	0	++	++++	No effect.	12
Ropinirole Requip	Tab 0.25, 0.5, 1, 2, 5 mg.	PO 0.25 mg tid initially, increasing in increments of 0.75 mg/day at weekly intervals for 4 weeks, then in increments of 1.5–3 mg/day at weekly intervals to a usual dosage of 3–12 mg/day in 3 divided doses.	0	++	+++	*Inhibits* CYP2D6	4–6

0 = none; 0/+ = minimal; + = mild; ++ = moderate; +++ = potent; ++++ = very potent.
^aErgot alkaloid.
From references 302, 303, 305, 306, and 308 and product information.

Ophthalmic Drugs for Glaucoma

Class Instructions. Ophthalmic Solutions. Proper instillation of eye drops improves absorption of the drug into the eye and minimizes systemic absorption and adverse effects. If you wear contact lenses, remove them. Wash your hands before instilling eye drops. Tilt the head back and pull down the lower lid. Place 1 drop into the lower lid. Once medication has been placed in the eye(s), close the eyes and press lightly on the inside corner of each eye. Keep the eyes closed and continue pressure to the inside corner of the eyes for 2–5 minutes. Wash your hands to remove medication. If you miss a dose, apply it as soon as possible. If it is almost time for your next dose, skip the missed dose and go back to your regular schedule. Do not double doses.[338] **Ophthalmic Ointments.** If you wear contact lenses, remove them. Wash your hands. Tilt the head back and pull down the lower lid. Unless told to use a different amount, squeeze a thin strip (about 0.5 cm) of ointment into the lower lid. Let go of the eyelid and close the eyes for 1–2 minutes. Wash your hands to remove any medication. To keep the medication as germ free as possible, do not touch the tip to any surface. Wipe the tip with a clean tissue before closing. If you miss a dose, take it as soon as possible. If it is almost time for your next dose, skip the missed dose and go back to your regular dosage schedule. Do not double doses.[338]

Pharmacology. The only medical treatment for primary open-angle glaucoma is to decrease intraocular pressure (IOP), the only treatable risk factor. Glaucoma drugs lower IOP by reducing production of aqueous humor, decreasing the resistance to outflow of aqueous humor through the trabecular meshwork, and improving flow through uveoscleral pathway.[339,340]

Administration and Dosage. The ocular cul-de-sac has a capacity of only about 7 μL. After instillation of an eye drop, this capacity temporarily increases to 30 μL.[341–343] Although manufacturers' package inserts often instruct an individual to instill a dose of 1 or 2 drops, the drop size of ophthalmic solutions, from about 26 μL for timolol to about 69 μL for carbachol, exceeds the capacity of the cul-de-sac.[344] Control dosage by changing the concentration of the solution rather than instilling multiple drops. Ophthalmic solutions are generally administered at a frequency that is determined by their duration of action. Gels and ocular inserts provide a sustained-release of active drug from the vehicle, allowing some products to be administered less frequently than solutions of the same drug. Because they are effective and have relatively fewer adverse effects, begin treatment with a β-adrenergic blocker with a goal of decreasing IOP by 30%.[339,340] To slow progression of visual field loss, patients with more severe glaucoma require greater reductions, possibly to as low as 7–12 mm Hg.[339,340,345] If the goal IOP cannot be reached, substitute a carbonic anhydrase inhibitor (CAI), latanoprost, or α₂-adrenergic agonist.[339,340,346] If monotherapy is not successful, use a rational combination of drugs.

Patient Instructions. One study found that, due to noncompliance, patients were without treatment for 30% of a 12-month follow-up period.[347] Because noncompliance is a major reason for treatment failure, persist in patient counseling. (*See* Class Instructions.)

Pharmacokinetics. In ocular therapeutics, the eye is considered a separate entity outside the body, with the aqueous humor considered the central compartment.[342] Absorption is the process by which a drug enters the aqueous humor, and bioavailability refers to the rate and extent of absorption into the aqueous humor. Distribution refers to the flow dynamics of partitioning and binding of the drug from the aqueous to surrounding tissues, such as the ciliary body.

Fate. In general, ophthalmic solutions must have lipid and aqueous solubility to penetrate the cornea and reach their sites of action in the ciliary body. The epithelium and endothelium of the cornea are lipophilic. The inner layer, the stroma, is hydrophilic. The lipophilic epithelium is penetrated by the undissociated drug. Then the stroma is penetrated by the dissociated, hydrophilic drug. Corneal penetration is enhanced when the epithelium is injured or otherwise compromised.[341–343] Drug that does not penetrate the cornea can be systemically absorbed through the conjunctival vessels or through nasolacrimal drainage. Most of an eye drop is drained within 15–30 sec of application and 80–85% of the drainage is through the nasolacrimal canal.[343,348] Drugs that are systemically absorbed after ophthalmic administration do not pass through the liver; therefore, a relatively small amount of absorbed drug can result in adverse systemic effects.[349] Nasolacrimal occlusion increases drug–corneal contact time, thereby enhancing ocular absorption and decreasing systemic absorption.[342,343,348,349] Drugs that pass through the cornea and reach their sites of action can be metabolized by esterases but mostly are eliminated from the eye by aqueous humor turnover, which is 1.5% of the anterior chamber volume per minute. Normally, very little drug reaches the vitreous or crosses the blood–ocular barrier. Because sampling the aqueous humor or ocular tissues would cause severe pain or injury, pharmacokinetic studies are not usually conducted in the eye.[342]

$t_{1/2}$. Half-life for ophthalmic solutions is determined primarily by tissue binding. For drugs that are not strongly bound to pigments in the iris or other tissues, half-life is determined by the aqueous humor turnover rate of 1.5%/min, which is consistent with a half-life of 46 min.[342]

Parameters to Monitor. (*See* specific drug class.) An ophthalmologist or optometrist should monitor IOP q 2 weeks during initial treatment and stabilization. Once target IOP has been reached, IOP, cup/disc ratios, and visual fields tests should be monitored by an ophthalmologist or optometrist q 3–12 months, depending on the severity of glaucoma and the progression of visual loss.[341,345] Pharmacist monitoring is limited to noncompliance and detection of adverse effects. When a patient presents with new systemic problems, always consider the ophthalmic drug as a potential cause.[339]

α₂-ADRENERGIC AGONISTS:

APRACLONIDINE HYDROCHLORIDE	Iopidine
BRIMONIDINE HYDROCHLORIDE	Alphagan

Pharmacology. Apraclonidine and brimonidine act at α₂-adrenergic sites in the ciliary body to inhibit norepinephrine release, causing a decrease in aqueous humor production.[346] Brimonidine also increases uveoscleral outflow.[350] Apraclonidine is more polar than clonidine, resulting in less permeability of the blood–brain barrier.[346] Apraclonidine has a high rate of tachyphylaxis, limiting it to short-term use. Brimonidine is more α_2-selective and more lipophilic than apraclonidine, allowing the use of lower concentrations.[346]

Administration and Adult Dosage. (Apraclonidine) **Ophth in laser surgery** 1 drop of 1% soln in the affected eye 1 hr before surgery and then 1 drop immediately after surgery to prevent the IOP spikes that occur. **Ophth in open-angle glaucoma as a short-term adjunct** 0.5% tid. (Brimonidine) **Ophth for primary open-angle glaucoma** 1 drop of 0.2% soln tid, about 8 hr apart. (*See* Notes.)

Special Populations. *Pediatric Dosage.* (Apraclonidine) same as adult dosage; (Brimonidine) (<12 yr) not recommended.[351]

Geriatric Dosage. Same as adult dosage.

Dosage Forms. (Apraclonidine) **Ophth Soln** 0.5, 1%. (Brimonidine) **Ophth Soln** 0.15, 0.2%.

Patient Instructions. (*See* Ophthalmic Solutions Class Instructions.)

Pharmacokinetics. *Onset and Duration* (Apraclonidine) onset 1 hr, peak 3 hr. (Brimonidine) onset 1 hr, peak 2 hr, duration about 6 hr.[346]

Fate. (*See* Ophthalmic Solutions Fate.) Brimonidine that is systemically absorbed is metabolized primarily in the liver; 74% is eliminated in the kidney within 120 hr.

$t_{1/2}$. (Apraclonidine) plasma half-life 8 hr. (Brimonidine) plasma half-life 3 hr. (*See* Ophthalmic Solutions $t_{1/2}$.)

Adverse Reactions. (Apraclonidine) causes adverse ocular effects in 15–48% of patients, especially allergic reactions and rarely upper eyelid retraction. Frequent systemic effects are dry mouth and dry nose. Cardiovascular effects have not been reported.[346] (Brimonidine) has similar but less frequent ocular adverse effects. Frequent ocular effects are blepharitis, blepharoconjunctivitis, conjunctival follicles, blurred vision, and headache. Like apraclonidine, it frequently causes dry mouth and dry nose. Brimonidine does not decrease heart rate. It can mildly decrease blood pressure in some patients, although it frequently causes lethargy.[350,352] Because it crosses the blood–brain barrier, it can cause mild hypotension in adults occasionally.[339] Several severe adverse systemic effects have been reported in children between 28 days and 3 months of age, including bradycardia, hypotension, hypothermia, hypotonia, apnea, dyspnea, hypoventilation, cyanosis, and lethargy. This is believed to be caused by immaturity of the blood–brain barrier and higher systemic concentrations because of low body weight.[351]

Precautions. (*See* Ophthalmic Solutions Precautions.)

Parameters to Monitor. Monitor for conjunctivitis and lethargy. (*See* Ophthalmic Solutions Parameters to Monitor.)

Notes. Brimonidine 0.15% preserved with an oxychloro complex (Alphagan P) is equivalent to the 0.2% solution preserved with benzalkonium chloride (Alphagan). Brimonidine bid is equivalent to **timolol** 0.5% in lowering IOP at peak, 6.5 vs 6.1 mm Hg, but much less effective in lowering trough IOP, 4.3 vs 6.3 mm Hg.[350] Brimonidine bid is more effective than **betaxolol** 0.25% suspension at peak and trough.[353] As adjunct therapy in patients who fail to reach target IOP with other therapy, brimonidine bid decreases IOP an additional 4.7 ± 5.3 mm Hg, or 20%.[351] (*See* Glaucoma Drugs Comparison Chart.)

β-ADRENERGIC BLOCKING DRUGS:	
BETAXOLOL HYDROCHLORIDE	Betoptic, Betoptic-S
CARTEOLOL HYDROCHLORIDE	Ocupress
LEVOBUNOLOL HYDROCHLORIDE	Betagan, Various
METIPRANOLOL	Optipranolol
TIMOLOL MALEATE	Timoptic, Timoptic-XE

Pharmacology. β-Adrenergic blocking drugs downregulate adenylate cyclase by blocking β$_2$-adrenergic receptors in the ciliary body, resulting in a decrease in aqueous production and intraocular pressure. Although **betaxolol** is a β$_1$-selective adrenergic blocker, it is effective in treating glaucoma. Betaxolol might have more β$_2$ activity than previously thought; small concentrations of β$_2$-blockade might be sufficient to curb aqueous production; β$_2$-receptors in the eye might be different from those in other tissues; or betaxolol's IOP-lowering effect might be caused by a calcium antagonistic effect.[346,354] **Carteolol** has intrinsic sympathomimetic activity (ISA) that theoretically makes it less likely to cause adverse pulmonary or cardiovascular effects and possibly provide increased blood flow to the retina.[355–358] ISA does not seem to make a difference in cardiac effects in most studies;[357,359] however, in one study night-time bradycardia was 4-fold greater in patients treated with **timolol** than in those treated with carteolol.[358] Retinal and optic nerve head circulations are improved by β-adrenergic blocking agents without ISA.[360]

Administration and Adult Dosage. (Betaxolol) **Ophth** 1 drop bid. (Carteolol) **Ophth** 1 drop bid. (Levobunolol) **Ophth** initiate treatment with 1 drop/day. (Metipranolol) **Ophth** 1 drop bid. (Timolol soln) **Ophth** 1 drop bid of 0.25% soln initially; if target IOP is not reached in 4 weeks, increase to 0.5%. (Timolol gel-forming soln) 1 drop/day of 0.25% soln initially; if target IOP is not reached in 4 weeks, increase to 0.5%. (*See* Notes.)

Special Populations. *Pediatric Dosage.* Same as adult dosage.

Geriatric Dosage. Same as adult dosage.

Dosage Forms. (Betaxolol) **Ophth Soln** 0.5%; **Ophth Susp** 0.25%. (Carteolol) **Ophth Soln** 1%. (Levobunolol) **Ophth Soln** 0.25, 0.5%. (Metipranolol) **Ophth Soln** 0.3%. (Timolol) **Ophth Gel-Forming Soln** 0.25, 0.5%; **Ophth Soln** 0.25, 0.5%.

Patient Instructions. (*See* Class Instructions.)

Pharmacokinetics. *Onset and Duration.* (Betaxolol) onset 30 min, peak 2 hr, duration 12 hr. (Carteolol) onset 1 hr, peak 2 hr, duration 12 hr. (Levobunolol) onset 1 hr, peak 2–6 hr, duration 24 hr. (Metipranolol) onset 30 min, peak 2 hr, duration 24 hr. (Timolol drops) onset 30 min, peak 1–2 hr, duration 24 hr.

Fate. (*See* Ophthalmic Solutions Fate.)

$t_{1/2}$. (Betaxolol) 12–20 hr; (carteolol) 3–7 hr; (levobunolol) 6 hr; (metipranolol) 3–4 hr; (timolol) 3–5 hr.[356] (*See* Ophthalmic Solutions $t_{1/2}$.)

Adverse Reactions. Frequent, but mild, ocular adverse effects include burning and stinging at instillation. Betaxolol ophthalmic suspension and timolol gel-forming solution frequently cause temporary blurred vision. Occasional, but serious, granulomatous anterior uveitis is caused by metipranolol.[361,362] Occasional, but serious, systemic reactions include bronchospasm, bradycardia, CHF, heart block, cerebral vascular ischemia, and depression.

Contraindications. Sinus bradycardia; greater than first-degree AV block; cardiogenic shock; overt cardiac failure. Nonselective drugs are also contraindicated in patients with histories of bronchial asthma or severe COPD.

Precautions. Diabetes mellitus; cerebrovascular insufficiency; myasthenia gravis.

Drug Interactions. Oral β-adrenergic blocking agents, calcium-channel blockers, and digoxin can cause additive effects on AV conduction. Quinidine can inhibit the metabolism of β-adrenergic blocking agents by CYP2D6, causing bradycardia.

Parameters to Monitor. (*See* Ophthalmic Solutions Parameters to Monitor.) Monitor for complaints of ocular adverse effects such as burning or stinging. Monitor pulse rate, shortness of breath, browache, nervousness, and depression.[341,355,363]

Notes. If target IOP is not reached with a β-blocker within 4 weeks, consider switching to a topical ophthalmic CAI, α_2-adrenergic agonist, or prostaglandin analogue rather than adding another drug. If monotherapy is not successful, a β-blocker can be combined with one of these drugs or **pilocarpine**. With the exception of betaxolol, β-blockers are not effective when combined with **epinephrine** or **dipivefrin**.[339,341,346] (*See* Glaucoma Drugs Comparison Chart.)

CARBONIC ANHYDRASE INHIBITORS:	
ACETAZOLAMIDE	Diamox
BRINZOLAMIDE	Azopt
DICHLORPHENAMIDE	Daranide
DORZOLAMIDE HYDROCHLORIDE	Trusopt
METHAZOLAMIDE	Naptazane

Pharmacology. CAIs inhibit the carbonic anhydrase II isoenzyme in the ciliary epithelium, thereby blocking the formation of bicarbonate. This causes a decrease in sodium and water outflow from the ciliary body. More than 99% of carbonic anhydrase must be inhibited to be effective. The result is a decrease of about 40% in aqueous humor production and a decrease in IOP of up to 30–35%.[341,364] Orally administered CAIs also inhibit carbonic anhydrase in the kidney, red blood cells, and other tissues, causing diuresis and often acidosis and other serious adverse effects that limit their use.[341,364,365]

Administration and Adult Dosage. Ophth for primary open-angle glaucoma (brinzolamide) 1 drop tid; (dorzolamide) 1 drop tid. When used adjunctively, dorzolamide is administered bid.[366] **PO for primary open-angle glaucoma** (acetazolamide) **SR cap** 500 mg bid has been better tolerated than tablets; **Tab** 125 mg q 4 hr to 250 mg qid. Dosages >1 g/day are no more effective. (Dichlorphenamide) 100–200 mg priming dose, followed by 100 mg q 12 hr until desired response is obtained, then 25–50 mg daily to tid. (Methazolamide) 50–100 mg bid-tid. **PO for prevention of altitude sickness** (acetazolamide) 750 mg/day.[367] (*See* Notes.)

Special Populations. *Pediatric Dosage.* Safety and efficacy not established. However, dorzolamide 2% ophthalmic solution is used in infantile glaucoma, and acetazolamide 5–10 mg/kg qid has been used when an oral CAI was necessary.[341,364,368]

Geriatric Dosage. Same as adult dosage.

Dosage Forms. (Acetazolamide) **Tab** 125, 250 mg; **SR Cap** 500 mg; **Inj** 500 mg. (Brinzolamide) **Ophth Susp** 1%. (Dichlorphenamide) **Tab** 50 mg. (Dorzolamide) **Ophth Soln** 2%. (Methazolamide) **Tab** 25, 50 mg.

Patient Instructions. (*See* Class Instructions.) **Dorzolamide** Tell your doctor if you experience itching, redness, swelling, or other sign of eye or eyelid irritation. This medication can cause you to have blurred vision for a short period. Make sure you know how to react to this medication before you drive, use a machine, or do anything else that might be dangerous if you cannot see properly. Dorzolamide can cause your eyes to become more sensitive to light. Wearing sunglasses and avoiding exposure to bright light can lessen the discomfort.[338]

Pharmacokinetics. *Onset and Duration.* (Acetazolamide) Tab peak IOP reduction 2–6 hr, duration 4–12 hr;[341,364] SR cap onset 2–4 hr, peak 4–8 hr, duration 12–24 hr.[341,364] (Brinzolamide) onset <2 hr, peak 2 hr, duration >12 hr.[369] (Dichlorphenamide) onset 30 min, peak 2 hr, duration 6 hr. (Dorzolamide) onset <2 hr, peak 2–4 hr, duration 6–8 hr.[341,370,371] (Methazolamide) onset 1–2 hr, peak 4–6 hr, duration 12–24 hr.[341]

Fate. For all oral CAIs there is a linear relationship between plasma concentration and dose. (Acetazolamide) virtually completely absorbed with a peak serum level of 30 mg/L occurring at 1 hr after a 500 mg dose of tablet; with SR Cap, serum levels remain >10 mg/L for 10 hr. 90% bound to plasma proteins; elimination is by active renal tubular secretion.[364] (Methazolamide) well absorbed and distributed in plasma, CSF, aqueous humor, red blood cells, bile, and extracellular fluid. Peak serum concentrations after 50 and 100 mg bid dosages are 5.1 and 10.7 mg/L, respectively. V_{dss} is 17–23 L. Renal clearance accounts for 20–25% of the total clearance, with about 25% of the drug eliminated in the urine unchanged. **Brinzolamide** and **dorzolamide** are systemically absorbed and bind to carbonic anhydrase in erythrocytes with terminal half-lives of 111 and 147 days, respectively; however, there is only a 21% decrease in baseline carbonic anhydrase activity, far below the 99% inhibition level necessary to induce systemic effects.[368] Laboratory values of patients receiving dorzolamide did not indicate metabolic acidosis or electrolyte imbalances such as those with long-term systemic CAIs.[370]

$t_{1/2}$. (Acetazolamide) 4 hr; (dichlorphenamide) 2 hr; (methazolamide) 14–15 hr.[341] (*See* Ophthalmic Solutions $t_{1/2}$.)

Adverse Reactions. Topical ophthalmic solutions frequently cause ocular burning, stinging, or allergic ocular reactions.[372] However, fewer patients discontinue dorzolamide than pilocarpine.[366,370,373] Frequent systemic effects of topical ophthalmic solutions consist of bitter taste, occasional headache, nausea, fatigue, and, rarely, urolithiasis and iridocyclitis. Oral administration frequently cause paresthesias, GI disturbances, anorexia, drowsiness, and confusion. Occasionally, metabolic acidosis, hypokalemia, or urolithiasis occurs. Attempt to treat acidosis with sodium acetate 90 mEq/day.[341] Rare, but possibly fatal, reactions include aplastic anemia, agranulocytosis, and thrombocytopenia.

Contraindications. (Oral) hypokalemia; hyponatremia; hyperchloremic acidosis; adrenocortical insufficiency; marked renal or hepatic impairment; severe COPD. Long-term use of oral CAIs is contraindicated in angle-closure glaucoma.

Precautions. Because all CAIs are sulfonamides, avoid their use in patients with histories of sulfonamide allergy. Japanese and Korean patients might be at greater risk for developing Stevens–Johnson syndrome.[374] Neither topical nor oral CAIs are recommended in patients with severe renal impairment. Caution in patients with hepatic impairment. Acidosis can cause sickling of RBC in patients with sickle cell anemia.

Drug Interactions. Do not use topical CAIs with oral CAIs because the combination is no more effective and adverse effects are additive, particularly in causing corneal endothelial dysfunction.[375] Oral CAIs can cause salicylate toxicity in patients taking high doses of aspirin, and salicylates can displace acetazolamide from plasma binding sites, causing acetazolamide toxicity and non–anion-gap hyperchloremic metabolic acidosis.[376] Diflunisal displaces acetazolamide from plasma binding sites. In one study, this resulted in a 5.6-fold increase in acetazolamide plasma levels.[377]

Parameters to Monitor. Malaise or fatigue, Cr_s, serum potassium, serum carbon dioxide. The value of monitoring CBC is controversial because the hematologic adverse effects can be immune mediated and idiosyncratic rather than dose related.[341,364,378] However, manufacturers recommend obtaining a baseline CBC and platelet count, with monitoring at regular intervals.

Notes. Because of their severe adverse effects and poor tolerability, use oral CAIs in primary open-angle glaucoma only as a last resort. Some clinicians consider laser surgery before using oral CAIs long term.[364] Use topical CAIs only if a topical β-blocker, prostaglandin analogue, or $α_2$-adrenergic agonist cannot be used or has failed to reach target IOP. If target IOP is not achieved with monotherapy, a topical CAI can be added to another topical treatment. Dorzolamide 2% tid as monotherapy lowers IOP 23% compared with 25% for **timolol** and 21% for **betaxolol**.[370] Added to timolol, dorzolamide 2% bid provides another 13–22% decrease in IOP, similar to that from adding acetazolamide.[368,379] Topical dorzolamide is as effective as oral acetazolamide.[371] (*See* Glaucoma Drug Comparison Chart.) For prophylaxis of acute altitude sickness, acetazolamide 500 mg/day is ineffective, but 750 mg/day is about as effective as **dexamethasone** 8–16 mg/day.[367]

CHOLINERGICS AND CHOLINESTERASE INHIBITORS:

CARBACHOL	Isopto Carbachol
DEMECARIUM	Humorsol
ECHOTHIOPHATE IODIDE	Phospholine Iodide
PILOCARPINE SALTS	Various

Pharmacology. Carbachol and pilocarpine are direct cholinergic agonists that act at acetylcholine receptors to stimulate the ciliary muscle. Carbachol is also a weak cholinesterase inhibitor. Cholinesterase inhibitors act indirectly by inhibiting AChE. Ciliary body contraction causes pupilary constriction and eases the restriction of outflow of aqueous humor through the trabecular meshwork. Demacarium and echothiophate are irreversible cholinesterase inhibitors with long durations of action.[380]

Administration and Adult Dosage. Ophth for glaucoma (carbachol) initiate at 1 drop tid of the 0.75% solution; (demecarium) 1 drop daily–bid of the 0.125–0.25% solution; (echothiophate) 1 drop daily–bid; (pilocarpine ophth soln) initiate with 1 drop of 1–2% solution q 6–8 hr. Most patients eventually require qid administration. Because pilocarpine is bound to pigments in the iris and the ciliary body, patients with dark eyes sometimes require 4% and occasionally 6% solutions; (pilocarpine gel) apply a thin strip hs; (pilocarpine inserts) place in conjunctival sac once weekly at hs. When switching to pilocarpine inserts, initiate therapy with Ocusert Pilo-20 because there is no correlation between dosage of solution and that of inserts. **Ophth for treatment of accommodative esotropia** (demecarium) 1 drop daily for 2–3 weeks and then q 2–3 days for 3–4 weeks; (echothiophate) 1 drop daily–q 2 days.

Special Populations. *Pediatric Dosage.* Same as adult dosage.

Geriatric Dosage. Same as adult dosage.

Dosage Forms. (Carbachol) **Ophth Soln** 0.75, 1.5, 2.25, 3%. (Demecarium) **Ophth Soln** 0.125, 0.25%. (Echothiophate Iodide) **Pwdr for reconstitution** 0.03, 0.06, 0.125, 0.25%. (Pilocarpine) **Ophth Gel** 4%; **Ocular therapeutic system (Ocusert Pilo)** 20, 40 μg/hr. (Pilocarpine HCl) **Ophth Soln** 0.25, 0.5, 1, 2, 3, 4, 5, 6, 8, 10%. (Pilocarpine Nitrate) **Ophth Soln** 1, 2, 4%.

Patient Instructions. (*See* Glaucoma Drugs Class Instructions.) Isoflurophate ophthalmic ointment is inactivated by moisture. Do not rinse the tip of the tube.

Pharmacokinetics. *Onset and Duration.* (Carbachol Ophth Soln) onset 13 ± 2.2 min, peak 4 hr, duration 8 hr. (Demecarium Ophth Soln) onset 2–4 hr, peak 24 hr, duration 5–9 days. (Echothiophate Soln) onset within minutes, peak 2–7 weeks, duration several weeks. (Isofluorophate Ophth Gel) onset 15 min, peak within 24 hr, duration 1–4 weeks. (Physostigmine Ophth Soln) onset 8 min, peak 1–2 hr, duration 4–6 hr. (Pilocarpine Ophth Soln) onset within min, peak 2 hr, duration

8 hr, (Pilocarpine Ophth Gel) 4% maintains IOP reductions of 30% or more for |24 hr.[381] (Pilocarpine Ocuserts) release drug constantly for 1 week.[382,383]

Fate. For absorption characteristics, *see* Glaucoma Drugs Fate. Cholinergic and cholinesterase inhibitors are hydrolyzed by acetylcholine.

t½. (*See* Ophthalmic Solutions $t_{1/2}$.)

Adverse Reactions. Reduced visual acuity in poor lighting occurs frequently. Occasional effects include ciliary spasm, headache, lacrimation, myopia, blurred vision, retinal detachment, and iris cysts. Adverse effects (eg, iris cysts) occur more often in children, especially with use of long-acting cholinesterase inhibitors. Cataracts occur in 30–50% of elderly patients using echothiophate or demecarium for at least 6 months.[341] Cholinergic syndrome consisting of weakness, nausea, diaphoresis, and dyspnea occurs rarely.[384,385] Because of their long duration of action, adverse systemic effects are more likely with long-acting cholinesterase inhibitors.[383] Patients with myopia of −6 diopters or greater and those with histories of retinal detachment are at greater risk of developing retinal detachment.[346]

Contraindications. Acute iritis and other conditions in which papillary constriction is undesirable.

Precautions. Pregnancy, lactation. Night driving or other activities in poor light. Use cholinesterase inhibitors cautiously in patients with histories of retinal detachment, asthma, bradycardia, hypotension, epilepsy, parkinsonism, recent MI, or patients using systemic cholinesterase inhibitors for myasthenia gravis.

Drug Interactions. Antihistamine, antidepressants, antipsychotics, and other anticholinergics can decrease the effects of cholinergics and cholinesterase inhibitors.

Parameters to Monitor. Intraocular pressure, cup/disc ratios, and visual field loss should be monitored by an ophthalmologist or optometrist. Miosis is an indication that cholinergic activity is present.[386] Monitor compliance, pulse for bradycardia, and complaints of visual blurring, nausea, vomiting, diarrhea, and headache.

Notes. (*See* Glaucoma Drugs Comparison Chart.) Use long-acting cholinesterase inhibitors in patients who are not controlled with pilocarpine. Longer-acting agents are also used to diagnose and treat accommodative esotropia.

PROSTAGLANDINS:	
BIMATOPROST	Lumigan
LATANOPROST	Xalatan
TRAVAPROST	Travatan
UNOPROSTONE ISOPROPYL	Rescula

Pharmacology. Latanoprost is an ester prologue analogue of prostaglandin $F_{2\alpha}$ that decreases IOP by increasing uveoscleral outflow by an unknown mechanism.[387] Latanoprost usually lowers IOP by 5–8 mm Hg regardless of baseline pressure.[388–391] This is important for patients with normal-tension glaucoma who do not respond as well to other drugs.[392] Unoprostone isopropyl is a docosanoid compound related to a metabolite of prostaglandin $F_{2\alpha}$.[393] Unoprostone lowers

IOP by about 5 mm Hg in patients with higher IOP[394] and about 2 mm Hg in patients with low-tension glaucoma.[393]

Administration and Adult Dosage. **Ophth for glaucoma** (Bimatoprost) 1 drop daily in the evening. (Latanoprost) 1 drop of 0.005% solution daily in the evening. Higher concentrations are not as effective as the 0.005% soln.[395] Once daily administration is more effective than bid and evening administration is more effective than morning administration.[392,395–397] (Travaprost) 1 drop daily in the evening. (Unoprostone) 1 drop bid.

Special Populations. *Pediatric Dosage.* Safety and efficacy not established.

Geriatric Dosage. Same as adult dosage.

Dosage Forms. **Ophth Soln** (Bimatoprost) 0.03%; (Latanoprost) 0.005%; (Travaprost) 0.004%; (Unoprostone) 0.15%.

Patient Instructions. (*See* Class Instructions.) If other eye drops are used with this drug, separate administrations by at least 5 min. Remove contact lenses before instilling drops. Lenses can be reinserted after 15 min.

Pharmacokinetics. *Onset and Duration.* (Bimatoprost) onset 4 hr, peak 8–12 hr, duration 24 hr; (Latanoprost) onset 3–4 hr, peak 8–12 hr, duration 24 hr; (Travaprost) onset 2 hr, peak 12 hr, duration 24 hr; (unoprostone) onset 30 min, peak 1–2 hr, duration 12 hr.[393]

Fate. (Bimatoprost) peak plasma level of 200 pmol/L is unlikely to produce systemic effects. (Latanaprost) is more lipophilic than its active metabolite, allowing excellent penetration of the cornea. Inside the aqueous, it is hydrolyzed to the active drug and reaches a peak concentration of 55 µg/L at 2–3 hr.[398] V_{dss} is 0.16 ± 0.02 L/kg. The active drug is not metabolized in the aqueous, but 77–88% is systemically absorbed within 3 min and 90% is bound to plasma proteins. A peak plasma level of 64 ng/L (about 10^{-10} mol/L) is reached within 40 min, a level too low to produce systemic effects. The active drug is metabolized by the liver and 88% of the metabolites are eliminated by the kidneys. Systemic Cl is 0.42 L/hr/kg. Systemic levels cannot be detected after 12 hr.[398] (Travaprost) peak plasma levels of 25 ng/L are reached in 30 min and rapidly eliminated. (Unoprostone) peak plasma concentration of 760 ng/L of the de-esterified metabolite of unoprostone is reached 15 min after ocular installation.[393]

$t_{1/2}$. (*See* Ophthalmic Solutions $t_{1/2}$.) Plasma half-lives are (latanoprost) 17 min; (unoprostone) 14 min.

Adverse Reactions. Ocular reactions frequently include burning, stinging, conjunctival hyperemia, foreign-body sensation, blurred vision. The major limitation is increased pigmentation of the iris in patients with green-brown, yellow-brown, and blue/gray-brown eyes that occurs after 3–17 months of use with latanoprost.[388,390,391,396,397,399,400] Unoprostone has been used primarily in Japanese patients who have dark irises; however, one case has been reported. Difference in the frequency of this reaction between the two prostoglandins might be caused by differences in the selectivity for prostaglandin receptors.[401,402] Flu symptoms occur frequently (6%) in patients receiving unoprostone. Diplopia occasionally occurs; retinal artery embolus, retinal detachment, and vitreous hemorrhage with latanaprost occur rarely. Occasional upper respiratory infection has been reported but cannot definitely be linked to latanaprost.[346,398]

Precautions. Infections occur from contamination of multiple-dose containers. Instruct patients to avoid touching the tip of the container to the eye. Patients with diabetic retinopathy or complicated ocular surgery have a greater risk of developing cystoid macular edema, anterior uveitis, or vitreous hemorrhage.[346,388]

Drug Interactions. Precipitate occurs when used with thimerosal-containing eye drops. Separate doses of different ophthalmic solutions by at least 5 min.

Parameters to Monitor. (*See also* Ophthalmic Solutions Parameters to Monitor.) Darkening of iris, eye pain.

Notes. In comparisons with **timolol**, patients receiving latanoprost have an equal or greater reduction in IOP.[388,391,396,397,399,403] Patients switched from timolol to latanoprost had an additional 1–5.5 mm Hg reduction in IOP.[388,404] Latanoprost is additive when added to another glaucoma treatment. Adding latanoprost to timolol results in an additional IOP reduction of 13–37%.[346,404] Latanoprost lowers IOP an additional 15% in patients receiving **acetazolamide**.[405] **Pilocarpine** given 1 hr before latanoprost does not provide further IOP reduction; however, pilocarpine given 10 min to 1 hr after latanoprost results in a further decrease in IOP of about 5 mm Hg.[406] (*See* Glaucoma Drugs Comparison Chart.)

SYMPATHOMIMETICS:

DIPIVEFRIN HYDROCHLORIDE	AKPro, Propine
EPINEPHRINE AND SALTS	Various

Pharmacology. Epinephrine stimulates α- and β$_2$-adrenergic receptors in the ciliary body, increasing outflow. Dipivefrin is an epinephrine prodrug that is enzymatically converted into epinephrine in the eye. IOP is reduced by 20–25%.[346,407]

Administration and Adult Dosage. *Ophth for glaucoma* (epinephrine) 1 drop (usually 2%) bid; (dipivefrin) 1 drop of 0.1% solution bid.

Special Populations. *Pediatric Dosage.* Same as adult dosage.

Geriatric Dosage. Same as adult dosage.

Dosage Forms. (Dipivefrin) **Ophth Soln** 0.1%; (epinephrine HCl) **Ophth Soln** 0.5, 1, 2%.

Patient Instructions. (*See* Class Instructions.)

Pharmacokinetics. *Onset and Duration.* Onset <45 min; peak 4–6 hr; duration 24 hr.[407]

Fate. Dipivefrin is absorbed 17 times more than epinephrine. Upon entry into the cornea, the two pivalic acid groups are removed by esterases, yielding epinephrine. Because of the better absorption, it can be administered as a 0.1% solution, decreasing the amount of epinephrine exposure to the conjunctiva and available for systemic absorption, thereby decreasing adverse effects.[342] Epinephrine that is absorbed systemically is metabolized by MAO and COMT.[407]

Adverse Reactions. Intolerance to ocular adverse effects leads to discontinuation of epinephrine in 80% of patients. Burning, tearing, reactive conjunctival hyperemia, allergic blepharoconjunctivitis, and mydriasis resulting in blurring of vision occur frequently.[338] Mydriasis is minimized when epinephrine is combined with pilocarpine and is more pronounced when used with β-adrenergic blockers.[407] Adrenochrome deposits in palpebral conjunctiva and the superficial cornea occur occasionally.[346,407] Rare systemic adverse effects include tachycardia, hypertension, anxiety, and arrhythmia.[346,349,407]

Precautions. Because epinephrine causes mydriasis, avoid use in patients with narrow-chamber angles because the lens prevents epinephrine from reaching the retina. About 30% of aphakic patients develop cystoid macular edema.[407]

Parameters to Monitor. IOP, cup/disk ratios, and visual fields tests should be performed by an ophthalmologist or optometrist q 3–12 mo, depending on the severity and progression of glaucoma. Monitor for blurring of vision, mydriasis, conjunctival irritation, hypertension and rapid pulse.

Notes. Do not use epinephrine solutions that are cloudy or have become pinkish or brownish.[338] Epinephrine provides no extra benefit when combined with β-adrenergic blockers except betaxolol.[346] (*See* Glaucoma Drugs Comparison Chart.)

GLAUCOMA DRUGS COMPARISON CHART[a]

DRUG CLASS AND DRUGS	DOSAGE FORMS	ADULT DOSAGE	ONSET	PEAK	DURATION
α₂-ADRENERGIC AGONISTS					
Apraclonidine HCl Iopidine	Ophth Soln 0.5, 1%.	0.5% tid short-term; 1% 1 hr before and immediately after surgery	1 hr	3 hr	——
Brimonidine Tartrate Alphagan Alphagan P	Ophth Soln 0.15%. (Alphagan P); 0.2% (Alphagan)	tid	1 hr	2 hr	6 hr
β-ADRENERGIC BLOCKERS					
Betaxolol HCl Betoptic Betoptic-S	Ophth Soln 0.5%. Ophth Susp 0.25%.	bid; bid	30 min 30 min	2 hr 2 hr	12 hr 24 hr
Carteolol HCl Ocupress	Ophth Soln 1%.	bid	1 hr	2 hr	12 hr
Levobunolol HCl Betagan Various	Ophth Soln 0.25, 0.5%.	daily-bid	1 hr	2–6 hr	24 hr
Metipranolol Optipranolol	Ophth Soln 0.3%.	bid	30 min	2 hr	24 hr
Timolol Maleate Timoptic Timoptic-XE	Ophth Soln 0.25, 0.5% Ophth Gel-Forming Soln 0.25, 0.5%.	bid daily	30 min 30 min	1–2 hr 1–2 hr	24 hr 24 hr

(continued)

GLAUCOMA DRUGS COMPARISON CHART[a] (continued)

DRUG CLASS AND DRUGS	DOSAGE FORMS	ADULT DOSAGE	ONSET	PEAK	DURATION
CAI TOPICAL					
Brinzolamide Azopt	Ophth Susp 1%.	tid	<2 hr	2 hr	>12 hr
Dorzolamide Trusopt	Ophth Soln 2%.	tid	<2 hr	2–4 hr	6–8 hr
CAI ORAL					
Acetazolamide Diamox	Tab 125, 250 mg;	125–250 mg q 4 hr to 250 mg qid	1–2 hr	2–4 hr	4–12 hr
Diamox Sequels	SR Cap 500 mg.	500 mg bid	2–4 hr	8 hr	12–24
Dichlorphenamide Daranide	Tab 50 mg.	25–50 mg daily-tid	30 min	2–4 hr	6–12 hr
Methazolamide Naptazane	Tab 25, 50 mg.	50–100 mg bid-tid	1–2 hr	4–6 hr	12–24 hr
CHOLINERGICS					
Carbachol Isopto Carbachol	Ophth Soln 0.75, 1.5, 2.25, 3%.	tid	13 min	4 hr	8 hr
Pilocarpine HCl Pilocar Various	Ophth Soln (HCl) 0.25, 0.5, 1, 2, 3, 4, 5, 6, 8, 10% Ophth Gel 4%	qid daily	minutes minutes	2 hr 2 hr	8 hr 24 hr
Pilocarpine Nitrate Pilagan	Ophth Soln (Nitrate) 1, 2, 4%.	qid	minutes	2 hr	8 hr *(continued)*

GLAUCOMA DRUGS COMPARISON CHART[a] (continued)

DRUG CLASS AND DRUGS	DOSAGE FORMS	ADULT DOSAGE	ONSET	PEAK	DURATION
Pilocarpine Ocular Therapeutic System Ocusert Pilo-20, 40	20, 40 µg/hr.	weekly	minutes	2 hr	7 days
CHOLINESTERASE INHIBITORS					
Demacarium Humorsol	Ophth Soln 0.125, 0.25%.	daily-bid	2–4 hr	24 hr	5–9 d
Echothiophate Iodide Phospholine Iodide	Pwdr 0.03, 0.06, 0.125, 0.25%.	daily-bid	minutes	2–7 weeks	several weeks
PROSTAGLANDIN ANALOGUES					
Bimatoprost Lumigan	Ophth Soln 0.03%.	p.m.	4 hr	8–12 hr	24 hr
Latanoprost Xalatan	Ophth Soln 0.005%.	p.m.	3–4 hr	8–12 hr	24 hr
Travaprost Travatan	Ophth Soln 0.004%.	p.m.	2 hr	12 hr	24hr
Unoprostone Rescula	Ophth Soln 0.15%.	bid	30 min	1–2 hr	12 hr
SYMPATHOMIMETICS					
Epinephrine Various	Ophth Soln 0.5, 1, 2%.	bid	<45 min	4–6 hr	24 hr
Dipivefrin Propine	Ophth Soln 0.1%.	bid	<45 min	4–6 hr	24 hr

CAI = carbonic anhydrase inhibitor.
[a]Dosages in this chart are for primary open-angle glaucoma.

516 CENTRAL NERVOUS SYSTEM DRUGS

REFERENCES

1. Anon. Drugs for epilepsy. *Med Lett Drugs Ther* 1995;37:37–40.
2. Levy RH et al., eds. *Antiepileptic drugs.* 4th ed. New York: Raven Press; 1995.
3. Cloyd JC et al. Antiepileptics in the elderly: pharmacoepidemiology and pharmacokinetics. *Arch Fam Med* 1994;3:589–98.
4. Bass J et al. Effects of enteral tube feedings on the absorption and pharmacokinetic profile of carbamazepine suspension. *Epilepsia* 1989;30:364–9.
5. Graves NM et al. Relative bioavailability of rectally administered carbamazepine suspension in humans. *Epilepsia* 1985;26:429–33.
6. Morrow JI, Richens A. Disposition of anticonvulsants in childhood. *Clin Pharmacokinet* 1989;17(suppl 1):89–104.
7. Bertilsson L et al. Autoinduction of carbamazepine metabolism in children examined by a stable isotope technique. *Clin Pharmacol Ther* 1980;27:83–8.
8. Mikati MA et al. Time course of carbamazepine autoinduction. *Neurology* 1989;39:592–4.
9. Theodore WH et al. Carbamazepine and its epoxide: relation of plasma levels to toxicity and seizure control. *Ann Neurol* 1989;25:194–6.
10. Greenblatt DJ et al. Clinical pharmacokinetics of anxiolytics and hypnotics in the elderly: therapeutic considerations (part I). *Clin Pharmacokinet* 1991;21:165–77.
11. Graves NM, Kriel RL. Rectal administration of antiepileptic drugs in children. *Pediatr Neurol* 1987;3:321–6.
12. Berlin A, Dahlstrom H. Pharmacokinetics of the anticonvulsant drug clonazepam evaluated from single oral and intravenous doses and by repeated oral administration. *Eur J Clin Pharmacol* 1975;9:155–9.
13. Specht U et al. Discontinuation of clonazepam after long-term treatment. *Epilepsia* 1989;30:458–63.
14. Pollack MH et al. Long-term outcome after acute treatment with alprazolam or clonazepam for panic disorder. *J Clin Psychopharmacol* 1993;13:257–63.
15. Herman JB et al. The alprazolam to clonazepam switch for the treatment of panic disorder. *J Clin Psychopharmacol* 1987;7:175–8.
16. Beauclair L et al. Clonazepam in the treatment of panic disorder: a double-blind, placebo-controlled trial investigating the correlation between clonazepam concentrations in plasma and clinical response. *J Clin Psychopharmacol* 1994;14:111–8.
17. Buchanan RA et al. Absorption and elimination of ethosuximide in children. *J Clin Pharmacol* 1969;9:393–8.
18. Goulet JR et al. Metabolism of ethosuximide. *Clin Pharmacol Ther* 1976;20:213–8.
19. Rho JM et al. Mechanism of action of the anticonvulsant felbamate: opposing effects on N-methyl-D-aspartate and γ-aminobutyric acid$_A$ receptors. *Ann Neurol* 1994;35:229–34.
20. Sachdeo R et al. Felbamate monotherapy: controlled trial in patients with partial onset seizures. *Ann Neurol* 1992;32:386–92.
21. Espe-Lillo J et al. Safety and efficacy of felbamate in treatment of infantile spasms. *Epilepsia* 1993;34:110.
22. Perhach JL et al. Felbamate. In, Meldrum BS, Porter RJ, eds. *New anticonvulsant drugs.* London: John Libby; 1986:117–23.
23. Wilensky AJ et al. Pharmacokinetics of W-554 (ADD 03055) in epileptic patients. *Epilepsia* 1985;26:602–6.
24. Pellock JM, Brodie MJ. Felbamate: 1997 update. *Epilepsia* 1997;38:1261–4.
25. Aweeka FT et al. Pharmacokinetics of fosphenytoin in patients with hepatic or renal disease. *Epilepsia* 1999;40:777–82.
26. Gerber N et al. Safety, tolerance and pharmacokinetics of intravenous doses of the phosphate ester of 3-hydroxymethyl-5,5-diphenylhydantoin: a new prodrug of phenytoin. *J Clin Pharmacol* 1988;28:1023–32.
27. Leppik IE et al. Pharamcokinetics and safety of a phenytoin prodrug given IV or IM in patients. *Neurology* 1990;40:456–60.
28. Jamerson BD et al. Venous irritation related to intravenous administration of phenytoin versus fosphenytoin. *Pharmacotherapy* 1994;14:47–52.
29. Wilder BJ et al. Safety and tolerance of multiple doses of intramuscular fosphenytoin substituted for oral phenytoin in epilepsy or neurosurgery. *Arch Neurol* 1996;53:764–8.
30. Fischer JH et al. Stability of fosphenytoin sodium with intravenous solutions in glass bottles, polyvinyl chloride bags, and polypropylene syringes. *Ann Pharmacother* 1997;31:553–9.
31. Crockett JG et al. Open-label follow-on study of gabapentin (GBP; Neurontin) monotherapy in patients with refractory epilepsy. *Epilepsia* 1995;36:69. Abstract.
32. McLean MJ. Clinical pharmacokinetics of gabapentin. *Neurology* 1994;44(suppl 5): S17–22.
33. Sivenius J et al. Double-blind study of gabapentin in the treatment of partial seizures. *Epilepsia* 1991;32:539–42.

34. Hooper WD et al. Lack of a pharmacokinetic interaction between phenobarbitone and gabapentin. *Br J Clin Pharmacol* 1991;31:171–4.
35. Ramsay RE. Clinical efficacy and safety of gabapentin. *Neurology* 1994;44(suppl 5):S23–30.
36. Asconape J, Collins T. Weight gain associated with the use of gabapentin. *Epilepsia* 1994;36(suppl 4):72. Abstract.
37. Wolf SM et al. Gabapentin toxicity in children manifesting as behavioral changes. *Epilepsia* 1996;36:1203–5.
38. Mikati M et al. Efficacy of gabapentin in children with refractory partial seizures. *Neurology* 1995;45(suppl 4):A201–2. Abstract.
39. Beydoun A et al. Gabapentin monotherapy: II. A 26-week, double-blind, dose-controlled, multicenter study of conversion from polytherapy in outpatients with refractory complex partial or secondarily generalized seizures. *Neurology* 1997;49:746–52.
40. Rowbotham M et al. Gabapentin for the treatment of postherpetic neuralgia: a randomized controlled trial. *JAMA* 1998;280:1837-42.
41. Backonja M et al. Gabapentin for the symptomatic treatment of painful neuropathy in patients with diabetes mellitus. *JAMA* 1998;280:1831-6.
42. Mao J, Chen LL. Gabapentin in pain management. *Anesth Analg* 2000;91:680–7.
43. Letterman L, Markowitz JS. Gabapentin: a review of published experience in the treatment of bipolar disorder and other psychiatric conditions. *Pharmacotherapy* 1999;19:565–72.
44. Btaiche IF, Woster PS. Gabapentin and lamotrigine: novel antiepileptic drugs. *Am J Health-Syst Pharm* 1995;52:61–9.
45. Rambeck B, Wolf P. Lamotrigine clinical pharmacokinetics. *Clin Pharmacokinet* 1993;25:433–43.
46. Jawad S et al. Lamotrigine: single-dose pharmacokinetics and initial 1 week experience in refractory epilepsy. *Epilepsy Res* 1987;1:194–201.
47. Besage FMC et al. Carbamazepine toxicity with lamotrigine: pharmacokinetic or pharmacodynamic interaction. *Epilepsia* 1998;39:183–7.
48. Motte J et al. Lamotrigine for generalized seizures associated with the Lennox-Gastaut syndrome. *N Engl J Med* 1997;337:1807–12.
49. Brodie MJ et al. Double-blind comparison of lamotrigine and carbamazepine in newly diagnosed epilepsy. *Lancet* 1995;345:476–9.
50. Cereghino JJ et al. Levetiracetam for partial seizures: results of a double-blind, randomized clinical trial. *Neurology* 2000;55:236–42.
51. Patsalos PN. Pharmacokinetic profile of levetiracetam: toward ideal characteristics. *Pharmacol Ther* 2000;85:77–85.
52. Schacter SC. Oxcarbazepine: current status and clinical applications. *Exp Opin Invest Drugs* 1999;8:1103–12.
53. Lloyd P et al. Clinical pharmacology and pharmacokinetics of oxcarbazepine. *Epilepsia* 1994;35(suppl 3):S10–3.
54. Dickinson RG et al. First dose and steady-state pharmacokinetics of oxcarbazepine and its 10-hydroxy metabolite. *Eur J Clin Pharmacol* 1989;37:69–74.
55. Beran R. Cross-reactive skin eruption with both carbamazepine and oxcarbazepine. *Epilepsia* 1993;34:163–5.
56. Working Group on Status Epilepticus. Treatment of convulsive status epilepticus. *JAMA* 1993;270:854–9.
57. Dunn DW. Status epilepticus in infancy and childhood. *Neurol Clin* 1990;8:647–57.
58. Scheuer ML, Pedley TA. The evaluation and treatment of seizures. *N Engl J Med* 1990;323:1468–74.
59. Graves NM et al. Relative bioavailability of rectally administered phenobarbital sodium parenteral solution. *DICP* 1989;23:565–8.
60. Alvin J et al. The effect of liver disease in man on the disposition of phenobarbital. *J Pharmacol Exp Ther* 1975;192:224–35.
61. Wilensky AJ et al. Kinetics of phenobarbital in normal subjects and epileptic patients. *Eur J Clin Pharmacol* 1982;23:87–92.
62. Heimann G, Gladtke E. Pharmacokinetics of phenobarbital in childhood. *Eur J Clin Pharmacol* 1977;12:305–10.
63. Meador KJ et al. Comparative cognitive effects of phenobarbital, phenytoin, and valproate in healthy adults. *Neurology* 1995;45:1494–99.
64. Mattson RH et al. Barbiturate-related connective tissue disorders. *Arch Intern Med* 1989;149:911–4.
65. Alldredge BK et al. Anticonvulsant hypersensitivity syndrome: in vitro and clinical observations. *Pediatr Neurol* 1994;10:169–71.
66. Ramsay RE. Pharmacokinetics and clinical use of parenteral phenytoin, phenobarbital, and paraldehyde. *Epilepsia* 1989;30(suppl 2):S1–3.
67. Dela Cruz FG et al. Efficacy of individualized phenytoin sodium loading doses administered by intravenous infusion. *Clin Pharm* 1988;7:219–24.

68. Blaser KU et al. Intravenous phenytoin: a loading scheme for desired concentrations. *Ann Intern Med* 1989;110:1029–31.

69. Bauer LA, Blouin RA. Age and phenytoin kinetics in adult epileptics. *Clin Pharmacol Ther* 1982;31:301–4.

70. Boucher BA et al. Phenytoin pharmacokinetics in critically ill trauma patients. *Clin Pharmacol Ther* 1988;44:675–83.

71. Levy RH, Yerby MS. Effects of pregnancy on antiepileptic drug utilization. *Epilepsia* 1985;26(suppl 1):S52–7.

72. Leppik IE et al. Altered phenytoin clearance with febrile illness. *Neurology* 1986;36:1367–70.

73. Tozer TN, Winter ME. Phenytoin. In, Evans WE et al., eds. *Applied pharmacokinetics: principles of therapeutic drug monitoring.* 3rd ed. Vancouver: Applied Therapeutics; 1992.

74. Goff DA et al. Absorption characteristics of three phenytoin sodium products after administration of oral loading doses. *Clin Pharm* 1984;3:634–8.

75. McCauley DL et al. Time for phenytoin concentration to peak: consequences of first-order and zero-order absorption. *Ther Drug Monit* 1989;11:540–2.

76. Browne TR et al. Estimation of the elimination half-life of a drug at any serum concentration when the K_m and V_{max} of the drug are known: calculations and validation with phenytoin. *J Clin Pharmacol* 1987;27:318–20.

77. Spengler RF et al. Severe soft-tissue injury following intravenous infusion of phenytoin—patient and drug administration risk factors. *Arch Intern Med* 1988;148:1329–33.

78. Smythe MA, Umstead GS. Phenytoin hepatotoxicity: a review of the literature. *DICP* 1989;23:13–8.

79. Delattre JY et al. Erythema multiforme and Stevens-Johnson syndrome in patients receiving cranial irradiation and phenytoin. *Neurology* 1988;38:194–8.

80. Haley CJ, Nelson J. Phenytoin-enteral feeding interaction. *DICP* 1989;23:796–8.

81. Sarkar M et al. The effects of storage and shaking on the settling properties of phenytoin suspension. *Neurology* 1989;39:207–9.

82. Mattson RH et al. Comparison of carbamazepine, phenobarbital, phenytoin and primidone in partial and secondarily generalized tonic-clonic seizures. *N Engl J Med* 1985;313:145–51.

83. Pisani F et al. Single dose kinetics of primidone in acute viral hepatitis. *Eur J Clin Pharmacol* 1984;27:465–9.

84. Cottrell PR et al. Pharmacokinetics of phenylethylmalonamide (PEMA) in normal subjects and in patients treated with antiepileptic drugs. *Epilepsia* 1982;23:307–13.

85. Rosenfeld WE. Topiramate: a review of preclinical, pharmacokinetic, and clinical data. *Clin Therapeutics* 1997;19:1294–308.

86. Markind JE. Topiramate: a new antiepileptic drug. *Am J Health-Syst Pharm* 1998;55:554–62.

87. Jansen JA et al. Absolute bioavailability of tiagabine. *Epilepsia* 1995;36(suppl 3):S159. Abstract.

88. Perucca E, Bialer M. The clinical pharmacokinetics of the newer antiepileptic drugs: focus on topiramate, zonisamide and tiagabine. *Clin Pharmacokinet* 1996;31:29–46.

89. Gustavson LE, Mengel HB. Pharmacokinetics of tiagabine, a γ-aminobutyric acid-uptake inhibitor, in healthy subjects after single and multiple doses. *Epilepsia* 1995;36:605–11.

90. Privitera M et al. Dose-ranging trial with higher doses of topiramate in patients with resistant partial seizures. *Epilepsia* 1995;36(suppl 4):33. Abstract.

91. Rosenfeld WE et al. Comparison of the steady-state pharmacokinetics of topiramate and valproate in patients with epilepsy during monotherapy and concomitant therapy. *Epilepsia* 1997;38:324–33.

92. Rosenfeld WE et al. Effect of topiramate on the pharmacokinetics of an oral contraceptive containing norethindrone and ethinyl estradiol in patients with epilepsy. *Epilepsia* 1997;38:317–23.

93. Sachdeo SK et al. Topiramate double-blind trial as monotherapy. *Epilepsia* 1996;36(suppl 4):33. Abstract.

94. Sachdeo RC et al. A double-blind, randomized trial of topiramate in Lennox-Gastaut syndrome. *Neurology* 1999;52:1882–7.

95. Brodie MJ, Dichter MA. Antiepileptic drugs. *N Engl J Med* 1996;334:168–75.

96. Zaccara G et al. Clinical pharmacokinetics of valproic acid—1988. *Clin Pharmacokinet* 1988;15:367–89.

97. Fischer JH et al. Effect of food on the serum concentration profile on enteric-coated valproic acid. *Neurology* 1988;38:1319–22.

98. Holmes GB et al. Absorption of valproic acid suppositories in human volunteers. *Arch Neurol* 1989;46:906–9.

99. Dreifuss FE et al. Valproic acid hepatic fatalities—II. US experience since 1984. *Neurology* 1989;39:201–7.

100. Mattson RH et al. A comparison of valproic acid with carbamazepine for the treatment of complex partial seizures and secondarily generalized tonic-clonic seizures in adults. *N Engl J Med* 1992;327:765–71.

101. APA Practice Guideline for the Treatment of Patients with Bipolar Disorder. *Am J Psychiatry* 1994;12(suppl):1–36.

102. Bowden CL et al. Efficacy of divalproex vs lithium and placebo in the treatment of mania. *JAMA* 1994;271:918–24.

103. Bowden CL. Predictors of response to divalproex and lithium. *J Clin Psychiatry* 1995;56(suppl 3):25–30.

104. Rothrock JF et al. A differential response to treatment with divalproex sodium in patients with intractable headache. *Cephalalgia* 1994;14:241–4.

105. Mathew NT et al. Migraine prophylaxis with divalproex. *Arch Neurol* 1995;52:281–6.

106. Oommen KJ, Mathews S. Zonisamide: a new antiepileptic drug. *Clin Neuropharmacol* 1999;22:192–200.

107. Davidson JRT, Connor KM. Bupropion sustained release: a therapeutic overview. *J Clin Psychiatry* 1998;59(suppl 4):25–31.

108. Cooper BR et al. Evidence that the acute behavioral and electrophysiological effects of bupropion (Wellbutrin) are mediated by a noradrenergic mechanism. *Neuropsychopharmacology* 1994;11:133–41.

109. Walker PM et al. Improvement in fluoxetine-associated sexual dysfunction in patients switched to bupropion. *J Clin Psychiatry* 1993;54:459–65.

110. Goldstein MG. Bupropion sustained release and smoking cessation. *J Clin Psychiatry* 1998;59(suppl 4):66-72.

111. Jermain DM et al. Pharmacotherapy of obsessive-compulsive disorder. *Pharmacotherapy* 1990;10:175–98.

112. Peters MD et al. Clomipramine: an antiobsessional tricyclic antidepressant. *Clin Pharm* 1990;9:165–78.

113. Stokes PE. Fluoxetine: a five-year review. *Clin Ther* 1993;15:216–43.

114. Monteiro WO et al. Anorgasmia from clomipramine in obsessive-compulsive disorder: a controlled trial. *Br J Psychiatry* 1987;151:107–12.

115. Sommi RW et al. Fluoxetine: a serotonin-specific second-generation antidepressant. *Pharmacotherapy* 1987;7:1–15.

116. Schweizer E et al. What constitutes an adequate antidepressant trial for fluoxetine? *J Clin Psychiatry* 1990;51:8–11.

117. Steiner M et al. Intermittent fluoxetine dosing in the treatment of women with premenstrual dysphoric disorder. *Psychopharmacol Bull* 1997;33:771–4.

118. Benet LZ et al. Design and optimization of dosage regimens: pharmacokinetic data. In, Hardman JG et al., eds. *Goodman and Gilman's the pharmacological basis of therapeutics/* 9th ed. New York: McGraw-Hill; 1996:1707–92.

119. Gutierrez MA, Stimmel GL. Management of and counseling for psychotropic drug-induced sexual dysfunction. *Pharmacotherapy* 1999;19:823–31.

120. Rothschild AJ. Sexual side effects of antidepressants. *J Clin Psychiatry* 2000;61(suppl 11):28–36.

121. Kinney-Parker JL et al. Fluoxetine and weight: something lost and something gained? *Clin Pharm* 1989;8:727–33.

122. Jefferson JW. Cardiovascular effects and toxicity of anxiolytics and antidepressants. *J Clin Psychiatry* 1989;50:368–78.

123. Tollefson GD et al. Absence of a relationship between adverse events and suicidality during pharmacotherapy for depression. *J Clin Psychopharmacol* 1994;14:163–9.

124. Feighner JP et al. Adverse consequences of fluoxetine-MAOI combination therapy. *J Clin Psychiatry* 1990;51:222–5.

125. Roose SP et al. Comparative efficacy of selective serotonin reuptake inhibitors and tricyclics in the treatment of melancholia. *Am J Psychiatry* 1994;151:1735–9.

126. Grimsley SR, Jann MW. Paroxetine, sertraline, and fluvoxamine: new selective serotonin reuptake inhibitors. *Clin Pharm* 1992;11:930–57.

127. Wilde MI et al. Fluvoxamine: an updated review of its pharmacology and therapeutic use in depressive illness. *Drugs* 1993;46:895–924.

128. Freeman CPL et al. Fluvoxamine versus clomipramine in the treatment of obsessive-compulsive disorder: a multi-center, randomized, double-blind, parallel group comparison. *J Clin Psychiatry* 1994;55:301–5.

129. Potter WZ et al. The pharmacologic treatment of depression. *N Engl J Med* 1991;325:633–42.

130. Preskorn SH. Recent pharmacologic advances in antidepressant therapy for the elderly. *Am J Med* 1993;94(suppl 5A):2S–12.

131. Baldessarini RJ. Current status of antidepressants: clinical pharmacology and therapy. *J Clin Psychiatry* 1989;50:117–26.

132. Frank E et al. Comparison of full-dose versus half-dose pharmacotherapy in the maintenance treatment of recurrent depression. *J Affect Disord* 1993;27:139–45.

133. Wright JM. Review of the symptomatic treatment of diabetic neuropathy. *Pharmacotherapy* 1994;14:689–97.

134. Max MB. Treatment of post-herpetic neuralgia: antidepressants. *Ann Neurol* 1994;35:S50–3.

135. Rappoport JL et al. Childhood enuresis II. Psychopathology, tricyclic concentration in plasma, and antienuretic effect. *Arch Gen Psychiatry* 1980;37:1146–52.

136. Puig-Antich J et al. Imipramine in prepubertal major depressive disorders. *Arch Gen Psychiatry* 1987;44:81–9.

137. Salzman C. Pharmacologic treatment of depression in the elderly. *J Clin Psychiatry* 1993;54(suppl 2):23–8.

138. Salzman C. Practical considerations in the pharmacologic treatment of depression and anxiety in the elderly. *J Clin Psychiatry* 1990;51(suppl 1):40–3.

139. Wisner KL, et al. Tricyclic dose requirements across pregnancy. *Am J Psychiatry* 1993;150:1541–2.

140. Preskorn SH. Pharmacokinetics of antidepressants. *J Clin Psychiatry* 1993;54(suppl 9):14–34.

141. DeVane CL. *Fundamentals of monitoring psychoactive drug therapy.* Baltimore: Williams & Wilkins; 1990.

142. Cole JO, Bodkin A. Antidepressant drug side effects. *J Clin Psychiatry* 1990;51(suppl 1):21–6.

143. Rosenstein DL et al. Seizures associated with antidepressants: a review. *J Clin Psychiatry* 1993;54:289–99.

144. Anon. Sudden death in children treated with a tricyclic antidepressant. *Med Lett Drugs Ther* 1990;32:53.

145. Stimmel GL et al. Mirtazapine: an antidepressant with noradrenergic and specific serotonergic effects. *Pharmacotherapy* 1997;17:10–21.

146. Stimmel GL et al. Mirtazapine safety and tolerability: analysis of the clinical trials database. *Primary Psychiatry* 1997;4:82–96.

147. Goodman WK, Charney DS. Therapeutic applications and mechanisms of action of monoamine oxidase inhibitors and heterocyclic antidepressant drugs. *J Clin Psychiatry* 1985;46(10, sec 2):6–22.

148. Cantú TG, Korek JS. Monoamine oxidase inhibitors and weight gain. *Drug Intell Clin Pharm* 1988;22:755–9.

149. Kahn D et al. The safety of switching rapidly from tricyclic antidepressants to monoamine oxidase inhibitors. *J Clin Psychopharmacol* 1989;9:198–202.

150. Brown CS, Bryant SG. Monoamine oxidase inhibitors: safety and efficacy issues. *Drug Intell Clin Pharm* 1988;22:232–5.

151. Shulman KI et al. Dietary restriction, tyramine, and the use of monoamine oxidase inhibitors. *J Clin Psychopharmacol* 1989;9:397–402.

152. Nierenberg AA, Amsterdam JD. Treatment-resistant depression: definition and treatment approaches. *J Clin Psychiatry* 1990;51(suppl 6):39–47.

153. Dopheide JA et al. Focus on nefazodone: a serotonergic drug for major depression. *Hosp Formul* 1995;30:205–12.

154. Fontaine R et al. A double-blind comparison of nefazodone, imipramine, and placebo in major depression. *J Clin Psychiatry* 1994;55:234–41.

155. Barbhaiya RH et al. Single-dose pharmacokinetics of nefazodone in healthy young and elderly subjects and in subjects with renal or hepatic impairment. *Eur J Clin Pharmacol* 1995;49:221–8.

156. Barbhaiya RH et al. Steady-state pharmacokinetics of nefazodone in subjects normal and impaired renal function. *Eur J Clin Pharmacol* 1995;49:229–35.

157. Voris JC et al. Nefazodone: single versus twice daily dose. *Pharmacotherapy* 1998;18:379–80.

158. DeWilde J et al. A double-blind, comparative, multicentre study comparing paroxetine with fluoxetine in depressed patients. *Acta Psychiatr Scand* 1993;87:141–5.

159. Dechant KL, Clissold SPP. Paroxetine. *Drugs* 1991;41:225–53.

160. DeVane CL. Pharmacokinetics of the selective serotonin reuptake inhibitors. *J Clin Psychiatry* 1992;53(suppl 2):13–20.

161. Tollefson GD et al. A multicenter investigation of fixed dose fluoxetine in the treatment of obsessive-compulsive disorder. *Arch Gen Psychiatry* 1994;51:559–67.

162. Greist J et al. Double-blind parallel comparison of three dosages of sertraline and placebo in outpatients with obsessive-compulsive disorder. *Arch Gen Psychiatry* 1995;52:289–95.

163. Johnson MR et al. Panic disorder: pathophysiology and drug treatment. *Drugs* 1995;49:328–44.

164. Sheehan DV, Harnett-Sheehan K. The role of SSRIs in panic disorder. *J Clin Psychiatry* 1996;57(suppl 10):51–8.

165. Montejo-Gonzalez AL et al. SSRI-induced sexual dysfunction: fluoxetine, paroxetine, sertraline, and fluvoxamine in a prospective, multicenter, and descriptive clinical study of 344 patients. *J Sex Marital Ther* 1997;23:176–94.

166. Gutierrez MA et al. Reboxetine: a selective norepinephrine reuptake inhibitor for the treatment of major depression. *Formulary* 1999;34:909–19.

167. Schatzberg AF. Clinical efficacy of reboxetine in major depression. *J Clin Psychiatry* 2000;61(suppl 10):31–8.

168. Heym J, Koe BK. Pharmacology of sertraline: a review. *J Clin Psychiatry* 1988;49(suppl 8):40–5.

169. Doogan DP, Caillard V. Sertraline: a new antidepressant. *J Clin Psychiatry* 1988;49(suppl 8):46–51.

170. Aguglia E et al. Double-blind study of the efficacy and safety of sertraline versus fluoxetine in major depression. *Int Clin Psychopharmacol* 1993;8:197–202.

171. Wisner KL et al. Serum sertraline and *N*-desmethylsertraline levels in breast-feeding mother-infant pairs. *Am J Psychiatry* 1998;155:690–2.

172. Bradley ME et al. Sertraline-associated syndrome of inappropriate antidiuretic hormone: case report and review of the literature. *Pharmacotherapy* 1996;16:680–3.

173. Cunningham LA. Once-daily venlafaxine extended release (XR) and venlafaxine immediate release (IR) in outpatients with major depression. *Ann Clin Psychiatry* 1997;9:157–64.

174. Schweizer E et al. Placebo-controlled trial of venlafaxine for the treatment of major depression. *J Clin Psychopharmacol* 1991;11:233–6.

175. Montgomery SA. Venlafaxine: a new dimension in antidepressant pharmacotherapy. *J Clin Psychiatry* 1993;54:119–26.

176. Cunningham LA et al. A comparison of venlafaxine, trazodone, and placebo in major depression. *J Clin Psychopharmacol* 1994;14:99–106.

177. Bryant SG, Ereshefsky L. Antidepressant properties of trazodone. *Clin Pharm* 1982;1:406–17.

178. Milne RJ, Goa KL. Citalopram. *Drugs* 1991;41:450–77.

179. Montgomery SA et al. The optimal dosing regimen for citalopram—a meta-analysis of nine placebo-controlled studies. *Int Clin Psychopharmacol* 1994;9(suppl 1):35–40.

180. Schatzberg AF. New indications for antidepressants. *J Clin Psychiatry* 2000;61(suppl 11):9-17.

181. Ereshefsky L et al. Pathophysiologic basis for schizophrenia and the efficacy of antipsychotics. *Clin Pharm* 1990;9:682–707.

182. Coyle JT. The clinical use of antipsychotic medications. *Med Clin North Am* 1982;66:993–1009.

183. Kane JM. The current status of neuroleptic therapy. *J Clin Psychiatry* 1989;50:322–8.

184. Heresco-Levy U et al. Trial of maintenance neuroleptic dose reduction in schizophrenic outpatients: two year outcome. *J Clin Psychiatry* 1993;54:59–62.

185. Brotman AW et al. A role for high-dose antipsychotics. *J Clin Psychiatry* 1990;51:164–6.

186. Rifkin A et al. Dosage of haloperidol for mania. *Br J Psychiatry* 1994;165:113–6.

187. Zaleon CR, Guthrie SK. Antipsychotic drug use in older adults. *Am J Hosp Pharm* 1994;51:2917–43.

188. Coryell W et al. Haloperidol plasma levels and dose optimization. *Am J Psychiatry* 1998;155:48–53.

189. Khot V et al. The assessment and clinical implications of haloperidol acute-dose, steady-state, and withdrawal pharmacokinetics. *J Clin Psychopharmacol* 1993;13:120–7.

190. Pearlman CA. Neuroleptic malignant syndrome: a review of the literature. *J Clin Psychopharmacol* 1986;6:257–73.

191. Gardos G et al. Ten year outcome of tardive dyskinesia. *Am J Psychiatry* 1994;151:836–41.

192. Ereshefsky L et al. Clozapine: an atypical antipsychotic agent. *Clin Pharm* 1989;8:691–709.

193. Lieberman JA et al. Clozapine: guidelines for clinical management. *J Clin Psychiatry* 1989;50:329–38.

194. Meltzer HY. An overview of the mechanism of action of clozapine. *J Clin Psychiatry* 1994;55(suppl 9):47–52.

195. Lieberman JA et al. Clinical effects of clozapine in chronic schizophrenia: response to treatment and predictors of outcome. *Am J Psychiatry* 1994;151:1744–52.

196. Jann MW et al. Pharmacokinetics and pharmacodynamics of clozapine. *Clin Pharmacokinet* 1993;24:161–76.

197. Alvir JMJ, Lieberman JA. Agranulocytosis: incidence and risk factors. *J Clin Psychiatry* 1994;55(suppl 9):137–8.

198. Miller DD. Review and management of clozapine side effects. *J Clin Psychiatry* 2000;61(suppl 8):14–7.

199. Chouinard G et al. A randomized clinical trial of haloperidol decanoate and fluphenazine decanoate in the outpatient treatment of schizophrenia. *J Clin Psychopharmacol* 1989;9:247–53.

200. Hemstrom CA et al. Haloperidol decanoate: a depot antipsychotic. *Drug Intell Clin Pharm* 1988;22:290–5.

201. Gerlach J. Oral versus depot administration of neuroleptics in relapse prevention. *Acta Psychiatr Scand* 1994;89(suppl 382):28–32.

202. Inderbitzin LB et al. A double-blind dose-reduction trial of fluphenazine decanoate for chronic, unstable schizophrenic patients. *Am J Psychiatry* 1994;151:1753–9.

203. Ereshefsky L et al. A loading-dose strategy for converting from oral to depot haloperidol. *Hosp Community Psychiatry* 1993;44:1155–61.

204. Foster RH, Goa KL. Olanzapine. *Pharmacoeconomics* 1999;15:611–40.

205. Bever KA, Perry PJ. Olanzapine: a serotonin-dopamine receptor antagonist for antipsychotic therapy. *Am J Health-Syst Pharm* 1998;55:1003–16.

206. Colvin CL, Tankanow RM. Pimozide: use in Tourette's syndrome. *Drug Intell Clin Pharm* 1985;19:421–4.

207. Tueth MJ, Cheong JA. Clinical uses of pimozide. *South Med J* 1993;86:344–9.

208. Ereshefsky L, Lacomb S. Pharmacological profile of risperidone. *Can J Psychiatry* 1993;38(suppl 3):S80–8.

209. Cohen LJ. Risperidone. *Pharmacotherapy* 1994;14:253–65.

210. Livingston MG. Risperidone. *Lancet* 1994;343:457–60.

211. Marder SR, Meibach RC. Risperidone in the treatment of schizophrenia. *Am J Psychiatry* 1994;151:825–35.

212. Heykants J et al. The pharmacokinetics of risperidone in humans: a summary. *J Clin Psychiatry* 1994;55(suppl 5):13–7.

213. Chou JCY, Serper MR. Ziprasidone—a new highly atypical antipsychotic. *Essent Psychopharmacol* 1998;2:463–85.

214. Allison DB et al. Antipsychotic-induced weight gain: a comprehensive research synthesis. *Am J Psychiatry* 1999;156:1686–96.

215. American Psychiatric Association. Practice guideline for the treatment of patients with schizophrenia. *Am J Psychiatry* 1997;154(suppl 4):1–63.

216. Beasley CM et al. Safety of olanzapine. *J Clin Psychiatry* 1997;58(suppl 10):13–7.

217. Small JG et al. Quetiapine in patients with schizophrenia. *Arch Gen Psychiatry* 1997;54:549–57.

218. Anon. Quetiapine for schizophrenia. *Med Lett Drugs Ther* 1997;39:117–8.

219. Arvanitis LA et al. Multiple fixed doses of Seroquel (quetiapine) in patients with acute exacerbation of schizophrenia: a comparison with haloperidol and placebo. *Biol Psychiatry* 1997;42:233–46.

220. Jonas JM, Cohon MS. A comparison of the safety and efficacy of alprazolam versus other agents in the treatment of anxiety, panic, and depression: a review of the literature. *J Clin Psychiatry* 1993;54(suppl 10):25–45.

221. Fawcett JA, Kravitz HM. Alprazolam: pharmacokinetics, clinical efficacy, and mechanism of action. *Pharmacotherapy* 1982;2:243–54.

222. Scavone JM et al. Alprazolam kinetics following sublingual and oral administration. *J Clin Psychopharmacol* 1987;7:332–4.

223. Kroboth et al. Alprazolam in the elderly: pharmacokinetics and pharmacodynamics during multiple dosing. *Psychopharmacology* 1990;100:477–84.

224. Patterson JF. Alprazolam dependency: use of clonazepam for withdrawal. *South Med J* 1988;81:830–2.

225. Dubovsky SL. Generalized anxiety disorder: new concepts and psychopharmacologic therapies. *J Clin Psychiatry* 1990;51(suppl 1):3–10.

226. Gorman JM, Papp LA. Chronic anxiety: deciding the length of treatment. *J Clin Psychiatry* 1990;51(suppl 1):11–5.

227. Kranzler HR, Orrok B. The pharmacotherapy of alcoholism. In, Tasman A et al., eds. *Review of psychiatry.* Vol. 8. Washington, DC: American Psychiatric Press; 1989:359–30.

228. Roy-Byrne PP, Cowley DS. *Benzodiazepines in clinical practice: risks and benefits.* Washington, DC: American Psychiatric Press; 1991:213–27.

229. Greenblatt DJ et al. Benzodiazepines: a summary of pharmacokinetic properties. *Br J Clin Pharmacol* 1981;11:11S–6.

230. Dietch JT, Jennings RK. Aggressive dyscontrol in patients treated with benzodiazepines. *J Clin Psychiatry* 1988;49:184–8.

231. Jann MW. Buspirone: an update on a unique anxiolytic agent. *Pharmacotherapy* 1988;8:100–16.

232. Sussman N. The uses of buspirone in psychiatry. *J Clin Psychiatry Monogr* 1994;12:3–19.

233. Gammans RE et al. Pharmacokinetics of buspirone in elderly subjects. *J Clin Pharmacol* 1989;29:72–8.

234. Gammans RE et al. Metabolism and disposition of buspirone. *Am J Med* 1986;80(suppl 3B):41–51.

235. Newton RE et al. Review of the side-effect profile of buspirone. *Am J Med* 1986;80(suppl 3B):17–21.

236. Schweizer E, Rickels K. New and emerging clinical uses for buspirone. *J Clin Psychiatry Monogr* 1994;12:46–54.

237. Brogden RN, Goa KL. Flumazenil. A preliminary review of its benzodiazepine antagonist properties, intrinsic activity and therapeutic use. *Drugs* 1988;35:448–67.

238. Longmire AW, Seger DL. Topics in clinical pharmacology: flumazenil, a benzodiazepine antagonist. *Am J Med Sci* 1993;306:49–52.

239. Hoffman EJ, Warren EW. Flumazenil: a benzodiazepine antagonist. *Clin Pharm* 1993;12:641–56.

240. Spivey WH. Flumazenil and seizures: analysis of 43 cases. *Clin Ther* 1992;14:292–305.

241. Kanto JH. Midazolam: the first water-soluble benzodiazepine. *Pharmacotherapy* 1985;5:138–55.

242. Bell GD et al. Intravenous midazolam for upper gastrointestinal endoscopy: a study of 800 consecutive cases relating dose to age and sex of patient. *Br J Clin Pharmacol* 1987;23:241–3.

243. Daneshmend TK, Logan RFA. Midazolam. *Lancet* 1988;1:389. Letter.

244. Saint-Maurice C et al. The pharmacokinetics of rectal midazolam for premedication in children. *Anesthesiology* 1986;65:536–8.

245. Yakabowich MR. Hypnotics in the elderly: appropriate usage guidelines. *J Geriatr Drug Ther* 1992;6:5–21.

246. Weiss KJ. Management of anxiety and depression syndromes in the elderly. *J Clin Psychiatry* 1994;55(suppl 2):5–12.

247. Garzone PD, Kroboth PD. Pharmacokinetics of the newer benzodiazepines. *Clin Pharmacokinet* 1989;16:337–64.

248. Robin DW et al. Triazolam in cirrhosis: pharmacokinetics and pharmacodynamics. *Clin Pharmacol Ther* 1993;54:630–7.

249. Scharf MB et al. Comparative amnestic effects of benzodiazepine hypnotic agents. *J Clin Psychiatry* 1988;49:134–7.

250. Roth T et al. Pharmacology and hypnotic efficacy of triazolam. *Pharmacotherapy* 1983;3:137–48.

251. Gillin JC, Byerley W. The diagnosis and management of insomnia. *N Engl J Med* 1990;322:239–48.

252. Treatment of sleep disorders of older people. *NIH Consensus Dev Conf Consens Statement* 1990;8:26–8.

253. Stimmel GL, Dopheide JA. Sleep disorders: focus on insomnia. *US Pharmacist* 2000;25:69–80.

254. Greenblatt DJ et al. Comparative kinetics and dynamics of zaleplon, zolpidem, and placebo. *Clin Pharmacol Ther* 1998;64:553–61.

255. Danjou P et al. A comparison of the residual effects of zaleplon and zolpidem following administration 5 to 2 h before awakening. *Br J Clin Pharmacol* 1999;48:367–74.

256. Scharf MB et al. A multi-center placebo-controlled study evaluating zolpidem in the treatment of chronic insomnia. *J Clin Psychiatry* 1994;55:192–9.

257. Jonas JM et al. Comparative clinical profiles of triazolam versus other shorter-acting hypnotics. *J Clin Psychiatry* 1992;53(suppl 12):19–31.

258. Langtry HD, Benfield P. Zolpidem: a review of its pharmacodynamic and pharmacokinetic properties and therapeutic potential. *Drugs* 1990;40:291–313.

259. Mitler MM. Evaluation of temazepam as a hypnotic. *Pharmacotherapy* 1981;1:3–13.

260. Kales A. Quazepam: hypnotic efficacy and side effects. *Pharmacotherapy* 1990;10:1–12.

261. Scherf MB et al. Estazolam and flurazepam: a multicenter, placebo-controlled comparative study in outpatients with insomnia. *J Clin Pharmacol* 1990;30:461–7.

262. Anon. Hypnotic drugs. *Med Lett Drugs Ther* 2000;42:71–2.

263. Breimer DD. Clinical pharmacokinetics of hypnotics. *Clin Pharmacokinet* 1977;2:93–109.

264. Post RM et al. Mechanisms of action of anticonvulsants in affective disorders: comparisons with lithium. *J Clin Psychopharmacol* 1992;12:23S–35.

265. Bowden CL. Efficacy of lithium in mania and maintenance therapy of bipolar disorder. *J Clin Psychiatry* 2000;61(suppl 9):35–40.

266. Kook KA et al. Accuracy and safety of a priori lithium loading. *J Clin Psychiatry* 1985;46:49–51.

267. Lobeck F. A review of lithium dosing methods. *Pharmacotherapy* 1988;8:248–55.

268. Gutierrez MA et al. Evaluation of a new steady-state lithium prediction method. *Lithium* 1991;2:57–9.

269. *USP-DI*, Vol I. Rockville, MD. The United States Pharmacopoeal Convention; 1996.

270. Hardy BG et al. Pharmacokinetics of lithium in the elderly. *J Clin Psychopharmacol* 1987;7:153–8.

271. Jefferson JW. Lithium: a therapeutic magic wand. *J Clin Psychiatry* 1989;50:81–6.

272. Jefferson JW. Lithium: the present and the future. *J Clin Psychiatry* 1990;51(suppl 8):4–8.

273. Gitlin MJ et al. Maintenance lithium treatment: side effects and compliance. *J Clin Psychiatry* 1989;50:127–31.

274. Salem RB. Recommendations for monitoring lithium therapy. *Drug Intell Clin Pharm* 1983;17:346–50.

275. Gitlin MJ. Lithium-induced renal insufficiency. *J Clin Psychopharmacol* 1993;13:276–9.

276. American Psychiatric Association. Practice guideline for the treatment of patients with bipolar disorder. *Am J Psychiatry* 1994;151(suppl 12):1–36.

277. Guay DRP. The emerging role of valproate in bipolar disorder and other psychiatric disorders. *Pharmacotherapy* 1995;15:631–47.

278. Bowden CL et al. Relation of serum valproate concentrations to response in mania. *Am J Psychiatry* 1996;153:765–70.

279. Snow B et al. The effect of amantadine on levodopa-induced dyskinesias in Parkinson's disease: a double-blind, placebo-controlled study. *Clin Neuropharmacol* 2000;23:82–5.

280. Stacy M. Pharmacotherapy for advanced Parkinson's disease. *Pharmacotherapy* 2000;20(1, pt 2):8S–16.

281. Koller WC et al. An algorithm for managing Parkinson's disease. *Neurology* 1994;44(suppl 1):S1–52.

282. Stern MB. Contemporary approaches to the pharmacotherapeutic management of Parkinson's disease: an overview. *Neurology* 1997;49(suppl 1):S2–9.

283. Aoki FY, Sitar DA. Clinical pharmacokinetics of amantadine hydrochloride. *Clin Pharmacokinet* 1988;14:35–51.

284. Hordam VW et al. Pharmacokinetics of amantadine hydrochloride in subjects with normal and impaired renal function. *Ann Intern Med* 1981;94(pt 1):454–8.

285. Aoki FY, Sitar DS. Amantadine kinetics in healthy elderly men: implications for influenza prevention. *Clin Pharmacol Ther* 1985;37:137–44.

286. Lang AE, Lozano AM. Parkinson's disease. *N Engl J Med* 1998;339:1130–43.

287. He H et al. Development of a sensitive and specific radioimmunoassay for benztropine. *J Pharm Sci* 1993;82:1027–32.

288. Nutt JG et al. The effect of carbidopa on the pharmacokinetics of intravenously administered levodopa: the mechanism of action in the treatment of parkinsonism. *Ann Neurol* 1985;18:537–43.

289. Juncos JL. Levodopa: pharmacology, pharmacokinetics, and pharmacodynamics. *Neurol Clin* 1992;10:487–509.

290. Yeh KC et al. Pharmacokinetics and bioavailability of Sinemet CR: a summary of human studies. *Neurology* 1989;39(suppl 2):S25–38.

291. LeWitt PA. Treatment strategies for extension of levodopa effect. *Neurol Clin* 1992;10:511–26.

292. Koller WC, Hubble JP. Levodopa therapy in Parkinson's disease. *Neurology* 1990;40(suppl 3):S40–7.

293. Cedarbaum JM. Pharmacokinetic and pharmacodynamic considerations in management of motor response fluctuations in Parkinson's disease. *Neurol Clin* 1990;8:31–49.

294. Hutton JT et al. Multicenter controlled study of Sinemet CR vs Sinemet (25/100) in advanced Parkinson's disease. *Neurology* 1989;39(suppl 2):S67–72.

295. Rogers SL, Friedhoff LT, and the Donepezil Study Group. The efficacy and safety of donepezil in patients with Alzheimer's disease. Results of a US multicentre, randomized, double-blind, placebo-controlled trial. *Dementia* 1996;7:293–303.

296. Rogers SL et al. A 24-week, double-blind, placebo-controlled trial of donepezil in patients with Alzheimer's disease. *Neurology* 1998;50:136–45.

297. Rogers SL et al. The pharmacokinetics and pharmacodynamics of E2020 (R,S)-1-benzyl-4-((5,6 dimethoxyl-1-indanon)-2 yl)-methylpiperidine hydrochloride, a novel inhibitor of acetylcholinesterase: implications for use in the treatment of Alzheimer's disease. *Neurobiol Aging* 1992;13:496.

298. Rogers SL, Friedhoff LT. The pharmacokinetic and pharmacodynamic profile of donepezil HCl (E2020) following single and multiple oral doses. *Clin Pharmacol Ther* 1997;61:181. Abstract.

299. Watts RL. The role of dopamine agonists in early Parkinson's disease. *Neurology* 1997;49(suppl 1):S34–48.

300. Goetz CG, Diederich NJ. Dopaminergic agonists for the treatment of Parkinson's disease. *Neurol Clin* 1992;10:527–40.

301. Piercey MF et al. Functional roles for dopamine-receptor subtypes. *Clin Neuropharmacol* 1995;18(suppl 1):S34–42.

302. Schran HF et al. The pharmacokinetics of bromocriptine in man. In, Goldstein M et al., eds. *Ergot compounds and brain function.* New York: Raven Press; 1980:125–39.

303. Friis ML et al. Pharmacokinetics of bromocriptine during continuous oral treatment of Parkinson's disease. *Eur J Clin Pharmacol* 1979;15:275–80.

304. Thalamas C et al. Effect of food on the pharmacokinetics of ropinirole in patients with Parkinson's disease. *Mov Disord* 1996;2(suppl 1):138. Abstract.

305. Gottwald MD et al. New pharmacotherapy for Parkinson's disease. *Ann Pharmacother* 1997;31:1205–17.

306. Rubin A et al. Physiologic disposition of pergolide. *Clin Pharmacol Ther* 1981;30:258–65.

307. McElvaney NG et al. Pleuropulmonary disease during bromocriptine treatment of Parkinson's disease. *Arch Intern Med* 1988;148:2231–6.

308. Langtry HD, Clissold SPP. Pergolide. A review of its pharmacological properties and therapeutic potential in Parkinson's disease. *Drugs* 1990;39:491–506.

309. Mizuno Y et al. Pergolide in the treatment of Parkinson's disease. *Neurology* 1995;45(suppl 3):S13–21.

310. Hubble JP et al. Pramipexole in patients with early Parkinson's disease. *Clin Neuropharmacol* 1995;18:338–47.

311. Parkinson Study Group. Safety and efficacy of pramipexole in early Parkinson disease. *JAMA* 1997;278:125–30.

312. Lieberman A et al. Clinical evaluation of pramipexole in advanced Parkinson's disease: results of a double-blind, placebo-controlled, parallel-group study. *Neurology* 1997;49:162–8.

313. Bonifati V, Meco G. New, selective catechol-*O*-methyltransferase inhibitors as therapeutic agents in Parkinson's disease. *Pharmacol Ther* 1999;81:1–36.

314. Keränen T et al. Inhibition of soluble catechol-*O*-methyltransferase and single-dose pharmacokinetics after oral and intravenous administration of entacapone. *Eur J Clin Pharmacol* 1994;46:151–7.

315. Scott LJ, Goa KL. Galantamine. A review of its use in Alzheimer's disease. *Drugs* 2000;60:1095–22.

316. Grutzendler J, Morris JC. Cholineserase inhibitors for Alzheimer's disease. *Drugs* 2000;61:41–52.

317. Bryson HM et al. Riluzole. A review of its pharmacodynamic and pharmacokinetic properties and therapeutic potential in amyotrophic lateral sclerosis. *Drugs* 1996;52:549–63.

318. Sanderink GJ et al. Involvement of human CYP1A isoenzymes in the metabolism and drug interactions of riluzole in vitro. *J Pharmacol Exp Ther* 1997;282:1465–72.

319. Bruno E et al. Population pharmacokinetics of riluzole in patients with amyotrophic lateral sclerosis. *Clin Pharmacol Ther* 1997;62:518–26.

320. Practice advisory on the treatment of amyotrophic lateral sclerosis with riluzole: report of the Quality Standards Subcommittee of the American Academy of Neurology. *Neurology* 1997;49:657–9.

321. Bensimon G et al. and the ALS/Riluzole Study Group. A controlled trial of riluzole in amyotrophic lateral sclerosis. *N Engl J Med* 1994;330:585–91.

322. Polinsky RJ. Clinical pharmacology of rivastigmine: a new-generation acetylcholinesterase inhibitor for the treatment of Alzheimer's disease. *Clin Ther* 1998;20;634–7.

323. Jann MW. Rivastigmine, a new-generation cholinesterase inhibitor for the treatment of Alzheimer's disease. *Pharmacotherapy* 2000;20:1–12.

324. Cutler NR et al. Dose-dependent CSF acetylcholinesterase inhibition by SDZ ENA 713 in Alzheimer's disease. *Acta Neurol Scand* 1998;97:244–50.

325. Youdim MBH, Finberg JPM. Pharmacological actions of l-deprenyl (selegiline) and other selective monoamine oxidase B inhibitors. *Clin Pharmacol Ther* 1994;56:725–33.

326. Mahmood I. Clinical pharmacokinetics and pharmacodynamics of selegiline. *Clin Pharmacokinet* 1997;33:99–102.

327. Olanow CW. Attempts to obtain neuroprotection in Parkinson's disease. *Neurology* 1997;49(suppl 1):S26–33.

328. The Parkinson Study Group. Effects of tocopherol and deprenyl on the progression of disability in early Parkinson's disease. *N Engl J Med* 1993;328:176–83.

329. The Parkinson Study Group. Effect of deprenyl on the progression of disability in early Parkinson's disease. *N Engl J Med* 1989;321:1364–71.

330. Parkinson Study Group. Impact of deprenyl and tocopherol treatment on Parkinson's disease in DATATOP patients requiring levodopa. *Ann Neurol* 1996;39:37–45.

331. Parkinson Study Group. Impact of deprenyl and tocopherol treatment on Parkinson's disease in DATATOP subjects not requiring levodopa. *Ann Neurol* 1996;39:29–36.

332. Heinonen EH et al. Pharmacokinetics and metabolism of selegiline. *Acta Neurol Scand* 1989;80(suppl 126):93–9.

333. Dingemanse J et al. Integrated pharmacokinetics and pharmacodynamics of the novel catechol-O-methyltransferase inhibitor tolcapone during first administration to humans. *Clin Pharmacol Ther* 1995;57:508–17.

334. Jorga KM et al. Optimizing levodopa pharmacokinetics with multiple tolcapone doses in the elderly. *Clin Pharmacol Ther* 1997;62:300–10.

335. Kurth MC et al. Tolcapone improves motor function and reduces levodopa requirement in patients with Parkinson's disease experiencing motor fluctuations: a multicenter, double-blind, randomized, placebo-controlled trial. *Neurology* 1997;48:81–7.

336. Waters CH. Tolcapone in stable Parkinson's disease: efficacy and safety of long-term treatment. The Tolcapone Stable Study Group. *Neurology* 1997;49:665–71.

337. Rajput AH et al. Tolcapone improves motor function in parkinsonian patients with the "wearing-off" phenomenon: a double-blind, placebo-controlled, multicenter trial. *Neurology* 1997;49:1066–71.

338. USP. *USP-DI. Volume II: advice for the patient: drug information in lay language.* 19th ed. Englewood, CO: Micromedex; 1999.

339. Alward WLM. Medical management of glaucoma. *N Engl J Med* 1998;339:1298–308.

340. Quigley HA. Open-angle glaucoma. *N Engl J Med* 1993;328:1097–106.

341. Stamper RL et al., eds. *Becker-Shaffer's diagnosis and therapy of the glaucomas.* St Louis: Mosby; 1999.

342. Schoenwald RD. Ocular pharmacokinetics. In, Zimmerman TJ et al., eds. *Textbook of ocular pharmacology.* Philadelphia: Lippincott-Raven; 1999:119–38.

343. Aritürk N et al. The effects of nasolacrimal canal blockage on topical medications for glaucoma. *Acta Ophthalmol Scand* 1996;74:411–3.

344. Fiscella RG. Costs of glaucoma medications. *Am J Health-Syst Pharm* 1998;55:272–5.

345. Coleman AL. Glaucoma. *Lancet* 1999;354:1803–10.

346. Hoyng PFJ, van Beek LM. Pharmacological therapy for glaucoma: a review. *Drugs* 2000;59:411–34.

347. Gurwitz JH et al. Treatment for glaucoma: adherence by the elderly. *Am J Public Health* 1993;83:711–6.

348. Zimmerman TJ et al. Therapeutic index of pilocarpine, carbachol, and timolol with nasolacrimal occlusion. *Am J Ophthalmol* 1992;114:1–7.

349. Everitt DE, Avorn J. Systemic effects of medications used to treat glaucoma. *Ann Intern Med* 1990;112: 120–5.

350. Schuman JS et al. A 1-year study of brimonidine twice daily in glaucoma and ocular hypertension. *Arch Ophthalmol* 1997;115:847–52.

351. Georg WS et al. Efficacy of brimonidine 0.2% as adjunctive therapy for patients with glaucoma inadequately controlled with otherwise maximal medical therapy. *Ophthalmology* 1999;106:1616–20.

352. Javitt JC et al. Clinical success and quality of life with brimonidine 0.2% or timolol 0.5% used twice daily in glaucoma or ocular hypertension: a randomized clinical trial. *J Glaucoma* 2000;9:224–34.

353. Serle JB, Brimonidine Study Group III. A comparison of the safety and efficacy of twice daily brimonidine 0.2% versus betaxolol 0.25% in subjects with elevated intraocular pressure. *Surv Ophthalmol* 1996;41(suppl 1):S39–47.

354. Allen RC et al. A double-masked comparison of betaxolol vs timolol in the treatment of open-angle glaucoma. *Am J Ophthalmol* 1996;101:535–41.

355. Sorensen SJ, Abel SR. Comparison of the ocular beta-blockers. *Ann Pharmacother* 1996;30:43–54.

356. James IM. Pharmacologic effects of beta-blocking agents used in the management of glaucoma (summary). *Surv Ophthalmol* 1989;33(suppl):453–4.

357. Stewart WC et al. Efficacy of carteolol hydrochloride 1% vs timolol maleate 0.5% in patients with increased intraocular pressure. *Am J Ophthalmol* 1997;124:498–505.

358. Netland PA et al. Cardiovascular effects of topical carteolol hydrochloride and timolol maleate in patients with ocular hypertension and primary open-angle glaucoma. *Am J Ophthalmol* 1997;123:465–77.

526   CENTRAL NERVOUS SYSTEM DRUGS

359. Diggory P et al. Topical beta-blockade with intrinsic sympathomimetic activity offers no advantage for the respiratory and cardiovascular function of elderly people. *Age Ageing* 1996;25:424–8.
360. Arend O et al. The acute effect of topical beta-adrenoreceptor blocking agents on retinal and optic nerve head circulation. *Acta Ophthalmol Scand* 1998;76:43–9.
361. Akingbehin T, Villada JR. Metipranolol-associated granulomatous anterior uveitis. *Br J Ophthalmol* 1991;75:519–23.
362. Akingbehin T et al. Metipranolol-induced adverse reactions: I. The rechallenge study. *Eye* 1992;6:277–9.
363. Gross RL, Pineyro A. Current use of ophthalmic beta blockers. *J Glaucoma* 1997;6:188–91.
364. Piper JG. Oral carbonic anhydrase inhibitors. In, Zimmerman TJ et al., eds. *Textbook of ocular pharmacology.* Philadelphia: Lippincott-Raven; 1999;277–85.
365. Palmberg P. A topical carbonic anhydrase inhibitor finally arrives. *Arch Ophthalmol* 1995;113:985–6. Editorial.
366. Strahlman ER et al. The use of dorzolamide and pilocarpine as adjunctive therapy to timolol in patients with elevated intraocular pressure. *Ophthalmology* 1996;103:1283–93.
367. Dumont L et al. Efficacy and harm of pharmacological prevention of acute mountainsickness: quantitative systematic review. *BMJ* 2000;321:267–72.
368. Donohue EK, Wilensky JT. Trusopt, a topical carbonic anhydrase inhibitor. *J Glaucoma* 1996;5:68–74.
369. Silver LH and the Brinzolamide Dose-Response Study Group. Dose-response evaluation of the ocular hypotensive effect of brinzolamide ophthalmic suspension (Azopt®). *Surv Ophthalmol* 2000;44(suppl 2):147–53.
370. Strahlman E et al. A double-masked, randomized 1-year study comparing dorzolamide (Trusopt), timolol, and betaxolol. *Arch Ophthalmol* 1995;113:1009–16.
371. Centofanti M et al. Comparative effects on intraocular pressure between systemic and topical carbonic anhydrase inhibitors: a clinical masked, cross-over study. *Pharmacol Res* 1997;35:481–5.
372. Lippa EA et al. MK-507 versus sezolamide: comparative efficacy of two topically active carbonic anhydrase inhibitors. *Ophthalmology* 1991;98:308–13.
373. Strohmaier K et al. A multicenter study comparing dorzolamide and pilocarpine as adjunctive therapy to timolol: patient preference and impact on daily life. *J Am Optom Assoc* 1998;69:441–51.
374. Shirato S et al. Stevens-Johnson syndrome induced by methazolamide treatment. *Arch Ophthalmol* 1997;115:550–3.
375. Epstein R et al. Combination of systemic acetazolamide and topical dorzolamide. *Ophthalmology* 1998;105:1581–2. Letter.
376. Rousseau P, Fuentevilla-Clifton A. Acetazolamide and salicylate interaction in the elderly: a case report. *JAGS* 1993;41:868–9.
377. Yablonski ME et al. Enhancement of the ocular hypotensive effect of acetazolamide by diflunisal. *Am J Ophthamol* 1998;106:332–6.
378. Fraunfelder FT, Fraunfelder FW. Short-term use of carbonic anhydrase inhibitors and hematologic side effects. *Arch Ophthalmol* 1992;110:446–7. Letter.
379. Hutzelmann JE et al. A comparison of the efficacy and tolerability of dorzolamide and acetazolamide as adjunctive therapy to timolol. *Acta Ophthalmol Scand* 1998;76:717–22.
380. Hammond RW. Understand what makes glaucoma agents work: a look at the drug mechanisms that lower IOP. *Rev Optom* 1994;131(suppl):2A–4A, 9A–20A.
381. Stewart RH et al. Long acting pilocarpine gel: a dose-response in ocular hypertensive subjects. *Glaucoma* 1984;6:182–5.
382. Hiett JA, Carlson DM. Ocular cholinergic agents. In, Onofrey BE, ed. *Clinical optometric pharmacology and therapeutics.* Philadelphia: Lippincott-Raven; 1997;Chap. 10:1–23.
383. Kaufman PL, Gabelt BT. Direct, indirect, and dual-action parasympathetic drugs. In, Zimmerman TJ et al., eds. *Textbook of ocular pharmacology.* Philadelphia: Lippincott-Raven; 1997:221–38.
384. Manoguerra A et al. Cholinergic toxicity resulting from ocular instillation of echothiophate iodide eye drops. *Clin Toxicol* 1995;33:463–5.
385. Kushnick H et al. Systemic pilocarpine toxicity from Ocusert leakage. *Arch Ophthalmol* 1996;114:1432. Letter.
386. Stelmack TR. Glaucoma medications: perspective. In, Onofrey BE, ed. *Clinical optometric pharmacology and therapeutics.* Philadelphia: Lippincott-Raven; 1997;Chap. 18:1–25.
387. Patel SS, Spencer CM. Latanoprost: a review of its pharmacological properties, clinical efficacy and tolerability in the management of primary open-angle glaucoma and ocular hypertension. *Drugs Aging* 1996;9:363–78.
388. Alm A, Widengard I. Latanoprost: experience of 2-year treatment in Scandinavia. *Acta Ophthalmol Scand* 2000;78:71–6.
389. Martin L. Clinical experience with latanoprost: a retrospective study of 153 patients. *Acta Ophthalmol Scand* 1999;77:336–9.

390. Camras CB et al. Latanoprost, a prostaglandin analog, for glaucoma therapy: efficacy and safety after 1 year of treatment in 198 patients. *Ophthalmology* 1996;103:1916–24.

391. Camras CB et al. Comparison of latanoprost and timolol in patients with ocular hypertension and glaucoma: a six-month, masked, multicenter trial in the United States. *Ophthalmology* 1996;103:138–47.

392. Greve EL et al. Reduced intraocular pressure and increased ocular perfusion pressure in normal tension glaucoma: a review of short-term studies with three dose regimens of latanoprost treatment. *Surv Ophthalmol* 1997;41(suppl 2):S89–92.

393. Haria M, Spencer CM. Unoprostone (isopropyl unoprostone). *Drugs Aging* 1996;9:213–8.

394. Yamomoto T et al. Clinical evaluation of UF-021 (Rescula; isopropyl unoprostone). *Surv Ophthalmol* 1997;41(suppl 2):S99–103.

395. Lusky M et al. A comparative study of two dose regimens of latanoprost in patients with elevated intraocular pressure. *Ophthalmology* 1997;104:1720–4.

396. Friström B. A 6-month, randomized, double-masked comparison of latanoprost with timolol in patients with open angle glaucoma or ocular hypertension. *Acta Ophthalmol Scand* 1996;74:140–4.

397. Alm A et al. Effects on intraocular pressure and side effects of 0.005% latanoprost applied once daily, evening or morning: a comparison with timolol. *Ophthalmology* 1995;102:1743–52.

398. Alm A. Prostaglandin derivates as ocular hypotensive agents. *Prog Retin Eye Res* 1998;17:291–312.

399. Watson P et al. A six-month, randomized, double-masked study comparing latanoprost with timolol in open-angle glaucoma and ocular hypertension. *Ophthalmology* 1996;103:126–37.

400. Wistrand PJ et al. The incidence and time-course of latanoprost-induced iridial pigmentation as a function of eye color. *Surv Ophthalmol* 1997;41(suppl 2):S129–38.

401. Yamamoto T, Kitazawa Y. Iris-color change developed after topical isopropyl unoprostone treatment. *J Glaucoma* 1997;6:430–2.

402. Eisenberg DL, Camras CB. A preliminary risk-benefit assessment of latanoprost and unoprostone in open-angle glaucoma and ocular hypertension. *Drug Saf* 1999;20:506–14.

403. Mishima HK et al. A comparison of latanoprost and timolol in primary open-angle glaucoma and ocular hypertension: a 12-week study. *Arch Ophthalmol* 1996;114:929–32.

404. Bucci MG et al. Intraocular pressure-lowering effects of latanoprost monotherapy versus latanoprost or pilocarpine in combination with timolol: a randomized, observer-masked multicenter study in patients with open-angle glaucoma. *J Glaucoma* 1999;8:24–30.

405. Rulo AH et al. Additive ocular hypotensive effect of latanoprost and acetazolamide: a short-term study in patients with elevated intraocular pressure. *Ophthalmology* 1997;104:1503–7.

406. Kent AR et al. Interaction of pilocarpine with latanoprost in patients with glaucoma and ocular hypertension. *J Glaucoma* 1999;8:257–62.

407. Hiett JA, Carlson DM. Ocular adrenergic agents. In, Onofrey BE, ed. *Clinical optometric pharmacology and therapeutics.* Philadelphia: Lippincott-Raven; 1997;Chap. 9:1–37.

Gastrointestinal Drugs

Acid-Peptic Therapy

ANTACIDS

Pharmacology. Antacids are weakly basic inorganic salts whose primary action is to neutralize gastric acid; pH >4 inhibits the proteolytic activity of pepsin. Aluminum-containing antacids suppress, but do not eradicate, *Helicobacter pylori* and can promote ulcer healing in peptic ulcer disease (PUD) by enhancing mucosal defense mechanisms.[1,2] Aluminum salts also bind phosphate and bile salts in the GI tract, decreasing serum phosphate and serum bile salt levels. Antacids can increase urine pH.

Administration and Adult Dosage. **PO for symptomatic relief of indigestion, nonulcer dyspepsia, epigastric pain in PUD, or heartburn in gastro-esophageal reflux disease (GERD)** 10–30 mL prn or 1 and 3 hr after meals and hs.[1,2] **PO for treatment of PUD** 100–160 mEq of acid-neutralizing capacity per dose, given 1 and 3 hr after meals and hs for 4–8 weeks or until healing is complete. Additional doses may be taken if epigastric pain persists. There is evidence that lower dosages can heal peptic ulcers.[1,2] **PO or NG for prevention or treatment of upper GI bleeding in critically ill patients** titrate to maintain intragastric pH >4.0.[3] **PO for phosphate binding in renal failure** (aluminum hydroxide) 1.9–4.8 g tid or qid or (calcium carbonate) 8–12 g/day; titrate dosage based on serum phosphate.[1]

Special Populations. *Pediatric Dosage.* **PO for treatment of PUD or GERD** (≤12 yr) at least 5–15 mL up to q 1 hr; (>12 yr) same as adult dosage.

Geriatric Dosage. Avoid using magnesium-containing antacids in renal impairment.

Other Conditions. Avoid using magnesium-containing antacids in patients with Cl$_{cr}$ <30 mL/min.

Dosage Forms. (*See* Antacid Products Comparison Chart.)

Patient Instructions. If antacids do not relieve symptoms of indigestion, upset stomach, or heartburn within 2 weeks, contact your health care practitioner. Diarrhea can occur with magnesium-containing antacids; decrease the daily dosage, alternate doses with, or switch to, an aluminum- or calcium-containing antacid. Constipation can occur with aluminum-containing antacids; decrease the daily dosage, alternate doses with, or switch to, a magnesium-containing antacid. Refrigerating liquid antacids or flavored antacids can improve their palatability. Antacids can interfere with other medications; take other medications 1 to 2 hours before or after antacids unless otherwise directed. If tablets are used, chew thoroughly before swallowing and follow with a glass of water.

Missed Doses. If your health care practitioner has told you to take this medicine on a regular schedule and you miss a dose, take it as soon as possible. If it is almost time for your next dose, skip the missed dose and return to your usual dosage schedule. Do not double doses.

Pharmacokinetics. *Onset and Duration.* Onset of acid neutralizing is immediate; duration is 30 ± 10 min in the fasted state and 1–3 hr if ingested with or within 1 hr after meals.[1]

Fate. Antacid cations are absorbed to different degrees. Sodium is highly soluble and readily absorbed; calcium absorption is generally less than 30% but can decrease with advancing age, intake, achlorhydria, and estrogen loss at menopause; magnesium is generally about 30% absorbed, but percentage of absorption changes inversely with intake; aluminum is slightly absorbed. Calcium, magnesium, and aluminum are excreted renally with normal renal function.[1] The unabsorbed portion is excreted in the feces.

Adverse Reactions. Long-term use of sodium- or calcium-containing antacids can cause systemic alkalosis. Hypercalcemia can occur with ingestion of large amounts of calcium; soluble antacids plus a diet high in milk products can result in milk-alkali syndrome, which can lead to nephrolithiasis and, in severe cases, neurologic abnormalities.[1] Magnesium-containing antacids cause dose-related laxative effects; hypermagnesemia occurs in patients with renal impairment.[1] Aluminum-containing antacids cause dose-related constipation, especially in the elderly. Prolonged administration or large dosages of aluminum hydroxide or carbonate can result in hypophosphatemia, particularly in the elderly and alcoholics; encephalopathy has been reported in dialysis patients receiving aluminum-containing antacids alone or with sucralfate.[1,2,4]

Precautions. Use caution with aluminum and calcium salts and avoid magnesium-containing products in patients with renal insufficiency. Use caution when using sodium bicarbonate in patients with chronic renal failure, edema, hypertension, or CHF. Because antacids are particulate and elevate intragastric pH, they can predispose critically ill patients to nosocomial pneumonia.[3]

Drug Interactions. Antacids reduce the absorption of numerous drugs by three different mechanisms: altering GI pH, altering urinary pH, and binding to drugs in the GI tract. Factors that affect the likelihood of drug interactions are the drug's dose, valence of cations (eg, tetracycline is polyvalent), and timing of the doses of antacid and drug. Some clinically important interactions include digoxin, oral iron, isoniazid, ketoconazole, oral quinolones, and oral tetracyclines. Antacids can reduce salicylate levels and increase quinidine levels because of urinary pH changes. Large dosages of calcium antacids can produce hypercalcemia in the presence of thiazides. Sodium polystyrene sulfonate resin can bind magnesium and calcium ions from the antacid in the gut, resulting in systemic alkalosis.

Parameters to Monitor. Monitor for relief of dyspepsia, epigastric pain or heartburn, and diarrhea or constipation. Monitor serum phosphate during long-term use of aluminum-containing products in patients with chronic renal impairment. Monitor for drug interactions.

Notes. Aggressive antacid therapy is at least as effective as the H_2-receptor antagonists or sucralfate when treating PUD or preventing stress-related mucosal bleeding; however, do not use antacids as first-line agents because large, frequent doses are inconvenient and associated with an increased risk of adverse effects.[1,2,4] Magaldrate is a chemical mixture of magnesium and aluminum hydroxides. **Alginic acid** has foaming and floating properties that can be beneficial in GERD. Most antacid products have been reformulated to contain low amounts of sodium; some antacid products contain considerable amounts of sugar or artificial sweetener. Antacid tablets, if chewed and swallowed, can be as effective as equivalent doses of liquid formulations. Although gastrin is stimulated by calcium, gastric acid rebound with calcium-containing antacids is of questionable clinical importance.[1]

ANTACID PRODUCTS COMPARISON CHART[a]

ANTACID	ORAL SUSPENSION		TABLETS	
	Acid Neutralizing Capacity mEq/5 mL	Sodium Content mg/5 mL[b]	Acid-Neutralizing Capacity mEq/Tablet	Sodium Content mg/Tablet[b]
Aluminum Carbonate, Basic				
Basaljel	11.5	3	12.5	2.8
Aluminum Hydroxide				
AlternaGEL	16	<2.5	—	—
Amphojel 300 mg	10	<2.3	8	1.4
Amphojel 600 mg	—	—	16	2.8
Aluminum Hydroxide with Magnesium Carbonate				
Gaviscon	4[d]	13	—	—
Gaviscon Extra Strength Relief Formula	14.3[d]	20.7	5–7.5[d,e]	29.9
Aluminum Hydroxide with Magnesium Hydroxide				
Maalox	13.3	<1.5	9.7	0.7
Maalox High Potency	27.2	<1	—	—
Aluminum Hydroxide with Magnesium Hydroxide and Simethicone				
Fast-Acting Mylanta	12.7	0.6	—	—
Fast-Acting Mylanta, Maximum Strength	25.4	0.05	—	—
Gelusil	—	—	11	<5
Maalox Plus	—	—	10.7	≤1
Maalox, Maximum Strength, Anti-Gas	29.8	<2.5	16.7	1.4
Mylanta	12.7	0.68	—	—
Mylanta, Maximum Strength	25.4	1.14	—	—

(continued)

531

ANTACID PRODUCTS COMPARISON CHART[a] (continued)

| | ORAL SUSPENSION | | TABLETS | |
ANTACID	Acid Neutralizing Capacity mEq/5 mL	Sodium Content mg/5 mL[b]	Acid-Neutralizing Capacity mEq/Tablet	Sodium Content mg/Tablet[b]
Aluminum Hydroxide with Magnesium Trisilicate and Sodium Bicarbonate				
Gaviscon (Chewable)[d]	—	—	0.5	18.4
Gaviscon-2 (Chewable)[d]	—	—	1	36.8
Calcium Carbonate				
Children's Mylanta Upset Stomach Relief	8	—	8	—
Maalox, Quick Dissolve	—	—	10.8	1
Maalox, Quick Dissolve Maximum Strength	—	—	18	2
Titralac	—	—	7.5	1.1
Tums	—	—	10	<2
Tums E-X	—	—	15	<2
Tums Ultra	—	—	20	≤4
Calcium Carbonate with Magnesium Hydroxide				
Di-Gel[c]	≥9	≤5	—	—
Fast-Acting Mylanta	24	0.3	12	0.3
Fast-Acting Mylanta, Maximum Strength	48	0.6	24	0.6
Fast-Acting Mylanta Supreme	12.6	0.7	—	—
Rolaids	—	—	14.8	<1

(continued)

ANTACID PRODUCTS COMPARISON CHART[a] (*continued*)

| | ORAL SUSPENSION | | TABLETS | |
ANTACID	Acid-Neutralizing Capacity mEq/5 mL	Sodium Content mg/5 mL[b]	Acid-Neutralizing Capacity mEq/Tablet	Sodium Content mg/Tablet[b]
Magaldrate				
Riopan	15	<0.3	—	—
Riopan Plus[c]	15	<0.3	13.5	0.1
Riopan Plus Double Strength[c]	—	—	30	≤0.5

[a]Products listed are representative of numerous brand and generic products on the market. Product formulations and, hence, neutralizing capacity and sodium content, are subject to change by the manufacturer.

[b]To determine the sodium content in mEq, multiply sodium content (mg) by 0.043.

[c]Contains simethicone.

[d]Contains alginate.

[e]Contains sodium bicarbonate.

BISMUTH PREPARATIONS
Pepto-Bismol, Tritec, Various

Pharmacology. Bismuth salts are used to treat nausea, indigestion, diarrhea, gastritis, and peptic ulcers. The precise method by which bismuth heals gastritis and ulcers is uncertain, but possible mechanisms are local gastroprotective effect, stimulation of endogenous prostaglandins, and antimicrobial activity against *Helicobacter pylori*. Given alone, bismuth salts suppress *H. pylori,* but long-term eradication requires combination therapy with antibiotics. **Bismuth subsalicylate** (BSS; Pepto-Bismol, various) is the bismuth salt used most frequently in the United States. **Ranitidine bismuth citrate** (RBC) is a complex of ranitidine, trivalent bismuth, and citrate.[1,2,5–7]

Administration and Adult Dosage. **PO for the control of nausea, abdominal cramps, and diarrhea** (BSS) 525 mg. Administer dosage q 30–60 min, if needed, to a maximum of 4.2 g/day. When given with antibiotics to eradicate *H. pylori*, treatment is usually limited to 1–2 weeks. (*See also* Eradication of *Helicobacter pylori* Infection.)

Special Populations. *Pediatric Dosage.* **PO for the control of nausea, abdominal cramps, and diarrhea** (BSS) (<3 yr) not recommended; (3–6 yr) 87 mg; (6–9 yr) 175 mg; (9–12 yr) 262 mg. Administer dosage q 30–60 min, if needed, to a maximum of 8 doses/day.

Geriatric Dosage. Same as adult dosage.

Dosage Forms. **Susp** (BSS) 17.5, 35 mg/mL; **Chew Tab** 262; **Tab** 262 mg; **Tab** (RBC) 400 mg (containing ranitidine 160 mg and bismuth citrate 240 mg) (Tritec).

Pharmacokinetics. After oral administration, BSS (58% bismuth, 42% salicylate) is converted in the GI tract to bismuth oxide and salicylic acid. Bismuth is less than 0.2% absorbed, with more than 99% of an oral dose excreted in the feces. Over 90% of the salicylate dose is absorbed and excreted in urine. RBC dissociates in intragastric fluid to ranitidine and soluble and insoluble forms of bismuth. Oral absorption of bismuth from RBC is variable.

Adverse Reactions. BSS and bismuth derived from RBC can temporarily darken the tongue and stool. Use BSS with caution in children; in the elderly; in patients with renal impairment, salicylate sensitivity, or bleeding disorders; in those receiving high-dosage salicylate therapy; or when potentially interacting medications are taken. Salicylic acid is less likely than aspirin to cause gastric mucosal damage and blood loss. Prolonged use, dosages higher than those recommended, and the use of other salts (subgallate and subnitrate) have been associated with neurotoxicity. Bismuth concentrations can be elevated in the elderly and patients with renal impairment because of decreased renal elimination. RBC should not be used as a single agent for the treatment of active duodenal or gastric ulcers. Use caution in children and teenagers who are experiencing or recovering from nausea and vomiting symptoms because these might be early sign of Reye's syndrome. Avoid BSS in patients who are hypersensitive to aspirin or nonaspirin salicylates.

HISTAMINE H$_2$-RECEPTOR ANTAGONISTS:	
CIMETIDINE	Tagamet, Various
FAMOTIDINE	Pepcid
NIZATIDINE	Axid
RANITIDINE	Zantac, Various

Pharmacology. Histamine H$_2$-receptor antagonists competitively inhibit the actions of histamine at the H$_2$ receptors of the parietal cell and reduce basal, nocturnal, pentagastrin-, and food-stimulated gastric acid.

	CIMETIDINE	FAMOTIDINE	NIZATIDINE	RANITIDINE
Ring structure	Imidazole	Thiazole	Thiazole	Furan
Relative potency	1	20–50	4–8	4–8

Administration and Adult Dosage. Tolerance to H$_2$-receptor antagonist can occur after 4 weeks of therapy, so higher-than-recommended doses might be required.[8–10]

INDICATION	CIMETIDINE	FAMOTIDINE	NIZATIDINE	RANITIDINE
PO for prevention or symptomatic relief of heartburn or indigestion (OTC)	200 mg/day or 200 mg bid.	10 mg/day or 10 mg bid.	75 mg/day or 75 mg bid.	75 mg/day or 75 mg bid.
PO for short-term treatment of active duodenal ulcer (4–8 weeks)	300 mg qid, 400 mg bid, 800 mg hs, or 1600 mg hs.[a]	20 mg bid or 40 mg hs.	150 mg bid or 300 mg hs.	150 mg bid or 300 mg hs.
PO for maintenance of healed duodenal ulcer	400 mg hs.	20 mg hs.	150 mg hs.	150 mg hs.
PO for short-term treatment of active benign gastric ulcer (6–8 weeks)	300 mg qid 400 mg bid or 800 mg hs	20 mg bid[b] or 40 mg hs.	150 mg bid or 300 mg hs.	150 mg bid or 300 mg hs.[b]

(continued)

INDICATION	CIMETIDINE	FAMOTIDINE	NIZATIDINE	RANITIDINE
PO for maintenance of healed gastric ulcer	400 mg hs[b] or 800 mg hs.	20 mg hs.[b]	150 mg hs.[b] or 300 mg hs.	150 mg hs. or 300 mg hs.
PO for symptomatic gastroesophageal reflux disease (6–12 weeks)	300 mg qid or 400 mg bid.	20 mg bid.	150 mg bid.	150 mg bid.
PO for healing of erosive esophagitis (6–12 weeks)	400 mg qid or 800 mg bid.	20 or 40 mg bid.	150 mg bid or 300 mg bid.[b]	150 mg qid or 300 mg bid.[b]
PO for maintenance of healed erosive esophagitis	300 mg qid,[b] 400 mg qid,[b] or 800 mg bid.[b]	20 mg bid[b] or 40 mg bid.[b]	150 mg bid[b] or 300 mg bid.[b]	150 mg bid or 300 mg bid.[b]
PO for pathological hypersecretory conditions	300 mg qid, up to 2.4 g/day; or adjust to patient needs.	20 mg q 6 hr, up to 160 mg q 6 hr; or adjust to patient needs.	[b]	150 mg bid, up to 6 g/day; or adjust to patient needs.
IM	300 mg q 6–8 hr.[c]	d	d	50 mg q 6–8 hr.[c]
IV intermittent	300 q 6–8 hr, up to 2.4 g/day.[c]	20 mg q 12 hr.[c]	d	50 mg q 6–8 hr, up to 400 mg/day.[c]
IV intermittent bolus	Dilute to 20 mL; inject over not less than 5 min.[c]	Dilute to 5–10 mL; inject over not less than 2 min.[c]	d	Dilute to 20 mL; inject over not less than 5 min.[c]
IV intermittent infusion	Dilute to 50 mL; infuse over 15–20 min.[c]	Dilute to 100 mL; infuse over 15–30 min.[c]	d	Dilute to 100 mL; infuse over 15–20 min.[c]
IV continuous infusion	37.5 mg/hr (900 mg/day); adjust to patient needs; up to 600 mg/hr has been given.[c,e]	1.67 mg/hr[b] (40 mg/day); adjust to patient needs.[c,e]	d	6.25 mg/hr (150 mg/day); adjust to patient needs; up to 220 mg/hr has been given.[c,e]

(continued)

IV for prevention of upper GI bleeding in critically ill patients (cimetidine) 50 mg/hr by continuous infusion;[e] (cimetidine, famotidine, or ranitidine) use standard dosages given by intermittent or continuous infusion.[b,e] In high-risk surgical patients, adjust the dose and/or frequency of intermittent IV therapy or the rate of continuous infusion to maintain the intragastric pH above 4.0.

[a]Heavy smokers with ulcers larger than 1 cm in diameter.
[b]Nonlabeled indication and dosage.
[c]Pathologic hypersecretory states, intractable ulcers, or patients unable to take oral medication.
[d]Nonlabeled route of administration.
[e]Loading dose can be given but appears to offer little advantage.
From references 2, 3, 8, and 11–15.

Special Populations. *Pediatric Dosage.* Except for ranitidine, the safety and efficacy are not well established.

	CIMETIDINE	FAMOTIDINE	NIZATIDINE	RANITIDINE
Neonates	5–10 mg/kg/day.	1–1.2 mg/kg/day.	Unknown.	0.5–3 mg/kg/day.
Children	20–40 mg/kg/day.	0.5–2 mg/kg/day.	6–10 mg/kg/day.	2–4 mg/kg/day.[a] 5–10 mg/kg/day.[b]

[a]Duodenal ulcer and gastric ulcer.
[b]Gastroesophageal reflux disease and esophagitis.
From references 3 and 16–19.

Geriatric Dosage. Reduce dosage based on renal function.
Other Conditions.

	CIMETIDINE	FAMOTIDINE	NIZATIDINE	RANITIDINE
Renal impairment[a]	Cl_{cr} 15–30 mL/min: 600 mg/day; <15 mL/min: 300–400 mg/day.	Cl_{cr} <10 mL/min: 20 mg/day or 20 mg every other day.	Cl_{cr} 20–50 mL/min: 150 mg/day; <20 mL/min: 150 mg every other day.	Cl_{cr} <50 mL/min: PO 150 mg/day or IM/IV 50 mg q 12–24 hr.

[a]Use the lowest dosage that permits an adequate response; further dosage reduction of cimetidine, famotidine, or ranitidine may be necessary with concomitant severe liver disease. Because only small amounts of H_2-receptor antagonists are removed by hemodialysis and peritoneal dialysis, additional doses may not be necessary; adjust dosage schedule so that the time of the scheduled dose coincides with the end of dialysis.
From references 11 and 13.

Dosage Forms.

	CIMETIDINE	FAMOTIDINE	NIZATIDINE	RANITIDINE
	Tab 100, 200, 300, 400, 800 mg.	Tab 10, 20, 40 mg. Chew Tab 10 mg Chew Tab 10 mg (Pepcid Complete)[b] Tab (rapid dissolving) 20, 40 mg.	Cap 150, 300 mg. Tab 75 mg.	Tab 75, 150, 300 mg. Tab (effervescent) 150 mg[a] Granules (effervescent) 150 mg[a] Cap 150, 300 mg.
	Soln 60 mg/mL. Inj 6 mg/mL (premixed) Inj 150 mg/mL.	Susp 8 mg/mL.[c] Inj. 0.4 mg/mL (premixed) Inj 10 mg/mL.[d]		Syrup 15 mg/mL Inj 0.5 (premixed), 25 mg/mL.

[a]Dissolve dose in approximately 180–240 mL (6–8 fl oz) of water before drinking.
[b]Contains calcium carbonate 800 mg and magnesium hydroxide 165 mg.
[c]Discard reconstituted suspension after 30 days.
[d]Store at 2–8°C (36–46°F).

Patient Instructions. The effectiveness of H_2-receptor antagonists in peptic ulcer disease might be decreased by cigarette smoking. Discontinue or decrease smoking or avoid smoking after the last dose of the day. Antacids can be used as needed for relief of epigastric pain. Even though ulcer or gastroesophageal reflux disease symptoms might improve, continue treatment for the duration of therapy unless instructed otherwise. If symptomatic relief is not obtained in 2 weeks with over-the-counter medication, contact your health care practitioner. Report any bleeding, vomiting, or severe esophageal or abdominal pain.

Missed Doses. If you miss a dose, take it as soon as possible. If it is almost time for your next dose, skip the missed dose and return to your usual dosage schedule. Do not double doses.

Pharmacokinetics.

	CIMETIDINE	FAMOTIDINE	NIZATIDINE	RANITIDINE
Onset.				
All agents have an oral onset of 1 hr and an IV onset of 15 min.				
Serum Levels.				
EC_{50}[a]	625 ± 375 µg/L	11 ± 2 µg/L	167 ± 13 µg/L	112 ± 52 µg/L
Fate.				
Oral bioavailability	60 ± 20%	41 ± 4%	95 ± 5%; 75% in renal failure.	55 ± 25%

(continued)

	CIMETIDINE	FAMOTIDINE	NIZATIDINE	RANITIDINE
V_d	1 ± 0.2 L/kg	1.2 ± 0.3 L/kg	1.4 ± 0.2 L/kg	1.6 ± 0.4 L/kg
Protein binding	20 ± 6%	16%	30 ± 5%	15%
Excreted unchanged in urine	75%	65–70%	70 ± 5%	68–79%
$t_{1/2}$				
Normal	1.9 ± 0.4 hr	3 ± 0.5 hr	1.4 ± 0.2 hr	2 ± 0.4 hr
Anuric	4.5 ± 0.5 hr	20+ hr	7.2 ± 1.3 hr	7 ± 3 hr

[a]EC_{50} is the serum concentration necessary to inhibit pentagastrin-stimulated secretion of acid by 50%.
From references 2, 11, 12, and 21.

Adverse Reactions. Adverse reactions are generally mild. The most frequent adverse events occur in 1–7% of patients and include headache, diarrhea, constipation, dizziness, drowsiness, and fatigue.[2,11–13] Reversible confusional states, depression, agitation, and other CNS manifestations can occur occasionally with all H_2-receptor antagonists, predominantly in severely ill patients or those with renal and/or hepatic disease or advanced age.[2,3,11] Reversible dose-dependent increases in ALT have been reported with IV cimetidine and IV ranitidine; administration over 15–30 min minimizes this effect. Rare cases of fatal hepatic disease with and without jaundice have been reported with cimetidine and ranitidine.[11] H_2-receptor antagonists do not markedly decrease hepatic blood flow.[11] Cardiac arrhythmias, tachycardia, and hypotension can occur after rapid IV bolus administration of cimetidine or ranitidine; bradycardia has been reported with IV and oral administration of cimetidine and ranitidine. Although a negative inotropic effect has been noted after oral administration of famotidine in healthy subjects and patients with CHF, refined hemodynamic monitoring failed to demonstrate a clinically important effect;[11] IV famotidine has been given safely to patients undergoing cardiac surgery.[20] Hematologic reactions occur occasionally with all H_2-receptor antagonists and include leukopenia, neutropenia, thrombocytopenia, and pancytopenia; agranulocytosis and aplastic anemia occur rarely.[2,11] Gynecomastia develops in fewer than 1% of all men receiving cimetidine but in 4% of men treated for pathologic hypersecretory states.[21] Dose-dependent increases in serum prolactin concentrations have been reported with cimetidine and ranitidine.[11] Hyperuricemia has been reported with nizatidine.

Precautions. Pregnancy; lactation. Dosage reduction might be required in severe renal and/or hepatic failure. Dosage reduction might not be required in patients treated with cimetidine because this drug can increase Cr_s by competing for renal tubular secretion.[13] This effect should not be interpreted as renal dysfunction. Symptomatic response to therapy does not preclude the possibility of gastric or esophageal malignancy.

Drug Interactions. Cimetidine inhibits hepatic CYP1A2, CYP2C8–10, CYP2D6, and CYP3A3–5; ranitidine inhibits CYP2D6 and CYP3A3–5 to a much lesser extent. Clinically important interactions with drugs metabolized by these isoenzymes can occur (the most important of which are carbamazepine, chlordiazepoxide, clozapine, diazepam, glipizide, lidocaine, phenytoin, propranolol, theophylline, tolbutamide, tricyclic antidepressants, quinidine, tacrine, and warfarin). Hepatic microsomal enzyme interactions with cimetidine are dose dependent.[22,23] Controversy remains about interactions with ranitidine, although in general they seem less likely and less severe than with cimetidine.[11,22,23] Cimetidine can inhibit the elimination of certain drugs secreted by renal tubules (eg, procainamide).[22,23] Nizatidine has been reported to increase serum salicylate concentrations in patients on high aspirin doses (3.9 g/day). Cimetidine, ranitidine, and nizatidine (but not famotidine) inhibit gastric mucosal alcohol dehydrogenase; the clinical importance of this interaction is uncertain.[24,25] Elevations in gastric pH can alter the rate or extent of absorption of ketoconazole, itraconazole, and other drugs whose dissolution and absorption are pH dependent.[22,23]

Parameters to Monitor. Improvement in epigastric pain or heartburn. However, pain relief in PUD and GERD does not correlate directly with endoscopic evidence of healing. Monitor Cr_s, CBC, AST, ALT, and CNS status periodically. In patients receiving IV doses of cimetidine (≥ 2.4 g/day) or ranitidine (≥ 400 mg/day), it is advisable to monitor serum transaminases routinely throughout IV therapy. When the drug is used to prevent upper GI bleeding in critically ill patients, measure the intragastric pH periodically. Monitor for potential drug interactions.

Notes. In general, the H_2-receptor antagonists are similar in efficacy when conventional dosages are prescribed for the treatment of gastric and duodenal ulcers and for maintenance of healing of duodenal ulcer. Ulcer healing rates are similar to those with **sucralfate** or aggressive **antacid** therapy.[2,12,13] The H_2-receptor antagonists are often used in combination with a number of antibiotics to eradicate *Helicobacter pylori* in peptic ulcer disease. (*See* Eradication of *Helicobacter pylori* Infection.) Usual dosages of H_2-receptor antagonists are less effective than **misoprostol** or **proton pump inhibitors** in preventing NSAID-induced gastric ulcer.[26,27] However, high-dose famotidine can be effective in preventing and healing NSAID-induced gastric and duodenal ulcers.[28–30] Although all H_2-receptor antagonists provide symptomatic relief and esophageal healing, higher dosages are required in patients with moderate to severe esophagitis than those used in patients with mild GERD symptoms.[8,12,15] Intermittent administration or continuous infusion of IV cimetidine, ranitidine, or famotidine is more effective than placebo in preventing upper GI bleeding in critically ill patients.[3] The maintenance of intragastric pH above 4.0 does not conclusively prevent upper GI bleeding.[3] Although it is easier to maintain the intragastric pH above 4.0 by continuous infusion, the superiority of continuous infusion of the H_2-receptor antagonists in preventing upper GI bleeding in the critically ill patient has not been established; intermittent administration and continuous infusion are at least as effective as sucralfate or aggressive antacid therapy.[3] Combination of an H_2-receptor antagonist with sucralfate provides two different mechanisms of drug action and might be beneficial. However, enhanced efficacy of two drugs compared with single-drug therapy has not been substantiated in controlled trials in patients with duodenal ulcer, gastric ulcer, or GERD or when used to prevent or treat upper GI bleeding. Coadministration of an H_2-receptor antagonist with a proton pump inhibitor is without established benefit and might compromise the action of the proton pump inhibitor.[2] Controlled trials have not demonstrated that H_2-receptor antagonists are of benefit in patients with active upper GI bleeding.[11] The relation of H_2-receptor antagonist therapy to the development of nosocomial pneumonia in critically ill patients is inconclusive.[3] (*See* Sucralfate.) Cimetidine can augment cell-mediated immunity by blockade of H_2-receptors on suppressor T lymphocytes; it remains difficult to determine whether this effect is clinically useful or potentially dangerous, especially after organ transplantation and in autoimmune disorders.[22] Cimetidine can reduce pain and hasten resolution of herpes zoster lesions.[31] Although it is not certain whether this immune system action is class specific or drug specific, it appears to be related to the cimetidine molecule. All H_2-receptor antagonists are stable in D5W, D10W, NS, LR, parenteral nutrition, or 5% sodium bicarbonate for 48 hr at room temperature.

MISOPROSTOL
Cytotec

Pharmacology. Misoprostol is a synthetic prostaglandin E_1 analogue that inhibits gastric acid secretion and enhances gastric mucosal defense. Antisecretory effects are dose dependent over the range of 50–200 μg; cytoprotective effects occur at doses of 200 μg or more. The gastric ulcer protective effect of misoprostol appears to plateau between 200 μg bid–tid, but no dose–response effect is apparent in preventing duodenal ulcers.[30,32] Cotherapy with misoprostol reduces the frequency of NSAID-induced complications, including GI perforation, obstruction, and bleeding, but its cost effectiveness remains controversial.[30,33] Misoprostol also causes uterine contraction.

Administration and Adult Dosage. **PO for GI protection during NSAID therapy** 200 μg qid with food; if this dosage is not tolerated, 100 μg qid can be used. Lower-dosage regimens of misoprostol 200 μg tid or bid appear similar in efficacy and better tolerated for protection against NSAID-induced gastric and duodenal ulcers than the 200 mg qid dosage. Dosage reduction is not required in renal impairment, hepatic failure, or the elderly. **PO or Vag for use with mifepristone for pregnancy termination** 400 μg 2 days after mifepristone dose. **Vag for cervical ripening at term** 25–100 μg.[34,35] **PO for cervical ripening at term** 100–200 μg.[34,36] (*See* Notes.)

Dosage Forms. **Tab** 100, 200 μg. Misoprostol is also available in combination with diclofenac in Arthrotec. (*See* Diclofenac.)

Pharmacokinetics. After oral administration, misoprostol is extensively absorbed and rapidly de-esterified to the active drug, misoprostol acid. Peak serum concentrations of misoprostol acid are reduced when the drug is taken with food. Plasma protein binding of misoprostol acid is <90%. Misoprostol acid undergoes further metabolism, but approximately 80% is excreted unchanged in urine.

Adverse Reactions. Diarrhea is reported to occur within 2 weeks of initiating therapy in 14–40% of patients on NSAIDs receiving 800 μg/day and less frequently with 400–600 μg/day. Diarrhea usually resolves in about 1 week with continued treatment; rarely, profound diarrhea occurs in patients with inflammatory bowel disease. Abdominal pain occurs in 13–20% of patients on NSAIDs receiving misoprostol 800 μg/day, but there is no consistent difference from placebo. Antacids (except those containing magnesium) can be used for abdominal pain relief. Nausea, flatulence, headache, dyspepsia, vomiting, and constipation occur occasionally. Women who receive misoprostol occasionally develop gynecologic disorders including cramps or vaginal bleeding.

Precautions. Advise patients (especially those receiving concurrent corticosteroids or anticoagulants) to report bleeding, vomiting, severe abdominal pain, and diarrhea. For GI protective uses, misoprostol is contraindicated in pregnancy because of the risk of abortion and women of childbearing potential should have a negative serum pregnancy test within 2 weeks of beginning therapy, should begin treatment on the second or third day of the next menstrual period, should comply with effective contraceptive measures, and should receive oral and written warnings of the hazards of misoprostol therapy and the risk of contraceptive failure. Warn patients not to give misoprostol to others.

Drug Interactions. Misoprostol does not affect the hepatic cytochrome P450 microsomal enzyme system and does not interfere with the beneficial effects of NSAIDs in rheumatoid arthritis.

Notes. In most trials of patients receiving long-term NSAID therapy for rheumatoid arthritis, misoprostol 200 μg qid was superior to the **H$_2$-receptor antagonists** or **sucralfate** in preventing NSAID-induced gastric ulcer; however, misoprostol did not relieve GI pain or discomfort associated with NSAID use.[26,30,33] **Omeprazole** 20 mg/day is associated with a lower relapse rate and is better tolerated than misoprostol 200 μg bid for prophylactic treatment. Misoprostol appears to be more effective than conventional methods of cervical ripenining at term;[34,35] oral and vaginal administrations appear to be equivalent in efficacy.[34]

PROTON PUMP INHIBITORS:	
LANSOPRAZOLE	Prevacid
OMEPRAZOLE	Prilosec
PANTOPRAZOLE	Protonix
RABEPRAZOLE	Aciphex

Pharmacology. Proton pump inhibitors (PPIs) are inactive substituted benzimidazoles that, when protonated in the secretory canaliculi of the parietal cells, covalently bind to H$^+$/K$^+$-ATPase (proton pump), which is the final pathway for acid secretion. PPIs produce a profound and prolonged antisecretory effect and inhibit basal, nocturnal, pentagastrin-, and food-stimulated gastric acid secretion. Serum gastric levels increase during treatment but return to pretreatment levels within 1–2 weeks of discontinuing therapy.

Administration and Adult Dosage. Administer the PPI at least 30–60 min before meals, preferable in the morning, because these agents inhibit only those proton pumps that are actively secreting acid. Infuse IV pantoprazole doses over 15 min via a dedicated line and the in-line filter provided. IV dosage is the same as PO dosage.

INDICATION	ESOMEPRAZOLE	LANSOPRAZOLE	OMEPRAZOLE	PANTOPRAZOLE	RABEPRAZOLE
Treatment of active duodenal ulcer (4 weeks)	—	15 mg/day.[a]	20 mg/day.[a]	40 mg/day.[b]	20 mg/day.[a]
Maintenance of duodenal ulcer healing (1 yr)	—	15 mg/day.[a]	20 mg/day.[b]	20 mg/day.[b]	20 mg/day.[b]
Treatment of active gastric ulcer (4–8 weeks)	—	30 mg/day.[a]	40 mg/day.[a]	40 mg/day.[b]	20–40 mg/day.[b]
Maintenance of gastric ulcer healing	—	15–30 mg/day.[b]	20–40 mg/day.[b]	40 mg/day.[b]	20–40 mg/day.[b]
Treatment of symptomatic gastroesophageal reflux disease (4–8 weeks)	20 mg/day.[a]	15 mg/day.[a]	20 mg/day.[a]	20 mg/day.[b]	20 mg/day.[a]
Treatment of erosive esophagitis (4–8 weeks)	20–40 mg/day.[a]	30 mg/day.[a]	20 mg/day.[a]	40 mg/day.[a]	20 mg/day.[a]
Maintenance of erosive esophagitis	20 mg/day.[a]	15 mg/day.[a]	20 mg/day.[a]	20–40 mg/day.[b]	20 mg/day.[a]
PO for treatment of pathologic hypersecretory conditions	—	60 mg/day,[a] up to 90 mg bid.[c]	60 mg/day,[a] up to 120 mg tid.[c]	80 mg/day.[b]	60 mg/day,[a] up to 120 mg tid.[c]
Helicobacter pylori eradication for reduction of the risk of duodenal ulcer recurrence	40 mg/day.[a,d]	30 mg bid[a,d] for 10 days.	20 mg bid[a,d] for 10 days.	20–40 mg bid[b,e,f] for 7 days.	40 mg bid[b,e] for 7 days.
Risk reduction of NSAID-induced gastric ulcers	—	15 mg/day.[a]	20 mg/day.[b]	40 mg/day.[b]	—

[a]FDA-approved regimen.
[b]Nonlabeled indication and dosage.
[c]Adjust dosage to patient's needs and continue as long as clinically indicated.
[d]Combined with clarithromycin 500 mg bid and amoxicillin 1 g bid for 10 days.
[e]Combined with clarithromycin 500 mg bid and amoxicillin 1 g bid for 7 days.
[f]Combined with clarithromycin 500 mg bid and metronidazole 400 mg bid for 7 days.
From references 2, 8, 15, and 38–48.

Special Populations. *Pediatric Dosage.* Safety and efficacy not well established. **PO for esophagitis** (omeprazole) (>10 months) 0.7 mg/kg/day initially, increasing as necessary up to 3.5 mg/kg/day; **PO for peptic ulcer disease in combination with antimicrobials for *H. pylori*** (<10 yr) 0.6 mg/kg/day or 20 mg/day; (>10 yr) 20 mg daily–bid.[49] Lansoprazole 0.45 mg/kg/day in 2 divided doses; up to 15 mg bid has been used for treatment of *H. pylori* in combination with antimicrobial therapy.[50]

Geriatric Dosage. Dosage reduction is not usually necessary; reduce only if the drug is not well tolerated.[53]

Other Conditions. Dosage adjustments of PPIs are unnecessary in renal impairment or mild to moderate liver disease. However, dosage reduction should be considered for chronic or severe hepatic impairment. Certain groups (ie, Asians) tend to be poor metabolizers, so a decrease in dose might be considered. PPIs are not readily dialyzable.

Dosage Forms.

LANSOPRAZOLE	OMEPRAZOLE	PANTOPRAZOLE	RABEPRAZOLE
Enteric-coated granules	Enteric-coated granules	Enteric-coated tablet	Delayed-release tablet
Cap 15, 30[a] mg.	Cap 10, 20, 40 mg.	Tab 40 mg Inj 40 mg.	Tab 20 mg.

[a]Prevpac for *Helicobacter pylori* therapy consists of 2 lansoprazole 30 mg capsules, 4 amoxicillin 500 mg capsules, and 2 clarithromycin 500 mg tablets in an individual daily administration pack.

Patient Instructions. Swallow capsule (lansoprazole, omeprazole) or tablet (pantoprazole, rabeprazole) whole; do not crush or chew. Take medication 30–60 minutes before meals, preferably in the morning. Capsules can be opened and the granules sprinkled on applesauce, yogurt, or apple or orange juice if you have difficulty swallowing. Do not chew, and do swallow the preparation immediately after sprinkling the content onto food. (*See* Notes.) The effectiveness of PPIs in peptic ulcer disease can be decreased by cigarette smoking. Even though symptoms can improve quickly, continue treatment for the duration of therapy unless instructed otherwise.

Missed Doses. If you miss a dose, take it as soon as possible. If it is almost time for the next dose, skip the missed dose and return to your usual dosage schedule. Do not double doses.

Pharmacokinetics. *Onset and Duration.* PO onset of antisecretory activity is 1–3 hr, with rabeprazole having the quickest onset and pantoprazole the slowest. Duration is dose dependent. Gastric acid inhibition increases with repeated daily doses, reaching a plateau after several days. Upon discontinuing the PPI, gastric secretory activity gradually returns to pretreatment level within 2–7 days. There is no indication that rebound gastric acidity occurs.

Pharmacokinetics.

	LANSOPRAZOLE	OMEPRAZOLE	PANTOPRAZOLE	RABEPRAZOLE
Oral Bioavailability (%)	80–85	30–40	77	52
Protein Binding (%)	97	95	98	96
Peak (hr)	1.7	0.5–3.5	2.4	2.9–3.8
V_d (L/kg)	0.4	0.13–0.35	0.15	0.34
$t_{1/2}$ (hr)	1.5–1.7	0.5–1	1–1.9	1–2
Urinary Excretion (%)	33	77	71	90

From references 2, 21, and 38–44.

Adverse Effects. All have similar short-term (<12 weeks) and long-term (>12 weeks) side effect profiles.[38] The most frequent short-term adverse effects are headache, diarrhea, nausea, and abdominal pain.[51–54] Flu-like symptoms, constipation, fatigue, malaise, muscle cramps, joint pain, myalgia, anxiety, skin rash, confusion, sleep disturbances, and taste perversion occur occasionally. Anaphylactic reactions, gynecomastia, hemolytic anemia, thrombocytopenia, and psychic disturbances occur rarely. Rare cases of severe skin reactions (eg, Stevens–Johnson syndrome, toxic epidermal necrolysis), hepatic failure, cholestatic jaundice, pancreatitis, interstitial nephritis, and agranulocytosis have occurred. Long-term use of PPIs have been thought to cause gastric cancer, gastric enterochromaffin cell hyperplasia, carcinoid tumors, bacterial overgrowth, atrophic gastritis, and decreased absorption of certain nutrients; however, recent studies have shown that the risk of such adverse effects is not increased.[38,51–53] Patients infected with *H. pylori* are at greater risk for atrophic gastritis.[51,53] Patients older than 65 yr have similar side effect profiles as younger individuals.

Precautions. Pregnancy; there are sporadic reports of congenital abnormalities in infants born to women who took omeprazole during pregnancy. Symptomatic response to PPI therapy does not preclude the possibility of gastric malignancy.

Drug Interactions. Elevations in gastric pH can increase the extent of absorption of ampicillin and pancreatic enzyme supplements and decrease the rate or extent of absorption of digoxin, itraconazole, iron salts, ketoconazole, and other drugs or dosage forms that are pH dependent.[38,53] PPIs are metabolized to different degrees via the CYP450 isoenzymes CYP3A4, CYP2C19, CYP1A2, and CYP2C9. Lansoprazole, pantoprazole, and rabeprazole do not increase diazepam, (R)-warfarin or phenytoin concentrations, but these medications are affected by omeprazole because of its extensive metabolism via the hepatic CYP2C19 isoenzyme.[38,53] Lansoprazole can increase the clearance of theophylline by 10%. Rabeprazole does not interact with phenytoin, warfarin, or theophylline; however, rabeprazole causes a 20% increase in serum digoxin trough levels. Pantoprazole has no interaction with warfarin, phenytoin, diazepam, or theophylline, even though it is metabolized via CYP2C19.[41] Absorption of PPIs is not affected by antacids.

Parameters to Monitor. Improvement in epigastric pain or heartburn; however, pain relief in PUD and GERD does not correlate directly with endoscopic evidence of healing. Monitor for potential drug interactions and adverse effects. Monitor laboratory values, including liver function tests, CBC, and SMA-7. Assess the indication, dosage, and duration of PPI therapy, especially as it relates to the need for treatment beyond 16 weeks. Monitor serum vitamin B_{12} concentrations every few years in patients on long-term PPI therapy, especially the elderly.[55]

Notes. PPIs are the drugs of choice for erosive esophagitis and Zollinger–Ellison syndrome. Standard dosages provide more rapid relief of symptoms and ulcer or esophageal healing than standard dosages of **H_2-receptor antagonists**.[8,15,38] Patients with gastric or duodenal ulcers or esophagitis refractory to H_2-receptor antagonists are likely to respond to PPIs, but the rate of recurrence after discontinuation is similar to that of H_2-receptor antagonists.[8,15,38] **NSAID**-induced gastric and duodenal ulcers can be prevented or treated by PPIs and are superior to and have a better side effect profile than **misoprostol** 200 μg bid or **ranitidine** 150 mg bid.[27,37,38,56] IV pantoprazole is no more effective than oral PPIs.

Coadministration of a PPI with an H_2-receptor antagonist or sucralfate is without established benefit. Lansoprazole and omeprazole are available as gelatin capsules that are formulated as enteric-coated granules from which the drug is released when pH rises above 6. It is important for patients not to chew or crush the capsules or enteric-coated granules because the protective enteric coating might be destroyed and thus decrease the drug's bioavailability.[57] Patients who have difficulty swallowing capsules or have feeding tubes can open the capsule and mix the granules with apple or orange juice. Granules also can be sprinkled onto applesauce for oral administration. Lansoprazole granules can be sprinkled onto Ensure pudding, cottage cheese, yogurt, or strained pears. Omeprazole and lansoprazole can be mixed with sodium bicarbonate to make a simplified suspension administered through feeding tubes.[57]

Esomeprazole magnesium (Nexium) is the (S)-isomer of omeprazole that is as effective as omeprazole in controlling pH and produces longer-lasting gastric acid suppression. Doses of 20–40 mg are effective for symptomatic relief of GERD, *H. pylori* infections, and erosive esophagitis healing and maintenance.[58–60] Side effects are similar to other PPIs and include diarrhea, abdominal pain, flatulence, headaches, and nausea. It is available as 20 and 40 mg delayed-release tablets.

SUCRALFATE
Carafate, Various

Pharmacology. Sucralfate is an aluminum hydroxide salt of a sulfated disaccharide. Its exact mechanism of action is not known. It forms an ulcer-adherent complex with proteinaceous exudates at the ulcer site, thereby protecting against further attack by acid, pepsin, and bile salts. Adherence to the ulcer crater is enhanced at pH <3.5. Sucralfate inhibits pepsin activity; a dose of 1 g has about 14–16 mEq of acid-neutralizing capacity. The aluminum moiety stimulates endogenous prostaglandins and binds bile salts and phosphate in the GI tract.[2,61,62]

Administration and Adult Dosage. **PO for short-term treatment of duodenal ulcer** 1 g qid on an empty stomach, 1 hr before meals and at bedtime, or 2 g bid for 4–8 weeks.[2,61,62] **PO for maintenance of healed duodenal ulcer** 1 g bid. **PO**

for short-term treatment of active benign gastric ulcer 1 g qid.[2,61,62] **PO for treatment of symptomatic GERD or erosive esophagitis** 1 g qid.[61,62] **PO or NG for prevention of upper GI bleeding in critically ill patients** 1 g q 4–6 hr.[3,61,62] **PO or NG for phosphate binding in renal failure** titrate dosage based on serum phosphate.[2,4,61]

Special Populations. *Pediatric Dosage.* Safety and efficacy not well established. PO 40–80 mg/kg/day in 4 divided doses. Alternatively, (<10 kg) 0.5 g q 6 hr; (>10 kg) 1 g q 6 hr.[63]

Geriatric Dosage. Dosage reduction usually not necessary.

Dosage Forms. **Tab** 1 g; **Susp** 100 mg/mL.

Patient Instructions. Take this drug with water on an empty stomach 1 hr before each meal and at bedtime. Antacids can be used as needed for pain relief but do not take them within 30 minutes before or after taking sucralfate. Take potentially interacting drugs 2 hours before taking sucralfate to avoid or minimize drug interactions. Even though symptoms can decrease, continue treatment for the duration of therapy unless instructed otherwise.

Missed Doses. If you miss a dose, take it as soon as possible. If it is almost time for your next dose, skip the missed dose and return to your usual dosage schedule. Do not double doses.

Pharmacokinetics. *Onset and Duration.* Onset (attachment of sucralfate to ulcer site) is within 1 hr; duration is about 6 hr.

Fate. Sucralfate is only minimally absorbed from the GI tract and is excreted primarily in the feces. About 3–5% (primarily aluminum) is absorbed and excreted in urine.[2,61] Aluminum excretion is decreased in uremia.

Adverse Reactions. Adverse reactions are usually minor and occur in about 5% of patients. Constipation occurs in about 2% of patients. Other effects, including diarrhea, nausea, gastric discomfort, indigestion, dry mouth, rash, pruritus, backache, dizziness, drowsiness, vertigo, and a metallic taste, occur occasionally. Aluminum accumulation and toxicity, including osteodystrophy, osteomalacia, encephalopathy, and seizures, have been reported in patients with chronic renal failure. Hypophosphatemia can develop in critically ill patients and those on prolonged sucralfate therapy. Bezoar formation in the esophagus and GI tract and intestinal obstruction and perforation have been reported.[3,61]

Precautions. Use with caution in patients receiving other aluminum-containing drugs or in chronic renal failure and dialysis. Avoid administration through feeding tubes because the drug can occlude the tube.

Drug Interactions. Sucralfate can inhibit the absorption of drugs including digoxin, ketoconazole, levothyroxine, phenytoin, quinidine, oral fluoroquinolones, tetracyclines, theophylline, and warfarin. In most cases, drug interactions can be avoided if the drug is given 2 hr before sucralfate administration, especially in patients receiving tube feedings.

Parameters to Monitor. Improvement in epigastric pain or heartburn; however, pain relief in PUD and GERD does not correlate directly with endoscopic evidence of healing. Monitor for constipation and signs of aluminum toxicity in the elderly, in chronic renal failure, or in patients receiving other aluminum-containing drugs. Obtain serum phosphate levels periodically in patients receiving concurrent aluminum-containing drugs or with prolonged use. Monitor for potential drug interactions.

Notes. Sucralfate is as effective as standard doses of the **H₂-receptor antagonists** in the short-term treatment and maintenance of healed duodenal ulcer.[2,61,62] Sucralfate can overcome the negative effect of cigarette smoking on duodenal ulcer healing and recurrence.[61] Its efficacy in healing erosive esophagitis and maintaining esophageal healing is inferior to the **H₂-receptor antagonists** or **proton pump inhibitors.** Sucralfate is effective in preventing stress-related mucosal bleeding and can be more cost effective than H₂-receptor antagonists.[3,62,64] Its efficacy as a single agent in preventing NSAID-induced gastric and duodenal ulcers, chemotherapy-induced stomatitis, and stress-related bleeding in high-risk critically ill surgical patients is unsubstantiated. Whether sucralfate is associated with a lower frequency of nosocomial pneumonia in critically ill patients than H₂-receptor antagonists or antacids remains controversial.[3,65] Although therapy with sucralfate and an H₂-receptor antagonist or PPI provides two different mechanisms of drug action, enhanced efficacy of two drugs has not been substantiated for any indication.

ERADICATION OF *HELICOBACTER PYLORI* INFECTION

One cause of peptic ulcer disease (PUD) is associated with *H. pylori* infections. Patients infected or colonized with *H. pylori* are at increased risk for developing PUD, gastric carcinoma, atrophic gastric and gastric mucosa-associated lymphoid tissue.[66,67] Thus, all patients who test positive for *H. pylori* should be treated.[67,68] The value of *H. pylori* eradication in patients with dyspepsia or nonulcer dyspepsia remains controversial.[69,70] The goal of therapy is to promote rapid ulcer healing and prevent relapse by eradicating the infection. Combination therapy that includes an antisecretory agent (PPI or ranitidine bismuth citrate) and two antimicrobial agents (amoxicillin and clarithromycin or metronidazole) for 10–14 days is effective in resolving the infection.[38,44,67] The use of any PPI combined with at least two antibiotics have achieved similar eradication rates against *H. pylori* infections.[38,44,47,48]

Factors to consider when choosing a *H. pylori* regimen include eradication rates, patient compliance, and minimizing drug resistance and adverse effects associated with the drug therapy. Dual therapy (PPI and one antibiotic) is rarely used because eradication rates are often poor (<70%), but triple therapy is used because it obtains an eradication rate of at least 80–90%. The eradication rate for quadruple therapy is >90%.[38] Even though quadruple therapy is effective in eliminating the infection, it is not ideal because of the complicated dosage regimen that can lead to decreased patient compliance. Adverse effects can decrease patient compliance, especially those treated with metronidazole.

When choosing antibiotics, resistance becomes an issue. Metronidazole resistance to *H. pylori* infections is most common, with a range of 7–80%, and is more frequent in women. Macrolide resistance is less common (1–10%) and is even less frequent with tetracycline and amoxicillin.[71] Quadruple therapy should be considered for patients who failed initial treatment.

Antibiotics should not be used for longer than 2 weeks. If treatment fails, a different antibiotic regimen should be considered. Although any PPI can be used in the various regimens, there are some substitutions that should not be done (eg, ampicillin for amoxicillin, doxycycline for tetracycline, azithromycin for clarithromycin, or an H_2-receptor antagonist for a PPI).[38,44,47,48]

DRUG TREATMENT REGIMENS USED TO ERADICATE *HELICOBACTER PYLORI*

DRUGS	DOSE	FREQUENCY	DURATION	EFFICACY[a]	ADVERSE EFFECTS[b]	COMPLIANCE[c]
Amoxicillin Omeprazole[d,e]	1 g 20 mg	bid–tid bid–tid	14 days 14 days	Poor–fair	Low–medium	Likely
Clarithromycin Omeprazole[d,e,f]	500 mg 40 mg	tid qd	14 days 14 days	Fair–good	Low–medium	Likely
Amoxicillin Lansoprazole[d,e,f,]	1 g 30 mg	tid tid	10–14 days 10–14 days	Poor–Fair	Low–medium	Likely
Clarithromycin RBC	500 mg 400 mg	tid bid	14 days 28 days	Fair–good	Low–Medium	Likely
Clarithromycin Metronidazole Omeprazole[d,e]	500 mg 500 mg 20 mg	bid bid bid	10–14 days 10–14 days 10–14 days	Good–excellent	Medium	Likely
Clarithromycin Amoxicillin Lansoprazole[d,e,f]	500 mg 1 g 30 mg	bid bid bid	10–14 days 10–14 days 10–14 days	Good–excellent	Low–medium	Likely
Amoxicillin Metronidazole Omeprazole[d,e]	1 g 500 mg 20 mg	bid bid bid	14 days 14 days 14 days	Fair–good	Medium	Likely

(continued)

DRUG TREATMENT REGIMENS USED TO ERADICATE *HELICOBACTER PYLORI* (continued)

DRUGS	DOSE	FREQUENCY	DURATION	EFFICACY[a]	ADVERSE EFFECTS[b]	COMPLIANCE[c]
Clarithromycin	500 mg	bid	14 days	Good	Medium	Unlikely
Metronidazole	500 mg	bid	14 days			
RBC	400 mg	bid	14–28 days			
BSS	525 mg	qid	14 days	Good–excellent	Medium–high	Unlikely
Metronidazole	150 mg	qid	14 days			
Tetracycline	500 mg	qid	14 days			
H₂RA[f]	Conventional ulcer healing dosage regimen for 28 days					
BSS	525 mg	qid	14 days	Fair–good	Medium–high	Unlikely
Metronidazole	250 mg	qid	14 days			
Amoxicillin	500 mg	qid	14 days			
H₂RA[f]	Conventional ulcer healing dosage regimen for 28 days					
BSS	525 mg	qid	7 days	Good–excellent	Medium–high	Unlikely
Metronidazole	500 mg	qid	7 days			
Tetracycline	500 mg	qid	7 days			
Omeprazole[d,e]	20 mg	bid	7 days			
BSS	525 mg	qid	7 days	Good–excellent	Medium–high	Unlikely
Metronidazole	500 mg	qid	7 days			
Clarithromycin	500 mg	bid	7 days			
Omeprazole[d,e]	20 mg	bid	7 days			

(continued)

DRUG TREATMENT REGIMENS USED TO ERADICATE *HELICOBACTER PYLORI* (continued)

DRUGS	DOSE	FREQUENCY	DURATION	EFFICACY[a]	ADVERSE EFFECTS[b]	COMPLIANCE[c]
BSS	525 mg	qid	7–14 days	Good–excellent	Medium	Unlikely
Clarithromycin	500 mg	tid	7–14 days			
Tetracycline	500 mg	qid	7–14 days			
Omeprazole[d,e]	20 mg	bid	7–14 days			

BSS = bismuth subsalicylate; H2RA = H2-receptor antagonist; PPI = proton pump inhibitor; RBC = ranitidine bismuth citrate.

[a]Efficacy (eradication rate): excellent >90%; good >80–90%; fair >70–80%; poor <70%.

[b]Adverse Effects = frequency of clinically important adverse effects.

[c]Compliance = estimate based on total number of tablets/capsules, frequency of administration, and clinically important adverse effects.

[d]Any PPI can be used (esomeprazole 40 mg, lansoprazole 30 mg, omeprazole 20 mg, pantoprazole 20–40 mg, rabeprazole 40 mg).

[e]PPI therapy can be extended to 28 days in patients with active ulcer.

[f]FDA-approved regimen.

Antiemetics

DOLASETRON MESYLATE
Anzemet

Pharmacology. Dolasetron and its active metabolite, hydrodolasetron, are selective serotonin$_3$ (5-HT$_3$) antagonists. Dolasetron is approved for the prevention of chemotherapy-induced nausea and vomiting and for the prevention and treatment of postoperative nausea and vomiting. Its use is similar to those of ondansetron and granisetron.[72] (*See* Antiemetic Drugs Comparison Chart.)

Adult Dosage. **PO or IV for chemotherapy-induced nausea and vomiting** 100 mg or 1.8 mg/kg. **IV for postoperative nausea and vomiting** 12.5 mg. **PO for postoperative nausea and vomiting** 100 mg. IV doses can be administered over a minimum of 30 sec or further diluted in 50 mL of NS or D5W and infused over a period of up to 15 min. In some dose-finding trials in adults, higher response rates were obtained with 200 mg PO and 2.4 mg IV than with lower doses by the respective routes.[72]

Pediatric Dosage. **PO or IV for chemotherapy-induced nausea and vomiting** (≤2 yr) safety and efficacy not established; (2–16 yr) 1.8 mg/kg, to a maximum of 100 mg. **IV for postoperative nausea and vomiting** (2–16 yr) 0.35 mg/kg, to a maximum of 12.5 mg. **PO for postoperative nausea and vomiting** (2–16 yr) 1.2 mg/kg, to a maximum of 100 mg.

Dosage Forms. **Inj** 20 mg/mL; **Tab** 50, 100 mg.

Pharmacokinetics. Approximately 75% of dolasetron mesylate is dolasetron base. The apparent absolute bioavailability of oral dolasetron is approximately 75%. Little dolasetron is detected in the plasma because of rapid conversion to hydrodolasetron by the ubiquitous enzyme, carbonyl reductase. Hydrodolasetron is partly metabolized in the liver and 61% is excreted unchanged in the urine. Hydrodolasetron has a V$_d$ of 5.8 ± 1.5 L/kg and Cl of 0.56 ± 0.16 L/hr/kg. Its half-life is 7.3 ± 1.8 hr.

Adverse Reactions. Acute, reversible ECG changes (PR and QT$_c$ prolongation, and QRS widening) have occurred in clinical trials and in healthy volunteers. Other adverse effects are similar to those of ondansetron and granisetron.

Notes. Dolasetron can be prepared extemporaneously as an oral solution by mixing the injectable form in apple or apple–grape juice. The diluted product can be kept up to 2 hr at room temperature before use.

DRONABINOL
Marinol

Pharmacology. Dronabinol (Δ-9-tetrahydrocannabinol) is an active antiemetic component of *Cannabis*. Its mechanism of action as an antiemetic is complex and poorly understood but it probably inhibits the chemoreceptor trigger zone in the medulla.

Administration and Adult Dosage. **PO as an antiemetic** 5 mg/m^2 1–3 hr before chemotherapy and then q 2–4 hr after chemotherapy, for a total of 4–6 doses/day. Dosage can be increased in 2.5 mg/m^2 increments, to a maximum of 15 mg/m^2/dose.[73–75] **PO for appetite stimulation** 2.5 mg before lunch and dinner or 2.5 mg at bedtime if unable to tolerate daytime administration. Dosage can be increased to a maximum of 20 mg/day.

Special Populations. *Pediatric Dosage.* **PO as an antiemetic during cancer chemotherapy** same as adult dosage in mg/m^2.

Geriatric Dosage. Same as adult dosage. (*See* Adverse Reactions.)

Dosage Forms. **Cap** 2.5, 5, 10 mg.

Patient Instructions. This drug can cause drowsiness or changes in mood. Until the extent of this effect is known, use caution when driving, operating machinery, or performing other tasks requiring mental alertness. Avoid excessive concurrent use of alcohol or other drugs that cause drowsiness. Store this medication in the refrigerator.

Missed Doses. Take this drug at regular intervals. If you miss a dose, take it as soon as you remember. If it is about time for the next dose, take that dose only. Do not double the dose or take extra.

Pharmacokinetics. *Onset and Duration.* Oral onset 30–60 min; peak 2–4 hr; duration is 4–6 hr but can be longer in those who have not previously used the drug.[76,77] *Cannabis* smoking onset 15 sec–2 min; peak 8–16 min; duration 3–12 hr.[78]

Fate. Bioavailability is 4–12% orally, 2–50% by smoking. About 95% bound to plasma proteins. V_d is 8.9 ± 4.2 L/kg; Cl is 0.21 ± 0.054 L/hr/kg. Primarily metabolized by hydroxylation to active and inactive metabolites. Ultimately, 35% of metabolites are found in feces and 15% in urine, with <1% excreted unchanged in urine.[79–81]

t½. Terminal phase 32 ± 12 hr, although time course of effects more closely parallels initial distribution phase.[79]

Adverse Reactions. Euphoria, dizziness, paranoia, or drowsiness occur frequently and might be accompanied by ataxia, loss of balance, and disorientation to the point of being disabling. Other frequent side effects are dry mouth, orthostatic hypotension, and conjunctival injection.[82] The "high" experienced by some is not always well tolerated, especially by older patients.[83]

Contraindications. Allergy to dronabinol, marijuana, or sesame oil; mentally ill patients.

Precautions. Avoid during lactation. Use with caution in patients with hypertension or heart disease. Use with caution in patients with epilepsy.[73]

Drug Interactions. Not well studied, but some apparent interactions have been reported after *Cannabis* use: additive or supra-additive sedation with alcohol and other CNS depressants; additive hypertension and/or tachycardia with anticholinergics, antihistamines, sympathomimetics, or tricyclic antidepressants; and hypomania with disulfiram or fluoxetine.

Parameters to Monitor. Observe for frequency of emesis, drowsiness, or disorientation.

Notes. Dronabinol is at least as effective as **phenothiazines** for chemotherapy-induced nausea and vomiting[75] but not as effective as **serotonin antagonists** or IV **metoclopramide**.[84,85] It is not particularly effective for cisplatin-induced nausea and vomiting. It might not be as effective as smoking *Cannabis,* which is easier to titrate.[85] (*See* Antiemetic Drugs Comparison Chart.)

GRANISETRON   Kytril

Pharmacology. Granisetron is a selective antagonist at the 5-HT$_3$ receptor used for the prevention of nausea and vomiting associated with cancer chemotherapy. Its use in cancer chemotherapy is similar to that of ondansetron, and its efficacy and side effects are comparable to those of ondansetron.[72,86] (*See* Antiemetic Drugs Comparison Chart.)

Adult Dosage. **IV for cancer chemotherapy-induced nausea and vomiting** 10 μg/kg administered in 20–50 mL NS or D5W over 5 min, 30 min before the start of chemotherapy. **PO for cancer chemotherapy-induced nausea and vomiting** 1 mg up to 1 hr before chemotherapy and additional 1 mg doses at 12-hr intervals thereafter while receiving chemotherapy.

Pediatric Dosage. **IV** (>2 yr) same as adult dosage, but this dosage might not be adequate for children.[86]

Dosage Forms. **Inj** 1 mg/mL; **Tab** 1 mg.

Pharmacokinetics. Oral absorption is approximately 60%. V$_d$ is 30 ± 1.5 L/kg; Cl is 0.060 ± 0.54 L/hr/kg. Elimination is mostly by hepatic metabolism, with 16 ± 14% appearing in the urine as unchanged drug. The half-life is 5.3 ± 3.5 hr (can be longer in cancer patients than in normals). The metabolism of granisetron might be changed by inducers or inhibitors of the cytochrome P450 system, but dosage adjustment is not recommended.

Adverse Reactions. (*See* Ondansetron).

ONDANSETRON HYDROCHLORIDE   Zofran

Pharmacology. Ondansetron is a selective antagonist at the 5-HT$_3$ receptor used for the prevention of nausea and vomiting associated with cancer chemotherapy, especially cisplatin, and for postoperative nausea and vomiting. It also is useful for radiotherapy-induced nausea and vomiting. Ondansetron is thought to block these receptors at both peripheral sites in the GI tract and within the area postrema in the CNS.[87] It is not a dopamine receptor antagonist, so it has no extrapyramidal side effects. (*See* Notes.)

Administration and Adult Dosage. **IV for chemotherapy-induced nausea or vomiting** 0.15 mg/kg for 3 doses (30 min before chemotherapy and then 4 and 8 hr after) or 0.45 mg/kg, to a maximum of 32 mg as a single dose or 8 mg IV as a single dose for cisplatin doses <100 mg/m^2.[72] (*See* Notes.) Infuse slowly over 15 min in 50 mL D5W or NS. **IV bolus for postoperative nausea or vomiting** 4 mg over 2–5 min before induction or postoperatively. **PO for chemotherapy-induced nausea or vomiting** 8 mg bid–tid or 24 mg once daily. **PO for radiotherapy-induced nausea or vomiting** 8 mg daily–tid. **PO for postoperative nausea or vomiting** 8–16 mg 1 hr before surgery.[72]

Special Populations. *Pediatric Dosage.* **IV for chemotherapy-induced nausea or vomiting** (<2 yr) safety and efficacy not established; (2–18 yr) same as adult dosage or 0.15 mg/kg for 2 doses for moderately emetogenic chemotherapy.[88–90]

IV for postoperative nausea or vomiting 0.05–0.1 mg/kg, to a maximum of 4 mg as a single dose over 30 sec before the surgical incision.[72] **PO for chemotherapy-induced nausea and vomiting** (4–11 yr) 4 mg q 8 hr. **PO for postoperative nausea or vomiting** 0.15 mg/kg 30–45 min before IV catheter placement.[91]

Geriatric Dosage. Same as adult dosage.

Other Conditions. In hepatic function impairment, do not exceed a single oral dose of 8 mg or a total daily IV dosage of 8 mg.

Dosage Forms. Inj 0.64, 2 mg/mL; **Tab** 4, 8, 24 mg; **Tab** (rapidly dissolving) 4, 8 mg; **Soln** 0.8 mg/mL.

Pharmacokinetics. *Fate.* Oral absorption is $62 \pm 15\%$. V_d is 1.9 ± 0.5 L/kg; Cl is 0.35 ± 0.16 L/hr/kg in adults and can be higher in children. The drug is extensively metabolized to glucuronide and sulfate conjugates. About 5% appears in urine as unchanged ondansetron.[79]

$t_{1/2}$. 3.5 ± 1.9 hr in normal adults, increased in the elderly.[79] However, the duration of activity is not related to the half-life.[72]

Adverse Reactions. Headache occurs frequently. Transient increased serum levels of hepatic enzymes also occur frequently, but these are probably caused by chemotherapy rather than by ondansetron.[72,92–94]

Contraindications. None known.

Precautions. Pregnancy; lactation; suspected ileus. Patients who are hypersensitive to other 5-HT$_3$ antagonists might cross-react with ondansetron.[95]

Drug Interactions. The metabolism of ondansetron can be changed by inducers or inhibitors of the cytochrome P450 system, but dosage adjustment is not recommended.

Parameters to Monitor. Frequency of vomiting.

Notes. Protect vials from light; inspect for discoloration and particulate matter before using.

　　Dexamethasone enhances the antiemetic effect of the 5-HT$_3$ antagonists;[72,96] the combination of ondansetron and dexamethasone is more effective than **metoclopramide** and dexamethasone for the acute component but not for the delayed phase of severely emetogenic chemotherapy.[72] Several studies have documented the lack of additional efficacy beyond that achieved with a total daily ondansetron dosage of 0.45 mg/kg.[96,97] (*See* Antiemetic Drugs Comparison Chart.)

PROCHLORPERAZINE SALTS　　　　　　　　　　Compazine, Various

Pharmacology. Prochlorperazine is a phenothiazine tranquilizer with antidopaminergic and weak anticholinergic activities. It suppresses the chemoreceptor trigger zone in the CNS and is used mainly for its antiemetic properties. It is not effective for the treatment of motion sickness or vertigo.

Administration and Adult Dosage. PO as an antiemetic 5–10 mg tid or qid; **PR as an antiemetic** 25 mg bid; **IM as an antiemetic** (deep in upper outer quadrant of buttock) 5–10 mg q 4–6 hr, to a maximum of 40 mg/day. **IM presurgically** (deep in upper outer quadrant of buttock) 5–10 mg 1–2 hr before induction, can repeat once before or after surgery; **IV presurgically** 5–10 mg 15–30 min before induction or as infusion (20 mg/L) started 15–30 min before induction. **SC** not recommended.

Special Populations. *Pediatric Dosage.* Not to be used in surgery or in patients <9 kg or <2 yr. **PO or PR as an antiemetic** (9–13 kg) 2.5 mg daily–bid; (14–18 kg) 2.5 mg bid–tid; (19–39 kg) 2.5 mg tid–5 mg bid. (*See* Notes.) **IM as an antiemetic** (deep in upper outer quadrant of buttock) 0.13 mg/kg. **SC** not recommended.

Geriatric Dosage. Use the lower end of the recommended dosage range in elderly patients.

Dosage Forms. **Inj** 5 mg/mL; **Supp** 2.5, 5, 25 mg; **Syrup** 1 mg/mL; **Tab** 5, 10, 25 mg. Larger-dose tablets are available for psychiatric use. Sustained-release products have no demonstrated advantage over rapid-release products.

Patient Instructions. This drug can cause drowsiness. Until the extent of this effect is known, use caution when driving, operating machinery, or performing other tasks requiring mental alertness. Avoid excessive concurrent use of alcohol or other drugs that cause drowsiness.

Missed Doses. Take this drug as prescribed. If you miss a dose, take it as soon as you remember. If it is about time for the next dose, take that dose only. Do not double the dose or take extra.

Pharmacokinetics. *Onset and Duration.* PO onset 30–40 min; PR onset 60 min; IM onset 10–20 min. Duration for all routes 3–4 hr.

Fate. The drug is well absorbed, but extensive and variable presystemic metabolism in the gut wall and liver limits bioavailability. Eliminated primarily by hepatic metabolism and biliary excretion.

$t_{\frac{1}{2}}$. 23 hr.[98]

Adverse Reactions. Extrapyramidal reactions, especially dystonias and dyskinesias, occur occasionally in adults and frequently in children (other extrapyramidal reactions are less likely because of the short duration of therapy when used as an antiemetic). Anticholinergic effects such as dry mouth, mydriasis, cycloplegia, urinary retention, decreased GI motility, and tachycardia occur occasionally. SC administration can cause local reactions at injection site.

Contraindications. Pediatric surgery; children <9 kg or <2 yr; coma or greatly depressed state caused by CNS depressants.

Precautions. Antiemetic action can mask signs and symptoms of overdose with other drugs and can mask the diagnosis and treatment of other conditions such as intestinal obstruction, brain tumor, or Reye's syndrome. Use with caution in conditions in which the drug's anticholinergic effects might be detrimental, in children with acute illnesses or dehydration, or in patients with histories of allergy to phenothiazine derivatives (eg, blood dyscrasias, jaundice). Avoid exposure to concentrate on hands or clothing because of the possibility of contact dermatitis.

Drug Interactions. Phenothiazines can decrease the efficacy of guanethidine or guanadrel or have additive hypotensive effects with hypotensive drugs. Phenothiazines can inhibit the antiparkinson activity of levodopa.

Parameters to Monitor. Monitor for extrapyramidal side effects and drug efficacy.

Notes. Protect the solution from light; a slight yellowish discoloration does not indicate altered potency, but markedly discolored solution should be discarded. Protect suppositories from heat. Prochlorperazine does not predictably reduce chemotherapy-induced nausea and vomiting in children and might be associated with an increase in symptoms.[99] (*See* Antiemetic Drugs Comparison Chart.)

ANTIEMETIC DRUGS COMPARISON CHART

| | | INITIAL DOSE[a,b] | | INDICATIONS | | |
DRUG	DOSAGE FORMS	Adult	Pediatric	Nausea and Vomiting	Motion Sickness	Vertigo
ANTIHISTAMINES						
Buclizine Bucladin-S	Chew Tab 50 mg.	PO 50 mg.	—		X	
Cyclizine Marezine	Tab 50 mg.	PO 50 mg.	PO (6–12 yr) 25 mg.		X	
Dimenhydrinate Dramamine Various	Tab 50 mg Chew Tab 50 mg Liquid 2.5, 3.1 mg/mL Inj 50 mg/mL.	PO 50–100 mg IM, IV 50 mg.	PO (2–6 yr) 12.5–25 mg, (6–12 yr) 25–50 mg. IM, IV (>2 yr) 1.25 mg/kg.	X	X	X
Diphenhydra-mine Benadryl Various	Cap 25, 50 mg Tab 25, 50 mg Chew Tab 12.5 mg Elxr 2.5 mg/mL Soln 1.25, 2.5 mg/mL Syrup 2.5 mg/mL Inj 50 mg/mL.	PO 50 mg IM, IV 10–50 mg.	PO (2–6 yr) 6.25 mg or 1.25 mg/kg, (6–12 yr) 12.5 mg IM, IV (>9 kg) 1.25 mg/kg.		X	
Meclizine Antivert Bonine Various	Cap 25, 30 mg Tab 12.5, 25, 50 mg Chew Tab 25 mg.	PO 25–50 mg.	—	X	X	c

(continued)

ANTIEMETIC DRUGS COMPARISON CHART (continued)

		INITIAL DOSE[a,b]		INDICATIONS		
DRUG	DOSAGE FORMS	Adult	Pediatric	Nausea and Vomiting	Motion Sickness	Vertigo
CANNABINOIDS						
Dronabinol (C-III)[d] Marinol	Cap 2.5, 5, 10 mg.	PO 5 mg/m².	PO 5 mg/m².	X		
PHENOTHIAZINES						
Chlorpromazine Thorazine Various	Tab 10, 25, 50 mg Liquid 30, 100 mg/mL Syrup 2 mg/mL Supp 25, 100 mg Inj 25 mg/mL.	PO 10–25 mg PR 50–100 mg IM 25 mg.	PO, IM (>6 months) 0.55 mg/kg PR (>6 months) 1 mg/kg.	X		
Perphenazine Trilafon	Tab 2, 4, 8, 16 mg Liquid 3.2 mg/mL Inj 5 mg/mL.	PO 2–4 mg IM 5 mg.	—	X		
Prochlorperazine Compazine Various	Tab 5, 10, mg Syrup 1 mg/mL Supp 2.5, 5, 25 mg Inj 5 mg/mL.	PO, IM 5–10 mg IV 2.5–10 mg PR 25 mg.	PO, PR (>9 kg or >2 yr) 2.5 mg IM (>9 kg or >2 yr) 0.13 mg/kg.	X		
Promethazine Phenergan Various	Syrup 1.25, 5 mg/mL Tab 12.5, 25, 50 mg Supp 12.5, 25, 50 mg Inj 25, 50 mg/mL.	PO, PR 25 mg IM, IV 12.5–25 mg.	PO, PR, IM (>2 yr) 0.25–0.5 mg/kg.	X	X	

(continued)

ANTIEMETIC DRUGS COMPARISON CHART (continued)

		INITIAL DOSE[a,b]		INDICATIONS		
DRUG	DOSAGE FORMS	Adult	Pediatric	Nausea and Vomiting	Motion Sickness	Vertigo
Thiethylperazine Torecan	Tab 10 mg Inj 5 mg/mL.	PO, IM 10 mg.	—	X		
Triflupromazine Vesprin	Inj 10, 20 mg/mL.	IM 5–15 mg IM (elderly) 2.5 mg IV 1 mg.	IM (>2.5 yr) 0.2–0.25 mg/kg.	X		
SEROTONIN 5-HT₃ ANTAGONISTS						
Dolasetron Anzemet	Tab 50, 100 mg Inj 20 mg/mL.	PO 100 mg IV 1.8 mg/kg.	PO 1.8 mg/kg IV 1.8 mg/kg.	X		
Granisetron Kytril	Tab 1 mg Inj 1 mg/mL.	PO 1 mg IV 10 µg/kg.	IV (>2 yr) 10 µg/kg.	X		
Ondansetron Zofran	Tab 4, 8, 24 mg Tab (rapidly dissolving) 4, 8 mg Soln 6.8 mg/mL Inj 0.64, 2 mg/mL.	PO 8 or 16 mg IV 0.15–0.45 mg/kg (max 32 mg).	PO (>4 yr) 4 mg IV (>2 yr) 0.15 mg/kg.	X		
MISCELLANEOUS						
Dexamethasone Decadron Various	Elxr 0.1 mg/mL Soln 0.1, 1 mg/mL Tab 0.25, 0.5, 0.75, 1, 1.5, 2, 4.6 mg Inj 4, 10, 20, 24 mg/mL.	PO, IV 10–20 mg.	PO, IV 10 mg/m².	e		

(continued)

ANTIEMETIC DRUGS COMPARISON CHART (*continued*)

DRUG	DOSAGE FORMS	INITIAL DOSE[a,b] Adult	INITIAL DOSE[a,b] Pediatric	INDICATIONS Nausea and Vomiting	INDICATIONS Motion Sickness	INDICATIONS Vertigo
Droperidol Inapsine	Inj 2.5 mg/mL	IM, IV 0.625–1.25 mg.	IV 0.015–0.075 mg/kg.	f		
Lorazepam (C-IV)[d] Ativan Various	Tab 0.5, 1, 2 mg Soln 2 mg/mL Inj 2, 4 mg/mL.	PO 1–2 mg.	PO 0.05 mg/kg.	e		
Methylprednisolone Solu-Medrol Various	Inj 40, 125, 500 mg.	IV up to 100 mg.	IV 2–4 mg/kg.	e		
Metoclopramide Reglan	Inj 5 mg/mL	IV 1–2 mg/kg.	IV 1–2 mg/kg.	X		
Scopolamine Scopace Transderm Scop	Transdermal Patch 1.5 mg (delivers 1 mg over 3 days). Tab 0.4 mg	1 disk behind ear over 3 days PO 0.4 mg	— —		X X	
Trimethobenzamide Tigan Various	Cap 100, 250 mg Supp 100, 200 mg Inj 100 mg/mL.	PO 250 mg PR 200 mg IM 200 mg.	PO (14–40 kg) 100–200 mg PR (<14 kg) 100 mg, (14–40 kg) 100–200 mg.	X		

[a]Initial dose only; check prescribing information for subsequent dosage.
[b]Doses of serotonin antagonists are for chemotherapy-induced nausea and vomiting. (*See* monograph for doses in postoperative nausea and vomiting.)
[c]Possibly effective.
[d]Controlled substance schedule designated in parentheses.
[e]Not labeled for this use; used as adjunctive for cancer chemotherapy-induced nausea and vomiting.
[f]Effective, but not labeled for this use.

Gastrointestinal Motility

BISACODYL
Dulcolax, Various

Pharmacology. Bisacodyl is a stimulant cathartic structurally similar to phenolphthalein that produces its effect by direct contact with colonic mucosa. It can inhibit water absorption in the small bowel and colon.[100,101]

Administration and Adult Dosage. PO as a laxative/cathartic 10–30 mg; **PR** 10 mg. Adjust dosage based on response.

Special Populations. *Pediatric Dosage.* PO (≤6 yr) safety and efficacy not established; (>6 yr) 5–10 mg or 0.3 mg/kg once daily; **PR** (≤6 yr) safety and efficacy not established; (6–12 yr) 5 mg; (>12 yr) 10 mg.

Geriatric Dosage. Same as adult dosage.

Dosage Forms. EC **Tab** 5 mg; **Enema** (adult) 10 mg; **Supp** 10 mg.

Patient Instructions. Swallow tablets whole (not chewed or crushed) and do not take within 1 hour of antacids or dairy products. Do not use oral products in children 6 years of age or less.

Pharmacokinetics. *Onset and Duration.* Onset PO 6–12 hr; PR 15 min–1 hr.[101,102]

Fate. Absorption is less than 5% by oral or rectal route, with subsequent conversion to the glucuronide salt and excretion in urine and bile. Rapidly converted in the gut by intestinal and bacterial enzymes to its active, but nonabsorbed, desacetyl metabolite.[103]

Adverse Reactions. Abdominal cramps occur frequently; with long-term use, metabolic acidosis or alkalosis, hypocalcemia, tetany, loss of enteric protein, and malabsorption occur occasionally; suppositories can cause proctitis and rectal inflammation and are not recommended for long-term use.

Drug Interactions. Antacids or milk can dissolve the enteric coating of oral bisacodyl tablets, causing drug release in the stomach and gastric irritation.

Contraindications. Acute surgical abdomen; nausea, vomiting, or other symptoms of appendicitis; fecal impaction; intestinal or biliary tract obstruction; abdominal pain of unknown origin.

Notes. Useful for preoperative or preradiographic bowel preparation. Bisacodyl has been used in combination with **polyethylene glycol (PEG) electrolyte lavage solution** to decrease the amount of solution required.[100,101,104] (*See* PEG Electrolyte Lavage Solution.)

DIPHENOXYLATE HYDROCHLORIDE AND ATROPINE SULFATE
Lomotil, Various

Pharmacology. Diphenoxylate is a synthetic meperidine congener without analgesic activity that slows GI motility. Because high doses of diphenoxylate (40–60 mg) cause systemic opioid activity, atropine is added in subtherapeutic amounts to decrease abuse potential.

Administration and Adult Dosage. PO for diarrhea 2 tablets or 10 mL qid initially and then, if control is achieved (usually within 48 hr), decrease to a **maintenance dosage** as low as 2 tablets or 10 mL daily prn. If chronic diarrhea is not controlled in 10 days at the full dosage, then symptoms are unlikely to be controlled by further administration.

Special Populations. *Pediatric Dosage.* **Use liquid only.** (<2 yr) Not recommended. **PO for diarrhea** 0.3–0.4 mg/kg/day of diphenoxylate in 4 divided doses initially, not to exceed adult dosage. Reduce dosage once diarrhea is controlled.

Geriatric Dosage. Same as adult dosage.

Dosage Forms. **Syrup** 500 μg diphenoxylate and 5 μg atropine/mL; **Tab** 2.5 mg diphenoxylate and 25 μg atropine.

Patient Instructions. This drug can cause dry mouth, blurred vision, drowsiness, or dizziness; use caution while driving or performing other tasks requiring alertness, coordination, or physical dexterity. Avoid alcohol and other CNS depressants. Seek medical attention if diarrhea persists or if fever, palpitations, or abdominal distention occurs.

Missed Doses. If you miss a dose, take it as soon as possible. If it is almost time for your next dose, skip the missed dose and return to your usual dosage schedule. Do not double doses.

Pharmacokinetics. *Onset and Duration.* Onset 45–60 min; duration 3–4 hr.

Fate. Diphenoxylate is well absorbed from the GI tract and metabolized to an active metabolite, diphenoxylic acid. Drug and metabolite attain peak serum levels in 2 hr. Diphenoxylate V_d is 3.8 ± 1.1 L/kg; Cl is 1.04 ± 0.14 L/hr/kg.[105] Conjugates of the drug and metabolite are excreted primarily in the urine.

$t_{1/2}$. (Diphenoxylate) 2.5 ± 0.6 hr; (diphenoxylic acid) 7.2 ± 0.7 hr.[106]

Adverse Reactions. Anticholinergic symptoms such as dry mouth, urinary retention, blurred vision, fever, or tachycardia occur frequently with high daily dosages and occasionally with usual dosages in children.[107] Drowsiness, dizziness, and headache occur occasionally.

Contraindications. Children <2 yr; obstructive jaundice; diarrhea associated with pseudomembranous enterocolitis or enterotoxin-producing bacteria. (*See* Notes.)

Precautions. Use with caution in children because of variable response and potential for toxicity (atropinism) with recommended dosages (particularly in children with Down's syndrome) and in patients with acute ulcerative colitis, hepatic dysfunction, or cirrhosis. (*See* Notes.)

Drug Interactions. Because of its chemical similarity to meperidine, avoid diphenoxylate use with MAOIs. Use with caution in combination with CNS depressants.

Parameters to Monitor. Frequency and volume of bowel movements; body temperature; blood in stool. Watch for signs of atropine toxicity. Monitor for abdominal distention.

Notes. In chronic diarrhea, diphenoxylate 5 mg is about equipotent with **loperamide** 2 mg or **codeine** 30–45 mg. It might provide temporary symptomatic relief of infectious traveler's diarrhea (although loperamide is preferred) if used cautiously with an antibiotic, but discontinue if fever occurs, symptoms persist beyond 48 hr, or blood or mucus appears in the stool.[108,109]

DOCUSATE SALTS   Various

Pharmacology. Docusate is an anionic surfactant that lowers the surface tension of the oil–water interface of the stool, allowing fecal material to be penetrated by water and fat, thereby softening the stool. The emulsifying action also enhances the absorption of many fat-soluble drugs and mineral oil. These agents also can cause subtle effects on fluid absorption and secretion in the GI tract.[100,101]

Administration and Adult Dosage. **PO as a stool softener** (sodium salt) 50–500 mg/day in single or divided doses (give solution/syrup in milk or fruit juice to mask taste); begin therapy with up to 500 mg/day and adjust after maximal effects occur (about 3 days);[103] (calcium salt) 240 mg/day; (potassium salt) 100–300 mg/day. Use of these agents in elderly, bedridden patients might be ineffective in altering the prevalence of constipation.[101] **PR as enema** 50–100 mg in water.

Special Populations. *Pediatric Dosage.* **PO** (sodium salt) (<3 yr) 10–40 mg/day; (3–6 yr) 20–60 mg/day; (6–12 yr) 40–120 mg/day; (>12 yr) same as adult dosage; give solution/syrup in milk, fruit juice, or formula to mask taste; (calcium salt) (≥6 yr) 50–150 mg/day; (potassium salt) (≥6 yr) 100 mg/day.

Geriatric Dosage. Same as adult dosage. (*See* Notes.)

Dosage Forms. (Sodium salt: Colace, various) **Cap** 50, 100, 240, 250 mg; **Soln** 10, 50 mg/mL; **Syrup** 3.3, 4 mg/mL; **Tab** 100 mg. (Calcium salt: Surfak, various) **Cap** 50, 240 mg. (Potassium salt: Dialose, various) **Cap** 240 mg; **Tab** 100 mg.

Patient Instructions. Take this with a full glass of fluid; take the liquid or solution forms in milk, fruit juice, or infant formula to mask the bitter taste.

Missed Doses. If you miss a dose, take it as soon as possible. If it is almost time for your next dose, skip the missed dose and return to your usual dosage schedule.

Pharmacokinetics. *Onset and Duration.* Onset of effect on stools is 2–3 days after first dose with continuous use.

Fate. Drug action is local to the gut, but docusate can be partially absorbed in the duodenum and jejunum and secreted in the bile.[107]

Adverse Reactions. Bitter taste, throat irritation, and nausea (more common with syrup and liquid) occur frequently, abdominal cramps occasionally. Docusate can change intestinal morphology and cellular function and cause fluid and electrolyte accumulation in the colon.[107]

Contraindications. Undiagnosed abdominal pain; intestinal obstruction; concomitant use with mineral oil.

Precautions. Rectal bleeding or failure to respond to therapy might indicate a serious condition and the need for medical attention.

Drug Interactions. Concomitant use with mineral oil can enhance mineral oil absorption.[100]

Parameters to Monitor. Frequency and consistency of stools; ease of defecation.

Notes. Surfactant stool softeners are useful for softening hard, dry stools, in painful anorectal conditions, and in cardiac and other conditions to lessen the strain of defecation. They are more useful in preventing than in treating constipation but they might not be effective for long-term prevention of constipation in institutionalized, elderly patients.[100,101,110]

LACTULOSE
Cephulac, Chronulac

Pharmacology. Lactulose is a synthetic disaccharide analogue of lactose that contains galactose and fructose and is metabolized by colonic bacteria to lactic and small amounts of acetic and formic acids. These acids result in acidification of colonic contents, decreased ammonia production and absorption, and an osmotic catharsis.[111]

Administration and Adult Dosage. PO as a cathartic 15–30 mL (10–20 g), to a maximum of 60 mL; **PO for hepatic encephalopathy** 30–45 mL (20–30 g) q 1 hr until laxation, then 30–45 mL tid or qid, titrated to produce about 2 or 3 soft stools/day. **PR for hepatic encephalopathy as an enema** 300 mL with 700 mL water or NS retained for 30–60 min, can repeat q 4–6 hr. Repeat immediately if evacuated too promptly.

Special Populations. *Pediatric Dosage.* **PO for hepatic encephalopathy** (infants) 2.5–10 mL/day in divided doses; (older children and adolescents) 40–90 mL/day in divided doses, titrated to produce 2 or 3 soft stools daily. If initial dose causes diarrhea, reduce dose immediately; if diarrhea persists, discontinue.

Geriatric Dosage. Same as adult dosage. (*See* Notes.)

Dosage Forms. **Syrup** 667 mg/mL.

Patient Instructions. This syrup can be mixed with fruit juice, water, or milk to improve its palatability. In the treatment of hepatic encephalopathy, 2–3 loose stools per day are common, but report any worsening of diarrhea. Report belching, flatulence, or abdominal cramps if they are bothersome.

Missed Doses. If you miss a dose, take it as soon as possible. If it is almost time for your next dose, skip the missed dose and return to your usual dosage schedule.

Pharmacokinetics. *Onset and Duration.* (Catharsis) onset 24–48 hr; duration 24–48 hr. (Hepatic encephalopathy) onset and duration variable; however, reversal of coma can occur within 2 hr of the first enema.

Fate. After oral administration, less than 3% is absorbed and most reaches the colon unabsorbed and unchanged. Unabsorbed drug is metabolized in the colon by bacteria to low-molecular-weight acids and carbon dioxide. The small amount of absorbed drug is excreted in the urine unchanged.[112]

Adverse Reactions. Flatulence, belching, and abdominal discomfort are frequent initially. Colonic dilation occurs occasionally. Excessive diarrhea and fecal water loss can result in hypernatremia.[113]

Contraindications. Patients who require a low-galactose diet.

Precautions. Use with caution in diabetics because the drug contains small amounts of free lactose and galactose. Rectal bleeding or failure to respond to therapy might indicate a serious condition and the need for medical attention.

Drug Interactions. Do not use other laxatives concomitantly because their induction of loose stools might confound proper lactulose dosage titration for hepatic encephalopathy. Nonabsorbable antacids can interfere with the colonic acidification of lactulose. Theoretically, some antibacterials might interfere with the intestinal bacteria that metabolize lactulose; however, oral neomycin has been used concurrently in hepatic encephalopathy.[112]

Parameters to Monitor. (Hepatic encephalopathy) observe for changes in hepatic encephalopathy and number of stools per day. Periodically obtain serum sodium, chloride, potassium, and bicarbonate levels during prolonged use, especially in elderly or debilitated patients.

Notes. Lactulose is effective in hepatic encephalopathy, but as a general laxative it offers no advantage over less expensive drugs.[113] One study of constipation in the elderly found that up to 60 mL/day of 70% **sorbitol** was equivalent in laxative effects and caused less nausea than the same dosage of lactulose syrup.[114]

LOPERAMIDE   Imodium

Pharmacology. Loperamide is a synthetic antidiarrheal structurally similar to haloperidol and without appreciable opiate activity that causes a dose-related inhibition of colonic motility and affects water and electrolyte movement through the bowel. Tolerance has not been observed.

Administration and Adult Dosage. **PO for acute diarrhea (℞) or traveler's diarrhea (over-the-counter [OTC])** 4 mg initially and then 2 mg after each unformed stool (often with an antibiotic for traveler's diarrhea), to a maximum of 16 mg/day (8 mg/day for no more than 2 days with OTC product).[108,109,115] **PO for chronic diarrhea (℞)** initiate therapy as above and then individualize dosage; **usual maintenance dosage** is 4–8 mg/day in single or divided doses. If clinical improvement does not occur after treatment with 16 mg/day for at least 10 days, symptoms are unlikely to be controlled by further use.

Special Populations. *Pediatric Dosage.* (<2 yr) safety and efficacy not established. **PO for acute diarrhea (℞)** (2–5 yr) up to 1 mg tid as liquid; (6–8 yr) 2 mg bid; (8–12 yr) 2 mg tid. After the first day of therapy, give 1 mg/10 kg after each loose stool, to a maximum daily dosage equal to the initial daily dosage. **PO for acute or traveler's diarrhea (OTC)** (2–5 yr) not recommended; (6–8 yr) 1 mg initially and then 1 mg after each loose stool, to a maximum of 4 mg/day for 2 days; (9–11 yr) 2 mg initially and then 1 mg after each loose stool, to a maximum of 6 mg/day for 2 days. **PO for chronic diarrhea** dosage not established.

Geriatric Dosage. Same as adult dosage.

Dosage Forms. **Cap** 2 mg; **Chew Tab** 2 mg; **Tab** 2 mg; **Liquid** 0.2, 1 mg/mL; **Chew Tab** 2 mg plus simethicone (Imodium Advanced).

Patient Instructions. This drug can cause drowsiness or dizziness. Until the severity of these reactions is known, use caution when performing tasks that require mental alertness. It can cause dry mouth. Drink plenty of clear fluids to prevent the dehydration that can accompany diarrhea. If diarrhea does not stop after a few days, or if abdominal pain, distention, or fever occurs, seek medical attention.

Missed Doses. If you miss a dose, take it as soon as possible. If it is almost time for your next dose, skip the missed dose and return to your usual dosage schedule.

Pharmacokinetics. *Onset and Duration.* Onset 45–60 min; duration 4–6 hr.

Fate. GI absorption is approximately 40%; ≥25% is excreted in the stool unchanged; <2% of a dose is recovered in the urine.[116,117]

$t_{1/2}$. 10.8 ± 1.7 hr.[116,117]

Adverse Reactions. Abdominal cramping, constipation, distention, headache, rash, tiredness, drowsiness, dizziness, and dry mouth occur frequently.[107]

Contraindications. (℞, OTC) patients who must avoid constipation; children <2 yr. (OTC) bloody diarrhea; body temperature above 38°C (101°F); diarrhea associated with pseudomembranous colitis; or enterotoxin-producing bacteria. (*See* Notes.)

Precautions. Use with caution in patients with ulcerative colitis. Discontinue if improvement is not observed within 48 hr. Use cautiously in patients with hepatic dysfunction.

Drug Interactions. Absorption of loperamide can be decreased by cholesterol-binding resins.

Parameters to Monitor. Frequency and volume of bowel movements; body temperature; blood in stool. Monitor for abdominal distention.

Notes. Adverse reactions might be less frequent and efficacy might be greater than with **diphenoxylate** with atropine. Loperamide can provide temporary symptomatic relief of infectious traveler's diarrhea if used cautiously with an antibiotic, but discontinue if fever occurs or other symptoms persist beyond 48 hr, or blood or mucus in stool develops.[108,109,111]

MAGNESIUM SALTS   Various

Pharmacology. Magnesium salts act as saline cathartics that inhibit fluid and electrolyte absorption by increasing osmotic forces in the gut lumen. Part of the action might be caused by cholecystokinin release, which stimulates small bowel motility and inhibits fluid and electrolyte absorption from the small intestine.[100,101,118]

Administration and Adult Dosage. **PO as a laxative/cathartic** (citrate) 240 mL; (sulfate) 20–30 mL of 50% solution (10–15 g) in a full glass of water; (hydroxide; milk of magnesia) 30–60 mL with liquid; (concentrate) 10–30 mL. (*See* Notes.)

Special Populations. *Pediatric Dosage.* **PO** (citrate) one-half the adult dosage; (sulfate) (2–5 yr) 2.5–5 g, (≥6 yr) 5–10 g in one-half glass or more of water; (hydroxide; milk of magnesia) 0.5 mL/kg.[100]

Geriatric Dosage. Same as adult dosage.

Other Conditions. Avoid use in patients with impaired renal function.[101,107,118]

Dosage Forms. **Soln** (citrate) 77 mEq/dL magnesium, 300 mL; (sulfate); **Susp** (hydroxide; milk of magnesia) 7–8.5%, many sizes, (*see* Notes) (also available as concentrates with 10 mL equivalent to 20 or 30 mL of susp); **Tab** (hydroxide; milk of magnesia) 311 mg; **Pwdr** (sulfate) 150, 240, 454 g.

Patient Instructions. Take milk of magnesia or magnesium sulfate with at least one full glass of liquid. You can take magnesium sulfate with fruit juice to partly mask its bitter taste. Refrigerating magnesium citrate improves its palatability.

Pharmacokinetics. *Onset and Duration.* Onset is dose dependent: (high end of dosage range) 0.5–3 hr; (low end of dosage range) 6–8 hr.[103]

Fate. Slow absorption of about 10% of a dose from the GI tract. Absorbed magnesium is rapidly excreted in the urine in normal renal function.[100,101]

Adverse Reactions. Abdominal cramping, excessive diuresis, nausea, vomiting, and diarrhea occur frequently. Excessive use can lead to electrolyte abnormalities; dehydration can occur if taken with insufficient fluids. Use in patients with renal impairment can lead to hypermagnesemia, CNS depression, and hypotension.[100,101,107,118]

Contraindications. Acute surgical abdomen; fecal impaction; intestinal obstruction; abdominal pain of unknown origin; nausea; vomiting.

Precautions. Rectal bleeding or failure to respond to therapy might indicate a serious condition and the need for medical attention. Avoid use in patients with impaired renal function.[100,101,107,118]

Drug Interactions. None known.

Parameters to Monitor. Periodically check serum magnesium levels in patients with impaired renal function who are receiving long-term daily administration.

Notes. Magnesium salts are useful for preparing the bowel for radiologic examination and surgical procedures. One regimen used magnesium citrate solution 300 mL 2 hr before PEG electrolyte lavage solution that was continued until the stool return was clear.[119] The following amounts of various magnesium salts are approximately equivalent to 80 mEq of magnesium: 100 mL citrate; 2.4 g (30 mL) milk of magnesia; and 10 g sulfate. The sulfate salt is the most potent but the least palatable cathartic. (*See also* Magnesium Salts in the Renal and Electrolyte sections.)

METOCLOPRAMIDE
Reglan, Various

Pharmacology. Metoclopramide stimulates the release of acetylcholine from the gastric myenteric plexus by antagonizing peripheral and central dopamine (D) receptors, specifically the D_2 subtype receptors. Metoclopramide also acts as a partial agonist at the $5\text{-}HT_4$ receptors, thereby facilitating the release of acetylcholine in the GI tract; however, it acts as an antagonist at the $5\text{-}HT_3$ receptor site.[120] It increases peristalsis of the gastric antrum, duodenum, and jejunum, relaxes the pyloric sphincter and duodenal bulb, and has little effect on the colon or gallbladder. In patients with GERD, metoclopramide produces a dose-dependent increase and duration of action in lower esophageal sphincter pressure. Its antiemetic action results from a direct antidopaminergic effect on the chemoreceptor trigger zone and vomiting center and from $5\text{-}HT_3$–receptor blocking effects. Metoclopramide increases prolactin secretion and serum prolactin. It also produces a transient increase in aldosterone secretion, thought to be related to direct stimulation of the adrenal gland via stimulation of the $5\text{-}HT_4$ receptor.[121]

Administration and Adult Dosage. PO for short-term treatment of symptomatic GERD in patients who fail to respond to conventional therapy up to 15 mg qid 30 min before each meal and hs for 4–12 weeks or intermittent single doses of up to 20 mg; **PO for symptomatic diabetic gastroparesis** 10 mg qid 30 min before each meal and hs for 2–8 weeks; **IM or IV for severe symptoms associated with gastroparesis** 10 mg qid for up to 10 days; **IV to facilitate small bowel intubation or to aid in radiologic examination** 10 mg over 1–2 min, 10-30 min before tube placement.[122,123] **PO to increase maternal milk supply** 10 mg tid for 10–14 days.[124] **PO, IM, or IV for the treatment of hiccups, PO** 10 mg q 6 hr for 10 days, or **IM, IV** 5–10 mg q 8 hr for 24–48 hr and then switch to PO.[125] **IV for prevention of chemotherapy-induced emesis** 2 mg/kg q 2–4 hr for 2–5 doses; **IV for delayed nausea and vomiting** 0.5 mg/kg or 30 mg IV q 4–6 hr for 3–5 days. **PO** 2 mg/kg q 2–4 hr for 2–5 doses; **PO for delayed nausea and vomiting** 0.5 mg/kg or 30 mg PO q 4–6 hr for 3–5 days.[72] **IM for prevention of postoperative nausea and vomiting** 10–20 mg near the end of surgery. **IV for treatment of postoperative nausea and vomiting** 10 mg q 4–6 hr prn postoperation.[72] Administer undiluted IV metoclopramide slowly (at least 1–2 min for a 10-mg dose); infuse diluted IV doses over at least 15 min (*See* Notes.)

Special Populations. *Pediatric Dosage.* IV to facilitate small bowel intubation or aid radiologic examination (<6 yr) 0.1 mg/kg; (6–14 yr) 2.5–5 mg; (>14 yr) same as adult dosage. **IV for postoperative nausea and vomiting** 0.1–0.2 mg/kg.[72]

Geriatric Dosage. Begin at one-half the initial dose (usually 5 mg) and increase or decrease based on efficacy and side effects.

Other Conditions. With Cl_{cr} <40 mL/min, begin at one-half the initial dose (usually 5 mg) and increase or decrease based on efficacy and side effects.

Dosage Forms. Tab 5, 10 mg; **Soln** 10 mg/mL; **Syrup** 1 mg/mL; **Inj** 5 mg/mL.

Patient Instructions. Take each dose 30 minutes before meals and at bedtime. This drug can cause drowsiness. Until the degree of drowsiness is known, use caution when driving, operating machinery, or performing other tasks requiring mental alertness. Avoid excessive concurrent use of alcohol or other drugs that cause drowsiness. Report any involuntary movements (eg, muscle spasms and jerky movements of the head and face) that occur, especially in children and the elderly.

Missed Doses. If you miss a dose, take it as soon as possible. If it is almost time for your next dose, skip the missed dose and return to your usual dosage schedule. Do not double doses.

Pharmacokinetics. *Onset and Duration.* (GI effects) PO onset 45 ± 15 min, IM 12.5 ± 2.5 min, IV 2 ± 1 min; duration 1–2 hr.

Fate. Bioavailabilities are PO 80 ± 15.5% and IM 85 ± 11%. Peak serum concentration after a PO dose occurs in 1–2 hr but can be delayed with impaired gastric emptying. The drug is about 30% bound to plasma proteins. V_d is 3.4 ± 1.3 L/kg, increased in uremia and in cirrhosis; Cl is 0.37 ± 0.08 L/hr/kg, decreased in uremia and in cirrhosis. About 85% of orally administered drug is recovered in the urine after 72 hr as unchanged drug; 20% of an IV dose is excreted unchanged in urine.[79]

$t_{1/2}$. α phase 5 min; β phase 5.5 ± 0.5 hr, increasing to about 14 hr in severe renal failure. Half-life also can be prolonged in cirrhosis.[79]

Adverse Reactions. Most side effects are related to dosage and duration of use. Drowsiness, restlessness, fatigue, and lassitude occur in 10% of patients with a dosage of 10 mg qid and in 70% with IV doses of 1–2 mg/kg. Acute dystonic reactions occur in 0.2% of patients receiving 30–40 mg/day, 2% in cancer chemotherapy-treated patients >35 yr receiving doses of 1–2 mg/kg, and 25% in cancer chemotherapy-treated children without prior diphenhydramine treatment. Parkinsonian symptoms, tardive dyskinesia, and akathisia occur less frequently. Rapid IV push produces transient, intense anxiety, and restlessness followed by drowsiness. Transient flushing of the face and/or diarrhea occur frequently after large IV doses. Hyperprolactinemia can occur, resulting in gynecomastia and impotence in males and galactorrhea and amenorrhea in females. Fluid retention can result from transient elevation of aldosterone secretion that occurs after parenteral, but not oral, administration.[121] Diarrhea, hypertension, and mental depression have been reported. Neuroleptic malignant syndrome is a rare, but potentially fatal, adverse effect reported to occur with metoclopramide.[126]

Contraindications. GI hemorrhage; mechanical obstruction or perforation; pheochromocytoma; epilepsy; concurrent use of drugs that cause extrapyramidal effects.

Precautions. Pregnancy; lactation. Use with caution in the elderly[127] and in patients with hypertension, renal failure, or Parkinson's disease, history of depression or attempted suicide, and after gut anastomosis. In patients with diabetic gastroparesis, insulin dosage or timing might require adjustment.

Drug Interactions. Absorption of drugs from the stomach or small bowel can be altered by metoclopramide (eg, digoxin and cimetidine absorption is decreased; cyclosporine absorption is increased). Anticholinergics and narcotics may antagonize GI effects of metoclopramide. Use with an MAOI can result in hypertension, and the combination should be avoided. Additive sedation can occur with alcohol or other CNS depressants.

Parameters to Monitor. Monitor periodically for CNS effects, extrapyramidal reactions, and changes in Cr_s, blood glucose, or blood pressure. (GERD or diabetic gastroparesis) observe for symptomatic relief.

Notes. Tolerance to the drug's gastrokinetic effect can develop with long-term therapy. Metoclopramide has been used in the treatment of neurogenic bladder, orthostatic hypotension, Tourette's syndrome, adynamic or chemotherapy-induced ileus, anorexia, and complications of scleroderma. If extrapyramidal symptoms occur, administer **diphenhydramine** 50 mg IM or **benztropine** 1–2 mg IM.

Cisapride (Propulsid—Janssen Pharmaceutica) was available for the symptomatic treatment of adults with nighttime heartburn due to GERD. Cisapride is no longer marketed in the United States, but will be available only through an Investigational Limited-Access Program because of serious cardiovascular effects (eg, prolonged QT interval, torsades de pointes) in patients taking interacting medications or with certain underlying health conditions. For patients to be considered for the Propulsid Investigational Limited-Access Program, they must have failed all standard therapies and have baseline laboratory tests and ECG, and undergone an appropriate diagnostic evaluation including radiologic examinations or endoscopy. Contact Janssen Pharmaceutica at 1-800-JANSSEN to determine whether a patient qualifies for the program.

Domperidone (Motilium—Janssen) is a prokinetic agent available outside the U.S. for the treatment of diabetic gastroparesis. It selectively blocks peripheral dopamine-D_2 receptors in the GI tract; it has antiemetic effects related to its action at the chemoreceptor trigger zone; and it stimulates pituitary prolactin release in humans but has no cholinergic activity. The drug does not cross the blood–brain barrier and thus does not produce CNS and extrapyramidal effects. Domperidone improves delayed gastric emptying and enhances antral and duodenal peristalsis but does not affect esophageal or colonic motility. PPIs, H_2- receptor antagonists, and antacids should not be coadministered with domperidone because the drug requires an acidic environment for activity. Dosages of 10–20 mg tid have been studied for dyspepsia and 20 mg qid is being studied for the treatment of diabetic gastroparesis. The most frequent side effects of domperidone are headache, dry mouth, anxiety, and elevation in serum prolactin concentrations.[128]

Erythromycin is a macrolide antibiotic that has prokinetic activity by acting as a motilin receptor agonist in the GI tract to stimulate GI contractility.[129] In gastroparesis, doses of 200–250 mg IV given over 15–30 min of the lactobionate salt, 250 mg PO tid of the ethylsuccinate salt, or 500 mg PO of the stearate salt 15–120 min before meals and at hs appears to be effective.[129,130] Erythromycin ethylsuccinate suspension formulation has a faster prokinetic action than erythromycin stearate tablets.[130]

PEG ELECTROLYTE LAVAGE SOLUTION GoLYTELY, Various

Pharmacology. Polyethylene glycol (PEG) electrolyte lavage solution is an isosmotic solution containing approximately 5.69 g/L sodium sulfate, 1.68 g/L sodium bicarbonate, 1.46 g/L sodium chloride, 745 mg/L potassium chloride, and 60 g/L PEG 3350; it is used for total bowel cleansing before GI examination. A solution lacking sodium sulfate, with a slight variation in other salts and PEG (NuLYTELY), and flavored solutions are available with improved palatability. PEG acts as an osmotic cathartic, and the electrolyte concentrations are such that there is little net fluid or electrolyte movement into or out of the bowel.[101,104,131]

Adult Dosage. **PO or NG** 200–300 mL orally q 10 min or by NG tube at a rate of 20–30 mL/min until about 4 L are consumed or the rectal effluent is clear. Use a 1-L trial before the full dosage in patients suspected of having bowel obstruction. Use the solution at least 4 hr before the examination, allowing the patient 3 hr for drinking and a 1-hr period to complete bowel evacuation. Another method is to give the solution the evening before the examination. Chilling the solution might improve its palatability but do not add other ingredients. Withhold solid food for 2 hr and medication for 1 hr before the solution is administered.

Pediatric Dosage. **PO or NG** 25–40 mL/kg/hr for 4–10 hr appear safe and useful for bowel evacuation.

Dosage Forms. Available as powder for reconstitution and oral solution.

Pharmacokinetics. The first bowel movement usually occurs after 1 hr, with total bowel cleansing 3–4 hr after starting.

Adverse Reactions. Frequent side effects are nausea, abdominal fullness, bloating (in up to 50% of patients), cramps, anal irritation, and vomiting. Urticaria, rhinorrhea, and dermatitis occur occasionally. Do not use PEG electrolyte lavage solution in patients with GI obstruction, gastric retention, toxic colitis, toxic megacolon, ileus, or bowel perforation; the solution seems to be safe for patients with liver, kidney, or heart disease.

Notes. This product is well suited for bowel cleansing before colonoscopy, but, because of some residual lavage fluid retained in the colon, other cleansng methods might be preferred before barium enema. Colonic cleaning with **bisacodyl** 15 mg orally followed by 2 L of PEG lavage solution 8 hr later has been found to be equally effective and more acceptable to patients than 4 L of solution used alone. Similar results were obtained using 300 mL of magnesium citrate solution 2 hr before PEG lavage solution that was continued until stool return was clear.[119] The drug might be useful as a GI evacuant in ingestions and overdoses with iron and some EC and SR drug products.[101,104,119,131,132]

PSYLLIUM HUSK

Konsyl, Metamucil, Various

Pharmacology. Psyllium is a bulk-forming cathartic that absorbs water and provides an emollient mass.

Administration and Adult Dosage. **PO for constipation** 2.5–12 g daily–tid, stirred in a full glass of fluid, followed by an additional glass of liquid. **PO for mild diarrhea** usual doses titrated to effect can be used to "firm up" effluent. **PO to lower cholesterol** 10–30 g/day in divided doses in combination with diet can decrease cholesterol in patients with mild to moderate hypercholesterolemia.[133,134]

Special Populations. *Pediatric Dosage.* **PO for constipation** (≤6 yr) safety and efficacy not established; (6–12 yr) 2.5–3 g (psyllium) daily–tid, with fluid as above.

Geriatric Dosage. Same as adult dosage.

Dosage Forms. **Pwdr** (sugar-free) Konsyl (containing 100% psyllium) 6 g packet, 200–660 g; Metamucil, Sugar-Free Orange Flavor (containing 65% psyllium); **Pwdr** (containing sugar) Metamucil Orange Flavor (50% or 65% sucrose), Konsyl-Orange (28% psyllium, 72% sucrose) 7, 11, 12 g packet, 210, 420, 538, 630, 960 g; **Wafer** Metamucil (containing 5 g fat) 3.4 g of psyllium per wafer.

Patient Instructions. Mix powder with a full glass of fluid before taking and follow with another glass of liquid.

Pharmacokinetics. *Onset and Duration.* Onset 12–24 hr, but 2–3 days might be required for full effect.[100]

Fate. Not absorbed from GI tract; eliminated unchanged in feces.

Adverse Reactions. Flatulence occurs frequently. Serious side effects are rare, but esophageal, gastric, intestinal, and rectal obstructions have been reported. Allergic reactions and bronchospasm have occurred after inhalation of dry powder.[100,101,135]

Contraindications. Acute surgical abdomen; fecal impaction; intestinal obstruction; abdominal pain of unknown origin; nausea; vomiting.

Precautions. Rectal bleeding or failure to respond to therapy might indicate a serious condition and the need for medical attention. Use with caution in patients who require fluid restriction because constipation can occur unless fluid intake is adequate. Psyllium can be hazardous in patients with intestinal ulcerations, stenosis, or disabling adhesions. Use effervescent Metamucil formulations (packet) with caution in patients who require potassium restriction (7.4 and 7.9 mEq potassium/packet). Use the noneffervescent formulations of Metamucil cautiously in diabetics because they contain 50% or 65% sucrose. Sugar-free preparations include Konsyl and Metamucil Sugar Free.

Drug Interactions. None known.

Notes. Psyllium is useful in lessening the strain of defecation and for inpatients who are on low-residue diets or constipating medications. It is safe to use during pregnancy.[100,101]

Miscellaneous Gastrointestinal Drugs

ACTIVATED CHARCOAL   Various

Pharmacology. Activated charcoal is a nonspecific GI adsorbent with a surface area of 900–2000 m^2/g that is used primarily in the management of acute poisonings.[136]

Administration and Adult Dosage. **PO or via gastric tube** 50–120 g dispersed in liquid as soon as possible after ingestion of poison (the Food and Drug Administration suggests 240 mL diluent/30 g activated charcoal). Repeat administration of activated charcoal after gastric lavage. (*See* Notes.)

Special Populations. *Pediatric Dosage.* **PO or via gastric tube** (≤12 yr) 25–50 g or 1–2 g/kg dispersed in liquid; (>12 yr) same as adult dosage.[137]

Geriatric Dosage. Same as adult dosage.

Dosage Forms. **Pwdr** plain or dispersed in water or sorbitol-water.

Patient Instructions. This drug causes stools to turn black.

Pharmacokinetics. *Onset and Duration.* Onset is immediate; duration is continual while it remains in the GI tract.

Fate. Not orally absorbed; eliminated unchanged in the feces.

Adverse Reactions. Black stools; gritty consistency can cause emesis in some patients.

Precautions. Insufficient hydration or use in patients with decreased bowel motility can result in intestinal bezoars.

Drug Interactions. Activated charcoal can decrease the oral absorption and efficacy of many drugs. (*See* Notes.)

Parameters to Monitor. Passage of activated charcoal in the stools. If sorbitol or other cathartics are administered, limit their dosages to prevent excessive fluid and electrolyte losses.

Notes. A suspension of activated charcoal in 25–35% **sorbitol** can increase palatability of the drug; total dosage of sorbitol should not exceed 1 g/kg. Substances *not* adsorbed by activated charcoal are mineral acids, alkalis, iron, cyanide, lithium and other small ions, and alcohols. Repeated oral doses of activated charcoal (eg, 15–30 g q 4–6 hr) have been used to enhance the elimination of some drugs, most notably **carbamazepine, phenobarbital, salicylates,** and **theophylline.**

ANTI-IRRITABLE BOWEL SYNDROME AGENTS

Alosetron (Lotronex) is a selective serotonin 5-HT$_3$ antagonist that was removed from the market after numerous reports of ischemic colitis and several deaths.[138–140] Several other drugs are being studied for use in treating irritable syndrome. **Tegaserod** (Zelnorm—Novartis) is a 5-HT$_4$-receptor partial agonist that appears to decrease abdominal pain and bloating and increase the frequency of bowel movements in patients with constipation-predominant irritable bowel syndrome. It also appears to be effective in alternating irritable bowel syndrome. The most effective dose is 6 mg bid, and the most common adverse effect is diarrhea with initial therapy, which eventually dissipates with continued treatment.[141] **Prucalopride** (Rezolor—Janssen) is being evaluated for patients with delayed small bowel and colonic motility. Patients with chronic constipation might benefit from this drug, which is a benzofurancarboxamide selective 5-HT$_4$-receptor agonist. In healthy subjects, prucalopride stimulates colonic activity; however, it has minimal effects on gastric and small bowel transit times.[142] Diarrhea, abdominal pain, headache, flatulence, and nausea are its most common side effects.[142,143] **Cilansetron** (Solvay) is a 5-HT$_3$-receptor antagonist similar to alosetron that is being evaluated for diarrhea-predominant irritable bowel syndrome. Cilansetron might have pharmacologic effects similar to those of alosetron.[144]

MESALAMINE PREPARATIONS

Pharmacology. Mesalamine (5-aminosalicylic acid [5-ASA]) is thought to be the active moiety of sulfasalazine. The mechanism of action of mesalamine in inflammatory bowel disease is unknown, but mesalamine seems to inhibit cyclooxygenase and 5-lipoxygenase, thereby downregulating the production of inflammatory prostaglandins in the colon. An immunomodulatory response also might occur because mesalamine inhibits and prevents the secretion of antibodies and lymphocytes during active disease. Mesalamine inhibits macrophage and neutrophil chemotaxis, reduces intestinal mononuclear cell production of immunoglobulin A and G antibodies, and is a scavenger of oxygen-derived free radicals, which are increased during active inflammatory bowel disease.[146–150] **Balsalazide** disodium is a prodrug that is cleaved by bacterial azoreductase in the colon to release mesalamine and the inactive carrier, 4-aminobenzoyl-β-alanine.[145] Balsalazide 750 mg is equivalent to 267 mg of mesalamine. Each molecule of **olsalazine** that reaches the colon is converted to 2 molecules of mesalamine.

Administration and Adult Dosage.

INDICATION	ASACOL	COLAZIDE	DIPENTUM	PENTASA	AXCAN, ROWASA
	Mesalamine	*Balsalazide*	*Olsalazine*	*Mesalamine*	*Mesalamine*
Short-term treatment of active mild to moderate ulcerative colitis.	PO 800 mg tid, or 1.6 g tid[a] for 6 weeks.	PO 2.25 g tid.	PO 500 mg tid,[a] 1 g bid,[a] or 1 g tid[a] for 3–6 weeks.	PO 1 g qid for 6–8 weeks.	PR 2 g hs,[a,b] or 4 g hs[b] for 3–6 weeks (enema).
Maintenance of ulcerative colitis remission.	PO 800 mg bid.	a	PO 500 mg bid.[c]	PO 1 g bid[a] or 1 g qid.[a]	PR 1–2 g hs[a,b] (enema).
Short-term treatment of active mild to moderate Crohn's disease.	PO 800 mg tid[a] or 1.6 g tid[a] for 8–16 weeks.	a	a	PO 1 g qid[a] for 8–16 weeks.	a
Maintenance of Crohn's disease remission.	PO 800 mg–1.6 g tid.[a]	a	a	PO 1 g bid[a] or 1 g qid.[a]	a
Treatment of active proctitis.	PO 800 mg tid.[a]	a	a	PO 1 g qid.[a]	PR 1–2 g hs,[a,b] 4 g hs[b] (enema); 500 mg bid or tid[d] (Axcan, Rowasa) suppository).

[a]Nonlabeled indication and dosage; optimal dosage regimen has not been determined.
[b]Retain enema for approximately 8 hr.
[c]Patients intolerant to sulfasalazine.
[d]Retain suppository for 1–3 hr or longer.
From references 146–149.

Special Populations. *Pediatric Dosage.* Safety and efficacy not established. Pediatric use has been reported. **PO mesalamine** (Asacol, Pentasa) 30–50 mg/kg/day in 3–4 divided doses (maximum dosages: Asacol 4.8 g/day, Pentasa 4 g/day); **PR mesalamine enema** 1–4 g q hs; **PR mesalamine suppository** 500 mg q hs or bid.[172,173]

Geriatric Dosage. No dosage reduction is necessary. Older patients are more likely to have renal impairment. (*See* Precautions.)

Other Conditions. Dosage reduction might be considered in severe renal and/or hepatic impairment.[146] (*See* Precautions.)

Dosage Forms.

DRUG	ASACOL	COLAZIDE	DIPENTUM	PENTASA	AXCAN, CANASA, ROWASA
	Mesalamine	*Balsalazide*	*Olsalazine*	*Mesalamine*	*Mesalamine*
Formulation.	Tablet enteric-coated pH dependent (pH 7), delayed release.	Capsule containing mesalamine prodrug cleaved by colonic bacterial azoreductases.	Capsule containing 5-ASA dimer; diazo bond is degraded by bacteria in colon.[a]	Capsule containing ethylcellulose-coated microgranules, controlled release.	Rectal suspension, suppository.
Site of action.	Distal ileum to colon.	Colon.	Colon.	Proximal jejunum to colon.	Rectum or splenic flexure (enema); rectum (suppository).
Dosage forms.	EC Tab 400 mg.	Cap 750 mg.	Cap 250 mg.	SR Cap 250 mg.	Enema 4 g/60 mL; (Rowasa) Supp 500 mg. (Axcan, Canasa, Rowasa)

5-ASA = 5-aminosalicylic acid.

[a]Each molecule of olsalazine that reaches the colon is converted to 2 molecules of mesalamine.

Patient Instructions. (Oral) take mesalamine with food and a full glass of water. Swallow tablets or capsules whole without breaking or chewing. The tablet core (Asacol) or small beads (Pentasa) might appear in the stool after mesalamine is released, but this does not mean there was a lack of effect. Report intact or partly intact tablets in the stool (Asacol) because this might indicate that the expected amount of mesalamine was not released from the tablet. Report nausea, vomiting, abrupt change in character or volume of stools, or skin rashes. (Rectal) empty bowel immediately before insertion of enema or suppository. Use enema at bedtime and retain for 8 hours, if possible. Retain suppository for at least 1 to 3 hours. Report signs of anal or rectal irritation. Rectal formulations can stain materials that come into direct contact with them.

Missed Doses. (Oral) if you miss a dose, take it as soon as possible. If it is almost time for your next dose, skip the missed dose and return to your usual dosage schedule. Do not double doses. (Rectal) if you miss a dose, use it as soon as possible if you remember it that same night. If you do not remember it until the next morning, skip the missed dose and return to your usual dosage schedule.

Pharmacokinetics. *Onset and Duration.* The onsets of action of Asacol, Dipentum, and Pentasa is delayed because of the release characteristics of their dosage forms; duration of action depends on intestinal transit time.[146] The onset of symptom relief is sooner with the balsalazide than with delayed-released mesalamine.

Fate. About $70 \pm 10\%$ of oral mesalamine is absorbed in the proximal small bowel when administered in an uncoated product or unbound to a carrier molecule; some absorption can occur in the distal small bowel, but mesalamine is poorly absorbed from the colon. Various oral dosage forms have been formulated to deliver mesalamine topically to the more distal sites of inflammation. (*See* Dosage Forms and Notes.) After oral administration, about 50% of mesalamine from Pentasa is released in the small bowel and 50% in the colon, although the amount released is patient specific.[150] About 20–30% of released mesalamine is absorbed after oral administration of Asacol or Pentasa; the remainder is excreted in the feces. About 98% of an oral olsalazine dose reaches the large bowel; less than 2% is absorbed. Mesalamine absorption from the enema is pH dependent; neutral solutions are better absorbed than acidic solutions.[146] Rowasa (at pH 4.5) is less than 15% rectally absorbed. Plasma protein binding: mesalamine (40%); N-acetylmesalamine (80%); olsalazine and olsalazine-O-sulfate (>99%).[146] Absorbed mesalamine is rapidly acetylated to N-acetyl-5-aminosalicylate (N-acetylmesalamine) in the intestinal mucosal wall and the liver. A small amount of olsalazine is metabolized to olsalazine-O-sulfate. N-acetylmesalamine is excreted in urine. Less than 1% of a dose of olsalazine is recovered unchanged in urine.

$t_{1/2}$. (Mesalamine) 1 ± 0.5 hr; (N-acetylmesalamine) 7.5 ± 1.5 hr; (olsalazine-O-sulfate) 7 days.[146]

Adverse Reactions. Adverse effects are usually less frequent than with oral sulfasalazine. Headache, flatulence, abdominal pain, diarrhea, dizziness, anorexia, and dyspepsia are the most frequent side effects reported with oral formulations and, to a lesser extent, rectal formulation.[146,149,151] An acute intolerance syndrome associated with mesalamine occurs in approximately 3% of patients. About 17%

of patients taking olsalazine 1 g/day experience secretory diarrhea. Dermatologic reactions include rash (1%), acne, pruritus, urticaria, alopecia, and photosensitivity. Renal insufficiency occurs in 0.2% of patients; renally impaired patients are at increased risk.[149] Rare adverse effects are oral, esophageal, and duodenal ulcerations; hepatotoxicity; jaundice; cholestasis; cirrhosis; liver failure; pancytopenia; leukopenia; agranulocytosis; and anemia.[149] Pericarditis, fatal myocarditis, hypersensitivity pneumonitis, pancreatitis, nephrotic syndrome, and interstitial nephritis occur rarely.[149,152] Allergic cross-reactions can occur in sulfasalazine-allergic patients.

Contraindications. Pyloric stenosis; intestinal obstruction; salicylate hypersensitivity.

Precautions. Mesalamine is considered safe in pregnancy; however, higher-than-normal doses have resulted in renal insufficiency in the fetus.[153,154] Monitor Cr_s periodically, especially in those with pre-existing renal impairments.[149,152] Use caution in impaired hepatic function. Patients who experience rash or fever with sulfasalazine might have the same reaction to mesalamine or olsalazine; oral desensitization is an option for those who are allergic to mesalamine.[155,156] Avoid Rowasa rectal suspension enemas in those with sulfite allergy.

Drug Interactions. In patients on warfarin, olsalazine can increase and mesalamine can decrease INR.[157] Omeprazole has no effect on mesalamine absorption.[149]

Parameters to Monitor. Improvement in abdominal cramping, diarrhea, and rectal bleeding. Monitor for adverse effects, including diarrhea (olsalazine), acute intolerance syndrome, and hypersensitivity reaction. Monitor BUN, Cr_s and urinalysis before and periodically during therapy. Monitor INR in patients taking concurrent warfarin.

Notes. The release characteristics of Pentasa are primarily time dependent, whereas those of Asacol are pH dependent; consequently, Asacol might not provide reliable site-specific release of 5-ASA if intestinal pH is inadequate. Balsalazide appears to more consistently distribute and liberate mesalamine in the colonic area, thus having greater effectiveness and less frequent side effects than sulfasalazine or olsalazine.[145,158] In 2–3% of patients taking Asacol intact or partly intact, tablets were found in the stools.

There appears to be no clinically important advantage of one oral mesalamine product over another, or over **sulfasalazine,** in treating or maintaining remission of mild to moderate ulcerative colitis.[146,149,159,160] A dose–response relationship exists when mesalamine is used to treat and maintain remission of mild to moderate ulcerative colitis.[149,161] A mesalamine preparation might be beneficial in the sulfasalazine-sensitive patient and men who wish to have children because mesalamine does not alter sperm count, morphology, or motility.[154] The enema is as effective as oral sulfasalazine or **hydrocortisone** enema in patients with active mild to moderate left-sided ulcerative colitis and proctitis and is associated with a more rapid response and fewer and milder adverse effects.[146,149,160] Patients refractory to oral sulfasalazine and oral or rectal hydrocortisone might respond to rectal mesalamine. Rectal mesalamine combined with oral sulfasalazine or **corticosteroids** can enhance induction and maintenance of remission in patients with mild to moderate ulcerative colitis, but the risk of adverse effects is increased.[162]

In Crohn's disease involving the ileum or proximal large bowel, oral formulations that deliver mesalamine to the small bowel and colon are preferable to sulfasalazine or olsalazine. Oral mesalamine preparations seem to be effective in treating active mild to moderate Crohn's disease[161] (including ileal or ilealcolonic) and maintaining remission.[149,160] Preventing recurrence after surgery with mesalamine prophylaxis in Crohn's disease is not effective.[163] Rectal mesalamine appears to be less effective in Crohn's disease, but efficacy depends on disease location and severity.[149,159,160]

OCTREOTIDE ACETATE   Sandostatin, Sandostatin LAR Depot

Pharmacology. Octreotide is a synthetic octapeptide with pharmacologic actions similar to those of somatostatin. The actions of somatostatin are regulated by somatostatin receptors (five known subtypes) located in regions of the brain, leptomeninges, anterior pituitary, endocrine and exocrine pancreas, GI mucosa, and cells of the immune system. Octreotide binds primarily to somatostatin-receptor subtype 2, to a lesser extent to subtype 5, and to an even lesser extent to subtype 3; it does not bind to subtypes 1 and 4. It suppresses the secretion of numerous substances including serotonin, gastrin, vasoactive intestinal peptide (VIP), cholecystokinin, insulin, glucagon, secretin, motilin, pancreatic polypeptide, and growth hormone (GH). It suppresses the luteinizing hormone response to gonadotropin-releasing hormone and the secretion of thyroid-stimulating hormone. It also decreases splanchnic and venous blood flow.[164,165]

Administration and Adult Dosage.   (*See also* Notes.)

INDICATION	OCTREOTIDE ACETATE IMMEDIATE	OCTREOTIDE ACETATE DEPOT
Metastatic carcinoid tumor	SC 100–600 μg/day in 2–4 doses × 2 weeks; dosages of 50–1500 μg/day (median 450 μg/day) have been used.	(Patients not currently receiving octreotide injection) initiate octreotide acetate injection for 2–4 weeks (see left for dosage). If tolerated and effective, then continue with depot formulation, as below.

(Patients currently receiving octreotide injection) IM intragluteally 20 mg initially q 4 weeks × 2 weeks. If symptoms do not resolve in 2 months, increase to 30 mg q 4 weeks. If symptoms resolve on 20 mg, then decrease to 10 mg q 4 weeks as a trial period. If symptoms worsen, then increase dose back to 20 mg IM q 4 weeks.[a] |
| VIP-secreting tumors (VIPomas) | SC 200–300 μg/day in 2–4 doses × 2 weeks. Dosages of 150–750 μg/day have been used (dosages >450 μg/day are usually not required). | Same as for metastatic carcinoid tumor. |
| Acromegaly | SC 50 μg tid, increasing q 2 weeks based on serum IGF-I level.[b,c] Most common dosage is 100 μg tid. Some require dosages up to 500 μg tid, but doses >300 μg/day usually do not have any added biochemical benefit. | (Patients not currently receiving octreotide injection) initiate octreotide acetate inj therapy for 2–4 weeks (see left for dosage). If tolerated and effective, continue with depot formulation (see below)

(Patients currently receiving octreotide injection) IM intragluteally 20 mg of depot formulation q 4 weeks × 3 months, then base dosage on serum GH level.[d,e] |

GH = growth hormone; IGF-I = insulin-like growth factor-I; VIP, vasoactive intestinal peptide.

[a]If the patient experiences exacerbation of symptoms, consider giving doses of octreotide acetate injection for a few days at the dose used before switching to the depot formulation.

[b]A more rapid titration can be obtained by drawing multiple GH levels during the 8 hr after the octreotide dose. The goal is to achieve GH <5 μg/L (or IGF-I <1.9 units/mL in men and <2.2 units/mL in women).

[c]Individuals who have received irradiation should discontinue octreotide for about 4 weeks each year. If symptoms worsen or laboratory results are abnormal, resume therapy.

[d]If GH ≤2.5 μg/L and symptoms are controlled, maintain dosage at 20 mg q 4 weeks; if GH >2.5 μg/L and symptoms not controlled, increase dosage to 30 mg q 4 weeks; if GH ≤1 μg/L and symptoms controlled, decrease dosage to 10 mg q 4 weeks; patients whose GH levels and symptoms are not controlled can increase dosage to 40 mg q 4 weeks; dosages >40 mg are not recommended.

[e]Individuals who have received pituitary irradiation should discontinue octreotide for about 8 weeks each year. If symptoms worsen or laboratory results are abnormal, resume therapy.

IV (immediate injection only) same dosage as SC, dilute in 50–200 mL of NS or D5W and infuse over 15–30 min or give by IV push over 3 min. In emergency situations (eg, carcinoid crisis), give by rapid IV bolus.

Special Populations. *Pediatric Dosage.* **SC (immediate)** (≥1 month) 1–10 μg/kg are well tolerated, and studies of various GI disorders have used widely different dosages in children 3 days–16 yr.[166] Octreotide has been studied in the treatment of hyperinsulinemic hypoglycemia in neonates in different dosages.[166,167] **SC for anti-VIP effects** 3.5 μg/kg/day divided q 8 hr.[168] **SC for chronic GI bleeding** 4–8 μg/kg/day.[169]

Geriatric Dosage. Dosage reduction is recommended because of decreased renal clearance, but specific guidelines are not established.

Other Conditions. The effect of hepatic disease on the disposition of octreotide is unknown. Reduction of maintenance dosages might be required in patients with renal impairment and those undergoing dialysis.[165]

Dosage Forms. **Inj (immediate)** 50, 100, 200, 500, 1000 μg/mL; **Inj (depot)** 2, 4, 6 mg/mL.

Patient Instructions. (Immediate-release) Instruct patient in sterile SC injection technique. Avoid multiple SC injections at the same site within a short period. Systematically rotate injection sites. Do not use solution if particulates and/or discoloration are present. Store medication in refrigerator but do not allow it to freeze; individual ampules can remain at room temperature for up to 24 hours. Octreotide is stable at room temperature for 14 days if protected from light. Pain at injection site can be minimized by using the smallest volume necessary to obtain the desired dose and by bringing the solution to room temperature before injection, but do not warm artificially. Stop medication and report if symptoms worsen or you have abnormal blood sugar levels or abnormal blood pressure. Inspect the vial for particulate matter or discoloration of the solution; do not use if either is present.

Missed Doses. (Immediate-release) If you miss a dose, take it as soon as possible. If it is almost time for your next dose, skip the missed dose and return to your usual dosage schedule. Do not double doses. Although you will not be harmed by forgetting a dose, the symptoms that you are trying to control might reappear. To control your symptoms, your doses should be evenly spaced over 24 hours.

Pharmacokinetics. *Onset and Duration.* (Immediate-release) SC peak concentrations occur in 0.4 hr (0.7 hr in acromegaly). Duration is up to 12 hr, depending on tumor type. (Depot) IM initial peak occurs at 1 hr and then slowly decreases over 3–5 days; a second peak appears 2–3 weeks postinjection. Duration is up to 2–3 weeks. Steady-state levels are usually attained after about 12 weeks.

Fate. Oral absorption is poor; SC and IV routes are bioequivalent. The drug is 65% protein bound (41% in acromegaly), primarily to lipoprotein and, to a lesser extent, albumin. V_d is 0.35 ± 0.22 L/kg; Cl is 0.16 ± 0.08 L/hr/kg. V_d and Cl are both increased in acromegaly; Cl is decreased in the elderly by 26% and in those with renal impairment. Octreotide exhibits nonlinear pharmacokinetics at dosages of 600 μg/day. About 32% is excreted unchanged in urine.

$t_{1/2}$. 1.5 ± 0.4 hr; increased by 46% in the elderly.

Adverse Reactions. Single doses of octreotide acetate can inhibit gallbladder contractility and decrease bile secretion. Approximately half of patients treated for at least 12 months experience cholesterol gallstones or sludge unrelated to age, sex, or dosage. About 22% of patients with acromegaly treated with the depot formulation developed new cholelithiasis, 7% of which were microstones. About 24% of patients with malignant carcinoid who received 18 months of depot therapy developed gallstones; 1% might require cholecystectomy. Five to 10 percent of nonacromegalic patients and 34–61% of acromegalics experience diarrhea, loose stools, nausea, and abdominal discomfort. The severity, but not frequency, is dose dependent and usually occurs with the initial dose, with the symptoms spontaneously resolving within 10–14 days.[164] Hypoglycemia (in 3%) and hyperglycemia (in 16%) are more common in acromegalics than in nonacromegalics. The frequencies of hypoglycemia (4%) and hyperglycemia (27%) are higher in carcinoid patients treated with the depot formulation. Octreotide suppresses secretion of TSH; alters the balance between insulin, glucagon, and GH; and might be responsible for cardiac conduction abnormalities, which are particularly frequent in acromegaly: bradycardia (25%), conduction abnormalities (10%), and arrhythmias (9%). Pain on injection occurs frequently with the immediate-release formulation and can be minimized by warming the solution before injection and using the smallest possible volume of solution to obtain the appropriate dose. Pain on injection is more frequent with the depot injection, from 2–11% in acromegalics to 20–50% in carcinoid patients. Flu-like symptoms, vomiting, flatulence, constipation, and headaches occur in 1–10%. Several cases of pancreatitis have been reported. Steatorrhea also can occur while on long-term therapy.[165] Abnormal Schilling's tests and decreased vitamin B_{12} levels have been reported.

Precautions. Pregnancy; lactation. Never give depot formulation by the IV or SC route. Use with caution in patients with diabetic gastroparesis because octreotide slows GI transit time;[170] insulin-dependent diabetics might require a reduction in insulin dosage.

Drug Interactions. In acromegaly, reducing the dosage of medications that cause bradycardia (eg, β-blockers) might be required. In all patients, the dosage of calcium-channel blocking drugs, diuretics, insulin, or oral hypoglycemics might require an adjustment with concurrent octreotide. Octreotide can decrease the absorption of some orally administered nutrients and drugs (eg, fat, cyclosporine).

Parameters to Monitor. Perform ultrasound of the gallbladder periodically during extended therapy. Obtain baseline and periodic total and/or free T_4 levels during long-term therapy. Monitor closely for hyper- or hypoglycemia, especially in diabetics. Periodically monitor vitamin B_{12} during long-term therapy. Evaluate cardiac function at baseline and periodically during therapy, especially in acromegalics. Monitor serum concentrations of drugs whose absorption might be affected by octreotide (eg, cyclosporine). To evaluate response, monitor GH or IGF-I concentrations in acromegalics; urinary 5-hydroxyindole acetic acid, plasma serotonin, plasma substance P in carcinoid patients; and plasma VIP in VIPoma patients.

Notes. The absorption of dietary fats can decrease while on octreotide therapy. Zinc levels should be monitored periodically in patients receiving parenteral nutrition and octreotide.

Store depot formulation at 2–8°C. Before administration, leave the drug at room temperature for 30–60 min. Octreotide must be administered immediately after mixing and should only be given IM intragluteally and not in the deltoid region to avoid injection site discomfort.

Store the immediate-release formulation at 2–8°C and protected from light. If stored at room temperature (20–30°C) and protected from light, the product is stable for 14 days. Before SC administration, the solution can be kept at room temperature to decrease injection site discomfort, but do not warm artificially. Octreotide 200 µg/mL is stable for up to 60 days in polypropylene syringes under refrigeration and protected from light.[171] Octreotide is not compatible with parenteral nutrition because of the formation of glycosyl octreotide conjugate.

SULFASALAZINE   Azulfidine, Various

Pharmacology. Sulfasalazine is a conjugate of sulfapyridine linked to mesalamine by an azo bond. This bond is cleaved by colonic bacteria to sulfapyridine and mesalamine, the active moiety. (*See* Mesalamine Preparations.)

Administration and Adult Dosage. **PO for short-term treatment of active mild to moderate ulcerative colitis or Crohn's disease** 4–6 g/day in equally divided doses; do not exceed an interval of 8 hr between nighttime and morning doses; administer with or after meals when feasible.[117,160] A lower initial dosage can decrease adverse GI effects. **PO for maintenance of remission of ulcerative colitis** 2–4 g/day in divided doses.[117,160] Dosages >4 g/day are associated with an increased frequency of adverse effects. Efficacy of sulfasalazine for Crohn's disease depends on the site of disease activity.[160] (*See* Notes.) **PO for desensitization of allergic patients** reinstitute sulfasalazine at a total daily dosage of 50–250 mg; thereafter, double the daily dosage q 4–7 days until the desired therapeutic effect is achieved. If symptoms of sensitivity recur, discontinue sulfasalazine. Do not attempt desensitization in patients who have histories of agranulocytosis or anaphylactic reactions during previous sulfasalazine therapy. Consider **mesalamine** instead of desensitization in sulfasalazine-sensitive patients.

Special Populations. *Pediatric Dosage.* (<2 yr) contraindicated; (≥2 yr) **PO for short-term treatment of active mild to moderate ulcerative colitis or Crohn's disease** 40–60 mg/kg/day in 3–6 equally divided doses. Dosages up to 75 mg/kg/day or up to 5 g/day in divided doses have been used.[172] Additional age-related information is available.[172,173] **PO for maintenance of remission of ulcerative colitis** 30 mg/kg/day in 4 equally divided doses.

Geriatric Dosage. No dosage reduction is necessary. However, older patients might have renal impairment.

Other Conditions. Consider dosage reduction in severe renal or hepatic impairment.[146]

Dosage Forms. **Tab** 500 mg; **EC Tab** 500 mg.

Patient Instructions. Take each dose after meals or with food and drink at least 1 full glass of water with each dose; drink several additional glasses of water daily. This medication must be taken continually to be effective. It is often necessary to continue medication even when symptoms such as diarrhea and abdominal cramping have been controlled. Report any nausea, vomiting, abrupt change in character or volume of stools, or skin rashes. Sulfasalazine can cause orange-yellow discoloration of the urine or skin. Reversible infertility can occur in males. Contact your physician or pharmacist if whole tablets appear in the stool.

Missed Doses. If you miss a dose, take it as soon as possible. If it is almost time for your next dose, skip the missed dose and return to your usual dosage schedule. Do not double doses.

Pharmacokinetics. *Onset and Duration.* Maximum effect is in 1–2 weeks; duration is 10 ± 2 hr after an oral dose.[117]

Fate. Sulfasalazine is 25–30% absorbed from the small intestine, but the absorbed drug is almost completely secreted unchanged in the bile. It is then metabolized in the large bowel by intestinal bacteria to **sulfapyridine** and mesalamine. Most of the sulfapyridine is absorbed from the bowel. Plasma protein binding: sulfasalazine (>99%); sulfapyridine (50%); mesalamine ($55 \pm 15\%$); N-acetylmesalamine (80%). Sulfapyridine is metabolized by acetylation to acetylsulfapyridine. Acetylsulfapyridine concentration depends on acetylator phenotype: slow acetylators have higher serum sulfapyridine concentrations, fast acetylators have lower serum sulfapyridine concentrations. After an oral dose of sulfasalazine, about 91% of sulfapyridine is recovered in the urine in 3 days as sulfapyridine, its metabolites, and small amounts of sulfasalazine. Mesalamine is eliminated primarily in the feces; only a small portion is absorbed, metabolized, and excreted in the urine as N-acetylmesalamine.[117]

$t_{1/2}$. (Sulfapyridine) 9 ± 4 hr, depending on acetylator phenotype.[117] (*See also* Mesalamine Preparations.)

Adverse Reactions. Anorexia, nausea, vomiting, dyspepsia, and headache occur in about one-third of patients and are related to serum sulfapyridine concentrations. These side effects usually resolve with dosage reduction.[174,175] Leukopenia occurs frequently. Mild allergic reactions such as rash, pruritus, and fever are common.[175] Decreased folate absorption leading to anemia can occur, so folic acid supplementation is recommended.[159,175] Rare toxic hypersensitivity reactions (caused by sulfapyridine) are neutropenia, agranulocytosis, hepatitis, pancreatitis, pericarditis, pneumonitis, peripheral neuropathy, and severe hemolytic anemia.[159,174,175] Sulfasalazine can cause orange-yellow discoloration of the urine or skin and precipitate acute attacks of porphyria. In men, sulfasalazine frequently leads to a reversible decrease in sperm count and abnormal sperm morphology and motility.[154,175]

Contraindications. Intestinal or urinary obstruction; porphyria; infants <2 yr; hypersensitivity to sulfasalazine, its metabolites, sulfonamides, or salicylates.

Precautions. Pregnancy, despite reports of safety; lactation. Use with caution in patients with renal or hepatic impairment, blood dyscrasias, slow acetylators, bronchial asthma, G-6-PD deficiency, or severe allergies.

Drug Interactions. Decreased digoxin bioavailability has been reported when sulfasalazine is concurrently administered.

Parameters to Monitor. Monitor therapeutic response (decrease in degree and frequency of diarrhea, rectal bleeding, abdominal cramping) and adverse effects (headache, anorexia, dyspepsia, nausea, hypersensitivity reactions). Obtain baseline and periodic serum electrolytes, liver function tests, CBC, reticulocyte counts, and urinalysis. Monitor serum folate periodically in patients on long-term therapy.[117] Monitor serum digoxin levels during initiation and after discontinuation of sulfasalazine.

Notes. There appears to be no important therapeutic advantage of sulfasalazine over oral **mesalamine** when used to treat or maintain remission of ulcerative colitis; however, the higher sulfasalazine dosages used to treat active disease are associated with an increased frequency of adverse effects.[149,160,175] Crohn's disease patients with involvement of the ileum do not respond as well to sulfasalazine as those with only large bowel disease.[149,174] Combining sulfasalazine with an oral or rectal **corticosteroid** or with rectal mesalamine might be beneficial in patients with ulcerative colitis who do not respond to single-drug therapy.[149,160,175] In ulcerative colitis patients receiving maintenance therapy, there was less absorption and greater acetylation of 5-ASA with sulfasalazine or olsalazine than with mesalamine (Asacol).[175] Sulfasalazine also has been used to treat ankylosing spondylitis and rheumatoid arthritis. Occasionally, the EC tablet can appear whole in the stool; if this occurs, consider switching the patient to the uncoated form of sulfasalazine or another mesalamine formulation. (*See also* Mesalamine Preparations.)

URSODIOL   Actigall, Urso, Various

Pharmacology. Ursodiol (ursodeoxycholic acid) is a hydrophilic bile acid used to dissolve small (<20 mm), noncalcified, radiolucent cholesterol gallstones in mildly symptomatic patients with functioning gallbladders who cannot undergo a cholecystectomy. It is also used to treat primary biliary cirrhosis. The exact mechanism of action of ursodiol is unclear, but it is thought to have a hepatocytoprotective effect by displacing accumulated toxic bile acids with hydrophilic bile acids, to promote secretion of toxic bile acid salts from the bile ducts and suppress the synthesis of chenodeoxycholic acid, and to act as an immunosuppressive agent by downregulating the antigen expression in hepatocytes in patients with primary biliary cirrhosis or primary sclerosing cirrhosis. Ursodiol improves liver function tests, liver histology, and certain immune markers; relieves pruritus in some patients; and can extend the period before death or to liver transplantation.[176,177] Ursodiol also appears to be effective in decreasing episodes of rejection and improving 1-yr survival rates after liver transplantation.[176] Patients undergoing bone marrow transplantation might benefit from ursodiol therapy through prevention of hepatic veno-occlusive disease.[178]

Administration and Adult Dosage. All doses should be administered with food. **PO for gallstone dissolution** 8–10 mg/kg/day in 2–3 divided doses. Complete gallstone dissolution usually requires 6–24 months of treatment, and treatment should be continued for at least 3 months after stones or sludge are not apparent on ultrasound. **PO for prevention of gallstones in patients with rapid weight loss** 300 mg bid. **PO for primary biliary cirrhosis** 13–15 mg/kg/day in 4 divided doses. **PO for prevention of hepatic veno-occlusive disease in bone marrow transplant** (<90 kg) 300 mg bid; (>90 kg) 300 mg tid (or 300 mg q AM and 600 mg q PM).[178] **PO as an adjunct to immunosuppressants after liver transplantation** 10–15 mg/kg/day in divided doses.[176,177]

Special Populations. *Pediatric Dosage.* Safety and efficacy not established; pediatric use has been reported. **PO for cystic fibrosis in patients with liver disease** 5–20 mg/kg/day in divided doses. Higher doses might be required in this patient population.[179] **PO for obese children with liver abnormalities** 10–12.5 mg/kg/day in 2 divided doses.[180]

Geriatric Dosage. No dosage reduction is necessary.

Dosage Forms. **Cap** 300 mg; **Tab** 250 mg. Ursodiol can be formulated into a suspension.[181,182]

Adverse Reactions. Ursodiol is relatively safe, with minimal side effects. The most common adverse effects are diarrhea, nausea, vomiting, dyspepsia, abdominal pain, and arthritis.

Drug Interactions. Bile acid sequestering agents (ie, cholestyramine, colestipol) and aluminum-containing antacids reduce ursodiol absorption; thus, the two drugs should be taken at least 2 hr apart. Oral contraceptives, estrogens, and lipid-lowering agents (eg, clofibrate) increase cholesterol secretion, thereby increasing the risk of developing cholesterol gallstones; using any of these agents can counteract the effectiveness of ursodiol.

REFERENCES

1. Pinson JB, Weart CW. Antacid products, H$_2$-receptor antagonists, antireflux and anti-flatulence products. In, Covington TR et al., eds. *Handbook of nonprescription drugs.* 11th ed. Washington, DC: American Pharmaceutical Association; 1996.
2. Del Valle J et al. Acid peptic disorders. In, Yamada T et al., eds. *Textbook of gastroenterology.* 3rd ed. Philadelphia: Lippincott Williams & Wilkins;1999:1370–444.
3. ASHP Therapeutic Guidelines on Stress Ulcer Prophylaxis. *Am J Health-Syst Pharm* 1999;15;56:347–79.
4. Maton PN, Burton ME. Antacids revisited: a review of their clinical pharmacology and recommended therapeutic use. *Drugs* 1999;57:855–70.
5. Lambert JR, Midolo P. The actions of bismuth in the treatment of *Helicobacter pylori* infection. *Aliment Pharmacol Ther* 1997;11(suppl 1):27–33.
6. Tillman LA et al. Review article: safety of bismuth in the treatment of gastrointestinal diseases. *Aliment Pharmacol Ther* 1996;10:459–67.
7. McColm AA et al. Ranitidine bismuth citrate: a novel anti-ulcer agent with different physiochemical characteristics and improved biological activity to a bismuth-citrate-ranitidine admixture. *Aliment Pharmacol Ther* 1996;10:241–50.
8. Earnest DL, Robinson M. Treatment advances in acid secretory disorders: the promise of rapid symptom relief with disease resolution. *Am J Gastroenterol* 1999;94(suppl 11):S17–24.
9. Sandvik AK et al. Review article: the pharmacological inhibition of gastric acid secretion-tolerance and rebound. *Aliment Pharmacol Ther* 1997;11:1013–8.
10. Mathot RA, Geus WP. Pharmacodynamic modeling of the acid inhibitory effect of ranitidine in patients in an intensive care unit during prolonged dosing: characterization of tolerance. *Clin Pharmacol Ther* 1999;66:140–51.
11. Feldman M, Burton ME. Histamine$_2$-receptor antagonists. Standard therapy for acid-peptic diseases (part I). *N Engl J Med* 1990;323:1672–80.

12. Feldman M, Burton ME. Histamine$_2$-receptor antagonists. Standard therapy for acid-peptic diseases (part II). *N Engl J Med* 1990;323:1749–55.

13. Lipsy RJ et al. Clinical review of histamine$_2$-receptor antagonists. *Arch Intern Med* 1990;150:745–51.

14. Amsden GW et al. Pharmacodynamics of bolus famotidine versus infused cimetidine, ranitidine, and famotidine. *J Clin Pharmacol* 1994;34:1191–8.

15. DeVault KR. Overview of medical therapy for gastroesophageal reflux disease. *Gastroenterol Clin North Am* 1999;28:831–45.

16. Orenstein SR . Management of supraesophageal complications of gastroesophageal reflux disease in infants and children. *Am J Med* 2000;108(suppl 4a):139S–43S.

17. Buck ML. Use of famotidine in infants and children. *Pediatr Pharmacother* 1998;4:1–6.

18. Mikawa K et al. Effects of oral nizatidine on preoperative gastric fluid pH and volume in children. *Br J Anaesth* 1994;73:600–4.

19. Simeone D et al. Treatment of childhood peptic esophagitis: a double-blind placebo-controlled trial of nizatidine. *J Pediatr Gastroenterol Nutr* 1997;25:51–5.

20. Wagner BKJ et al. Famotidine pharmacokinetics in patients undergoing cardiac surgery. *Drug Invest* 1994; 8:271–7.

21. Shamburek RD, Schubert ML. Control of gastric acid secretion. Histamine H$_2$-receptor antagonists and H+K(+)-ATPase inhibitors. *Gastroenterol Clin North Am* 1992;21:527–50.

22. Smallwood RA. Safety of acid suppressing drugs. *Dig Dis Sci* 1995;40(suppl):63S–80S.

23. Humphries TJ, Merritt GJ. Review article: drug interactions with agents used to treat acid-related diseases. *Aliment Pharmacol Ther* 1999;13(suppl 3):18–26.

24. Zimatkin SM, Anichtchik OV. Alcohol-histamine interactions. *Alcohol Alcohol* 1999;34:141–7.

25. Gugler R. H2-antagonists and alcohol. Do they interact? *Drug Saf* 1994;10:271–80.

26. Porro GB et al. Double-blind, double-dummy endoscopic comparison of the mucosal protective effects of misoprostol versus ranitidine on naproxen-induced mucosal injury to the stomach and duodenum in rheumatic patients. *Am J Gastroenterol* 1997;92:663–7.

27. Yeomans ND et al. A comparison of omeprazole with ranitidine for ulcers associated with nonsteroidal antiinflammatory drugs. Acid Suppression Trial: Ranitidine versus Omeprazole for NSAID-associated Ulcer Treatment (ASTRONAUT) Study Group. *N Engl J Med* 1998;338:719–26.

28. Taha AS et al. Famotidine for the prevention of gastric and duodenal ulcers caused by nonsteroidal anti-inflammatory drugs. *N Engl J Med* 1996;334:1435–9.

29. Hudson N et al. Famotidine for healing and maintenance in nonsteroidal anti-inflammatory drug–associated gastroduodenal ulceration. *Gastroenterology* 1997;112:1817–22.

30. Wallace JL. Nonsteroidal anti-inflammatory drugs and gastroenteropathy; the second hundred years. *Gastroenterology* 1997;112:1000–16.

31. Burnakis TG. The histamine receptor antagonist cimetidine in the treatment of herpes zoster. *Hosp Pharm* 1997;32:1162–7.

32. Raskin JB et al. Misoprostol dosage in the prevention of nonsteroidal anti-inflammatory drug-induced gastric and duodenal ulcers: a comparison of three regimens. *Ann Intern Med* 1995;123:344–50.

33. Schoenfeld P et al. Review article: nonsteroidal anti-inflammatory drug-associated gastrointestinal complications—guidelines for prevention and treatment. *Aliment Pharmacol Ther* 1999;13:1273–85.

34. Wing DA et al. A randomized comparison of oral and intravaginal misoprostol for labor induction. *Obstet Gynecol* 2000;95(6, pt 1):905–8.

35. Hofmeyr GJ, Gulmezoglu AM. Vaginal misoprostol for cervical ripening and labour induction in late pregnancy. *Cochrane Database Syst Rev* 2000(2):CD000941.

36. Bartha JL et al. Oral misoprostol and intracervical dinoprostone for cervical ripening and labor induction: a randomized comparison. *Obstet Gynecol* 2000;96:465–9.

37. Hawkey CJ et al. Omeprazole compared with misoprostol for ulcers associated with nonsteroidal anti-inflammatory drugs. *N Engl J Med* 1998;338:727–34.

38. Welage LS, Berardi RR. Evaluation of omeprazole, lansoprazole, pantoprazole, and rabeprazole in the treatment of acid-related diseases. *J Am Pharm Assoc* 2000;40:52–62.

39. Langtry HD, Wilde MI. Lansoprazole. *Drugs* 1997;54:473–500.

40. Fitton A, Wiseman L. Pantoprazole. A review of its pharmacological properties and therapeutic use in acid-related disorders. *Drugs* 1996;51:460–82.

41. Smith C. Pantoprazole. A new benzimidazole proton pump inhiitor for oral and IV administration. *Formulary* 2000;35:28–37.

42. Humphries TJ, Barth J. Review article: rabeprazole's profile in patients with gastrointestinal diseases. *Aliment Pharmacol Ther* 1999;13(suppl 5):25–32.

43. Langtry HD, Markham A. Rabeprazole. A review of its use in acid-related gastrointestinal disorders. *Drugs* 1999;58:725–42.

44. Klotz U. Pharmacokinetic considerations in the eradication of *Helicobacter pylori*. *Clin Pharmacokinet* 2000;38:243–70.

45. Katz PO. Treatment of gastroesophageal reflux disease: use of algorithms to aid in management. *Am J Gastroenterol* 1999;94(suppl 11):S3–10.

46. Huang J, Hunt RH. Treatment of acute gastric and duodenal ulcer. In, Wolfe MM et al., eds. *Therapy of digestive disorders*. 1st ed. Philadelphia: WB Saunders; 2000:113–26.

47. Stack WA et al. Safety and efficacy of rabeprazole in combination with four antibiotic regimens for the eradication of *Helicobacter pylori* in patients with chronic gastritis with or without peptic ulceration. *Am J Gastroenterol* 1998;93:1909–13.

48. Dajani AI et al. One-week triple regime therapy consisting of pantoprazole, amoxicillin and clarithromycin for cure of *Helicobacter pylori* associated upper gastrointestinal diseases. *Digestion* 1999;60:298–304.

49. Walters JK et al. The use of omeprazole in the pediatric population. *Ann Pharmacother* 1998;32:478–81.

50. Shashidhar H et al. A prospective trial of lansoprazole triple therapy for pediatric *Helicobacter pylori* infection. *J Pediatr Gastroenterol Nutr* 2000;30:276–82.

51. Klinkenberg-Knol EC et al. Long-term omeprazole treatment in resistant gastroesophageal reflux disease: efficacy, safety, and influence on gastric mucosa. *Gastroenterology* 2000;118:661–9.

52. Freston JW et al. Safety profile of lansoprazole: the US clinical trial experience. *Drug Saf* 1999;20:195–205.

53. Reilly JP. Safety profile of the proton-pump inhibitors. *Am J Health-Syst Pharm* 1999;56(suppl 4):S11–7.

54. Kahrilas PJ. Tolerability of rabeprazole. *Pharm Times* 2000;13–6.

55. Richter JE. Gastroesophageal reflux disease in the older patient: presentation, treatment, and complications. *Am J Gastroenterol* 2000;95:368–73.

56. La Corte R et al. Prophylaxis and treatment of NSAID-induced gastroduodenal disorders. *Drug Saf* 1999;20:527–43.

57. Sharma VK. Comparison of 24-hour intragastric pH using four liquid formulations of lansoprazole and omeprazole. *Am J Health-Syst Pharm* 1999;56(suppl 4):S18–21.

58. Lind T et al. Esomeprazole provides improved acid control vs omeprazole in patients with symptoms of GERD. *Gastroenterology* 2000;118(suppl 4)A:334. Abstract.

59. Kahrilas PJ et al. Comparison of esomeprazole, a novel PPI, vs omeprazole in GERD patients with erosive esophagitis (EE). *Gastroenterology* 2000;118(suppl 4)A:1224. Abstract.

60. Fennerty MB et al. Esomeprazole based triple therapy is more effective than dual therapy for eradication of *H pylori*. *Gastroenterology* 2000;118(suppl 4)A:266. Abstract.

61. McCarthy DM. Sucralfate. *N Engl J Med* 1991;325:1017–25.

62. Jensen SL, Funch Jensen P. Role of sucralfate in peptic disease. *Dig Dis* 1992;10:153–61.

63. Crill CM, Hak EB. Upper gastrointestinal tract bleeding in critically ill pediatric patients. *Pharmacotherapy* 1999;19:162–80.

64. Ben-Menachem T et al. Prophylaxis for stress-related gastric hemorrhage in the medical intensive care unit. A randomized, controlled, single-blind study. *Ann Intern Med* 1994;121:568–75.

65. Ephgrave KS et al. Effects of sucralfate vs antacids on gastric pathogens: results of a double-blind clinical trial. *Arch Surg* 1998;133:251–7.

66. Scheiman JM, Cutler AF. *Helicobacter pylori* and gastric cancer. *Am J Med* 1999;106:222–6.

67. Howden CW. Clinical expressions of *Helicobacter pylori* infection. *Am J Med* 1996;100(5A):27S–32S.

68. Blaser MJ. In a world of black and white, *Helicobacter pylori* is gray. *Ann Intern Med* 1999;130:695–7.

69. Talley NJ. How should *Helicobacter pylori* positive dyspeptic patients be managed? *Gut* 1999;45(suppl 1):I28–31.

70. Stanghellini V et al. How should *Helicobacter pylori* negative patients be managed? *Gut* 1999;45(suppl 1):I32–5.

71. Peitz U et al. A practical approach to patients with refractory *Helicobacter pylori* infection, or who are re-infected after standard therapy. *Drugs* 1999;57:905–20.

72. ASHP Commission on Therapeutics. ASHP therapeutic guidelines on the pharmacologic management of nausea and vomiting in adult and pediatric patients receiving chemotherapy or radiation therapy or undergoing surgery. *Am J Health-Syst Pharm* 1999;56:729–64.

73. Poster DS et al. Δ^9-tetrahydrocannabinol in clinical oncology. *JAMA* 1981;245:2047–51.

74. Cocchetto DM et al. A critical review of the safety and antiemetic efficacy of delta-9-tetrahydrocannabinol. *Drug Intell Clin Pharm* 1981;15:867–75.

75. Voth EA, Schwartz RH. Medicinal applications of delta-9-tetrahydrocannabinol and marijuana. *Ann Intern Med* 1997;126:791–8.

76. Lemberger L et al. Delta-9-tetrahydrocannabinol. Temporal correlation of the psychologic effects and blood levels after various routes of administration. *N Engl J Med* 1972;286:685–8.

77. Hollister LE et al. Do plasma concentrations of Δ^9-tetrahydrocannabinol reflect the degree of intoxication? *J Clin Pharmacol* 1981;21(suppl 8–9):171S–7S.

78. Huestis MA et al. Characterization of the absorption phase of marijuana smoking. *Clin Pharmacol Ther* 1992;52:31–41.

79. Benet LZ et al. Design and optimization of dosage regimens; pharmacokinetic data. In, Hardman JG et al., eds. *Goodman and Gilman's the pharmacological basis of therapeutics.* 9th ed. New York: McGraw-Hill; 1996:1707–92.

80. Wall ME et al. Metabolism, disposition, and kinetics of delta-9-tetrahydrocannabinol in men and women. *Clin Pharmacol Ther* 1983;34:352–63.

81. Agurell S et al. Pharmacokinetics and metabolism of Δ^1-tetrahydrocannabinol and other cannabinoids with emphasis in man. *Pharmacol Rev* 1986;38:21–43.

82. Devine ML et al. Adverse reactions to delta-9-tetrahydrocannabinol given as an antiemetic in a multicenter study. *Clin Pharm* 1987;6:319–22.

83. Anon. Synthetic marijuana for nausea and vomiting due to cancer chemotherapy. *Med Lett Drugs Ther* 1985; 27:97–8.

84. Gralla RJ et al. Antiemetic therapy: a review of recent studies and a report of a random assignment trial comparing metoclopramide with delta-9-tetrahydrocannabinol. *Cancer Treat Rep* 1984;68:163–72.

85. Doblin RE, Kleiman MAR. Marijuana as antiemetic medicine: a survey of oncologists' experiences and attitudes. *J Clin Oncol* 1991;9:1314–9.

86. Adams VR, Valley AW. Granisetron: the second serotonin-receptor antagonist. *Ann Pharmacother* 1995;29: 1240–51.

87. Freeman AJ et al. Selectivity of 5-HT$_3$ receptor antagonists and anti-emetic mechanisms of action. *Anticancer Drugs* 1992;3:79–85.

88. Holdsworth MT et al. Assessment of chemotherapy-induced emesis and evaluation of a reduced-dose intravenous ondansetron regimen in pediatric outpatients with leukemia. *Ann Pharmacother* 1995;29:16–21.

89. Billett AL, Sallan SE. Antiemetics in children receiving cancer chemotherapy. *Support Care Cancer* 1994; 2:279–85.

90. Foot ABM, Hayes C. Audit of guidelines for effective control of chemotherapy and radiotherapy induced emesis. *Arch Dis Child* 1994;71:475–80.

91. Rose JB et al. Preoperative oral ondansetron for pediatric tonsillectomy. *Anesth Analg* 1996;82:558–62.

92. Blackwell CP, Harding SM. The clinical pharmacology of ondansetron. *Eur J Cancer Clin Oncol* 1989; 25(suppl 1):S21–4.

93. Hesketh PJ et al. GR 38032F (GR-C507/75): a novel compound effective in the prevention of acute cisplatin-induced emesis. *J Clin Oncol* 1989;7:700–5.

94. Grunberg SM et al. Dose ranging phase I study of the serotonin antagonist GR38032F for prevention of cisplatin-induced nausea and vomiting. *J Clin Oncol* 1989;7:1137–41.

95. Kataja V, de Bruijn KM. Hypersensitivity reactions associated with 5-hydroxytryptamine$_3$-receptor antagonists: a class effect? *Lancet* 1996;347:584–5.

96. Chaffee BJ, Tankanow RM. Ondansetron—the first of a new class of antiemetic agents. *Clin Pharm* 1991; 10:430–46.

97. Grunberg SM et al. Randomized double-blind comparison of three dose levels of intravenous ondansetron in the prevention of cisplatin-induced emesis. *Cancer Chemother Pharmacol* 1993;32:268–72.

98. Vozeh S et al. Pharmacokinetic drug data. *Clin Pharmacokinet* 1988;15:254–82.

99. Zeltzer L et al. Paradoxical effects of prophylactic phenothiazine antiemetics in children receiving chemotherapy. *J Clin Oncol* 1984;2:930–6.

100. Covington TR et al., eds. *Handbook of nonprescription drugs.* 11th ed. Washington, DC: American Pharmaceutical Association; 1996.

101. Schiller LR. Clinical pharmacology and use of laxatives and lavage solutions. *J Clin Gastroenterol* 1999;28: 11–8.

102. Anon. Laxative drug products for over-the-counter human use; tentative final monograph. *Fed Regist* 1985;50:2124–58.

103. Brunton LL. Agents affecting gastrointestinal water flux and motility; emesis and antiemetics; bile acids and pancreatic enzymes. In, Hardman JG et al., eds. *Goodman and Gilman's the pharmacological basis of therapeutics.* 9th ed. New York: McGraw-Hill; 1996:917–36.

104. Adams WJ et al. Bisacodyl reduces the volume of polyethylene glycol solution required for bowel preparation. *Dis Colon Rectum* 1994;37:229–33.

105. Karim A et al. Pharmacokinetics and metabolism of diphenoxylate in man. *Clin Pharmacol Ther* 1972;13: 407–19.

106. Jackson LS, Stafford JE. The evaluation and application of a radioimmunoassay for the measurement of diphenoxylic acid, the major metabolite of diphenoxylate hydrochloride (Lomotil), in human plasma. *J Pharmacol Methods* 1987;18:189–97.

107. Gattuso JM, Kamm MA. Adverse effects of drugs used in the management of constipation and diarrhea. *Drug Saf* 1994;10:47–65.

108. Ansdell VE, Ericsson CD. Prevention and empiric treatment of traveler's diarrhea. *Med Clin North Am* 1999;83:945–73.

109. Ryan ET, Kain KC. Health advice and immunizations for travelers. *N Engl J Med* 2000;342:1716–25.

110. Castle SC et al. Constipation prevention: empiric use of stool softeners questioned. *Geriatrics* 1991;46:84–6.

111. Clausen MR, Mortensen PB. Lactulose, disaccharides and colonic flora: clinical consequences. *Drugs* 1997;53:930–42.

112. Crossley JR, Williams R. Progress in the treatment of chronic portasystemic encepahalopathy. *Gut* 1984;25: 85–98.

113. Kot TV, Pettit-Young NA. Lactulose in the management of constipation: a current review. *Ann Pharmacother* 1992;26:1277–82.

114. Lederle FA et al. Cost-effective treatment of constipation in the elderly: a randomized double-blind comparison of sorbitol and lactulose. *Am J Med* 1990;89:597–601.

115. Anon. Advice for travelers. *Med Lett Drugs Ther* 1999;41:39–41.

116. Killinger JM et al. Human pharmacokinetics and comparative bioavailability of loperamide hydrochloride. *J Clin Pharmacol* 1979;19:211–8.

117. Lauritsen K et al. Clinical pharmacokinetics of drugs used in gastrointestinal disease (part II). *Clin Pharmacokinet* 1990;19:94–125.

118. Swain R, Kaplan-Machlis B. Magnesium for the next millennium. *South Med J* 1999;92:1040–7.

119. Sharma VK et al. Randomized, controlled study of pretreatment with magnesium citrate on the quality of colonoscopy preparation with polyethylene glycol electrolyte lavage solution. *Gastrointest Endosc* 1997;46:541–3.

120. Hasler WL. Disorders of gastric emptying. In, Yamada T et al., eds. *Textbook of gastroenterology*. 3rd ed. Philadelphia: Lippincott Williams & Wilkins; 1999:1341–69.

121. Rizzi CA et al. Regulation of plasma aldosterone levels by metoclopramide: a reappraisal of its mechanism from dopaminergic antagonism to serotonergic agonism. *Neuropharmacology* 1997;36:763–8.

122. Heiselman DE et al. Enteral feeding tube placement success with intravenous metoclopramide administration in ICU patients. *Chest* 1995;107:1686–8.

123. Paz HL et al. Motility agents for the placement of weighted and unweighted feeding tubes in critically ill patients. *Intensive Care Med* 1996;22:301–4.

124. Anderson PO, Valdés V. Increasing breast milk supply. *Clin Pharm* 1993;12:479–80.

125. Friedman NL. Hiccups: a treatment review. *Pharmacotherapy* 1996;16:986–95.

126. Nonino F, Campomori A. Neuroleptic malignant syndrome associated with metoclopramide. *Ann Pharmacother* 1999;33:644–5.

127. Stewart RB et al. Metoclopramide: an analysis of inappropriate long-term use in the elderly. *Ann Pharmacother* 1992;26:977–9.

128. Barone JA. Domperidone: a peripherally acting dopamine2-receptor antagonist. *Ann Pharmacother* 1999;33:429–40.

129. Weber FH et al. Erythromycin: a motilin agonist and gastrointestinal prokinetic agent. *Am J Gastroenterol* 1993;88:485–90.

130. Ehrenpreis ED et al. Which form of erythromycin should be used to treat gastroparesis? A pharmacokinetic analysis. *Aliment Pharmacol Ther* 1998;12:373–6.

131. Goodale EP, Noble TA. Pediatric bowel evacuation with a polyethylene glycol and iso-osmolar electrolyte solution. *DICP* 1990;23:1008–9.

132. Shannon M. Ingestion of toxic substances by children. *N Engl J Med* 2000;342:186–91.

133. Chan EK, Schroeder DJ. Psyllium in hypercholesterolemia. *Ann Pharmacother* 1995;29:625–6.

134. Anderson JW et al. Long-term cholesterol-lowering effects of psyllium as an adjunct to diet therapy in the treatment of hypercholesterolemia. *Am J Clin Nutr* 2000;71:1433–8.

135. Freeman GL. Psyllium hypersensitivity. *Ann Allergy* 1994;73:490–2.

136. Cooney DO. *Activated charcoal in medical applications*. New York: Marcel Dekker; 1995.

137. Palatnick W, Tennenbein M. Activated charcoal in the treatment of drug overdose. *Drug Saf* 1992;7:3–7.

138. Balfour JA et al. Alosetron. *Drugs* 2000;59:511–8.

139. Gunput MD. Review article: clinical pharmacology of alosetron. *Aliment Pharmacol Ther* 1999;13(suppl 2):70–6.

140. GlaxoWellcome decides to withdraw lotronex from the market. FDA Talk Paper, November 28, 2000. www.fda.gov/bbs/topics/answers/ans01058.htm

141. Scott LJ, Perry CM. Tegaserod. *Drugs* 1999;58:491–6.

142. Bouras EP et al. Selective stimulation of colonic transit by the benzofuran 5HT4 agonist, prucalopride, in healthy humans. *Gut* 1999;44:682–6.

143. Poen AC et al. Effect of prucalopride, a new enterokinetic agent, on gastrointestinal transit and anorectal function in healthy volunteers. *Aliment Pharmacol Ther* 1999;13:1493–7.

144. Stacher G et al. Effects of the 5-HT3 antagonist cilansetron vs placebo on phasic sigmoid colonic motility in healthy man: a double-blind crossover trial. *Br J Clin Pharmacol* 2000;49:429–36.

145. Prakash A, Spencer CM. Balsalazide. *Drugs* 1998;56:83–9.

146. Small RE, Schraa CC. Chemistry, pharmacology, pharmacokinetics, and clinical applications of mesalamine for the treatment of inflammatory bowel disease. *Pharmacotherapy* 1994;14:385–98.

147. Goldenberg MM. Critical drug appraisal: mesalamine in the treatment of inflammatory bowel disease. *P & T* 1997;(October):498–510.

148. Bonapace CR, Mays DA. The effect of mesalamine and nicotine in the treatment of inflammatory bowel disease. *Ann Pharmacother* 1997;31:907–13.

149. Prakash A, Markham A. Oral delayed-release mesalazine: a review of its use in ulcerative colitis and Crohn's disease. *Drugs* 1999;57:383–408.

150. Elton E, Hanauer SB. Review article: the medical management of Crohn's disease. *Aliment Pharmacol Ther* 1996;10:1–22.

151. Sands BE. Therapy of inflammatory bowel disease. *Gastroenterology* 2000;118(2, suppl 1):S68–82.

152. Corrigan G, Stevens PE. Review article: interstitial nephritis associated with the use of mesalazine in inflammatory bowel disease. *Aliment Pharmacol Ther* 2000;14:1–6.

153. Connell W, Miller A. Treating inflammatory bowel disease during pregnancy: risks and safety of drug therapy. *Drug Saf* 1999;21:311–23.

154. Subhani JM, Hamiliton MI. Review article: The management of inflammatory bowel disease during pregnancy. *Aliment Pharmacol Ther* 1998;12:1039–53.

155. Stelzle RC, Squire EN. Oral desensitization to 5-aminosalicylic acid medications. *Ann Allergy Asthma Immunol* 1999;83:23–4.

156. Gonzalo MA et al. Desensitization after fever induced by mesalazine. *Allergy* 1999;54:1224–5.

157. Marinella MA. Mesalamine and warfarin therapy resulting in decreased warfarin effect. *Ann Pharmacother* 1998;32:841–2.

158. Green JR et al. Balsalazide is more effective and better tolerated than mesalamine in the treatment of acute ulcerative colitis. *Gastroenterology* 1998;114:15–22.

159. Hanauer SB, Meyers S. Management of Crohn's disease in adults. *Am J Gastroenterol* 1997;92:559–66.

160. Stein RB, Hanauer SB. Medical therapy for inflammatory bowel disease. *Gastroenterol Clin North Am* 1999;28:297–321.

161. Singleton JW et al. Mesalamine capsules for the treatment of active Crohn's disease: results of a 16-week trial. Pentasa Crohn's Disease Study Group. *Gastroenterology* 1993;104:1293–301.

162. d'Albasio G et al. Combined therapy with 5-aminosalicylic acid tablets and enemas for maintaining remission in ulcerative colitis: a double-blind study. *Am J Gastroenterol* 1997;97:1143–7.

163. Lochs H et al. Prophylaxis of postoperative relapse in Crohn's disease with mesalamine: European Cooperative Crohn's Disease Study VI. *Gastroenterology* 2000;118:264–73.

164. Lamberts SWJ et al. Octreotide. *N Engl J Med* 1996;334:246–54.

165. Beglinger C, Drewe J. Somatostatin and octreotide: physiological background and pharmacological application. *Digestion* 1999;60(suppl 2):2–8.

166. Tauber MT et al. Clinical use of the long acting somatostatin analogue octreotide in pediatrics. *Eur J Pediatr* 1994;153:304–10.

167. Barrons RW. Octreotide in hyperinsulinism. *Ann Pharmacother* 1997;31:239–41.

168. Colon AR. Drug therapy in pediatric gastrointestinal disease. In, Lewis JH, ed. *A pharmacologic approach to gastrointestinal disorders.* Baltimore: Williams & Wilkins; 1994:519–34.

169. Zellos A, Schwarz KB. Efficacy of octreotide in children with chronic gastrointestinal bleeding. *J Pediatr Gastroenterol Nutr* 2000;30:442–6.

170. Chen JD et al. Effects of octreotide and erythromycin on gastric myoelectrical and motor activities in patients with gastroparesis. *Dig Dis Sci* 1998;43:80–9

171. Ripley RG et al. Stability of octreotide acetate in polypropylene syringes at 5 and 20°C. *Am J Health-Syst Pharm* 1995;52:1910–1.

172. Baldassano RN, Piccoli DA. Inflammatory bowel disease in pediatric and adolescent patients. *Gastroenterol Clin North Am* 1999;28:445–58.

173. Wyllie R, Sarigol S. The treatment of inflammatory bowel disease in children. *Clin Pediatr* 1998;37:421–5.

174. Allgayer H. Sulfasalazine and 5-ASA compounds. *Gastroenterol Clin North Am* 1992;2:643–58.

175. Stretch GL et al. 5-amino salicylic acid absorption and metabolism in ulcerative colitis patients receiving maintenance sulphasalazine, olsalazine or mesalazine. *Aliment Pharmacol Ther* 1996;10:941–7.

176. Kowdley KV. Ursodeoxycholic acid therapy in hepatobiliary disease. *Am J Med* 2000;108:481–6.

177. Trauner M, Graziadei IW. Review article: mechanisms of action and therapeutic applications of ursodeoxy-cholic acid in chronic liver diseases. *Aliment Pharmacol Ther* 1999;13:979–96.

178. Essell JH et al. Ursodiol prophylaxis against hepatic complications of allogeneic bone marrow transplantation. *Ann Intern Med* 1998;128(12, pt 1):975–81.

179. Colombo C et al. Ursodeoxycholic acid therapy in cystic fibrosis-associated liver disease: a dose-response study. *Hepatology* 1992;16:924–30.

180. Vajro P et al. Lack of efficacy of ursodeoxycholic acid for the treatment of liver abnormalities in obese children. *J Pediatr* 2000;136:739–43.

181. Johnson CE, Nesbitt J. Stability of ursodiol in an extemporaneously compounded oral liquid. *Am J Health-Syst Pharm* 1995;52:1798–800.

182. Mallett MS et al. Stability of ursodiol 25 mg/ml in an extemporaneously prepared oral liquid. *Am J Health-Syst Pharm* 1997;54:1401–4.

Hematologic Drugs

Coagulants and Anticoagulants

ABCIXIMAB ReoPro

Pharmacology. Abciximab is a chimeric human-murine monoclonal antibody Fab fragment that binds to and irreversibly inhibits the platelet glycoprotein IIb/IIIa receptor. Blockade of the glycoprotein IIb/IIIa receptor prevents fibrinogen from binding, thereby inhibiting platelet aggregation. Abciximab also binds to the vitronectin receptor found on platelets, endothelial cells, monocytes, and smooth muscle cells; the clinical relevance of this is unknown. Abciximab inhibits platelet aggregation and prolongs bleeding time in a dose-dependent manner.[1,2]

Administration and Adult Dosage. **IV for percutaneous coronary intervention** 0.25 mg/kg as a bolus 10–60 min before starting percutaneous coronary intervention and then 0.125 µg/kg/min (up to 10 µg/min) by continuous infusion for 12 hr. **IV for unstable angina and planned percutaneous intervention within 24 hr** 0.25 mg/kg as a bolus and then 0.125 µg/kg/min (up to 10 µg/min) by continuous infusion for 18–24 hr, concluding 1 hr after the percutaneous coronary intervention. (*See* Parameters to Monitor and Notes.)

Special Populations. *Geriatric Dosage.* Same as adult dosage.

Dosage Forms. **Inj** 2 mg/mL.

Pharmacokinetics. *Onset and Duration.* Rapid inhibition of platelet function after IV administration. Platelet function gradually recovers after discontinuation of the IV infusion; bleeding time approaches baseline values within 24 hr and ex vivo platelet aggregation approaches baseline levels within 48 hr. Low levels of glycoprotein IIb/IIIa inhibition are detectable for up to 14 days after administration.[1]

Fate. Abciximab is rapidly cleared from the plasma after administration by rapid binding to the glycoprotein IIb/IIIa receptor.

$t_{1/2}$. α phase <10 min; β phase 30 min.[1]

Adverse Reactions. Bleeding, particularly from vascular access sites, occurs frequently. To minimize bleeding complications, care of the femoral artery access site is important and lower doses of unfractionated heparin are necessary during the percutaneous coronary intervention. (*See* Notes.) If serious bleeding complications occur, discontinue abciximab and transfuse platelets, if needed, to restore platelet function. Thrombocytopenia (<100,000/µL) has been reported in 2.6–5.6% of patients; severe thrombocytopenia (<50,000/µL) has occurred in 0.9–1.7% of patients. Thrombocytopenia can occur rapidly after administration and might require platelet transfusions if reversal is necessary.[1]

Contraindications. Active internal bleeding; recent (within 6 weeks) clinically significant GI or GU bleeding; history of CVA within 2 yr or CVA with significant residual neurologic deficit; bleeding diathesis; administration of oral anticoagulants within 7 days unless PT ≤1.2 times control; thrombocytopenia (<100,000/μL); recent (within 6 weeks) major surgery or trauma; intracranial neoplasm, AV malformation, or aneurysm; severe uncontrolled hypertension; presumed or documented history of vasculitis; use or planned use of IV dextran before or during percutaneous coronary intervention.

Precautions. Use with caution in patients being treated concomitantly with other antithrombotic drugs including thrombolytics, unfractionated heparin, low-molecular-weight heparin, oral anticoagulants; NSAIDs; and other drugs that increase bleeding risk.

Parameters to Monitor. Monitor CBC including platelet count; prothrombin time; aPTT; and activated clotting time at baseline. Maintaining the activated clotting time at 200–300 sec during percutaneous coronary intervention minimizes the risk of bleeding complications.[1,3] Monitor platelet count 2–4 hr after the IV bolus and again at 24 hr or before hospital discharge, whichever occurs first. If prolonged infusion of unfractionated heparin is necessary after percutaneous coronary intervention, maintain aPTT at 60–85 sec.

Notes. Abciximab must be filtered using a sterile, nonpyrogenic, low-protein-binding 0.2 or 0.22 μ filter either at admixture or during administration with an in-line filter. To minimize the risk of bleeding complications, the following care for the arterial access site is recommended: maintain patient on complete bed rest with the affected limb restrained in a straight position while vascular sheaths are in place; discontinue unfractionated heparin immediately after percutaneous coronary intervention; remove vascular sheaths within 6 hr of completing the procedure if aPTT ≤50 sec or activated clotting time ≤175 sec; after sheath removal, apply pressure to the femoral artery for at least 30 min with manual compression or a mechanical device; and maintain bed rest for 6–8 hr after sheath removal. To minimize bleeding complications, the following periprocedural heparin dosage is recommended: if baseline activated clotting time ≤150 sec, administer 70 units/kg heparin IV bolus; if 150–199 sec, administer 50 units/kg heparin IV bolus; if ≥200 sec, do not administer heparin. During percutaneous coronary intervention, administer 20 units/kg heparin IV boluses as necessary to maintain activated clotting time at 200–300 sec.[1,3]

ALTEPLASE   Activase

Pharmacology. Alteplase (recombinant tissue-type plasminogen activator [rt-PA]) is a 1-chain tissue plasminogen activator (fibrinolytic) produced by recombinant DNA technology. It has a high affinity for fibrin-bound plasminogen, allowing activation on the fibrin surface. Most plasmin formed remains bound to the fibrin clot, minimizing systemic effects.[4–6]

Administration and Adult Dosage. Accelerated IV infusion for clot lysis after MI (preferred) 15 mg as a bolus, followed by 0.75 mg/kg (up to 50 mg) over 30 min, and then 0.5 mg/kg (up to 35 mg) over the next 60 min. Start heparin infusion (titrated to an aPTT of 1.5–2.0 times control) with or at completion of the alteplase infusion and continue for at least 48 hr. (*See* Notes.) **Alternatively, IV infusion for clot lysis after MI** 60 mg over 1 hr (6–10 mg in the first 1–2 min) and then 20 mg/hr for 2 hr to a total of 100 mg (for patients <65 kg, administer a dose of 1.25 mg/kg over 3 hr). Begin as soon as possible after acute MI symptoms. Adjunctive heparin is also recommended.[5,7,8] **IV infusion for pulmonary embolism** 100 mg over 2 hr. Institute heparin infusion immediately after alteplase infusion when the aPTT or thrombin time returns to 2 times normal. Alternatively, 0.6 mg/kg as a single dose over 2 min in addition to heparin infusion has been used successfully.[9] **IV infusion for acute ischemic stroke** 0.9 mg/kg, to a maximum of 90 mg; give 10% initially as a bolus, with the remainder given over the next 60 min. Avoid anticoagulants or antiplatelet drugs for 24 hr after treatment.[10,11] **IV for catheter clearance** slowly inject 0.5 mg (1 mL) into the occluded catheter port. If catheter volume exceeds 1 mL, slowly inject a sufficient volume of NS to fill the catheter. Allow the solution to dwell for 60 min and then aspirate and flush the catheter with NS. If unsuccessful, repeat with escalating doses of alteplase (eg, 1 mg, 2 mg) to a maximum of 2 mg.[12]

Special Populations. *Pediatric Dosage.* Safety and efficacy not established.

Geriatric Dosage. Same as adult dosage.

Dosage Forms. **Inj** 50, 100 mg.

Pharmacokinetics. *Onset and Duration.* Duration is several hours because of binding with fibrin. However, rethrombosis after reperfusion appears to be inversely proportional to serum half-life.[5]

Fate. There is rapid uptake by hepatocytes and fibrin binding. V_c is 3.8–6.6 L and $V_{d\beta}$ is 0.1 ± 0.01 L/kg; Cl is 0.6 ± 0.24 L/hr/kg.[5,13]

t½. α phase 4.8 ± 2.4 min; β phase 26 ± 10 min.[13]

Adverse Reactions. Bleeding from GI and GU tracts and ecchymoses occur frequently. Retroperitoneal or gingival bleeding or epistaxis occur occasionally. Superficial bleeding from trauma sites also can occur. The overall risk of intracranial hemorrhage is 0.1–0.75%.[10] In ISIS-3, the rates for definite or possible cerebral bleed were: rt-PA (**duteplase,** a 2-chain form of alteplase), 0.5%; **streptokinase,** 0.2%; **anistreplase,** 0.7%.[14] Independent risk factors for thrombolytic-induced intracranial hemorrhage with alteplase are age >65 yr, body weight <70 kg, and hypertension on hospitalization.[7]

Contraindications. Active internal bleeding; history of CVA; recent (within 2 months) intracranial or intraspinal surgery or trauma; intracranial neoplasm, AV malformation, or aneurysm; bleeding diathesis; severe uncontrolled hypertension.

Precautions. Use with caution in the following: pregnancy; recent (within 10 days) major surgery, trauma, GI or GU bleeding; cerebrovascular disease; systolic blood pressure ≥180 mm Hg, diastolic blood pressure ≥110 mm Hg; high likelihood of left heart thrombus; acute pericarditis; subacute bacterial endocarditis; hemostatic defects; significant liver dysfunction; septic thrombophlebitis; age >75 yr; concurrent oral anticoagulants. Avoid IM injections and noncompressible arterial punctures; minimize arterial and venous punctures and excessive patient handling. Stop immediately if severe bleeding or anaphylactoid reaction occurs.

Drug Interactions. Preliminary data from a nonrandomized study suggest that concurrent IV nitroglycerin therapy impairs the thrombolytic effect of alteplase in acute MI.[15] Anticoagulants or antiplatelet drugs can increase the risk of bleeding.

Parameters to Monitor. For short-term thrombolytic therapy of MI, laboratory monitoring is of little value. No correlation has been made between clotting test results and likelihood of hemorrhage or efficacy.[5]

Notes. Other than cerebral hemorrhage, no clear differences in bleeding risk have been observed with the various thrombolytics.[5,7] Data from the ISIS-3 trial show the 5-week mortalities for **duteplase, streptokinase,** and **anistreplase** to be virtually identical.[14] Based on the GUSTO trial, some investigators have suggested that the accelerated alteplase regimen be used for patients <75 yr with anterior or large infarctions presenting within 4 hr of symptoms. The absolute survival advantage over streptokinase was 0.9%, representing a 14% risk reduction.[8,16] Double-bolus alteplase (50 mg IV over 1–3 min followed by 40–50 mg IV 30 min later) was compared with accelerated infusion alteplase to shorten and simplify administration. The double-bolus method was associated with a slightly higher rate of intracranial hemorrhage and is not recommended.[17] In a study on catheter clearance, 96.5% of catheters were cleared successfully, 86.2% with a dose of 0.5 mg, 8.6% with 1 mg, and 1.7% with 2 mg.[12]

ANISTREPLASE   Eminase

Pharmacology. Anistreplase (anisoylated plasminogen-streptokinase activator complex) is an acylated form of the streptokinase–plasminogen complex that is temporarily inactive. After deacylation, the streptokinase–plasminogen complex promotes thrombolysis by converting plasminogen to the proteolytic enzyme plasmin. Thrombolysis occurs through the action of plasmin on fibrin.[7,10,13,18,19]

Adult Dosage. IV for post-MI clot lysis 30 units over 2–5 min as a single injection. Adjunctive IV heparin is associated with higher bleeding rates than aspirin alone in anistreplase-treated patients and offers no additional improvement in outcome.

Dosage Forms. Inj 30 units.

Pharmacokinetics. Deacylation and thrombolysis begin immediately after injection. Duration of fibrinolytic activity is 4–6 hr. Anistreplase undergoes deacylation and local inactivation in the circulation by inhibitor complex formation and proteolysis and, to a lesser extent, is metabolized rapidly by the liver. V_d is 0.084 ± 0.027 L/kg, with a Cl of 0.055 ± 0.02 L/hr/kg and half-life of 1.2 ± 0.4 hr.

Adverse Reactions. Data from ISIS-3 indicated that bleeding was slightly more common with anistreplase than with streptokinase or rt-PA; however, major bleeding rates were similar. In ISIS-3 the rates for definite or possible cerebral bleeding were: **anistreplase,** 0.7%; **streptokinase,** 0.2%; rt-PA (**duteplase,** a 2-chain form of alteplase), 0.5%.[14] Allergic reactions similar to those reported with streptokinase are rash, erythema, bronchoconstriction, and, rarely, anaphylaxis. Precautions and monitoring parameters are the same as those for streptokinase.

Notes. Ease of administration (30 units given over 2–5 min as a single IV injection) is a potential advantage of anistreplase for the emergent treatment of acute MI in some settings (eg, in the field). However, anistreplase is more expensive than streptokinase, has the same allergy profile, offers no efficacy advantage, and might be associated with a slightly higher bleeding risk.

ARGATROBAN
Acova

Pharmacology. Argatroban is a modified amino acid that is a reversible, competitive, direct thrombin inhibitor used as an anticoagulant in patients with heparin-induced thrombocytopenia.[20]

Administration and Adult Dosage. **IV as an anticoagulant** 2–10 µg/kg/min, titrating aPTT to 1.5–3 times control. Dosage might need to be reduced in renal or hepatic impairment.

Dosage Forms. **Inj** 100 mg/mL.

Pharmacokinetics. *Onset and Duration.* Onset <10 min after a bolus or 1–3 hr after start of infusion without a bolus; the effect dissipates with a half-life of 18–41 min after cessation.[21]

Fate. The drug is metabolized in the liver to three metabolites that are excreted renally.

Adverse Reactions. Bleeding is the most frequent complication but is usually minor. No specific reversal agent exists. Dose-related prolongation of PT occurs.[20] Other common side effects include dyspnea, hypotension, and fever. Repeat exposure does not appear to predispose to immunologic reactions or excessive anticoagulation.

Parameters to Monitor. Monitor aPTT 2 hr after initiation of therapy or dosage adjustment and then once daily after stable anticoagulation has been achieved.

Notes. To initiate **warfarin** therapy, add the desired PT elevation to the argatroban-induced PT elevation (not to exceed 30 sec) and begin warfarin. Once this PT is achieved, stop argatroban. Argatroban has been used as an anticoagulant during extracorporeal circulation[22] and percutaneous coronary intervention.

CLOPIDOGREL BISULFATE
Plavix

Pharmacology. Clopidogrel is an antiplatelet agent that prevents platelet aggregation by direct inhibition of ADP binding to receptor sites, inhibiting subsequent activation of the glycoprotein IIb/IIIa complex. This action is irreversible; therefore, platelets exposed to clopidogrel are inhibited for their life spans.

Adult Dosage. **PO for reduction of stroke, MI, or vascular death** 75 mg once daily. A loading dose of 300 mg on the first day is often used to hasten the onset of action.

Dosage Forms. **Tab** 75 mg.

Pharmacokinetics. Clopidogrel is rapidly absorbed; bioavailability is about 50%; 98% is bound to plasma proteins. The parent compound has no platelet-inhibiting activity and undergoes extensive hepatic metabolism to a carboxylic acid derivative (main metabolite) and an unidentified active metabolite. The half-life of the carboxylic acid metabolite is about 8 hr.

Adverse Reactions. The most frequent side effects are diarrhea in 4.5%, rash in 4.2%, GI hemorrhage in 2%, and GI ulcers in 0.7% of patients. Serious, but less frequent, side effects are intracranial hemorrhage in 0.4% and severe neutropenia in 0.04%. Clopidogrel has been associated with the development of thrombotic thrombocytopenia purpura.[23] The drug is contraindicated in active bleeding as in patients with peptic ulcer or intracranial hemorrhage. Use with caution in patients at increased risk of bleeding from trauma, surgery, or other conditions. Clopidogrel should be discontinued 7 days before elective surgery if an antiplatelet effect is not desired.

Drug Interactions. Use with caution in patients receiving anticoagulants or drugs that inhibit platelet function including NSAIDs.

Notes. The overall risk reduction for clopidogrel was 8.7% greater than that for **aspirin** in the CAPRIE study in patients at risk for ischemic events.[24]

DALTEPARIN	Fragmin

Pharmacology. Dalteparin is a low-molecular-weight heparin (average mass 3000–8000 daltons) prepared by depolymerization and chromatographic purification of unfractionated porcine intestinal mucosa heparin. Other pharmacologic properties are similar to those of enoxaparin.[25] (*See* Low-Molecular-Weight Heparins Comparison Chart.)

Adult Dosage. SC for prevention of ischemic complications in unstable angina and non–Q-wave MI 120 IU/kg (to a maximum of 10,000 IU) q 12 hr with concurrent oral aspirin 81–160 mg once daily. Continue treatment until patient is clinically stable, usually 5–8 days. **SC for prevention of DVT and PE after abdominal surgery** 2500 IU 1–2 hr before surgery and once daily for 5–10 days. **SC for prevention of DVT and PE after abdominal surgery in high-risk patients (eg, with malignancy)** 5000 IU the evening before surgery and then once daily postoperatively, or 2500 IU 1–2 hr before surgery, 2500 IU 4–8 hr postoperatively, and then 5000 IU once daily for 5–10 days. **SC for prevention of DVT and PE after hip replacement surgery** 2500 IU 2 hr before and 12 hr after surgery, and then 5000 IU once daily for 6–13 days; or 5000 IU 10–14 hr before surgery, 5000 IU 4–8 hr postoperatively, and then 5000 IU once daily thereafter. For postoperative initiation, give 2500 IU 4–8 hr postoperatively and then 5000 IU once daily.

Dosage Forms. **Inj** 2500 IU/0.2 mL, 5000 IU/0.2 mL; 95,000 IU.

Pharmacokinetics. Bioavailability after SC injection is about 87 ± 6%. After SC doses V_d is 0.04–0.06 L/kg; after a single IV dose Cl is 0.025 ± 0.0054 L/hr/kg and the terminal half-life is 2.1 ± 0.3 hr; after SC administration the apparent half-life is 3–5 hr. Dalteparin is eliminated primarily by the kidney.

Adverse Reactions. Overall, rates of major and minor bleeding complications are similar to those with unfractionated **heparin.** Hematoma or pain at the injection site occurs frequently. Thrombocytopenia occurs in fewer than 1% of patients; however, dalteparin should be used with extreme caution in patients with histories of heparin-induced thrombocytopenia (in vitro platelet testing is recommended before use). Rash, fever, skin necrosis, and anaphylactoid reactions occur rarely.

Contraindications. (*See* Enoxaparin Sodium.) Patients undergoing regional anesthesia should not receive dalteparin for unstable angina or non–Q-wave MI.

Precautions. (*See* Enoxaparin.)

ENOXAPARIN SODIUM   Lovenox

Pharmacology. Enoxaparin is a low-molecular-weight heparin (average mass 3500–5500 daltons) prepared by depolymerization of unfractionated porcine intestinal mucosa heparin. Like unfractionated **heparin,** enoxaparin binds with antithrombin III, accelerating the rate at which antithrombin III neutralizes several activated clotting factors. However, enoxaparin has many biologic properties that differ from those of unfractionated heparin. Enoxaparin has a higher ratio of antifactor Xa to antifactor IIa activity, reduced interactions with platelets, and less lipoprotein lipase–releasing activity. It also has a lower affinity for platelet factor 4, von Willebrand factor (VIIIR), and vascular endothelium. At recommended dosages, single injections do not markedly affect platelet aggregation, prothrombin time, or aPTT.[26–29] (*See* Low-Molecular-Weight Heparins Comparison Chart.)

Administration and Adult Dosage. **SC for prevention of DVT and PE after hip or knee replacement surgery** 30 mg bid for 7–10 days started 12–24 hr postoperatively. **SC for prevention of DVT and PE after abdominal surgery** 40 mg once daily for 7–10 days started 2 hr before surgery. **SC for active DVT treatment with and without PE** 1 mg/kg q 12 hr initiated with warfarin therapy; continue for at least 5 days and until a warfarin target INR of 2.0 is achieved on 2 consecutive days. **SC for unstable angina or non–Q-wave MI** 1 mg/kg q 12 hr with concurrent aspirin 100–325 mg once daily. Continue treatment for at least 2 days or until patient is clinically stable, usually 2–8 days.

Special Populations. *Pediatric Dosage.* **SC for treatment** (neonates) 1.6 mg/kg bid; (older infants and children) 1 mg/kg bid dosages have been used.

Geriatric Dosage. Elderly patients might have reduced elimination; use with caution in these patients.

Other Conditions. Elimination can be delayed in renal insufficiency; use with caution in these patients.

Dosage Forms. **Inj** 30 mg/0.3 mL; 40 mg/0.4 mL; 60 mg/0.6 mL; 80 mg/0.8 mL; 100 mg/1 mL.

Pharmacokinetics. *Onset and Duration.* Peak antifactor Xa occurs 3–5 hr after SC injection and persists for about 12 hr after a 40 mg SC injection.

Fate. Mean absolute bioavailability after SC injection is about 92%. V_d is about 6 L and Cl is about 1.5 L/hr after IV administration. Some hepatic desulfation and depolymerization occur, but most of the drug is eliminated renally.

$t_{1/2}$. The apparent half-life after SC administration is 4.5 hr.

Adverse Reactions. Overall, rates of major and minor bleeding complications in comparative studies with unfractionated heparin are similar. In clinical trials of enoxaparin in hip replacement surgery, major bleeding occurred in 4% of patients compared with 6% of patients treated with unfractionated heparin. Thrombocytopenia, fever, pain on injection, asymptomatic increases in transaminase levels, hypochromic anemia, and edema occur frequently. Skin necrosis occurs occasionally.

Contraindications. Hypersensitivity to heparin or pork-derived products; active major bleeding; thrombocytopenia associated with positive in vitro testing for antiplatelet antibody in the presence of a low-molecular-weight heparin.

Precautions. If epidural or spinal anesthesia or spinal puncture is used, patients receiving low-molecular-weight heparins for prevention of thromboembolic complications are at risk for developing epidural or spinal hematoma, which can result in permanent paralysis. The risk of these events can increase when postoperative indwelling epidural catheters are used. Use with caution in patients with renal impairment.

Drug Interactions. Use with caution in patients receiving oral anticoagulants or drugs that inhibit platelet function, including NSAIDs.

Parameters to Monitor. Monitor CBC, including platelet count, and stool for occult blood periodically; aPTT monitoring is not required.

LOW-MOLECULAR-WEIGHT HEPARINS COMPARISON CHART

DRUG	DOSAGE FORMS	ADULT DOSAGE	AVERAGE MASS (DALTONS)	AF-XA[a] (IU/MG)	AF-XA/AF-IIA[b] RATIO	HALF-LIFE (HR)
Dalteparin Fragmin	Inj 2500, 5000, IU/0.2 mL, 10,000 IU/mL.	SC for DVT prophylaxis 2500–5000 IU/day SC for DVT treatment, unstable angina or non-Q-wave MI 120 IU/kg bid.	3000–8000	160	4:1	2.8–4
Danaparoid[c] Orgaran	Inj 750 units/ 0.6 mL.	SC for DVT prophylaxis 750 units bid SC for DVT treatment 2000 units q 12 hr.	6500	—	3.35:1	18.3
Enoxaparin Lovenox	Inj 30 mg/0.3 mL, 40 mg/0.4 mL, 60 mg/0.6 mL, 80 mg/0.8 mL, 100 mg/1 mL.	SC for DVT prophylaxis 30 mg bid; SC post-abdominal surgery 40 mg/day SC for DVT treatment unstable angina or non-Q-wave MI 1 mg/kg q 12 hr.	3500–5500	100	2.7:1	3.5–5.9

(continued)

603

LOW-MOLECULAR-WEIGHT HEPARINS COMPARISON CHART (continued)

DRUG	DOSAGE FORMS	ADULT DOSAGE	AVERAGE MASS (DALTONS)	AF-XA[a] (IU/MG)	AF-XA/AF-IIA[b] RATIO	HALF-LIFE (HR)
Fondaparinux Arixtra (Investigational— Sanofi)	—	SC for DVT prophylaxis 1.5–3 mg once daily. SC for DVT treatment 7.5 mg once daily.	1800	700	d	15–20
Nadroparin Fraxiparin (Investigational— Sanofi)	—	SC for DVT prophylaxis 4400 IU once daily SC for DVT treatment 90–92 IU/kg bid.	4500	85	3.2:1	2.3–5
Tinzaparin Innohep	Inj 20,000 IU/mL.	SC for DVT prophylaxis 50–75 IU/kg once daily SC for DVT treatment 175 IU/kg once daily.	4900	86	1.9:1	1.85

[a]Antifactor Xa activity.
[b]Antifactor Xa:antifactor IIa ratio. The ratio for unfractionated heparin is 1.
[c]A heparinoid; mixture of low-molecular-weight sulfated nonheparin glycosaminoglycans: heparan sulfate (84%), dermatan sulfate (12%), and chondroitin sulfate (4%).
[d]Fondaparinux is a pure XA inhibitor.
From references 5, 25, 26, 28, 30, and 31.

EPTIFIBATIDE
Integrilin

Pharmacology. Eptifibatide is a synthetic, cyclic heptapeptide that reversibly binds to and inhibits the platelet glycoprotein IIb/IIIa receptor. Inhibition of the glycoprotein IIb/IIIa receptor prevents fibrinogen from binding, thereby preventing platelet aggregation. Eptifibatide inhibits platelet aggregation and prolongs bleeding time in a dose-dependent manner.[1]

Administration and Adult Dosage. **IV for unstable angina or non–Q-wave MI (acute coronary syndrome)** 180 µg/kg as a bolus and then 2 µg/kg/min by continuous infusion. Continue infusion for up to 72 hr, until hospital discharge or CABG surgery, whichever occurs first. Should percutaneous coronary intervention be performed, continue infusion for 18–24 hr after completing procedure (up to 96 hr total duration). Concomitant heparin therapy is recommended. (*See* Notes.) **IV for percutaneous intervention** 180 µg/kg as a bolus and then 2 µg/kg/min continuous infusion for 20–24 hr. Give a second bolus of 180 µg/kg 10 min after the first.

Special Populations. *Other Conditions.* In patients with renal insufficiency: for Cr_s 2–4 mg/dL, give 180 µg/kg as a bolus and then 1 µg/kg/min continuous infusion. For percutaneous intervention, give a second bolus of 180 µg/kg 10 min after the first.

Dosage Forms. **Inj** 0.75, 2 mg/mL.

Pharmacokinetics. *Onset and Duration.* Rapid inhibition of platelet function occurs after IV administration. Platelet function recovers soon after discontinuation of the IV infusion; bleeding time returns to baseline within 30 min and ex vivo platelet aggregation approaches baseline levels within 2–4 hr.[1]

Fate. Renal elimination accounts for about 50% of the total body clearance of eptifibatide. Cl is 0.055–0.058 L/kg/hr.

$t_{1/2}$. 1.5–2.5 hr.[1]

Adverse Reactions. Bleeding, particularly from vascular access sites, occurs frequently. Oropharyngeal, GI, and GU bleeding also can occur. The frequency of thrombocytopenia is equal to that of placebo.[1,32,33]

Contraindications. Active internal bleeding within previous 30 days; history of CVA within 30 days or any history of hemorrhagic CVA; bleeding diathesis; thrombocytopenia (<100,000/µL); recent (within 6 weeks) major surgery or trauma; severe uncontrolled hypertension; current or planned use of another parenteral glycoprotein IIb/IIIa inhibitor; dependency on hemodialysis.

Precautions. (*See* Abciximab.) Use caution in elderly patients because eptifibatide clearance might be reduced, increasing risk of bleeding.

Parameters to Monitor. Monitor CBC (including platelet count), PT, aPTT, and activated clotting time (if percutaneous coronary intervention performed). In clinical trials, the target activated clotting time (ACT) for patients treated with eptifibatide and undergoing percutaneous coronary intervention was 300–350 sec.[32] If concomitant administration of unfractionated heparin is necessary, maintain aPTT at 50–70 sec.[33]

Notes. (*See* Abciximab, Notes for vascular access site care after percutaneous coronary intervention.) To minimize bleeding complications, use the following heparin dosages: **continuous IV heparin infusion** (≥70 kg) 5000 units as a bolus and then 1000 units/hr; (<70 kg) 60 units/kg as a bolus and then 12 units/kg/hr.[33] **Initial IV heparin boluses during percutaneous coronary intervention** (baseline ACT ≤150 sec) 100 units/kg (up to 10,000 units); (baseline ACT 151–225 sec) 75 units/kg; (baseline ACT 226–299 sec) 50 units/kg; (baseline ACT ≥300 sec) do not administer heparin; then **IV boluses during percutaneous coronary intervention as needed to maintain ACT of 300–350 sec** (ACT 275–299 sec) 25 units/kg; (ACT <275 sec) 50 units/kg.[32]

HEPARIN SODIUM Various

Pharmacology. A heterogeneous, unfractionated group of mucopolysaccharides derived from the mast cells of animal tissues. It binds with antithrombin III, accelerating the rate at which antithrombin III neutralizes *activated forms* of factors XII, XI, IX, X, VII, and II. It is active in vitro and in vivo.

Administration and Adult Dosage. Express dosage in units only; dosage must be individually titrated to desired effect (usually 1.5–2.5 times aPTT).[4,8,34] Weight-based nomograms and computer-assisted dosages of heparin are effective, safe, and superior to "standard care" or empiric approaches.[35–37] **IV for thrombophlebitis or PE** (continuous infusion) 50–100 units/kg initially and then 15–25 units/hr/kg; alternatively, 5000 units initially and then 1000 units/hr; (intermittent) 75–125 units/kg q 4 hr.[4,8,34,38] Duration of therapy for thrombophlebitis or PE is 7–10 days, followed by oral anticoagulation (preferably initiated during the first 24 hr of heparin therapy).[34,39] A 5-day course of heparin has been shown to be as effective as a 10-day course in treating DVT.[40] **SC for thrombophlebitis or PE** 10,000–20,000 units initially (preceded by a 5000-unit IV loading dose) and then 8000–10,000 units q 8 hr or 15,000–20,000 units q 12 hr. **SC for prophylaxis of DVT (low dose)** 5000 units 2 hr before surgery, repeated q 8–12 hr for 5–7 days or until patient is ambulatory.[41] **IV for heparin lock flush** inject sufficient solution (of 10 or 100 units/mL) into injection hub to fill the entire set after each heparin lock use. Some institutions reserve the 100 units/mL solution for flushing triple-lumen central catheters and use NS for all other catheters.

Special Populations. *Pediatric Dosage.* Same as adult dosage in units/kg.

Geriatric Dosage. Same as adult dosage.

Other Conditions. Patients with PE might require larger heparin doses than patients with thrombophlebitis.[38] (*See* Administration and Adult Dosage.) Patients with severe renal dysfunction might require lower dosages.[5] There is no good evidence that liver disease appreciably affects dosage requirements.

Dosage Forms. **Inj** 1000, 2000, 2500, 5000, 7500, 10,000, 20,000, 40,000 units/mL; 2, 50, 100 units/mL (prediluted); **Heparin Lock Flush** 10, 100 units/mL.

Patient Instructions. This drug is potentially harmful when taken with nonprescription or prescription drugs. Consult your physician or pharmacist when considering the use of other medications, in particular aspirin-containing products.

Pharmacokinetics. *Onset and Duration.* Onset immediate after IV administration.

Serum Levels. The relation between heparin serum concentrations and aPTT response can change between reagents and reagent lots. Each laboratory should establish a therapeutic aPTT range corresponding to heparin serum concentrations of 0.2–0.4 unit/mL using protamine titration.[5] Circadian variation in heparin activity can occur, and aPTT response can change during the day at a given infusion rate.[42]

Fate. SC bioavailability is 20–40% and is dose dependent.[5] There is no biotransformation in plasma or liver; transfer and storage in reticuloendothelial cells have been suggested.[34,43] V_d is 0.058 ± 0.011 L/kg (approximates plasma volume).[13] Cl is dose dependent; Cl can be increased in PE, but this has not been a consistent finding.[34]

$t_{1/2}$ (Pharmacologic) 90 ± 60 min, dose related; higher doses lead to increased half-life; half-life can decrease in PE, but this has not been a consistent finding.[34,38,43,44] Shorter half-life has been reported in smokers vs nonsmokers.[5]

Adverse Reactions. Bleeding occurs in 3–20% of patients receiving short-term, high-dose therapy.[34,45] Bleeding risk is increased by 3-fold when the aPTT is 2.0–2.9 and by 8-fold when the aPTT >3.0 times the control.[34] Heparin administration by continuous IV infusion can cause a lower frequency of bleeding complications than intermittent IV administration.[34] Renal dysfunction, liver disease, and other factors (serious cardiac illness, malignancy, age >60 yr, and maximum aPTT >2.2 times control) can increase bleeding risk.[5,43,45] (*See* Precautions.) Thrombocytopenia occurs frequently (usually 1–5%) and might be more common with heparin derived from bovine lung. (*See* Notes.) However, recent studies have suggested little difference and an overall decline in prevalence.[34,46,47] The decline might be related to improved manufacturing techniques and reduced therapy duration.[46] Osteoporosis and bone fractures occur rarely with doses of 15,000 units/day or more for longer than 5 months.[34] Patients receiving prolonged therapy or with diabetes or renal dysfunction rarely develop marked hyperkalemia.[48]

Contraindications. Active bleeding; thrombocytopenia; threatened abortion; subacute bacterial endocarditis; suspected intracranial hemorrhage; regional or lumbar block anesthesia; severe hypotension; shock; and after eye, brain, or spinal cord surgery.

Precautions. Risk factors for hemorrhage are IM injections, trauma, recent surgery, age >60 yr, malignancy, peptic ulcer disease, potential bleeding sites, and acquired or congenital hemostatic defects.[34]

Drug Interactions. Anticoagulants or antiplatelet drugs including aspirin and other NSAIDs can increase risk of bleeding.

Parameters to Monitor. Baseline aPTT, PT/INR, hematocrit, and platelet count. Obtain aPTT (therapeutic range 1.5–2.5 times control) 3 or 4 times (or until therapeutic range is achieved) on day 1 and at least daily thereafter. Monitor platelets and hematocrit every other day and signs of bleeding (melena, hematuria, ecchymoses, hematemesis, epistaxis) daily.[4,8,34]

Notes. Heparin-induced thrombocytopenia is a potentially serious, and sometimes fatal, complication of heparin therapy. **Lepirudin** is approved for management of heparin-induced thrombocytopenia (*see* Lepirudin monograph). Other agents including **danaparoid, ancrod** (Venacil, compassionate use—Knoll), **dextran,** and **argatroban** also have been used successfully in these patients.[49]

LEPIRUDIN Refludan

Pharmacology. Lepirudin is a recombinant hirudin analogue that binds to thrombin in a 1:1 stoichiometric complex, thereby inhibiting the thrombogenic activity of thrombin, including clot-bound thrombin. Inhibition of thrombin occurs independently of antithrombin III.[50]

Administration and Adult Dosage. **IV for heparin-induced thrombocytopenia and associated thromboembolic disease** 0.4 mg/kg (up to 44 mg) as a bolus and then 0.15 mg/kg/hr (up to 16.5 mg/hr) by continuous infusion for 2–10 days or longer, if necessary. **IV in patients being treated concomitantly with thrombolytics** 0.2 mg/kg as a bolus and then 0.1 mg/kg/hr by continuous infusion. **Adjust dosage based on aPTT as follows:** for supratherapeutic aPTT, hold infusion for 2 hr and then reduce infusion rate by 50%; for subtherapeutic aPTT, increase infusion in 20% increments, not to exceed 0.21 mg/kg/hr.

Special Populations. *Other Conditions.* In renal insufficiency (Cr_s >1.5 mg/dL or Cl_{cr} <60 mL/min), reduce the IV bolus to 0.2 mg/kg and base the initial IV infusion on renal function: Cl_{cr} 45–60 mL/min or Cr_s 1.6–2 mg/dL, give 0.075 mg/kg/hr; Cl_{cr} 30–44 mL/min or Cr_s 2.1–3 mg/dL, give 0.045 mg/kg/hr; Cl_{cr} 15–29 mL/min or Cr_s 3.1–6 mg/dL, give 0.0225 mg/kg/hr; Cl_{cr} <15 mL/min or Cr_s >6 mg/dL, not recommended.

Dosage Forms. **Inj** 50 mg.

Pharmacokinetics. *Fate.* About 45% of the administered dose is eliminated in the urine, largely as unchanged drug (35%). Clearance is approximately 25% lower in women than in men and is also reduced about 20% in the elderly.

$t_{1/2}$. α phase 10 min; β phase 1.3 hr.

Adverse Reactions. Bleeding complications are the most frequent adverse reactions. Hypersensitivity reactions, primarily allergic skin reactions, occur frequently.

Contraindications. Hypersensitivity to hirudins.

Precautions. Use with caution in patients with active internal bleeding, history of recent major bleeding, or known bleeding diathesis; history of CVA or any history of intracranial hemorrhage; history of intracranial neoplasm, AV malformation, or aneurysm; recent puncture of large blood vessel or organ biopsy; recent (within 1 month) major surgery or trauma; severe uncontrolled hypertension; bacterial endocarditis; poor renal function; receiving concomitant antithrombotic therapy including thrombolytics. Up to 40% of patients with heparin-induced thrombocytopenia treated with lepirudin develop antihirudin antibodies, which can increase the anticoagulant effects of lepirudin, necessitating strict monitoring of aPTT values.

Parameters to Monitor. Monitor aPTT 4 hr after initiating lepirudin therapy, 4 hr after each change in infusion rate, and daily once target aPTT has been achieved. Maintain aPTT approximately 1.5–2.5 times the control aPTT.

Notes. **Desirudin** (Revasc—Aventis) is a recombinant hirudin that is being studied for use in DVT prevention after hip replacement.

PHYTONADIONE
AquaMephyton, Mephyton

Pharmacology. Vitamin K is a required cofactor for the hepatic microsomal enzyme system that carboxylates glutamyl residues in precursor proteins to γ-carboxyglutamyl residues. These proteins are present in vitamin K–dependent clotting factors (II, VII, IX, and X), anticoagulation proteins (proteins C and S), bone (osteocalin), some plasma proteins (protein Z), and the proteins of several organs (kidney, lung, and testicular tissue).[51–53]

Administration and Adult Dosage. The normal daily nutritional requirement is about 0.03–1.5 μg/kg.[52,54,55] The adult RDAs are 70 μg/day for men 19–24 yr and 80 μg/day for men >25 yr and 60 μg/day for women 19–24 yr and 65 μg/day for women >25 yr.[56] **PO, SC, or IM to reverse bleeding** 2.5–10 mg up to 25 mg initially. A single dose of 1–5 mg is usually sufficient to normalize PT during anticoagulant therapy, but in severe bleeding, 20–50 mg might be needed.[52,56–58] The initial dose can be repeated, based on PT and clinical response, after 12–48 hr if given PO and 6–8 hr if given parenterally. Use the smallest dosage possible to reverse anticoagulants and obviate possible refractoriness to additional anticoagulant therapy.[52,59] **IV** do not give AquaMephyton intravenously unless it is *absolutely essential* (eg, INR >20, serious warfarin overdose or life-threatening bleeding). Give IV in 10 mg doses at infusion rates no greater than 1 mg/min.[57] The drug can be diluted in preservative-free dextrose or saline solution just before IV use. **PO for antenatal use in pregnant women receiving anticonvulsants** 20 mg/day throughout the last 4 weeks of pregnancy.[53]

Special Populations. *Pediatric Dosage.* RDAs are (<6 months) 5 μg/day; (6 months–1 yr) 10 μg/day; (1–3 yr) 15 μg/day; (4–6 yr) 20 μg/day; (7–10 yr) 30 μg/day; (11–14 yr) 45 μg/day; (15–18 yr) 55 μg/day for females, 65 μg/day for males.[56] **IM for prophylaxis of hemorrhagic disease of the newborn** 0.5–1 mg within 1 hr of birth. **SC or IM for treatment of hemorrhagic disease of the newborn** 1 mg; more if mother has been receiving an oral anticoagulant.

Geriatric Dosage. (>55 yr) RDAs are 65 μg/day for women and 80 μg/day for men.[56]

Dosage Forms. **Tab** (Mephyton) 5 mg; **Inj** (AquaMephyton) 2, 10 mg/mL.

Pharmacokinetics. *Onset and Duration.* Reversal of anticoagulant effect is variable among individuals; parenteral onset is often within 6 hr; peak and duration differ across individuals and doses. A 5 mg IV dose usually returns PT to normal in 24–48 hr.[60] Large doses can cause prolonged refractoriness to oral anticoagulants.[52,59]

Fate. Absorbed from the GI tract via intestinal lymphatics only in the presence of bile; well absorbed after parenteral administration. Metabolized in the liver to hydroquinone and epoxide forms, which are interconvertible with the quinone.[51] Little storage occurs in the body. Without bile, hypoprothrombinemia develops over several weeks.[52,59,61]

Adverse Reactions. The drug itself appears to be nontoxic, but severe reactions (eg, flushing, dyspnea, chest pain) and, occasionally, deaths have occurred after IV administration of AquaMephyton, possibly caused by the emulsifying agents.[52,55,62] This product should rarely be used IV, and only when other routes of administration are not feasible. A transient flushing sensation, peculiar taste, and pain and swelling at the injection site can occur. Large parenteral doses in neonates have caused hyperbilirubinemia.

Precautions. Temporary refractoriness to oral anticoagulants can occur, especially with large doses of vitamin K. Reversal of anticoagulant activity can restore previous thromboembolic conditions. No effect or worsening of hypoprothrombinemia can occur in severe liver disease, and repeated doses are not warranted if response to the initial dose is unsatisfactory.[52,62]

Drug Interactions. Mineral oil and cholesterol-binding resins can impair phytonadione absorption.

Parameters to Monitor. Monitor PT before and at intervals after administration of the drug; the interval depends on the route of administration, the condition being treated, and the patient's status. (*See* Administration and Adult Dosage.)

Notes. Always protect the drug from light. Phytonadione reverses the effects of oral anticoagulant therapy but has no antagonist activity against heparin.

RETEPLASE Retavase

Pharmacology. Reteplase (recombinant plasminogen activator) is a nonglycosylated mutant of wild-type tissue plasminogen activator. In animals, this modification results in less high-affinity fibrin binding, longer half-life, and greater thrombolytic potency than **alteplase** (rt-PA).

Administration and Adult Dosage. **IV for post-MI clot lysis** two 10 IU boluses 30 min apart, with adjunctive IV heparin given as a 5000 unit bolus followed by 1000 units/hr (aPTT target 1.5–2.0 times control) for at least 24 hr.

Dosage Forms. **Inj** 10.8 IU.

Pharmacokinetics. *Onset and Duration.* Onset of fibrinolytic activity is immediate after IV administration; duration is about 48 hr as assessed by fibrinogen levels.

Fate. V_d is about 6 L. Elimination is primarily by the liver and kidneys.

$t_{1/2}$. α phase 14 ± 0.7 min (range 11–19 min); β phase 173 ± 33 min.[63]

Adverse Reactions. (*See* Alteplase.)

Contraindications. (*See* Alteplase.)

Precautions. (*See* Alteplase.)

Notes. In the Reteplase Angiographic Phase II International Dose-finding study (RAPID) open-label MI trial, reteplase achieved more rapid, complete, and sustained thrombolysis than did standard-dose rt-PA, with comparable bleeding risk.[64] The RAPID trial did not have sufficient power to detect differences in mortality between the groups. The GUSTO-III trial found reteplase equivalent to accelerated-infusion **alteplase** in MI for the combined endpoints of death or nonfatal, disabling stroke.[65] The International Joint Efficacy Comparison of Thrombolytics (INJECT) trial suggested that reteplase mortality rates were similar to those observed with streptokinase.[66]

STREPTOKINASE   Streptase

Pharmacology. A bacterial protein derived from group C β-hemolytic streptococci. It acts indirectly by forming a streptokinase–plasminogen activator complex that activates another plasminogen and converts it to the proteolytic enzyme plasmin. Plasmin then hydrolyzes fibrin, fibrinogen, factors II, V, and VIII, complement, and kallikreinogen.

Administration and Adult Dosage. IV for post-MI clot lysis 1.5 million IU over 60 min. **IV for PE, DVT, arterial thrombosis, or embolism** 250,000 IU over 30 min, followed by 100,000 IU/hr for 24–72 hr (72 hr if DVT suspected).[67] Institute heparin therapy. (*See* Notes and Parameters to Monitor.) **For arteriovenous cannula occlusion** slowly instill 250,000 IU in 2 mL solution into each occluded limb of cannula; clamp for 2 hr, aspirate contents, and flush with NS. **Selective intra-arterial infusion** (investigational) 5000 IU/hr for 5–48 hr.[68,69] (*See* Notes.)

Special Populations. *Pediatric Dosage.* Safety and efficacy not established.

Geriatric Dosage. Same as adult dosage.

Dosage Forms. Inj 250,000, 750,000, 1.5 million IU.

Pharmacokinetics. *Onset and Duration.* Onset of fibrinolytic activity immediately after IV administration; duration 8–24 hr after discontinuation of the infusion.[70]

Fate. V_d is 0.08 ± 0.04 L/kg; Cl is 0.1 ± 0.04 L/hr/kg.[13] Clearance results in part from formation of an antigen–antibody complex that remains soluble and is rapidly removed.[5] Local inactivation in the circulation by inhibitor complex formation and proteolysis occurs. It is postulated that the reticuloendothelial system also contributes to clearance.[71]

$t_{1/2}$. α phase averages 18–23 min and is related to antigen–antibody formation; β phase averages 83 min and appears to be related to clearance by the reticuloendothelial system.[5,71]

Adverse Reactions. Surface bleeding complications occur frequently and usually follow invasive procedures (eg, venous cutdowns, arterial punctures, and sites of surgical intervention). Severe internal bleeding is reported occasionally, but its prevalence is no greater than with other thrombolytics or standard anticoagulant therapy. Transient hypotension occurs occasionally. In ISIS-3 the rates for definite or possible cerebral bleeding were: streptokinase, 0.2%; rt-PA (**duteplase**, a 2-chain form of alteplase), 0.5%; **anistreplase**, 0.7%.[14] Occasional allergic reactions are fever, urticaria, itching, flushing, and musculoskeletal pain. Anaphylactoid reactions occur rarely with preparations now in use.[5,72]

Contraindications. (*See* Alteplase.)

Precautions. (*See* Alteplase.) Prior exposure to anistreplase or streptokinase within the last 12 months.

Drug Interactions. Anticoagulants or antiplatelet drugs can increase risk of bleeding.

Parameters to Monitor. For short-term thrombolytic therapy of MI, laboratory monitoring is of little value. For IV continuous infusion, monitor thrombin time, aPTT, or PT to detect activation of the fibrinolytic system, performed 3–4 hr after initiating therapy and q 12 hr throughout treatment.[72] No correlation has been made between clotting test results and likelihood of hemorrhage or efficacy; however, prolongation of the thrombin time to 2–5 times normal control value has been recommended.

Notes. In addition to post-MI clot lysis, streptokinase is recommended for treatment of thrombosis involving the axillary–subclavian system, the popliteal vein or deep veins of the thigh and pelvis, and for patients in whom massive pulmonary emboli have caused obstruction of blood flow to one or more lung segments or when clinical shock is present.[72] The risk of stroke and intracranial bleeding appears to be less with streptokinase (by a difference of ≤0.5%) than with other thrombolytic agents.[73] Thrombolytic therapy can help prevent venous valvular damage and the development of venous or pulmonary hypertension.[74] The recommended fixed dosage schedule results in sufficient activation of plasminogen in 95% of patients.[75] However, consider using **alteplase** in those patients exposed to streptokinase or anistreplase within the last 12 months.[7] The benefits of instituting anticoagulant therapy with **heparin** after completion of the thrombolytic infusion are not clear. However, it is recommended that heparin infusion (to an aPTT of 1.5–2.0 times control) be given only when there is high risk for systemic or venous thromboembolism (eg, anterior MI, CHF, previous embolus, atrial fibrillation). Heparin is initiated without a bolus 4 hr after the start of streptokinase infusion (or when aPTT is less than twice control) and continued for at least 48 hr.[7,10]

TENECTEPLASE

TNKase

Pharmacology. Tenecteplase is a recombinant tissue plasminogen activator, modified from human tissue plasminogen activator (t-PA). Genetic mutations of human t-PA resulted in greater thrombolytic potency, enhanced fibrin-specificity, decreased systemic activation of plasminogen, resistance to plasminogen activator inhibitor 1, and a longer half-life compared with t-PA.[76]

Administration and Adult Dosage. IV bolus for myocardial infarction (<60 kg) 30 mg; (60–69 kg) 35 mg; (70–79 kg) 40 mg; (80–89 kg) 45 mg; (≥90 kg) 50 mg. Give tenecteplase in combination with continuous IV heparin infusion. (*See* Notes.)

Dosage Forms. Inj 50 mg.

Pharmacokinetics. *Onset and Duration.* Rapid onset of thrombolysis occurs after IV administration.

Fate. Hepatic metabolism is the primary mode of clearance. Cl is 5.94–7.14 L/hr. $t_{½}$. α phase 18–24 min; β phase 90–130 min.[76]

Adverse Reactions. (*See* Alteplase.)

Contraindications. (*See* Alteplase.)

Precautions. (*See* Alteplase.)

Parameters to Monitor. (*See* Alteplase.) Monitor aPTT while on concomitant heparin therapy; target aPTT is 50–75 sec.[77]

Notes. In ASSENT-2, patients also were given concomitant IV heparin therapy as follows: (>67 kg) 4000 units as a bolus and then 800 units/hr by continuous infusion; (>67 kg) 5000 units as a bolus and then 1000 units/hr by continuous infusion. Heparin therapy was continued for 48–72 hr. This study demonstrated comparable patency rates, mortality, intracranial hemorrhage, and stroke compared with front-loaded **alteplase**.[77]

TICLOPIDINE   Ticlid

Pharmacology. Ticlopidine is an antiplatelet agent that inhibits most known stimuli (eg, ADP, collagen, epinephrine) for platelet aggregation. It prolongs bleeding time, normalizes shortened platelet survival, suppresses platelet growth factor release, and might block von Willebrand factor and fibrinogen interactions with platelets.[78–80]

Adult Dosage. PO for thrombotic stroke reduction in patients with stroke or stroke precursors, patients with unstable angina, or those undergoing coronary artery bypass graft or coronary angioplasty 250 mg bid.

Dosage Forms. **Tab** 250 mg.

Pharmacokinetics. The onset of clinical effect is delayed, with maximum efficacy being achieved in 3–8 days. Approximately 80% of the drug is absorbed orally, with peak serum concentrations occurring in about 2 hr. Ticlopidine undergoes extensive liver metabolism to possibly active metabolites, with only 2% excreted unchanged in urine. Half-life is 4–5 days with repeated dosages.

Adverse Reactions. Diarrhea and rash occur frequently. Minor bleeding such as bruising, petechiae, epistaxis, and hematuria occur occasionally. Severe neutropenia occurs in about 0.8% of patients and mild to moderate neutropenia in about 1.6% of patients during the first 3 months of therapy; neutropenia usually resolves within 3 weeks of discontinuation, although sepsis and death have been reported. Thrombocytopenia, thrombotic thrombocytopenic purpura, and cholestasis occur rarely.[80,81] Obtain CBC and differential counts q 2 weeks during the first 3 months of therapy; more frequent monitoring is recommended if the ANC is consistently declining or is less than 30% of the baseline value or if patients demonstrate signs and symptoms of thrombotic thrombocytopenic purpura (weakness, pallor, petechiae, or purpura), dark urine, jaundice, or neurologic changes.

Notes. The Ticlopidine Aspirin Stroke Study trial found a 12% risk reduction in nonfatal stroke or cardiovascular death with ticlopidine compared with aspirin in high-risk (previous TIA or minor stroke) men and women. For secondary stroke prevention, the Canadian American Ticlopidine Study trial found that the risk of stroke, MI, or cardiovascular death was reduced by 23% with ticlopidine over placebo. Ticlopidine also was shown to markedly reduce MI, cardiovascular death, and ECG evidence of ischemia in patients with unstable angina.[82,83] Reserve ticlopidine for patients intolerant to aspirin and clopidogrel.

TIROFIBAN
Aggrastat

Pharmacology. Tirofiban is a nonpeptide, tyrosine derivative that reversibly binds to and inhibits the platelet glycoprotein IIb/IIIa receptor. Inhibition of the glycoprotein IIb/IIIa receptor prevents fibrinogen from binding, thereby preventing platelet aggregation. Tirofiban inhibits platelet aggregation and prolongs bleeding time in a dose-dependent manner.[1]

Administration and Adult Dosage. **IV for unstable angina or non–Q-wave MI (acute coronary syndrome)** 0.4 μg/kg/min infusion for 30 min and then 0.1 μg/kg/min by continuous infusion. Continue infusion until patient has clinically stabilized; infusion can be continued for up to 108 hr. Tirofiban can be administered to patients who undergo percutaneous coronary intervention. Should percutaneous coronary intervention be performed during tirofiban therapy, continue infusion for 12–24 hr after completing the procedure. Give tirofiban in combination with continuous IV heparin infusion. (*See* Notes.)

Special Populations. *Other Conditions.* (Cl$_{cr}$ <30 mL/min) reduce maintenance infusion rate by 50%.

Dosage Forms. **Inj** 50, 250 μg/mL.

Pharmacokinetics. *Onset and Duration.* Rapid inhibition of platelet function occurs after IV administration. Platelet function recovers soon after discontinuation of the IV infusion; bleeding time and ex vivo platelet aggregation return to near baseline levels within 3–8 hr.[1]

Fate. Renal elimination accounts for 39–69% of the total body clearance. About 65% of a dose is excreted in the urine, largely as unchanged drug; about 25% of an administered dose is excreted in the feces. Cl is 9.12–18.84 L/hr.

t$_{½}$. 1.5–2 hr.[1]

Adverse Reactions. Bleeding complications are the most frequent adverse reactions. Use care to minimize the risk of bleeding by minimizing vascular and other trauma and providing proper care of vascular access sites in patients having percutaneous coronary interventions performed. Thrombocytopenia occurs in <2% of patients and is reversible at discontinuation of the drug.[84]

Contraindications. Active internal bleeding or bleeding diathesis within the previous 30 days; history of CVA within 30 days or any history of intracranial hemorrhage; history of intracranial neoplasm, AV malformation, or aneurysm; thrombocytopenia; recent (within 1 month) major surgery or trauma; history, symptoms, or findings suggestive of aortic dissection; severe uncontrolled hypertension; current or planned use of another parenteral glycoprotein IIb/IIIa inhibitor; acute pericarditis.

Precautions. (*See* Abciximab.)

Parameters to Monitor. Monitor CBC (including platelet count), prothrombin time, aPTT, and activated clotting time (if percutaneous coronary intervention performed). Maintain aPTT approximately 2 times control aPTT.[84]

Notes. (*See* Abciximab for vascular access site care after percutaneous coronary intervention.) **IV heparin during therapy** 5000 units as a bolus and then

1000 units/hr continuous infusion adjusted to maintain aPTT 2 times control. **IV heparin if percutaneous coronary intervention was performed** discontinue IV infusion and give 5000–7500 units of heparin as a bolus and then 1000 units/hr by continuous infusion.[84]

UROKINASE
Abbokinase

Pharmacology. Urokinase is a proteolytic enzyme produced by renal parenchymal cells that act to directly convert plasminogen to plasmin, with effects similar to those of streptokinase.[5]

Administration and Adult Dosage. **IV for pulmonary emboli** 4400 IU/kg loading dose over 10 min, followed by 4400 IU/kg/hr for 12 hr. Heparin therapy is initiated without a loading dose after discontinuation of the thrombolytic when the thrombin time or other coagulation test no longer exceeds 2 times normal control. **Selective intracoronary infusion** 6000 IU/min for up to 2 hr. **IV for catheter clearance** attach a 1 mL tuberculin syringe filled with 5000 IU reconstituted solution (Open-Cath) and slowly inject an amount equal to the catheter volume; aspirate and repeat q 5 min as necessary. If not successful, allow urokinase to remain in the catheter for 30–60 min before attempting to aspirate. For central venous catheters whose functions have not been restored by the bolus method, a 6- or 12-hr infusion of 40,000 IU/hr (5000 IU/mL at 8 mL/hr) in adults might be useful.[85]

Dosage Forms. **Inj** 5000, 9000, 250,000 IU.

Pharmacokinetics. The drug's half-life is about 10–20 min.

Adverse Reactions. Side effects, contraindications, and precautions are similar to those of streptokinase, although allergic reactions occur much less frequently.

WARFARIN SODIUM
Coumadin, Various

Pharmacology. Warfarin prevents the conversion of vitamin K back to its active form from vitamin K epoxide. This impairs formation of the vitamin K–dependent clotting factors II, VII, IX, and X (prothrombin) and proteins C and S (physiologic anticoagulants). The (S)-warfarin enantiomer is approximately 4-fold more potent an anticoagulant than (R)-warfarin.[5,86]

Administration and Adult Dosage. **PO or IV** 5–7.5 mg/day (range 2–10 mg/day), titrating dosage to an INR of 2.0–3.0 for treatment or prophylaxis of venous thrombosis, PE, systemic embolism, tissue heart valves, valvular heart disease, atrial fibrillation (except patients <60 yr with "lone atrial fibrillation"), and recurrent systemic embolism. Adjust dosage to an INR of 2.5–3.5 for management of mechanical prosthetic valves (upper end of range for caged-ball, tilting-disk, and mitral position valves);[87] adding **aspirin** 100 mg/day offers additional protection but increases the risk of mild bleeding.[7,34] For post-MI patients who are at increased risk of systemic or pulmonary embolism, maintain a warfarin dosage that achieves an INR of 2.5–3.5 for up to 3 months. Low-dose warfarin (1 mg/day) without measurable changes in PT/INR begun 3 days before central venous catheter placement and continued while the catheter remains in place is recommended to reduce the risk of axillary–subclavian venous thrombosis.[8,88] (*See* Notes.)

Special Populations. *Pediatric Dosage.* (<18 yr) safety and efficacy not established. However, when used, dosage is titrated based on INR as in adult dosage.

Geriatric Dosage. Same as adult dosage. (*See also* Precautions.)

Other Conditions. Large variability in response requires that dosage be carefully individualized to each patient. Patients with liver disease, CHF, hyperthyroidism, or fever might be particularly sensitive to warfarin. Renal failure does not enhance the hypoprothrombinemic response to warfarin, but these patients might have compromised hemostatic mechanisms that predispose to bleeding.[89]

Dosage Forms. **Tab** 1, 2, 2.5, 3, 4, 5, 6, 7.5, 10 mg; **Inj** 2 mg.

Patient Instructions. This drug is potentially harmful when taken with nonprescription or prescription drugs. Consult your physician or pharmacist when considering the use of other medications, in particular aspirin-containing products.

Missed Doses. Take this drug at the same time each day. It is important that you not miss any doses. If you do miss a dose, take it as soon as you remember. If it is about time for the next dose, take that dose only. Do not double the dose or take extra.

Pharmacokinetics. *Onset and Duration.* Peak PT effect is in 36–72 hr;[90] at least 4–6 days of warfarin therapy are required before full therapeutic effect is achieved.[4,34] Duration after discontinuation depends on resynthesis of vitamin K–dependent clotting factors II, VII, IX, and X (which requires about 4–5 days).

Fate. Completely absorbed orally; well absorbed after small bowel resection;[91] 99 ± 1% is bound to plasma proteins.[13] V_d (racemic) is 0.14 ± 0.06 L/kg; Cl (racemic) is 0.0027 ± 0.0014 L/hr/kg.[13] It undergoes oxidative P450 enzyme biotransformation in the liver: (R)-warfarin, CYP1A2; (S)-warfarin, CYP2C subfamily,[92] producing warfarin alcohols, which have minor anticoagulant activity.[93,94] Less than 2% is excreted unchanged in urine.[13]

$t_{1/2}$. 37 ± 15 hr,[13,95] unchanged in acute hepatic disease.[96] Enantiomer half-lives: (R)-warfarin 43 ± 14 hr; (S)-warfarin 32 ± 12 hr.[13]

Adverse Reactions. Bleeding (major and minor) occurs frequently (6–29%); fatal or life-threatening hemorrhage has been reported in 1–8% of patients. Risk factors for increased bleeding are PT ratio >2.0, age >60 yr, and other comorbid conditions. Skin necrosis (occurring early in therapy and involving the breast, buttocks, thigh, or penis), purple-toe syndrome (occurring after 3–8 weeks of therapy), and alopecia rarely occur.[4,34,45,97,98]

Contraindications. Pregnancy; threatened abortion; blood dyscrasias; bleeding tendencies; unsupervised patients with senility, alcoholism, psychosis, or lack of cooperation; anticipated spinal puncture procedure; regional or lumbar anesthesia.

Precautions. Avoid all IM injections because of the risk of hematoma. Several other factors can influence response: diet, travel, and environment. Monitor patients with liver disease, CHF, atrial fibrillation, hyperthyroidism, or fever especially carefully. The elderly have a greater risk of major trauma (eg, hip fractures) and physiologic changes in subcutaneous tissues and joint spaces, which can allow bleeding to expand unchecked.[98]

Drug Interactions. There are many important interactions that have potential clinical importance. Careful monitoring and appropriate dosage adjustment are recommended when any potential interacting drug is added or discontinued. Some agents commonly associated with increased warfarin effect are amiodarone, cimetidine, ciprofloxacin, clofibrate, erythromycin, fluconazole, fluvoxamine, lovastatin, metronidazole, quinidine, and trimethoprim-sulfamethoxazole. Some agents commonly associated with decreased warfarin effect are barbiturates, carbamazepine, cholestyramine, griseofulvin, and rifampin. (*See* references 99 and 100 for more comprehensive information regarding warfarin drug interactions.)

Parameters to Monitor. Monitor PT/INR daily while hospitalized and then weekly to monthly for therapeutic effect; hematocrit; stool guaiac; urinalysis (for hematuria) for toxicity. Also monitor for ecchymoses, hemoptysis, and epistaxis.

Notes. Loading dose has no therapeutic advantage and might be unsafe because of excessive depression of factor VII.[34] Predictive techniques using small loading doses (eg, 10 mg/day for 2–3 days) were developed with a therapeutic range target much higher than current recommendations. With the current narrow and lower therapeutic target, the predictive error of these techniques might be unacceptable.[34] **Phytonadione** begins to restore the PT toward normal within 4–8 hr, although large doses can induce subsequent resistance to anticoagulant effect lasting ≥1 week.[101] A small oral dose (eg, 2.5 mg) or small slow IV injection (0.5–1 mg) of phytonadione can be used to bring an elevated PT/INR back into target range without resulting resistance.[7] Treat the first episode of venous thrombosis for 6 weeks in patients with reversible risk factors and 6 months in others. Consider continuing warfarin for an indefinite period in patients with active cancer or recurrent venous thrombosis.[102]

Hematopoietics

EPOETIN ALFA
Epogen, Procrit

Pharmacology. Epoetin alfa (erythropoietin) is a recombinant human glycoprotein produced from mammalian cells and stimulates production of RBC. The product contains the identical amino acid sequence and produces the same biologic effects as natural erythropoietin.[103–106]

Administration and Adult Dosage. **IV or SC for dialysis or nondialysis chronic renal failure patients** 50–100 units/kg 3 times/week initially, increasing or decreasing by 25 units/kg to maintain a target hematocrit of 30–36%. When the target hematocrit is reached (or when the increase >4% in any 2-week period), reduce the dosage to 25 units/kg 3 times/week. If at any time the hematocrit exceeds 36%, discontinue epoetin until the target hematocrit is achieved and then resume at a lower dosage. Individualize the maintenance dosage to maintain the target hematocrit. **IV or SC for zidovudine-treated or HIV-infected patients** 100 units/kg 3 times/week for 8 weeks initially, increasing or decreasing by 50–100 units/kg based on response; maximum effective dosage is 300 units/kg 3 times/week. If hematocrit exceeds 40%, discontinue epoetin until the hematocrit returns to 36% and then reduce dosage by 25%; adjust dosage to maintain desired hematocrit target. Patients with initial erythropoietin levels >500 units/L are unlikely to respond to epoetin. **SC for anemia in chemotherapy-treated cancer patients** 150 units/kg 3 times/week for 8 weeks initially, increasing to 300 units/kg 3 times/week if there is an unsatisfactory reduction in transfusion requirement or an unsatisfactory increase in hematocrit. If hematocrit exceeds 40%, discontinue epoetin until the hematocrit returns to 36% and then reduce dosage by 25%; adjust dosage to maintain desired hematocrit target. **SC for reduction of allogenic blood transfusion in surgery patients** 300 units/kg/day for 10 days before surgery, on day of surgery, and 4 days after surgery; alternatively, 600 units/kg/week 21, 14, and 7 days before surgery and on day of surgery. For use in anemic patients (hemoglobin >10 g/dL and ≤13 g/dL) undergoing noncardiac, nonvascular surgery with an anticipated large blood loss.

Special Populations. *Pediatric Dosage.* Safety and efficacy not established. **SC for anemia of prematurity** (preterm neonates) 200 units (140 units/kg) every other day for 10 doses;[107] alternatively, 250 units/kg 3 times/week.[106] **SC or IV for anemia of end-stage renal disease** (newborn–18 yr) 50 units/kg 3 times/week has been used.[108,109]

Geriatric Dosage. Same as adult dosage.

Dosage Forms. **Inj** 2000, 3000, 4000, 10,000, 20,000, 40,000 units/mL.

Pharmacokinetics. *Onset and Duration.* In response to administration 3 times/week, reticulocyte count increases within 10 days followed by increases in RBC count, hematocrit, and hemoglobin in about 2–6 weeks.

Fate. Not orally bioavailable. Peak serum levels occur 5–24 hr after SC administration. V_d is 0.033–0.055 L/kg; Cl is about 0.00282 L/hr/kg.[103]

$t_{1/2}$. 9.3 ± 3.3 hr initially; 6.2 ± 1.8 hr during long-term therapy.[103]

Adverse Reactions. Hypertension, headache, tachycardia, nausea, vomiting, clotted vascular access, shortness of breath, hyperkalemia, and diarrhea occur frequently. Seizures occur occasionally; CVA, TIA, and MI occur rarely.[103–106]

Contraindications. Uncontrolled hypertension. Hypersensitivity to mammalian cell-derived products or albumin.

Precautions. Pregnancy. Use cautiously with a known history of seizure or underlying hematologic diseases such as sickle cell anemia, myelodysplastic syndromes, and hypercoagulable states.

Drug Interactions. None known.

Parameters to Monitor. Evaluate iron stores before and during therapy. Supplemental iron might be required to maintain a transferrin saturation of at least 20% and ferritin levels of at least 100 μg/L. Determine hematocrit twice a week for 2–6 weeks or until stabilized in the target range; monitor at regular intervals thereafter. Monitor CBC with differential platelet count, BUN, Cr_s, serum uric acid, serum phosphorus, and serum potassium at regular intervals.

Notes. **Darbopoetin** (Aranesp—Amgen) is a highly glycosylated form of erythropoetin that is absorbed slowly and can be given once weekly or every 2 weeks. The weekly dose in μg/kg equals the total weekly dosage of epoetin alfa in IV/week divided by 200.

FERROUS SALTS

Various

Pharmacology. Ferrous salts are soluble forms of iron, an essential nutrient that functions primarily as the oxygen-binding core of heme in red blood cells (as hemoglobin) and muscles (as myoglobin) and in the respiratory enzyme cytochrome C.

Administration and Adult Dosage. PO as a dietary supplement RDAs are 10 mg/day for men (19–51 yr) and 15 mg/day for women (19–51 yr).[56] **PO for treatment of iron deficiency** 2–3 mg/kg/day of elemental iron in divided doses. (*See* Ferrous Salts Comparison Chart for usual dosage ranges for individual salts.) Dose-related adverse effects can be decreased by using suboptimal dosages, increasing the daily dosage gradually, or administering with a small amount of food (although this latter method reduces absorption). After hemoglobin is normalized, continue oral therapy for 3–6 months to replenish iron stores.

Special Populations. *Pediatric Dosage.* PO for prophylaxis RDA (infants) 6 mg/day; (1–10 yr) 10 mg/day; (11–18 yr, males) 12 mg/day; (11–18 yr, females) 15 mg/day.[56] **PO for treatment** (infants) 10–25 mg of elemental iron in 3–4 divided doses; (6 months–2 yr) up to 6 mg/kg/day of elemental iron in 3–4 divided doses; (2–12 yr) 3 mg/kg/day of elemental iron in 3–4 divided doses.

Geriatric Dosage. Same as adult dosage, except dosage in women older than 51 yr is 10 mg/day of elemental iron.

Other Conditions. Iron requirement during pregnancy is approximately twice that of the normal, nonpregnant woman because of an expanding blood volume and the demands of the fetus and placenta. The RDA in pregnancy is 30 mg/day, and a prophylactic dose of 15–30 mg/day of elemental iron during the second and third trimesters has been recommended to prevent depletion of maternal iron stores. Iron-deficient patients might need higher doses.

Dosage Forms. (*See* Ferrous Salts Comparison Chart.)

Patient Instructions. Take this drug with a full glass of water on an empty stomach (1 hour before or 2 hours after meals) for best absorption. Take liquid preparations in water or juice and drink with a straw to minimize tooth staining. If gastric distress or nausea occurs, a small quantity of food can be taken with the drug but do not take with antacids because absorption is decreased. Iron preparations can cause constipation and black stools. Keep all iron products out of the reach of children.

Missed Doses. Take this drug at regular intervals. If you miss a dose, take it as soon as you remember. If it is about time for the next dose, take that dose only. Do not double the dose or take extra.

Pharmacokinetics. *Onset and Duration.* Responses to equivalent amounts of oral or parenteral therapy are essentially the same. Reticulocytes increase within 4–7 days and reach a peak on about the 10th day. An increase in hemoglobin of at least 2 g/dL and a 6% increase in hematocrit should occur in about 3–4 weeks. Three to 6 months of therapy are generally required for restoration of iron stores.[110,111]

Serum Levels. Normal levels are 65–170 µg/dL (12–30 µmol/L) in men, 50–170 µg/dL (9–30 µmol/L) in women, and 50–120 µg/dL (9–21 µmol/L) in children. A decrease in the transferrin saturation (serum iron ÷ total iron-binding capacity $\times$ 100) indicates preanemic iron deficiency. A transferrin saturation <16% or plasma ferritin concentration <12 μg/L indicates probable iron deficiency.[110,111] In overdosage, toxicity can occur at iron levels >350 μg/dL (63 μmol/L). Chelation therapy is indicated at these levels, especially if the patient is symptomatic.[110]

Fate. Iron is absorbed primarily from the duodenum at a rate that depends on the amount of iron in storage sites. About 10% of dietary iron is absorbed in normal subjects, 20% in iron-deficient patients, and as much as 70% of medicinal iron is absorbed during marked iron deficiency or increased erythropoiesis. In the plasma, iron is oxidized to the ferric state, combined with transferrin, and used or stored as ferritin (mostly in the reticuloendothelial system and hepatocytes). The average loss in the healthy adult male is about 1 mg/day. GI loss of extravasated red cells, iron in bile, and exfoliated mucosal cells accounts for two-thirds of this iron. The other one-third is lost in the skin and urine. Menstruating women have an additional loss of about 0.5 mg/day.

Adverse Reactions. Side effects are related primarily to the dose of elemental iron. Frequent GI irritation, constipation, and stained teeth (liquid preparations only—dilute and use a drinking straw). An increased risk of cancer associated with excessive iron stores has been reported.[112]

Contraindications. Hemochromatosis; hemosiderosis; hemolytic anemias in which no true iron deficiency exists.

Precautions. Use with caution in patients with peptic ulcer, regional enteritis, or ulcerative colitis. Serious acute poisoning (which can be fatal) occurs frequently in children: doses as low as 20 mg/kg of elemental iron can cause toxicity; 40 mg/kg is considered serious; and >60 mg/kg is potentially lethal.[113]

Drug Interactions. Food, calcium carbonate, sodium bicarbonate, and possibly magnesium trisilicate can reduce iron absorption. Vitamin E can reduce utilization of iron in iron-deficiency anemia. Iron salts can reduce oral absorption of carbidopa/levodopa, methyldopa, penicillamine, quinolones, tetracyclines, and thyroid hormones.

Parameters to Monitor. Periodic reticulocyte count, hemoglobin, and hematocrit. (*See* Onset and Duration.)

Notes. Ferrous salts are used to prevent and treat iron-deficiency anemias. Such anemias occur most frequently with exceptional blood losses (eg, pathologic bleeding, menstruation) and during periods of rapid growth (eg, infancy, adolescence, pregnancy). Iron is ineffective in hemoglobin disturbances not caused by iron deficiency. Concurrent administration of high doses of **vitamin C** can enhance absorption (particularly when given with SR formulations), but cost/benefit might not warrant its use. Wide variations in dissolution and absorption exist among SR and EC products, and the frequency of adverse effects, although negligible, probably reflects the small amount of ionic iron available for absorption because of transport of the iron past the duodenum and proximal jejunum.[114]

FERROUS SALTS COMPARISON CHART

DRUG	SOLID DOSAGE FORMS[a]	ADULT DOSAGE (CAP OR TAB/DAY)	ELEMENTAL IRON/CAP OR TAB (%)	(mg Fe)	OTHER DOSAGE FORMS[a]
Carbonyl Iron	Cap 50 mg iron.	3	100	50	Susp 12 mg/mL iron.
Ferrous Fumarate	Chew Tab 100 mg	1–4	33	33	Drp 75 mg/mL
	Tab 63, 200, 324, 325, 350 mg.	1–4	33	20, 66	Susp 20 mg/mL.
		1–2	33	106, 106, 115	
Ferrous Gluconate	Tab 240, 325 mg.	3–6	11	27, 36	Elxr 60 mg/mL.
Ferrous Sulfate Exsiccated	SR Tab 160 mg	1–2	30	50	
	Tab 187, 200 mg.	3–4	30	60, 65	
Ferrous Sulfate Hydrous	SR Cap/Tab various	—	20	—	Drp 125 mg/mL
	Cap 250 mg	3	20	50	Elxr 44 mg/mL
	Tab 195, 300, 324 mg.	3–6	20	39	Syrup 18 mg/mL.
		3	20	60, 65	
Polysaccharide-Iron Complex	Cap 150 mg iron	1–2	—	150	Elxr 20 mg/mL iron.
	Tab 50 mg iron.	2–4	—	50	

[a]Doses listed represent total iron salt, not elemental iron, except for carbonyl iron and polysaccharide-iron complex.

FILGRASTIM
Neupogen

Pharmacology. Filgrastim is an *Escherichia coli*–derived (nonglycosylated) re-combinant human granulocyte colony-stimulating factor (G-CSF). G-CSF is one of many glycoprotein hormones that regulate the proliferation and differentiation of hematopoietic progenitor cells and the function of mature blood cells. Specifically, G-CSF promotes proliferation and maturation and enhances the function and migration of neutrophil granulocytes. G-CSF also promotes pre–B-cell activation and growth and acts in synergy with interleukin-3 to support megakaryocyte and platelet production.[104,115]

Administration and Adult Dosage. SC or IV for myelosuppressive cancer chemotherapy 5 μg/kg/day as a single injection. The drug is usually discontinued once the postnadir ANC reaches 1500–2000/μL. Based on severity of ANC nadir, dosage can be increased in 5 μg/kg/day increments for each chemotherapy cycle. **SC continuous infusion for chemotherapy-induced febrile neutropenia** 12 μg/kg/day beginning within 12 hr of empiric antibiotic therapy and continued until ANC is >5000/μL and the patient is afebrile for 4 days.[116] **IV or SC for bone marrow transplant patients** 10 μg/kg/day infused IV over 4 or 24 hr or as a continuous SC infusion and then decreasing to 5 μg/kg/day when ANC is >1000/μL for 3 consecutive days. Discontinue therapy if the ANC remains >1000/μL for 3 more consecutive days; resume at a dosage of 5 μg/kg/day when ANC becomes <1000/μL. **SC for severe chronic neutropenia** (congenital) 6 μg/kg bid; (idiopathic or cyclic) 5 μg/kg/day. Target ANC range is 1500–10,000/μL; decrease dosage if ANC is persistently >10,000/μL. **SC with erythropoietin to decrease hematologic toxicity from zidovudine** 3.6 μg/kg/day initially, increasing or decreasing weekly by 1 μg/kg/day to maintain a target ANC of 1500–5000/μL.[117]

Special Populations. *Pediatric Dosage.* Safety and efficacy not established. **IV or SC** adult dosages in μg/kg are well tolerated.

Geriatric Dosage. Same as adult dosage.

Dosage Forms. Inj 300, 600 μg/mL.

Patient Instructions. Your pharmacist or physician should instruct you on proper dosage, administration, and disposal. Store vials in the refrigerator but do not freeze. Vials are designed for single use only; discard any unused portion. Bring vial to room temperature before administration; do not shake.

Pharmacokinetics. *Onset and Duration.* Increase in neutrophilic band forms occurs within about 60 min after administration. After therapy is discontinued, neutrophil counts return to baseline values in about 4 days.[115]

Fate. Not orally bioavailable. V_d is about 0.15 L/kg; Cl is 0.03–0.042 L/hr/kg.

t½. 3.5–3.85 hr.

Adverse Reactions. Mild to moderate bone pain responsive to non-narcotic analgesics is reported frequently. Transient decreases in blood pressure occur occasionally. During long-term therapy, splenomegaly occurs frequently; occasional exacerbation of skin disorders, alopecia, hematuria, proteinuria, thrombocytopenia, and osteoporosis also are reported. Other adverse effects occur during administration of filgrastim that are likely the consequence of the underlying malignancy or cytotoxic chemotherapy. Acute reactions to sargramostim (eg, febrile episodes, flushing, hypotension, tachycardia, and hypoxia) appear to be more common than with filgrastim.[104,115,117,118]

Contraindications. History of hypersensitivity to *E. coli*–derived proteins. Do not use 24 hr before and 24 hr after administration of cytotoxic chemotherapy.

Precautions. Use with caution in any malignancy with myeloid characteristics because of the possibility of tumor growth. The efficacy of filgrastim has not been established in patients receiving nitrosoureas, mitomycin, fluorouracil, or cytarabine.

Drug Interactions. None known.

Parameters to Monitor. Perform CBC and platelet counts before chemotherapy and twice a week during filgrastim therapy. Regular monitoring of WBC count at the time of recovery from the postchemotherapy nadir is recommended to avoid excessive leukocytosis.

Notes. Other potential uses for filgrastim include AIDS-related neutropenia, myelodysplastic syndromes, and drug-induced neutropenia or aplastic anemia. Further clinical trials are needed to prove that use of filgrastim for these and other indications is beneficial, safe, and cost effective.

IRON DEXTRAN
DexFerrum, InFeD, Various

Pharmacology. (*See* Ferrous Salts.) The overall response to parenteral iron is no more rapid or complete than the response to orally administered iron, so iron dextran is indicated only when oral iron therapy is determined to be ineffective or impossible.

Administration and Adult Dosage. The total cumulative amount required for restoration of hemoglobin (Hb) in g/dL and body stores of iron can be approximated using lean body weight (LBW) in kg (or actual body weight if less than LBW) from the formula:

$$\text{Total mg Iron} = (0.0442 \times [\text{Desired Hb} - \text{Observed Hb}] \times \text{LBW} + [0.26 \times \text{LBW}]) \times 50$$

To calculate dose in mL, divide the result by 50. Usual Hb target for adults is 14.8 g/dL. The dose of iron required secondary to blood loss can be estimated from the formula:

$$\text{Total mg Iron} = \text{Blood Loss (mL)} \times \text{Hematocrit (observed, as decimal fraction)}$$

Deep IM (in upper outer quadrant of buttock only with the Z-track technique) 25 mg (0.5 mL) test dose the first day and then, if no adverse reaction occurs, administer a maximum daily dose of 100 mg (2 mL) until the total calculated amount is reached. **Slow IV** test dose of 25 mg (0.5 mL) over at least 30 sec the first day; if no adverse reaction occurs after at least 1 hr, proceed (until the total calculated amount is reached) by daily increments over 2–3 days, to a maximum dose of 100 mg/day at a rate not to exceed 50 mg/min.[117] **IV in erythropoietin-treated dialysis patients** 100–200 mg/week after dialysis. **Total dose IV infusion** is an off-label use and is discouraged by the FDA but is widely used. The total calculated dose of iron dextran is diluted in 500 mL of NS (dextrose solutions increase local phlebitis) and infused at a rate of 6 mg/min after a 30 mL test dose is delivered over 2 min.[119]

Special Populations. *Pediatric Dosage.* (<4 months) safety and efficacy not established; (5–15 kg) total cumulative amount required for restoration of Hb (in g/dL) and body stores of iron can be estimated using body weight (W) in kg from the formula:

$$\text{Total mg Iron} = (0.0442 \times [\text{Desired Hb} - \text{Observed Hb}] \times W + [0.26 \times W]) \times 50$$

To calculate dose in mL, divide the result by 50. Usual Hb target for children ≤15 kg is 12 g/dL. Maximum daily dose is (infants <5 kg) 25 mg (0.5 mL), (children <10 kg) 50 mg (1 mL), (children >15 kg) same as adult dosage.

Geriatric Dosage. Same as adult dosage.

Dosage Forms. **Inj** 50 mg elemental iron/mL.

Pharmacokinetics. *Onset and Duration.* Hematologic response is the same as with oral therapy, although total body stores of iron are replaced when the above dosage regimens are used.

Serum Levels. (*See* Ferrous Salts.)

Fate. After IV administration, the inert complex is gradually cleared from the plasma by the reticuloendothelial cells of the liver, spleen, and bone marrow. With doses >500 mg, the rate of uptake is 10–20 mg/hr. Iron dextran is then dissociated and released as free ferric iron (at a rate controlled by the serum iron level), which combines with transferrin and is incorporated into hemoglobin within the bone marrow.[119–121] Although all iron is eventually released in this manner, many months often are required for this process to be completed.[110]

Adverse Reactions. Hypotension and peripheral vascular flushing occur with too-rapid IV administration. Mild, transient reactions including flushing, fever, myalgia, arthralgia, and lymphadenopathy usually occur only occasionally but have occurred in 80–90% of patients with active rheumatoid arthritis or active SLE. Immediate anaphylactoid reactions, which can be life-threatening, occur in 0.1–0.6% of patients.[122] A predictive test for predisposition to anaphylaxis is not available. IM administration has been associated with variable degrees of soreness, sterile abscess formation, tissue staining, and sarcoma formation.[120] Total dose infusion appears to be tolerated as well as divided doses.[119]

Contraindications. Anemias other than iron-deficiency anemia; hemochromatosis; hemosiderosis; SC administration.

Precautions. Pregnancy. Use with extreme caution with serious liver impairment. Patients with rheumatoid arthritis might have an acute exacerbation or reactivation of joint pain and swelling after administration. History of allergies and/or asthma. Because of the potential for anaphylactoid reactions, have epinephrine, diphenhydramine, and methylprednisolone immediately available during iron dextran administration. Use parenteral iron only in patients in whom an iron-deficient state has been clearly established and who are not amenable to oral therapy.

Drug Interactions. None known.

Parameters to Monitor. (*See* Ferrous Salts.)

Notes. **Sodium ferric gluconate complex** (Ferrlecit) is an injectable iron product containing 12.5 mg/mL of elemental iron. It is indicated for iron-deficiency anemia in chronic hemodialysis patients receiving epoetin alfa. A test dose is not required, but a test dose of 2 mL in 50 mL of NS given IV over 1 hr has been used. The standard dose is 10 mL/100 mL NS infused over 1 hr. Most patients require a total dosage of 1 g of elemental iron in 8 doses on sequential dialysis sessions to replete iron stores. It might be better tolerated than iron dextran, but it is much more expensive. It is a good alternative in patients intolerant to iron dextran.

Iron sucrose (Venofer) is an injectable iron product containing 20 mg/mL of elemental iron. It is indicated for iron-deficiency anemia in chronic hemodialysis patients receiving epoetin alfa. A test dose is not required, but a test dose of 2.5 mL in 50 mL of NS over 3–10 min has been used. The drug can be given by direct IV injection at a rate of 1 mL (20 mg of iron) per minute or by slow infusion by diluting one vial (100 mg iron) in no more than 100 mL of NS and infusing it over at least 15 min. The recommended dosage is 100 mg of iron (1 vial) no more than 3 times per week to a total of 1 g in 10 doses. This regimen can be repeated if necessary.

SARGRAMOSTIM
Leukine

Pharmacology. Sargramostim is a yeast-derived (glycosylated) recombinant human granulocyte–macrophage colony-stimulating factor (GM-CSF). GM-CSF is one of many glycoprotein hormones that regulate the proliferation and differentiation of hematopoietic progenitor cells and the function of mature blood cells. Specifically, GM-CSF promotes proliferation, maturation, and function of neutrophils, eosinophils, monocytes, and macrophages. GM-CSF also stimulates production of cytokines such as interleukin-1 and tumor necrosis factor.[115,118,123]

Administration and Adult Dosage. **IV after autologous bone marrow infusion** 250 µg/m^2/day given as a 2-hr infusion beginning 2–4 hr after the autologous bone marrow infusion. Give the first dose no sooner than 24 hr after the last chemotherapy dose or 12 hr after the last dose of radiotherapy. Continue sargramostim until the ANC is >1500/µL for 3 consecutive days. **IV for bone marrow transplantation failure or delay in engraftment** 250 µg/m^2/day for 14 days as a 2-hr infusion; repeat in 7 days if engraftment has not occurred. If there is no improvement, a third course with 500 µg/m^2/day given for 14 days can be tried. **IV for induction chemotherapy in acute myelogenous leukemia** 250 µg/m^2/day over 4 hr starting 4 days after completion of chemotherapy if bone marrow is hypoplastic (<5% blasts). Continue until ANC is >1500/µL for 3 consecutive days or at most 42 days. Discontinue or reduce dosage by 50% if ANC is >20,000/µL. Discontinue if leukemic regrowth occurs. **SC for AIDS patients receiving ganciclovir** 1–15 µg/kg/day has been used investigationally.

Dosage Forms. Inj 250, 500 µg.

Adverse Reactions. Acute reactions (eg, febrile episodes, flushing, hypotension, tachycardia, and hypoxia) appear to be more common than with filgrastim. Other adverse reactions that occur frequently with sargramostim are bone pain, lethargy, rash, and fluid retention.

Parameters to Monitor. Obtain CBC with differential twice weekly. In patients with renal or hepatic insufficiency, monitor renal and hepatic functions q 2 weeks.

Notes. Sargramostim is indicated for myeloid reconstitution after autologous bone marrow transplantation. It has also been used with some success to maintain normal neutrophil counts in AIDS patients receiving **ganciclovir.** Other potential uses for sargramostim are AIDS-related neutropenia, myelodysplastic syndromes, and congenital, chronic, or drug-induced neutropenia, and aplastic anemia. Controlled clinical trials are needed to prove that use for these and other indications is beneficial, safe, and cost effective. Clinical and laboratory evidence suggest that sargramostim enhances the effect of **zidovudine** against HIV.[104,115,118,123–125]

REFERENCES

1. Dobesh PP, Latham KA. Advancing the battle against acute ischemic syndromes: a focus on the GP IIb–IIIa inhibitors. *Pharmacotherapy* 1998;18:663–85.
2. LeBreton H et al. Role of platelets in restenosis after percutaneous coronary revascularization. *J Am Coll Cardiol* 1996;28:1643–51.
3. The EPILOG Investigators. Platelet glycoprotein IIb/IIIa receptor blockade and low-dose heparin during percutaneous coronary revascularization. *N Engl J Med* 1997;336:1689–96.
4. Hyers TM et al. Antithrombotic therapy for venous thromboembolic disease. *Chest* 1995;108:335S–51.
5. Lutomski DM et al. Pharmacokinetic optimisation of the treatment of embolic disorders. *Clin Pharmacokinet* 1995;28:67–92.
6. International Society and Federation of Cardiology and World Health Organization Task Force on Myocardial Reperfusion. Reperfusion in acute myocardial infarction. *Circulation* 1994;90:2091–102.
7. Becker RC, Ansell J. Antithrombotic therapy: an abbreviated reference for clinicians. *Arch Intern Med* 1995;155:149–61.
8. The GUSTO Investigators. An international randomized trial comparing four thrombolytic strategies for acute myocardial infarction. *N Engl J Med* 1993;329:673–82.
9. Levine LZ et al. A randomized trial of a single bolus dosage regimen of recombinant tissue plasminogen activator in patients with acute pulmonary embolism. *Chest* 1990;98:1473–9.
10. Cairns JA et al. Coronary thrombolysis. *Chest* 1995;108:401S–23.
11. The National Institute of Neurological Disorders rt-PA Stroke Study Group. Tissue plasminogen activator for acute ischemic stroke. *N Engl J Med* 1995;333:1581–7.
12. Davis SN et al. Activity and dosage of alteplase dilution for clearing occlusions of venous access devices. *Am J Health-Syst Pharm* 2000;57:1039–45.
13. Benet LZ et al. Design and optimization of dosage regimens; pharmacokinetic data. In, Hardman JG et al., eds. *Goodman and Gilman's the pharmacological basis of therapeutics.* 9th ed. New York: McGraw-Hill; 1996:1707–92.
14. Third International Study of Infarct Survival Collaborative Study. ISIS-3: a randomized comparison of streptokinase vs tissue plasminogen activator vs anistreplase and of aspirin plus heparin vs aspirin alone among 41,299 cases of suspected acute myocardial infarct. *Lancet* 1992;339:753–70.
15. Nicolini FA et al. Concurrent nitroglycerin therapy impairs tissue-type plasminogen activator-induced thrombolysis in patients with acute myocardial infarction. *Am J Cardiol* 1994;74:662–6.
16. Fuster V. Coronary thrombolysis—a perspective for the practicing physician. *N Engl J Med* 1993;329:723–4.
17. The Continuous Infusion Versus Double-Bolus Administration of Alteplase (COBALT) Investigators. A comparison of continuous infusion of alteplase with double-bolus administration for acute myocardial infarction. *N Engl J Med* 1997;337:1124–30.
18. Munger MA, Forrence EA. Anistreplase: a new thrombolytic for the treatment of acute myocardial infarction. *Clin Pharm* 1990;9:530–40.

19. O'Connor CM et al. A randomized trial of intravenous heparin in conjunction with anistreplase (anisoylated plasminogen streptokinase activator complex) in acute myocardial infarction: the Duke University Clinical Cardiology Study (DUCCS) 1. *J Am Coll Cardiol* 1994;23:11–8.

20. Januzzi JL Jr, Jang I-K. Heparin induced thrombocytopenia: diagnosis and contemporary antithrombin management. *J Thromb Thrombol* 1999;7:259–64.

21. Swan SK et al. Comparison of anticoagulant effects and safety of argatroban and heparin in healthy subjects. *Pharmacotherapy* 2000;20:756–70.

22. Kawada T et al. Clinical application of argatroban as an alternative anticoagulant for extracorporeal circulation. *Hematol Oncol Clin North Am* 2000;14:445–7.

23. Bennet CL et al. Thrombotic thrombocytopenic purpura associated with clopidogrel. *N Engl J Med* 2000;342:1773–7.

24. CAPRIE Steering Committee. A randomised, blinded, trial of clopidogrel versus aspirin in patients at risk for ischaemic events (CAPRIE). *Lancet* 1996;348:1329–39.

25. Howard PA. Dalteparin: a low-molecular-weight heparin. *Ann Pharmacother* 1997;31:192–203.

26. Green D et al. Low molecular weight heparin: a critical analysis of clinical trials. *Pharmacol Rev* 1994;46:89–109.

27. Noble S et al. Enoxaparin. A reappraisal of its pharmacology and clinical applications in the prevention and treatment of thromboembolic disease. *Drugs* 1995;49:388–410.

28. Levine M et al. A comparison of low-molecular-weight heparin administered primarily at home with unfractionated heparin administered in the hospital for proximal deep-vein thrombosis. *N Engl J Med* 1996;334:677–81.

29. Lensing AWA et al. Treatment of deep venous thrombosis with low-molecular-weight heparins. A meta-analysis. *Arch Intern Med* 1995;155:601–7.

30. Verstraete M. Pharmacotherapeutic aspects of unfractionated and low molecular weight heparins. *Drugs* 1990;40:498–530.

31. de Valk HW et al. Comparing subcutaneous danaparoid with intravenous unfractionated heparin for the treatment of venous thromboembolism. A randomized controlled trial. *Ann Intern Med* 1995;123:1–9.

32. The IMPACT-II Investigators. Randomised placebo-controlled trial of effect of eptifibatide on complications of percutaneous coronary intervention: IMPACT-II. *Lancet* 1997;349:1422–8.

33. The PURSUIT Trial Investigators. Inhibition of platelet glycoprotein IIb/IIIa with eptifibatide in patients with acute coronary syndromes. *N Engl J Med* 1998;339:436–43.

34. Carter BL. Therapy of acute thromboembolism with heparin and warfarin. *Clin Pharm* 1991;10:503–18.

35. Raschke RA et al. The weight-based heparin dosing nomogram compared with a "standard care" nomogram. A randomized controlled trial. *Ann Intern Med* 1993;119:874–81.

36. Kershaw B et al. Computer-assisted dosing of heparin. Management with pharmacy-based anticoagulation service. *Arch Intern Med* 1994;154:1005–11.

37. Gunnarsson PS et al. Appropriate use of heparin. Empiric vs nomogram-based dosing. *Arch Intern Med* 1995;155:526–32.

38. Simon TL et al. Heparin pharmacokinetics: increased requirements in pulmonary embolism. *Br J Haematol* 1978;39:111–20.

39. Kruchoski ME, Emory CE. Initiating heparin and warfarin therapy concurrently. *Hosp Pharm* 1986;21:174.

40. Hull RD et al. Heparin for 5 days as compared with 10 days in the initial treatment of proximal venous thrombosis. *N Engl J Med* 1990;322:1260–4.

41. Melamed AJ, Suarez J. Detection and prevention of deep venous thrombosis. *Drug Intell Clin Pharm* 1988;22:107–14.

42. Cooke HM, Lynch A. Biorhythms and chronotherapy in cardiovascular disease. *Am J Hosp Pharm* 1994;51:2569–80.

43. Estes JW. Clinical pharmacokinetics of heparin. *Clin Pharmacokinet* 1980;5:204–20.

44. Hirsh J et al. Heparin kinetics in venous thrombosis and pulmonary embolism. *Circulation* 1976;53:691–5.

45. Landefeld CS et al. A bleeding risk index for estimating the probability of major bleeding in hospitalized patients starting anticoagulant therapy. *Am J Med* 1990;89:569–78.

46. Bailey RT et al. Heparin-associated thrombocytopenia: a prospective comparison of bovine lung heparin, manufactured by a new process, and porcine intestinal heparin. *Drug Intell Clin Pharm* 1986;20:374–8.

47. Becker PS, Miller VT. Heparin-induced thrombocytopenia. *Stroke* 1989;20:1449–59.

48. Oster JR et al. Heparin-induced aldosterone suppression and hyperkalemia. *Am J Med* 1995;98:575–86.

49. Gupta AK et al. Heparin-induced thrombocytopenia. *Ann Pharmacother* 1998;32:55–9.

50. Verstraete M. Direct thrombin inhibitors: appraisal of the antithrombotic/hemorrhagic balance. *Thromb Haemost* 1997;78:357–63.

51. Uotila L. The metabolic functions and mechanism of action of vitamin K. *Scand J Clin Lab Invest* 1990;201(suppl):109–17.

52. Hardman JG et al., eds. *Goodman and Gilman's the pharmacological basis of therapeutics.* 9th ed. New York: McGraw-Hill; 1996:1583–5.

53. Thorp JA et al. Current concepts and controversies in the use of vitamin K. *Drugs* 1995;49:376–87.

54. Frick PG et al. Dose response and minimal daily requirement for vitamin K in man. *J Appl Physiol* 1967;23:387–9.

55. Mattea EJ, Quinn K. Adverse reactions after intravenous phytonadione administration. *Hosp Pharm* 1981;16:224–35.

56. Food and Nutrition Board, NRC. *Recommended dietary allowances.* 10th ed. Washington, DC: National Academy Press; 1989.

57. Hirsch J et al. Oral anticoagulants. Mechanism of action, clinical effectiveness, and optimal therapeutic range. *Chest* 1998;114(suppl):445S.

58. Patel RJ et al. Randomized, placebo-controlled trial of oral phytonadione for excessive anticoagulation. *Pharmacotherapy* 2000;20:1159–66.

59. Koch-Weser J, Sellers EM. Drug interactions with coumarin anticoagulants (2 parts). *N Engl J Med* 1971;285:487–9,547–58.

60. Zieve PD, Solomon HM. Variation in the response of human beings to vitamin K. *J Lab Clin Med* 1969;73:103–10.

61. Woolf IL, Babior BM. Vitamin K and warfarin. *Am J Med* 1972;53:261–7.

62. O'Reilly RA et al. Intravenous vitamin K1 injections: dangerous prophylaxis. *Arch Intern Med* 1995;155:2127.

63. Noble S, McTavish D. Reteplase. A review of its pharmacological properties and clinical efficacy in the management of acute myocardial infarction. *Drugs* 1996;52:589–605.

64. Lopez LM. Clinical trials in thrombolytic therapy, Part 2: The open-artery hypothesis and RAPID-1 and RAPID-2. *Am J Health-Syst Pharm* 1997;54(suppl 1):S27–30.

65. The Global Use of Strategies To Open Occluded Coronary Arteries (GUSTO III) Investigators. A comparison of reteplase with alteplase for acute myocardial infarction. *New Engl J Med* 1997;337:1118–23.

66. Randomised, double-blind comparison of reteplase double-bolus administration with streptokinase in acute myocardial infarction: trial to investigate equivalence. International Joint Efficacy Comparison of Thrombolytics (INJECT). *Lancet* 1995;346:329–36.

67. Rogers LQ, Lutcher CL. Streptokinase therapy for deep vein thrombosis: a comprehensive review of the English literature. *Am J Med* 1990;88:389–95.

68. Katzen BT, van Breda A. Low dose streptokinase in the treatment of arterial occlusion. *AJR* 1981;136:1171–8.

69. Belkin M et al. Intra-arterial fibrinolytic therapy. *Arch Surg* 1986;121:769–73.

70. Fletcher AP et al. The maintenance of a sustained thrombolytic state in man. I. Induction and effects. *J Clin Invest* 1959;38:1096–110.

71. Fletcher AP et al. The clearance of heterologous protein from the circulation of normal and immunized man. *J Clin Invest* 1958;37:1306–15.

72. Sherry S et al. Thrombolytic therapy in thrombosis: a National Institutes of Health consensus development conference. *Ann Intern Med* 1980;93:141–4.

73. Levine MN et al. Hemorrhagic complications of thrombolytic therapy in the treatment of myocardial infarction and venous embolism. *Chest* 1995;108:291S–301.

74. Goldhaber SZ. Contemporary pulmonary embolism thrombolysis. *Chest* 1995;107(suppl):45S–51.

75. Marder VJ. The use of thrombolytic agents: choice of patient, drug administration, laboratory monitoring. *Ann Intern Med* 1979;90:802–8.

76. Smalling RW. A fresh look at the molecular pharmacology of plasminogen activators: from theory to test tube to clinical outcomes. *Am J Health-Syst Pharm* 1997;54:S17–22.

77. ASSENT-2 Investigators. Single-bolus tenecteplase compared with front-loaded alteplase in acute myocardial infarction: the ASSENT-2 double-blind randomised trial. *Lancet* 1999;354:716–22.

78. Haynes RB et al. A critical appraisal of ticlopidine, a new antiplatelet agent. Effectiveness and clinical indications for prophylaxis of atherosclerotic events. *Arch Intern Med* 1992;152:1376–80.

79. Matchar DB et al. Medical treatment for stroke prevention. *Ann Intern Med* 1994;121:41–53.

80. Carlson JA, Maesner JE. Fatal neutropenia and thrombocytopenia associated with ticlopidine. *Ann Pharmacother* 1994;28:1236–8.

81. Cassidy LJ et al. Probable ticlopidine-induced cholestatic hepatitis. *Ann Pharmacother* 1995;29:30–2.

82. Hass WK et al. A randomized trial comparing ticlopidine hydrochloride with aspirin for the prevention of stroke in high-risk patients. *N Engl J Med* 1989;321:501–7.

83. Gent M et al. The Canadian American Ticlopidine Study (CATS) in thromboembolic stroke. *Lancet* 1989;1:1215–20.

84. The PRISM-PLUS Study Investigators. Inhibition of the platelet glycoprotein IIb/IIIa receptor with tirofiban in unstable angina and non-Q-wave myocardial infarction. *N Engl J Med* 1998;338:1488–97.

85. Haire WD, Lieberman RP. Thrombosed central venous catheters: restoring function with 6-hour urokinase infusion after failure of bolus urokinase. *JPEN* 1992;16:129–32.

86. Breckenridge A et al. Pharmacokinetics and pharmacodynamics of the enantiomers of warfarin in man. *Clin Pharmacol Ther* 1974;15:424–30.

87. Fihn SD. Aiming for safe anticoagulation. *N Engl J Med* 1995;333:54–5. Editorial.

88. Bern MM et al. Very low doses of warfarin can prevent thrombosis in central venous catheters. *Ann Intern Med* 1990;112:423–8.

89. O'Reilly RA, Aggeler PM. Determinants of the response to oral anticoagulant drugs in man. *Pharmacol Rev* 1970;22:35–96.

90. Nagashima R et al. Kinetics of pharmacologic effects in man: the anticoagulant action of warfarin. *Clin Pharmacol Ther* 1969;10:22–35.

91. Lutomski DM et al. Warfarin absorption after massive small bowel resection. *Am J Gastroenterol* 1985;80:99–102.

92. Slaughter RL, Edwards DJ. Recent advances: the cytochrome P450 enzymes. *Ann Pharmacother* 1995;29:619–24.

93. Yacobi A et al. Serum protein binding as a determinant of warfarin body clearance and anticoagulant effect. *Clin Pharmacol Ther* 1976;19:552–8.

94. Lewis RJ et al. Warfarin metabolites: the anticoagulant activity and pharmacology of warfarin alcohols. *J Lab Clin Med* 1973;81:925–31.

95. O'Reilly RA et al. Studies on the coumarin anticoagulant drugs: the pharmacodynamics of warfarin in man. *J Clin Invest* 1963;42:1542–51.

96. Williams RL et al. Influence of acute viral hepatitis on disposition and pharmacologic effect of warfarin. *Clin Pharmacol Ther* 1976;20:90–7.

97. Hirsh J. Drug therapy: oral anticoagulant drugs. *N Engl J Med* 1991;324:1865–75.

98. Landefeld CS, Goldman L. Major bleeding in outpatients treated with warfarin: incidence and prediction by factors known at the start of outpatient therapy. *Am J Med* 1989;87:144–52.

99. Hansten PD, Horn JR. *Drug interactions and updates quarterly.* Vancouver, WA: Applied Therapeutics; 2001. Updated quarterly.

100. Tatro DS, ed. *Drug interaction facts.* Philadelphia: JB Lippincott; 2001. Updated quarterly.

101. Deykin D. Warfarin therapy (second of two parts). *N Engl J Med* 1970;283:801–3.

102. Hirsh J. The optimal duration of anticoagulant therapy for venous thrombosis. *N Engl J Med* 1995;332:1710–1. Editorial.

103. Schwenk MH, Halstenson CE. Recombinant human erythropoietin. *DICP* 1989;23:528–36.

104. Petersdorf SH, Dale DC. The biology and clinical applications of erythropoietin and the colony-stimulating factors. *Adv Intern Med* 1995;40:395–428.

105. Erslev AJ. Erythropoietin. *N Engl J Med* 1991;324:1339–44.

106. Zachée P. Controversies in selection of epoetin dosages. Issues and answers. *Drugs* 1995;49:536–47.

107. Ohis RK, Christensen RD. Recombinant erythropoietin compared with erythrocyte transfusion in the treatment of anemia of prematurity. *J Pediatr* 1991;119:781–8.

108. Ongkingco JR et al. Use of low-dose subcutaneous recombinant human erythropoietin in end-stage renal disease: experience with children receiving continuous cycling peritoneal dialysis. *Am J Kidney Dis* 1991;18:446–50.

109. Rigden SP et al. Recombinant human erythropoietin therapy in children maintained by haemodialysis. *Pediatr Nephrol* 1990;4:618–22.

110. Hardman JG et al., eds. *Goodman and Gilman's the pharmacological basis of therapeutics.* 9th ed. New York: McGraw-Hill; 1996.

111. Koeller JM, Van Den Berg C. Anemias. In, Koda-Kimble MA, Young LY, eds. *Applied therapeutics: the clinical use of drugs.* 6th ed. Vancouver, WA: Applied Therapeutics; 1995:88.3–88.17.

112. Stevens RG. Iron and the risk of cancer. *Med Oncol Tumor Pharmacother* 1990;7:177–81.

113. Olson KR, ed. *Poisoning and drug overdose.* Norwalk, CT: Appleton & Lange; 1990.

114. Middleton EJ et al. Studies on the absorption of orally administered iron from sustained-release preparations. *N Engl J Med* 1966;274:136–9.

115. Anon. G-CSF and GM-CSF: white blood cell growth factors. *Hosp Pharm* 1990;25:881–2.

116. Maher DW et al. Filgrastim in patients with chemotherapy-induced febrile neutropenia. *Ann Intern Med* 1994;121:492–501.

117. Miles SA et al. Combined therapy with recombinant granulocyte colony-stimulating factor and erythropoietin decreases hematologic toxicity zidovudine. *Blood* 1991;77:2109–17.

118. Demuynck H et al. Comparative study of peripheral blood progenitor cell collection in patients with multiple myeloma after single-dose cyclophosphamide combined with rhGM-CSF or rhG-CSF. *Br J Haematol* 1995;90:384–92.

119. Auerbach M et al. A randomized trial of three iron dextran infusion methods for anemia in EPO-treated dialysis patients. *Am J Kidney Dis* 1998;31:81–6.

120. Kumpf VJ, Holland EG. Parenteral iron dextran therapy. *DICP* 1990;24:162–6.

121. Wood JK et al. The metabolism of iron-dextran given as a total-dose infusion to iron deficient Jamaican subjects. *Br J Haematol* 1968;14:119–29.

122. Novey HS et al. Immunologic studies of anaphylaxis to iron dextran in patients on renal dialysis. *Ann Allergy* 1994;72:224–8.

123. Hogan KR, Peters MD. Granulocyte-macrophage colony-stimulating factor in neutropenia. *DICP* 1991;25:32–5.

124. Grossberg HS, Bonnem EM. GM-CSF with ganciclovir for the treatment of CMV retinitis in AIDS. *N Engl J Med* 1989;320:1560. Letter.

125. Groopman JE. Granulocyte-macrophage colony-stimulating factor in human immunodeficiency virus disease. *Semin Hematol* 1990;27(suppl 3):8–14.

Hormonal Drugs

Adrenal Hormones

Class Instructions. Corticosteroids. (Systemic use) these drugs may be taken with food, milk, or an antacid to minimize stomach upset. Take single daily doses or alternate-day doses in the morning before 9 AM. Take multiple daily doses at evenly spaced intervals during the day. Report unusual weight gain, lower extremity swelling, muscle weakness, black tarry stools, vomiting of blood, facial swelling, menstrual irregularities, prolonged sore throat, fever, cold, infection, serious injury, fatigue, anorexia, nausea, vomiting, diarrhea, weight loss, dizziness, or low blood sugar. Consult your physician during periods of increased stress. If you are diabetic, you may have increased requirements for insulin or oral hypoglycemics. Carry appropriate identification if you are taking long-term corticosteroid therapy. Do not discontinue this medication without medical approval; tell any new health care provider that you are taking a corticosteroid. Avoid immunizations with live vaccines.

Missed Doses. If a dose is missed and the proper schedule is *every other day,* take it as soon as possible and resume the schedule unless it is past noon. In that case, wait until the next morning and resume every-other-day administration. If the proper schedule is *once a day,* take the dose as soon as possible. If you do not remember until the next day, do not double that day's dose; skip the missed dose. If the proper schedule is *several times a day,* take the dose as soon as possible and resume the normal schedule. If you do not remember until the next dose is due, then take the regular and missed doses and resume the normal dosage schedule.

COSYNTROPIN
Cortrosyn

Pharmacology. Cosyntropin is a synthetic polypeptide containing the first 24 of the 39 amino acids of natural **corticotropin (adrenocorticotropic hormone; ACTH)** and retaining the full activity of corticotropin with decreased antigenicity. Cosyntropin 250 μg is pharmacologically equivalent to corticotropin 25 units. Cosyntropin stimulates the adrenal cortex to produce and secrete gluco- and mineralocorticoids and androgens similar to corticotropin. Cosyntropin is used as a diagnostic agent to detect adrenocortical insufficiency but can be used therapeutically as a substitute for corticotropin.

Adult Dosage. IM or IV for diagnostic use hold all exogenous corticosteroids (except dexamethasone) on the test day because of assay cross-reactivity and, if the patient is not taking spironolactone or an estrogen, a baseline cortisol level (which should exceed 5 μg/dL) is drawn in the morning just before the dose. Then, cosyntropin 250 μg in 1 mL of NS is given IM, or 250 μg in 2–5 mL NS is given IV push over 2 min. Normal cortisol levels are >18 μg/dL (500 nmol/L)

631

30 min after the injection and ≥7 μg/dL (190 nmol/L) above baseline. If the cortisol level is drawn 60 min postadministration, then an approximate doubling of the baseline cortisol value indicates a normal response. Alternatively, give an infusion of 250 μg in D5W or NS over 6 hr in the morning, with serum cortisol levels drawn before and after. The second cortisol level should be >18 μg/dL (500 nmol/L) and ≥7 μg/dL (190 nmol/L) above baseline. **IV for therapeutic use** 250 μg infused IV over 8 hr elicits maximal adrenocortical secretion.[1,2]

Pediatric Dosage. IM or IV as a diagnostic agent (≤2 yr) 125 μg given as above.

Geriatric Dosage. Same as adult dosage.

Dosage Forms. Inj 250 μg.

Adverse Reactions. (Diagnostic use) rare reports of hypersensitivity. (Therapeutic use) salt and water retention, and virilization occur.

DEXAMETHASONE	Decadron, Hexadrol, Various

Pharmacology. Dexamethasone is a potent, long-acting glucocorticoid lacking sodium-retaining activity with low to moderate doses. (*See* Prednisone Pharmacology and the Oral Corticosteroids Comparison Chart.)

Administration and Adult Dosage. Total daily dosage is variable depending on the clinical disorder and patient response. Not recommended for alternate-day administration because of prolonged duration of activity. **PO, IM, or IV for acute, self-limited allergic disorders or exacerbation of chronic allergic disorders** 4–8 mg on the first day in one dose, then taper over 5 days; give tapering dosage in 2 divided doses for 3 days, once daily for 2 days, then discontinue. **IV for cerebral edema** 10 mg (as the sodium phosphate) initially, followed by 4 mg IM or IV q 6 hr for several days until maximal response occurs; then decrease the dosage over 5–7 days and discontinue. **PO, IM, or IV for palliative management of recurrent or inoperable brain tumors** 2 mg bid-tid. **PO or IV as an antiemetic with cancer chemotherapy** (usually in combination with other antiemetics) 10–20 mg immediately before therapy; optionally, up to 40 mg may be given after chemotherapy.[3,4] **PO as the dexamethasone suppression test to screen for Cushing's disease** 1 mg at 11 PM; a measured serum cortisol at 8 AM the next morning <5 μg/dL (140 nmol/L) indicates a normal response.[5] Alternatively, PO 0.5 mg q 6 hr for 48 hr (8 doses), with a 24-hr urine collected for 17-hydroxycorticosteroids (17-OHCs) during the second 24-hr period. A normal response is ≤2.5 mg (6.9 μmol) of 17-OHCs during the second 24-hr period.[5] **PO as a Cushing's syndrome test to distinguish pituitary origin from other causes** 2 mg q 6 hr for 48 hr (8 doses). A normal response is a 24-hr urine concentration of <2.5 mg (6.9 μmol) of 17-OHCs.[5] (*See* Notes.) **IM (aqueous) in the mother for antenatal prevention of neonatal distress syndrome** starting 24 hr or more before premature delivery, give 6 mg q 12 hr for 4 doses; however, betamethasone may be the preferred agent.[6,7] (*See* Notes.) **IV for septic shock** not recommended because of a lack of efficacy and a possible increase in mortality.[8] **IM (depot) for prolonged systemic effect** 8–16 mg q 1–3 weeks. (*See also* Inhaled Corticosteroids Comparison Chart in the Respiratory Drugs section.)

Special Populations. *Pediatric Dosage.* **PO, IM, or IV for airway edema** 0.25–0.5 mg/kg/dose q 6 hr prn for croup or beginning 24 hr before planned extubation, then for 4–6 doses; **PO, IM, or IV as an anti-inflammatory or immunosuppressive** 0.03–0.15 mg/kg/day divided q 6–12 hr; **PO, IM, or IV for cerebral edema** 1.5 mg/kg once, then 1.5 mg/kg/day divided q 4–6 hr for 5 days, then taper over the next 5 days and discontinue. **IV to prevent hearing loss and other neurologic sequelae in** *Haemophilus influenzae* **bacterial meningitis** (>2 months) 0.15 mg/kg q 6 hr, beginning no sooner than 20 min before (or with) the first dose of antibiotics and continued for 4 days.[8–10]

Geriatric Dosage. Consider using a lower dosage for decreased body size.

Patient Instructions. (*See* Class Instructions: Corticosteroids.)

Dosage Forms. **Elxr** 0.1 mg/mL; **Soln** 0.1, 1 mg/mL; **Tab** 0.25, 0.5, 0.75, 1, 1.5, 2, 4, 6 mg; **Inj** 4, 10, 20, 24 mg/mL (as sodium phosphate); **Depot Inj** 8, 16 mg/mL (as acetate).

Pharmacokinetics. *Onset and Duration.* (*See* Oral Corticosteroids Comparison Chart.)

Serum Levels. Serum concentration is not directly correlated with therapeutic effect.[11]

Fate. After oral administration, 78 ± 14% is absorbed; 68% is plasma protein bound. V_d is 0.82 ± 0.22 L/kg. The drug is eliminated primarily by hepatic metabolism, with about 2.6 ± 0.6% excreted unchanged in urine.[2,12,13]

$t_{1/2}$. (Males) 3.5 ± 0.87 hr; (females) 2.4 ± 0.16 hr.[2,12,13]

Adverse Reactions. (*See* Prednisone Adverse Reactions.) Perineal itching or burning can occur after IV administration.[14]

Contraindications. Systemic fungal infections (except as maintenance therapy in adrenal insufficiency); administration of live virus vaccines to patients receiving an immunosuppressive dosage of dexamethasone; IM use in idiopathic thrombocytopenic purpura.

Precautions. (*See* Prednisone.)

Parameters to Monitor. (*See* Prednisone.)

Notes. The dexamethasone suppression test for diagnosis of depression is of unproven value.[15,16] Variations of the dexamethasone suppression test (for Cushing's disease screening) have been used.[5] Betamethasone appears to be the corticosteroid of choice for prevention of neonatal distress; the maternal dosage is 12 mg IM q 24 hr for 2 doses (usually as Celestone Soluspan).[6,7]

METHYLPREDNISOLONE SODIUM SUCCINATE   Solu-Medrol, Various

Pharmacology. Methylprednisolone sodium succinate is an injectable glucocorticoid that has about 1.25 times greater anti-inflammatory potency than prednisone or prednisolone and a similar duration of biologic activity. (*See* Prednisone Pharmacology, Oral Corticosteroids Comparison Chart.) It is commonly used when oral therapy is not possible and in situations in which large parenteral doses are necessary.

Administration and Adult Dosage. **IV initial dosage** 10–40 mg given over one to several minutes; dosages up to 30 mg/kg q 4–6 hr (high-dose therapy) for up to 48–72 hr are used for severe, acute conditions. Infuse large doses (≥500 mg) slowly (eg, over 30–60 min) because arrhythmias and sudden death have occurred with rapid infusions.[17] **IV for acute spinal cord injury** 30 mg/kg over 15 min, begun within 8 hr of injury, followed 45 min later by a continuous IV infusion of 5.4 mg/kg/hr for 23 hr.[18,19] (*See* Notes.)

Special Populations. *Pediatric Dosage.* IV as an anti-inflammatory or immunosuppressive 0.16–0.8 mg/kg/day in 2–4 divided doses.[9]

Geriatric Dosage. In the elderly, consider using lower dosages for decreased body size.

Dosage Forms. **Inj** 40, 125, 500 mg, 1, 2 g; **Depot Inj** (as acetate) 20, 40, 80 mg/mL. (*See also* Oral Corticosteroids Comparison Chart.)

Pharmacokinetics. Plasma protein binding is 78 ± 3%. V_d is 1.2 ± 0.2 L/kg; Cl is 0.37 ± 0.054 L/hr/kg. The drug is extensively metabolized, with 4.9 ± 2.3% excreted unchanged in urine. The serum half-life is 2.2 ± 0.5 hr and is not affected by renal function.[2,13]

Adverse Reactions. Side effects are similar to prednisone in equivalent dosages.

Drug Interactions. Ketoconazole and some macrolide antibiotics reduce methylprednisolone elimination, possibly leading to excessive corticosteroid effect. (*See also* Prednisone Drug Interactions.)

Notes. Evidence of efficacy in improving the outcome of septic shock is lacking, and, because of increased mortality in some patient groups, the use of methylprednisolone in septic shock is not recommended.[8] Small, early studies in patients with acute spinal cord injury treated with high-dose methylprednisolone within 8 hr appeared to show improved neurologic recovery,[2,18,20] although the bulk of evidence indicates no such benefit.[21]

PREDNISONE
Deltasone, Orasone, Various

Pharmacology. Prednisone is a synthetic glucocorticoid with less sodium-retaining activity than hydrocortisone. Prednisone is inactive until converted into **prednisolone.** At the cellular level, glucocorticoids appear to act by controlling the rate of protein synthesis mediated through gene transcription. Clinically, these drugs are used primarily for their anti-inflammatory and immunosuppressant effects.[22]

Administration and Adult Dosage. Total daily dosage is variable and must be individualized depending on the clinical disorder and patient response.[2,5] Daily divided high-dose therapy for initial control of more severe disease states may be necessary until satisfactory control is obtained, usually 4–10 days for many allergic and collagen diseases. Administration of a short- or intermediate-acting preparation given as a single dose in the morning (before 9 AM) is likely to produce fewer side effects and less pituitary–adrenal suppression than a divided dosage regimen with the same agent or an equivalent dosage of a long-acting agent. Alternate-day therapy (ie, total 48-hr dosage administered every other morning) with intermediate-acting agents (eg, prednisone) further reduces the prevalence and degree of side effects. However, it might not be uniformly effective in treating all disease states, unless large doses are used (eg, 40–60 mg every other day for adults requiring long-term corticosteroid therapy for asthma). Complete adrenal suppression might not occur with single daily doses given in the morning if the prednisone dose is ≤15 mg, but Cushing's syndrome can still occur and patients should receive supplemental corticosteroids during periods of unusual stress.[5,20] **In times of stress** (eg, surgery, severe trauma, serious illness), patients on long-term corticosteroid therapy (>5 mg/day prednisone or equivalent) should receive supplemental IV **hydrocortisone** 100–300 mg/day or PO prednisone 25–75 mg/day in divided doses for 1–3 days.[1,2,5,20] Guidelines for withdrawal from glucocorticoid therapy have been published.[1,5]

Common initial doses are: **PO for acute asthma exacerbations in adults and adolescents** 40–60 mg/day in 1 or 2 doses for 3–10 days; hospitalized patients may require a parenteral preparation and a larger dosage (eg, methylprednisolone 120–180 mg/day in 3–4 divided doses for 48 hr, then 60–80 mg/day).[23] Reduce dosage to minimum effective maintenance dosage as soon as possible; **PO as an adjunct therapy for** *Pneumocystis carinii* **pneumonia** (with an arterial PO_2 ≤70 mm Hg or an arterial–alveolar gradient ≥35 mm Hg) 40 mg bid for 5 days begun with antimicrobial therapy, then 20 mg bid for 5 days, then 20 mg/day for the duration of antimicrobial therapy;[22,24] **PO for rheumatoid arthritis** 5–7.5 mg/day;[2] **PO for collagen diseases** 1 mg/kg/day in divided doses;[2] **PO for acute gout** 30–50 mg/day, gradually decreasing over 10 days;[25] **PO for nephrotic syndrome** 1–2 mg/kg/day;[2] **PO for skin disorders** 40 mg/day, up to 120 mg/day in pemphigus;[2] **PO for ulcerative colitis** 10–30 mg/day or, if severe, 60–120 mg/day;[2] **PO for thrombocytopenia** 0.5 mg/kg/day;[2] **PO for organ transplantation** (in combination with other immunosuppressants) 50–100 mg once, then taper dosage and make further dosage adjustments based on the clinical situation;[2] **PO for acute exacerbations of multiple sclerosis** 200 mg/day for 1 week, then 80 mg every other day for 1 month.

Special Populations. *Pediatric Dosage.* Dosage depends on disease state and patient response rather than strict adherence to age or body weight. *Common initial doses are:* **PO for acute asthma** 1–2 mg/kg/day, to a maximum of 60 mg/day in 1–2 divided doses for 3–10 days; hospitalized patients may require a parenteral preparation and a larger dosage (eg, methylprednisolone 1 mg/kg q 6 hr for 48 hr, then 1–2 mg/kg/day, to a maximum of 60 mg/day, in 2 divided doses).[23] **PO for inflammation or immunosuppression** 0.5–2 mg/kg/day in 1–4 divided doses.[26]

Geriatric Dosage. Consider using lower dosages for decreased body size.

Dosage Forms. **Soln** 1, 5 mg/mL; **Syrup** 1 mg/mL; **Tab** 1, 2.5, 5, 10, 20, 50 mg.

Patient Instructions. (*See* Class Instructions: Corticosteroids.)

Pharmacokinetics. *Onset and Duration.* (*See* Oral Corticosteroids Comparison Chart.)

Serum Levels. Serum concentration is not directly correlated with therapeutic effect.[5,11] A timed prednisolone serum drug level can be useful for estimating clearance and identifying abnormalities in absorption, elimination, or patient compliance.[27]

Fate. Bioavailability is 80 ± 11%, prednisone is about 75% plasma protein bound and prednisolone is 90–95% plasma protein bound, depending on serum concentration.[2] Prednisone is metabolized in the liver to its active form, prednisolone.[11] Liver disease does not impair conversion to active metabolite. In fact, patients with liver disease and hypoalbuminemia are more likely to suffer major side effects of prednisone as a result of decreased protein binding and reduced prednisolone clearance.[11,28,29] V_d of prednisolone is 1.5 ± 0.2 L/kg; 3 ± 2% of a dose of prednisone is excreted unchanged in urine, with an additional 15 ± 5% excreted as prednisolone.[2]

t₁/₂. (Prednisone) 3.6 hr; (prednisolone) 2.2 hr.[2] Biologic half-life exceeds serum half-life. (*See* Oral Corticosteroids Comparison Chart.)

Adverse Reactions. Dose- and duration-related side effects include fluid and electrolyte disturbances (with possible edema and hypertension), hyperglycemia and glycosuria, spread of herpes conjunctivitis, activation of tuberculosis, osteoporosis, bone fractures, myopathy, menstrual irregularities, behavioral disturbances (increasing with dosages >40 mg/day), poor wound healing, ocular cataracts, glaucoma, arrest of growth (in children), hirsutism, pseudotumor cerebri (primarily in children), and Cushing's syndrome (moon face, buffalo hump, central obesity, easy bruising, acne, hirsutism, and striae).[2,11,30–32] Prolonged therapy can lead to suppression of pituitary–adrenal function. Too rapid withdrawal of long-term therapy can cause acute adrenal insufficiency (eg, fever, myalgia, arthralgia, and malaise); adrenally suppressed patients cannot respond to stress.

Contraindications. Systemic fungal infections (except as maintenance therapy in adrenal insufficiency); administration of live virus vaccines in patients receiving immunosuppressive doses of corticosteroids.

Precautions. Pregnancy. Use with caution in diabetes mellitus; osteoporosis; peptic ulcer; esophagitis; tuberculosis; and other acute and chronic bacterial, viral, and fungal infections; hypertension or other cardiovascular diseases; hypothyroidism; immunizations; hypoalbuminemia; psychosis; and liver disease. Suppression of PPD and other skin test reactions can occur.

Drug Interactions. Corticosteroids can increase serum glucose levels, and an increase in the dosage of antidiabetic drugs might be required. Corticosteroids can decrease isoniazid and salicylate serum levels. Amphotericin B and loop and thiazide diuretics can enhance corticosteroid-induced potassium depletion. Carbamazepine, phenobarbital (and possibly other barbiturates), phenytoin (best documented with dexamethasone), rifampin, and possibly aminoglutethimide increase the metabolism of corticosteroids.

Parameters to Monitor. Observe for behavioral disturbances and signs or symptoms of Cushing's syndrome. With short-term, high-dose therapy, frequently monitor serum potassium and glucose and blood pressure. With long-term therapy, monitor these parameters occasionally and perform periodic eye examinations and possibly stool guaiac. Monitor growth in infants and children on prolonged therapy.

Notes. Other, more expensive glucocorticoids offer minimal advantages over prednisone in most clinical situations.[2] Dosage ranges for **prednisolone** are the same as those for prednisone. Patients who have received daily glucocorticoid therapy for less than 2 weeks *do not* require dosage tapering to prevent acute adrenal insufficiency; however, dosage tapering may be required to maintain an adequate clinical response.[1,2,5] Efficacy in patients with stable COPD is controversial.[31,33,34]

ORAL CORTICOSTEROIDS COMPARISON CHART

DURATION AND DRUG	DOSAGE FORMS	EQUIVALENT ANTI-INFLAMMATORY DOSE (MG)[a]	RELATIVE ANTI-INFLAMMATORY POTENCY[a]	RELATIVE MINERALO-CORTICOID ACTIVITY	SERUM HALF-LIFE (HR)	COMMENTS
SHORT-ACTING GLUCOCORTICOIDS (BIOLOGIC ACTIVITY 8–12 HR)						
Cortisone Various	Tab 5, 10, 25 mg.	25	0.8	2	0.5	Must be metabolized to active form (hydrocortisone).
Hydrocortisone Various	Tab 5, 10, 20 mg Susp (as cypionate) 2 mg/mL.	20	1	2	1.5	Daily secretion in adults is 20 mg.
INTERMEDIATE-ACTING GLUCOCORTICOIDS (BIOLOGIC ACTIVITY 18–36 HR)						
Methylprednisolone Medrol Various	Tab 2, 4, 8, 16, 24, 32 mg.	4	5	0	2.2	Minimal sodium-retaining activity.
Prednisolone Various	Tab 5 mg Syrup 1, 3 mg/mL.	5	4	1	2.2	Minimal sodium-retaining activity.
Prednisone Various	Tab 1, 2.5, 5, 10, 20, 50 mg Soln 1, 5 mg/mL Syrup 1 mg/mL.	5	4	1	3.6	Must be metabolized to active form (prednisolone).
Triamcinolone Aristocort Kenacort Various	Tab 4, 8 mg Syrup 0.8 mg/mL.	4	5	0	2.6	

(continued)

ORAL CORTICOSTEROIDS COMPARISON CHART (continued)

DURATION AND DRUG	DOSAGE FORMS	EQUIVALENT ANTI-INFLAMMATORY DOSE (MG)[a]	RELATIVE ANTI-INFLAMMATORY POTENCY[a]	RELATIVE MINERALO-CORTICOID ACTIVITY	SERUM HALF-LIFE (HR)	COMMENTS
LONG-ACTING GLUCOCORTICOIDS (BIOLOGIC ACTIVITY 36–54 HR)						
Betamethasone Celestone	Tab 0.6 mg Syrup 0.12 mg/mL.	0.6–0.75	25	0	5+	Minimal sodium-retaining activity, but with high doses, retention may occur.
Dexamethasone Decadron Hexadrol Various	Tab 0.25, 0.5, 0.75, 1, 1.5, 2, 4, 6 mg Elxr 0.1 mg/mL Soln 0.1, 1 mg/mL.	0.75	25	0	Males 3.5 Females 2.4	No sodium-retaining activity with low to moderate doses.
MINERALOCORTICOID (BIOLOGIC ACTIVITY 18–36 HR)						
Fludrocortisone Florinef	Tab 100 μg.	—	10	125	3.5+	Mineralocorticoid used in Addison's disease.

[a]Anti-inflammatory potency does not correlate with immunosuppressive effects.[35]
From references 2, 12, 13, and 36.

TOPICAL CORTICOSTEROIDS

Pharmacology. Topical corticosteroids have nonspecific, local anti-inflammatory effects in the dermal and epidermal skin layers that probably occur by inhibiting mediators in the arachidonic acid pathway in cells, by suppressing DNA synthesis at the cellular level, and by decreasing the influx of WBCs into the local area. Potency is dependent on the characteristics and concentration of the drug and the vehicle used and is usually measured by the assessment of the relative degree of skin blanching (vasoconstrictor assay).[37–41]

Administration and Adult Dosage. Uses for the nonprescription hydrocortisone preparations include relief of itching, inflammation, and rashes caused by eczema; insect bites; poison oak, ivy, or sumac; soaps, detergents, or cosmetics; jewelry; seborrheic dermatitis, psoriasis; and external genital or anal itching. Prescription indications include relief of inflammatory and pruritic manifestations of corticosteroid-responsive dermatoses including contact or atopic dermatitis; nummular, stasis, or asteatotic eczema; lichen planus; lichen simplex chronicus; insect and arthropod bite reactions; and first- and second-degree localized burns and sunburns. These products are usually applied sparingly in a light film, 2–4 times/day; however, with continuous use, a repository effect may make 1–2 applications/day as effective. High-potency agents should be reserved for short-term or intermittent use only but may be more effective and cause fewer adverse effects than continuous therapy with lower potency products. Treatment with very high-potency agents should not exceed 2 consecutive weeks and the total dosage should not exceed 50 g/week because of the hypothalamic-pituitary-adrenal (HPA) axis suppressing potential.[37–41]

Dosage Forms. (*See* Topical Corticosteroids Comparison Chart.)

Patient Instructions. Avoid prolonged use around the eyes (or contact with the eyes); in the genital and rectal areas; on the face, armpits, and in skin creases. Do not use with occlusive dressings unless directed.

Missed Doses. Apply a missed dose as soon as you remember unless it is almost time for the regular schedule. If it is almost time for the regular application, then continue on the regular schedule. Do not apply a double dose.

Pharmacokinetics. The absorption of these drugs depends on the physical properties of the drug itself, the surface area of use, the thickness of the skin (greater absorption from the face, in skin folds, in the perineum, and on denuded skin; lesser absorption from the palms and soles), skin temperature or hydrational state (greater with increased skin temperature or increased hydration), the age of the patient (children have a greater surface area:mass ratio and increased systemic effects), the use of occlusive dressings, the vehicle, application frequency, and length of treatment. Approximately 12–30 g is sufficient to cover the adult body one time. (*See* Topical Corticosteroids Comparison Chart.)

Adverse Reactions. Adverse reactions occur more frequently with increasing product potency and include local burning, itching, irritation, erythema, dryness, folliculitis, hypertrichosis, acneiform eruptions, hypopigmentation, rosacea, skin atrophy, striae, telangiectasias, purpura, perioral dermatitis, overgrowth of skin bacteria and fungi, allergic contact dermatitis, and cataracts or glaucoma with prolonged application around the eye. Systemically, there can be enough absorption of potent steroids to cause suppression of the HPA axis, causing symptoms of Cushing's syndrome, and growth retardation, particularly in young children.

TOPICAL CORTICOSTEROIDS COMPARISON CHART

CLASS AND DRUG	BRAND NAMES	DOSAGE FORMS	STRENGTHS
LOW-POTENCY AGENTS (Modest anti-inflammatory effects. Safest for chronic application, face and intertriginous areas, use under occlusion, and use on young children and infants.)			
Aclometasone Dipropionate	Aclovate	Cream, Ointment	0.05%
Desonide	Tridesilon, Various	Cream, Ointment	0.05%
Fluocinolone Acetonide	Various	Cream, Ointment	0.01%
Hydrocortisone	Hytone, Various	Cream, Lotion, Ointment, Solution, Spray	0.5–2.5%
Hydrocortisone Acetate	Various	Cream, Ointment	0.5, 1%
MEDIUM-POTENCY AGENTS (Effective for moderate inflammatory dermatoses [eg, chronic eczematous dermatoses]. May be used for a limited duration of time on the face and intertriginous areas.)			
Betamethasone Valerate	Valisone, Various	Cream Foam Lotion Ointment	0.01–0.1% 0.12% 0.1% 0.1%
Desoximetasone	Topicort, Various	Cream, Gel	0.05%
Fluocinolone Acetonide	Synalar, Various	Cream, Ointment, Solution	0.01, 0.025% 0.01%
Hydrocortisone Valerate	Westcort	Cream, Ointment	0.2%
Mometasone Furoate	Elocon	Cream, Lotion, Ointment	0.1%
Triamcinolone Acetonide	Aristocort, Kenalog	Cream, Lotion, Ointment	0.025%, 0.1%
HIGH-POTENCY AGENTS (May be used for more severe eczematous dermatoses [eg, lichen simplex chronicus, psoriasis]. May be used for intermediate duration, with the exception of areas of thickened skin and chronic conditions. May be used on the face or in intertriginous areas for short periods of time.)			
Amcinonide	Cyclocort	Cream, Lotion,	0.1%
Betamethasone	Diprosone,	Ointment	0.05%
Dipropionate	Various	Cream, Lotion, Ointment, Aerosol	0.1%

(continued)

TOPICAL CORTICOSTEROIDS COMPARISON CHART (*continued*)

CLASS AND DRUG	BRAND NAMES	DOSAGE FORMS	STRENGTHS
Desoximetasone	Topicort	Cream, Ointment	0.25%
Diflorasone Diacetate	Psorcon, Various	Cream, Ointment	0.05%
Fluocinolone Acetonide	Synalar-HP	Cream	0.2%
Fluocinonide	Lidex, Various	Cream, Gel, Ointment, Solution	0.05%
Halcinonide	Halog	Cream, Ointment, Solution	0.1%
Triamcinolone Acetonide	Aristocort, Kenalog	Cream, Ointment	0.5%

VERY–HIGH-POTENCY AGENTS (Used primarily as an alternative to systemic corticosteroids when local areas are involved. Used on thick, chronic lesions of psoriasis, lichen simplex chronicus, or discoid lupus erythematosus. Skin atrophy is likely. Use for short duration on small areas. Do not use with occlusive dressings.)

Betamethasone Dipropionate, Augmented	Diprolene	Cream, Gel, Lotion, Ointment	0.05%
Clobetasol Propionate	Temovate, Various	Cream, Gel	0.05%
Diflorasone Diacetate	Psorcon	Ointment	0.05%
Halobetasol Propionate	Ultravate	Cream, Ointment	0.05%

From references 37–41.

Antidiabetic Drugs

ACARBOSE   Precose

Pharmacology. Acarbose is an oral α-glucosidase inhibitor indicated for the management of hyperglycemia caused by type 2 diabetes mellitus. Inhibition of this gut enzyme system effectively reduces the rate of complex carbohydrate digestion and the subsequent absorption of glucose, thereby lowering postprandial glucose excursions in type 2 diabetes.[42] In obese and nonobese patients with type 2 diabetes, acarbose monotherapy is associated with a 0.5–1% decrease in hemoglobin A_{1c}.[43]

Administration and Adult Dosage. **PO for type 2 diabetes** (as monotherapy or with a sulfonylurea) 25 mg, tid initially, just before meals. Increase to 50 mg tid after 4–8 weeks and, if necessary, to 100 mg tid after 4–8 additional weeks. Dosages >100 mg tid are not recommended because of increased risk of hepatotoxicity, and patients weighing ≤60 kg should not receive >50 mg tid.

Special Populations. *Pediatric Dosage.* Safety and efficacy not established.

Geriatric Dosage. Same as adult dosage.

Dosage Forms. **Tab** 25, 50, 100 mg.

Patient Instructions. Take acarbose at the beginning of each meal. When a meal is skipped, also skip taking this medication. If a dose is missed, do not take it unless it is just before the next meal. If hypoglycemia occurs, dextrose (glucose) needs to be ingested; sucrose (table sugar) is not effective.

Pharmacokinetics. *Fate.* The drug is poorly absorbed from the GI tract (<2%). It undergoes extensive metabolism in the GI tract via intestinal flora and digestive enzymes. The clinical effect is not dependent on the serum level achieved. All absorbed acarbose and metabolites are renally excreted. In patients with renal impairment, plasma acarbose concentrations are elevated in relation to the degree of renal dysfunction.

$t_{\frac{1}{2}}$. About 2 hr with normal renal function.

Adverse Reactions. The major side effects of acarbose are flatulence, diarrhea, and abdominal pain. Acarbose monotherapy is not associated with hypoglycemia; however, patients managed with combination therapy (with a sulfonylurea or insulin) can experience hypoglycemia secondary to the other drug. In this setting, manage hypoglycemia with oral glucose (if the patient is conscious) or IV glucose or glucagon (if the patient is unconscious) rather than with a complex carbohydrate (eg, sucrose). Attempting to manage hypoglycemia with oral sugar sources other than glucose is not effective in acarbose-treated patients and might have grave consequences.

Contraindications. Inflammatory bowel disease; colonic ulceration; obstructive bowel disorders; cirrhosis; type 1 diabetes; history of diabetic ketoacidosis.

Precautions. Use with caution in patients with disorders of digestion or absorption or with medical conditions that might deteriorate with increased intestinal gas formation. Not recommended in patients with Cr_s >2 mg/dL.

Drug Interactions. Charcoal and other intestinal adsorbents as well as digestive preparations containing amylase, pancreatin, and related enzymes should not be taken concurrently with acarbose.

Parameters to Monitor. Monitor clinical symptoms of hyperglycemia (mainly polyphagia, polyuria, polydipsia, or numbing or tingling of feet) or hypoglycemia (hunger, nervousness, sweating, palpitations, headaches, confusion, drowsiness, anxiety, or blurred vision) when taken concurrently with insulin or insulin secretagogues (eg, sulfonylureas). Self-monitoring of fasting and selected postprandial blood glucose levels by the patient is also helpful. (*See* Blood Glucose Monitors Comparison Chart.) Long-term diabetic control may best be monitored using hemoglobin A_{lc}.[44]

Notes. **Miglitol** (Glyset—Bayer) is an α-glucosidase inhibitor that has similar indications, uses, and side effects as acarbose. The dosage of the two drugs is the same. The clinical benefits, if any, of miglitol over acarbose have not been determined. **Voglibose** (Takeda America) is another α-glucosidase inhibitor in clinical trials.

ALDOSE REDUCTASE INHIBITORS

Prolonged hyperglycemia causes excess flux of glucose into tissues, and glucose is shunted to the polyol pathway, resulting in excess sorbitol production. Excess intracellular sorbitol causes a reduction in the uptake of myoinositol and ultimately a down-regulation in the Na^+/K^+-ATPase system. This process is thought to be one of the biochemical mechanisms leading to the development of neuropathy, collagen disorders, cataracts, and possibly retinopathy in patients with diabetes. Because aldose reductase is the rate-limiting enzyme in this pathway, aldose reductase inhibitors are being studied as a possible means of decreasing the sorbitol-linked sequelae of diabetes.[45] Although this is a promising class of drugs, the side effects, dosage regimens, and long-term benefits are to be determined. Aldose reductase inhibitors currently under investigation are **fidarestat** and **zopolrestat** (Alond—Pfizer).[46]

GLUCAGON   Glucagon Emergency Kit, Glucagon Diagnostic Kit

Pharmacology. Glucagon is a counterregulatory hormone that increases blood glucose levels by induction of glycogenolysis. It is indicated for the treatment of the unconscious hypoglycemic patient but is effective only in patients with adequate hepatic glycogen stores. Glucagon also has been used as a bowel relaxant during diagnostic procedures and in overdosage with **β-blockers** or **calcium-channel blockers**.[47]

Adult Dosage. IM, SC, or IV for hypoglycemia 0.5–1 mg. Response is usually observed in 10–20 min.

Dosage Forms. Inj 1 mg.

Adverse Reactions. Glucagon occasionally causes nausea and vomiting, so position patients to prevent aspiration. Administration of glucagon rarely results in generalized allergic reactions such as urticaria, respiratory distress, and hypotension. Glucagon can precipitate hypertensive crisis in the patient with underlying pheochromocytoma (secondary to release of catecholamines).

INSULINS

Pharmacology. Insulin promotes cellular uptake of glucose, fatty acids, and amino acids and their conversion to glycogen, triglycerides, and proteins. Beef and pork insulins are extracted and purified from the animal's pancreas. Human insulin is produced by recombinant DNA technology or enzymatic conversion of pork insulin. No differences in side effects or long-term control of diabetes have been observed between human insulin and highly purified pork insulin.

Administration and Adult Dosage. SC for type 1 diabetes usual initial dosage ranges of 0.6–0.75 unit/kg/day in divided doses.[48] During the first week of therapy, the dosage requirement might escalate to 1 unit/kg/day in divided doses because of insulin resistance and the usual age group (adolescents) being treated. The dosage requirement can temporarily decrease to 0.1–0.5 unit/kg/day if the patient experiences a "honeymoon phase." Dosage adjustments are made on the basis of clinical symptoms, blood glucose levels, and hemoglobin A_{1c} values. Insulin can be administered by various methods depending on a number of factors. Single daily SC injections of intermediate-acting insulin are often used but should not usually be relied on to adequately control blood glucose levels in the type 1 patient because they are not sufficient to prevent long-term complications even though they can offer protection from diabetic ketoacidosis. Intensive forms of insulin therapy, which may provide better glycemic control, include the split-and-mixed regimen (2 SC injections daily of mixed short- and long-acting insulin), multiple daily SC doses of short-acting insulin in combination with a single injection of long-acting insulin, and insulin pump therapy. **IV, SC, or IM for diabetic ketoacidosis (IV preferred for patients in shock)** 0.1 unit/kg, followed by a continuous infusion of 0.1–0.2 unit/kg/hr. If the serum glucose does not change in the first hour, double the insulin rate, with further adjustments in insulin dosage based on glucose levels.[49] Fluid and electrolyte repletion must accompany insulin therapy. **SC for type 2 diabetes** (patients unresponsive to oral agent therapy or with extreme hyperglycemia: fasting serum glucose >200–225 mg/dL) may need as little as 5–10 units/day or >100 units/day.[49] Patients who require <30 units/day may be well controlled with 1 injection/day of intermediate-acting insulin; patients who require >30 units/day should be treated with ≥2 injections/day. Insulin resistance in the type 2 population is usually associated with obesity. Weight reduction and improved glycemic control usually improve insulin response.

Special Populations. *Pediatric Dosage.* (See Administration and Adult Dosage.) **Common maintenance dosages** are 0.6–0.9 unit/kg/day in divided doses in prepubertal children, up to 1.5 units/kg/day during puberty, and <1 unit/kg/day after puberty. Requirements occasionally can be as high as 200 units/day during growth spurts.

Geriatric Dosage. Same as adult dosage.

Other Conditions. Insulin requirements may be decreased in patients with renal or hepatic impairment or hypothyroidism. Requirements may be increased during pregnancy (especially in the second and third trimesters), in patients with high fever, hyperthyroidism, or severe infections; and after trauma or surgery.

Dosage Forms. (*See* Insulins Comparison Chart.)

Patient Instructions. Instruct patients in the following areas: use of insulin syringes and needles; storage, mixing, and handling of insulin; urine ketone testing; blood glucose testing; adherence to proper diet and regular meals; personal hygiene (especially the feet); and recognition and treatment of hypoglycemia and hyperglycemia. (*See* Sulfonylurea Agents.)

Pharmacokinetics. *Onset and Duration.* Human insulin is more soluble than animal-source insulins and may have a shorter onset and duration of action. (*See* Insulins Comparison Chart.)

Serum Levels. Patients with diabetes vary widely in their responses to insulin, and serum levels are not normally monitored clinically.

Fate. The rate of absorption depends on the insulin type. (*See* Insulins Comparison Chart.) Serum levels are affected by obesity, diet, degree of activity, pancreatic β-cell activity, growth hormone, and circulating antibodies. Insulin is metabolized primarily in the liver, although the kidneys are responsible for the metabolism of up to 40% of the daily insulin output.[50]

$t_{\frac{1}{2}}$. (Regular insulin) 4–5 min after IV administration.

Adverse Reactions. Hypoglycemia is dose related. Patients being treated with intensive insulin regimens of ≥3 injections/day are more prone to hypoglycemic episodes than are patients treated with the conventional 1–2 injections/day.[51] Local allergic reactions, with an onset of 15 min–4 hr, are usually caused by insulin impurities; 70% of these patients have histories of interrupted treatment. Immune or nonimmune insulin resistance occurs occasionally. Lipohypertrophy at the injection site can occur, especially with repeated use of the same site. Lipoatrophy also can occur at the injection site and be less frequent with the highly purified animal or human insulins. Allergy, resistance, and lipoatrophy can be overcome by switching to a more highly purified product (eg, human insulin). In general, pork insulin is less antigenic than beef-pork or pure beef insulin (neither is available in the United States) because it is structurally more similar to human insulin, which is the least immunogenic.[52]

Contraindications. Hypoglycemic episodes.

Precautions. Use with caution in patients with renal or hepatic disease or hypothyroidism. Insulin requirements can change with exercise or infection, or when switching animal sources or to more purified products.

Drug Interactions. Alcohol can produce hypoglycemia, especially in fasting patients; moderate increases in blood glucose can occur in nonfasting patients. Oral contraceptives, corticosteroids, furosemide, niacin (large doses), diazoxide, thiazide diuretics, and thyroid hormones (large doses) can increase insulin requirements. Anabolic steroids can decrease the insulin requirement. Avoid MAOIs in patients with diabetes because they can interfere with the normal adrenergic response to hypoglycemia by prolonging the action of antidiabetic agents. β-Blockers prolong hypoglycemic episodes and inhibit tachycardia and tremors, which are signs of hypoglycemia (sweating is not inhibited); hypertension can occur during hypoglycemia; cardioselective β-blockers (eg, atenolol, metoprolol) are less likely than nonselective types (eg, nadolol, propranolol) to cause problems.

Parameters to Monitor. Monitor blood glucose routinely. (*See* Blood Glucose Monitors Comparison Chart.) Long-term diabetic control is best monitored using hemoglobin A_{1c}.[44] The patient should continually watch for subjective symptoms of hypoglycemia and hyperglycemia. Observe for signs of lipoatrophy, lipohypertrophy, and allergic reactions.

Notes. Human insulin is the insulin of choice for patients with insulin resistance, pregnancy, or allergy; new insulin-dependent patients; or any patient taking insulin intermittently. Insulin is stable for 1–2 months at constant room temperature and up to 24 months under refrigeration. Insulin is adsorbed by glass and plastic IV infusion equipment, with little difference between glass and plastic; maximal adsorption occurs within 15 sec. Adsorption can be minimized by the addition of small amounts (1–2%) of **albumin** to the infusion container; however, this may be costly and unnecessary because patient response is generally adequate without addition of albumin. Variation can be minimized by flushing all new IV administration equipment with 50 mL of the insulin-containing solution (thereby saturating "binding sites") before it is used.[53]

Pump devices are available to deliver insulin depending on or independent of a measured serum glucose level. "Open-loop" devices can deliver insulin at a constant rate and be manually controlled. "Closed-loop" devices (the "artificial pancreas") can deliver insulin at variable rates in response to serum glucose but are used only in experimental settings.

Novel forms of insulin delivery are currently under investigation, with inhaled insulin showing the most promise. Pulmonary tissue provides a large absorptive surface for insulin. Insulin can be delivered effectively as an inhaled aerosol and in one study had an onset of action that was 23 min earlier than SC regular insulin and sustained its action for >3 hr. Ninety-nine units of inhaled insulin was metabolically equivalent to 10 units of SC insulin.[54] Pulmonary-delivered insulins are currently in clinical trials.

INSULIN ANALOGUES

Insulin injected SC does not result in serum insulin concentrations that mimic normal physiologic insulin response. More than 30 human insulin analogues with different pharmacokinetic profiles have been produced using recombinant DNA technology. The goal of insulin analogue research is to produce a human insulin analogue with a rapid action (to provide bolus postprandial insulin) and a slow, extended release pattern (to provide basal insulin). **Insulin lispro** (Humalog) is a rapid-acting analogue with a pharmacokinetic profile between that of IV and SC regular human insulin. It has an onset in ≤15 min, a peak at 1–2 hr, and a duration of 2–4 hr. Insulin lispro offers a pharmacokinetic profile that is superior to regular human insulin when used to cover postprandial glycemic excursions. Another short-acting analogue, **insulin aspart** (Novolog), has a pharmacokinetic profile similar to that of insulin lispro.[55] The long-acting analogue, **insulin glargine** (Lantus), has an onset of action of approximately 1 hr, with a sustained peak activity beginning at 4–5 hr and persisting for 24 hr. Insulin glargine is a basal insulin that is administered once daily at bedtime; it must be used in combination with a rapid-acting premeal insulin such as insulin lispro to achieve optimum results.[55,56]

INSULINS COMPARISON CHART[a]		
PRODUCT	MANUFACTURER	STRENGTH
RAPID-ACTING (ONSET, <0.25 HR; PEAK, 1–2 HR; DURATION 2–4 HR)		
Biosynthetic		
NovoLog (Aspart)	Novo Nordisk	U-100
Humalog (Lispro)	Lilly	U-100
SHORT-ACTING (ONSET, 0.5–2 HR; PEAK, 3–4 HR; DURATION, 4–8 HR)		
Pork		
Iletin II Regular	Lilly	U-100
Purified Pork Regular	Novo Nordisk	U-100
Human		
Humulin R	Lilly	U-100, U-500
Novolin R	Novo Nordisk	U-100
Velosulin	Novo Nordisk	U-100

(*continued*)

INSULINS COMPARISON CHART[a] (*continued*)

PRODUCT	MANUFACTURER	STRENGTH
INTERMEDIATE-ACTING (ONSET, 2–4 HR; PEAK, 8–14 HR; DURATION, 14–24 HR)		
Pork		
Iletin II Lente	Lilly	U-100
Iletin II NPH	Lilly	U-100
Purified Pork Lente	Novo Nordisk	U-100
Purified Pork NPH	Novo Nordisk	U-100
Human		
Humulin L (Lente)	Lilly	U-100
Humulin N (NPH)	Lilly	U-100
Novolin L (Lente)	Novo Nordisk	U-100
Novolin N (NPH)	Novo Nordisk	U-100
LONG ACTING (ONSET, 6–14 HR; PEAK, NONE; DURATION, 20–30 HR)		
Human		
Humulin U (Ultralente)	Lilly	U-100
Lantus (Glargine)[b]	Aventis	U-100
FIXED COMBINATIONS (ONSET, 0.5–1 HR; PEAK, 3–10 HR; DURATION, 14–18 HR)		
Human		
Humalog Mix 75/25[b,c]	Lilly	U-100
Humulin 70/30[b]	Lilly	U-100
Novolin 70/30[b]	Novo Nordisk	U-100
Humulin 50/50[b]	Lilly	U-100

[a]There can be variations within the ranges of onset, peak, and duration among manufacturers. Onset and duration may be prolonged in long-standing diabetes, and large doses may have prolonged durations of action. Site of injection, depth of injection, and whether site is exercised, massaged, or has heat applied to it also affect rate of insulin absorption. Human insulins have a slightly more rapid onset and a shorter duration of action than animal-derived insulins.

[b]These products contain isophane and regular insulin in the specified proportions; the first number designates the percentage of isophane insulin and the second designates the percentage of regular insulin.

[c]Suspension of insulin lispro protamine and soluble insulin lispro. Onset is within 0.25 hr.

From references 51, and 57, and product information.

METFORMIN   Glucophage

Pharmacology. Metformin is a biguanide antihyperglycemic agent used in the management of type 2 diabetes mellitus. It does not affect insulin secretion; rather, it reduces hepatic glucose production and enhances glucose utilization by muscle. Reported increases in glucose utilization in muscle are 7–35%. In addition to blood glucose reductions (mean 53 mg/dL), metformin may have beneficial effects on serum lipids.[58] (*See* Notes.)

Administration and Adult Dosage. **PO for type 2 diabetes** (immediate-release) initiate 500 mg tablets with a dosage of 1 tablet bid with morning and evening meals. Increase dosage in 500 mg/day increments at weekly intervals, to a maximum of 2.5 g/day. Initiate 850 mg tablets with 1 tablet/day before the morning meal. Increase dosage in 850 mg/day increments q 2 weeks, to a maximum of 850 mg tid. Individualize maintenance dosage based on glycemic response. Give all dosages up to 2 g/day in 2 divided doses; larger dosages require a tid regimen to reduce GI discomfort. **PO** (SR Tab) 500 mg/day with the evening meal initially, increasing in 500 mg/day increments at weekly intervals to a maximum of 2 g/day with the evening meal. To switch from the immediate-release to the SR formulation, give the same daily dosage of SR as a single dose with the evening meal.

Special Populations. *Pediatric Dosage.* Safety and efficacy not established.

Geriatric Dosage. Initial and maintenance dosages should be lower in the elderly. Avoid usual maximum adult dosage. Do not start metformin in patients ≥80 yr unless renal function is normal.

Dosage Forms. **Tab** 500, 850, 1000 mg; **SR Tab** 500 mg (Glucophage XR); **Tab** 250 mg with glyburide 1.25 mg, 500 mg with glyburide 2.5 or 5 mg (Glucovance).

Patient Instructions. Take metformin just before meals to reduce gastrointestinal side effects (diarrhea, nausea, and heartburn). Contact your physician if gastrointestinal side effects persist. Do not take metformin if you develop a serious medical condition such as myocardial infarction, stroke, or serious infection; require surgery; consume excessive amounts of alcohol; or require x-ray procedures with contrast dyes. Discontinue metformin and contact your health care provider immediately if hyperventilation, muscle pain, malaise, unexplained drowsiness, or other unusual symptoms occur that might indicate the development of lactic acidosis.

Missed Doses. Take as soon as possible, unless the time for the next dose is near. Do not double doses.

Pharmacokinetics. *Fate.* Absorption half-life is 0.9–2.6 hr for immediate-release tablets; peak levels occur at 4–8 hr (median 7 hr) with the SR formulation. Absolute bioavailability is 50–60% for both products. With immediate-release tablets, peak serum levels are 1–2 mg/L in patients with type 2 diabetes; with the SR formulation, peak levels are 20% lower. Plasma protein binding is negligible; V_d is 654 ± 358 L after a single 850 mg oral dose; Cl is proportional to renal function. Metformin is excreted in the urine unchanged.[58]

$t_{1/2}$. (Immediate-release) 1.7–4.5 hr with normal renal function.[58]

Adverse Reactions. Acute side effects occur in as many as 30% of patients treated with metformin. Side effects include primarily GI complaints, such as diarrhea, abdominal discomfort, nausea, anorexia, and metallic taste. GI side effects are usually transient and dose related and can be mitigated by giving the drug just before meals, initiating therapy with small doses and slowly increasing the dosage. Metformin reduces serum **vitamin B_{12}** levels in approximately 7% of patients but is rarely associated with anemia. Vitamin B_{12} deficiency anemia can be treated with vitamin B_{12} supplementation or by discontinuing metformin. Diminished vitamin B_{12} absorption and transport can be improved with oral **calcium** supplementation.[59] Lactic acidosis has been reported; however, almost all cases occur in patients in whom metformin was contraindicated or in patients who attempted suicide by overdose. Lactic acidosis occurs in 0.03 case/1000 patient-yr, with fatalities in about 50% of cases.[58]

Contraindications. Acute or chronic metabolic acidosis; patients undergoing radiographic studies requiring contrast media (withhold metformin just before the radiographic study and do not reinstate for 48 hr after contrast media administration and upon documentation of normal renal function); abnormal Cl_{cr} or Cr_s >1.5 mg/dL in males or >1.4 mg/dL in females; any disease that can cause hypoxia and result in accumulation of lactate (eg, CHF requiring pharmacologic treatment, MI, severe infections, stroke); hepatic dysfunction.

Precautions. Avoid in pregnancy and lactation.

Drug Interactions. Furosemide and nifedipine increase serum levels of metformin, the clinical relevance of which is unknown. Cimetidine reduces the tubular secretion of metformin and can increase peak serum concentrations by as much as 60%.[60] (*See also* Insulin Drug Interactions.)

Parameters to Monitor. Monitor renal function, hepatic function, and CBC before initiation of therapy and at least annually thereafter. Monitor renal function more closely in the elderly because of the age-related changes in renal function and greater risk for acute renal failure. (*See* Contraindications.) The goal of therapy is to reduce fasting blood glucose and glycosylated hemoglobin levels to normal or near normal by using the lowest effective dosage of the drug.

Notes. Because of its effect on weight and lipids, metformin is an appropriate choice for initial monotherapy in obese, new-onset type 2 diabetic patients, whereas **sulfonylureas** are usually a better choice for nonobese patients. In patients who do not respond to metformin monotherapy, combination therapy with a sulfonylurea or a thiazolidinedione might be effective. Weight loss has been associated with metformin therapy (mean 0.8 kg); weight gain (mean 2.8 kg) has been found in patients treated with sulfonylureas.[61] Reductions in total cholesterol, LDL cholesterol, and triglycerides of 5%, 8%, and 16%, respectively, and an increase of 2% in HDL cholesterol have been reported.

NATEGLINIDE Starlix

Pharmacology. Nateglinide is a meglitinide similar to repaglinide that is a rapid-acting oral insulin secretagogue that stimulates insulin secretion in relation to serum blood glucose levels.

Adult Dosage. **PO for type 2 diabetes** (alone or in combination with metformin) 120 mg tid before each meal. For patients near their HbA_{1c} goals, a dose of 60 mg can be used. Dosage adjustment is not necessary in the elderly or those with mild to severe renal impairment or mild to moderate hepatic impairment.

Dosage Forms. **Tab** 60, 120 mg.

Pharmacokinetics. Oral bioavailability is 72%. Peak plasma concentrations occur within 0.5–1.9 hr. Plasma protein binding is 97%; Cl is 8.4 L/hr. The drug is metabolized in the liver primarily by CYP3A4 and somewhat by CYP2C9, with 80% of the parent drug and glucuronide metabolites eliminated in the urine. Mild to moderate hepatic cirrhosis does not markedly alter single-dose pharmacokinetics of nateglinide. Half-life is 1.4 hr.[62] Administration with metformin does not alter the pharmacokinetics of either drug.[63]

Adverse Reactions. The most frequent side effect is mild hypoglycemia manifested by increased sweating, tremor, dizziness, and increased appetite. Headache has occurred. Because of nateglinide's hepatic metabolism and extensive protein binding, interactions with other drugs affecting CYP3A4 and CYP2C9 or drugs extensively protein bound might result in pharmacokinetic interactions.

Contraindications, Precautions, and Parameters to Monitor. (*See* Repaglinide.)

REPAGLINIDE	Prandin

Pharmacology. Repaglinide is a meglitinide agent that stimulates insulin release from the pancreas, although it is structurally unrelated to sulfonylureas. Compared with the sulfonylureas, repaglinide has a quicker onset and shorter duration of action, resulting in a lower risk of prolonged hypoglycemia.[64]

Administration and Adult Dosage. **PO for type 2 diabetes** newly treated patients with HbA_{1c} <8% should start with 0.5 mg within 30 min before each meal. Patients previously treated with antidiabetic agents should start with 1 or 2 mg within 30 min before each meal. Increase dosage based on glycemic response, to a maximum of 4 mg/dose or 16 mg/day. Starting doses of repaglinide are unchanged when taken concurrently with metformin.

Special Populations. *Pediatric Dosage.* Safety and efficacy not established.

Geriatric Dosage. Dosage adjustment is not needed unless renal function is compromised. However, the elderly are more sensitive to hypoglycemia and should be monitored closely with initiation of therapy.

Other Conditions. No adjustment of the initial dosage is required in renal impairment but use caution with subsequent dosage increases. In patients with hepatic abnormalities, wait longer before increasing the dosage.

Dosage Forms. **Tab** 0.5, 1, 2 mg.

Patient Instructions. Take each dose 0 to 30 minutes before each meal, usually 15 minutes. Recognize signs and symptoms of hypoglycemia and treat accordingly. Skip your dose if you will miss a meal. Add a dose when you eat an extra meal.

Missed Doses. If you miss a dose, take your regular dose at your next scheduled meal. Do not double the dose.

Pharmacokinetics. *Fate.* Oral bioavailability is 56%. Peak plasma concentrations occur within 1 hr; food reduces mean peak concentration by 20%, although time to peak concentration is not altered. Serum concentrations are higher and prolonged in those with liver impairment. Plasma protein binding is >98%. V_d is 31 L; Cl is 38 L/hr. The drug is metabolized primarily in the liver by CYP3A4 to inactive metabolites excreted in the feces.

$t_{1/2}$. About 1 hr.

Adverse Reactions. The most frequent side effect is hypoglycemia. Upper respiratory infections, sinusitis, nausea, diarrhea, constipation, arthralgia, and headache have been reported, but their frequencies are equal to or only slightly higher than that of placebo.

Contraindications. Diabetic ketoacidosis; type 1 diabetes.

Precautions. Pregnancy; lactation. Use cautiously in patients with renal impairment and those at increased risk of hypoglycemia, including those with hepatic or adrenal insufficiency and in debilitated, elderly, or malnourished patients. Hypoglycemia is more frequent in treatment of previously untreated patients and those with HbA_{1c} <8%.[65]

Drug Interactions. Inhibitors of CYP3A4 (eg, ketoconazole, miconazole, erythromycin) inhibit the metabolism of repaglinide. CYP3A4 inducers (eg, rifampin, barbiturates, carbamazepine) might reduce serum levels of repaglinide.

Parameters to Monitor. Monitor fasting and selected postprandial blood glucose levels regularly and HbA_{1c} periodically.

SULFONYLUREA AGENTS

Pharmacology. Sulfonylureas enhance insulin secretion from pancreatic β-cells and potentiate insulin action on several extrahepatic tissues. Long-term, sulfonylureas increase peripheral utilization of glucose, suppress hepatic gluconeogenesis, and possibly increase the sensitivity and/or number of peripheral insulin receptors. Second-generation sulfonylureas (eg, **glyburide, glipizide, glimeperide**) are more potent than first-generation agents and are used in much smaller dosages, with lower resultant blood levels. These lower serum concentrations decrease the likelihood of protein-binding displacement and hepatic metabolic interference.

Administration and Adult Dosage. (*See* Sulfonylurea Agents Comparison Chart.)

Special Populations. *Pediatric Dosage.* Safety and efficacy not established.

Geriatric Dosage. Start at the lower end of the dosage range and slowly titrate upward if needed. Observe precautions with renal or hepatic impairment.

Other Conditions. Dosage alterations may be necessary with all sulfonylureas in patients with severe hepatic dysfunction. With renal disease, especially in geriatric patients, there is an increased duration of action with **chlorpropamide, acetohexamide,** and possibly **glyburide.**[66]

Dosage Forms. (*See* Sulfonylurea Agents Comparison Chart.)

Patient Instructions. Eat a recommended diet consistently on a day-to-day basis. Take this medication at the same time each day (in the morning for once-daily medications). Report factors that might alter blood glucose levels (eg, infection, fasting states) and any side effects.

Missed Doses. Take a missed dose as soon as you remember unless it is near time of the next dose. Do not double doses.

Pharmacokinetics. (*See* Sulfonylurea Agents Comparison Chart.)

Adverse Reactions. Hypoglycemic reactions (especially with **chlorpropamide**), anorexia, nausea, vomiting, diarrhea, allergic skin reactions, and cholestatic jaundice occur occasionally. Hematologic disorders, mild disulfiram-like reaction to alcohol, hyponatremia (most common with **chlorpropamide** but can occur with **tolbutamide**), and bone marrow suppression occur rarely.[67]

Contraindications. Pregnancy; type 1 diabetes; juvenile, unstable, or brittle diabetes; diabetes complicated by acidosis, ketosis, diabetic coma, major surgery, severe infection, or severe trauma.

Precautions. Patients sensitive to one sulfonylurea might experience cross-sensitivity to other sulfonylureas. **Chlorpropamide** can cause hyponatremia, particularly in elderly women taking diuretics.[68]

Drug Interactions. Drugs that have been reported to enhance sulfonylurea effects include chloramphenicol (chlorpropamide and tolbutamide), dicumarol, fluconazole (glipizide, glyburide, tolbutamide, and possibly others), sulfonamides, and high-dose salicylates. Rifampin stimulates the metabolism of tolbutamide and possibly other sulfonylureas. Drugs that impair glucose tolerance include oral contraceptives, corticosteroids, thiazide diuretics, furosemide, thyroid hormones (large doses), and niacin.[69] Acute ingestion of alcohol in combination with sulfonylureas can produce severe hypoglycemia. (*See also* Insulin Drug Interactions.)

Parameters to Monitor. Monitor clinical symptoms of hyperglycemia (mainly polyphagia, polyuria, polydipsia, or numbing or tingling of feet) or hypoglycemia (hunger, nervousness, warmth, sweating, palpitations, headaches, confusion, drowsiness, anxiety, blurred vision, or paresthesias of lips). Monitor fasting serum glucose levels frequently at the initiation of therapy to gauge the adequacy of the dosage. Self-monitoring of fasting and selected postprandial blood glucose levels by the patient is also helpful. (*See* Blood Glucose Monitors Comparison Chart.) Long-term diabetic control may best be monitored using hemoglobin A_{lc}.

Notes. Sulfonylureas are usually an appropriate choice for nonobese, new-onset type 2 diabetic patients, whereas **metformin** is more appropriate for obese type 2 patients.[70] Individualize the choice of sulfonylurea based on the patient's characteristics (eg, renal function, hepatic function, likelihood of hypoglycemia) and the pharmacokinetics of the drugs. Glyburide, glipizide, glimepiride, and chlorpropamide are more effective at lowering blood glucose than acetohexamide, tolazamide, or tolbutamide.[52] Acetohexamide, tolazamide, and tolbutamide probably should be reserved for mild hyperglycemia or in those likely to develop hypoglycemia (eg, the elderly). In patients who do not respond to sulfonylurea monotherapy, combination therapy with **insulin, metformin, rosiglitazone, pioglitazone,** or **acarbose** may be effective.[71] **Glimeperide** is the most potent sulfonylurea agent, has the lowest rate of hypoglycemia, and does not affect potassium channels in the heart.[72]

SULFONYLUREA AGENTS COMPARISON CHART

DRUG	DOSAGE FORMS	DAILY DOSAGE	FATE	DURATION (HR)	COMMENTS
FIRST-GENERATION					
Acetohexamide Dymelor Various	Tab 250, 500 mg.	250 mg–1.5 g in 2 divided doses.	65% converted to an active metabolite (hydroxyhexamide).	12–18	May be useful in the elderly and others prone to hypoglycemia but avoid in patients with renal dysfunction.
Chlorpropamide Diabinese Various	Tab 100, 250 mg.	100–500 mg in a single dose.	Metabolized, and 20% excreted unchanged.	24–72	Avoid in elderly and in patients with renal dysfunction. Causes disulfiram-like reaction in 30% of patients.
Tolazamide Tolinase Various	Tab 100, 250, 500 mg.	100 mg–1 g in 1–2 divided doses.	Converted to weakly active metabolites.	16–24	Delayed onset of action (≤4 hr). May be useful in the elderly and others prone to hypoglycemia.
Tolbutamide Orinase Various	Tab 500 mg.	500 mg–3 g in 2–3 divided doses.	Converted to inactive compounds.	6–12	May be useful in the elderly and others prone to hypoglycemia.

(continued)

SULFONYLUREA AGENTS COMPARISON CHART (*continued*)

DRUG	DOSAGE FORMS	DAILY DOSAGE	FATE	DURATION (HR)	COMMENTS
SECOND-GENERATION					
Glimepiride Amaryl	Tab 1, 2, 4 mg.	1–8 mg in a single dose.	Converted to inactive and active metabolites.	24	Similar to glyburide. Lowest rate of hypoglycemia and does not affect cardiac potassium channels.
Glipizide Glucotrol Glucotrol XL	Tab 5, 10 mg SR Tab 2.5, 5, 10 mg.	Non-SR 5–40 mg in 1–2 divided doses. SR 5–20 mg in a single dose.	Converted to inactive metabolites.	10–24 (non-SR) 18–24 (SR)	Take non-SR product on an empty stomach.
Glyburide DiaBeta Glynase Micronase Various	Tab 1.25, 2.5, 5 mg Tab (micronized) 1.5, 3, 4.5, 6 mg.	Nonmicronized 1.25–20 mg in 1–2 divided doses Micronized 0.75–12 mg in 1–2 divided doses.	Converted to inactive and active metabolites.	18–24	The micronized product (Glynase, various) offers no advantage over the nonmicronized products.
COMBINATION PRODUCT					
Glyburide and Metformin Glucovance	Tab 1.25 mg glyburide plus 250 mg metformin, 2.5 mg or 5 mg glyburide plus 500 mg metformin.	1.25 mg/250 mg daily-bid initially, to a maximum of 20 mg/2000 mg daily in 1–2 divided doses.	(See individual agents.)	18–24	

From references 67, and 68 and product information.

PIOGLITAZONE
Actos

Pharmacology. Pioglitazone is a thiazolidinedione antihyperglycemic agent used to improve insulin sensitivity in patients with type 2 diabetes. Insulin-dependent glucose disposal in skeletal muscle is improved and hepatic glucose production is decreased; both actions contribute to pioglitazone's glucose-lowering effects. Pioglitazone is only effective in the presence of insulin; by itself it does not lead to hypoglycemia and does not increase insulin secretion. Because insulin is required for its action, pioglitazone should not be used in patients with type 1 diabetes. **Rosiglitazone** (Avandia) is another thiazolidinedione antidiabetic agent that acts similarly to pioglitazone.

Administration and Adult Dosage. PO for type 2 diabetes (monotherapy) 15–30 mg once daily with food; after a 4-week trial dosage can be increased to a maximum of 45 mg/day. If no response occurs at the maximum dose of 45 mg/day, other therapeutic options should be considered; **(combination therapy with insulin, sulfonylurea, or metformin)** 15–30 mg once daily initially, increasing q 4 weeks to a maximum of 45 mg/day. Dosages of insulin or sulfonylurea may need to be decreased based on the glucose-lowering response. For those on **insulin,** decrease the insulin dosage when fasting plasma glucose levels are <100 mg/dL or if hypoglycemic symptoms occur.

Special Populations. *Pediatric Dosage.* Safety and efficacy not established.

Geriatric Dosage. (>65 yr) no differences in efficacy or safety; dosage adjustments are not required.

Other Conditions. No dosage adjustment is required in renal impairment.

Dosage Forms. Tab 15, 30, 45 mg.

Patient Instructions. Take once daily without regard to meals. If you are taking insulin, a sulfonylurea, or other glucose-lowering agent, you should understand the signs and symptoms of hypoglycemia and its appropriate treatment. Report nausea, vomiting, abdominal pain, loss of appetite, or dark urine immediately to your health care provider. Because pioglitazone's effect on oral contraceptives has not been established, other means of contraception may be required.

Missed Doses. If you forget to take a dose, take your regular dose the next day. Do not double the dose on the next day.

Pharmacokinetics. *Fate.* Oral absorption is rapid, with the peak plasma concentration in 2 hr. Steady-state serum levels are achieved in 7 days. Extensively bound to serum albumin (>99%). V_d is 10.5–26.5 L/kg. Metabolized extensively by hydroxylation and oxidation in the liver and principally by CYP2C8 and CYP3A4. Renal elimination is negligible (15–30%), with most of the oral dose believed to be excreted into the bile unchanged or as metabolites and subsequently eliminated in the feces.

$t_{1/2}$. 16–24 hr.

Adverse Reactions. Mild to moderate hypoglycemia when used concurrently with a sulfonylurea or insulin. Headache, anemia (mean hemoglobin value decrease of 2–4%), edema, weight gain.[73]

Contraindications. Active liver disease or ALT levels exceeding 2.5 times the upper limit of normal.

Precautions. Premenopausal anovulatory individuals might resume ovulation, placing them at risk for pregnancy. Use cautiously in patients with edema.

Drug Interactions. Ethinyl estradiol and norethindrone plasma concentrations might be reduced, resulting in possible loss of contraceptive efficacy. Ketoconazole and possibly other drugs that inhibit CYP3A4 might inhibit the metabolism of pioglitazone. Additionally, CYP3A4-metabolized drugs such as calcium-channel blockers, corticosteroids, cyclosporine, and HMG-CoA reductase inhibitors have not been specifically studied but might affect the metabolism of pioglitazone.

Parameters to Monitor. Monitor serum ALT levels at the start of therapy, q 2 months for the first 12 months, and then periodically. If ALT is elevated 1–2.5 times the upper limit of normal at any time (before initiation or during therapy), the cause of the enzyme elevation should be determined. If ALT levels exceed 3 times the upper limit of normal, pioglitazone should be discontinued. Monitor fasting blood sugars and HbA$_{1c}$. (*See* Sulfonylureas.)

Notes. In patients with type 2 diabetes on insulin therapy, pioglitazone often results in a decreased requirement for **insulin.** Patients on concomitant therapy with insulin or **sulfonylureas** should not alter the doses of the latter medications until positive changes in fasting plasma glucose levels are obtained (fasting blood sugars <100 mg/dL) or if symptoms of hypoglycemia are experienced. (*See* Thiazolidinedione Comparison Chart.)

THIAZOLIDINEDIONE COMPARISON CHART

DRUG	MONOTHERAPY INITIATION DOSE	COMBINATION INITIATION DOSE	MAXIMUM DOSE	COMMENTS
Pioglitazone Actos	15–30 mg once daily.	15–30 mg once daily.	45 mg once daily.	Approved for use with insulin, a sulfonylurea, or metformin. May improve lipid profile.
Rosiglitazone Avandia	2 mg bid or 4 mg once daily.	2 mg bid or 4 mg once daily.	4 mg bid or 8 mg once daily.	Approved for use with a sulfonylurea or metformin. May increase LDL and HDL cholesterol.[74]

BLOOD GLUCOSE MONITORS COMPARISON CHART

NAME MANUFACTURER	TEST STRIP USED	RANGE (MG/DL)	TEST TIME (SEC)	FEATURES
Accu-Chek Advantage (Roche Diagnostics)	Advantage or Comfort Curve	10–600	40	No cleaning, wiping, or timing; touchable test strips; time and date; large target area; 100-value memory; PC down loading.
Accu-Chek Complete (Roche Diagnostics)	Advantage or Comfort Curve	10–600	40	2-step procedure; pushbutton selection; stores and analyzes up to 1000 values.
Accu-Chek Instant (Roche Diagnostics)	Instant Glucose	20–500	12	No wiping or timing; 9-value memory; Spanish version available.
Accu-Chek Simplicity (Roche Diagnostics)	Simplicity or Comfort Curve	20–500	25–30	Large target area requires small blood sample; 30-value memory.
Accu-Chek Voice Mate (Roche Diagnostics)	Comfort Curve	10–600	40	For visually impaired and the blind; voice guidance; no need to clean.
Assure (Chronimed)	Assure	30–550	35	Large touch-screen display; 180-test memory.
AtLast Blood Glucose System (Amira Medical)	AtLast	40–400	15	Sample taken from the forearm, upper arm, thigh; 10-test memory with 14-day average.
CheckMate Plus (Questar Medical)	CheckMate Plus	25–500	15–70	Display provides words for guidance; no wiping or timing; 6 language prompts; data port allows downloading to a PC.
ExacTech (Abbott Laboratories)	ExacTech	40–450	30	Credit-card size and shape; no wiping, timing, or cleaning; last reading recall.
ExacTech RSG (Abbott Laboratories)	ExacTech RSG	40–450	30	No calibration required; no cleaning or maintenance.
FastTake (LifeScan)	FastTake	20–600	15	Very small blood sample needed; compact; 150-test memory; warning to test ketones when range is 240–600; PC downloading.

(continued)

BLOOD GLUCOSE MONITORS COMPARISON CHART (*continued*)

NAME MANUFACTURER	TEST STRIP USED	RANGE (MG/DL)	TEST TIME (SEC)	FEATURES
Glucometer DEX (Bayer Diagnostics)	Glucometer DEX Test Sensors	10–600	30	10-test cartridge; 100-test memory; PC downloading.
Glucometer Elite Diabetes Care System (Bayer Diagnostics)	Elite	20–600	30	No buttons; turns on when test strip inserted; blood touched to tip of test strip is automatically drawn; lancing device included; videotape available; 20-test memory.
Glucometer Elite XL (Bayer Diagnostics)	Elite	20–600	30	No buttons; 120-test memory; 14-day average; lancing devices and lancets included; 120-test memory; video available.
Glucometer Encore Diabetes Care System (Bayer Diagnostics)	Encore	20–600	15	Automatic 3-min shutoff; 10-test memory; Spanish instructions available.
Medisense 2 Card (Abbott Laboratories)	Medisense 2 or Precision Q.I.D.	20–600	20	No cleaning, wiping, timing; individually wrapped test strips; credit-card size; large display window.
Medisense 2 Pen (Abbott Laboratories)	Medisense 2 or Precision Q.I.D.	20–600	20	No cleaning, wiping, timing; individually wrapped test strips; pen size.
One Touch Basic (LifeScan)	Genuine One Touch	0–600	45	75-test memory; large easy-to-handle test strips; single-button coding.
One Touch FastTake (LifeScan)	FastTake	20–600	15	Very small blood sample; warning to test ketones when range is 240–600; 150-test memory; PC downloading.
One Touch Profile (LifeScan)	One Touch	0–600	45	No timing, wiping or blotting; large display in English, Spanish, and 17 other languages; time and date; cleaning notification; 250-test memory; 14- and 30-day test averages.

(continued)

BLOOD GLUCOSE MONITORS COMPARISON CHART (*continued*)

NAME MANUFACTURER	TEST STRIP USED	RANGE (MG/DL)	TEST TIME (SEC)	FEATURES
One Touch SureStep (LifeScan)	SureStep	0–500	15–30	Large display; touchable test strips; 150-test memory; PC downloading.
Precision Extra (Abbott Laboratories)	Precision Extra	20–600	20	Also measures ketones; 450-test memory.
Precision Q.I.D. (Abbott Laboratories)	Precision Q.I.D.	20–600	20	Automatic start when small blood sample applied; OK to touch strip; compact size; large display; 150-test memory; data-downloading capacity.
Precision Q.I.D. Pen (Abbott Laboratories)	Precision Q.I.D.	20–600	20	Same features as Precision Q.I.D.; pen shape for portability.
Prestige (Home Diagnostics)	Prestige	25–600	10	Nonwipe system; blood applied to strip outside the monitor; large display; universal symbols guide user; English and Spanish videos available.
Prestige XL (Home Diagnostics)	Prestige	25–600	10	365-test memory; large display; English and Spanish videos available.
Select GT (Chronimed)	Select GT	30–600	50	Large display; blood application inside or outside the meter, 100-test memory; universal symbols.
Supreme II (Chronimed)	Supreme	30–600	50	Large display; blood application inside or outside the meter; 100-test memory; universal symbols.
SureStep (LifeScan)	SureStep	0–500	15–30	Large display; touchable test strip; 10-test memory; PC downloading.

Adapted from reference 75.

BLOOD GLUCOSE TEST STRIPS COMPARISON CHART: STRIPS FOR VISUAL READING

NAME (MANUFACTURER)	COLOR CHART INCREMENTS (MG/DL)	PROCEDURE
Chemstrip bG (Roche Diagnostics)	20, 40, 80, 120, 180, 240, 400, 800.	Wipe after 1 min, read after 2 min.
Glucostix Reagent Strips (Roche Diagnostics)	20, 40, 70, 110, 140, 180, 250, 400, 800.	Blot after 30 sec, read 90 sec later.
Select GT Strips (Chronimed)	Low, 40, 70, 120, 180, 240, 400, high.	Wait 60 sec, turn strip over and read.
Supreme Strips (Chronimed)	Low, 40, 70, 120, 180, 240, 400, high.	Wait 60 sec, turn strip over and read.

Adapted from reference 75.

Contraceptives

Class Instructions. Oral Contraceptives. Take this drug at approximately the same time each day for maximum efficacy. This drug may be taken at bedtime or with food, milk, or an antacid if stomach upset occurs. Use an additional form of contraception concurrently during the first 7 days of the oral progestin-only products or if you do not start your oral contraceptives on day 1 of menses. If spotting occurs and no oral doses have been missed, continue to take tablets even if spotting continues. Report immediately if any of the following occur: new severe or persistent headache; blurred or loss of vision; shortness of breath; severe leg, chest, or abdominal pain; or any abnormal vaginal bleeding. Hormonal contraceptives do not protect against HIV infection or other sexually transmitted diseases.

COMBINATION ORAL CONTRACEPTIVES

Pharmacology. These products contain an estrogen, ethinyl estradiol or mestranol, and one of several 19-nortestosterone progestins, which are taken in a cyclic fashion, usually 21 of 28 days. As contraceptives, estrogens suppress follicle-stimulating hormone (FSH) and luteinizing hormone (LH) to inhibit ovulation, cause edematous endometrial changes that are hostile to implantation of the fertilized ovum, accelerate ovum transport, and produce degeneration of the corpus luteum (luteolysis). Progestins inhibit ovulation by suppression of LH, inhibit sperm capacitation, slow ovum transport, produce a thinning endometrium that hampers implantation, and cause cervical mucus changes that are hostile to sperm migration. Induction of a pseudopregnancy state and anovulation improves symptoms of endometriosis. Anovulatory dysfunctional uterine bleeding caused by unopposed estrogen or estrogen withdrawal responds to progestins. (*See* Contraception Efficacy, Risks and Benefits of Oral Contraceptives Comparison Charts.)

Administration and Adult Dosage. **PO for contraception** (monophasic combinations) 1 tablet daily beginning on the first day of menses and continue for 21 days;

stop for 7 days and start the next cycle of 21 tablets. Combination 28-day products (7 inert or iron tablets) are taken, 1 tablet daily continuously; (multiphasic combinations) 1 tablet daily beginning on the first day of menses (Triphasil only) or manufacturer states first Sunday after the beginning of menstruation (if menstruation begins on Sunday, take first tablet on that day), although day-1 start is most effective, then 1 tablet daily for 21 or 28 days as above. **PO for contraception postpartum** start 6 weeks postpartum if not breastfeeding; lactation prolongs period of infertility. **PO for contraception postabortion** start immediately if gestation is terminated at 12 weeks or earlier; start in 1 week if gestation is terminated at 13–28 weeks. **PO for emergency postcoital contraception** (Ovral, Preven) 2 tablets taken as soon as possible after coitus and 2 more tablets taken 12 hr later, but within 72 hr after coitus; or (Lo-Ovral) 4 tablets taken as soon as possible after coitus and 4 more taken 12 hr later, but within 72 hr after coitus.[76-78] (*See* Notes.) **PO for dysfunctional uterine bleeding (anovulatory cycles)** (any combination agent) 1 tablet daily to qid for 5–7 days for acute bleeding, then 1 tablet daily cyclically as for contraception for 3 months to prevent further bleeding.[79] **PO for dysmenorrhea or endometriosis** (any combination tablet) 1 tablet daily continuously for 15 weeks, followed by 1 drug-free week; repeat 16-week cycle for 6–12 months to induce a pseudopregnant state.[80]

Special Populations. *Geriatric Dosage.* Same as adult dosage.

Other Conditions. Discontinue oral contraceptives at least 2 weeks before elective major surgery and do not reinstitute until at least 2 weeks afterward. Stop immediately in patients undergoing emergency surgery or immobilization for long periods; institute low-dose SC heparin or other appropriate thromboembolytic prophylaxis in the postoperative period and restart cycle 4 weeks after returning to normal activities.[78] Start with an agent containing at least 50 μg estrogen in women receiving rifampin or any cytochrome P450–inducing anticonvulsant.[76-78]

Dosage Forms. (*See* Oral Contraceptive Agents Comparison Chart.)

Patient Instructions. (*See* Class Instructions: Oral Contraceptives.) (Contraception) any menstrual irregularities and bothersome side effects should diminish after the first 3–4 cycles. Report if no menses occur for 2 months. (Acute anovulatory bleeding) expect heavy and severely cramping flow 2–4 days after stopping therapy, with normal periods thereafter.

Missed Doses. If you miss 1 active dose, take it as soon as you remember it and take the next tablet at the correct time even if you take 2 tablets on the same day or at the same time. If you miss 2 active doses in week 1 or 2, take 2 tablets on the day you remember and 2 tablets the next day. If you miss 2 active doses in week 3 or miss 3 or more active tablets, then (if you start on day 1) start a new pack the same day or (if you start on Sunday) take 1 tablet daily until Sunday and then start a new pack that day. Use an alternative form of contraception for the next 7 days after you miss 2 or more active doses in weeks 1, 2, or 3 or abstain from sex for the next 7 days.

Pharmacokinetics. *Onset and Duration.* Onset of contraception after 1 week of oral regimen. Dysfunctional uterine bleeding should decrease within 12–24 hr of starting the regimen.[79]

Serum Levels. No correlation of estradiol or mestranol serum levels with pharmacologic activity.

Fate. There are marked intra- and interpatient variabilities in the pharmacokinetics of all these agents. All are concentrated in body fat and endometrium and penetrate poorly into breast milk.[81–90] **Desogestrel** is a prodrug that undergoes extensive first-pass and possibly gut-wall metabolism to its active form, 3-ketodesogestrel. Bioavailability is 63 ± 7%; 65% bound to albumin and 35% to sex hormone–binding globulin (SHBG); SHBG increases by about 200% during long-term use. V_d is 2.4 ± 1.1 L/kg; Cl is 0.2 ± 0.1 L/hr/kg. About 45% is recovered in urine as glucuronides (38–61%), sulfates (23–29%), and unconjugated forms (14–28%); 31% is recovered in feces.[81,82,91–93]

Ethinyl estradiol is rapidly absorbed, with peak concentrations in 60 ± 30 min; bioavailability is 59 ± 13%.[81,86,87] It undergoes extensive small intestine and hepatic first-pass metabolism and conjugation to sulfates and hydroxylation to active 2-hydroxylethinyl estradiol and other hydroxylated metabolites. Ethinyl estradiol is 98.5% bound to albumin and not bound to SHBG. V_d is 5 ± 2 L/kg; reported Cl has ranged from 0.4 ± 0.2 to 1 ± 0.3 L/hr/kg. About 23–59% is excreted in urine, 30–53% in feces as glucuronides and sulfates, and 28–43% undergoes enterohepatic circulation with a rebound in estradiol levels 10–14 hr after administration.[78,81,83–87,91,93] (*See* Estradiol and Its Esters monograph for estrogen replacement.)

Ethynodiol diacetate undergoes rapid absorption and hydrolysis to norethindrone and its metabolites in vivo. (*See* Progestin-Only Contraceptives.) **Mestranol** is approximately 54% demethylated to ethinyl estradiol; serum levels of ethinyl estradiol after oral administration of 50 μg of mestranol are equivalent to those after 35 μg of ethinyl estradiol.[87,90] **Norgestrel/levonorgestrel, norethindrone, and norethindrone acetate** (*see* Progestin-Only Contraceptives). **Norethynodrel** is rapidly converted to norethindrone in vitro.[83,90] **Norgestimate** undergoes hepatic and gut metabolism to levonorgestrel (15.4 ± 5.4%), norgestrel acetate (9.5 ± 1.7%), norgestrel oxime (10.6 ± 1.8%), and 8.1 ± 4.5% as other conjugated metabolites.[84] It is not bound to sex hormone-binding globulin. From 35% to 49% is excreted in urine (57% conjugated sulfates and glucuronides and 12% unconjugated) and 16–49% in feces.

$t_{1/2}$. (Desogestrel) 24 ± 5 hr;[91,92] (ethinyl estradiol) 15 ± 3 to 33 ± 10 hr;[81,91] (levonorgestrel) 31.4 ± 18.5 hr;[80–86,89,90] (norgestimate) 16 hr, (norethindrone) 7.6 ± 1.9 hr.[81–85,90,94]

Adverse Reactions. The risk of major congenital malformations is not increased if oral contraceptives are taken during pregnancy.[95,96] Most of the risks of oral contraceptives are minimal with the lower dosages of estrogens and progestins currently available.[78,96–100] (*See* Risks and Benefits of Oral Contraceptives and Hormone Excess and Deficiency Symptomatology Comparison Charts.)

Contraindications. Known or suspected pregnancy; presence or history of thrombophlebitis or thromboembolic disorders; presence or history of carcinoma of breast or genitals, or other estrogen-dependent tumors; cerebral vascular or coronary artery disease; uncontrolled hypertension; focal migraine; markedly impaired liver function; hepatic adenoma or carcinoma; cholestatic jaundice of pregnancy or jaundice with prior oral contraceptive use; undiagnosed abnormal genital bleeding; malabsorption syndrome, heavy smoking (>15 cigarettes/day) in women ≥35 yr;[78,98] polycythemia vera because of greater tendency for deep vein thrombosis. (*See* Notes.)

Precautions. Use with caution in patients with hyperlipidemia, diabetes, conditions that might be aggravated by fluid retention (eg, hypertension, convulsions, migraine, and cardiac or renal dysfunction), or severe varicosities, in adolescents in whom regular menses are not established, and during lactation.

Drug Interactions. Oral contraceptives might be less effective, resulting in increased breakthrough bleeding or pregnancy, when given with some antibiotics (eg, ampicillin, griseofulvin, metronidazole, nitrofurantoin, neomycin, penicillin, rifampin, tetracycline), or anticonvulsants (eg, barbiturates, carbamazepine, phenytoin). Administer doses of vitamin C ≥1 g/day at least 4 hr before or after oral contraceptives to avoid increasing the bioavailability of ethinyl estradiol; use caution if long-term vitamin C intake is discontinued.[78,101]

Parameters to Monitor. Complete pretreatment physical examination with special reference to blood pressure, breasts, abdomen, pelvic organs, and Pap smear at least q 1–2 yr.

Notes. The initial oral contraceptive prescribed should be a combined product (eg, Ovcon-35, Ortho-Cept, Desogen, Ortho-Novum 7/7/7, Tri-Norinyl, Ortho-Cyclen) containing the smallest effective dose of estrogen (≤35 μg ethinyl estradiol) and progestin (≤0.15 mg desogestrel or levonorgestrel, ≤1 mg norethindrone, or ≤0.25 mg norgestimate) that provides an acceptable pregnancy rate and minimizes side effects.[76,78] Prescribing oral contraceptives to smokers ≥35 yr requires adequate informed consent because of a doubled risk of cardiovascular disease.[97,99] The health risks of pregnancy in healthy, nonsmoking women in their forties is greater than the risks of taking sub-50 μg estrogen or progestin-only contraceptives.[96,99] (*See* Risks and Benefits of Oral Contraceptives Comparison Chart.) For emergency postcoital contraception, 2 doses of a combination contraceptive might be somewhat less effective than high-dose estrogens.[102]

PROGESTIN-ONLY CONTRACEPTIVES:	
LEVONORGESTREL/NORGESTREL	Norplant, Ovrette, Plan B
MEDROXYPROGESTERONE ACETATE	Depo-Provera
NORETHINDRONE	Micronor, Nor-Q.D.

Pharmacology. Norgestrel and norethindrone are 19-nortestosterone derivatives; only the L-isomer of norgestrel (levonorgestrel) is active. Medroxyprogesterone acetate is a 17α-acetoxyprogesterone derivative with greater progestational activity and oral efficacy than native progesterone. These compounds share the actions of progestins, although progestin-only contraceptives suppress ovulation in only about 50% of cycles. (*See* Combination Oral Contraceptives.)

Administration and Adult Dosage. **PO for contraception** (norethindrone) 0.35 mg/day or (norgestrel) 0.075 mg/day continuously at the same time each day, starting on the first day of menses or immediately postpartum. **IM** (medroxyprogesterone acetate) 150 mg q 3 months, starting within 5 days of menses or immediately postabortion or postpartum (within 5 days to 6 weeks of delivery). In breastfeeding mothers, the first dose is recommended at 6 weeks postpartum, although some clinicians give it 3–6 weeks postpartum.[76,103–107] **PO for emergency postcoital contraception** (Plan B) 1 tablet taken as soon as possible after coitus and 1 more tablet taken 12 hr later, but within 72 hr after coitus; **Subdermal** (levonorgestrel) 216 mg (6 Norplant implants) q 5 yr; insert within 7 days of onset of menstruation, immediately postabortion, or no earlier than 6 weeks postpartum if breastfeeding; insertion and removal require a simple surgical procedure performed by trained personnel.[108] (*See also* Progesterone.)

Dosage Forms. **Tab** (norethindrone) 0.35 mg (Micronor, Nor-Q.D.); (norgestrel) 0.075 mg (Ovrette); (levonorgestrel) 0.75 mg (Plan B). **Implant Pellet** (levonorgestrel) kit of 6 capsules, each containing 36 mg (Norplant). **Inj** (medroxyprogesterone acetate) use only the 150 mg/mL dosage form of Depo-Provera for contraception.

Patient Instructions. (*See* Class Instructions: Oral Contraceptives.) Spotting and breakthrough bleeding occur more frequently than with the combination oral contraceptives during the first few months of use; notify prescriber if this persists through the third month.[76,96,108] (Plan B) If you vomit within 1 hour of taking a tablet, call your health care provider to discuss whether to repeat the dose. You might experience spotting during use of this medication, and your next menstrual period might be delayed. If it is delayed more than 7 days, you might be pregnant. (Depo-Provera) use an alternative form of contraception for the first 2 weeks if your first injection is more than 5 days after the start of menses. Cessation of menses is common after 1 to 2 years. (Norplant) use an alternative form of contraception for the first 24 hours if inserted more than 7 days after the start of menses. Irregular bleeding patterns should become more regular 9 to 12 months after insertion. The implants may be visible under the skin. Removal at 5 years must be done by trained personnel.

Missed Doses. (Oral contraceptives) If you miss a dose, even if it is taken only 3 hours late, use an additional backup method for the next 48 hours. Take the missed dose as soon as you remember. If menses do not occur within 45 days, discontinue the contraceptive, use an alternate nonhormonal method of contraception, and make sure you are not pregnant. Because of the higher risk of failure if 1 tablet is missed every 1 to 2 cycles, consider changing the time of tablet taking or using a different contraceptive.

Pharmacokinetics. *Onset and Duration.* (Oral contraceptives) onset after 1 week; duration 24 hr. (Depo-Provera) onset is within 24 hr if given within 5 days of menses; the drug prevents ovulation the first month of use; ovulation is inhibited for at least 14 weeks after 150 mg IM; mean interval before return of ovulation after last injection is 9 months; 70% of former users conceive within the first 12 months after stopping.[82,103,104] (Norplant) onset is within 24 hr after subdermal implantation if inserted within 7 days of menses; immediately reversible once removed, normal ovulatory cycles return during the first month after removal.

Serum Levels. (Ovulation inhibition) levonorgestrel 0.2 μg/L (0.64 nmol/L); medroxyprogesterone >0.1 μg/L (0.25 nmol/L);[101–104] norethindrone 0.4 μg/L (1.34 nmol/L).[108]

Fate. **Levonorgestrel** is completely absorbed orally with no first-pass metabolism.[81–86,89] Peak serum levels occur in 1.1 ± 0.4 hr, are dose dependent, and exhibit considerable interindividual variations. Oral administration of 30 μg yields peak levels of 0.9 ± 0.7 μg/L (2.9 ± 2.2 nmol/L); 150 μg yields 3.6 ± 0.5 μg/L (11.5 ± 1.6 nmol/L); 250 μg yields 5 ± 0.5 μg/L (16 ± 1.6 nmol/L). Within 24 hr after implantation of Norplant, levonorgestrel produces serum levels >0.3 μg/L (0.96 nmol/L). Release of 80 μg/day of levonorgestrel during the first 6–12 months yields levels of 0.4 ± 0.1 μg/L (1.1 ± 0.4 nmol/L); thereafter, release of 25–35 μg/day yields levels that remain above 0.28 ± 0.16 μg/L (0.9 ± 0.5 nmol/L) for the remainder of the 5 yr. Levels are unmeasurable within 48 hr after removal of the implant.[108] Levonorgestrel is concentrated in body fat and endometrium but penetrates poorly into breast milk (approximately 10% of serum levels); it is bound 69.4% to sex hormone-binding globulin and 30% to albumin. V_d is 1.5 ± 0.4 L/kg; Cl is 0.05 ± 0.01 L/hr/kg. Conjugated glucuronides, sulfates, and unconjugated levonorgestrel and its metabolites are excreted 45% in urine and 32% in feces.[84,89] (*See* Medroxyprogesterone Acetate and Norethindrone.)

t½. (Levonorgestrel) 31.4 ± 18.5 hr;[81–86,89,90] (medroxyprogesterone acetate) about 50 days, reflecting slow IM absorption from depot; (norethindrone) 6.4 ± 3 hr.[81–85,90,94]

Adverse Reactions. (Oral contraceptives) menstrual irregularities, including spotting, breakthrough bleeding, prolonged cycles, and amenorrhea, are frequent. Because ovulation is suppressed in only about 50% of cycles, functional ovarian cysts might occur. Most resolve spontaneously within 4 weeks, and surgical intervention is usually not necessary. Ectopic pregnancy occurs in 6% of all pregnancies. Low doses of progestins have minimal effects on the following: serum glucose, insulin or lipid levels; coagulation; liver or thyroid function; blood pressure; or cardiovascular complications.[76,96,103,104,108] (Plan B) nausea, abdominal pain, fatigue, headache and menstrual changes occur frequently. (Depo-Provera) menstrual irregularities, spotting, and breakthrough bleeding are frequent in the first 12 months after IM injection; amenorrhea (after 1 yr), infertility (up to 18 months), and weight gain of 1–1.5 kg also occur. Reversible reduced bone density changes occur with >5 yr of use as contraceptive, but there is no clinical evidence of fractures. Long-term use (>5 yr) does not increase the overall risk of ovarian, liver, breast, or cervical cancer but reduces the risk of endometrial cancer for at least 8 yr after stopping.[96,103,104,109] (Norplant) the most frequent adverse effects are irregular menstrual bleeding, headaches, weight gain, mood changes and depression, premenstrual bilateral mastalgia, galactorrhea (especially after discontinuation of lactation), acne, outbreaks of genital herpes in patients with a history. Rarely, rash, implant expulsions, and local complications (eg, infection, hematoma formation, irritation, allergic reactions to adhesives) occur.[108–111]

Contraindications. Thrombophlebitis or history of deep vein thrombophlebitis or thromboembolic disorders; known or suspected carcinoma of the breast or endometrium, or other estrogen-dependent tumors; undiagnosed abnormal genital bleeding. Known or suspected pregnancy is a contraindication, but the risk of congenital malformations is not increased when progestin-only contraceptives are taken during pregnancy.[96,105] Although acute liver disease, benign or malignant liver tumors, history of cholestatic jaundice of pregnancy, or jaundice with prior hormonal contraceptive use are listed as contraindications by manufacturers, liver disease is not considered by others to be a contraindication to progestin-only contraceptives.[96]

Precautions. Use with caution in patients with histories of depression, diabetes, gestational diabetes, coronary artery disease, cerebrovascular disease, hyperlipidemia, liver disease, or hypertension. Although progestins are not harmful to the fetus during the first 4 months of pregnancy, confirm a negative pregnancy test before reinjecting women >2 weeks late for their IM injection.[96,105] Progestin-only contraceptives used during breastfeeding pose no risk to the infant,[96,103–107] and they usually do not decrease breastmilk production if begun ≥6 weeks postpartum.

Drug Interactions. Rifampin and cytochrome P450–inducing anticonvulsants can decrease efficacy. Long-term use of griseofulvin can increase menstrual irregularities.[76,96,103,104,108]

Parameters to Monitor. Complete pretreatment physical examination with special reference to blood pressure, breasts, abdomen, pelvic organs, and Pap smear at least q 1–2 yr.

Notes. Progestin-only contraceptives are the hormonal contraceptives of choice during breastfeeding or in patients with contraindications to estrogen therapy (eg, hypertension, diabetes, hyperlipidemia, smokers).[76,96,103,104] Long-term noncontraceptive benefits of IM medroxyprogesterone acetate are decreases in menstrual blood loss, anemia, candidal vulvovaginitis, pelvic inflammatory disease, and endometrial cancer. A 30% reduction in seizure frequency was observed in a small group of women with uncontrolled seizures who became amenorrheic with medroxyprogesterone.[103,104]

CONTRACEPTION EFFICACY COMPARISON CHART

METHOD	AVERAGE PREGNANCY RATES PER 100 WOMAN-YR
Oral Monophasic Combination	
<30 µg ethinyl estradiol (EE)[a]	0.75
35–49 µg EE	0.27
50 µg EE	0.16
Oral Multiphasic Combination	0.33
Oral Progestin Only[a]	
Age 25–30 yr	3.1
Age 30–34 yr	2.0
Age 35–39	1.0
Age ≥40 yr	0.3
Lactating	0.3
Subdermal Progestin Implant	0.2
Injectable Depot Progestin	0.3
Emergency Postcoital (within 72 hr of intercourse)	
Ovral 2 tablets q 12 hr for 2 doses	0.2–2.5[b]
Ethinyl estradiol 5 mg/day for 5 days	0.5–1.6[b]
Intrauterine Device	
Copper T 380	0.5
Progestasert	2.9
Barrier Method	
Diaphragm	1.9
Condom[c]	3.6
Vaginal Sponge	10
Cervical Cap	13
Vaginal Spermicide (cream, foam, jelly)	11.9
Other	
Tubal Sterilization	<1
Coitus Interruptus	6.7
Rhythm	15.5
Abstinence Method	70

[a]Mestranol 50 µg is approximately equal to 35 µg of ethinyl estradiol.
[b]Postcoital contraception numbers represent the percentage of women in whom pregnancies occur.
[c]Protects against most sexually transmitted diseases.
From references 76, 77, 95, 96, 104, 108, and 112–114.

ORAL CONTRACEPTIVE AGENTS COMPARISON CHART

MONOPHASIC COMBINATION AGENTS CONTAINING <50 µg OF ESTROGEN

PRODUCT	CYCLE[a]	ESTROGEN[b]	PROGESTIN[c]	POTENCY[d] Estrogenic[e]	Progestational[f]	Androgenic[g]	BREAKTHROUGH BLEEDING AND SPOTTING (%)[h]
Alesse, Levlite	21, 28	Ethinyl estradiol 20 µg.	Levonorgestrel 0.1 mg.	+	+	+	8
Loestrin 1/20	21, 28	Ethinyl estradiol 20 µg.	Norethindrone acetate 1 mg.	+	++	++	25
Desogen, Ortho-Cept	21, 28	Ethinyl estradiol 30 µg.	Desogestrel 0.15 mg.	+	+	±	4
Loestrin 1.5/30	21, 28	Ethinyl estradiol 30 µg.	Norethindrone acetate 1.5 mg.	+	+++	+++	31
Levlen, Levora 0.15/30, Nordette	21, 28	Ethinyl estradiol 30 µg.	Levonorgestrel 0.15 mg.	+	+	++	14
Lo/Ovral, Low-Ogestrel	21, 28	Ethinyl estradiol 30 µg.	Norgestrel 0.3 mg.	+	+	++	10
Yasmin	28	Ethinyl estradiol 30 µg.	Drospirenone 3 mg.[j]	+	+	0	–
Brevicon, ModiCon, Various	21, 28	Ethinyl estradiol 35 µg.	Norethindrone 0.5 mg.	++	+	+	15
Ovcon-35	21, 28	Ethinyl estradiol 35 µg.	Norethindrone 0.4 mg.	++	+	+	19
Demulen 1/35, Zovia 1/35E	21, 28	Ethinyl estradiol 35 µg.	Ethynodiol diacetate 1 mg.	+	++	+	38

(continued)

ORAL CONTRACEPTIVE AGENTS COMPARISON CHART (continued)

PRODUCT	CYCLE[a]	ESTROGEN[b]	PROGESTIN[c]	Estrogenic[e]	Progestational[f]	Androgenic[g]	BREAKTHROUGH BLEEDING AND SPOTTING (%)[h]
					POTENCY[d]		
Norinyl 1+35, Ortho-Novum 1/35, Various	21, 28	Ethinyl estradiol 35 μg.	Norethindrone 1 mg.	++	++	+	15
Ortho-Cyclen	21, 28	Ethinyl estradiol 35 μg.	Norgestimate 0.25 mg.	++	++	+	11
BIPHASIC[i] COMBINATION PRODUCTS CONTAINING <50 μG OF ESTROGEN							
Jenest-28	28	Ethinyl estradiol 35 μg (days 1–21).	Norethindrone 0.5 mg (days 1–7); 1 mg (days 8–21).	++	+	+	7
Mircette	28	Ethinyl estradiol 20 μg (days 1–21); 10 μg (days 24–28).	Desogestrel 0.15 mg (days 1–21).	+	+	±	12
Neocon 10/11, Nelova 10/11, Ortho-Novum 10/11 Various	21, 28	Ethinyl estradiol 35 μg (days 1–21).	Norethindrone 0.5 mg (days 1–10); 1 mg (days 11–21).	++	+	+	20

(continued)

ORAL CONTRACEPTIVE AGENTS COMPARISON CHART (*continued*)

TRIPHASIC[c] COMBINATION PRODUCTS CONTAINING <50 µG OF ESTROGEN

PRODUCT	CYCLE[a]	ESTROGEN[b]	PROGESTIN[c]	POTENCY[d] Estrogenic[e]	POTENCY[d] Progestational[f]	POTENCY[d] Androgenic[g]	BREAKTHROUGH BLEEDING AND SPOTTING (%)[h]
Cyclessa	28	Ethinyl estradiol 25 µg (days 1–21).	Desogestrel 0.1 mg (days 1–7); 0.125 mg (days 8–14); 0.15 mg (days 15–21).	+	+	±	—
Estrostep	21, 28	Ethinyl estradiol 20 µg (days 1–5); 30 µg (days 6–12); 35 µg (days 13–21).	Norethindrone acetate 1 mg (days 1–21).	+	+	+	—
Ortho-Novum 7/7/7	21, 28	Ethinyl estradiol 35 µg (days 1–21).	Norethindrone 0.5 mg (days 1–7); 0.75 mg (days 8–14); 1 mg (days 15–21).	++	+	+	12
Ortho Tri-Cyclen	21, 28	Ethinyl estradiol 35 µg (days 1–21).	Norgestimate 0.18 mg (days 1–7); 0.215 mg (days 8–14); 0.25 mg (days 15–21).	++	+	±	9

(continued)

671

ORAL CONTRACEPTIVE AGENTS COMPARISON CHART (continued)

				POTENCY[d]			BREAKTHROUGH BLEEDING AND SPOTTING (%)[h]
PRODUCT	CYCLE[a]	ESTROGEN[b]	PROGESTIN[c]	Estrogenic[e]	Progestational[f]	Androgenic[g]	
Tri-Norinyl	21, 28	Ethinyl estradiol 35 μg (days 1–21).	Norethindrone 0.5 mg (days 1–7); 1 mg (days 8–16); 0.5 mg (days 17–21).	++	+	+	15
Tri-Levlen, Triphasil, Trivora-28	21, 28	Ethinyl estradiol 30 μg (days 1–6); 40 μg (days 7–11); 30 μg (days 12–21).	Levonorgestrel 0.05 mg (days 1–6); 0.075 mg (days 7–11); 0.125 mg (days 12–21).	+	+	+	15

MONOPHASIC COMBINATION AGENTS CONTAINING 50 μG OF ESTROGEN

Norinyl 1 + 50, Ortho–Novum 1/50, Various	21, 28	Mestranol 50 μg.	Norethindrone 1 mg.	++	++	+	11
Demulen 1/50, Zovia 1/50E	21, 28	Ethinyl estradiol 50 μg.	Ethynodiol diacetate 1 mg.	+	++	+	13

(continued)

ORAL CONTRACEPTIVE AGENTS COMPARISON CHART (*continued*)

PRODUCT	CYCLE[a]	ESTROGEN[b]	PROGESTIN[c]	POTENCY[d] Estrogenic[e]	POTENCY[d] Progestational[f]	POTENCY[d] Androgenic[g]	BREAKTHROUGH BLEEDING AND SPOTTING (%)[h]
Ovcon-50	21, 28	Ethinyl estradiol 50 μg.	Norethindrone 1 mg.	++	++	++	12
Ovral	21, 28	Ethinyl estradiol 50 μg.	Norgestrel 0.5 mg.	++	+++	+++	5
PROGESTIN ONLY							
Micronor, Nor-Q.D.	Continuous	None.	Norethindrone 0.35 mg.	0	+++	+	42
Ovrette	Continuous	None.	Norgestrel 0.075 mg.	0	+	+	35
POSTCOITAL							
Plan B	2 doses of 1 tablet each (*see monograph*)	—	Levonorgestrel 0.75 mg.	—	—	—	—
Preven	2 doses of 2 tablets each (*see monograph*)	Ethinyl estradiol 50 μg.	Levonorgestrel 0.25 mg.	—	—	—	—

+++ = High; ++ = Moderate; + = Low; ± = Very Low; 0 = None.
[a]28-day cycles contain 7 inert or iron tablets to complete the 28-day cycle.
[b]Estrogen equivalent potency: ethinyl estradiol is about 1.5 times as potent as mestranol. Inhibition of ovulation requires 50 μg of ethinyl estradiol or 80 μg of mestranol.

(*continued*)

ORAL CONTRACEPTIVE AGENTS COMPARISON CHART (*continued*)

cMost products contain either norethindrone or norgestrel. Norethindrone may be preferred over norgestrel, which has a marked adverse effect on lipid profile (decreased HDL, increased LDL). Only levonorgestrel is biologically active and exists in newer preparations. Older preparations contain norgestrel, which also has an inactive D-isomer. Desogestrel and norgestimate have positive effects on lipids.

dPotency designations are based on laboratory tests of individual components. Applicability of these methods for combination products used clinically has been questioned.

eOverall estrogenic effect as modified by antiestrogenic or estrogenic effect of progestational component. Relative estrogenic potency as measured by affinity for estrogen receptor (all are relatively weak): norethynodrel > ethynodiol diacetate > norethindrone acetate > norethindrone > levonorgestrel/norgestimate/desogestrel. Antiestrogenic potency: norethindrone acetate > levonorgestrel > norethindrone > ethynodiol diacetate > norethynodrel > norgestimate > desogestrel.

fProgestational potency as measured by delay of menses test. Relative progestogenic potency: norgestimate > desogestrel > levonorgestrel > norethindrone > norethindrone acetate > ethynodiol diacetate > norethynodrel.

gRelative androgenic potency (prostate growth in rats): levonorgestrel > norethindrone > norethindrone acetate > ethynodiol diacetate > norethynodrel > norgestimate > desogestrel. Drospirenone is antiandrogenic.

hPrevalence of breakthrough bleeding (BTB) decreases from the first cycle to third cycle by 50–66% per cycle; these figures represent data submitted to FDA on prevalence of BTB in the third cycle of use. BTB can result from either estrogen or progestin deficiency. Bleeding decreases after the first 6 months of use regardless of the formulation used.

iBi- and triphasic compounds are overall estrogen dominant.

jDrospirenone is a spironolactone analogue that has antiandrogenic and antimineralocorticoid activity. As such, it can cause mild diuresis and potassium retention. Use with caution in patients predisposed to potassium retention (eg, renal insufficiency, ACE inhibitors, angiotensin receptor blockers, potassium-sparing diuretics).

From references 76, 78, 85, and 97.

RISKS AND BENEFITS OF ORAL CONTRACEPTIVES COMPARISON CHART

CONDITION	CLINICAL INFORMATION	COMMENTS
RISKS		
Breast Cancer	Controversial. Overall, lifetime risk is not increased. A meta-analysis of 27 studies indicates a relative risk of 1.16 after 4–12 yr of use. The relative risk is increased to 3 if started in teenage years and duration is >10 yr.	Further information required regarding risk with progestin-only contraceptives.
Cerebrovascular Accidents	Risk of hemorrhagic stroke is increased 2.5-fold compared with nonusers; ever-users have a 1.5-fold risk compared with never-users. Risk is mostly in heavy smokers ≥35 yr and with pre-disposing risk factors (eg, hypertension, diabetes, hyperlipidemia). Odds ratio is 2.9 with combined oral contraceptives (OCs) containing 50 μg of estrogen, 1.8 for combined OCs with 30–40 μg estrogen, and 0.9 for progestin-only products.	Related to both the estrogen and progestin components. Minimal risk with 35 μg/day and progestin-only preparations.
Cervical Cancer	Increased risk of cervical erosions, eversions, dysplasias, and conversion to cancer in situ. Relative risk is 1.8–2.1 times that of nonusers and increased with duration of use >5 yr; other risk factors include multiple sexual partners and early sexual activity.	May increase risk of herpes or papillomavirus infection, which accelerate progression of preinvasive lesions.
Gallbladder Disease	Relative risk of 1.36 for gallstones in users compared to nonusers only during the first 4 yr of use, then risk returns to baseline.	Estrogens increase cholesterol saturation.
Hepatic Tumors	Both benign and malignant tumors reported. Relative risk is 2.6 for users; 9.6 with duration of use >5 yr. Shock can result from rupture of mass. Surgical intervention may be needed, because tumors are not always reversible after discontinuation. Risk is greater in smokers and those with a history of hepatitis B infection or diabetes.	Unknown, although mestranol and higher-dosage formulations are implicated. Progestin-only contraceptives not implicated.

(continued)

675

RISKS AND BENEFITS OF ORAL CONTRACEPTIVES COMPARISON CHART (*continued*)

CONDITION	CLINICAL INFORMATION	COMMENTS
Hyperglycemia	Abnormal glucose tolerance found in predisposed individuals (eg, subclinical or gestational diabetes) and rare cases of diabetic ketoacidosis reported. These effects are minimal with combinations containing ≤35 µg/day of ethinyl estradiol or newer progestins. Norgestrel has greatest insulin-antagonizing activity.	Hyperinsulinemia with relative insulin resistance caused by progestins with minimal effect from estrogens.
Hyperlipidemia	Elevated triglycerides; can precipitate pancreatitis in patients with underlying hyperlipidemia; adverse effects on lipids are greatest with progestin-dominant products, especially levonorgestrel and ethynodiol diacetate, and lowest with norgestimate and desogestrel.	Estrogens increase triglycerides and HDL; progestins increase LDL and decrease HDL. Minimal effect with progestin-only products.
Hypertension	Mild BP elevations of 4 mm Hg systolic and 1 mm Hg diastolic, usually reversible upon drug discontinuation, occur in 1–5% of users. Rare with low-dose products. More common in older women and in those with a family history of hypertension.	Related to both estrogen and progestin components. Consider progestin-only contraceptives.
Infertility	Little risk of permanent sterility. Conception rate after discontinuation may temporarily lag behind that of nonusers for a few months.	Risk concentrated in older women with a long history of contraceptive use.
Myocardial Infarction	No increased risk in healthy nonsmokers; risk is increased 2.8 times that of nonusers in smokers ≥35 yr with presence of other predisposing factors (eg, hyperlipidemia, diabetes, hypertension). Relative risk of 1.9 for current and past users of low-dose products.	Questionably thromboembolic because risk reverses after drug discontinuation.

(continued)

RISKS AND BENEFITS OF ORAL CONTRACEPTIVES COMPARISON CHART (*continued*)

CONDITION	CLINICAL INFORMATION	COMMENTS
Postpill Amenorrhea	Prevalence is 0.2–2.6% after use; check for pituitary tumor in presence of galactorrhea.	Risk is increased if menses were irregular prior to starting. Unrelated to duration or dose.
Pulmonary Embolism	Risk or fatal pulmonary embolism is 9.6-fold that of nonusers.	Risk appears related to progestin. Cyproterone, desogestrel and gestodene carry a 2- to 3-fold greater risk than levonorgestrel.
Thromboembolism and Thrombophlebitis	Risk is increased 2.8-fold that of nonuser; risk is greatest in smokers, sedentary females >50 yr, those with hypertension, and duration of use >5 yr. Desogestrel-containing products have a 2-fold risk compared with other progestins and 4- to 5-fold that of nonusers. Minimal risk with progestin-only products.	Related to desogestrel and to estrogen dose. Estrogens decrease antithrombin III and increase coagulation factors and platelet aggregation. A history of venous thrombosis might be a reason to avoid combination products. Factor V Leiden is also a risk factor.
Teratogenesis	No increased risk of congenital cardiac, limb, or other malformations if oral or progestin-only contraceptives taken during pregnancy. Reports of masculinization of female genitalia reported when high doses of progestin were used for threatened abortion.	Exhaustive review of 18 prospective studies and meta-analysis of 12 prospective cohorts show relative risk of 0.99–1.04.
BENEFITS[a]		
Breast Disease	A 50–75% reduction in fibrocystic disease and fibroadenoma with >2 yr of use.	Protection greatest with progestin-dominant products. Does not prevent breast cancer.
Endometrial Cancer	A 54–72% reduction in endometrial cancer with ≥2 yr of continuous use. Benefit persists for as long as 15 yr after drug discontinuation. Greatest effects in nulliparous women.	Progestin component protective against endometrial adenomatous hyperplasia (precursor to adeno cancer) by opposing estrogen effect.

(continued)

RISKS AND BENEFITS OF ORAL CONTRACEPTIVES COMPARISON CHART (*continued*)

CONDITION	CLINICAL INFORMATION	COMMENTS
Ovarian Cancer	A 30% risk reduction with duration of use ≤4 yr, 60% risk reduction with >5 yr, 80% risk reduction with >12 yr of use compared to nonusers. Protection persists for 10 yr after drug discontinuation.	Mechanism unknown.
Ovarian Cysts	An 80–90% risk reduction.	Less protection with triphasics and low-dose products.
Pelvic Inflammatory Disease/Ectopic Pregnancy	Risk reduction of 50–70% with >1 yr of use and beneficial reduction of ectopic pregnancy rate.	Does not protect against gonorrhea or chlamydial cervicitis.
Menstrual Cycle Effects	A 90% improvement in dysmenorrhea and 50% reduced risk of iron deficiency anemia. Reduction in premenstrual symptoms (eg, anxiety, depression, and headache).	Decrease in menstrual flow and menstrual fluid prostaglandins.
Acne	Combined oral contraceptives lower serum testosterone levels with improvement of acne.	Use least androgenic progestins (eg, desogestrel, norgestimate) or antiandrogen (ie, drospirenone) for greatest effect. Progesterone attenuates immune response.
Rheumatoid Arthritis	A 50% reduction in frequency.	

[a]Most risks and benefits have been documented with the higher-dose estrogen products (>50 µg/day).
From references 76, 78, 95–100, and 112–118.

HORMONE EXCESS AND DEFICIENCY SYMPTOMATOLOGY COMPARISON CHART

CONDITION	SYMPTOMATOLOGY
Estrogen Excess[a]	Estrogen excess also can be a result of progestin deficiency. Symptoms include nausea, vomiting, vertigo, leukorrhea, increase in leiomyoma size, uterine cramps, breast tenderness with fluid retention, cystic breast changes, cholasma, edema, and fluid retention resulting in abdominal or leg pain with cyclic weight gain, headaches on pill days, and hypertension.
Estrogen Deficiency	Estrogen deficiency also can be a result of progestin excess. Symptoms include irritability, nervousness, decreased libido, hot flashes, early and midcycle breakthrough bleeding and spotting (days 1–7), atrophic vaginitis, dyspareunia, no withdrawal bleeding with continued contraceptive use, and decreased amount of withdrawal bleeding.
Progestin Excess	Progestin excess also can be a result of estrogen deficiency. Symptoms include increased appetite and weight gain on nonpill days, tiredness, fatigue, weakness, depression, decreased libido, decreased length of menstrual flow, *Candida* vaginitis, headaches on nonpill days, and breast tenderness on nonpill days.
Progestin Deficiency	Progestin deficiency also can be a result of estrogen excess. Symptoms include late breakthrough bleeding (days 8–21), heavy menstrual flow and clots, dysmenorrhea, and delayed onset of menses following last pill.
Androgen Excess	Symptoms include increased appetite and weight gain, oily scalp, acne, and hirsutism.

[a]Less likely with preparations containing <50 µg/day ethinyl estradiol.
From references 76 and 96–98.

Female Sex Hormones

ESTRADIOL AND ITS ESTERS   Alora, Climara, Combi Patch, Delestrogen, Estinyl, Estrace, Estraderm, Estring, Vagifem, Vivelle, Various

Pharmacology. Estradiol (17β-estradiol; E_2) is the most potent of the naturally occurring estrogens and the major estrogen secreted during the reproductive years. Estradiol and other estrogens produce characteristic effects on specific tissues (such as breast), cause proliferation of vaginal and uterine mucosa, increase calcium deposition in bone, and accelerate epiphyseal closure after initial growth stimulation. Addition of the ethinyl radical results in an orally active compound that is 200 times more potent than estradiol. (*See* Notes.)

Administration and Adult Dosage. For patients with an intact uterus, continuous daily or monthly (at least 10–12 days) administration of a progestin is recommended to induce endometrial sloughing and decrease the risk of endometrial cancer; administration of progestin quarterly (14 days of progestin q 3 months) also might be effective.[119–121] **PO for postmenopausal symptoms and atrophic**

vaginitis administer daily or, if uterus is present, continuous daily or cyclic regimen of 3 weeks on followed by 1 week off, using the smallest effective dosage; (micronized estradiol) 0.5–2 mg/day initially, adjusted as necessary to control symptoms; (ethinyl estradiol) 0.02 mg/day or every other day, to a maximum of 0.05 mg/day; severe cases may require 0.05 mg tid initially until improvement, then decrease to 0.05 mg/day; administer as with micronized estradiol; (micronized estradiol plus norgestimate) 1 tablet daily per packaging (*see* Dosage Forms) (Ortho-Prefest); (ethinyl estradiol plus norethindrone) 1 tablet daily and re-evaluate at 3–6 months (fcmhrt 1/5). **Top patch for postmenopausal symptoms or osteoporosis** initiate with a 25 or 50 μg/day patch; patch is changed once (Climara) or twice (Estraderm, Vivelle) weekly and administered continuously or cyclically (eg, for 3 weeks followed by 1 week without patch). Dosage can be increased if symptoms are not controlled. Combi Patch can be used continuously or sequentially, in which a 50 μg/day estradiol-only patch is used for the first 14 days and Combi Patch is used for the second 14 days of a 28-day cycle. Start either method with the 0.14 mg norethindrone patch and change the patch twice weekly. (*See* Notes.) **Vag for postmenopausal vasomotor symptoms and atrophic vaginitis** (micronized estradiol cream) 200–400 μg/day for 1–2 weeks, then reduce to 100–200 μg/day for 1–2 weeks, then to maintenance of 100 μg 1–3 times/week; (estradiol hemihydrate vaginal tablet) 1 tablet vaginally daily for 2 weeks, then 1 tablet vaginally twice weekly (Vagifem). **Vag for symptoms of postmenopausal urogenital atrophy** (Estring) insert one 2 mg ring into the upper vagina q 3 months. **PO for prevention of osteoporosis** use minimum effective dosage of 2 mg/day micronized estradiol; 20 μg/day of ethinyl estradiol or equivalent; or ethinyl estradiol 5 μg/day plus 1 mg norethindrone acetate (femhrt 1/5). **PO for dysfunctional uterine bleeding** 0.05–0.1 mg/day of micronized estradiol or 10–20 μg/day of ethinyl estradiol for 10–20 days with addition of progestin the third week.[79] **PO for palliation of breast cancer in postmenopausal women** (ethinyl estradiol) 1 mg tid, or (micronized estradiol) 10 mg tid for at least 3 months. **PO for palliation of advanced inoperable prostatic cancer** (ethinyl estradiol) 0.15–2 mg/day, or (micronized estradiol) 1–2 mg tid. **IM for postmenopausal symptoms and prevention of osteoporosis** when oral or vaginal therapy does not provide expected response, is poorly tolerated, or when noncompliance occurs (estradiol cypionate) 1–5 mg q 3–4 weeks; (estradiol valerate) 10–20 mg q 4 weeks. **IM for dysfunctional uterine bleeding** (estradiol valerate) 20 mg initially, then 5 mg q 2 weeks with addition of progestin. **IM for palliation of advanced inoperable prostatic cancer** (polyestradiol phosphate) 40 mg q 2–4 weeks; (estradiol valerate) 30 mg or more q 1–2 weeks depending on patient response.

Special Populations. *Geriatric Dosage.* Same as adult dosage.

Other Conditions. Because estrogens can increase the risk of postsurgery thromboembolic complications, discontinue estrogens at least 4 weeks before surgery, if feasible.

Dosage Forms. **Tab** (micronized estradiol) 0.5, 1, 1.5, 2 mg; (ethinyl estradiol) 0.02, 0.05, 0.5 mg; **Tab** micronized estradiol 1 mg plus norethindrone acetate 0.5 mg (Activella); micronized estradiol 1 mg 3 tablets followed by micronized estradiol 1 mg plus norgestimate 90 μg 3 tablets (Ortho-Prefest); ethinyl estradiol 5 μg plus norethindrone acetate 1 mg (femhrt 1/5); **SR Patch** (estradiol) 25, 37.5, 50, 75, 100 μg/day; **SR Patch** (estradiol) 50 μg/day plus norethindrone acetate 140 or 250 μg/day (Combi Patch). (*See* Notes.) **Vag Crm** (estradiol) 100 μg/g; **Vag Ring** (estradiol) 2 mg (Estring); **Inj** (estradiol cypionate in oil) 5 mg/mL; 2 mg/mL with testosterone cypionate 50 mg/mL (DepoTestadiol, various); (estradiol valerate in oil) 10, 20, 40 mg/mL; 2 mg/mL with testosterone enanthate 90 mg/mL.

Patient Instructions. Report immediately if any of the following occur: new severe or persistent headache or vomiting; blurred or lost vision; speech impairment; calf, chest, or abdominal pain; weakness or numbness of extremities; or any abnormal vaginal bleeding. This (oral) drug may be taken with food, milk, or an antacid to minimize stomach upset. (Patch) discard the protective liner and apply the patch to a clean, dry, and intact area of skin, preferably on the abdomen. Avoid excessively hairy, oily, or irritated areas. Apply immediately after opening and press the patch firmly in place with the palm of your hand for about 10 seconds to ensure good contact, particularly around the edges. Do not apply to the breasts or the waistline. To minimize irritation, rotate sites with an interval of at least 1 week between applications to a particular site.

Pharmacokinetics. *Onset and Duration.* (Menopausal symptoms) onset of therapeutic E_2 levels after oral or vaginal administration is 0.5–1 hr, with peak levels at 5 hr and progressive decline toward baseline by 12–24 hr. Onset of relief of menopausal symptoms occurs within days of the first cycle of therapy. Reductions of LH and FSH levels occur within 3 hr and 6 hr, respectively, with a duration of 24 hr.[91,122] Peak E_2 levels after IM products are (valerate) 2.2 days, (cypionate) 4 days. Duration of depot products is variable after IM injection; (valerate) 14–21 days, (cypionate) 14–28 days, (polyestradiol phosphate) 14–28 days.[122,123] (Cancer) response to estradiol therapy should be apparent within 3 months after initiation of oral therapy.

Serum Levels. (Relief of menopausal symptoms) E_2 levels: apparent at >40 ng/L (147 pmol/L); 80% relief with 68 ng/L (250 pmol/L); 100% relief with 112 ng/L (411 pmol/L).[82,102,119,120,122,124,125] (Prevention of osteoporosis) 60 ng/L (220 pmol/L).

Fate. (Ethinyl estradiol) PO administration of 20 μg yields ethinyl estradiol levels of 25 ng/L (84 pmol/L); 30 μg yields 60 ng/L (202 pmol/L). (*See* Combination Oral Contraceptives.)

(Estradiol) oral bioavailability of micronized estradiol (E_2) is 4.9 ± 5% because of extensive and rapid first-pass metabolism.[123] Topical absorption is affected by skin thickness and site of patch application: 100% (abdomen) and 85% (thigh).[100,122] Oral or vaginal administration results in unphysiologic levels of estrone ($E_1 > E_2$; E_1 is less after Vag than PO administration).[82,102,119,122–126] Patch yields levels of $E_2 > E_1$ (minor E_1 elevations).[102,119,122–126] Steady-state E_2 level after PO administration of 1 mg estradiol is 35 ± 5 ng/L (128 ± 18 pmol/L) or an increase of 25 ng/L (92 pmol/L) over baseline; after 2 mg, 63 ± 11 ng/L (231 ± 40 pmol/L) or 40 ng/L (147 pmol/L) over baseline; after 4 mg, 121 ± 15 ng/L (444

± 55 pmol/L) or 50 ng/L (183 pmol/L) over baseline; after 6 mg, 207 ± 200 ng/L (760 ± 734 pmol/L).[82,122] (Vag) 0.2 mg estradiol yields 80 ± 19 ng/L (293 ± 7 pmol/L) of E_2.[122] (Patch) 25 μg yields 25 ng/L (92 pmol/L); 50 μg yields 38 ± 10 ng/L (138 ± 36 pmol/L); 100 μg yields 89 ± 82 ng/L (327 ± 302 pmol/L) of E_2.[102,125] (See Notes.)

Estradiol is about 60% bound to albumin, 38% to sex hormone-binding globulin, and 3% unbound. It is widely distributed and concentrated in fat. V_d is 10.9 ± 2.9 L; Cl is 24.2 ± 7 L/hr/m^2 or 0.77 L/hr/kg.[82,122,123] Estradiol and its esters are converted in the liver, endometrium, and intestine, 15% to estrone (active), 65% to estrone sulfate and its conjugates (primarily sulfates and glucuronides with reconversions of 5% estrone and 1.4% estrone sulfate back to E_2). E_2 is excreted 50% in urine and 10% in feces, with some enterohepatic circulation. Less than 1% is excreted unchanged in urine and 50–80% as conjugates: estrone 20%, estriol 20%, estradiol glucuronide 7%.[82,122,123] (Estradiol valerate and cypionate) these are slowly hydrolyzed to E_2 and their respective free acids. (Polyestradiol phosphate) slowly hydrolyzed to E_2.

$t_{1/2}$. (Estradiol) 1 hr;[82,122,123] (ethinyl estradiol) 15 ± 3 to 33 ± 10 hr.[81–91]

Adverse Reactions. (See Postmenopausal Hormone Replacement Risks and Benefits Comparison Chart.) Nausea, vomiting, bloating, breast tenderness, and spotting occur frequently. (See Hormone Excess and Deficiency Symptomatology Comparison Chart.) Hypercalcemia occurs occasionally in patients with breast cancer. Thromboembolism, thrombophlebitis, diabetes, hypertension, and gallbladder disease are less likely to occur with hormone replacement dosages than with oral contraceptive dosages. Pain at injection site occurs frequently. Occasional redness and irritation at application site with patch; rash rarely.

Contraindications. Pregnancy; history or presence of estrogen-dependent cancer (except in appropriate patients treated for metastatic disease); undiagnosed abnormal genital bleeding; history or presence of thromboembolism or severe thrombophlebitis. A history of breast cancer might not be an absolute contraindication to estrogen therapy in women with severe menopausal symptoms.[119,127] Active or severe chronic liver disease is a contraindication for combinations with testosterone.

Precautions. Use with caution in patients with disease states that could be exacerbated by increased fluid retention (eg, asthma; epilepsy; migraine; and cardiac, hepatic, or renal dysfunction); in women with strong family histories of breast cancer or presence of fibrocystic disease, fibroadenoma, or abnormal mammogram; in women with fibromyomata, cardiovascular disease, diabetes, hypertriglyceridemia, severe liver disease, or history of jaundice during pregnancy; and in young patients in whom bone growth is not complete. Oral estrogen can increase thyroid-binding globulin and cause false elevations in total T_4 and T_3 and false depression of resin T_3 uptake while the thyroid index, thyroid-stimulating hormone, and the patient remain euthyroid. Estrace 2 mg and Estinyl 0.02 mg contain tartrazine, which may cause allergic reactions, including bronchospasm, in susceptible individuals.

Drug Interactions. Estrogens can reduce the effects of tricyclic antidepressants and warfarin and increase the effects of corticosteroids by increasing their half-lives. Barbiturates, rifampin, and other cytochrome P450 inducers can decrease estrogen levels.

Parameters to Monitor. Signs and symptoms of side effects, especially abnormal bleeding. Pretreatment and physical examination with reference to blood pressure, breasts, abdomen, pelvic organs, and Pap smear. Baseline laboratory tests should include glucose, triglycerides, cholesterol, LFTs, and calcium. Repeat physical examination annually; repeat laboratory tests only if abnormal at baseline.

Notes. Estradiol has been advocated as the estrogen replacement of choice because it is the principal estrogen of the reproductive years; however, advantages over other estrogens have not been established. Synthetic 17α-alkylated estrogens (eg, ethinyl estradiol) are generally not recommended in menopausal replacement therapy because of their potent hepatic effects. The combination of an **androgen** with estrogen is indicated for moderate to severe vasomotor symptoms in patients not improved by estrogen alone. Potential benefits include increased libido and psychological well-being. An alternative to estrogens for hot flashes is **megestrol acetate** 20 mg bid, which reduced hot flashes by 50% during 4 weeks of use in one study.[128] The combination of **norethindrone acetate** and estradiol in a single patch (Combi Patch) results in less endometrial hyperplasia than an estradiol-only patch.

Nonoral estradiol administration (eg, patch, vaginal, implant, injection), avoids first-pass effect and theoretically results in a preferable premenopausal physiologic serum level ratio of $E_2 > E_1$. Oral administration results in an unphysiologic ratio of $E_2 < E_1$ (E_1 levels are not directly related to efficacy).[82,102,122,123,125,129] Avoiding the first-pass effect allows a smaller dosage to be used and prevents undesirable changes from liver stimulation (ie, increases in renin substrate, sex hormone-binding globulin, thyroxine-binding globulin, coagulation factors, transferrin, growth hormone levels, and cortisol-binding globulin and a reduction in insulin-like growth factor) and their sequelae (ie, gallbladder disease, hypertension, and hypercoagulable states in some women).[102,125,129,130] Hepatic stimulation varies with oral preparations, with ethinyl estradiol > conjugated estrogens > E_2. Enhanced liver action is also responsible for the cardioprotective effects on lipids and occurs even with vaginal estrogens.[131] Transdermal administration appears to exert favorable effects on serum lipoproteins (ie, elevation of HDLs and depression of LDLs) after >4 months of use and protects against bone loss and fractures similarly to oral estrogens.[102,125,129,130]

Postmenopausal women most likely to develop osteoporosis are whites and Asians; blacks are at less risk.[119,129,132] Numerous estrogens and other drugs are available for the prevention and treatment of postmenopausal osteoporosis.[133] In women in whom estrogen replacement therapy is intolerable or contraindicated, oral bisphosphonates have increased bone mass and reduced vertebral fractures, vertebral deformities, and loss of height. (*See* Alendronate). **Calcitonin salmon** (Miacalcin) 200 IU/day intranasally has increased bone mass in women >5 yr postmenopausal with low bone mass who cannot take estrogens.[134] Slow-release **fluoride** (Slow Fluoride) appears to be useful in a dosage of 25 mg/day for up to 4 yr, but immediate-release products are not useful because the drug is irritating to the GI tract and the new bone formed is brittle and subject to fracture.[135]

ESTROGENS, CONJUGATED	Cenestin, Premarin, Various
ESTROGENS, ESTERIFIED	Estratab, Menest, Various

Pharmacology. Conjugated estrogens contain a mixture of 50–65% sodium estrone sulfate, 20–35% sodium equilin sulfate, and other estrogenic substances obtained from the urine of pregnant mares. Esterified estrogens are a combination of 75–85% sodium estrone sulfate and 6.5–15% sodium equilin sulfate prepared from Mexican yams. (*See* Estradiol and Its Esters.)

Administration and Adult Dosage. For patients with intact uteri, continuous daily or monthly (for at least 10–12 days) administration of a progestin is recommended to induce endometrial sloughing and decrease the risk of endometrial cancer; administration of progestin quarterly (14 days of progestin q 3 months) also might be effective.[119–121] **PO for postmenopausal symptoms and atrophic vaginitis** use smallest effective dosage in the range of 0.3–1.25 mg/day continuously or, if uterus is present, in cycles of 21–25 days/month. **PO for prevention of postmenopausal osteoporosis** use minimum effective dosage of 0.625 mg/day continuously, or cyclically if uterus is present, or 0.3 mg/day if 1.5 g/day of elemental calcium is also used; higher dosages of 1.25 mg/day may be necessary after fractures caused by osteoporosis.[119,133] For women experiencing migraine or other symptoms during the withdrawal period, a 5-day/week regimen or a shorter withdrawal period may be used. **Vag for postmenopausal symptoms and/or atrophic vaginitis** 1.25–2.5 mg/day; (atrophic vaginitis) 0.3 mg 3 times/week might be effective.[124] **PO for dysfunctional uterine bleeding** 1.25–2.5 mg/day for 10 days.[79] **IV (preferred) or IM for rapid cessation of dysfunctional uterine bleeding** 25 mg of conjugated estrogens, may repeat in 6–12 hr prn, to a maximum of 3 doses.[79] **IV for bleeding from uremia** 0.6 mg/kg/day diluted in 50 mL of NS and infused over 30–40 min for 5 days; dosages as high as 60 mg/day IV have been used.[136,137] **PO for palliation of breast cancer** (patients should be ≥5 yr postmenopausal) 10 mg tid. **PO for palliation of prostatic cancer** 1.25–2.5 mg tid.

Special Populations. *Geriatric Dosage.* Same as adult dosage.

Dosage Forms. **Tab** (conjugated) 0.3, 0.625, 0.9, 1.25, 2.5 mg (Cenestin, Premarin, various); 0.625 mg with medroxyprogesterone acetate 2.5, 5 mg (Prempro); 0.625 mg with medroxyprogesterone acetate 5 mg (Premphase); (esterified) 0.3, 0.625, 1.25, 2.5 mg; 0.625 mg with testosterone 1.25 mg (Estratest H.S.); 1.25 mg with testosterone 2.5 mg (Estratest); **Inj** (conjugated) 25 mg; **Vag Crm** (conjugated) 0.625 mg/g.

Patient Instructions. Report immediately if any of the following occur: new severe or persistent headache or vomiting; blurred or loss of vision; speech impairment; calf, chest, or abdominal pain; weakness or numbness of extremities; or any abnormal vaginal bleeding. This (oral) drug may be taken with food, milk, or an antacid to minimize stomach upset.

Pharmacokinetics. *Onset and Duration.* (Menopausal symptoms) PO peak onset of equilin sulfate is 4 hr; onset of estrone is 3 hr, with a peak at 5 hr; duration is >24 hr. After vaginal administration, onset of therapeutic estradiol levels is 3 hr and peak occurs in 6 hr, with decline over 24 hr to baseline values. Gonadotropin suppression occurs within 1 month of therapy, although suppression to pre-menopausal levels might not occur.[125] (Uremia) improvement in bleeding time occurs within 6 hr after starting estrogens; maximum improvement occurs within 2–5 days after initiation of estrogens; effects last 3–10 days after drug discontinuation.[136,137]

Serum Levels. (*See* Estradiol and Its Esters.)

Fate. Conjugated equilin and estrone sulfate are rapidly absorbed and hydrolyzed to unconjugated forms when given orally or vaginally. Oral administration of 0.3 mg yields steady-state estradiol (E_2) levels of 48 ± 12 ng/L (175 ± 45 pmol/L) or an increase of 20 ng/L (73 pmol/L) over baseline; 0.625 mg yields 103 ± 33 ng/L (378 ± 120 pmol/L) or 50 ng/L (184 pmol/L) over baseline; 1.25 mg yields 125 ± 66 ng/L (460 ± 243 pmol/L) or 70 ng/L (257 pmol/L) over baseline. Vaginal administration of 0.3 mg yields steady-state E_2 levels of 7 ± 22 ng/L (26 ± 81 pmol/L); 0.625 mg yields 36 ± 16 ng/L (131 ± 57 pmol/L); 1.25 mg yields 94 ± 44 ng/L (344 ± 161 pmol/L).[82,122,123] (Estrone sulfate) V_d is 38 ± 13 L; Cl is 3.9 ± 1.2 L/hr/m^2.[138,139] Estrone sulfate is rapidly converted to estrone and estradiol. (Equilin sulfate) Cl is 7.3 ± 4 L/hr/m^2. Approximately 30% of equilin sulfate is metabolized to active 17α-dihydroequilin sulfate and 2% to active 17α-dihydroequilin.[138] Inactivation of estrogens occurs mainly in the liver, with degradation to less active estrogenic products (eg, estrone). Metabolites are conjugated with sulfate and glucuronic acid; urinary recovery is 70–88% within 5 days after oral administration. (*See* Estradiol and Its Esters.)

$t_{\frac{1}{2}}$. (Estrone sulfate) 4–5 hr. (Equilin) 19–27 min. (Equilin sulfate) 190 min. (17α-dihydroequilin) 45 ± 5 min. (17α-dihydroequilin sulfate) 2.5 ± 0.6 hr.[138]

Adverse Reactions, Contraindications, Precautions, Drug Interactions, Parameters to Monitor. (*See* Estradiol and Its Esters.)

Notes. Oral and vaginal administrations result in an unphysiologic $E_1 > E_2$ ratio, although higher E_2 levels occur orally than vaginally.[122–125] (*See* Estradiol Notes, Postmenopausal Hormone Replacement Risks and Benefits Comparison Chart.)

ESTROPIPATE   Ogen, Various

Pharmacology. Estropipate is estrone sulfate stabilized with inert piperazine. Estrone (E_1) is the major estrogen produced in the postmenopausal period. It is one-half as potent as estradiol (E_2) and shares the actions of other estrogens. (*See* Estradiol and Its Esters.)

Administration and Adult Dosage. For patients with intact uteri, continuous daily or monthly administration (minimum of 10–12 days) of progestin is recommended to induce endometrial sloughing and decrease the risk of endometrial cancer; administration of progestin quarterly (14 days of progestin q 3 months) also might be effective.[119–121] **PO for postmenopausal symptoms and prevention of osteoporosis** use the smallest effective dosage in the range of 0.625–5 mg/day continuously or in cycles of 21–25 days/month; administer as with conjugated estrogens. **Vag for postmenopausal symptoms and/or atrophic vaginitis** 3–6 mg/day. **PO for palliation of inoperable advanced prostatic cancer** 3–6 mg tid.

Special Populations. *Geriatric Dosage.* Same as adult dosage.

Dosage Forms. Tab (as conjugated estrogens equivalent) 0.625, 1.25, 2.5, 5 mg; **Vag Crm** 1.5 mg/g.

Patient Instructions. Report immediately if any of the following occur: new severe or persistent headache or vomiting; blurred or loss of vision; speech impairment; calf, chest, or abdominal pain; weakness or numbness of extremities; or any abnormal vaginal bleeding. This (oral) drug may be taken with food, milk, or an antacid to minimize stomach upset.

Pharmacokinetics. Estrone is not orally active because of enzymatic degradation in the gut and liver. Addition of a piperazine moiety increases oral absorption such that E_2 levels are similar to those after administration of estradiol. Oral administration of 0.6 mg estropipate yields E_2 serum levels of 34 ng/L (124 pmol/L); 1.2 mg yields 42 ng/L (154 pmol/L).[82,122,123] Estrone is hydroxylated to α-hydroxyestrone, estriol, and 2-hydroxyestrone. The half-life of estrone is estimated to be 12 hr in serum; however, this does not reflect events in peripheral tissues. The half-life of estrone sulfate is 4–5 hr.[82,122,123,126] (*See* Estradiol and Its Esters.)

Adverse Reactions, Contraindications, Precautions, Drug Interactions, Parameters to Monitor, Notes. (*See* Estradiol and Its Esters.)

ESTROGENS COMPARISON CHART

DRUG	DOSAGE FORMS	EQUIPOTENT PHYSIOLOGIC DOSE[a,b]	COMMENTS
STEROIDAL AGENTS			
Conjugated Estrogens Premarin Various	Tab 0.3, 0.625, 0.9, 1.25, 2.5 mg Vag Crm 0.625 mg/g Inj 25 mg.	0.625 mg.	Mixture of 50–65% sodium estrone sulfate, 20–35% equilin sulfate, and other estrogenic substances from the urine of pregnant mares. Expensive; nausea is rare.
Esterified Estrogens Estratab Menest Various	Tab 0.3, 0.625, 1.25, 2.5 mg	0.625 mg.	Similar to conjugated estrogens. Mixture of 75–85% sodium estrone sulfate and 6.5–15% sodium equilin sulfate obtained from Mexican yams.
Estradiol, Micronized Estrace	Tab 0.5, 1, 1.5, 2 mg Vag Crm 100 mg/g Vag Ring 2 mg.	1 mg.	Moderate cost; some nausea with oral; estradiol is the major estrogen secreted during the reproductive years.
Estradiol Climara Estraderm Vivelle	SR Patch 25, 37.5, 50, 75, 100 μg/day.	50 μg/day.	Estraderm contains alcohol; Climara and Vivelle do not contain alcohol and may be less irritating to the skin.
Estradiol Cypionate Depo-Estradiol Various	Inj (in oil) 5 mg/mL.	—	Pain at injection site; variable onset with a duration of 14–28 days.

(continued)

687

ESTROGENS COMPARISON CHART (continued)

DRUG	DOSAGE FORMS	EQUIPOTENT PHYSIOLOGIC DOSE[a,b]	COMMENTS
Estradiol Valerate Delestrogen Various	Inj (in oil) 10, 20, 40 mg/mL.	1 mg.	Pain at injection site; variable onset with a duration of 14–21 days.
Ethinyl Estradiol Estinyl Feminone	Tab 0.02, 0.05, 0.5 mg.	5 μg.	Not recommended for estrogen replacement because of its potent hepatic effects. (See Estradiol Notes.)
Estrone Various	Inj 2, 5 mg/mL.	0.9 mg.	No advantage over conjugated/esterified estrogens; estrone is the major estrogen of the postmenopausal years.
Estropipate Ogen Various	Tab 0.625, 1.25, 2.5, 5 mg Vag Crm 1.5 mg/g.	0.625 mg.	Ogen 0.625 mg = 0.75 mg estropipate. Ogen 1.25 mg = 1.5 mg estropipate. Ogen 2.5 mg = 3 mg estropipate. Ogen 5 mg = 6 mg estropipate.
NONSTEROIDAL AGENTS			
Dienestrol Various	Vag Crm 0.01%.	—	

[a]Potency of estrogens: estradiol > estrone. Potency is based on the effects on the liver.
[b]See monographs or product information for exact dosage regimens for various uses.

POSTMENOPAUSAL HORMONE REPLACEMENT RISKS AND BENEFITS COMPARISON CHART

RISKS/BENEFITS	CLINICAL INFORMATION	COMMENTS
Cancer, Breast	Controversial; no association with <5 yr duration of use to relative risk of 1.25–1.45 among current users with >5 yr duration of use; highest risk of 1.7 reported among long-term users >60 yr. No risk found in past users, regardless of duration of use. Two meta-analyses show minimal risk with >15 yr of use.	Addition of progestin does not reduce risk. Regular mammography is recommended. Consider limiting duration of treatment to <5 yr if risks of cancer outweigh cardioprotective benefits.
Cancer, Colon	A 46% decrease in colon cancer risk; no effect on rectal cancer.	In slender women, risk is reduced by up to 75%.
Cancer, Endometrial	Relative risk of 8.2 with unopposed estrogen use; risk increases with higher dosage and duration >5 yr; 34% risk after 3 yr; 20% lifetime probability of needing a hysterectomy with un-opposed estrogen therapy.	Relative risk of 1 with the concurrent addition of a minimum of 10–14 days of progestin. No increased risk of estrogen hyperplasia or need for hysterectomy with concurrent progestin therapy.
Cardiovascular Disease	Three meta-analyses and a cohort study suggest a 40–50% re-duction in the risk of coronary and fatal heart disease with unopposed estrogens; benefits may be greater in those with heart disease and >15 yr duration of use. Decreased lifetime probability of developing coronary artery disease. Hormone replacement for ≥1 yr associated with a 52% decreased risk of peripheral arterial disease. Unknown protection against stroke.	Combination with progestin may be protective, but data are insufficient. May be related to estrogen's effects on lipids or direct effect of re-laxing blood vessel walls.
Hypertension	Estrogens can reduce BP.	Hormone replacement is not contraindicated in hypertension.
Lipids	Unopposed oral estrogens reduce LDL and increase HDL by 10–15%; however, estrogens can increase triglyceride levels.	Progesterone antagonizes beneficial estrogen lipid effects less than medroxyprogesterone. Most favorable effects on lipids occur with estrogen alone. Nonoral estrogens (eg, patch, vaginal) produce less HDL beneficial effects.

(continued)

POSTMENOPAUSAL HORMONE REPLACEMENT RISKS AND BENEFITS COMPARISON CHART (*continued*)

RISKS/BENEFITS	CLINICAL INFORMATION	COMMENTS
Gallbladder Disease	Estrogen treatment is associated with a 2.1 relative risk (RR). RR of 2.6 with >10 yr of use; RR of 2.4 for users of 1.25 mg or more of conjugated/estrified estrogen.	Mortality unaffected; may require cholecystectomy.
Osteoporosis	Inhibits bone resorption and prevents bone loss; 15–50% increase in bone density if begun within 3 yr of menopause. Osteoporosis risk increased in Caucasian and Asian ethnic groups, in sedentary lifestyle, in smokers, with low calcium and vitamin D intake, and excessive alcohol or thyroxine intake.	Alendronate (Fosamax) orally, intranasal calcitonin (Miacalcin), etidronate (Didronel), and slow-release fluoride also may be effective. (See Estradiol Notes.)
Fractures	One-half as many fractures of spinal and hip bones with >5 yr of use; 28% reduction with 10 yr use; 40% with 15 yr use; and 55% with 20 yr. Risk returns near baseline 6 yr or more after cessation of therapy. Decreased lifetime probability of osteoporotic fracture. Risk increases 4-fold for each 1 SD decrease in bone density at the hip; 66% of femoral neck fractures occur when bone density is below the lowest quartile.	Bone densitometry can identify women at highest risk.
Vaginal Bleeding	Unpredictable bleeding occurs in 35–40% of women with uteruses yearly.	Amenorrhea usually occurs after 6–8 months of combination estrogen/progestin therapy.

From references 119, 121, 127, 130, 132, 139, and 157–164.

MEDROXYPROGESTERONE ACETATE Depo-Provera, Provera, Various

Pharmacology. Medroxyprogesterone is a 17α-acetoxyprogesterone derivative with greater progestational effects and oral efficacy than progesterone. Progesterone transforms an estrogen-primed proliferative endometrium into a secretory endometrium.

Administration and Adult Dosage. **PO for secondary amenorrhea, or abnormal uterine bleeding, or to induce withdrawal bleeding after postmenopausal estrogen replacement therapy** 5–10 mg/day for 5–10 days, depending on the degree of endometrial stimulation desired, beginning on the presumed 16th or 21st day of the cycle for abnormal uterine bleeding. In secondary amenorrhea, therapy can be started at any time. **PO for postmenopausal symptoms and osteoporosis** (combined with continuous estrogen) 2.5–5 mg/day.[140,141] (*See* Notes.) **PO for relief of vasomotor symptoms** 20 mg/day; **IM for relief of vasomotor symptoms** 150 mg/day.[142] (*See* Notes.) **IM for endometrial or renal carcinoma** 400 mg–1 g/week initially for a few weeks, then, if improvement occurs, reduce to maintenance dosage of 400 mg/month. (*See also* Progestin-Only Contraceptives.)

Special Populations. *Geriatric Dosage.* Same as adult dosage.

Dosage Forms. **Tab** 2.5, 5, 10 mg; **Inj** 150, 400 mg/mL.

Patient Instructions. Report immediately if any of the following occur: new severe or persistent headache; blurred vision; calf, chest, or abdominal pain; or any abnormal vaginal bleeding. This (oral) drug may be taken with food, milk, or an antacid to minimize stomach upset. (Dysfunctional uterine bleeding) expect heavy and severely cramping flow 2–4 days after stopping therapy; expect a normal period after a few days.

Pharmacokinetics. *Onset and Duration.* Withdrawal bleeding (in estrogen-primed endometrium) occurs 3–7 days after the last dose.[103,104] Onset of symptomatic relief of hot flashes within 4–7 days; maximum relief after 1 month; duration 8–20 weeks after discontinuation.[142]

Serum Levels. Inhibition of ovulation and tumor response occurs with medroxyprogesterone levels >0.1 μg/L (0.25 nmol/L).[101,103,104,143]

Fate. Medroxyprogesterone acetate (MPA) is rapidly absorbed orally with no first-pass metabolism; oral bioavailability is 5.7 ± 3.8%; IM bioavailability is 2.5 ± 1.7%, with a large interpatient variation in serum levels after oral or IM administration.[82,143] Higher concentration depot formulation is associated with lower serum concentrations but equivalent bioavailability.[144] Peak concentrations occur in 2–7 hr and are 2–10 times higher after oral than after IM depot injection. PO 10 mg yields peak levels of 3–4 μg/L (7.5–10 nmol/L), declining to 0.3–0.6 μg/L (0.8–1.5 nmol/L) by 24 hr; PO 100 mg yields 13 ± 7 μg/L (34 ± 18 nmol/L), declining to 2 μg/L (5 nmol/L) by 24 hr; PO 500 mg yields 13 ± 8 μg/L (34 ± 21 nmol/L). After 150 mg IM of the 150 mg/mL formulation, peak levels of 8.3 ± 3.2 μg/L (21 ± 8 nmol/L) occur within a few days, declining to levels of 0.8 ± 0.7 μg/L (2 ± 1.8 nmol/L) for 92 ± 44 days. After 400 mg IM of the 400 mg/mL formulation, peak serum levels of 6.2 ± 2.3 μg/L (16 ± 6 nmol/L) are achieved after 16.3 ± 15.6 days.[82,94,103,104,144] The drug is stored in fat; >90% is protein bound to albumin; 83% of a dose is present in serum as the parent drug and conjugated medroxyprogesterone; it is hydroxylated to 6-α-hydroxy-MPA and 21-hydroxy-MPA, which both have unknown activities. From 15% to 20% of a dose is excreted in urine as glucuronide and sulfate conjugates; 45–80% is excreted in feces.[94]

$t_{1/2}$. 50 days, reflecting slow IM absorption from depot.

Adverse Reactions. Frequent breast tenderness, weight gain, and depression occur. Adverse lipid effects (increased LDL, decreased HDL) occur with dosages ≥10 mg/day; dosages of 2.5–5 mg/day have negligible effects.[121,140,144] (*See also* Progestin-Only Contraceptives, Postmenopausal Hormone Replacement Risks and Benefits Comparison Chart, and Hormone Excess and Deficiency Symptomatology Comparison Chart.)

Contraindications. Known or suspected pregnancy or as a diagnostic test for pregnancy. Thrombophlebitis, history of deep vein thrombophlebitis, or thromboembolic disorders; known or suspected carcinoma of the breast or endometrium, or other estrogen-dependent tumors; undiagnosed abnormal genital bleeding. Although acute liver disease, benign or malignant liver tumors, and history of cholestatic jaundice of pregnancy or jaundice with prior hormonal contraceptive use are listed as contraindications by manufacturers, liver disease is not considered by others to be a contraindication to progestin-only contraceptives.[96]

Precautions. Use with caution in patients with histories of depression, diabetes, gestational diabetes, coronary artery disease, cerebrovascular disease, hyperlipidemia, liver disease, or hypertension. Although progestins are not harmful to the fetus during the first 4 months of pregnancy; confirm a negative pregnancy test before reinjecting a woman >2 weeks late for her IM injection.[96,105] Progestin-only contraceptives used during breastfeeding pose no risk to the infant,[96,103–107] and they usually do not decrease breastmilk production if begun after 6 weeks postpartum.

Drug Interactions. Rifampin and cytochrome P450–inducing anticonvulsants can increase progestin metabolism. Long-term use of griseofulvin can increase menstrual irregularities.[76,96,103,104,108]

Parameters to Monitor. Complete pretreatment physical examination with special reference to blood pressure, breasts, abdomen, pelvic organs, and Pap smear yearly.

Notes. Continuous administration of low-dose progestin and estrogen combinations in postmenopausal syndrome causes amenorrhea in >50% of women and does not appear to negatively influence blood lipids when compared with cyclic therapy.[121,140,141,145] Concurrent administration of estrogen with progestin for amenorrhea might be associated with less breakthrough bleeding than with progestin alone. There is no evidence that progestins are effective in preventing habitual abortion or treating threatened abortion.

MIFEPRISTONE Mifeprex

Pharmacology. Mifepristone (RU-486) is a synthetic steroid with antiprogestational effects.

Adult Dosage. PO for pregnancy termination through day 49 of pregnancy 600 mg as a single dose, followed in 2 days by misoprostol 200 mg PO. Patients should return on day 14 to assess efficacy of the procedure and bleeding.

Dosage Forms. Tab 200 mg.

Pharmacokinetics. Oral bioavailability is 69% with a 20 mg dose. It is 98% bound to albumin and α_1-acid glycoprotein. It is metabolized primarily by CYP3A4 to three major metabolites. Most of drug is eliminated in feces, with 9% of the drug and metabolites eliminated in urine. Clearance is dose dependent, with 50% eliminated between 12 and 72 hr; the remaining drug is eliminated with a half-life of 18 hr.

Adverse Reactions. Vaginal bleeding and cramping are expected effects of the drug (plus misoprostol) and occur mostly on day 3. Bleeding is generally heavier than a normal menstrual period. Other frequent effects are nausea, vomiting, diarrhea, headache, dizziness, and fatigue. Drugs that affect CYP3A4 can alter mifepristone metabolism. The metabolism of drugs metabolized by CYP3A4 might be affected.

Contraindications. Confirmed or suspected ectopic pregnancy or undiagnosed abdominal mass; IUD in place; chronic adrenal failure; concurrent long-term corticosteroid use; allergy to mifepristone, misoprostol or other prostaglandin; hemorrhagic disorder; anticoagulant therapy; inherited porphyria.

Notes. Pregnancy termination should be conducted only in a setting where a qualified physician can assess the gestational age of the fetus, diagnose ectopic pregnancies, and provide surgical intervention in case of incomplete abortion or severe bleeding (or have made plans to provide such care through others).

NORETHINDRONE ACETATE   Aygestin

Pharmacology. Norethindrone acetate is a 19-nortestosterone derivative that shares the actions of progestins. It has oral efficacy, greater progestational activity than progesterone, and less androgenic activity than androgens. (*See also* Medroxyprogesterone Acetate, Progesterone.)

Administration and Adult Dosage. PO for withdrawal bleeding after postmenopausal estrogen replacement therapy or combined for estrogen replacement therapy 2.5–10 mg/day starting on days 15–20 of the cycle and continuing for 5–10 days, or 0.5–1 mg/day continuously combined with estrogen.[140,141,145] (*See* Medroxyprogesterone Acetate Notes.) PO for amenorrhea or abnormal uterine bleeding 2.5–10 mg/day starting on day 5 and ending on day 25 of menses. In cases of secondary amenorrhea, therapy can be started at any time.[79] PO for endometriosis 5 mg/day for 2 weeks, increasing in 2.5 mg/day increments q 2 weeks until a maintenance dosage of 15 mg/day is reached.[80]

Special Populations. *Geriatric Dosage.* Same as adult dosage.

Dosage Forms. Tab 5 mg.

Patient Instructions. Report immediately if any of the following occur: new severe or persistent headache; blurred vision; calf, chest, or abdominal pain; or any abnormal vaginal bleeding. This (oral) drug may be taken with food, milk, or an antacid to minimize stomach upset. (Dysfunctional uterine bleeding) expect heavy and severely cramping flow 2 to 4 days after stopping therapy; expect a normal period after a few days.

Pharmacokinetics. *Onset and Duration.* (Uterine bleeding) after oral administration, acute bleeding should decrease in 1–2 days and stop in 3–4 days. (Withdrawal bleeding) onset 3–7 days after last oral dose.[81]

Fate. Norethindrone acetate is rapidly and completely absorbed, with a mean bioavailability of 64 ± 16% because of first-pass metabolism.[81–85,94] Norethindrone acetate is rapidly converted to norethindrone in vivo.[81,85,87,90] Norethindrone is 36% bound to sex hormone-binding globulin and 61% bound to albumin. It is concentrated in body fat and endometrium; breast milk levels are 10% of maternal serum levels. V_d is 4.3 ± 9 L/kg; Cl is 0.5 ± 1.5 L/hr/kg. Over 50% is eliminated in urine and 20–40% in feces as conjugated glucuronides and sulfates; <5% of norethindrone acetate is excreted as unchanged norethindrone.[81–85,90,94]

$t_{1/2}$. (Norethindrone) 6.4 ± 3 hr.[81–85,90,94]

Adverse Reactions. (*See* Medroxyprogesterone Acetate, Postmenopausal Hormone Replacement Risks and Benefits Comparison Chart, and Hormone Excess and Deficiency Symptomatology Comparison Chart.)

Contraindications. (*See* Medroxyprogesterone Acetate, Postmenopausal Hormone Replacement Risks and Benefits Comparison Chart.)

Precautions. (*See* Medroxyprogesterone Acetate, Postmenopausal Hormone Replacement Risks and Benefits Comparison Chart, and Hormone Excess and Deficiency Symptomatology Comparison Chart.)

Drug Interactions, Parameters to Monitor, Notes. (*See* Medroxyprogesterone Acetate.)

PROGESTERONE	Crinone, Progestasert, Prometrium, Various
HYDROXYPROGESTERONE CAPROATE	Duralutin, Various

Pharmacology. Progesterone is the natural hormone that induces secretory changes in the endometrium, relaxes uterine smooth muscle, and maintains pregnancy. Hydroxyprogesterone is a natural progestin with minimal progestational activity; esterification with caproic acid produces a progestational compound more potent than progesterone with a prolonged duration of activity.

Administration and Adult Dosage. **PO to prevent endometrial hyperplasia during postmenopausal estrogen replacement therapy** (micronized progesterone) 200 mg/day for 12 days of cycle.[118] **IM for secondary amenorrhea or dysfunctional uterine bleeding** (progesterone) 5–10 mg/day for 6–8 days or (only for amenorrhea) 100–150 mg as a single dose; (hydroxyprogesterone caproate) 375 mg, may repeat in 4 weeks prn. **IM for palliation of metastatic endometrial cancer** (hydroxyprogesterone caproate) 500 mg–1 g 2–3 times/week. **Intrauterine for contraception** (progesterone) 38 mg q 12 months, releases 68 μg/day; insert at any time during menstrual cycle or within 7 days of onset of menses, immediately postabortion, or no earlier than 6 weeks postpartum if breastfeeding; insertion and removal are done by trained personnel. **Vag for progesterone supplementation** (progesterone) 90 mg daily. (*See* Notes.)

Special Populations. *Geriatric Dosage.* Same as adult dosage.

Dosage Forms. **Cap** (micronized progesterone) 100, 200 mg (Prometrium); **Inj** (progesterone in oil) 50 mg/mL; (hydroxyprogesterone caproate in oil) 125, 250 mg/mL; **Intrauterine** (progesterone) 38 mg (Progestasert); **Vag Gel** (progesterone 8%) 90 mg/applicatorful (Crinone).

Patient Instructions. Report immediately if any of the following occur: new severe or persistent headache; blurred vision; calf, chest, or abdominal pain; or any abnormal vaginal bleeding. (Dysfunctional uterine bleeding) expect heavy flow and severe cramping 2 to 4 days after injection; expect a normal period after a few days. (Progestasert only) you might experience increased menstrual flow, cramping, and spotting. Check the position of the strings monthly after each period or after abnormal cramping to ensure proper placement of the IUD. Contact your prescriber immediately if the strings are missing, if you miss a menstrual period, or if you have fever, pelvic pain, severe cramping, unusual vaginal bleeding, or any signs of infection.

Pharmacokinetics. *Onset and Duration.* (Amenorrhea) onset of withdrawal bleeding occurs 48–72 hr after last dose of IM progesterone and 2 weeks after IM hydroxyprogesterone caproate; (dysfunctional uterine bleeding) onset within 6 days of IM progesterone.[79] Duration is 12–24 hr with oral progesterone, 9–17 days with IM hydroxyprogesterone caproate. (Contraception) onset within 24 hr after insertion of Progestasert.

Serum Levels. (Endometrial progestational activity [luteal phase]) 15 µg/L (48 nmol/L) of progesterone.

Fate. (Progesterone) bioavailability of oral progesterone is incomplete because of first-pass metabolism, with wide interpatient variations; micronized forms are somewhat better absorbed.[82,121,145,146] Higher levels of progesterone and active metabolites occur after IM, vaginal, or rectal administration because first-pass effect is avoided. Serum levels of progesterone after oral and IM increase rapidly to reach luteal-phase values within 2.4 ± 1.1 hr and remain elevated for <12 hr after oral administration and 48 hr after IM administration. (PO) 100 mg micronized progesterone yields peak progesterone levels of 7 ± 3.4 µg/L (23 ± 11 nmol/L); 200 mg yields 28 ± 19 µg/L (89 ± 59 nmol/L); (IM) 100 mg yields 60 µg/L (192 nmol/L); (Vag) 200 mg bid yields 19 ± 2 µg/L (61 ± 7 nmol/L); (Vag) 400 mg once daily yields 29 ± 53 µg/L (93 ± 188 nmol/L).[82,145,147] Oral progesterone V_d is 850 ± 265 L/kg; Cl is 19 ± 38 L/hr/kg.[145] Progesterone circulates 80% bound to albumin and 17% to corticosteroid-binding globulin and distributes into fat. It undergoes rapid gut and hepatic metabolism, with formation of active metabolites: 20α-dihydroprogesterone (25–50% of the progestational activity of progesterone), 17-hydroxyprogesterone, and 11-deoxycorticosterone (a potent mineralocorticoid).[82,148,149] Hydroxyprogesterone caproate is cleaved to form 17-hydroxyprogesterone in the body; 17-hydroxyprogesterone, whether formed from progesterone or exogenously administered, is further metabolized to 11-deoxycortisol and then cortisol. Urinary excretion of progesterone is 50–60%

as 5α-pregnanediol glucuronide and other conjugated glucuronic acid or sulfate metabolites; 5–10% excreted in feces.

$t_{1/2}$. (Progesterone) 32.6 ± 9.3 hr.[145]

Adverse Reactions. Local reactions and swelling at the site of progesterone injection. The beneficial effects of estrogen-increased HDL levels are not reversed by progesterone.[121] (*See* Postmenopausal Hormone Replacement Risks and Benefits Comparison Chart, Hormone Excess and Deficiency Symptomatology Comparison Chart.) (Progestasert) intermenstrual spotting and menstrual bleeding irregularities, expulsion, ectopic pregnancy, uterine perforation, pelvic inflammatory disease, cramping, and pain. Intrauterine administration of contraceptive doses of progesterone has no systemic effects.[76]

Contraindications. (*See* Medroxyprogesterone Acetate.) **Progestasert** pregnancy; active, recent, or recurrent pelvic infections, including gonorrhea or *Chlamydia* infection.

Precautions. (*See* Medroxyprogesterone Acetate, Postmenopausal Hormone Replacement Risks and Benefits Comparison Chart, and Hormone Excess and Deficiency Symptomatology Comparison Chart.) Patients allergic to peanuts should not use Prometrium.

Drug Interactions. (*See* Medroxyprogesterone Acetate.)

Parameters to Monitor. Complete pretreatment and annual physical examinations with special reference to blood pressure, breasts, abdomen, pelvic organs, and Pap smear.

Notes. Progesterone is widely used in the treatment of premenstrual syndrome; however, in double-blind, controlled trials, oral micronized and vaginal progesterone were no better than placebo.[150,151]

RALOXIFENE	Evista

Pharmacology. Raloxifene is a selective estrogen receptor modulator similar to tamoxifen. It acts like an estrogen in the bone and like an estrogen antagonist on the breast and uterus. Raloxifene increases bone mineral density and decreases serum LDL cholesterol levels but does not stimulate endometrial growth.[152,153]

Administration and Adult Dosage. **PO for prevention of postmenopausal osteoporosis** 60 mg once daily with supplemental calcium.

Dosage Forms. **Tab** 60 mg.

Pharmacokinetics. Oral bioavailability is 2% because of an extensive first-pass effect. It is highly bound to albumin and α_1-acid glycoprotein and has a V_d of 2348 L/kg. Cl is 40–60 L/hr/kg. The drug is metabolized to glucuronide metabolites, some of which undergo enterohepatic recycling, and can be converted back to the parent drug. Metabolites are excreted primarily in feces. The half-life is about 28 hr.

Adverse Reactions. Hot flashes occur in 25–30% of women; leg cramps also are frequent. It increases the risk of venous thrombosis and is a teratogen.

Contraindications. Women who might become pregnant or who have a history of venous thrombotic events.

Drug Interactions. Cholestyramine (and presumably colestipol) binds raloxifene and reduces its absorption and enterohepatic recirculation. The drugs should not be coadministered. Raloxifene decreases the effect of warfarin, and PT should be monitored carefully when they are given together.

Notes. Raloxifene increases bone mineral density, decreases the risk of vertebral fracture,[154] and decreases the risk of invasive breast cancer.[155] It also favorably alters cardiovascular risk factors (eg, LDL-c, lipoprotein-a, HDL-c), but protection against cardiovascular disease is not established.[156]

Thyroid and Antithyroid Drugs

IODIDES   Various

Pharmacology. Iodide inhibits the synthesis and release of thyroid hormone and preoperatively decreases the size and vascularity of the hyperplastic thyroid gland. Large doses block the uptake of radioactive iodine by the thyroid gland.

Administration and Adult Dosage. **PO for hyperthyroidism, as an adjunct to antithyroid agents or for preoperative thyroidectomy preparation** 100–200 mg (5 drops of saturated solution of potassium iodide [SSKI] or 10–15 drops of Lugol's solution) q 8 hr diluted in a glass of water, milk or juice; dosages as high as 500 mg/day have been used. However, administration of smaller doses of 30–50 mg iodine and continued suppression with doses of 15–50 mg/day also may be effective in patients with mild disease.[165] Use for 7–10 days before surgery. **PO for thyroid storm** 200 mg q 6 hr. **PO for prophylaxis in radiation emergency** 100 mg iodine immediately before or within 1–2 hr after exposure and daily for 3–7 days, to a maximum of 10 days after exposure.

Special Populations. *Pediatric Dosage.* **PO for thyrotoxicosis** 300 mg (6 drops SSKI) q 8 hr diluted as above. **PO for prophylaxis in a radiation emergency** (<1 yr) 50 mg iodine immediately before or after exposure and daily for 3–7 days, to a maximum of 10 days after exposure; (>1 yr) same as adult dosage.

Geriatric Dosage. Same as adult dosage.

Dosage Forms. **Soln** (SSKI) 50 mg/drop iodide (1 g/mL); (Lugol's or strong iodine) 8 mg/drop iodide (50 mg/mL iodine plus 100 mg/mL potassium iodide); **Tab** 100 mg iodide (130 mg potassium iodide); **EC Tab** not recommended.

Patient Instructions. Dilute solution in a glass (8 fluid ounces) of liquid before taking; it may be taken with food, milk, or an antacid to minimize stomach upset. Do not use if solution turns brownish-yellow. If crystals form in the solution, they can be dissolved by warming the closed container in warm water. Dissolve tablets in one-half glass of water or milk before taking. Do not use if you are breastfeeding; advise your physician if you are pregnant. Discontinue use and report if fever, skin rash, epigastric pain, or joint swelling occur.

Pharmacokinetics. *Onset and Duration.* Onset 24–48 hr in hyperthyroidism; maximum effect in 10–15 days. (*See* Notes.)

Serum Levels. (Iodide) >50 μg/L (0.4 mmol/L) inhibits iodide binding by thyroid in hyperthyroidism; >200 μg/L (1.6 mmol/L) inhibit iodide uptake by normal thyroid.[166]

Fate. Iodide is well absorbed throughout the GI tract and concentrated in the thyroid, stomach, salivary glands, and breastmilk. Renal clearance is 1.8 L/hr/kg; approximately 100 μg of iodine is excreted in urine daily; fecal excretion of iodine is negligible.[166]

Adverse Reactions. Any adverse reaction warrants drug discontinuation. Goiter, hypothyroidism, and hyperthyroidism occur frequently in euthyroid patients with a history of a thyroid disorder.[167–171] Iodism occurs with prolonged use and is indicated by metallic taste, GI upset, soreness of teeth and gums, coryza, frontal headaches, painful swelling of salivary glands, diarrhea, acneiform skin eruptions, and erythema of face and chest. Rarely, hypersensitivity occurs and is manifested by angioedema, cutaneous hemorrhages, and symptoms resembling serum sickness. (*See* Precautions.)

Contraindications. Pulmonary tuberculosis; pulmonary edema; multinodular goiters.[165,167–170]

Precautions. Pregnancy, because fetal goiter, asphyxiation, and death can occur; lactation. Use iodides with caution in patients with untreated Hashimoto's thyroiditis, in iodide-deficient patients, in children with cystic fibrosis, and in euthyroid patients with histories of postpartum thyroiditis, subacute thyroiditis, amiodarone or lithium-induced thyroid disease, or previously treated Graves' disease because they can be particularly sensitive to iodide-induced hypothyroidism.[167–171] Patients with nontoxic multinodular goiters might be prone to development of hyperthyroidism. Avoid iodides entirely in patients with toxic nodular goiter or toxic nodules because thyrotoxicosis can be further aggravated.[165,167–170] Iodides are not recommended for use as expectorants because of their potential to induce acneiform eruptions, exacerbate existing lesions, and adversely affect the thyroid. Small-bowel lesions are associated with enteric-coated potassium-containing tablets, which can cause obstruction, hemorrhage, perforation, and possible death. This dosage form is not recommended.

Drug Interactions. Iodide prevents uptake of ^{131}I for several weeks and delays onset of thioamide action if given before the thioamide. Lithium can potentiate the antithyroid action of iodide. Serum iodine can be elevated if potassium-sparing diuretics are taken with potassium iodide.

Parameters to Monitor. Monitor for signs of iodism (*see* Adverse Reactions), hypothyroidism, hyperthyroidism, and parotitis occasionally during long-term use. Monitor thyroid function tests at least q 6–12 months during long-term use in patients with family histories of thyroid disease or goiter. Monitor serum potassium frequently in patients who are taking other drugs that might affect serum potassium (eg, diuretics).

Notes. Iodide has the most rapid onset of any treatment for hyperthyroidism. In thyroid storm, iodide theoretically should be given 1 hr after the thioamide dose but should not be withheld if oral thioamides cannot be given. The therapeutic effects of iodide are variable and transient, with "escape" occurring after 10–14 days; do not use iodide alone in the therapy of hyperthyroidism.[165] Pharmacologic amounts of iodide can be present in serum from **radiographic contrast agents** and vaginal douches such as **povidone-iodine.**[167–170]

LEVOTHYROXINE SODIUM   Levothroid, Levoxyl, Synthroid, Unithroid, Various

Pharmacology. Levothyroxine is a synthetic hormone identical to the thyroid hormone T_4. Thyroid hormones are responsible for normal growth, development, and energy metabolism.

Administration and Adult Dosage. **PO for replacement in hypothyroidism <6 months duration** full replacement dosage of 1.6–1.7 μg/kg/day initially, increasing if needed and tolerated in 25–50 μg/day increments at 6–8 week intervals to a maintenance dosage that normalizes thyroid-stimulating hormone (TSH).[172–174] **Usual maintenance dosages** 75–100 μg/day for women and 100–150 μg/day for men. Higher mean replacement dosages are required in patients with spontaneous hypothyroidism (1.7–1.8 μg/kg/day) than in those with iatrogenic hypothyroidism after radioiodine therapy for Graves' disease (1.5–1.6 μg/kg/day).[172–175] Once-weekly replacement therapy can be effective.[176] **PO for replacement of subclinical hypothyroidism** same as adult dosage. The desirability of treatment is controversial; benefits are greatest in those with TSH >10 μIU/mL, hypercholesterolemia, and subtle symptoms of hypothyroidism. Replacement reduces levels of homocysteine and may lower the risk of clinical cardiovascular disease (eg, MI, aortic atherosclerosis.)[177–179] **PO for suppression therapy of nodules** 100–150 μg/day initially, increasing, if necessary and tolerated, in 25–50 μg/day increments at 6–8 week intervals to suppress TSH to below normal, detectable limits to prevent further thyroid growth. Dosages are usually higher than those required for replacement therapy and risks must be assessed, especially in patients with cardiac disease. If no improvement after 1 yr, consider stopping therapy.[180,181] **PO for suppression therapy of thyroid cancer after thyroidectomy** 2.11 μg/kg/day initially, increasing, if needed and tolerated, in 25–50 μg/day increments at 6–8 week intervals to a dosage of 150–250 μg/day to suppress the TSH level to undetectable levels.[172–175] **IV for myxedema coma** 400–500 μg or 300 μg/m² to increase serum T_4 levels by 3–5 μg/dL (39–65 nmol/L), then 50–100 μg/day until oral administration is possible; use smaller dosages in cardiovascular disease.[182,183] **IM** indicated only for replacement therapy if the patient cannot take oral medication; parenteral dosage is about 80% of the oral dosage because of bioavailability differences.[172,173]

Special Populations. *Pediatric Dosage.* **PO for hypothyroidism** (preterm infants and full-term neonates to 1 yr) 10–15 μg/kg/day to normalize T_4 to >10 μg/dL (129 nmol/L) within 3–4 weeks; (>1 yr) 3–5 μg/kg/day (average 3.5).[172,184] Adjust maintenance dosage on the basis of growth, development, and T_4 and TSH values. Replacement by at least 24 months of age corrects short stature by age 5 yr. Syrup can be formulated from tablets, with a stability of 15 days.[185]

Geriatric Dosage. **PO for hypothyroidism** (>50 yr) start with 25–50 μg/day initially, then increase if tolerated in 12.2–25 μg/day increments at 6–8 week intervals to a maintenance dosage necessary to normalize TSH; (>65 yr) <1 μg/kg/day may be required.[172–175] **IV for myxedema coma** (>55 yr) <500 μg initially to improve outcome, then same as adult dosage.[182] Poorly compliant elderly patients (mean age 86 yr) have been maintained on a twice-weekly dosing regimen; however, this regimen might be dangerous in cardiac patients.[186]

Other Conditions. In patients with cardiovascular disease or severe, long-standing (>6 months) myxedema, **PO** 12.5–25 μg/day initially, increasing, if tolerated, at 6–8 week intervals by 12.5–25 μg/day increments to a maintenance dosage necessary to normalize TSH.[172–175] In patients with cardiovascular disease, particularly angina, dosage increments should be balanced between exacerbation of angina and maintenance of euthyroidism. In some patients with severe coronary disease, incomplete control of hypothyroidism might be necessary to prevent further exacerbation of angina. During pregnancy, a 20–50% increase in dosage might be required to maintain a normal TSH level.[172–175] In those with continued mood disturbances on sole T4 therapy, *see* Liothyronine.

Dosage Forms. Tab 25, 50, 75, 88, 100, 112, 125, 137, 150, 175, 200, 300 μg; Inj 200, 500 μg.

Patient Instructions. This medication must be taken regularly to maintain proper hormone levels in the body. Report immediately if chest pain (especially in elderly patients), palpitations, sweating, nervousness, or other signs of overactivity occur.

Missed Doses. Take any missed dose as soon as it is remembered, but if more than 1 dose is missed, do not double dosage.

Pharmacokinetics. *Onset and Duration.* PO onset 3–5 days; peak effect 3–4 weeks; duration after cessation of therapy 7–10 days. IV onset in myxedema coma 6–8 hr, maximum effect in 1 day.[172,182,183]

Serum Levels. (Physiologic and therapeutic during levothyroxine therapy) free T4 6–21 ng/L (12–26 pmol/L); total T4 50–120 μg/L (65–155 nmol/L). Peak free T4 levels can be 12.7 ± 2.6%, and total T4 levels 8.1 ± 1.2% higher than trough levels or levels obtained 10 hr after a dose.[187,188] Many drugs and pathologic and physiologic states affect binding and hence can affect results of some serum level determinations.[166,167,169,171,174]

Fate. Oral bioavailability ranges from 74 ± 11% to 93 ± 25% and can be decreased by many factors (eg, malabsorption, concurrent food, and drugs; *see* Drug Interactions).[167,189] A dose of 500 μg IV increases serum T4 levels by 3–5 μg/dL (39–65 nmol/L).[172,183] Only 0.03% is unbound in plasma. V_d is (hypothyroid) 0.17 ± 0.22 L/kg; (euthyroid) 0.16 ± 0.09 L/kg; (hyperthyroid) 0.23 ± 0.44 L/kg. Turnover is (hypothyroid) 9.2 ± 1.7%/day; (euthyroid) 11.2 ± 1.7%/day; (hyperthyroid) 21 ± 4.9%/day. Cl is (hypothyroid) 0.0008 ± 0.0033 L/hr/kg; (euthyroid) 0.00074 ± 0.0017 L/hr/kg; (hyperthyroid) 0.002 ± 0.0007 L/hr/kg.[190] About 80% is deiodinated in the body; 35% is peripherally converted to the more active T3 and 45% to inactive reverse T3.[166] Another 15–20% is conjugated in the liver to form glucuronides and sulfates, which undergo enterohepatic recirculation with reabsorption or excretion in the feces.

$t_{1/2}$. (Hypothyroid) 7.5 ± 7.1 days; (euthyroid) 6.2 ± 4.7 days; (hyperthyroid) 3.2 ± 1.7 days.[190] Protein binding affects half-life (increased binding retards elimination and decreased binding increases elimination).

Adverse Reactions. Most are dose related and can be avoided by increasing the initial dosage slowly to the minimum effective maintenance dosage. Signs of overdosage are headache, palpitations, chest pain, heat intolerance, sweating, leg cramps, weight loss, diarrhea, vomiting, nervousness, and other symptoms of hyperthyroidism. Long-term thyroid administration that results in TSH suppression can predispose to ventricular hypertrophy, atrial fibrillation, osteoporosis, and increased fracture risk by increasing bone resorption in postmenopausal women with a history of hyperthyroidism.[172–175,191]

Contraindications. Thyrotoxicosis; uncorrected adrenal insufficiency.

Precautions. Initiate and increase dosage with caution in patients with cardiovascular disease, the elderly, and in long-standing hypothyroidism. In myxedema coma, give a corticosteroid concurrently.[183] The status of other metabolic diseases, including diabetes, adrenal insufficiency, hyperadrenalism, and panhypopituitarism, can be affected by changes in thyroid status.

Drug Interactions. Bran, fiber, cholesterol-binding resins, sodium polystyrene sulfonate, iron, aluminum-containing products, and calcium carbonate can decrease oral absorption. Phenytoin, carbamazepine, and other enzyme inducers; sertraline and possibly other serotonin reuptake inhibitors, and ritonavir can increase levothyroxine requirements.[167,169,189,192] The action of some drugs (eg, digoxin, warfarin, insulin, sympathomimetics, theophylline) can be altered by changing thyroid status.[169,174]

Parameters to Monitor. (Adults) TSH, free T_4 or free T_4 index, and clinical status of the patient q 6–8 weeks initially. Monitor trough levels or obtain levels at least 10 hr after tablet ingestion to avoid transient peak effects.[187,188] After stabilization, monitor free T_4 or free T_4 index, TSH, and clinical status at 6–12 month intervals. (Children) Monitor the parameters above q 4 weeks initially and q 3–4 months after stabilization. In congenital hypothyroidism, monitor T_4 because TSH can remain elevated despite adequate replacement doses.[184] (>50 yr) Evaluate the replacement dosage annually and adjust downward as necessary because dosage requirements decrease with age.[172–175]

Notes. Levothyroxine is the drug of choice for thyroid replacement because of purity, long half-life, and close simulation to normal physiologic hormone levels. Protect from light and moisture. Concerns about tablet potency prompted the FDA to require that all manufacturers submit a new drug application for levothyroxine by August 2001. Unithroid is the first levothyroxine tablet to obtain FDA approval. Bioequivalence is reported between Synthroid, Levothroid, and Levoxyl.[173,188,193] Use of adjunctive thyroid hormones for depression may be effective; T_3 is used instead of T_4 (*see* Liothyronine).[194] Physiologic dosages of thyroid hormones in euthyroid patients are ineffective for weight reduction, obesity, or premenstrual tension; larger dosages might result in toxicity.[175] (*See* Thyroid Replacement Products Comparison Chart.)

LIOTHYRONINE SODIUM
Cytomel, Triostat, Various

Pharmacology. Liothyronine is a synthetic hormone identical to the thyroid hormone T_3, which is 4 times as potent by weight as T_4. (*See* Levothyroxine.)

Administration and Adult Dosage. **PO for replacement in hypothyroidism <6 months in duration** 25 μg/day initially, increasing, if needed and tolerated, in 12.5–25 μg/day increments at 1–2 week intervals to a maintenance dosage of 25–100 μg/day to normalize TSH. **PO for severe hypothyroidism** 5 μg/day initially, increasing in 5–10 μg/day increments at 1–2 week intervals until 25 μg/day is reached, then increase in 12.5–25 μg/day increments at 1–2 week intervals until euthyroid. Dividing daily dosage into 2–3 doses can prevent wide serum level fluctuations. **PO for augmentation of tricyclic therapy for depression** 25–50 μg daily.[194,195] No data are available in combination with serotonin reuptake inhibitors. **IV for myxedema coma** 25–50 μg initially, then 10–12.5 μg q 4–6 hr to a minimum of 10–15 μg q 12 hr until PO administration is possible; use smaller dosages of 10–20 μg IV initially in cardiovascular disease. Some suggest that T_3 is preferable in myxedema coma when impairment of T_4 to T_3 conversion is suspected or in cardiac disease because adverse effects will dissipate faster.[182,183] Limited experience exists with IV dosages >100 μg/day. **PO for T_3 suppression test** 75–100 μg/day in 2–3 divided doses for 7 days, then repeat ^{131}I thyroid uptake test.

Special Populations. *Pediatric Dosage.* **PO for congenital hypothyroidism** 5 μg/day initially, increasing in 5 μg/day increments at 3–4 day intervals until the desired effect is obtained. **Usual maintenance dosage** (<1 yr) 20 μg/day; (1–3 yr) 50 μg/day; (>3 yr) 25–100 μg/day. Levothyroxine is the drug of choice in congenital hypothyroidism.[184]

Geriatric Dosage. Not recommended because of greater potential for cardiotoxicity. **PO** if used, start at PO 5 μg/day and increase in 5 μg/day increments at 2-week intervals, if tolerated, until desired response is obtained. (*See* Levothyroxine.)

Other Conditions. Not recommended in those with cardiovascular disease but, if used, start at PO 5 μg/day and increase in 5 μg/day increments at 2-week intervals, if tolerated, until desired response is obtained. (*See* Levothyroxine.) For those with continued mood disturbances on sole T_4 therapy, substitution of T_3 5 μg bid for 50 μg of levothyroxine of the total daily T_4 replacement dosage has been advocated.[196]

Dosage Forms. **Tab** 5, 25, 50 μg; **Inj** 10 μg/mL.

Patient Instructions. This medication must be taken regularly to maintain proper hormone levels in the body. Report immediately if chest pain (especially in elderly patients), palpitations, sweating, nervousness, or other signs of overactivity occur.

Missed Doses. Take any missed dose as soon as it is remembered, but if more than 1 dose is missed, do not double dosage.

Pharmacokinetics. *Onset and Duration.* PO onset 1–3 days; duration after cessation of therapy 3–5 days.

Serum Levels. During T_3 replacement, T_4 is maintained at ≤ 10 μg/L (13 nmol/L).[197]

Fate. Oral absorption is usually complete but can decrease in CHF. With a typical replacement dosage, T_3 has a peak of 4.5–7 μg/L (7–11 nmol/L) 1–2 hr postdose, returning to 0.88–1.6 μg/L (1.4–2.5 nmol/L) before the next dose 24 hr later.[197] V_d is (hypothyroid) 0.53 ± 0.04 L/kg; (euthyroid) 0.52 ± 0.03 L/kg; (hyperthyroid) 0.94 ± 0.07 L/kg. Turnover is (hypothyroid) 50 ± 5%/day; (euthyroid) 68 ± 11%/day; (hyperthyroid) 110 ± 22%/day. Cl is (hypothyroid) 0.012 ± 0.002 L/hr/kg; (euthyroid) 0.02 ± 0.003 L/hr/kg; (hyperthyroid) 0.043 ± 0.013 L/hr/kg.[190,198] Excreted in urine as deiodinated metabolites and their conjugates.

$t_{½}$. (Hypothyroid) 38 ± 6 hr; (euthyroid) 25 ± 3 hr; (hyperthyroid) 17 ± 4.7 hr.[190]

Adverse Reactions. (*See* Levothyroxine.) Dose-related adverse effects are more likely and appear more rapidly than with levothyroxine because regulation of dosage is more difficult. Liothyronine and its mixtures (eg, desiccated thyroid, liotrix) cause "unphysiologic" toxic peaks in serum T_3 levels not found during levothyroxine replacement therapy.[172,174,175]

Contraindications. (*See* Levothyroxine)

Precautions. (*See* Levothyroxine.)

Drug Interactions. Normal serum T_3 levels are age related and can be decreased by a wide variety of pharmacologic agents (eg, amiodarone, iodinated contrast dyes, corticosteroids, propylthiouracil) or clinical circumstances (eg, malnutrition, chronic renal, hepatic, pulmonary, or cardiac disease; or acute sepsis) which impair peripheral or pituitary T_4 to T_3 conversion.[166,167,174] (*See also* Levothyroxine Drug Interactions.)

Parameters to Monitor. Serum TSH and T_3 levels. (*See* Levothyroxine.)

Notes. Liothyronine is not considered the drug of choice for replacement therapy in hypothyroidism because of its shorter half-life (necessitating more frequent administration), greater potential for cardiotoxicity, the greater difficulty of monitoring, and its greater expense.[172–174] **Liothyronine** is the preparation of choice when thyroid supplements must be stopped before isotope scanning. After scanning, maintenance therapy with **levothyroxine** is recommended. The use of IV T_3 after cardiopulmonary bypass might improve postoperative recovery and cardiac function in adults, children, and infants.[199–201] (*See* Thyroid Replacement Products Comparison Chart.)

THYROID REPLACEMENT PRODUCTS COMPARISON CHART

DRUG	DOSAGE FORMS	EQUIVALENT DOSAGE	CONTENTS	RELATIVE ONSET AND DURATION[a]	COMMENTS
Levothyroxine Levothroid Levoxyl Synthroid Unithroid Various	Tab 25, 50, 75, 88, 100, 112, 125, 137, 150, 175, 200, 300 μg. Inj 200, 500 μg.	60 μg	T_4	Long	Preparation of choice. T_4 content is now standardized using HPLC, and bioequivalence among products is likely.
Liothyronine Cytomel Triostat Various	Tab 5, 25, 50 μg Inj 10 μg/mL.	25 μg	T_3	Short	Expensive; difficult to monitor. Preparation of choice if thyroid supplements are to be stopped for isotope scanning.
Liotrix Thyrolar	Tab 1/4, 1/2, 1, 2, 3.[b]	#1 Tab[c]	T_4 and T_3 in 4:1 ratio	Intermediate	No advantages; more costly and suffers from T_3 content. (See Thyroid, Desiccated.)
Thyroid, Desiccated Various	Tab 15, 30, 60, 90, 120, 180, 240, 300 mg.	60 mg	T_4 and T_3 in variable ratio	Intermediate	Inexpensive; allergy to animal protein rarely occurs; supraphysiologic elevations in T_3 and T_3 toxicosis may occur.

[a]With equivalent dosages.
[b]Numbers represent equivalent dosage of thyroid in grains (ie, 15, 30, 60, 120, 180 mg, respectively).
[c]Thyrolar-1 contains T_4 50 μg and T_3 12.5 μg; other strengths are in the same proportion.
From references 172–174.

METHIMAZOLE   Tapazole

Pharmacology. Methimazole is a thioamide antithyroid drug that interferes with the synthesis of thyroid hormones by inhibiting iodide organification. Unlike propylthiouracil (PTU), methimazole does not block peripheral conversion of T_4 to T_3. Titers of thyroid receptor–stimulating antibody (TRab) decline during therapy, suggesting an immunosuppressive effect. Methimazole is 10 times more potent than PTU on a weight basis.

Administration and Adult Dosage. **PO for hyperthyroidism** 30–40 mg/day as a single dose. If GI intolerance occurs, divide dosage q 8 hr initially until euthyroid (usually 6–8 weeks), then decrease by 33–50% over several weeks to a maintenance dosage of 5–15 mg/day in a single dose. Severe disease might require 2 divided doses. The addition of levothyroxine is not recommended because remission rates have not shown improvement.[202] **PO for thyroid storm** 40–120 mg/day, divided q 8 hr until euthyroid. Traditional treatment duration for hyperthyroidism is 1–2 yr, although shorter courses of 8 months might be effective in mild disease.[165] Treatment may be continued indefinitely, if necessary, to control the disease and if no toxicity occurs. **PR** methimazole can be formulated for rectal administration.[203]

Special Populations. *Pediatric Dosage.* **PO** 0.5-0.7 mg/kg/day or 15–20 mg/m^2/day, to a maximum of 30–60 mg/day given in 1–2 divided doses, with a maintenance dosage of 50% of the initial dosage.[204]

Geriatric Dosage. Same as adult dosage.

Other Conditions. In pregnancy, dosages should be as low as possible to maintain maternal T_4 levels in approximately the upper normal to mildly thyrotoxic range. Initially give a maximum of 20–30 mg/day orally in single or 3 divided doses for 4–6 weeks, then decrease to 5–15 mg/day in a single dose. The intellectual development and growth of children exposed to methimazole in utero appear to be similar to unexposed siblings.[205]

Dosage Forms. **Tab** 5, 10 mg.

Patient Instructions. Report sore throat, fever, or oral lesions immediately because they might be early signs of a rare, but severe, blood disorder. Also report any skin rashes, itching, or yellowing of eyes and skin. Be sure to take at prescribed dosage intervals.

Missed Doses. If you miss a dose, take it as soon as possible. If it is time for the next dose, take both doses.

Pharmacokinetics. *Onset and Duration.* **PO** onset about 2–3 weeks, which is consistent with the elimination of existing T_4 stores. Duration intrathyroidally 40 hr.[165,206]

Serum Levels. <0.2 mg/L (1.8 μmol/L) inhibits iodide organification.[206]

Fate. Well absorbed orally. Considerable interindividual variations in pharmacokinetic parameters. Peak serum levels occur at 2.3 ± 0.8 hr; the peak after 30 mg orally is 0.8 ± 0.2 mg/L (6.8 ± 1.9 μmol/L); after 60 mg orally, 1.5 ± 0.5 mg/L (14 ± 4 μmol/L); after 60 mg rectally, 1.1 ± 0.5 mg/L (10 ± 5 μmol/L).[203,206,207] The drug is actively concentrated in the thyroid gland, with peak intrathyroidal levels of 0.11–1.1 mg/L (1–10 μmol/L) within 1 hr;[206] there is minimal plasma protein binding; it is distributed into breast milk 10 times greater than PTU.[165] V_d is 1.4 ± 0.6 L/kg; Cl is 0.072 ± 0.018 L/hr/kg. There are no active metabolites; 7–12% is excreted unchanged in urine, 6% excreted as inorganic sulfate, 1.5% as sulfur metabolites, and 50% as unknown metabolites.[206,207]

$t_{1/2}$. α phase 3 ± 1.4 hr; β phase 18.5 ± 13 hr in normal and hyperthyroid patients, increased to 21 hr in cirrhosis.[206] Intrathyroidal half-life is 20 hr.

Adverse Reactions. Maculopapular skin rashes and itching occur frequently and can disappear spontaneously with continued treatment; urticaria requires drug discontinuation.[165,175] Methimazole can be given to patients who develop only a nonurticarial maculopapular rash on PTU. Mild transient leukopenia occurs frequently in untreated Graves' disease, does not predispose to agranulocytosis, and is not an indication to discontinue the drug.[165,175] Agranulocytosis occurs occasionally, usually in the first 3 months of therapy. Risk increases with dosages >40 mg/day in patients >40 yr; granulocyte colony-stimulating factors (eg, **filgrastim**) can hasten recovery.[165,175] Rarely, fever, arthralgias, cholestatic or hepatocellular toxicity, vasculitis, lupus-like syndrome, hypoprothrombinemia, aplastic anemia, thrombocytopenia, nephrotic syndrome, loss of taste, and spontaneous appearance of circulating antibodies to insulin or glucagon occur.[165,175,208] Rare teratogenic risk of scalp defects.[205]

Contraindications. Manufacturer states that breastfeeding is a contraindication, but most experts feel that breastfeeding can be performed with dosages of ≤10 mg/day and careful monitoring of infant thyroid function.[165]

Precautions. Although methimazole crosses the placenta at rates 4 times greater than **propylthiouracil** and has been associated with scalp defects (aplasia cutis), recent reports indicate methimazole can be given in pregnant patients intolerant to PTU.[165,205] Use with caution during lactation and in patients with severe allergic reactions to other thioamides. A low prevalence of cross-sensitivity occurs between thioamide compounds for nonurticarial skin rashes, so if these occur, another thioamide can be substituted. However, a 50% chance of cross-sensitivity exists for severe reactions (eg, agranulocytosis, hepatitis), so do not substitute another thioamide.[165,175]

Drug Interactions. Iodide given before a thioamide delays the response to the thioamide, especially in thyroid storm. Changes in thyroid status can alter pharmacodynamics and pharmacokinetics of digoxin, warfarin, theophylline, β-blockers, and insulin.

Parameters to Monitor. Monitor clinical status; serum free T_4 or T_4 index, and TSH monthly initially until euthyroid, then q 3–6 months. Obtain occasional LFTs and CBC with differential (but these are not recommended routinely because they are not predictive of toxicity, and transient leukopenia and elevations in LFTs can occur). Obtain AST, ALT, total bilirubin, and alkaline phosphatase if patient reports signs of hepatitis; WBC and differential counts if patient reports signs of agranulocytosis such as fever, sore throat, or malaise.

Notes. Methimazole is the drug of choice for treatment of uncomplicated hyperthyroidism because it is better tolerated and fewer tablets can be given once daily, improving patient compliance.[165] Remission rates of 20–40% are common after cessation of therapy. Favorable remission rates correlate with longer duration of therapy, higher dosages, mild disease, shrinkage of goiter size with therapy, disappearance of thyroid receptor–stimulating antibodies, and initial presentation with T_3 toxicosis.[165] Most patients eventually require surgery or radioiodine; however, a trial of a thioamide is worthwhile in patients with minimal thyroid enlargement or very mild hyperthyroidism. Adjunctive therapy with **cholestyramine** 4 g tid can lower thyroid hormone levels more rapidly.[209] Methimazole rather than PTU may be preferred during radioactive iodine therapy because it does not interfere with the thyroid uptake of iodine like PTU.[210] In thyroid storm, PTU is the drug of choice.

PROPYLTHIOURACIL Various

Pharmacology. Propylthiouracil (PTU) is a thioamide antithyroid drug that blocks the synthesis of thyroid hormones and, at dosages >450 mg/day, decreases the peripheral conversion of T_4 to T_3. Titers of thyroid receptor stimulating antibody decline during therapy, consistent with an immunosuppressive effect.

Administration and Adult Dosage. **PO for hyperthyroidism** 100–200 mg (depending on the severity of hyperthyroidism) q 6–8 hr initially until euthyroid (usually 6–8 weeks), then decrease by 33–50% over several weeks to a maintenance dosage of 50–150 mg/day in a single dose. Rarely, initial dosages of 1–1.2 g/day (maximum dosage) in 3–6 doses might be necessary.[165] **PO for thyroid storm** 200–250 mg q 6 hr until euthyroid; maintenance dosage is determined by patient response. Traditional treatment duration for hyperthyroidism is 1–2 yr, although shorter courses of 8 months might be effective in mild disease.[165,174] Treatment may be continued indefinitely, if necessary, to control the disease and if no toxicity occurs. The addition of levothyroxine is not recommended because remission rates have not shown improvement.[202] **PR** PTU can be formulated for rectal administration.[211,212]

Special Populations. *Pediatric Dosage.* Give orally in 3 divided doses. **PO** 150–300 mg/m^2/day. Alternatively, (6–10 yr) 5–10 mg/kg/day or 50–150 mg/day initially; (≥10 yr) 150–300 mg/day initially.[204] Maintenance dosage is determined by patient response.

Geriatric Dosage. Same as adult dosage.

Other Conditions. In pregnancy, the dosage should be as small as possible to maintain a mildly hyperthyroid maternal state; initially 300 mg/day orally in 3 divided doses for 4–6 weeks, then decrease to 50–150 mg/day in a single dose. The intellectual development and growth of children exposed to PTU in utero appear to be similar to unexposed siblings.[205]

Dosage Forms. **Tab** 50 mg.

Patient Instructions. Report sore throat, fever, or oral lesions immediately because they may be an early sign of a severe, but rare, blood disorder. Also report any skin rashes, itching, or yellowing of eyes and skin. Be sure to take at prescribed dosage intervals.

Missed Doses. If you miss a dose, take it as soon as possible. If it is time for the next dose, take both doses.

Pharmacokinetics. ***Onset and Duration.*** PO onset of therapeutic effect 2–3 weeks, consistent with the elimination of existing thyroxine stores.

Serum Levels. Peak PTU levels >4 mg/L (24 μmol/L) produce antithyroid activity; 3 mg/L (18 μmol/L) reduces organification by 50%; 0.8 mg/L (5 μmol/L) reduces peripheral conversion activity by 50%.[207,213]

Fate. Oral bioavailability is 77 ± 13%. Peak levels occur 2 ± 0.3 hr after oral administration and 4.7 ± 1 hr after rectal administration. Peak serum level after an oral dose of 50 mg is 1 ± 0.2 mg/L (6 ± 1.2 μmol/L); after 200 mg, 4.5 ± 0.7 mg/L (26 ± 4 μmol/L); after 300 mg, 7 ± 0.8 mg/L (42 ± 5 μmol/L); after 400 mg rectally, 3 ± 0.8 mg/L (18 ± 5 μmol/L).[211,212] PTU is actively concentrated in the thyroid gland, 40% as unknown metabolite, 32% as sulfate, and 20% as unchanged PTU; peak intrathyroidal levels of 0.17 ± 1.7 mg/L (1–10 μmol/L) occur within 1 hr.[207] The drug is 80% plasma protein bound; it distributes poorly into breast milk.[165] V_d is 0.29 ± 0.06 L/kg; Cl is 0.23 ± 0.04 L/hr/kg. About 85% is excreted in 24 hr, 61% as glucuronides, 8–9% as inorganic sulfates, 8–10% as unknown sulfur metabolites, and <10% excreted unchanged in urine.[207,213]

$t_{1/2}$. 1.3 ± 0.6 hr.[207,213]

Adverse Reactions. (*See* Methimazole.) Agranulocytosis is not more prevalent at higher doses as it is with methimazole. Rarely, hepatitis occurs; hepatocellular toxicity is more frequent than cholestatic jaundice.[165,175,214] Transient transaminase elevations can occur in asymptomatic individuals, which normalize within 3 months with continued drug administration.

Contraindications. Manufacturer states that breastfeeding is a contraindication, but it can be used with infant thyroid monitoring because of low milk levels and lack of effect on infants.[165,205]

Precautions. (*See* Methimazole.) Although it crosses the placenta poorly (25% that of methimazole), it can cause fetal hypothyroidism and goiter.[205] Thyroid dysfunction can diminish as pregnancy progresses, allowing a reduction in dosage and, in some cases, a withdrawal of therapy 2–3 weeks before delivery. Adjunctive thyroid hormone therapy prevents maternal hypothyroidism but, because of minimal placental transfer, has little effect on the fetus.[205] Use with caution before surgery or during treatment with anticoagulants because of hypoprothrombinemic effect.[175]

Drug Interactions. (*See* Methimazole.)

Parameters to Monitor. (*See* Methimazole.) INR monitoring is advisable, particularly before surgery.

Notes. Because propylthiouracil decreases peripheral conversion of T_4 to T_3, it is considered the thioamide of choice in treating thyroid storm. Some prefer PTU rather than methimazole in pregnancy and breastfeeding, although either can be used.[165,205] Patients pretreated with PTU might require a 25% higher dosage of radioactive iodine for efficacy.[210]

REFERENCES

1. Walsh JP, Dayan CM. Role of biochemical assessment in management of corticosteroid withdrawal. *Ann Clin Biochem* 2000;37:279–88.

2. Schimmer BP, Parker KL. Adrenocorticotropic hormone: adrenocortical steroids and their synthetic analogs; inhibitors of the synthesis and action of adrenal hormones. In, Hardman JG et al., eds. *Goodman and Gilman's the pharmacological basis of therapeutics*. 9th ed. New York: McGraw-Hill; 1996:1459–85.

3. The Italian Group for Antiemetic Research. Dexamethasone, granisetron, or both for the prevention of nausea and vomiting during chemotherapy for cancer. *N Engl J Med* 1995;332:1–5.

4. Grunberg SM, Hesketh PJ. Control of chemotherapy-induced emesis. *N Engl J Med* 1993;329:1790–6.

5. Orth DN et al. The adrenal cortex. In, Wilson JD, Foster DW, eds. *Williams textbook of endocrinology*. 9th ed. Philadelphia: WB Saunders; 1998:517–664.

6. Chen B, Yancey MK. Antenatal corticosteroids in preterm premature rupture of membranes. *Clin Obstet Gynecol* 1998;41:832–41.

7. Baud O et al. Antenatal glucocorticoid treatment and cystic periventricular leukomalacia in very premature infants. *N Engl J Med* 1999;341:1190–6.

8. McGowan JE et al. Guidelines for the use of systemic glucocorticoids in the management of selected infections. *J Infect Dis* 1992;165:1–13.

9. Benitz WE, Tatro DS. *The pediatric drug handbook*. 2nd ed. Chicago: Year Book; 1988.

10. Prober CG. The role of steroids in the management of children with bacterial meningitis. *Pediatrics* 1995; 95:29–31.

11. Baxter JD. Minimizing the side effects of glucocorticoid therapy. *Adv Intern Med* 1990;35:173–94.

12. Tsuei SE et al. Disposition of synthetic glucocorticoids. I. Pharmacokinetics of dexamethasone in healthy adults. *J Pharmacokinet Biopharm* 1979;7:249–64.

13. Gustavson LE, Benet LZ. Pharmacokinetics of natural and synthetic glucocorticoids. In, Anderson DC, Winter JSD, eds. *Butterworth's international medical reviews: clinical endocrinology*. Vol. 4, Adrenal cortex. London: Butterworth; 1985:235–81.

14. Baharav E et al. Dexamethasone-induced perineal irritation. *N Engl J Med* 1986;314:515–6. Letter.

15. Health and Public Policy Committee, American College of Physicians. The dexamethasone suppression test for the detection, diagnosis, and management of depression. *Ann Intern Med* 1984;100:307–8.

16. Nierenberg AA, Feinstein AR. How to evaluate a diagnostic marker test: lessons from the rise and fall of dexamethasone suppression test. *JAMA* 1988;259:1699–702.

17. Kamm GL, Hagmeyer KO. Allergic-type reactions to corticosteroids. *Ann Pharmacother* 1999;33:451–60.

18. Anon. Drugs for acute spinal cord injury. *Med Lett Drugs Ther* 1993;35:72–3.

19. Lesar TS. Standardized dosing tables to reduce errors involving high-dose methylprednisolone for acute spinal cord injury. *Hosp Pharm* 1994;29:935–8.

20. Lamberts SW et al. Corticosteroid therapy in severe illness. *N Engl J Med* 1997;337:1285–92.

21. Short DJ et al. High dose methylprednisolone in the management of acute spinal cord injury—a systematic review from a clinical perspective. *Spinal Cord* 2000;38:273–86.

22. Jantz MA, Sahn SA. Corticosteroids in acute respiratory failure. *Am J Respir Crit Care Med* 1999;160: 1079–100.

23. National Institutes of Health. *Highlights of the expert panel report 2: guidelines for the diagnosis and management of asthma*. NIH Publication No. 97-4051A; 1997.

24. The National Institutes of Health-University of California Expert Panel for Corticosteroids as Adjunctive Therapy for Pneumocystis Pneumonia. Consensus statement of the use of corticosteroids as adjunctive therapy for Pneumocystis pneumonia in the acquired immunodeficiency syndrome. *N Engl J Med* 1990;323: 1500–4.

25. Groff GD et al. Systemic steroid therapy for acute gout: a clinical trial and review of the literature. *Semin Arthritis Rheum* 1990;19:329–36.

26. Taketomo CK et al., eds. *Pediatric dosage handbook*. 6th ed. Cleveland: Lexi-Comp; 1999–2000.

27. Hill MR et al. Monitoring glucocorticoid therapy: a pharmacokinetic approach. *Clin Pharmacol Ther* 1990;48:390–8.

28. Gambertoglio JG et al. Pharmacokinetics and bioavailability of prednisone and prednisolone in healthy volunteers and patients: a review. *J Pharmacokinet Biopharm* 1980;8:1–52.

29. Lewis GP et al. Prednisone side-effects and serum-protein levels. *Lancet* 1971;2:778–81.

30. Saag KG et al. Low dose long-term corticosteroid therapy in rheumatoid arthritis: an analysis of serious adverse events. *Am J Med* 1994;96:115–23.

31. McEvoy CE, Niewoehner DE. Adverse effects of corticosteroid therapy for COPD. A critical review. *Chest* 1997;111:732-43.

32. J. Patten SB, Neutel CI. Corticosteroid-induced adverse psychiatric effects: incidence, diagnosis and management. *Drug Saf* 2000;22:111–22.

33. Callahan CM et al. Oral corticosteroid therapy for patients with stable chronic obstructive pulmonary disease: a meta-analysis. *Ann Intern Med* 1991;114:216–23.

34. Weinberger SE. Recent advances in pulmonary medicine. *N Engl J Med* 1993;328:1389–97.

35. Mukwaya G. Immunosuppressive effects and infections associated with corticosteroid therapy. *Pediatr Infect Dis J* 1988;7:499–504.

36. Derendorf H et al. Pharmacokinetics of triamcinolone acetonide after intravenous, oral, and inhaled administration. *J Clin Pharmacol* 1995;35:302–5.

37. United States Pharmacopeial Convention. *USP DI: Drug information for the health care professional.* 20th ed. Rockville, MD: World Color Book Services; 2000.

38. Guzzo CA et al. Dermatological pharmacology. In, Goodman LS et al., eds. *Goodman and Gilman's the pharmacological basis of therapeutics.* 9th ed. New York: McGraw-Hill; 1996:1593–616.

39. Maddin S, Ho VC. Dermatologic therapy. In, Moschella SL, Hurley HJ, eds. *Dermatology.* 3rd ed. Philadelphia: WB Saunders; 1992:2187–215.

40. Stoughton RB, Cornell RC. Corticosteroids. In, Fitzpatrick TB et al., eds. *Dermatology in general medicine.* 4th ed. New York: McGraw-Hill; 1993:2846–50.

41. Hepburn H et al. Topical steroid treatment in infants, children, and adolescents. In, Schachner LA, ed. *Advances in dermatology.* St Louis: Mosby-Year Book; 1994:225–54.

42. Mooradian AD, Thurman JE. Drug therapy of postprandial hyperglycaemia. *Drugs* 1999;57:19–29.

43. Lebovitz HE. α-Glucosidase inhibitors in the treatment of hyperglycemia. In, Lebovitz HE, ed. *Therapy for diabetes mellitus and related disorders.* 2nd ed. Alexandria, VA: American Diabetes Association; 1994.

44. Anon. Tests of glycemia in diabetes. *Diabetes Care* 1999;22(suppl 1):S77–9.

45. Steele JW et al. Epalrestat: a review of its pharmacology, and therapeutic potential in late-onset complications of diabetes mellitus. *Drugs Aging* 1993;3:532–5.

46. Campbell RK, White JR. New products in development for patients with diabetes. In, *Medications for the treatment of diabetes.* Alexandria, VA: American Diabetes Association; 2000:160–73.

47. White CM. A review of potential cardiovascular uses of intravenous glucagon administration. *J Clin Pharmacol* 1999;39:442–7.

48. Skyler JS. Insulin treatment. In, Lebovitz HE, ed. *Therapy for diabetes mellitus and related disorders.* 3rd ed. Alexandria, VA: American Diabetes Association; 1998:186–203.

49. Genuth S. Diabetic ketoacidosis and hyperosmolar hyperglycemic nonketotic syndrome in adults. In, Lebovitz HE, ed. *Therapy for diabetes mellitus and related disorders.* 3rd ed. Alexandria, VA: American Diabetes Association; 1998:83–96.

50. Kahn SE et al. Insulin secretion in the normal and diabetic human. In, Alberti KGMM et al., eds. *International textbook of diabetes mellitus.* 2nd ed. New York: John Wiley & Sons; 1997:337–53.

51. The Diabetes Control and Complications Trial Research Group. The effect of intensive treatment of diabetes on the development and progression of long-term complications in insulin-dependent diabetes mellitus. *N Engl J Med* 1993;329:977–86.

52. White JR Jr, Campbell RK. Pharmacologic therapies in the management of diabetes mellitus. In, Haire-Joshu D, ed. *Management of diabetes mellitus. Perspectives of care across the life span.* St. Louis: Mosby-Year Book; 1994:119–48.

53. Peterson L et al. Insulin adsorbance to polyvinylchloride surfaces with implications for constant-infusion therapy. *Diabetes* 1976;25:72–4.

54. Heinemann L et al. Time-action profile of inhaled insulin. *Diabet Med* 1997;14:63–72.

55. Setter SM et al. Insulin aspart: a new rapid-acting insulin analog. *Ann Pharmacother* 2000;34:1423–31.

56. Rosskamp RH, Park G. Long-acting insulin analogs. *Diabetes Care* 1999;22(suppl 2):B109–13.

57. Santiago JV, ed. *Medical management of insulin-dependent (type I) diabetes.* 2nd ed. Alexandria, VA: American Diabetes Association; 1993.

58. Bailey CJ, Turner RC. Metformin. *N Engl J Med* 1996;334:574–9.

59. Bauman WA et al. Increased intake of calcium reverses vitamin B_{12} malabsorption induced by metformin. *Diabetes Care* 2000;23:1227–31.

60. Somogyi A et al. Reduction of metformin tubular secretion by cimetidine in man. *Br J Clin Pharmacol* 1987;23:545–51.

61. Hermann LS et al. Therapeutic comparison of metformin and sulfonylurea, alone and in various combinations. *Diabetes Care* 1994;17:1100–8.

62. Choudhury S et al. Single-dose pharmacokinetics of nateglinide in subjects with hepatic cirrhosis. *J Clin Pharmacol* 2000;40:634–40.

63. Hirschberg Y et al. Improved control of mealtime glucose excursions with coadministration of nateglinide and metformin. *Diabetes Care* 2000;23:349–53.

64. Wolffenbuttel BHR, Landgraf R, Dutch and German Repaglinide Study Group. A 1-year multicenter randomized double-blind comparison of repaglinide and glyburide for the treatment of type 2 diabetes. *Diabetes Care* 1999;22:463–7.
65. Levien TL, Baker DE. *Drug evaluation—repaglinide.* Dana Point, CA: The Formulary Monograph Service; April 1998.
66. Gossain VV et al. Management of diabetes in the elderly: a clinical perspective. *J Assoc Acad Minor Phys* 1996;5:22–31.
67. Davidson MB. Rational use of sulfonylureas. *Postgrad Med* 1992;92:69–85.
68. Gerich JE. Oral hypoglycemic agents. *N Engl J Med* 1989;321:1231–45.
69. White JR Jr, Campbell RK. Drug/drug and drug/disease interactions and diabetes. *Diabetes Educ* 1995;21:283–9.
70. White JR. The pharmacologic management of patients with type II diabetes mellitus in the era of oral agents and insulin analogs. *Diabetes Spectrum* 1996;9:227–34.
71. DeFronzo RA. Pharmacologic therapy for type 2 diabetes mellitus. *Ann Intern Med* 1999;131:281–303.
72. Campbell RK, White JR. Overview of medications used to treat type 2 diabetes. In, *Medications for the treatment of diabetes.* Alexandria, VA: American Diabetes Association; 2000:23–43.
73. Campbell RK, White JR. Glitazones. In, *Medications for the treatment of diabetes.* Alexandria, VA: American Diabetes Association; 2000:71–86.
74. Olgihara T et al. Enhancement of insulin sensitivity by troglitazone lowers blood pressure in diabetic hypertensives. *Am J Hypertens* 1995;8:316–20.
75. Anon. Blood glucose meters and data management. In, *Resource guide January 2001.* Supplement to Diabetes Forecast. Alexandria, VA: American Diabetes Association; 2001.
76. Hatcher RA et al. *Contraceptive technology.* 16th rev. ed. New York: Irvington; 1994.
77. Van Look PFA, von Hertzen H. Emergency contraception. *Br Med Bull* 1993;49:158–70.
78. Weisberg E. Prescribing oral contraceptives. *Drugs* 1995;49:224–31.
79. Bayer SR, DeCherney AH. Clinical manifestations and treatment of dysfunctional uterine bleeding. *JAMA* 1993;269:1823–8.
80. Lu PY, Ory SJ. Endometriosis: current management. *Mayo Clin Proc* 1995;70:453–63.
81. Shenfield GM, Griffin JM. Clinical pharmacokinetics of contraceptive steroids. An update. *Clin Pharmacokinet* 1991;20:15–37.
82. Kuhl H. Pharmacokinetics of oestrogens and progestogens. *Maturitas* 1990;12:171–97.
83. Stanczyk FZ, Roy S. Metabolism of levonorgestrel, norethindrone, and structurally related contraceptive steroids. *Contraception* 1990;42:67–93.
84. Kuhnz W et al. Systemic availability of levonorgestrel after single oral administration of norgestimate-containing combination oral contraceptive to 12 young women. *Contraception* 1994;49:255–63.
85. Fotherby K. Potency and pharmacokinetics of gestagens. *Contraception* 1990;41:533–50.
86. Back DJ et al. Comparative pharmacokinetics of levonorgestrel and ethinyloestradiol following intravenous, oral, and vaginal administration. *Contraception* 1987;36:471–9.
87. Goldzieher JW. Selected aspects of the pharmacokinetics and metabolism of ethinyl estrogens and their clinical implications. *Am J Obstet Gynecol* 1990;163:318–22.
88. Goldzieher JW. Pharmacokinetics and metabolism of ethinyl estrogens. In, Goldzieher JW, Fotherby K, eds. *Pharmacology of the contraceptive steroids.* New York: Raven Press; 1994:140–51.
89. Kuhnz W et al. Pharmacokinetics of levonorgestrel and ethinylestradiol in 14 women during three months of treatment with a tri-step combination oral contraceptive: serum protein binding of levonorgestrel and influence of treatment on free and total testosterone levels in the serum. *Contraception* 1994;50:563–79.
90. Orme ML'E et al. Clinical pharmacokinetics of oral contraceptive steroids. *Clin Pharmacokinet* 1983;8: 95–136.
91. Archer DF et al. Pharmacokinetics of a triphasic oral contraceptive containing desogestrel and ethinyl estradiol. *Fertil Steril* 1994;61:645–51.
92. McClamrock HD, Adashi EY. Pharmacokinetics of desogestrel. *Am J Obstet Gynecol* 1993;168:1021–8.
93. Orme M et al. The pharmacokinetics of ethinylestradiol in the presence and absence of gestodene and desogestrel. *Contraception* 1991;43:305–17.
94. Fotherby K. Pharmacokinetics and metabolism of progestins in humans. In, Goldzieher JW, Fotherby K, eds. *Pharmacology of the contraceptive steroids.* New York: Raven Press; 1994:99–126.
95. Kubba A, Guillebaud J. Combined oral contraceptives: acceptability and effective use. *Br Med Bull* 1993;49:140–57.
96. McCann MF, Potter LS. Progestin-only oral contraception: a comprehensive review. *Contraception* 1994;50: S138–48.
97. Speroff L et al. Evaluation of a new generation of oral contraceptives. *Obstet Gynecol* 1993;81:1034–47.
98. Thorogood M, Villard-Mackintosh L. Combined oral contraceptives: risks and benefits. *Br Med Bull* 1993;49:124–39.

99. Upton GV, Corbin A. Contraception for the transitional years of women older than 40 years of age. *Clin Obstet Gynecol* 1992;35:855–64.
100. Schlesselman JJ. Net effect of oral contraceptive use on the risk of cancer in women in the United States. *Obstet Gynecol* 1995;85:793–801.
101. Shenfield GM. Oral contraceptives: are drug interactions of clinical significance. *Drug Saf* 1993;9:21–37.
102. Corson SL. A decade of experience with transdermal estrogen replacement therapy: overview of key pharmacologic and clinical findings. *Int J Fertil* 1993;38:79–91.
103. Kaunitz AM. Long-acting injectable contraception with depot medroxyprogesterone acetate. *Am J Obstet Gynecol* 1994;170:1543–9.
104. Kaunitz AM, Rosenfield A. Injectable contraception with depot medroxyprogesterone acetate. Current status. *Drugs* 1993;45:857–65
105. Pardthaisong T et al. The long-term growth and development of children exposed to Depo-Provera during pregnancy or lactation. *Contraception* 1992;45:313–24.
106. World Health Organization Task Force for Epidemiological Research on Reproductive Health; Special Programme of Research, Development and Research Training in Human Reproduction. Progestogen-only contraceptives during lactation: I: infant growth. *Contraception* 1994;50:35–53.
107. World Health Organization Task Force for Epidemiological Research on Reproductive Health; Special Programme of Research, Development and Research Training in Human Reproduction. Progestogen-only contraceptives during lactation: II: infant development. *Contraception* 1994;50:55–68.
108. Darney PD. Hormonal implants: contraception for a new century. *Am J Obstet Gynecol* 1994;170:1536–43.
109. Skegg DCG et al. Depot medroxyprogesterone acetate and breast cancer. A pooled analysis of the World Health Organization and New Zealand Studies. *JAMA* 1995;273:799–804.
110. Wysowski DK, Green L. Serious adverse events in Norplant users reported to the Food and Drug Administration's Med Watch spontaneous reporting system. *Obstet Gynecol* 1995;85:538–42.
111. Dunson TR et al. Complications and risk factors associated with the removal of Norplant implants. *Obstet Gynecol* 1995;85:543–48.
112. Bagshaw S. The combined oral contraceptive. Risks and adverse effects in perspective. *Drug Saf* 1995;12:91–6.
113. Anon. After the morning after and the morning after that. *Lancet* 1995;345:1381–2. Editorial.
114. Hannaford PC et al. Oral contraception and stroke. Evidence from the Royal College of General Practitioners' Oral Contraception Study. *Stroke* 1994;25:935–42.
115. Lidegaard O. Decline in cerebral thromboembolism among young women after introduction of low-dose oral contraceptives: an incidence study for the period 1980–1993. *Contraception* 1995;52:85–92.
116. Goldzieher JW, Zamah NM. Oral contraceptive side effects: where's the beef? *Contraception* 1995;52:327–35.
117. Vandenbroucke JP et al. Oral contraceptives and the risk of venous thrombosis. *N Engl J Med* 2001;344:1527–35.
118. Parkin L et al. Oral contraceptives and fatal pulmonary embolism. *Lancet* 2000;355:2133–4.
119. Belchetz PE. Hormonal treatment of postmenopausal women. *N Engl J Med* 1994;330:1062–71.
120. Ettinger B et al. Cyclic hormone replacement therapy using quarterly progestin. *Obstet Gynecol* 1994;83:693–700.
121. The Postmenopausal Estrogen/Progestin Interventions (PEPI) Trial. Effects of estrogen or estrogen/progestin regimens on heart disease risk factors in postmenopausal women. *JAMA* 1995;273:199–208.
122. Lobo RA, Cassidenti DL. Pharmacokinetics of oral 17β-estradiol. *J Reprod Med* 1992;37:77–84.
123. Anderson F. Kinetics and pharmacology of estrogens in pre- and postmenopausal women. *Int J Fertil* 1993;38(suppl 1):53–64.
124. Handa VL et al. Vaginal administration of low-dose conjugated estrogens: systemic absorption and effects on the endometrium. *Obstet Gynecol* 1994;84:215–8.
125. Pang SC et al. Long-term effects of transdermal estradiol with and without medroxyprogesterone acetate. *Fertil Steril* 1993;59:76–82.
126. Kuhnz W et al. Pharmacokinetics of estradiol free and total estrone, in young women following single intravenous and oral administration of 17 beta-estradiol. *Arzneimittelforschung* 1993;43:966–73.
127. Cobleigh MA et al. Estrogen replacement therapy in breast cancer survivors: a time for change. *JAMA* 1994;272:540–5.
128. Loprinzi CL et al. Megestrol acetate for the prevention of hot flashes. *N Engl J Med* 1994;331:347–52.
129. Campagnoli C et al. Long-term hormone replacement treatment in menopause: new choices, old apprehensions, recent findings. *Maturitas* 1993;18:21–46.

130. Lufkin EG et al. Treatment of postmenopausal osteoporosis with transdermal estrogen. *Ann Intern Med* 1992;117:1–9.
131. Walsh BW et al. Effects of postmenopausal estrogen replacement on the concentrations and metabolism of plasma lipoproteins. *N Engl J Med* 1991;325:1196–204.
132. Lindsay R. Prevention and treatment of osteoporosis. *Lancet* 1993;341:801–5.
133. Anon. Drugs for prevention and treatment of postmenopausal osteoporosis. *Med Lett Drugs Ther* 2000; 42:97–100.
134. Overgaard K et al. Effect of calcitonin given intranasally on bone mass and fracture rates in established osteoporosis: a dose-response study. *BMJ* 1992;305:556–61.
135. Anon. New drugs for osteoporosis. *Med Lett Drugs Ther* 1996;38:1–3.
136. McCarthy ML, Stoukides CA. Estrogen therapy of uremic bleeding. *Ann Pharmacother* 1994;28:60–2.
137. Zachee P et al. Hematologic aspects of end-stage renal failure. *Ann Hematol* 1994;69:33–40.
138. Bhavnani BR, Cecutti A. Pharmacokinetics of 17β-dihydroequilin sulfate and 17β-dihydroequilin in normal postmenopausal women. *J Clin Endocrinol Metab* 1994;78:197–204.
139. Steinberg KK et al. A meta-analysis of the effect of estrogen replacement therapy on the risk of breast cancer. *JAMA* 1991;265:1985–90. {Erratum *JAMA* 1991:266:1362.}
140. Udoff L et al. Combined continuous hormone replacement therapy: a critical review. *Obstet Gynecol* 1995; 86:306–16.
141. Archer DF et al. Bleeding patterns in postmenopausal women taking continuous combined or sequential regimens of conjugated estrogens with medroxyprogesterone acetate. Menopause Study Group. *Obstet Gynecol* 1994;83:686–92.
142. Ravnikar V. Physiology and treatment of hot flushes. *Obstet Gynecol* 1995;75:3S–8.
143. Etienne MC et al. Improved bioavailability of a new oral preparation of medroxyprogesterone acetate. *J Pharm Sci* 1991;80:1130–2.
144. Wright CE et al. Effect of injection volume on the bioavailability of sterile medroxyprogesterone acetate suspension. *Clin Pharm* 1983;2:435–8.
145. Norman TR et al. Comparative bioavailability of orally and vaginally administered progesterone. *Fertil Steril* 1991;56:1034–9.
146. Munk-Jensen N et al. Continuous combined and sequential estradiol and norethindrone acetate treatment of postmenopausal women: effect of plasma lipoproteins in a two-year placebo-controlled trial. *Am J Obstet Gynecol* 1994;171:132–8.
147. Nahoul K et al. Profiles of plasma estrogens, progesterone and their metabolites after oral or vaginal administration of estradiol or progesterone. *Maturitas* 1993;16:185–202.
148. Padwick M et al. Absorption and metabolism of oral progesterone when administered twice daily. *Fertil Steril* 1986;46:402–7.
149. Ottoson UB et al. Serum levels of progesterone and some of its metabolites including deoxycorticosterone after oral and parenteral administration. *Br J Obstet Gynaecol* 1984;91:1111–9.
150. Freeman EW et al. A double-blind trial of oral progesterone, alprazolam, and placebo in treatment of severe premenstrual syndrome. *JAMA* 1995;274:51–7.
151. Freeman E et al. Ineffectiveness of progesterone suppository treatment of premenstrual syndrome. *JAMA* 1990;264:349–53.
152. Anon. Raloxifene for postmenopausal osteoporosis. *Med Lett Drugs Ther* 1998;40:29–30.
153. Ashworth LE. Focus on raloxifene. *Formulary* 1998;33:305–17.
154. Ettinger B et al. Reduction of vertebral fracture risk in postmenopausal women with osteoporosis treated with raloxifene. *JAMA* 1999;282:637–45.
155. Cummings SR et al. The effect of raloxifene on risk of breast cancer in postmenopausal women. *JAMA* 1999;281;2189–97.
156. Walsh BW et al. Effects of raloxifene on serum lipids and coagulation factors in healthy postmenopausal women. *JAMA* 1998;279:1445–51.
157. Grady D et al. Hormone therapy to prevent disease and prolong life in postmenopausal women. *Ann Intern Med* 1992;117:1016–37.
158. American College of Physicians. Guidelines for counseling postmenopausal women about preventive hormone therapy. *Ann Intern Med* 1992;117:1038–41.
159. Lip GYH et al. Hormone replacement therapy and blood pressure in hypertensive women. *J Hum Hypertens* 1994;8:491–4.
160. Colditz GA et al. The use of estrogens and progestins and the risk of breast cancer in postmenopausal women. *N Engl J Med* 1995;332:1589–93.
161. Stanford JL et al. Combined estrogen and progestin hormone replacement therapy in relation to risk of breast cancer in middle-aged women. *JAMA* 1995;274:137–42.

162. Dupont WD, Page DL. Menopausal estrogen replacement therapy and breast cancer. *Arch Intern Med* 1991; 151:67–72.

163. Ettinger B et al. Reduced mortality associated with long-term postmenopausal estrogen therapy. *Obstet Gynecol* 1996;87:6–12.

164. Westendorp ICD et al. Hormone replacement therapy and peripheral arterial disease. *Arch Intern Med* 2000; 160:2498–502.

165. Cooper DS. Antithyroid drugs for the treatment of hyperthyroidism caused by Graves' disease. *Endocrinol Metab Clin North Am* 1998;27:225–47.

166. Braverman LE, Utiger RD. *Werner & Ingbar's the thyroid: a fundamental and clinical text*. 8th ed. Philadelphia: Lippincott Williams & Wilkins; 2000.

167. Dong BJ. How medications affect thyroid function. *West J Med* 2000;172:102–6.

168. Dunn JT et al. The prevention and management of iodine-induced hyperthyroidism and its cardiac features. *Thyroid* 1998;8:101–6.

169. Surks MI, Sievert R. Drugs and thyroid function. *N Engl J Med* 1995;333:1688–94.

170. Gittoes NJL, Franklyn JA. Drug-induced thyroid disorders. *Drug Saf* 1995;13:46–55.

171. Harjai KJ, Licata AA. Effects of amiodarone on thyroid function. *Ann Intern Med* 1997;126:63–73.

172. Mandel SJ et al. Levothyroxine therapy in patients with thyroid disease. *Ann Intern Med* 1993; 119:492–502.

173. Lindsay RS, Toft AD. Hypothyroidism. *Lancet* 1997;349:413–7.

174. Singer PA et al. Treatment guidelines for patients with hyperthyroidism and hypothyroidism. *JAMA* 1995;273:808–12.

175. Bartalena L et al. Adverse effects of thyroid hormone preparations and antithyroid drugs. *Drug Saf* 1996;15:53–63.

176. Grebe SKG et al. Treatment of hypothyroidism with once weekly thyroxine. *J Clin Endocrinol Metab* 1997;82:870–5.

177. Ayala AR et al. When to treat mild hypothyroidism. *Endocrinol Metab Clin North Am* 2000;29:399–415.

178. Hak AE et al. Subclinical hypothyroidism is an independent risk factor for atherosclerosis and myocardial infarction in elderly women: the Rotterdam study. *Ann Intern Med* 2000;132:270–8.

179. Hussein WI et al. Normalization of hyperhomocyteinemia with L-thyroxine in hypothyroidism. *Ann Intern Med* 1999;131:348–51.

180. Zelmanovitz F et al. Suppressive therapy with levothyroxine for solitary thyroid nodules: a double-blind controlled clinical study and cumulative meta-analyses. *J Clin Endocrinol Metab* 1998;83:3881–5.

181. Gharib H, Mazzaferri EL. Thyroxine suppressive therapy in patients with nodular thyroid disease. *Ann Intern Med* 1998;128:386–94.

182. Yamamoto T el al. Factors associated with mortality of myxedema coma: report of eight cases and literature survey. *Thyroid* 1999;9:1167–74.

183. Nicoloff JT, LoPresti JS. Myxedema coma. A form of decompensated hypothyroidism. *Endocrinol Metab Clin North Am* 1993;22:279–90.

184. LaFranchi S. Congenital hypothyroidism: etiologies, diagnosis, and management. *Thyroid* 1999;9:735–40.

185. Alexander KS et al. Stability of an extemporaneously formulated levothyroxine sodium syrup compounded from commercial tablets. *Int J Pharm Compound* 1997;1:60–4.

186. Taylor J et al. Twice-weekly dosing for thyroxine replacement in elderly patients with primary hypothyroidism. *J Int Med Res* 1994;22:273–7.

187. Ain KA et al. Thyroid hormone levels affected by time of blood sampling in thyroxine-treated patients. *Thyroid* 1993;3:81–5.

188. Dong BJ et al. Bioequivalence of generic and brand-name levothyroxine products in the treatment of hypothyroidism. *JAMA* 1997;277:1205–13.

189. Singh N et al. Effect of calcium carbonate on the absorption of levothyroxine. *JAMA* 2000;283:2822–5.

190. Nicoloff JT et al. Simultaneous measurement of thyroxine and triiodothyronine peripheral turnover kinetics in man. *J Clin Invest* 1972;51:473–83.

191. Greenspan SL, Greenspan FS. The effect of thyroid hormone on skeletal integrity. *Ann Intern Med* 1999; 130:750–8.

192. Tseng A, Fletcher D. Interaction between ritonavir and levothyroxine. *AIDS* 1998;12:2235–6.

193. Escalante DA et al. Assessment of interchangeability of two brands of levothyroxine preparation with a third-generation TSH assay. *Am J Med* 1995;98:374–8.

194. Jackson IMD. The thyroid axis and depression. *Thyroid* 1998;8:951–6.

195. Fava M. New approaches to the treatment of refractory depression. *J Clin Psychiatry* 2000;61(suppl 1):26–32.

196. Bunevicius R et al. Effects of thyroxine as compared with thyroxine plus triiodothyronine in patients with hypothyroidism. *N Engl J Med* 1999;340:424–9.

197. Salter DR et al. Triiodothyronine (T$_3$) and cardiovascular therapeutics: a review. *J Card Surg* 1992;7:363–74.

198. Zaninovich AA et al. Multicompartmental analysis of triiodothyronine kinetics in hypothyroid patients treated orally or intravenously with triiodothyronine. *Thyroid* 1994;4:285–93.

199. Bettendorf M et al. Tri-iodothyronine treatment in children after cardiac surgery: a double-blind, randomised, placebo-controlled study. *Lancet* 2000;356:529–34.

200. Mullis-Jansson SL et al. A randomized double-blind study of the effect of triiodothyronine on cardiac function and morbidity after coronary bypass surgery. *J Thorac Cardiovasc Surg* 1999;117:1128–34.

201. Portman MA et al. Triiodothyronine repletion in infants during cardiopulmonary bypass for congenital heart disease. *J Thorac Cardiovasc Surg* 2000;120:604–8.

202. Toft A. Thyroxine suppression therapy in Graves' disease. *Baillieres Clin Endocrinol Metab* 1997;11:537–48.

203. Nabil N et al. Methimazole: an alternative route of administration. *J Clin Endocrinol Metab* 1982;54:180–1.

204. Zimmerman D, Lteif AN. Thyrotoxicosis in children. *Endocrinol Metab Clin North Am* 1998;27:109–26.

205. Masiukiewicz US, Burrow GN. Hyperthyroidism in pregnancy: diagnosis and treatment. *Thyroid* 1999;9:647–52.

206. Cooper DS et al. Methimazole pharmacology in man: studies using a newly developed radioimmunoassay for methimazole. *J Clin Endocrinol Metab* 1984;58:473–9.

207. Kampmann JP, Hansen JM. Clinical pharmacokinetics of antithyroid drugs. *Clin Pharmacokinet* 1981;6:401–28.

208. Arab DM et al. Severe cholestatic jaundice in uncomplicated hyperthyroidism treated with methimazole. *J Clin Endocrinol Metab* 1995;80:1083–5.

209. Mercado M et al. Treatment of hyperthyroidism with a combination of methimazole and cholestyramine. *J Clin Endocrinol Metab* 1996;81:3191–3.

210. Kaplan MM et al. Treatment of hyperthyroidism with radioactive iodine. *Endocrinol Metab Clin North Am* 1998;27:205–23.

211. Walter RM, Bartle WR. Rectal administration of propylthiouracil in the treatment of Graves' disease. *Am J Med* 1990;88:69–70.

212. Bartle WR et al. Rectal absorption of propylthiouracil. *Int J Clin Pharmacol Ther Toxicol* 1988;26:285–7.

213. Cooper DS et al. Acute effects of propylthiouracil (PTU) on a thyroidal iodide organification and peripheral iodothyronine deiodination: correlation with serum PTU levels measured by radioimmunoassay. *J Clin Endocrinol Metab* 1982;54:101–7.

214. Williams KV et al. Fifty years of experience with propylthiouracil-associated hepatotoxicity: what have we learned? *J Clin Endocrinol Metab* 1997;82:1727–33.

Renal and Electrolytes

Diuretics

Class Instructions. Diuretics. If you are taking more than one dose a day, take the last dose in the afternoon or early evening to avoid having to void urine during the night. Avoid heavily salted foods, but rigid salt restriction is not necessary. Avoid excessive water intake. Report any dizziness or lightheadedness (especially when arising from sitting or lying), muscle cramps, weakness, lethargy, dry mouth, thirst, or low urine output.

Missed Doses. Take this drug at regular intervals. If you miss a dose, take it as soon as you remember. If it is about time for the next dose, take that dose only. Do not double the dose or take extra.

AMILORIDE HYDROCHLORIDE
Midamor, Various

Pharmacology. Amiloride is a potassium-sparing diuretic with a mechanism and site of action resembling triamterene. It has mild antihypertensive activity and a longer duration of action than triamterene.[1-3]

Adult Dosage. PO 10 mg/day in 1–2 doses, to a maximum of 20 mg/day, although a dosage >10 mg/day is seldom necessary.

Dosage Forms. Tab 5 mg; **Tab** 5 mg with hydrochlorothiazide 50 mg (Moduretic 5-50, various).

Pharmacokinetics. Onset within 2 hr; maximum effect 6–10 hr after an oral dose; duration about 24 hr. The drug is about 50% orally absorbed, decreasing to 30% when taken with food. Half the absorbed drug is excreted unchanged in urine. Half-life is 6–9 hr in normal renal function, increasing up to 144 hr in renal failure.

Adverse Reactions. Adverse reactions are generally similar to triamterene; however, in contrast to triamterene, renal stone formation has not been reported with amiloride.

BUMETANIDE
Bumex, Various

Pharmacology. Bumetanide is a loop diuretic with renal pharmacology similar to furosemide. Bumetanide is estimated to be approximately 40 times as potent as furosemide on a weight basis.[1-6]

Administration and Adult Dosage. PO for diuresis 0.5–2 mg as a single dose and repeat q 4–5 hr as needed, to a maximum of 10 mg/day. **IV or IM dose** is 0.5–1 mg, IV given over 1–2 min. Repeat doses may be administered as needed q 2–3 hr, to a maximum of 10 mg/day. For long-term control of edema, intermittent regimens are recommended as alternate daily doses or daily doses for 3–4 days with 1–2 day drug holidays. **IV infusion** 1 mg IV bolus, followed by (Cl_{cr} >75 mL/min) 0.5 mg/hr; (Cl_{cr} 25–75 mL/min) 0.5–1 mg/hr; or (Cl_{cr} <25 mL/min) 1–2 mg/hr.[3]

Special Populations. *Pediatric Dosage.* 0.015–0.1 mg/kg/dose q 6–24 hr, to a maximum of 10 mg/day.

Geriatric Dosage. Start with a low initial dose and titrate to response.

Other Conditions. No adjustment is necessary for renal impairment, hemodialysis, or chronic ambulatory peritoneal dialysis.

Dosage Forms. **Tab** 0.5, 1, 2 mg; **Inj** 0.25 mg/mL.

Patient Instructions. (*See* Class Instructions: Diuretics.)

Pharmacokinetics. *Onset and Duration.* Onset is within 30–60 min after oral administration and within minutes after IV administration. Durations of diuresis are 4–6 hr orally and 2–3 hr IV.[5,6]

Serum Levels. Site of action is within the renal tubule and not the serum; therefore, serum concentrations do not reflect diuretic activity.

Fate. Bioavailability is 80–96%.[5,6] V_{dss} is 0.16–0.24 L/kg in normal subjects. Protein binding to albumin is 94–97%. Renal excretion of unchanged drug accounts for 50% of administered drug, with hepatic metabolism and biliary excretion accounting for the remainder. The metabolites are inactive.

$t_{1/2}$. 0.3–1.5 hr; 1.9 ± 0.1 hr in renal insufficiency; 2.3 ± 0.4 hr in cirrhosis.[5,6]

Adverse Reactions. Hypokalemia, hyponatremia, and hyperuricemia occur frequently. Muscle cramps, dizziness, hypotension, headache, and nausea occur occasionally. The ototoxic potential of bumetanide is believed to be less than that of furosemide and most likely associated with rapid IV administration, high-dose therapy, or use in renal impairment.

Contraindications. Anuria; hepatic coma; coexisting severe electrolyte depletion.

Precautions. (*See* Furosemide.)

Drug Interactions. Aminoglycoside-related ototoxicity risk can be increased with concomitant bumetanide therapy. Cardiac glycoside toxicity is enhanced with diuretic-induced hypokalemia and hypomagnesemia. Concomitant use with other loop or thiazide diuretics enhances diuresis.

Parameters to Monitor. (*See* Furosemide.)

FUROSEMIDE   Lasix, Various

Pharmacology. Furosemide is a loop diuretic that is actively secreted via the nonspecific organic acid transport system into the lumen of the thick ascending limb of Henle's loop, where it decreases sodium reabsorption by competing for the chloride site on the Na^+-K^+-$2Cl^-$ cotransporter.[1,2] Medullary hypertonicity is diminished, thereby decreasing the kidney's ability to reabsorb water. Excretion of sodium, chloride, potassium, hydrogen ion, calcium, magnesium, ammonium, bicarbonate, and possibly phosphate is enhanced. IV furosemide increases venous capacitance independent of diuretic effect, producing rapid improvement in pulmonary edema.[1]

Administration and Adult Dosage. **PO for edema** 20–80 mg as a single dose initially; double successive doses q 6–8 hr until response is obtained. The maximum single oral dose depends on the disease state: 80 mg for hepatic cirrhosis with preserved renal function,[3] 240 mg for nephrotic syndrome,[3] 80–160 mg for CHF (with normal kidney function);[3] however, dosages up to 2500 mg/day have been recommended in refractory CHF.[7] After response, effective dosage is given in 1–3 doses daily; usual daily maintenance dosage depends on the single dose to which the patient responded. **PO for chronic renal failure** 80 mg initially, increasing in 80 mg/day increments until response is obtained, to a maximum of 160 mg and 400 mg for Cl_{cr} <20 mL/min.[8] (*See* Special Populations.) **PO for hypertension** 40 mg bid. **IV** should be used only when oral administration is not feasible. IV doses may be given over 1–2 min, except the rate should not exceed 4 mg/min when large doses are given. **IM or IV for edema** use one-half the dose of PO furosemide (as outlined above);[8] may double the dose q 2 hr or more until desired response is obtained. This dosage is then given in 1–2 doses daily for maintenance. Dosages up to 4 g/day IV have been used in refractory CHF.[7] **IV for acute pulmonary edema** 40 mg initially, may repeat in 30–60 min with 80 mg, if necessary (assuming relatively normal kidney function). For patients with renal impairment, the initial and subsequent doses must be adjusted based on renal function. For example, if Cl_{cr} is 50 mL/min (about one-half normal), the dose must be doubled; if Cl_{cr} is 25 mL/min, the dose must be quadrupled. **Continuous IV infusion for edema** 40 mg loading dose followed by (Cl_{cr} 75 mL/min) 10 mg/hr; (Cl_{cr} 25–75 mL/min) 10–20 mg/hr; (Cl_{cr} <25 mL/min) 20–40 mg/hr.[3]

Special Populations. *Pediatric Dosage.* **PO for edema** 2 mg/kg in 1 dose initially, increasing by 1–2 mg/kg in 6–8 hr, if necessary, to a maximum of 6 mg/kg/day. **IM or IV** 1 mg/kg in 1 dose initially, increasing by 1 mg/kg q 2 hr or more until desired response is obtained, or to a maximum of 6 mg/kg/day. Maximum single dose depends on renal function. (*See* Notes.)

Geriatric Dosage. Start with a low initial dose and titrate to response.

Other Conditions. For Cl_{cr} <20 mL/min, maximal response is attained with single IV doses of 200 mg (400 mg PO). Hence, there appears to be no need to administer larger single doses to such patients.[8] A diminished response can occur in severe decompensated CHF, caused in part by alterations in oral absorption[9] and decreased renal blood flow (despite relatively normal GFR), resulting in decreased delivery of furosemide to the renal tubule; IV administration circumvents absorption problems. However, decompensated CHF usually affects only the rate rather than the extent of oral furosemide absorption.[10] In addition, high-dose therapy might be beneficial in severe, refractory CHF.[9] (*See* Administration and Adult Dosage.) For patients with cirrhosis, dosage is based on renal function.

Dosage Forms. **Soln** 8, 10 mg/mL; **Tab** 20, 40, 80 mg; **Inj** 10 mg/mL.

Patient Instructions. (*See* Class Instructions: Diuretics.)

Pharmacokinetics. *Onset and Duration.* (Venous capacitance) IV onset 5 min, duration >1 hr. (Diuresis) PO onset 30–60 min, peak 1–2 hr, duration 6 hr; IV onset 15 min, peak 30–60 min, duration 1–2 hr; duration might be prolonged in severe renal impairment. (Hypertension) maximum effect on BP might not occur for several days.

Serum Levels. Site of action is within the renal tubules and not the serum; therefore, serum concentrations do not reflect diuretic activity. High serum levels can be associated with ototoxicity.[11]

Fate. Pharmacokinetics are variable and absorption is erratic; 61 ± 17% (range 20–100) is bioavailable in normals, 30–100% in renal failure.[11,12] The rate, but not the extent, of absorption might be decreased in patients with edematous bowel caused by decompensated CHF;[10] 96–99% is plasma protein bound, reduced in CHF, renal disease, or cirrhosis.[12] V_d is 0.11 L/kg; Cl is 0.12 ± 0.24 L/hr/kg; V_d and Cl depend on protein binding.[11,12] Two possible inactive metabolites exist: a glucuronide, which is excreted primarily in urine (and to a lesser extent in the feces by passive diffusion into the GI lumen), and saluamine, which could be a true metabolite or an analytical artifact. Renal clearance is primarily by active secretion; 50–80% (IV) and 20–55% (PO) are excreted unchanged in urine. Renal clearance is decreased in renal failure, consistent with decreased renal blood flow, a reduction of functioning nephrons, and the presence of competitive inhibitors for secretion.[12]

$t_{1/2}$. 92 ± 7 (range 30–120) min in normals, can be extended in cirrhosis to 81 ± 8 min or CHF to 122 min, and markedly prolonged in end-stage renal disease to 9.7 hr, and in multiorgan failure to 20–24 hr. Mean residence time has been proposed as a more appropriate estimate of duration: 51.4 min (IV); 135–195 min (PO).[11,12]

Adverse Reactions. Dehydration, hypotension, hypochloremic alkalosis, and hypokalemia are frequent. Hyperglycemia and glucose intolerance occur as with thiazides. (*See* Hydrochlorothiazide.) With high-dose therapy (>250 mg/day), hyperuricemia occurs frequently. Tinnitus and hearing loss, occasionally permanent, occur frequently in association with rapid IV injection of large doses in patients with renal impairment.[8,12,13] Rarely, thrombocytopenia, neutropenia, jaundice, pancreatitis, and a variety of skin reactions occur.

Contraindications. Anuria (except for single dose in acute anuria).

Precautions. Use with caution in patients with severe or progressive renal disease; discontinue if renal function worsens. Use with caution in liver disease (can precipitate hepatic encephalopathy), history of diabetes mellitus or gout, and in patients allergic to other sulfonamide derivatives. Use with caution in patients with hypokalemia, hypomagnesemia, or hypocalcemia.

Drug Interactions. Cholestyramine and colestipol decrease furosemide absorption, and NSAIDs can decrease the diuretic effect of furosemide. Aminoglycoside ototoxicity can be enhanced in renally impaired patients. IV furosemide can produce flushing, sweating, and BP variations in patients taking chloral hydrate.

Parameters to Monitor. Monitor serum potassium closely, other electrolytes periodically, and serum glucose, uric acid, BUN, and Cr_s occasionally. Observe for clinical signs of fluid or electrolyte depletion such as dry mouth, thirst, weakness, lethargy, muscle pains or cramps, hypotension, oliguria, tachycardia, and GI upset.

Notes. Furosemide is light sensitive; oral solution should be stored at 15–30°C and protected from light. In severe proteinuria (>3.5 g/day), urinary albumin binds furosemide and reduces its effectiveness, explaining the higher dosage required to achieve adequate free drug concentrations.[10] In general, clinical nonresponders tend to have a decreased fraction of loop diuretics excreted in the urine. For these patients and those with CHF and renal impairment, larger doses may force more drug into the tubule; however, the risk of ototoxicity must be considered. Alternatively, combined use with a **thiazide** or **metolazone** orally can be effective by blocking sodium reabsorption at multiple tubule sites; however, these agents (especially metolazone) have a slow onset of action. Alternative treatment regimens include IV **acetazolamide** and low-dose dopamine given with the loop diuretic.[4,7,14] (*See* Loop Diuretics Comparison Chart.)

LOOP DIURETICS COMPARISON CHART

DRUG	DOSAGE FORMS	ADULT DOSAGE[a]	PEDIATRIC DOSAGE[a]	DOSAGE IN RENAL IMPAIRMENT	COMMENTS
Bumetanide Bumex Various	Tab 0.5, 1, 2 mg Inj 0.25 mg/mL.	PO for edema 0.5–2 mg/day, to a maximum of 10 mg/day. IM or IV over 1–2 min 0.5–1 mg, to a maximum of 10 mg/day IV continuous infusion 1 mg, then 1–2 mg/hr.	PO, IM, or IV 0.01–0.02 mg/kg, to a maximum of 0.4 mg/kg or 10 mg total daily dosage.	For Cl_{cr} <15 mL/min, maximal response is attained with single PO or IV doses of 8–10 mg; IV infusion of 12 mg over 12 hr may be more effective and less toxic.	1 mg PO or IV = 40 mg IV furosemide.
Ethacrynic Acid Edecrin	Tab 25, 50 mg. Inj 50 mg.	PO minimal dose in the range of 50–200 mg/day initially, to a maximum of 200 mg bid IV 50 mg or 0.5–1 mg/kg, to a maximum of 100 mg.	PO (infants) not established; (children) 25 mg or 1 mg/kg initially, increased in 25 mg increments to desired effect; IV not established; 1 mg/kg has been used.	Not recommended with Cl_{cr} <10 mL/min; for Cl_{cr} of 10–50 mL/min, increase interval to q 8–12 hr.	Nonsulfonamide. Reliable potency data not available; however, 50 mg IV is about equal to furosemide 35 mg IV.
Furosemide Lasix Various	Tab 20, 40, 80 mg Soln 8, 10 mg/mL. Inj 10 mg/mL.	(See monograph.)	(See monograph.)	Maximum response occurs with 200 mg IV or an average of 400 mg PO, although quite variable.	IV dose averages 50% of PO dose, with great variability.
Torsemide Demadex	Tab 5, 10, 20, 100 mg Inj 10 mg/mL.	(See monograph.)	(See monograph.)	Maximal response occurs with PO or IV dose of 50–100 mg.	5–10 mg PO or IV = 20 mg IV furosemide.

[a]Higher doses needed for patients with CHF, liver cirrhosis, and nephrotic syndrome.
From references 5–7, 13, and 14, and product information.

HYDROCHLOROTHIAZIDE   Esidrix, HydroDIURIL, Oretic, Various

Pharmacology. Thiazides increase sodium and chloride excretion by interfering with their reabsorption in the cortical diluting segment of the nephron; a mild diuresis of slightly concentrated urine results.[1,2] Excretion of potassium, bicarbonate, magnesium, phosphate, and iodide excretion is increased; calcium excretion is decreased. Decreases in interstitial fluid volume, reductions in intracellular calcium secondary to a fall in smooth muscle sodium concentration, and a change in the affinity of cell surface receptors to vasoconstrictive hormones are thought to be among the mechanisms for the hypotensive effect of the thiazides. Urine output is paradoxically decreased in diabetes insipidus.[1]

Administration and Adult Dosage. PO for edema 25–200 mg/day in 1–3 doses initially; 25–100 mg/day or intermittently for maintenance, to a maximum of 200 mg/day. **PO for hypertension** 12.5–50 mg/day. Maintenance dosages >50 mg/day provide little additional benefit in controlling essential hypertension and can increase the frequency of dose-related biochemical abnormalities.[15]

Special Populations. *Pediatric Dosage.* PO (<6 months) up to 3.3 mg/kg/day in 2 divided doses; (>6 months) 2–2.2 mg/kg/day in 2 divided doses.

Geriatric Dosage. Start with a low initial dose and titrate to response.

Other Conditions. At a Cl_{cr} <30 mL/min, usual dosages of thiazides and most related drugs are not very effective as diuretics but may be used in conjunction with loop diuretics.[16]

Dosage Forms. **Tab** 25, 50, 100 mg; **Cap** 12.5 mg; **Soln** 10 mg/mL.

Patient Instructions. (*See* Class Instructions: Diuretics.) If stomach upset occurs, take drug with meals. Report persistent anorexia, nausea, or vomiting.

Pharmacokinetics. *Onset and Duration.* Onset of diuresis within 2 hr; peak in 4–6 hr; duration 6–12 hr. Onset of hypotensive effect in 3–4 days; duration ≤1 week after discontinuing therapy.

Serum Levels. The site of diuretic action is within the renal tubules and not the serum; therefore, serum concentrations do not reflect diuretic activity.

Fate. Oral bioavailability is 71 ± 15% in healthy individuals, increased when given with an anticholinergic, and decreased by one-half in CHF and after intestinal shunt surgery. There are no differences in absorption among single-entity formulations. The drug is 58 ± 17% plasma protein bound; V_d is 0.83 ± 0.31 L/kg; Cl is 0.29 ± 0.07 L/hr/kg. Over 95% is excreted unchanged in urine by filtration and secretion. In severe renal impairment, renal clearance is prolonged 5-fold, with nonrenal clearance (mechanism as yet unidentified) playing a larger role in elimination.[11,17]

$t_{1/2}$. 2.5 ± 0.2 hr; prolonged in uncompensated CHF or renal impairment.[11,17,18]

Adverse Reactions. Hypokalemia is frequent; however, its treatment in otherwise healthy hypertensive patients is usually unnecessary. Potassium supplements or potassium-sparing diuretics (*see* Notes) may be indicated in patients with arrhythmias, MI, or severe ischemic heart disease; those with chronic liver disease; elderly eating poor diets; patients taking digoxin, a corticosteroid, or drugs that interfere with ventricular repolarization such as phenothiazines and heterocyclic antidepressants; and those whose serum potassium level fall below 3 mEq/L. Hyperuricemia occurs frequently but is reversible, and treatment is unnecessary unless the patient has renal impairment or a history of gout.[19] Hyperglycemia and alterations in glucose tolerance (usually reversible), loss of diabetic control, or precipitation of diabetes mellitus occur occasionally. Decreased glucose tolerance might increase in prevalence after several years of therapy.[20,21] Thrombocytopenia and pancreatitis occur rarely. Elevation of serum cholesterol and triglycerides occurs; the clinical importance is unknown but can increase the risk of coronary heart disease.

Contraindications. Anuria; pregnancy, unless accompanied by severe edema; allergy to sulfonamide derivatives.

Precautions. Use with caution in patients with renal function impairment, liver disease (can precipitate hepatic encephalopathy), history of diabetes mellitus, or gout. Use with caution in patients with diabetes mellitus because thiazides might worsen glucose intolerance.[20,21]

Drug Interactions. Cholestyramine and colestipol decrease oral absorption of thiazides, and NSAIDs can decrease the diuretic effect of thiazides. Anticholinergics can increase oral bioavailability. Dosage of potent hypotensive agents might have to be reduced if a thiazide is added to the regimen. Concurrent calcium-containing antacids can cause hypercalcemia. Long-term thiazides can reduce lithium excretion.

Parameters to Monitor. Monitor serum potassium weekly to monthly initially; q 3–6 months when stable. Monitor other serum electrolytes periodically. Monitor all electrolytes more closely when other losses occur (eg, vomiting, diarrhea). Observe for clinical signs of fluid or electrolyte depletion such as dry mouth, thirst, weakness, lethargy, muscle pains or cramps, hypotension, oliguria, tachycardia, and GI upset. Monitor BP periodically during antihypertensive therapy and serum glucose in patients with diabetes mellitus.

Notes. For the prevention of hypokalemia during thiazide therapy, a **potassium-sparing diuretic** may be preferred over potassium supplements in alkalotic patients because these agents decrease hydrogen ion loss, which can correct alkalosis and drive more potassium extracellularly.[22] Potassium-sparing diuretics also may be preferred for patients predisposed to hypomagnesemia and for those with serum potassium <3 mEq/L because potassium supplements rarely correct hypokalemia of this severity. (*See* Thiazides and Related Diuretics Comparison Chart.) JNC-VI guidelines recommend diuretics and β-blockers as initial drugs of choice for patients with hypertension based on demonstrated reductions in morbidity and mortality.

THIAZIDES AND RELATED DIURETICS COMPARISON CHART[a]

DRUG	DOSAGE FORMS	ORAL DIURETIC DOSAGE RANGE (MG/DAY)[b]	EQUIVALENT DIURETIC DOSAGE (MG)	PEAK EFFECT (HR)	DURATION OF DIURESIS (HR)
Bendroflumethiazide Naturetin	Tab 5, 10 mg.	2.5–15	5	4	6–12
Benzthiazide Exna Various	Tab 50 mg.	50–150	50	4–6	12–18
Chlorothiazide Diuril Various	Tab 250, 500 mg Susp 50 mg/mL Inj 500 mg.[c]	500–2000	500	4 (PO) 0.5 (IV)	6–12 (PO) 2 (IV)
Chlorthalidone[d] Hygroton Thalitone Various	Tab (Thalitone)[e] 15, 25 mg Tab 25, 50, 100 mg.	100–200 60–120 (Thalitone)	50	2	24–72
Hydrochlorothiazide Various	Cap 12.5 mg Tab 25, 50, 100 mg Soln 10, mg/mL.	25–100	50	4–6	6–12
Hydroflumethiazide Diucardin Saluron Various	Tab 50 mg.	25–200	50	3–4	12–24
Indapamide[d] Lozol Various	Tab 1.25, 2.5 mg.	2.5–5	2.5	2	up to 36

(continued)

THIAZIDES AND RELATED DIURETICS COMPARISON CHART[a] (*continued*)

DRUG	DOSAGE FORMS	ORAL DIURETIC DOSAGE RANGE (MG/DAY)[b]	EQUIVALENT DIURETIC DOSAGE (MG)	PEAK EFFECT (HR)	DURATION OF DIURESIS (HR)
Methyclothiazide Aquatensen Enduron Various	Tab 2.5, 5 mg.	2.5–10	5	6	24
Metolazone[d] Mykrox Zaroxolyn	Tab (Mykrox)[e] 0.5 mg Tab 2.5, 5, 10 mg.	5–20 0.5–1 (Mykrox)	5 (Zaroxolyn)	2	12–24
Polythiazide Renese	Tab 1, 2, 4 mg.	1–4	2	6	24–48
Quinethazone[d] Hydromox	Tab 50 mg.	50–200	50	6	18–24
Trichlormethiazide Metahydrin Naqua Various	Tab 2, 4 mg.	2–4	2	6	24

[a]From USP-DI and product informtion; patients unresponsive to maximal dosage of one agent are unlikely to respond to another agent.
[b]Dosages are for edema.
[c]There is no therapeutic advantage in giving the drug parenterally.
[d]Not a thiazide, but similar in structure and mechanism of action.
[e]Thalitone and Mykrox are more bioavailable than other formulations of the respective drugs.

| **MANNITOL** | Osmitrol, Various |

Pharmacology. Mannitol and other osmotic diuretics do not act on specific receptors but rather on tubular fluid composition after filtration at the glomerulus. Mannitol inhibits sodium and chloride reabsorption in the proximal tubule and ascending loop of Henle predominantly. Excretion of sodium, potassium, calcium, and phosphate is increased. Renal blood flow is increased, the GFR of superficial nephrons is increased, and that of deep nephrons is decreased.[23] Mannitol increases serum osmolality by expanding intravascular volume and decreasing intraocular and intracranial pressures.[1,3,23]

Administration and Adult Dosage. *Never administer IM or SC or add to whole blood for transfusion.* **IV as diagnostic evaluation of acute oliguria** (if BP and CVP are normal and *after* cardiac output is maximized) give test dose of 12.5 g as a 15–20% solution over 3–5 min (often given with **furosemide** 80–120 mg IV), may repeat in 1 hr if urine output is <50 mL/hr. If no response after 2 doses, give no more mannitol and treat for acute tubular necrosis. If response occurs, look for underlying cause of oliguria (eg, hypovolemia). **IV for prevention of acute renal failure** give test dose as above to a total dose of ≥50 g in 1 hr as a loading dose, then maintain urine output at 50 mL/hr with continuous infusion of 5% solution, plus 20 mEq/L sodium chloride and 1 g/L calcium gluconate. **IV for reduction of intracranial or intraocular pressure** 1.5–2 g/kg over 30–60 min as a 15–20% solution. **IV to decrease nephrotoxicity of cisplatin** 12.5 g IV push just before cisplatin, then 10 g/hr for 6 hr as a 20% solution. Replace fluids with 0.45% sodium chloride with 20–30 mEq/L potassium chloride at 250 mL/hr for 6 hr. Maintain urine output >100 mL/hr with mannitol infusion.[24,25] (*See* Notes.)

Special Populations. *Pediatric Dosage.* **IV for oliguria or anuria** give test dose of 20 mg/kg as above; the therapeutic dose is 2 g/kg over 2–6 hr as a 15–20% solution. **IV for reduction of intracranial or intraocular pressure** 2 g/kg over 30–60 min as a 15–25% solution. **IV for intoxications** 2 g/kg as 5–10% solution as needed to maintain a high urinary output. (*See* Notes.)

Geriatric Dosage. Start with a low initial dose and titrate to response.

Dosage Forms. **Inj** 5, 10, 15, 20, 25%.

Pharmacokinetics. *Onset and Duration.* (Diuresis) onset 1–3 hr, duration depends on half-life. (Decrease in intraocular pressure) onset in 30–60 min, duration 4–6 hr. (Decrease in intracranial pressure) onset within 15 min, peak 60–90 min, duration 3–8 hr after stopping infusion.[26]

Serum Levels. The site of diuretic action is within the renal tubules and not the serum; therefore, serum concentrations do not reflect diuretic activity.

Fate. About 17% is absorbed orally. IV doses of 1 and 2 g/kg increase serum osmolality by 11 and 32 mOsm/kg, decrease serum sodium by 8.7 and 20.7 mEq/L, and decrease hemoglobin by 2.2 and 2.5 g/dL, respectively.[27] V_c is 0.074 L/kg; $V_{d\beta}$ is 0.23 L/kg; Cl is 0.086 L/hr/kg.[28] Mannitol is eliminated almost completely unchanged in urine.

$t_{1/2}$. α phase 0.11 ± 0.12 hr; β phase 2.2 ± 1.3 hr.[28]

Adverse Reactions. Most serious and frequent reactions are fluid and electrolyte imbalance, in particular symptoms of fluid overload (eg, pulmonary edema, hypertension, water intoxication, and CHF). Acute renal failure has been reported occasionally with high doses, especially in patients with renal impairment.[29,30] Dermal necrosis can occur if solution extravasates. Anaphylaxis has been reported rarely.

Contraindications. Patients with well-established anuria caused by severe renal disease or impaired renal function who do not respond to test dose; severe pulmonary congestion, frank pulmonary edema, or severe CHF; severe dehydration; edema not caused by renal, cardiac, or hepatic disease associated with abnormal capillary fragility or membrane permeability; active intracranial bleeding except during craniotomy.

Precautions. Pregnancy. Observe solution for crystals before administering. (*See* Notes.) Water intoxication can occur if fluid input exceeds urine output. Masking of inadequate hydration or hypovolemia can occur by drug-induced sustaining of diuresis. If extravasation occurs, aspirate any accessible extravasated solution, remove the IV catheter, and apply a cold compress to the area. Mannitol should not be added to whole blood for transfusion.

Drug Interactions. None known.

Parameters to Monitor. Monitor urine output closely and discontinue drug if output is low. Monitor serum electrolytes closely, taking care not to misinterpret low serum sodium as a sign of hypotonicity. (*See* Fate.) If serum sodium is low, measure serum osmolality. Observe for clinical signs of fluid or electrolyte depletion such as dry mouth, thirst, weakness, lethargy, muscle pains or cramps, hypotension, oliguria, tachycardia, and GI upset.

Notes. Mannitol can crystallize out of solution at concentrations >15%. The crystals can be redissolved by warming containers in hot water and shaking or by autoclaving; cool to body temperature before administration. Administer concentrated solutions through an inline filter. Addition of electrolytes to solutions of ≥20% concentration can cause precipitation.

SPIRONOLACTONE
Aldactone, Various

Pharmacology. Spironolactone is a steroidal competitive aldosterone antagonist that acts from the interstitial side of the distal and collecting tubular epithelium to block sodium–potassium exchange, producing a delayed and mild diuresis. The diuretic effect is maximal in states of hyperaldosteronism. Excretion of sodium and chloride excretion is increased; excretion of potassium and magnesium is decreased.[31–33] Spironolactone has mild antihypertensive activity and has demonstrated a beneficial effect in class III and IV CHF.[34]

Administration and Adult Dosage. **PO for edema** 25–200 mg/day (usually 100 mg) in 2–4 divided doses initially, adjusting dosage after 5 days. If response is inadequate, add a thiazide or loop diuretic to the regimen. **PO for essential hypertension** 50–100 mg/day initially, adjusting dosage after 2 weeks. **PO for ascites** 100 mg/day initially, increasing to 200–400 mg/day in 2–4 divided doses. Restrict sodium to ≤2 g/day and, if necessary, fluid to 1 L/day. To eliminate delay in onset, a loading dose of 2–3 times the daily dosage may be given on the first day of therapy.[35] **PO for Class III or IV CHF** 12.5–25 mg/day.

Special Populations. *Pediatric Dosage.* **PO** (neonates) 1–3 mg/kg/day q 12–24 hr; (older children) 1.5–3.3 mg/kg/day in divided doses q 6–24 hr.[36]

Geriatric Dosage. Start with a low initial dose and titrate to response.

Dosage Forms. **Tab** 25, 50, 100 mg; **Tab** 25 mg with hydrochlorothiazide 25 mg (Aldactazide, various); **Tab** 50 mg with hydrochlorothiazide 50 mg (Aldactazide 50/50).

Patient Instructions. (*See* Class Instructions: Diuretics.) Avoid excessive amounts of high-potassium foods or salt substitutes.

Pharmacokinetics. *Onset and Duration.* Onset 1–2 days, peak 2–3 days with continued administration; onset can be hastened by giving loading dose; duration 2–3 days after cessation of therapy.

Serum Levels. Not established and not used clinically.

Fate. Bioavailability is about 90%;[31] food promotes absorption and possibly decreases first-pass effect.[37] Spironolactone undergoes rapid and extensive metabolism to canrenone (active metabolite), 7α-thiomethylspironolactone (major metabolite), and other sulfur-containing metabolites; together with the parent drug, these metabolites contribute to the overall antimineralocorticoid activity.[31,38] Metabolites are eliminated primarily renally, with minimal biliary excretion. Little or no parent drug is excreted unchanged in urine.[37,38]

$t_{1/2}$. (Spironolactone) 1.4 ± 0.5 hr; (7α-thiomethylspironolactone) 13.8 ± 6.4 hr; (canrenone) 16.5 ± 6.3 hr.[38]

Adverse Reactions. Hyperkalemia can occur, most frequently in patients with renal function impairment (especially those with diabetes mellitus) and those receiving potassium supplements or concomitant ACE inhibitors. Dehydration and hyponatremia occur occasionally, especially when the drug is combined with other diuretics. In patients receiving high dosages, frequent estrogen-like side effects such as gynecomastia, decreased libido, and impotence in males occur; menstrual irregularities and breast tenderness occur in females. These effects are reversible after drug discontinuation.[39,40]

Contraindications. Anuria; acute renal insufficiency; rapidly deteriorating renal function; severe renal failure; serum potassium >5.5 mEq/L or development of hyperkalemia while taking the drug; hypermagnesemia.

Precautions. Pregnancy. Patients with renal impairment, especially those with diabetes mellitus and/or receiving an ACE inhibitor, are at risk for developing hyperkalemia. Use with caution in patients with hepatic disease. Do not use with triamterene or amiloride. Give potassium supplements only to patients with demonstrated hypokalemia who are taking a proximally acting diuretic and a corticosteroid concurrently with spironolactone or only for very short periods in treating cirrhosis and ascites.

Drug Interactions. Use with ACE inhibitors increases risk of hyperkalemia, especially in renal impairment. Spironolactone increases serum concentration of digoxin by reducing renal clearance. In addition, spironolactone and its metabolites cross-react with digoxin-binding antibody in some digoxin immunoassays.

Parameters to Monitor. Monitor serum electrolytes, in particular potassium, periodically, especially early in the course of therapy. Monitor BUN and/or Cr_s periodically. In ascites, also obtain daily weight and urinary electrolytes and maintain weight loss at no greater than 0.5–1 kg/day and urinary Na^+/K^+ ratio at >1. Observe for clinical signs of fluid or electrolyte depletion such as dry mouth, thirst, weakness, lethargy, muscle pains or cramps, hypotension, oliguria, tachycardia, and GI upset.

Notes. Spironolactone is used in the diagnosis of primary aldosteronism and may be useful in the management of the condition in patients unable to undergo surgery.

TORSEMIDE   Demadex

Pharmacology. Torsemide is a loop diuretic similar to furosemide. Over the normal dosage range, its diuretic potency by weight is about 2–4 times that of furosemide. Onset of diuresis is similar but duration is longer (up to 8–12 hr orally).[41–43]

Adult Dosage. **PO for hypertension** 5–10 mg/day orally. **Initial PO or IV for edema or chronic renal failure** 20 mg/day; dosage may be doubled until the desired response is obtained, to a usual maximum of 200 mg/day; or, IV by continuous infusion, give 20 mg loading dose, then 10–20 mg/hr. **PO or IV for cirrhosis** 5–10 mg/day initially with a potassium-sparing diuretic, to a usual maximum of 40 mg/day. (*See* Furosemide Notes and Loop Diuretics Comparison Chart.)

Dosage Forms. **Tab** 5, 10, 20, 100 mg; **Inj** 10 mg/mL.

Pharmacokinetics. Oral bioavailability is 79–91% (median 80); V_d is 0.14–0.19 L/kg. In healthy individuals, the elimination half-life of torsemide is dose dependent, ranging from 2.2 to 3.8 hr. Nonrenal Cl remains essentially constant over a dosage range of 5–20 mg, but renal Cl and fraction excreted decrease, suggesting saturable renal clearance. Further studies are needed to clarify whether torsemide undergoes dose-dependent renal elimination. Renal impairment (Cl_{cr} <60 mL/min) does not appreciably alter pharmacokinetic parameters; hemodialysis and hemofiltration do not markedly influence serum clearance.

Adverse Reactions. Although the potential for hypokalemia exists, torsemide's kaliuretic potency is less than that of furosemide, suggesting that it is less potassium wasting during long-term therapy; the clinical relevance of this observation is unknown. Precautions and monitoring parameters are the same as those for furosemide.

TRIAMTERENE   Dyrenium

Pharmacology. Triamterene acts directly from the distal tubular lumen on active sodium exchange for potassium and hydrogen, producing a mild diuresis that is independent of aldosterone concentration. Excretion of sodium, chloride, calcium, and possibly bicarbonate excretion is increased; excretion of potassium and possibly magnesium excretion is decreased. Antihypertensive activity is inconsistent and less pronounced than with thiazides or spironolactone.[32,33]

Administration and Adult Dosage. **PO** initially 100 mg bid after meals if used alone, lower dosage if used with another diuretic. Adjust the maintenance dosage to the needs of the patient, which can range from 100 mg/day to 100 mg every other day, to a maximum of 300 mg/day.

Special Populations. *Pediatric Dosage.* **PO** 2–4 mg/kg/day initially, may increase to 6 mg/kg/day in 1–2 doses after meals, to a maximum of 300 mg/day. Decrease dosage if used with another diuretic.

Geriatric Dosage. Start with a low initial dose and titrate to response.

Dosage Forms. **Cap** 50, 100 mg; **Cap** 50 mg with hydrochlorothiazide 25 mg (Dyazide, various); **Tab** 75 mg with hydrochlorothiazide 50 mg (Maxzide, various); 37.5 mg with hydrochlorothiazide 25 mg (Maxzide-25, various).

Patient Instructions. (*See* Class Instructions: Diuretics.) This drug may be taken with food or milk to minimize stomach upset. Report persistent loss of appetite, nausea, or vomiting. Avoid eating excessive amounts of high-potassium foods or salt substitutes.

Pharmacokinetics. *Onset and Duration.* Onset 2–4 hr; full therapeutic effect might not occur for several days; duration 7–9 hr.

Serum Levels. The site of diuretic action is within the renal tubules and not the serum; therefore, serum concentrations do not reflect diuretic activity.

Fate. Variable absorption, depending on formulation,[44,45] bioavailability is $52 \pm 22\%$.[45] When the total urinary excretion of triamterene and its pharmacologically active metabolite are considered, the bioavailability value of triamterene reaches $83.2 \pm 25.9\%$.[45] Triamterene undergoes marked first-pass metabolism with rapid hydroxylation followed by immediate conjugation to the sulfate ester, which is the predominant form in plasma and urine.[45] The sulfate conjugate is nearly equipotent with the parent in causing sodium excretion and sparing of potassium.[46,47] Triamterene is 50–55% plasma protein bound,[34,35] and its sulfate conjugate is 91% protein bound.[45] After oral administration, serum concentrations of triamterene and its sulfate conjugate undergo a rapid decline over the first 6–8 hr after administration, followed by a slower terminal phase.[46] Both are eliminated renally by filtration and secretion. The fraction of a dose excreted as the parent is $3 \pm 2\%$; that for the sulfate conjugate is $34 \pm 8\%$.[46] The sulfate conjugate can accumulate in renal impairment.[47]

$t_{1/2}$. β phase (healthy adults) 4.3 ± 0.7 hr for triamterene and 3.1 ± 1.2 hr for sulfate;[45] up to 12 hr in cirrhosis.[48] Half-lives might be prolonged in the elderly.[49]

Adverse Reactions. Nausea, vomiting, diarrhea, and dizziness occur occasionally. Dehydration and hyponatremia with an increase in BUN occur occasionally, especially when the drug is combined with other diuretics. Triamterene renal stones occur occasionally. Hyperkalemia occurs occasionally, especially in diabetics and those with renal impairment; metabolic acidosis has been reported. Megaloblastic anemia can occur in alcoholic cirrhosis.

Contraindications. Severe or progressive renal disease or dysfunction (except possibly nephrosis); severe renal failure; severe hepatic disease; serum potassium >5.5 mEq/L or development of hyperkalemia while taking the drug; hypermagnesemia.

Precautions. Pregnancy. Patients with renal impairment, especially those with diabetes mellitus and/or receiving an ACE inhibitor, are at risk for developing hyperkalemia. Can elevate serum uric acid in patients predisposed to gout. Do not use with spironolactone or amiloride.

Drug Interactions. Use with ACE inhibitors increases risk of hyperkalemia, especially in renal impairment. Indomethacin (and probably other NSAIDs) can reduce renal function when combined with triamterene.

Parameters to Monitor. Monitor serum electrolytes, in particular potassium, periodically, especially early in the course of therapy. Monitor BUN and/or Cr_s periodically. Observe for clinical signs of fluid or electrolyte depletion such as dry mouth, thirst, weakness, lethargy, muscle pains or cramps, hypotension, oliguria, tachycardia, and GI upset.

DIURETICS OF CHOICE COMPARISON CHART[a]

CONDITION	LOOP DIURETICS	OSMOTIC DIURETICS	THIAZIDES	POTASSIUM-SPARING AGENTS	COMMENTS
Relative potency	>15%	10–15%	5–10%	<5%	Values refer to maximum fraction of filtered sodium excreted after maximally effective dose of drug.
Hypertension	A	—	A	D	Sustained antihypertensive effect of thiazides exhibits a flat dose-response curve and occurs at doses below the threshold for diuresis. Loop diuretics are diuretics of choice with Cl$_{cr}$ <30 mL/min.
Congestive heart failure	A	—	A	A (spironolactone)	Begin with thiazide with low dosage; if ineffective, substitute a loop diuretic. Loop diuretics are diuretics of choice with Cl$_{cr}$ <30 mL/min. Spironolactone reduces morbidity and mortality in NYHA Class III and IV CHF.
Pulmonary edema	A (IV)	—	—	—	Prompt venodilation precedes diuretic effect.
Hepatic ascites	B	—	—	A	Spironolactone is the agent of choice; urine Na:K ratio <1 indicates need for higher dosage (200–1000 mg/day). Rate of diuresis should not exceed 750 mL/day (no peripheral edema), or up to 2 L/day (if edema is present).
Renal failure	A	C	—	—	A loop diuretic plus a thiazide (in a high dose) can evoke a clinically useful diuresis even when Cl$_{cr}$ is <15 mL/min; however, provocative diuretic challenges in oliguric patients can be potentially hazardous, especially if the cause of renal failure is uncertain.

(continued)

DIURETICS OF CHOICE COMPARISON CHART[a] (*continued*)

CONDITION	LOOP DIURETICS	OSMOTIC DIURETICS	THIAZIDES	POTASSIUM-SPARING AGENTS	COMMENTS
Diabetes insipidus	—	—	A	—	Thiazides are most useful in the nephrogenic form; a long-acting agent is preferred. In pituitary form, oral diuretics may be a useful alternative for patients who prefer oral therapy to the use of intranasal or IV desmopressin.
Hypercalcemia	A	—	—	—	High-dose furosemide (IV 80–100 mg q 1–2 hr) with IV saline for forced diuresis to promote calcium excretion.
Hypercalciuria	—	—	A	—	Thiazides cause marked reduction in urinary calcium excretion; they also appear effective in preventing calcium stone formation irrespective of whether urinary calcium is abnormally elevated.

A = diuretic of choice; B = diuretic of second choice if patient is unresponsive to first choice; C = useful in some circumstances; D = useful as an adjunct to a more potent diuretic to reduce potassium loss and possibly enhance therapeutic effect.

[a]This table is a guide to the selection of the most appropriate diuretic for the condition listed but is not an all-inclusive guide to therapy.
From references 32, 33, and 50–52.

Electrolytes

Class Instructions. Oral Electrolytes. Take oral products with (tablets) or diluted in (liquids and powders) 6 to 8 fluid ounces of water or juice to avoid gastrointestinal injury or laxative effect. However, if you are undergoing hemodialysis, you may need to limit the volume of water you take. This medication may be taken with food or after meals if upset stomach occurs.

CALCIUM SALTS   Various

Pharmacology. Calcium plays an important role in neuromuscular activity, pancreatic insulin release, gastric hydrogen secretion, blood coagulation, and platelet aggregation; as a cofactor for some enzyme reactions; and in bone and tooth metabolism.[53]

Administration and Adult Dosage. PO as dietary supplement (elemental calcium) recommended intake is (19–50 yr, including pregnant and lactating women) 1000 mg/day; (≥50 yr) 1200 mg/day.[54,55] **PO to lower serum phosphate in endstage renal disease (ESRD)** (calcium carbonate) 650 mg with each meal initially, adjust dosage to decrease serum phosphate to <6 mg/dL;[56] (calcium acetate) 1334 mg with each meal initially, adjust dosage to decrease serum phosphate to < 6 mg/dL. (*See* Notes.) **IV for emergency elevation of serum calcium** (calcium gluconate) 15 mg/kg in NS or D5W infused over 8–10 hr (typically raises serum calcium by 2–3 mg/dL);[57] may repeat q 1–3 days depending on response; (calcium gluceptate) 1.1–1.4 g infused at a rate not to exceed 36 mg/min of elemental calcium. **IV for hypocalcemic tetany** 10–20 mL calcium gluconate infused over 10 min, may repeat until tetany is controlled. *Faster IV infusion rates can result in cardiac dysfunction.*[58]

Special Populations. *Pediatric Dosage.* **PO as dietary supplement** (elemental calcium) adequate intake is (0–6 months) 210 mg/day; (7–12 months) 270 mg/day; (1–3 yr) 500 mg/day; (4–8 yr) 800 mg/day; (9–18 yr) 1300 mg/day.[54] **PO for hypocalcemia** (elemental calcium) (neonates) 50–150 mg/kg/day in 4–6 divided doses, to a maximum of 1 g/day; (children) 20–65 mg/kg/day in 4 divided doses. **IV for emergency elevation of serum calcium** (infants) <1 mEq, may repeat q 1–3 days depending on response; (children) 1–7 mEq, may repeat q 1–3 days depending on response. **IV for hypocalcemic tetany** (infants) 2.4 mEq/day in divided doses; (children) 0.5–0.7 mEq/kg tid–qid, or more until tetany controlled.

Geriatric Dosage. Postmenopausal women have a requirement of 1200 mg/day, including those on estrogen replacement or a bisphosphonate.[55] Lower dosage might be required in some patients because of the age-related decrease in renal function; conversely, requirements might increase with advanced renal insufficiency.

Other Conditions. Adolescence, renal impairment, and pregnancy might increase requirements; base maintenance dosage on serum calcium, serum phosphate, and diet.[53,54]

Dosage Forms. (*See* Oral Calcium Products Comparison Chart.) **Inj** (chloride) 1 g/10 mL (contains 273 mg or 13.6 mEq Ca); (gluconate) 1 g/10 mL (contains 93 mg or 4.65 mEq Ca); (gluceptate) 1.1 g/5 mL (contains 90 mg or 4.5 mEq Ca).

Patient Instructions. (*See* Class Instructions: Oral Electrolytes.) Do not take within 2 hours of taking oral tetracycline or fluoroquinolone products. Take calcium tablets with food to maximize absorption. If used as a phosphate binder, calcium must be taken with food. Allow effervescent tablets to degas in a glass of water (about 4 minutes) before taking.

Missed Doses. Take this drug at regular intervals. If you miss a dose, take it as soon as you remember and then return to your normal dosage schedule.

Pharmacokinetics. *Serum Levels.* Normal serum total calcium is 8.4–10.2 mg/dL (2.1–2.6 mmol/L) for an adult with a serum albumin of 4 g/dL. Because a lesser fraction of calcium is protein bound in hypoalbuminemia, the patient's value must be corrected based on serum albumin:

Corrected Serum Calcium = Serum Calcium in mg/dL + (0.8 × [4 – Serum Albumin in g/dL]).

Fate. Oral calcium absorption is about 30% and depends on vitamin D and parathyroid hormone. Absorption decreases with age, high intake, achlorhydria, and estrogen loss at menopause;[54] absorption increases when taken with food[55,58] or in divided doses.[59] Bioavailability from various salt forms does not appear to differ substantially in normals;[60] however, differences in disintegration and dissolution among commercial formulations exist.[56,58] About 99% of total body calcium is found in bone and teeth; of the 1% in extracellular fluid, 40–45% is plasma protein bound (mostly to albumin); 8–10% is complexed to citrate, phosphate, and other anions; and 45–50% is diffusible and physiologically active. About 135–155 mg/day are secreted into the GI tract, with 85% reabsorbed. Fecal loss of unabsorbed dietary calcium and endogenous excretion is 100–130 mg/day, urine loss is 150 mg/day, and sweat loss is 15 mg/day.[59]

Adverse Reactions. IV calcium solutions, especially calcium chloride, are extremely irritating to the veins.[57] Constipation or flatulence occurs frequently, especially with high dosages; the frequency probably does not differ markedly among salt forms.[55] Calcium overload caused by oral calcium supplements is rare; immobilization, dosages in excess of 3–4 g/day, vitamin D therapy, and renal impairment can contribute to hypercalcemia, hypercalciuria, or nephrolithiasis during oral supplementation. Symptoms of calcium intolerance include nausea, intestinal bloating, excess gas, vomiting, constipation, abdominal pain, dry mouth, and polyuria.

Contraindications. Hypercalcemia; sarcoidosis; severe cardiac disease; digitalis glycoside therapy; calcium nephrolithiasis; calcium-phosphate product >60–70 in the setting of uremia is associated with calcification in extraosseous tissues and should be avoided. To determine calcium–phosphate product, multiply the serum phosphate value (in mg/dL) by the serum calcium value (in mg/dL).

Precautions. Avoid extravasation of parenteral calcium products. If extravasation occurs, aspirate any accessible extravasated solution, remove IV catheter, and apply a cold compress to the area.

Drug Interactions. Concomitant thiazide diuretic therapy and sodium depletion or metabolic acidosis can increase tubular reabsorption of calcium. Calcium reduces oral absorption of fluoroquinolones, tetracyclines, and iron salts. Concomitant use with sodium polystyrene sulfonate can lead to metabolic alkalosis and compromised activity of the binding resin.

Parameters to Monitor. Serum calcium regularly, with frequency determined by patient's condition; BUN and/or Cr_s, serum phosphate, magnesium, and serum albumin (especially if low) periodically.

Notes. Calcium supplementation also can be achieved by dietary measures: skim milk provides 300 mg calcium/8 fluid ounces, 300 mg/8 fluid ounces of low-fat yogurt, 272 mg/ounce of Swiss cheese, and 200 mg/6 fluid ounces of calcium-fortified orange juice.[55] Calcium carbonate is inexpensive and a good first-line agent. However, dissolution of calcium from phosphate and carbonate salts is pH dependent. These salts might not be optimal calcium sources for patients with elevated GI pH, such as the elderly or those with achlorhydria. Calcium carbonate as a chewable tablet or nougat or the use of an alternative calcium salt have been recommended.[58] In ESRD, use calcium salts when serum phosphate is <8 mg/dL; when serum phosphate is >8 mg/dL, use aluminum hydroxide. Calcium acetate binds about twice the amount of phosphorus for the same quantity of calcium absorbed;[56] however, the frequency of hypercalcemia does not seem to be diminished. (*See* Oral Calcium Products Comparison Chart.)

ORAL CALCIUM PRODUCTS COMPARISON CHART

PRODUCT	PERCENTAGE CALCIUM	ELEMENTAL CALCIUM CONTENT
Calcium Acetate	25	667 mg Tab = 169 mg
Calphron		667 mg Tab = 169 mg
PhosLo		
Calcium Carbonate	40	5 mL Susp = 500 mg
Calciday-667		650 mg Tab = 260 mg
Cal-Sup		667 mg Tab = 267 mg
Caltrate 600		750 mg Tab = 300 mg
Os-Cal		1250 mg Tab = 500 mg
Titralac		1500 mg Tab = 600 mg
Tums		
Calcium Citrate	21.1	950 mg Tab = 200 mg
Citracal Tablets		2376 mg Tab = 500 mg
Citracal Liquitabs		
Calcium Glubionate	6.5	5 mL Syrup = 115 mg
Neo-Calglucon		
Calcium Gluconate	9.3	500 mg Tab = 45 mg
Various		650 mg Tab = 58.5 mg
		975 mg Tab = 87.8 mg
		1000 mg Tab = 90 mg
Calcium Lactate	13	325 mg Tab = 42.3 mg
Various		650 mg Tab = 84.5 mg
Calcium Phosphate, Tribasic	39	1565 mg Tab = 600 mg
Posture		
Dairy Products	—	Cheese 28 g = 300–400 mg
		Skim milk 250 mL = 300 mg
		Yogurt 28 g = 43 mg

From references 54–57 and product information.

MAGNESIUM SALTS   Various

Pharmacology. Magnesium is the second most abundant intracellular cation, with an essential role in neuromuscular function and protein and carbohydrate enzymatic systems; it functions as a cofactor for enzymes involved in transfer, storage, and utilization of intracellular energy. Magnesium also is an integral component of bone matrix.[61]

Administration and Adult Dosage. PO as dietary supplement (elemental magnesium) RDA is (≥11 yr) 410–420 mg/day for males and 320–360 mg/day for nonpregnant, nonlactating women.[54] **PO for symptomatic chronic deficiency** (elemental magnesium) 12–24 mg/kg in divided doses.[62] A renal threshold for magnesium excretion exists, so replacement is best accomplished slowly, usually over 5 days. **IV for prevention of negative balance** (elemental magnesium) 100–200 mg/day in parenteral nutrition solution.[62] **IM for mild deficiency** 1 g MgSO4 q 4–6 hr until serum magnesium is normalized or signs and symptoms abate.[62] **IM for severe hypomagnesemia** 2 g MgSO$_4$ as a 50% solution q 8 hr until serum magnesium is normalized or signs and symptoms abate; because IM injections are painful, continuous IV infusions might be preferred.[63] **IV infusion for severe hypomagnesemia** 48 mEq/day (6 g MgSO$_4$) for 3–7 days by continuous infusion.[63] **IV for life-threatening hypomagnesemia (acute arrhythmias and seizures)** 8–16 mEq (1–2 g MgSO$_4$) over 5–10 min, followed by continuous infusion of 48 mEq magnesium/day.[63] **IV for pre-eclampsia or eclampsia** 4–6 g MgSO$_4$, then 1–2 g/hr by continuous infusion to maintain target serum level. (*See* Notes.)

Special Populations. *Pediatric Dosage.* **IV for hypomagnesemia** 25 mg/kg MgSO$_4$ as a 25% solution over 3–5 min q 6 hr for 3–4 doses. **IM for seizures** 20–40 mg/kg MgSO$_4$ as a 20% solution as needed. **IV for severe seizures** 100–200 mg/kg MgSO$_4$ as a 1–3% solution infused slowly with close monitoring of blood pressure. Administer one-half the dose during the initial 15–20 min and the total dose within 1 hr.

Geriatric Dosage. Lower dosage might be required in some patients because of the age-related decrease in renal function.

Other Conditions. Base maintenance dosage on serum magnesium and diet. Renal impairment decreases requirement. In severe renal failure, reduce dosage by at least 50% of the recommended amount and monitor serum magnesium after each dose.[64] Concomitant administration of potassium and calcium may be necessary because many causes of hypomagnesemia also lead to hypocalcemia and hypokalemia.[62]

Dosage Forms. (*See* Magnesium Products Comparison Chart.)

Patient Instructions. (*See* Oral Electrolytes Class Instructions.)

Missed Doses. Take this drug at regular intervals. If you miss a dose, take it as soon as you remember. Do not double the dose or take extra.

Pharmacokinetics. *Onset and Duration.* Peak levels are achieved immediately after IV, 1 hr after IM. Duration (anticonvulsant) is 30 min with IV, 3–4 hr post-onset with IM.

Serum Levels. (Normal) 1.3–2.1 mEq/L (0.65–1.1 mmol/L); (pre-eclampsia or eclampsia) 4–6 mEq/L (2–3 mmol/L).[61] Intracellular and extracellular concentrations can vary independently; hence, serum magnesium levels might not be indicative of total body stores.

Fate. Oral absorption varies inversely with intake; in general, 24–76% is absorbed,[65] principally in upper small intestine. Total body content is about 24 g,[61] 60% of which is in bone, 39% in tissues, and 1% in extracellular fluid; 30% is plasma protein bound. Elimination is primarily by the kidneys, with only 1–2% in feces. Raising the serum concentration above normal exceeds the maximum tubular reabsorption capacity with subsequent excretion of excess.

Adverse Reactions. Serum concentration related: (3–5 mEq/L; 1.5–2.5 mmol/L) hypotension; (5–10 mEq/L; 2.5–5 mmol/L) PR interval changes, QRS prolongation, peaked T waves; (10 mEq/L; 5 mmol/L) areflexia; (15 mEq/L; 7.5 mmol/L) respiratory paralysis; (25 mEq/L; 12.5 mmol/L) cardiac arrest.[65] Pain on IM injection occurs very frequently.[64]

Contraindications. Hypermagnesemia; heart block; myocardial damage; severe renal failure.

Precautions. Use with caution in patients with renal impairment (Cl_{cr} <30 mL/min) and those concurrently taking a digitalis glycoside. With bolus $MgSO_4$ administration, 1 g of 10% calcium gluconate IV should be available in case apnea or heart block occurs.[65]

Drug Interactions. IV magnesium can potentiate neuromuscular blocking agents.

Parameters to Monitor. Serum magnesium regularly, frequency determined by condition of patient; BUN and/or Cr_s, serum potassium, and calcium periodically. Deep tendon reflexes, respiratory rate, BP, and ECG periodically.

Notes. For mild deficiencies, dietary supplementation may be sufficient to normalize magnesium stores; sources are cereals, nuts, green vegetables, meat, and fish.[65] Magnesium gluconate is preferred for oral replacement and supplementation because it is possibly better absorbed and potentially causes less diarrhea.[62] Patients on long-term diuretic therapy who are prone to hypomagnesemia may benefit from using the minimally effective dose of diuretic and 20–30 mEq/day of magnesium orally or changing to a magnesium-sparing agent (ie, amiloride, spironolactone, or triamterene).[66] Drugs known to produce hypomagnesemia are aminoglycoside antibiotics, amphotericin B, diuretics, alcohol, and cisplatin.[63,66] Coadministration of 3 g $MgSO_4$ IV with high-dose **cisplatin** chemotherapy has been recommended.[66] The role of IV magnesium for acute MI remains unresolved.[67] Correction of refractory hypocalcemia and hypokalemia with concurrent hypomagnesemia requires magnesium replacement to restore mineral balance.[62] To avoid precipitation when $MgSO_4$ and calcium chloride are added to parenteral nutrition mixtures, use of calcium gluceptate has been recommended because it reacts more slowly than calcium chloride and a precipitate does not form.[68] (*See* Magnesium Products Comparison Chart.)

MAGNESIUM PRODUCTS COMPARISON CHART

PRODUCT	MAGNESIUM CONTENT[a] (MEQ/G)	DOSAGE FORMS[b]	COMMENTS
Magnesium, Chelated Chelated magnesium	8.3	Tab 500 mg = 100 mg Mg.	Amino acid chelate; sodium free; oral use only.
Magnesium Chloride Slo-Mag Various	9.8	SR Tab 535 mg = 64 mg Mg Inj 200 mg/mL = 23.6 mg/mL Mg.	Alternative to parenteral $MgSO_4$.
Magnesium Citrate Various	4.4	Soln 60 mg/mL = 3.2 mg/mL Mg.	Oral use only.
Magnesium Gluconate Almora Magatrate Magonate	4.5–4.8	Tab 500 mg = 27–29 mg Mg Soln 11 mg/mL = 0.63 mg/mL Mg.	Very soluble; well absorbed; produces no diarrhea.
Magnesium Hydroxide Milk of Magnesia	34	Susp 40 mg/mL = 16.3 mg/mL Mg Susp 80 mg/mL = 32.6 mg/mL Mg Tab 300 mg = 122 mg Mg Tab 600 mg = 244 mg Mg.	Readily available in combination antacid formulations. Start with 5 mL Susp or 1 Tab, increase as tolerated to qid. Requires gastric acid for absorption. Inexpensive.

(continued)

MAGNESIUM PRODUCTS COMPARISON CHART (*continued*)

PRODUCT	MAGNESIUM CONTENT[a] (MEQ/G)	DOSAGE FORMS[b]	COMMENTS
Magnesium Oxide	49.6	Cap 140 mg = 84 mg Mg. Tab 400 mg = 238 mg Mg.	Poorly soluble; net absorption low, especially in malabsorptive states.
Magnesium Sulfate Epsom salt	8.1	Inj 10% = 9.6 mg/mL Mg. Inj 12.5% = 12 mg/mL Mg. Inj 50% = 48 mg/mL Mg. Pwdr 1 g = 97.2 mg Mg.	Use IV, IM, or PO.

[a] 1 mEq = 12 mg = 0.5 mmol Mg.
[b] Magnesium products exhibit variable oral absorption; increase dosage incrementally until no further rise in serum magnesium occurs or until diarrhea occurs.

PHOSPHATE SALTS   Various

Pharmacology. Phosphate is a structural element of bone and is involved in carbohydrate metabolism, energy transfer, and muscle contraction, and as a buffer in the renal excretion of hydrogen ion.[56] Many of the factors that influence serum calcium concentration also influence serum phosphate directly or indirectly.

Administration and Adult Dosage. The RDA is 700 mg/day.[54] **PO for phosphate replacement** 250–500 mg (8–16 mmol) of phosphorus tid–qid; **IV replacement (recent and uncomplicated hypophosphatemia)** 0.08 mmol/kg, to a maximum of 0.2 mmol/kg; (prolonged and multiple causes) 0.16 mmol/kg, to a maximum of 0.24 mmol/kg. Infuse doses over 6 hr and additional dosage guided by serum concentrations.[69] **IV for symptomatic hypophosphatemia** patients with phosphorus levels of 1.6–1.9 mg/dL have received 15 mmol over 2 hr[70] and those with phosphorus <1.24 mg/dL have received 30 mmol over 3 hr[71] with success (both without regard to weight). Reassess at completion of infusion to determine need for additional therapy. When serum concentration reaches 2 mg/dL (0.67 mmol/L) and the patient can eat a normal diet, change to oral administration and a phosphate-rich diet.[72,73] (*See* Phosphate Products Comparison Chart)

Special Populations. *Pediatric Dosage.* The RDAs are (0–6 months) 100 mg/day; (7–12 months) 275 mg/day; (1–8 yr) 460–500 mg/day; (9–18 yr) 1250 mg/day.[54] **PO for replacement** (<4 yr) 250 mg (8 mmol) of phosphorus qid initially; (<4 yr) same as adult dosage. **IV replacement** (serum phosphate 0.5–1 mg/dL) 0.05–0.08 mg/kg (0.15–0.25 mmol/kg) per dose over 4–6 hr; (serum phosphate <0.5 mg/dL) 0.08–0.12 mg/kg (0.25–0.35 mmol/kg) per dose over 6 hr.[60] Repeat doses as needed to achieve desired serum concentration. Actual dosage depends on signs, symptoms, and serum phosphate concentration.

Geriatric Dosage. Lower dosage might be required in some patients because of the age-related decrease in renal function.

Other Conditions. Renal impairment decreases requirement. Choose the appropriate salt form based on the patient's sodium and potassium requirements. Requirement is increased during alcohol withdrawal, diabetic ketoacidosis, respiratory alkalosis, aluminum antacid therapy, burns, postsurgical status, and nutritional repletion.

Dosage Forms. (*See* Phosphate Products Comparison Chart.)

Patient Instructions. (*See* Class Instructions: Oral Electrolytes.) Do not take capsules whole; instead, dissolve contents in 3/4 glass of water before taking. Powder in packets must be dissolved in 1 gallon of water before using. Chilling solution may improve palatability. Do not take with calcium-containing products.

Missed Doses. Take this drug at regular intervals. If you miss a dose, take it as soon as you remember. Do not double the dose or take extra.

Pharmacokinetics. *Serum Levels.* (As phosphorus) adults 2.7–4.5 mg/dL (0.9–1.5 mmol/L); children 4.5–5.5 mg/dL (1.5–1.8 mmol/L). Normal serum phosphorus concentrations can differ by as much as 0.6 mg/dL throughout the day because of changes in transcellular distribution. Concentrations <1.5 mg/dL indicate severe hypophosphatemia and require replacement therapy.[74]

Fate. Normal adult dietary intake is 1–1.8 g/day, 60–70% of which is absorbed, primarily in the duodenum and jejunum.[56] Most of the absorbed phosphorus is excreted in urine.[69]

Adverse Reactions. Diarrhea and stomach upset occur frequently with oral administration.[69,75] Dose-related hyperphosphatemia, metastatic calcium deposition, dehydration, hypotension, hypomagnesemia, and hyperkalemia or hypernatremia (depending on salt used) can occur.

Contraindications. Hyperphosphatemia; hypocalcemia; hyperkalemia (potassium salt); hypernatremia (sodium salt); severe renal failure.

Precautions. Use cautiously in patients with renal impairment and those with hypercalcemia. Dilute IV forms before use and administer slowly.

Drug Interactions. None known.

Parameters to Monitor. Serum phosphorus regularly, frequency determined by condition of patient; BUN and/or Cr_s, serum calcium, and magnesium periodically.[76] Monitor serum sodium and/or potassium periodically, depending on salt form used.

Notes. Phosphate salts can precipitate in the presence of calcium salts in IV solutions; add no more than 40 mmol of phosphate and 5 mEq of calcium per liter. Calcium supplementation may be necessary to prevent hypocalcemic tetany during phosphate repletion. IV calcium gluconate or calcium chloride may be given until tetany subsides. Inorganic phosphorus exists in the body as mono- and dibasic forms, the relative proportions of which are pH dependent. It is therefore preferable to report concentrations as mg/dL or mmol/L rather than mEq/L.[69] (*See* Phosphate Products Comparison Chart.)

PHOSPHATE PRODUCTS COMPARISON CHART

PRODUCT	DOSAGE FORMS[a]	PHOSPHORUS CONTENT[b]		CATION CONTENT
		mg	mmol	
POTASSIUM SALTS				
K-Phos Original	Tab.	114	3.6	3.7 mEq K$^+$/tablet.
Neutra-Phos K	Pwdr Packet.	250 (per packet)	8	14.3 mEq K$^+$/packet.
Potassium Phosphate	Inj.	94 (per mL)	3	4.4 mEq K$^+$/mL.
SODIUM SALTS				
Fleet's Phospho-Soda	Soln.	128 (per mL)	4.1	111 mg (4.8 mEq) Na$^+$/mL.
Sodium Phosphate	Inj.	94 (per mL)	3	93 mg (4 mEq) Na$^+$/mL.
SODIUM-POTASSIUM SALTS				
K-Phos Neutral	Tab.	250 (per tablet)	8	298 mg (13 mEq) Na$^+$ and 1.1 mEq K$^+$/tablet.
Neutra-Phos Plain	Pwdr Packet.	250 (per packet)	8	164 mg (7 mEq) Na$^+$ and 7 mEq K$^+$/packet.
Skim Milk	Liquid.	931 (per quart)	30	510 mg (22 mEq) Na$^+$ and 37 mEq K$^+$/quart.

[a]Contents of capsules, tablets, and powders must be diluted in water before administration.
[b]31.25 mg = 1 mmol.
From references 69, 72, and 73 and product information.

744

POTASSIUM SALTS   Various

Pharmacology. Potassium is the major cation of the intracellular space, where its major role is regulating muscle and nerve excitability. Another role is controlling intracellular volume (similar to sodium's control of extracellular volume), protein synthesis, enzymatic reactions, and carbohydrate metabolism.[77] The chloride salt is preferred for most uses because concomitant chloride loss and metabolic alkalosis frequently accompany hypokalemia. Nonchloride salts are preferred in acidosis (eg, secondary to amphotericin B or carbonic anhydrase inhibitor therapy and in chronic diarrhea with bicarbonate loss).[78,79]

Administration and Adult Dosage. Variable, must be adjusted to needs of patient. **PO for prophylaxis with diuretic therapy** prevention of hypokalemia can generally be accomplished by giving 20 mmol/day of KCl, whereas treatment requires as much as 40–100 mmol/day.[80] For nonedematous, ambulatory patients with uncomplicated hypertension, the goal should be to achieve a serum potassium of ≥4 mmol/L, and concentrations ≤3.4 mmol/L should be treated.[80] For edematous patients (eg, with CHF), consider routine supplementation with KCl even if the potassium is normal (eg, 4 mmol/L).[80] In those with mild potassium deficits, 40–80 mEq/day is recommended; with severe deficit, 100–120 mEq/day is indicated with careful monitoring of serum potassium.[81] **IV administration in peripheral vein** (serum potassium >2.5 mEq/L) may be infused at 10–20 mEq/hr;[79] reserve rates faster than 20 mEq/hr for emergency situations; may repeat q 2–3 hr as needed; do not exceed a maximum concentration of 40 mEq/L. **IV administration in central vein** (serum potassium <2.5 mEq/L) 30–60 mEq/hr may be administered[79]; do not exceed a maximum concentration of 80 mEq/L. Infusion into a central vein requires use of a volume control device. Potassium concentration should not exceed 60 mEq/L unless the infusion site is through a large vein distal to the heart (eg, femoral vein) or more than one IV line is available, in which case the potassium dose may be delivered through two different ports; however, more concentrated solutions (200 mEq/L) infused at slow rates (20 mEq/hr) have been used with relative safety.[82] (*See* Special Populations, Other Conditions.)

Special Populations. *Pediatric Dosage.* **PO** 1–2 mEq/kg/day during diuretic therapy.

Geriatric Dosage. Lower dosage might be required in some patients because of the age-related decrease in renal function.

Other Conditions. Base maintenance dosage on serum potassium; renal impairment decreases requirement. For patients with renal impairment or any form of heart block, decrease infusion rate by one-half and do not exceed 5–10 mEq/hr.[79]

Dosage Forms. **PO.** (*See* Potassium Products Comparison Chart.) **Inj** (potassium chloride) 2 mEq/mL; (potassium acetate) 2, 4 mEq/mL; (potassium phosphate) 4.4 mEq/mL of potassium and 3 mmol/mL of phosphate. (*See* Potassium Products Comparison Chart.)

Patient Instructions. (*See* Class Instructions: Oral Electrolytes.) Do not chew or crush tablets. The expanded wax matrix of sustained-release forms may be found in the stool, but this does not imply a lack of absorption.

Missed Doses. Take this drug at regular intervals. If you miss a dose, take it as soon as you remember and then return to your normal dosage schedule. Do not double the dose or take extra.

Pharmacokinetics. *Onset and Duration.* Peak elevation of serum potassium concentrations after SR preparations is slightly delayed (median of 2 hr) compared with the liquid form (median of 1 hr). Effect on serum potassium is most pronounced in the first 3 hr after administration.[83]

Serum Levels. Differs depending on laboratory. Normal serum levels are (newborn) 5–7.5 mEq/L, (child) 3.4–4.7 mEq/L, and (adult) 3.5–5.1 mEq/L. Total body stores are about 50 mEq/kg or 3500 mEq. As a general rule, a decrease of 1 mEq/L in serum potassium reflects a 10–20% total body deficit; however, there is considerable variation;[81] signs of hypokalemia appear <2.5 mEq/L; concentrations >7 mEq/L or <2.5 mEq/mL are dangerous. Clinical signs of hypokalemia or hyperkalemia are not reliable indicators of serum concentrations. Alkalosis decreases concentrations, and acidosis increases concentrations. Any hypokalemia-induced change in ECG must be treated as a medical emergency with IV potassium. Likewise, hyperkalemia-induced changes in ECG must be treated as a medical emergency.

Fate. When initially administered, the rates of absorption and excretion are more rapid with the liquid than with the SR forms; however, bioavailability is the same (78–90%) during long-term administration.[83,84] About 10 mEq/day is eliminated in feces, 60–90 mEq/day in urine, and 7.5 mEq/L in sweat.

Adverse Reactions. Bad taste, nausea, vomiting, diarrhea, and abdominal discomfort occur frequently with oral liquids. Do not use enteric-coated tablets because they can cause small-bowel and occasionally gastric ulceration.[81] Local tissue necrosis can occur if IV solution extravasates. Hyperkalemia can occur occasionally. Patients with diabetic nephropathy are at increased risk for hyperkalemia.[85]

Contraindications. Severe renal impairment; untreated Addison's disease; adynamia episodica hereditaria; acute dehydration; heat cramps; hyperkalemia; concurrent ACE inhibitor or potassium-sparing diuretic in patients with renal impairment.[81] In addition, all solid dosage forms (including SR products) are contraindicated in patients in whom delay or arrest of the tablet through the GI tract can occur.

Precautions. Use with caution (if at all) in patients receiving potassium-sparing diuretics or ACE inhibitors and those with digitalis-induced atrioventricular conduction disturbances or renal failure. Avoid extravasation of parenteral potassium products. If extravasation occurs, aspirate any accessible extravasated solution, remove IV catheter, and apply a cold compress to the area.

Drug Interactions. Use with an ACE inhibitor or potassium-sparing diuretic can result in hyperkalemia.

Parameters to Monitor. Serum potassium weekly to monthly initially, q 3–6 months when stable, BUN and/or Cr_s periodically. For supplementation in patients on long-term diuretic therapy, obtain pretreatment serum levels of potassium and magnesium and reassess after 2–3 weeks and then monthly to determine pattern of potassium loss. Once steady state or normokalemia is achieved, assess quarterly or as condition requires.[81]

Notes. Place the patient on a cardiac monitor before starting IV potassium.[79] A potassium-sparing diuretic may be preferable to potassium supplementation when large supplements are needed, aldosterone concentrations are elevated, enhanced diuretic response is desired, or magnesium loss is of concern. If large doses of potassium fail to correct hypokalemia, suspect hypomagnesemia because potassium balance is strongly dependent on magnesium homeostasis.[78,86] If a hypokalemic patient is also hypomagnesemic, as occurs with **amphotericin B** therapy, the patient might not respond to potassium replacement therapy unless magnesium balance is restored. (*See* Potassium Products Comparison Chart.)

POTASSIUM PRODUCTS COMPARISON CHART

PRODUCT	DOSAGE FORMS	COMMENTS
Potassium Acetate Various	Inj 2, 4 mEq/mL.	Useful in metabolic acidosis; avoid in metabolic alkalosis.
Potassium Acetate/ Bicarbonate/ Citrate Trikates Tri-K	Soln 3 mEq/mL.[a]	Preferred form in patients with delayed GI transit time or metabolic acidosis; avoid nonchloride salts in metabolic alkalosis.
Potassium Chloride K-Lyte/Cl Adolph's Morton No Salt NuSalt	Inj 2 mEq/mL Soln 20, 30, 40, 45 mEq/15 mL[a] Pwdr Packet 20, 25, 50 mEq[b] SR Cap/Tab 6.7, 8, 10, 20 mEq[b] Salt Substitutes 50–70 mEq/tsp.	Ideal for hypochloremic metabolic alkalosis.
Potassium Bicarbonate/ Citrate K-Lyte	Tab, Effervescent 25, 50 mEq.	Preferred form in patients with delayed GI transit time or metabolic acidosis; avoid nonchloride salts in metabolic alkalosis.
Potassium Gluconate Kaon	Soln 1.33 mEq/mL.[a]	Preferred form in patients with metabolic acidosis; avoid nonchloride salts in metabolic alkalosis.

[a]Liquids have rapid absorption, low frequency of GI ulceration, and unpleasant taste.
[b]Bioequivalent to liquid forms; avoid in patients with delayed GI transit time.
From references 78, 79, 81 and product information.

ORAL REHYDRATION SOLUTIONS   Various

Pharmacology. Oral rehydration solutions supply sodium, chloride, potassium, and water to prevent or replace mild to moderate fluid loss (5–10% dehydration) in diarrhea or postoperative states or when food and liquid intakes are temporarily discontinued. A carbohydrate (usually 2–2.5% glucose) is present to aid in sodium transport and subsequent water absorption.[87,89]

Administration and Adult Dosage. PO 1900–2850 mL (2–3 quarts)/day. Give only enough solution to supply the calculated water loss plus daily requirement.

Special Populations. *Pediatric Dosage.* Depends primarily on estimated fluid and electrolyte losses.[90] **PO for mild dehydration (3–5%)** 50 mL/kg of oral rehydration plus replacement of ongoing losses (10 mL/kg for each diarrheal stool and replace estimated emesis) over 4 hr.[90] Reassess patient q 2 hr. **PO for moderate dehydration (6–9%)** 100 mL/kg or oral rehydration fluid plus replacement of ongoing losses over 4 hr.[90] Reassess hydration status of patient hourly. **Severe dehydration (10% or greater)** IV replacement fluids are indicated.

Geriatric Dosage. Lower dosage might be required because of the age-related decrease in renal function.

Other Conditions. Adjust intake based on fluid status and serum electrolytes. When electrolyte-containing foods are restarted, adjust solution intake accordingly.

Dosage Forms. (*See* Oral Rehydration Solutions Comparison Chart.)

Patient Instructions. These products are not for fluid replacement in prolonged or severe diarrhea. Reconstitute powdered products in tap water; do not mix with milk or fruit juices. If additional fluids are desired, drink water or other nonelectrolyte-containing fluids to quench thirst.

Adverse Reactions. Hypernatremia, hyperkalemia, and acid–base disturbances can occur occasionally, especially in renal insufficiency or if errors occur in reconstituting bulk powders.

Contraindications. Intractable vomiting; adynamic ileus; intestinal obstruction; perforated bowel; shock; renal dysfunction (anuria, oliguria); monosaccharide malabsorption.[88]

Precautions. Use parenteral replacement to correct electrolyte imbalances caused by severe fluid loss (10–15% of body weight), inability to take oral fluids, severe gastric distention, or severe vomiting. Errors in reconstituting or diluting commercial powders can have severe consequences.

Drug Interactions. None known.

Parameters to Monitor. Serum sodium, potassium, chloride, and bicarbonate regularly, with frequency determined by condition of patient; BUN and/or Cr_s or urine-specific gravity periodically; input and output, weight, and signs and symptoms of dehydration daily.

Notes. To prevent dehydration early in the course of diarrhea or maintain hydration after parenteral replacement in adults and children, 90 mEq/L of sodium is acceptable. For infants who have higher insensible water losses, diluted solutions containing 50–60 mEq/L of sodium are suggested.[92] Alternatively, solutions of higher sodium concentration may be used in a ratio of 2:1 with additional free water.[87] Vomiting does not preclude use of oral replacement solutions; spooning small quantities into the mouth of the child who is experiencing some vomiting usually results in the administration of sufficient fluid to correct dehydration.[88] (*See* Oral Rehydration Solutions Comparison Chart.)

ORAL REHYDRATION SOLUTIONS COMPARISON CHART

| SOLUTION | DOSAGE FORMS | ELECTROLYTES (MEQ/L)[a] | | | | | CARBOHYDRATE |
		Na+	K+	Cl-	Base	Other	
Infalyte	Soln 1000 mL.	50	25	45	34 Citrate	—	Rice syrup solids 3%.
Pedialyte	Soln 237, 946 mL.	45	20	35	30 Citrate	—	Dextrose 2.5%.
Rehydralyte	Soln 237 mL.	75	20	65	30 Citrate	—	Dextrose 2.5%.
Resol	Soln 960 mL.	50	20	50	34 Citrate	4 Ca++ 4 Mg++ 5 HPO4	Glucose 2%.
WHO Oral Rehydration Salts[c]	Powder.[b]	90	20	80	30 Bicarbonate	—	Glucose 2%.

[a]Optimal solution (mEq/L): Na+ 75–100, K+ 20–30, Cl- 65–100, base 20–30, carbohydrate 1.5–2%.
[b]Reconstitute powder in tap water; do not mix with milk or fruit juices.
[c]WHO = World Health Organization; available from Jianas Brothers Packaging, 2533 SW Boulevard, Kansas City, MO; tel (816) 421–2880.
From references 89–92 and product information.

SEVELAMER HYDROCHLORIDE   Renagel

Pharmacology. Sevelamer is a polymer that binds phosphate in the GI tract. It is used in patients with end-stage renal disease to lower serum phosphate.

Adult Dosage. PO for hyperphosphatemia dosage is based on serum phosphate: for serum phosphate of (>6 and ≤7.5 mg/dL) 800–806 mg tid; (≥7.5 and <9 mg/dL) 1200-1209 mg tid; (≥9 mg/dL) 1600–1612 mg tid.

Pediatric Dosage. Safety and efficacy not established.

Dosage Forms. Cap 403 mg; **Tab** 400, 800 mg.

Patient Instructions. Take the dosage form whole with meals. Do not chew tablet or capsule or take capsule apart. Take any other medications one hour or more before or 3 hours after taking this medication.

Pharmacokinetics. Sevelamer is not absorbed from the GI tract. It is eliminated in the feces.

Adverse Reactions. Well tolerated. Occasional nausea, dyspepsia, diarrhea, flatulence and constipation reported.

Contraindications. Hypophosphatemia; bowel obstruction.

Precautions. Use with caution in patients with dysphagia, swallowing disorders, GI motility disorders or major GI tract surgery.

Drug Interactions. Sevelamer might bind with concomitantly administered drugs and decrease their absorption.

SODIUM POLYSTYRENE SULFONATE   Kayexalate, Various

Pharmacology. A cation exchange resin that exchanges potassium for sodium. Each gram of resin binds up to 1 mEq of potassium and liberates 1–2 mEq of sodium.[93] Sorbitol is present in some products to induce diarrhea and reduce the potential for fecal impaction. (*See* Notes.)

Administration and Adult Dosage. PO 15–20 g, may repeat as often as q 2 hr,[79] although doses up to 40 g have been recommended;[94] total dosage and duration of therapy depend on patient response. If suspension does not contain sorbitol, give powder with, or suspended in, a sorbitol solution (eg, 15 mL of 70% sorbitol). **PR as enema** 50 g retained for 30 min, if possible, may repeat as often as q 45 min.[79] Follow enema by an irrigation of up to 2 L of nonsodium-containing fluid to remove resin from bowel.

Special Populations. *Pediatric Dosage.* For small children and infants, calculate dosage on the basis of 1 g of resin binding 1 mEq of potassium.

Geriatric Dosage. Lower dosage might be required in some patients because of the age-related decrease in renal function.

Other Conditions. In severe situations, such as ongoing tissue damage or rapidly rising serum potassium in renal failure, a dosage of 80–100 g for every mEq/L of potassium above 5 mEq/L has been recommended.[94] However, under such circumstance, other forms of therapy may be considered.

Dosage Forms. Pwdr 454 g; **Susp** (containing sorbitol) 15 g/60 mL.

Pharmacokinetics. *Onset and Duration.* PO onset 1–2 hr; PR retention enema lowers potassium within 0.5–1 hr.[79]

Fate. Not absorbed from GI tract; binds potassium and liberates sodium as it passes through the intestine.

Adverse Reactions. Anorexia, nausea, and vomiting occur frequently with large doses; gastric irritation, constipation, and fecal impaction (especially in the elderly) occur occasionally. These effects can be avoided with enema. However, intestinal necrosis caused by enema has been reported. Use of **sorbitol** in the enema and failure to follow it with a cleansing enema can predispose uremic patients to potentially fatal intestinal necrosis.[93]

Precautions. Use with caution in patients who cannot tolerate any additional sodium load (eg, severe CHF, severe hypertension, marked edema). In addition to potassium, other cations (eg, magnesium, calcium) can bind to the resin, causing electrolyte imbalances. If rapid potassium lowering is required, give **insulin** with or without glucose.

Drug Interactions. None known.

Parameters to Monitor. Serum potassium at least daily and more frequently if indicated; serum magnesium and calcium periodically; ECG and patient signs and symptoms are useful in evaluating status.

Notes. On average, 50 g of resin will lower serum potassium by 0.5–1 mEq/L.[95,96] Although sodium polystyrene sulfonate is used because of its ability to bind potassium, it also exchanges sodium for other di- and trivalent ions (eg, calcium, magnesium, iron). Rectal administration is less effective than oral use. Heating can alter the exchange properties of the resin. Sodium polystyrene sulfonate–induced constipation may be treated with 70% **sorbitol** in oral doses (ie, 10–20 mL/2 hr) sufficient to produce 1 or 2 watery stools/day.

Bisphosphonates

ALENDRONATE SODIUM   Fosamax

Pharmacology. Alendronate is a nitrogen-containing bisphosphonate that is 100–1000 times as potent as etidronate in inhibiting bone resorption in the rat.[97] Bisphosphonates are cleared rapidly from the circulation and localized to hydroxyapatite bone mineral surfaces where they influence osteoclast function. Postulated cellular mechanisms of action include inhibition of osteoclast formation/recruitment, inhibition of osteoclast activation, inhibition of mature osteoclast activity, and induction of osteoclast apoptosis.[98] Alendronate's action on osteoclast function is hypothesized to be related to the inhibition of the intracellular mevalonate pathway.[99]

Administration and Adult Dosage. PO for prevention of osteoporosis in postmenopausal women 5 mg/day or 35 mg once weekly;[100,101] **PO for treatment of osteoporosis in postmenopausal women** 10 mg/day or 70 mg once weekly;[101–104] **PO for osteoporosis in men** 10 mg/day;[105] **PO for glucocorticoid-induced**

osteoporosis in men and women 5 mg/day, except for postmenopausal women not receiving estrogen, for whom the recommended dosage is 10 mg/day;[106] **PO for Paget's disease of bone in men and women** 40 mg/day for 6 months.[107]

Special Populations. *Pediatric Dosage.* (<18 yr) Safety and efficacy not established.

Geriatric Dosage. Same as adult dosage.

Other Conditions. Dosage adjustment is unnecessary in patients with hepatic impairment or Cl_{cr} >35 mL/min.

Dosage Forms. **Tab** 5, 10, 35, 40, 70 mg.

Patient Instructions. Take alendronate with 180–240 mL (6 to 8 fluid ounces) of water on an empty stomach in the morning at least 30 minutes before any food, beverage, or other medicines. Food and beverages, including mineral water, coffee, tea, or juice, decrease alendronate absorption. Antacids or calcium or vitamin supplements also decrease the absorption of alendronate. Do not lie down for 30 minutes after taking alendronate.

Missed Doses. If you miss a dose of this medicine, resume your usual schedule the next morning. Do not double doses. If you are taking your dose once weekly and miss a scheduled dose, take your weekly dose the next day. Do not take two tablets on the same day.

Pharmacokinetics. *Fate.* Oral bioavailability is 0.9–1.8% in animals.[108,109] Plasma protein binding to albumin is 70–80% in animals; V_d is 28 L exclusive of bone distribution. It is excreted renally.

$t_{1/2}$. Plasma concentrations fall by >95% within 6 hr after IV administration. The terminal half-life in humans is estimated to exceed 10 yr, reflecting skeletal release of alendronate.

Adverse Reactions. Mild, transient falls in serum calcium and phosphate have been reported. Dose-related abdominal pain, dyspepsia, constipation, diarrhea, esophageal ulcer, dysphagia, and abdominal distention can occur. Postmarketing surveillance showed an increased risk of erosive esophagitis, some with ulcerations, primarily in patients who did not comply with recommended administration guidelines.[110–112] Ulcerations are occasionally severe, necessitating hospitalization.[110]

Contraindications. Abnormalities of the esophagus that delay esophageal emptying such as stricture or achalasia; inability to stand or sit upright for at least 30 min; hypocalcemia.

Precautions. The drug must be taken with 180–240 mL of water and patients must not lie down for at least 30 min after oral administration. Avoid use with Cl_{cr} <35 mL/min.

Drug Interactions. Concomitant calcium-containing products interfere with alendronate absorption and should be administered no sooner than 30 min after a dose. Concomitant use with IV randitidine results in a 2-fold increase in bioavailability. Avoid concomitant ingestion with food, orange juice, or caffeine.

Parameters to Monitor. Monitor serum calcium, phosphorus, and creatinine. In osteoporosis, monitor bone mineral density by dual x-ray absorptiometry and for radiologic evidence of fractures. For evidence of active Paget's disease, monitor urinary hydroxyproline and creatinine. Assess pain in patients with Paget's disease who present with pain. (*See* Bisphosphonates Comparison Chart.)

PAMIDRONATE DISODIUM   Aredia

Pharmacology. Pamidronate is a nitrogen-containing bisphosphonate that is about 100 times as potent as etidronate in inhibiting bone resorption in the rat.[97] (*See* Alendronate.)

Administration and Adult Dosage. **IV for hypercalcemia of malignancy** (moderate hypercalcemia: corrected serum calcium of 12–13.5 mg/dL) 60–90 mg.[113] The 60 mg dose is given as an initial, single-dose infusion over at least 4 hr, and the 90 mg dose must be given by an initial, single-dose infusion over 24 hr; (severe hypercalcemia: corrected serum calcium >13.5 mg/dL) 90 mg as an initial, single-dose infusion over 24 hr.

Corrected Serum Calcium = Serum Calcium in mg/dL + (0.8 × [4 – Serum Albumin in g/dL]).

IV for Paget's disease 30 mg/day as a 4-hr infusion on 3 consecutive days for a total of 90 mg. **IV for osteolytic bone lesions of multiple myeloma** 90 mg once monthly as a 4-hr infusion.[114] **IV for osteolytic bone metastases of breast cancer** 90 mg q 3–4 weeks as a 2-hr infusion.[115,116]

Special Populations. *Pediatric Dosage.* Safety and efficacy not established.

Geriatric Dosage. Same as adult dosage.

Other Conditions. Although pharmacokinetic data are lacking, dosage adjustment appears unnecessary in patients with hepatic impairment. Renal clearance is correlated with Cl_{cr} and renally impaired patients excrete less unchanged drug.[117] In patients receiving intermittent therapy, dosage adjustment is probably unnecessary.

Dosage Forms. Inj 30, 90 mg.

Pharmacokinetics. *Fate.* Oral bioavailability is estimated to be 0.3%.[109] Pamidronate is not metabolized and eliminated exclusively by renal excretion. About 46 ± 16% of the drug is excreted unchanged in the urine within 120 hr.

$t_{\frac{1}{2}}$. 2.5 hr.

Adverse Reactions. Generalized malaise has occurred. Hypocalcemia has been reported in patients with hypercalcemia and Paget's disease. Abdominal pain, anorexia, constipation, nausea, and vomiting have been reported in at least 15% of patients receiving pamidronate for hypercalcemia and 5% of patients with Paget's disease. Transient mild temperature elevation (1°C) has occurred. Redness, swelling/induration, and pain on palpation can occur at the IV insertion site.

Precautions. Obtain laboratory tests at the start of therapy. (*See* Parameters to Monitor.) Use with caution in patients with Cl_{cr} >5 mg/dL.

Parameters to Monitor. Monitor serum potassium, calcium, phosphate, creatinine, albumin, and complete blood count and temperature in patients with hypercalcemia of malignancy. In Paget's disease, reductions in serum alkaline phosphatase and urinary hydroxyproline excretion are indicative of a therapeutic response. Assessment pain in patients with Paget's disease who present with pain.

Notes. Do not mix pamidronate with any calcium-containing products. (*See* Bisphosphonates Comparison Chart.)

BISPHOSPHONATES COMPARISON CHART

DRUG	DOSAGE FORMS	INDICATIONS	DOSAGE
Alendronate Sodium Fosamax	Tab 5, 10, 35, 40, 70 mg.	Osteoporosis treatment and prevention; corticosteroid-induced osteoporosis; Paget's disease.	(*See* monograph.)
Etidronate Disodium Didronel	Tab 200, 400 mg Inj 300 mg.	Hypercalcemia of malignancy; Paget's disease; heterotropic ossification.	IV for hypercalcemia 7.5 mg/kg/day over ≥2 hr for 3 days, followed by PO 20 mg/kg/day for 30 days prn. PO for Paget's disease 5–10 mg/kg/day for up to 6 months or 11–20 mg/kg/day for up to 3 months. PO for heterotropic ossification 20 mg/kg/day for 1 month before and 3 months after hip replacement or, if caused by spinal cord injury, 20 mg/kg/day for 2 weeks, then 10 mg/kg/day for 10 weeks.
Pamidronate Disodium Aredia	Inj 30, 90 mg.	Hypercalcemia of malignancy; Paget's disease; osteolytic bone lesions and metastases.	(*See* monograph.)
Risedronate Actonel	Tab 5, 30 mg.	Treatment and prevention of osteoporosis; Paget's disease.	PO for osteoporosis 5 mg/day. PO for Paget's disease 30 mg/day for 2 months.
Tiludronate Skelid	Tab 240 mg (200 mg of free acid).	Paget's disease.	PO 400 mg qid for 3 months.
Zolendronate Zometa (Investigational— Novartis)	Injection.	Hypercalcemia of malignancy; osteolytic bone lesions of metastatic breast cancer and multiple myeloma; Paget's disease.	IV for hypercalcemia of malignancy 0.02–0.04 mg/kg; IV for osteolytic bone lesions 1–3 mg; IV for Paget's disease 0.2–0.4 mg.

From references 101–107, 109, 113–116, and 118–127.

Gout Therapy

ALLOPURINOL
Zyloprim, Various

Pharmacology. Allopurinol, a structural analogue of the purine base hypoxanthine, competitively inhibits xanthine oxidase. This reduces serum and urinary uric acid levels by blocking the conversion of hypoxanthine and xanthine to uric acid and decreasing urine synthesis.[128–130]

Administration and Adult Dosage. **PO for control of gout** 100 mg/day initially, increasing in 100 mg/day increments at weekly intervals until a serum uric acid level of ≤6 mg/dL is attained. **PO for maintenance of mild gout** 200–300 mg/day in single or divided doses; **PO for maintenance of moderately severe tophaceous gout** 400–600 mg/day, to a maximum of 800 mg/day for resistant cases. Give dosages that exceed 300 mg/day in divided doses. Give prophylactic colchicine 0.5–1.2 mg/day and/or an NSAID starting before allopurinol and continuing for 1 to several months after initiation of therapy because of an initial increased risk of gouty attacks.[128–131] A fluid intake sufficient to yield a daily urinary output of at least 2 L and the maintenance of a neutral or slightly alkaline urine are desirable. In transferring from a uricosuric agent to allopurinol, reduce the uricosuric dosage over several weeks while gradually increasing the dosage of allopurinol. **PO or IV for secondary hyperuricemia associated with vigorous treatment of malignancies** 600–800 mg/day for 2–3 days is advisable with a high fluid intake and then reduce to 300 mg/day. Start at least 2–3 days (preferably 5 days) before initiation of cancer therapy. Discontinue when the potential for uric acid overproduction is no longer present.[132,133] IV should be used only in those who do not tolerate PO allopurinol. **PO for recurrent calcium oxalate stones in hyperuricosuria** 200–300 mg/day adjusted based on control of hyperuricosuria.

Special Populations. *Pediatric Dosage.* **PO for secondary hyperuricemia associated with malignancies** (<6 yr) 150 mg/day; (6–10 yr) 300 mg/day; alternatively, 2.5 mg/kg q 6 hr, to a maximum of 600 mg/day. Start at least 2–3 days (preferably 5 days) before cancer therapy.[132] Evaluate response 48 hr after cancer therapy is started and adjust dosage as needed.

Geriatric Dosage. Lower dosage might be required in some patients because of the age-related decrease in renal function.

Other Conditions. In renal impairment, reduce initial dosage as follows: (Cl_{cr} 80 mL/min) 250 mg/day; (Cl_{cr} 60 mL/min) 200 mg/day; (Cl_{cr} 40 mL/min) 150 mg/day; (Cl_{cr} 20 mL/min) 100 mg/day; (Cl_{cr} 10 mL/min) 100 mg q 2 days; (Cl_{cr} <10 mL/min) 100 mg q 3 days.[134] Base subsequent dosage adjustment on serum uric acid levels.

Dosage Forms. **Tab** 100, 300 mg; **Inj** 500 mg.

Patient Instructions. This drug may be taken with food, milk, or an antacid to minimize stomach upset. Adults should drink at least 10–12 full glasses (each containing 8 fluid ounces) of fluid each day. Avoid large amounts of alcohol (can increase uric acid in blood) or vitamin C (can increase the possibility of kidney stones by making the urine more acidic). Report any skin rash, painful urination, blood in urine, eye irritation, swelling of lips or mouth, itching, chills, fever, sore throat, nausea, or vomiting while taking this drug. Allopurinol can cause drowsiness; use caution while driving or performing other tasks requiring alertness, coordination, or physical dexterity.

Missed Doses. Take this drug at regular intervals. If you miss a dose, take it as soon as you remember. Do not double the dose or take extra.

Pharmacokinetics. *Onset and Duration.* A measurable decrease in uric acid occurs in 2–3 days; normal serum uric acid is achieved in 1–3 weeks.

Fate. Well absorbed orally (67–81%) but rectal absorption is poor (0–6% of oral bioavailability). Rapidly oxidized to oxypurinol, an active, but less potent, inhibitor of xanthine oxidase. Protein binding of allopurinol or oxypurinol is negligible.[165] Allopurinol V_d is 1.5 ± 0.7 L/kg, Cl is 0.77 ± 0.22 L/hr/kg; oxypurinol V_d is about 1.6 L/kg.[135,165] Oxypurinol and allopurinol are excreted unchanged in urine in a ratio of about 10:1.[165]

$t_{1/2}$. (Allopurinol) 1.4 ± 0.4 hr; (oxypurinol) 19.7 ± 7.3 hr with normal renal function, 5–10 days in renal failure.[165]

Adverse Reactions. A mild maculopapular skin rash occurs in about 2% of patients, but the percentage increases to about 20% with concurrent ampicillin. These rashes might not recur if allopurinol is stopped and restarted at a lower dosage and oral desensitization to minor rashes from allopurinol in patients has been effective.[130,136,137] Exfoliative, urticarial, purpuric, and erythema multiform lesions also are reported occasionally. These more severe reactions require drug discontinuation because severe hypersensitivity reactions such as vasculitis, toxic epidermal necrolysis, Stevens–Johnson syndrome, renal impairment, and hepatic damage can result. An occasional hypersensitivity syndrome (frequently marked by fever, rash, hepatitis, renal failure, and eosinophilia) has a mortality rate reportedly as high as 27%. It can begin 1 day–2 yr (average 6 weeks) after start of therapy and appears related to pre-existing renal dysfunction, elevated oxypurinol serum levels, or concurrent thiazide or other diuretic therapy.[134,138,139] Occasionally, nausea, vomiting, abdominal pain, and drowsiness occur. Rarely, alopecia, cataract formation, hepatotoxicity, bone marrow depression, leukopenia, leukocytosis, or renal xanthine stones occur.[140]

Contraindications. Children (except for hyperuricemia secondary to malignancy). Do not restart the drug in patients who have developed severe reactions. (*See* Adverse Reactions.)

Precautions. Pregnancy; lactation. Use with caution and in reduced dosage in renal impairment. Adjust dosage conservatively in patients with impaired renal function who are on a diuretic concomitantly.[134,139]

Drug Interactions. Diuretics can contribute to allopurinol toxicity, although a cause-and-effect relationship has not been established. Allopurinol markedly increases the toxicity of oral azathioprine and mercaptopurine. Allopurinol can increase the risk of hypersensitivity reactions to captopril, ampicillin skin rashes, bone marrow suppression caused by cyclophosphamide, neurotoxicity of vidarabine, and nephrotoxicity of cyclosporine. Allopurinol also can increase the effect of some oral anticoagulants but probably not that of warfarin. Large doses (600 mg/day) of allopurinol can increase theophylline serum levels. Concurrent use of salicylate for its antirheumatic effect does not compromise the action of allopurinol. Uricosuric agents can increase the excretion and decrease the effect of oxypurinol.

Parameters to Monitor. Monitor serum uric acid levels; pretreatment 24-hr urinary uric acid excretion.[128–130] Periodically determine liver function (particularly in patients with pre-existing liver disease). Monitor renal function tests and CBC, especially during the first few months of therapy. Renal function is particularly important in patients on concurrent diuretic therapy.[134,139]

Notes. Allopurinol is the drug of choice for patients with impaired renal function who respond poorly to uricosuric agents; however, these patients should be monitored closely because of increased frequency of adverse reactions.[128–131,134] Current data do not support the routine treatment of asymptomatic hyperuricemia in patients other than those receiving vigorous treatment of malignancies and in marked overexcreters.[128–130] Allopurinol has been used investigationally to reduce tissue damage during coronary artery bypass surgery, for organ transplantation storage solutions, and in the treatment of leishmaniasis.[147] Because of limited studies showing very poor or no absorption of extemporaneously compounded allopurinol suppositories, this dosage form is not recommended.[165] Although preliminary reports indicated that extemporaneously prepared allopurinol mouthwash might be effective in protecting against fluorouracil-induced mucositis, one well-controlled clinical trial found it ineffective for this indication, and it is not recommended.[141]

COLCHICINE Various

Pharmacology. Colchicine is an anti-inflammatory agent relatively specific for gout, with activity probably because of the impairment of leukocyte chemotaxis, mobility, adhesion and phagocytosis, and a reduction of the lactic acid production resulting from a decrease in urate crystal deposition.[130]

Administration and Adult Dosage. PO for acute gout 1–1.2 mg initially at the first warning of an attack, then 0.5–1.2 mg q 1–2 hr until pain is relieved or GI toxicity occurs (ie, nausea, vomiting, stomach pain, or diarrhea), to a maximum total dosage of 4–8 mg. Pain and swelling typically abate within 12 hr and usually are gone in 24–48 hr. An interval of 3 days is advised if a second course is required. **PO for prophylaxis in chronic gout** 0.5–1.8 mg/day or every other day depending on severity; divided doses are preferred with higher dosages. **PO for surgical prophylaxis in patients with gout** 0.5–0.6 mg tid, 3 days before and after surgery. **Slow IV for acute gout** (if patient cannot take oral preparation) 1–2 mg initially, diluted (if desired) in nonbacteriostatic NS, over 2–5 min, then 0.5 mg q 6–24 hr prn, to a maximum of 4 mg in 24 hr, or a maximum 4 mg for a single course of treatment.[130,142] Some clinicians recommend a single IV dose of 3 mg over 5 min; others recommend an initial dose of ≤1 mg, then 0.5 mg 1–2 times daily prn. If pain recurs, give IV 1–2 mg/day for several days; however, no more colchicine should be given by any route for at least 7 days after a full course (4 mg) of IV therapy.[130,142] IV colchicine is very irritating and extravasation must be avoided to prevent tissue and nerve damage; change to oral therapy as soon as possible. **Do not administer by SC or IM routes.** (*See* Notes.)

Special Populations. *Geriatric Dosage.* Reduce the maximum IV colchicine dosage to 2 mg, with at least 3 weeks between courses, and lower the dosage further if previously maintained on oral colchicine.[142]

Other Conditions. Reduce the total IV and PO dosage of colchicine in renal impairment in proportion to the remaining renal function.[142,143] The dosage of prophylactic colchicine should not exceed 0.5 mg/day with $Cl_{cr} \leq 50$ mL/min, because of increased risk of peripheral neuritis and myopathy.[144] Not recommended in patients who require hemodialysis.[144]

Dosage Forms. **Tab** 500, 600 μg; **Inj** 500 μg/mL.

Patient Instructions. You should always have a supply of this drug at hand, and you should take it promptly at the earliest symptoms of a gouty attack. Relief of gout pain or occurrence of nausea, vomiting, stomach pain, or diarrhea indicate that the full therapeutic dosage has been attained and no more drug should be taken. After treatment of an attack, do not take any more colchicine for at least 3 days. Immediately report black tarry stools or bright red blood in the stools, which can indicate gastrointestinal bleeding. Report any tiredness, weakness, numbness, or tingling. Also immediately report sore throat, fever, oral lesions, or unusual bleeding that can be an early sign of a severe, but rare, blood disorder.

Missed Doses. If you are taking this drug at regular intervals, such as daily, and you miss a dose, take it as soon as you remember. If it is about time for the next dose, take that dose only. Do not double the dose or take extra.

Pharmacokinetics. *Fate.* Rapidly but variably absorbed after oral administration (healthy young adults, 44 ± 17%; elderly, 45 ± 19%), with partial hepatic deacetylation. Plasma protein binding is approximately 50%; extensive leukocyte uptake occurs with levels found for up to 9 days. Distribution after IV administration is triphasic; V_d of the terminal phase is 6.7 ± 1.4 L/kg for healthy young adults and 6.3 ± 2.3 L/kg for the elderly. Cl is 0.15 ± 0.02 L/hr/kg for healthy young adults and 0.12 ± 0.01 L/hr/kg for the elderly. Urinary (about 10% unchanged), biliary, and fecal elimination occur.[143,145,146]

$t_{\frac{1}{2}}$. (Healthy young adults) second phase 1.2 ± 0.2 hr; terminal phase 30 ± 6 hr; (elderly) second phase 1.2 ± 0.1 hr; terminal phase 34 ± 8 hr.[145]

Adverse Reactions. Nausea, vomiting, stomach pain, and diarrhea are frequent and can occur several hours after oral or IV drug administration; discontinue drug at first signs. Prolonged administration occasionally can cause bone marrow depression with agranulocytosis or thrombocytopenia, aplastic anemia, and purpura. Peripheral neuritis and myopathy with characteristically elevated creatine kinase occur occasionally. This reaction is associated with standard (unadjusted) dosage in renal insufficiency and usually resolves in 3–4 weeks after drug withdrawal.[130,142–144,147] Alopecia, reversible malabsorption of vitamin B_{12}, and reversible azoospermia occur. Tissue and nerve damage can occur with IV extravasation. Overdosage can cause hemorrhagic gastroenteritis, vascular damage leading to shock, nephrotoxicity, and paralysis. As little as 7 mg has proved fatal, but much larger dosages have been survived.[143,148–150]

Contraindications. Serious GI, renal, hepatic, or cardiac disorders; combined hepatic, and renal dysfunction;[143,144] blood dyscrasias.

Precautions. Use with great caution in elderly or debilitated patients, especially those with early manifestations of hepatic, renal, GI, or heart disease. Reduce dosage if weakness, anorexia, nausea, vomiting, stomach pain, or diarrhea occurs.[143,151]

Drug Interactions. None known.

Notes. Colchicine is most effective when used early in the attack before most WBC chemotaxis takes place.[128–130] For acute gout, an **NSAID** or a **corticosteroid** (systemically or intra-articularly) may be preferred, but daily colchicine often is given for prophylaxis against recurrent gouty attacks before and during the first one to several months of allopurinol or uricosuric treatment.[128–130] Continuous prophylactic colchicine therapy can be effective in suppressing the acute attacks and renal dysfunction of familial Mediterranean fever.[143,150] Colchicine therapy also might be effective for primary biliary cirrhosis and certain inflammatory dermatoses.[143,150,151]

PROBENECID
Benemid, Various

Pharmacology. Probenecid, a sulfonamide, is an organic acid that inhibits renal tubular reabsorption of urate, thereby increasing the urinary excretion of uric acid and lowering serum urate. Probenecid also interferes with renal tubular secretion of many drugs, causing an increase or prolongation in their serum levels. (*See* Notes.)

Administration and Adult Dosage. **PO for chronic gout** 250 mg bid for 1 week, then 500 mg bid (not to be started during an acute attack). **Colchicine** 0.5–1.2 mg/day or an NSAID started before and continued for 1 to several months after initiation of uricosuric treatment diminishes exacerbation of uricosuric-induced gouty attacks.[128–130] To prevent hematuria, renal colic, costovertebral pain, and urate stone formation, liberal fluid intake and alkalinization of the urine with 3–7.5 g/day sodium bicarbonate or 7.5 g/day potassium citrate are recommended, at least until serum uric acid levels normalize and tophaceous deposits disappear. If an acute gouty attack is precipitated during therapy, increase the dosage of colchicine or add a corticosteroid or an NSAID to control the attack.[128–130] (*See* Precautions.) Decrease daily dosage by 500 mg q 6 months if no acute attacks occur, adjusted to maintain normal serum uric acid levels. **PO to prolong penicillin or cephalosporin action** 2 g/day in 4 divided doses, except with known renal impairment. **PO with procaine penicillin G for uncomplicated gonorrhea** 1 g as a single dose. **PO with procaine penicillin G for neurosyphilis** 2 g/day in 4 divided doses for 10–14 days.[152] **PO with cefoxitin for outpatient treatment of pelvic inflammatory disease** 1 g as a single dose.[152]

Special Populations. *Pediatric Dosage.* (<2 yr) contraindicated. **PO to prolong penicillin or cephalosporin action** (<50 kg) 25 mg/kg initially, then maintain at 40 mg/kg/day or 1.2 g/m^2/day in 4 divided doses; (>50 kg) same as adult dosage.

Geriatric Dosage. Same as adult dosage unless renal impairment is present.

Other Conditions. For chronic gout in renal impairment (although probably ineffective when $Cl_{cr} \leq 30$ mL/min), increase initial dosage of 500 mg bid in 500 mg/day increments q 4 weeks to the dosage that maintains normal serum uric acid levels, to a maximum of 2 g/day in divided doses. Reduce dosage for prolonging penicillin or cephalosporin action in patients with renal impairment.

Dosage Forms. **Tab** 500 mg.

Patient Instructions. This drug may be taken with food, milk, or an antacid to minimize stomach upset. Drink a large amount (10 to 12 full glasses) of fluids each day and avoid the use of aspirin- or salicylate-containing products unless directed otherwise.

Missed Doses. If you are taking this drug at regular intervals, such as daily, and you miss a dose, take it as soon as you remember. If it is about time for the next dose, take that dose only. Do not double the dose or take extra.

Pharmacokinetics. *Fate.* Rapidly and completely absorbed from the GI tract; 74–99% plasma protein bound (decreasing with increasing dose), mostly to albumin.[153] V_d is 0.17 ± 0.03 L/kg.[11] Probenecid is extensively metabolized or conjugated, exhibiting Michaelis–Menten elimination; about 40% is excreted in urine as the monoacylglucuronide, <5% as unchanged drug, and the remainder as hydroxylated metabolites, which can have uricosuric activity.[154,155]

$t_{1/2}$. Dose dependent (increases with increasing dose): 4.5 ± 0.6 hr with 0.5 g; 12 hr with 2 g.[11,156]

Adverse Reactions. Headache, nausea, vomiting, urinary frequency, rash, and dizziness occur frequently. Exacerbation of gout, hematuria, renal colic, costovertebral pain, and uric acid stones can occur. Nephrotic syndrome, hepatic necrosis, aplastic anemia, hemolytic anemia (possibly related to G-6-PD deficiency), and severe allergic reactions occur rarely.

Contraindications. Children <2 yr; known blood dyscrasias or uric acid kidney stones; initiation during an acute gouty attack.

Precautions. Hypersensitivity reactions require drug discontinuation. Use with caution in patients with histories of sulfonamide allergy, peptic ulcer, or G-6-PD deficiency. (*See* Notes.)

Drug Interactions. Salicylates and pyrazinamide antagonize the uricosuric action of probenecid. Probenecid can increase the serum concentration of many drugs, including acyclovir, benzodiazepines, some β-lactams, clofibrate, dapsone, methotrexate, NSAIDs, penicillamine, sulfonamides, sulfonylureas, thiopental, and zidovudine. NSAID clearance might be decreased by competitively inhibiting formation or renal excretion of acylglucuronide metabolites.[157]

Parameters to Monitor. Serum uric acid weekly until stable when treating hyperuricemia; pretreatment 24-hr urinary uric acid excretion. If alkali is administered, periodically determine acid–base balance.

Notes. Current data do not support the treatment of patients with asymptomatic hyperuricemia caused by *undersecretion* of uric acid.[128,130,131] Most useful in symptomatic patients with reduced urinary excretion of urate: <800 mg/day on an unrestricted diet or <600 mg/day on a purine-restricted diet.[128] Ineffective in prolonging the half-life of β-lactams that do not undergo renal tubular secretion (eg, ceftazidime, ceftriaxone).[158]

SULFINPYRAZONE   Anturane, Various

Pharmacology. Sulfinpyrazone is an analogue of phenylbutazone that lacks anti-inflammatory and analgesic properties. It is a uricosuric agent with a mechanism and site of action resembling those of probenecid. Sulfinpyrazone, like probenecid, interferes with the renal tubular secretion of many drugs. It also has antiplatelet and antithrombotic activities but currently is not used clinically for these indications.[128–130,159]

Adult Dosage. PO as a uricosuric 200–400 mg/day orally in 2 divided doses with meals or milk, increasing over 1 week to a maximum of 800 mg/day with adequate fluid intake and alkalization of the urine. Reduce to the lowest dosage needed to control serum uric acid (as low as 200 mg/day). In elderly, azotemic cardiovascular patients, initiate therapy with 200 mg/day and increase in 200 mg/day increments q 4 days or keep constant for another 4 days depending on Cr_s and serum uric acid, to a maximum maintenance dosage of 800 mg/day.[160]

Dosage Forms. Tab 100 mg; **Cap** 200 mg.

Pharmacokinetics. Oral absorption is rapid and complete, with peak serum levels occurring in 1–2 hr. V_d is 0.73 ± 0.23 L/kg; Cl of the parent compound is 0.14 ± 0.044 L/hr/kg. Hepatic metabolism yields four metabolites. The parent compound is mainly responsible for uricosuric activity; the sulfide metabolite produces the antiplatelet effect. Half-lives are 10 ± 1.3 hr (sulfinpyrazone) and 14.3 ± 4.5 hr (sulfide metabolite).[161,162]

Adverse Reactions. Adverse effects are similar to those of probenecid, with occasional acute renal insufficiency, possibly caused by precipitation of uric acid in renal tubules or decrease in prostaglandin synthesis.[163,164] **Colchicine** 0.5–1.2 mg/day started before and continued for 1 to several months after initiation of uricosuric treatment diminishes exacerbation of uricosuric-induced gouty attacks. Treat acute exacerbations of gout by increasing the colchicine dosage or adding an NSAID or a corticosteroid. Sulfinpyrazone is contraindicated in patients with peptic ulcers, symptoms of GI inflammation or ulceration, and blood dyscrasias. Avoid sulfinpyrazone in renal insufficiency because it might not be effective. Salicylates can antagonize the action of sulfinpyrazone.

REFERENCES

1. Brater DC. Pharmacology of diuretics. *Am J Med Sci* 2000;319:38–50.
2. Hebert SC. Molecular mechanisms. *Semin Nephrol* 1999;19:504–23.
3. Brater DC. Diuretic therapy. *N Engl J Med* 1998;339:387–95.
4. Ellison DH. Diuretic drugs and the treatment of edema: from clinic to bench and back again. *Am J Kidney Dis* 1994;23:623–43.
5. Ward A, Heel RC. Bumetanide. A review of its pharmacodynamic and pharmacokinetics properties and therapeutic use. *Drugs* 1984;28:426–64.
6. Brater DC. Disposition and response to bumetanide and furosemide. *Am J Cardiol* 1986;57:20A–5A.
7. Gerlag PG, van-Meijel JJ. High-dose furosemide in the treatment of refractory congestive heart failure. *Arch Intern Med* 1988;148:286–91.

8. Brater DC. Resistance to diuretics: mechanisms and clinical implications. *Adv Nephrol Necker Hosp* 1993;22:349–69.

9. Vasko MR et al. Furosemide absorption altered in decompensated congestive heart failure. *Ann Intern Med* 1985;102:314–8.

10. Van Meyel JJ et al. Absorption of high dose furosemide (frusemide) in congestive heart failure. *Clin Pharmacokinet* 1992;22:308–18.

11. Benet LZ et al. Design and optimization of dosage regimens; pharmacokinetic data. In, Hardman JG et al., eds. *Goodman and Gilman's the pharmacological basis of therapeutics.* 9th ed. New York: McGraw-Hill; 1996:1707–92.

12. Ponto LL, Schoenwald RD. Furosemide (frusemide): a pharmacokinetic/pharmacodynamic review (part I). *Clin Pharmacokinet* 1990;18:381–408.

13. Ponto LL, Schoenwald RD. Furosemide (frusemide): a pharmacokinetic/pharmacodynamic review (part II). *Clin Pharmacokinet* 1990;18:460–71.

14. Ellison DH. Diuretic resistance: physiology and therapeutics. *Semin Nephrol* 1999;19:581–97.

15. Kaplan NM. Diuretics: correct use in hypertension. *Semin Nephrol* 1999;19:569–74.

16. Aronoff GR et al. *Drug prescribing in renal failure. Dosing guidelines for adults.* 4th ed. Philadelphia: ACCP; 1999.

17. Beermann B, Groschinsky-Grind M. Clinical pharmacokinetics of diuretics. *Clin Pharmacokinet* 1980;5:221–45.

18. Welling PG. Pharmacokinetics of the thiazide diuretics. *Biopharm Drug Dispos* 1986;7:501–35.

19. Greenberg A. Diuretic complications. *Am J Med Sci* 2000;319:10–24.

20. O'Bryne S, Feely J. Effects of drugs on glucose tolerance in non-insulin–dependent diabetes (part II). *Drugs* 1990;40:203–19.

21. O'Bryne S, Feely J. Effects of drugs on glucose tolerance in non-insulin–dependent diabetes (part I). *Drugs* 1990;40:6–18.

22. Womack PL, Hart LL. Potassium supplements vs. potassium-sparing diuretics. *DICP* 1990;24:710–1.

23. Lang F. Osmotic diuresis. *Renal Physiol* 1987;10:160–73.

24. Hoffman DM, Grossano D. Use of mannitol diuresis to reduce cis-platinum nephrotoxicity. *Drug Intell Clin Pharm* 1978;12:489–90. Letter.

25. Anand AJ, Bashey B. Newer insights into cisplatin nephrotoxicity. *Ann Pharmacother* 1993;27:1519–25.

26. Nissenson AR. Mannitol. *West J Med* 1979;131:277–84.

27. Manninen PH et al. The effect of high-dose mannitol on serum and urine electrolytes and osmolality in neuro-surgical patients. *Can J Anaesth* 1987;34:442–6.

28. Anderson P et al. Use of mannitol during neurosurgery: interpatient variability in the plasma and CSF levels. *Eur J Clin Pharmacol* 1988;35:643–9.

29. Dorman HR et al. Mannitol-induced acute renal failure. *Medicine* (Baltimore) 1990;69:153–9.

30. Horgan KJ et al. Acute renal failure due to mannitol intoxication. *Am J Nephrol* 1989;9:106–9.

31. Skluth HA, Gums JG. Spironolactone: a re-examination. *DICP* 1990;24:52–9.

32. Lant A. Diuretics: clinical pharmacology and therapeutic use (part II). *Drugs* 1985;29:162–88.

33. Lant A. Diuretics: clinical pharmacology and therapeutic use (part I). *Drugs* 1985;29:57–87.

34. Pitt B et al. The effect of spironolactone on morbidity and mortality in patients with severe heart failure. *N Engl J Med* 1999;341:709–17.

35. Sadee W et al. Multiple dose kinetics of spironolactone and canrenoate–potassium in cardiac and hepatic failure. *Eur J Clin Pharmacol* 1974;7:195–200.

36. Taketomo CK et al. *Pediatric dosage handbook.* 6th ed. Hudson, OH: Lexi-Comp; 2000.

37. Overdiek HW, Merkus FW. Influence of food on the bioavailability of spironolactone. *Clin Pharmacol Ther* 1986;40:531–6.

38. Gardiner P et al. Spironolactone metabolism: steady-state serum levels of the sulfur-containing metabolites. *J Clin Pharmacol* 1989;29:342–7.

39. Overdiek JW, Merkus FW. Spironolactone metabolism and gynaecomastia. *Lancet* 1986;1:1103. Letter.

40. Jeunemaitre X et al. Efficacy and tolerance of spironolactone in essential hypertension. *Am J Cardiol* 1987;60:820–5.

41. Friedel HA, Buckley MM. Torsemide: a review of its pharmacological properties and therapeutic potential. *Drugs* 1991;41:81–103.

42. Brater DC et al. Clinical pharmacology of torsemide, a new loop diuretic. *Clin Pharmacol Ther* 1987;42:187–92.

43. Gehr TW et al. The pharmacokinetics of intravenous and oral torsemide in patients with chronic renal insufficiency. *Clin Pharmacol Ther* 1994;56:31–8.

44. Sharoky M et al. Comparative efficacy and bioequivalence of a brand-name and a generic triamterene-hydrochlorothiazide combination product. *Clin Pharm* 1989;8:496–500.

45. Gilfrich H et al. Pharmacokinetics of triamterene after IV administration to man: determination of bioavailability. *Eur J Clin Pharmacol* 1983;25:237–41.

46. Muirhead MR et al. Effect of cimetidine on renal and hepatic drug elimination: studies with triamterene. *Clin Pharmacol Ther* 1986;40:400–7.

47. Knauf H et al. Delayed elimination of triamterene and its active metabolite in chronic renal failure. *Eur J Clin Pharmacol* 1983;24:453–6.

48. Mutschler E et al. Pharmacokinetics of triamterene. *Clin Exp Hypertens* 1983;5:249–69.

49. Sica DA, Gehr TW. Triamterene and the kidney. *Nephron* 1989;51:454–61.

50. Brater DC. Use of diuretics in cirrhosis and nephrotic syndrome. *Semin Nephrol* 1999;19:575–80.

51. Friedman PA, Bushinsky DA. Diuretic effects on calcium metabolism. *Semin Nephrol* 1999;19:551–6.

52. Sica DA, Gehr TWB. Diuretic combinations in refractory oedema states. Pharmacokinetic-pharmacodynamic relationships. *Clin Pharmacokinet* 1996;30:229–49.

53. Weaver CM, Heaney RP. Calcium. In, Shils ME et al., eds. *Modern nutrition in health and disease*. 9th ed. Baltimore: Williams & Wilkins; 1999:141–55.

54. Food and Nutrition Board, Institute of Medicine. *Dietary reference intakes for calcium, phosphorus, magnesium, vitamin D and fluoride*. Washington, DC: National Academy Press; 1997.

55. Anon. Calcium supplements. *Med Lett Drugs Ther* 2000;42:29–31.

56. Delmez JA, Slatopolsky E. Hyperphosphatemia: its consequences and treatment in patients with chronic renal disease. *Am J Kidney Dis* 1992;19:303–17.

57. Tohme JF, Bilezikian JP. Hypocalcemic emergencies. *Endocrinol Metab Clin North Am* 1993;22:363–75.

58. Carr CJ, Shangraw RF. Nutritional and pharmaceutical aspects of calcium supplementation. *Am Pharm* 1987;2:49–50, 54–7.

59. Blanchard J, Aeschlimann JM. Calcium absorption in man: some dosing recommendations. *J Pharmacokinet Biopharm* 1989;17:631–44.

60. Sheikh MS et al. Gastrointestinal absorption of calcium from milk and calcium salts. *N Engl J Med* 1987;317:532–6.

61. Shils ME. Magnesium. In, Shils ME et al., eds. *Modern nutrition in health and disease*. 9th ed. Baltimore: Williams & Wilkins; 1999:169–92.

62. Al-Ghandi SMG et al. Magnesium deficiency: pathophysiologic and clinical overview. *Am J Kidney Dis* 1994;5:737–52.

63. Rude RK. Magnesium metabolism and deficiency. *Endocrinol Metab Clin North Am* 1993;22:377–95.

64. Montgomery P. Treatment of magnesium deficiency. *Clin Pharm* 1987;6:834–5.

65. Reinhart RA. Magnesium metabolism: a review with special reference to the relationship between intracellular content and serum levels. *Arch Intern Med* 1988;148:2415–20.

66. Berkelhammer C, Bear RA. A clinical approach to common electrolyte problems: hypomagnesemia. *Can Med Assoc J* 1985;132:360–8.

67. Oto A. Magnesium treatment in acute myocardial infarction: an unresolved consensus. *Eur Heart J* 1999;20:86–8. Editorial.

68. Chernow B et al. Hypomagnesemia: implications for the critical care specialist. *Crit Care Med* 1982;10:193–6.

69. Lloyd CW, Johnson CE. Management of hypophosphatemia. *Clin Pharm* 1988;7:123–8.

70. Rosen GH et al. Intravenous phosphate repletion regimen for critically ill patients with moderate hypophosphatemia. *Crit Care Med* 1995;23:1204–10.

71. Perreault MM et al. Efficacy and safety of intravenous phosphate replacement in critically ill patients. *Ann Pharmacother* 1997;31:683–8.

72. Hodgson SF, Hurley DL. Acquired hypophosphatemia. *Endocrinol Metab Clin North Am* 1993;22:397–409.

73. Rubin MF, Narins RG. Hypophosphatemia: pathophysiological and practical aspect of its therapy. *Semin Nephrol* 1990;10:536–45.

74. Subramanian R et al. Severe hypophosphatemia. Pathophysiologic implications, clinical presentations, and treatment. *Medicine* (Baltimore) 2000;79:1–8.

75. Peppers MP et al. Endocrine crises: hypophosphatemia and hyperphosphatemia. *Crit Care Clin* 1991;7:201–14.

76. Kingston M, Al-Siba'i MB. Treatment of severe hypophosphatemia. *Crit Care Med* 1985;13:16–8.

77. Martin ML et al. Potassium. *Emerg Med Clin North Am* 1986;4:131–44.

78. Krishna GG. Hypokalemic states: current clinical issues. *Semin Nephrol* 1990;10:515–24.

79. Zull DN. Disorders of potassium metabolism. *Emerg Med Clin North Am* 1989;7:771–94.

80. Cohn JN et al. New guidelines for potassium replacement in clinical practice: a contemporary review by the National Council on Potassium in Clinical Practice. *Arch Intern Med* 2000; 160:2429–36.

81. Stanaszek WF, Romankiewicz JA. Current approaches to management of potassium deficiency. *Drug Intell Clin Pharm* 1985;19:176–84.

82. Kruse JA, Carlson RW. Rapid correction of hypokalemia using concentrated intravenous potassium chloride infusions. *Arch Intern Med* 1990;150:613–7.

83. Toner JM, Ramsay LE. Pharmacokinetics of potassium chloride in wax-based and syrup formulations. *Br J Clin Pharmacol* 1985;19:489–94.

84. Skoutakis VA et al. The comparative bioavailability of liquid, wax-matrix, and microencapsulated preparations of potassium chloride. *J Clin Pharmacol* 1985;25:619–21.

85. Breyer JA. Diabetic nephropathy in insulin-dependent patients. *Am J Kidney Dis* 1992;20:533–47.

86. Freedman BI, Burkart JM. Endocrine crises: hypokalemia. *Crit Care Clin* 1991;7:143–53.

87. Finch MH, Younoszai KM. Oral rehydration therapy. *South Med J* 1987;80:609–13.

88. Balistreri WF. Oral rehydration in acute infantile diarrhea. *Am J Med* 1990;88(6A):30S–3S.

89. Grisanti KA, Jaffe DM. Dehydration syndromes: oral rehydration and fluid replacement. *Emerg Med Clin North Am* 1991;9:565–88.

90. American Academy of Pediatrics, Provisional Committee on Quality Improvement, Subcommittee on Acute Gastroenteritis. Practice parameter: the management of acute gastroenteritis in young children. *Pediatrics* 1996;97:424–35.

91. Swedberg J, Steiner JF. Oral rehydration therapy in diarrhea: not just for Third World children. *Postgrad Med* 1983;74:335–41.

92. Anon. Oral rehydration solutions. *Med Lett Drugs Ther* 1983;25:19–20.

93. Lillemoe KD et al. Intestinal necrosis due to sodium polystyrene (Kayexalate) in sorbitol enemas: clinical and experimental support for the hypothesis. *Surgery* 1987;101:267–72.

94. Elms JJ. Potassium imbalance: causes and prevention. *Postgrad Med* 1982;72:165–71.

95. Alvo M, Warnock DG. Hyperkalemia. *West J Med* 1984;141:666–71.

96. Greenberg A. Hyperkalemia: treatment options. *Semin Nephrol* 1998;18:46–57.

97. Fleisch H. Bisphosphonates: mechanisms of action. *Endocr Rev* 1998;19:80–100.

98. Rodan GA. Mechanisms of action of bisphosphonates. *Annu Rev Pharmacol Toxicol* 1998;38:375–88.

99. Rogers MJ et al. Cellular and molecular mechanisms of action of bisphosphonates. *Cancer* 2000;88:2961–78.

100. Hosking D et al. Prevention of bone loss with alendronate in postmenopausal women under 60 years of age. *N Engl J Med* 1998;338:485–92.

101. Schnitzer T et al. Therapeutic equivalence of alendronate 70 mg once-weekly and alendronate 10 mg daily in the treatment of osteoporosis. *Aging Clin Exp Res* 2000;12:1–12.

102. Cummings SR et al. Effect of alendronate on risk of fracture in women with low bone density but without vertebral fractures. Results from the Fracture Intervention Trial. *JAMA* 1998;280:2077–82.

103. Black DM et al. Randomised trial of effect of alendronate on risk of fracture in women with existing vertebral fractures. *Lancet* 1996;348:1535–41.

104. Liberman UA et al. Effect of oral alendronate on bone mineral density and the incidence of fractures in postmenopausal osteoporosis. *N Engl J Med* 1995;333:1437–41.

105. Orwoll E et al. Alendronate for the treatment of osteoporosis in men. *N Engl J Med* 2000;343:604–10.

106. Saag KG et al. Alendronate for the prevention and treatment of glucocorticoid-induced osteoporosis. *N Engl J Med* 1998;339:292–9.

107. Lombardi A. Treatment of Paget's disease of bone with alendronate. *Bone* 1999;24:59S–61S.

108. Porras AG et al. Pharmacokinetics of alendronate. *Clin Pharmacokinet* 1999;36:315–28.

109. Lin JH. Bisphosphonates: a review of their pharmacokinetic properties. *Bone* 1996;18:75–85.

110. de Groen PC et al. Esophagitis associated with the use of alendronate. *N Engl J Med* 1996;335:1016–21.

111. Liberman UA, Hirsch LJ. Esophagitis and alendronate. *N Engl J Med* 1996;335:1069–70. Letter.

112. Bauer DC et al. Upper gastrointestinal tract safety profile of alendronate. The Fracture Intervention Trial. *Arch Intern Med* 2000;160:517–25.

113. Nussbaum SR et al. Single-dose intravenous therapy with pamidronate for the treatment of hypercalcemia of malignancy: comparison of 30-, 60-, and 90-mg dosages. *Am J Med* 1993;95:297–304.

114. Berenson JR et al. Efficacy of pamidronate in reducing skeletal events in patients with advanced multiple myeloma. *N Engl J Med* 1996;334:488–93.

115. Hillner BE et al. American Society of Clinical Oncology guideline on the role of bisphosphonates in breast cancer. *J Clin Oncol* 2000;18:1378–91.

116. Hortobagyi GN et al. Efficacy of pamidronate in reducing skeletal complications in patients with breast cancer and lytic bone metastases. *N Engl J Med* 1996;335:1785–91.

117. Berenson JR et al. Pharmacokinetics of pamidronate disodium in patients with cancer with normal or impaired renal function. *J Clin Pharmacol* 1997;37:285–90.

118. Singer FR et al. Treatment of hypercalcemia of malignancy with intravenous etidronate. A controlled, multicenter study. *Arch Intern Med* 1991;151:471–6.

119. Khairi MRA et al. Treatment of Paget disease of bone (osteitis deformans). Results of a one-year study with sodium etidronate. *JAMA* 1974;230:562–7.

120. Harris ST et al. Effects of risedronate treatment on vertebral and nonvertebral fractures in women with postmenopausal osteoporosis. A randomized controlled trial. *JAMA* 1999;282:1344–52.

121. Reginster J-Y et al. Randomized trial of the effects of risedronate on vertebral fractures in women with established postmenopausal osteoporosis. *Osteoporos Int* 2000;11:83–91.

122. Siris ES et al. Risedronate in the treatment of Paget's disease of bone: an open label, multicenter study. *J Bone Miner Res* 1998;13:1032–8.

123. Fraser WD et al. A double-blind, multicentre, placebo-controlled study of tiludronate in Paget's disease of bone. *Postgrad Med J* 1997;73:496–502.

124. McClung MR et al. Tiludronate therapy for Paget's disease of bone. *Bone* 1995;17(5 suppl):493S–6S.

125. Body JJ et al. A dose-finding study of zoledronate in hypercalcemic cancer patients. *J Bone Miner Res* 1999;14:1557–61.

126. Lipton A. Zoledronate in the treatment of osteolytic bone metastases. *Br J Clin Prac* 1996;87(suppl):21S–2S.

127. Siris E. Zoledronate in the treatment of Paget's disease. *Br J Clin Pract* 1996;87(suppl):19S–20S.

128. Star VL, Hochberg MC. Prevention and management of gout. *Drugs* 1993;45:212–22.

129. Conaghan PG, Day RO. Risks and benefits of drugs used in the management and prevention of gout. *Drug Safety* 1994;11:252–8.

130. Emmerson BT. The management of gout. *N Engl J Med* 1996;334:445–51.

131. Campbell SM. Gout: how presentation, diagnosis, and treatment differ in the elderly. *Geriatrics* 1988;43(11):71–7.

132. Conger JD. Acute uric acid nephropathy. *Med Clin North Am* 1990;74:859–71.

133. Smalley RV et al. Allopurinol: intravenous use for prevention and treatment of hyperuricemia. *J Clin Oncol* 2000;18:1758–63.

134. Hande KR et al. Severe allopurinol toxicity: description and guidelines for prevention in patients with renal insufficiency. *Am J Med* 1984;76:47–56.

135. Walter-Sack I et al. Disposition and uric acid lowering effect of oxipurinol: comparison of different oxipurinol formulations and allopurinol in healthy individuals. *Eur J Clin Pharmacol* 1995;49:215–20.

136. Fam AG et al. Desensitization to allopurinol in patients with gout and cutaneous reactions. *Am J Med* 1992;93:299–302.

137. Tanna SB et al. Desensitization to allopurinol in a patient with previous failed desensitization. *Ann Pharmacother* 1999;33:1180–3.

138. Roujeau JC, Stern RS. Severe adverse cutaneous reactions to drugs. *N Engl J Med* 1994;331:1272–85.

139. Arellano F, Sacristán JA. Allopurinol hypersensitivity syndrome: a review. *Ann Pharmacother* 1993;27:337–43.

140. Pascual E. Gout update: from lab to the clinic and back. *Curr Opin Rheumatol* 2000;12:213–8.

141. Loprinzi CL et al. A controlled evaluation of an allopurinol mouthwash as prophylaxis against 5-fluorouracil-induced stomatitis. *Cancer* 1990;65:1879–82.

142. Wallace SL, Singer JZ. Review: systemic toxicity associated with the intravenous administration of colchicine—guidelines for use. *J Rheumatol* 1988;15:495–9.

143. Levy M et al. Colchicine: a state-of-the-art review. *Pharmacotherapy* 1991;11:196–211.

144. Wallace SL et al. Renal function predicts colchicine toxicity: guidelines for the prophylactic use of colchicine in gout. *J Rheumatol* 1991;18:264–9.

145. Rochdi M et al. Pharmacokinetics and absolute bioavailability of colchicine after IV and oral administration in healthy human volunteers and elderly subjects. *Eur J Clin Pharmacol* 1994;46:351–4.

146. Jusko WJ, Gretch M. Plasma and tissue protein binding of drugs in pharmacokinetics. *Drug Metab Rev* 1976;5:43–140.

147. Day RO. New uses for allopurinol. *Drugs* 1994;48:339–44.

148. Hood RL. Colchicine poisoning. *J Emerg Med* 1994;12:171–7.

149. Mullins ME et al. Fatal cardiovascular collapse following acute colchicine ingestion. *Clin Toxicol* 2000;38:51–4.

150. Ben-Chetrit E, Levy M. Colchicine: 1998 update. *Semin Arthritis Rheum* 1998;28:48–59.

151. Sullivan TP et al. Colchicine in dermatology. *J Am Acad Dermatol* 1998;39:993–9.

152. Anon. Drugs for sexually transmitted infections. *Med Lett Drugs Ther* 1999;41:85–90.

153. Emanuelsson BM et al. Non-linear elimination and protein binding of probenecid. *Eur J Clin Pharmacol* 1987;32:395–401.

154. Israili ZH et al. Metabolites of probenecid. Chemical, physical, and pharmacological studies. *J Med Chem* 1972;15:709–13.

155. Perel JM et al. Identification and renal excretion of probenecid metabolites in man. *Life Sci* 1970;9:1337–43.

156. Dayton PG et al. The physiological disposition of probenecid, including renal clearance, in man, studied by an improved method for its estimation in biological material. *J Pharmacol Exp Ther* 1963;140:278–86.

157. Smith PC et al. Effect of probenecid on the formation and elimination of acyl glucuronides: studies with zomepirac. *Clin Pharmacol Ther* 1985;38:121–7.
158. Brown GR. Cephalosporin-probenecid drug interactions. *Clin Pharmacokinet* 1993;24:289–300.
159. Patrono C et al. Platelet-active drugs. The relationships among dose, effectiveness, and side effects. *Chest* 1998;114:470S–88S.
160. Palummeri E et al. Sulphinpyrazone in cardiovascular elderly azotemic patients: a proposal of a guided incremental dose schedule. *J Int Med Res* 1984;12:271–6.
161. Mahoney C et al. Kinetics and metabolism of sulfinpyrazone. *Clin Pharmacol Ther* 1983;33:491–7.
162. Schlicht F et al. Pharmacokinetics of sulfinpyrazone and its major metabolites after a single dose and during chronic treatment. *Eur J Clin Pharmacol* 1985;28:97–103.
163. Orlandini G, Brognoli M. Acute renal failure and treatment with sulfinpyrazone. *Clin Nephrol* 1983;20:161–2.
164. Rosenkranz B et al. Effects of sulfinpyrazone on renal function and prostaglandin formation in man. *Nephron* 1985;39:237–43.
165. Murrell GAC, Rapeport WG. Clinical pharmacokinetics of allopurinol. *Clin Pharmacokinet* 1986;11:343–53.

Respiratory Drugs

Antiasthmatics

Class Instructions. Antiasthmatic Inhalers. (Aerosols) Remove inhaler cap and hold inhaler upright. Shake inhaler. Tilt your head back and breathe out slowly. To position inhaler, open your mouth with the inhaler 1 to 2 inches away or in your mouth. (For young children and corticosteroid inhalers, use a spacer or holding chamber.) Press down on inhaler to release medication as you start to breathe slowly. Breathe slowly for 3 to 5 seconds. Hold your breath for 10 seconds to allow the medication to reach deep into the lungs. Repeat as directed. (Dry Powder) Close your mouth tightly around the mouthpiece and inhale rapidly. Hold the device horizontally (parallel to the ground) after it has been activated. Do not exhale into the device.

Do not exceed the prescribed dosage. Report if symptoms do not completely clear or the inhaler is required more than prescribed. Clean the mouthpiece weekly with hot water and soap. Store away from heat and direct sunlight. Bronchodilators can cause nervousness, tremors (especially with terbutaline or albuterol), or rapid heart rate. Report if these effects continue after dosage reduction; if chest pain, dizziness, or headache occur; or if asthmatic symptoms are not relieved.

Missed Doses. Take missed doses as soon as possible. However, if it is almost time for your next dose, skip the missed dose and go back to your regular schedule. Do not double doses.

ALBUTEROL SULFATE
Proventil, Ventolin, Volmax, Various

Pharmacology. Albuterol is a selective β_2-adrenergic agonist that produces bronchodilation, vasodilation, uterine relaxation, skeletal muscle stimulation, peripheral vasodilation, and tachycardia.[1]

Administration and Adult Dosage. Inhal for asthma (metered-dose inhaler) 90–180 µg (1–2 puffs) q 4–6 hr prn and just before exercise; (inhalation solution) 2.5 mg by nebulization tid–qid; (inhalation capsule) 1–2 inhalation capsules q 4–6 hr or 1 capsule 15 min before exercise. **Inhal for severe bronchospasm** nebulized by compressed air or oxygen 2.5–5 mg (0.5–1 mL of 0.5% in 2–3 mL NS) q 4–6 hr prn (q 1–2 hr under medical supervision). **PO for asthma** 2–4 mg q 6–8 hr, increase as tolerated to a maximum of 32 mg/day; **SR Tab** 4–8 mg q 12 hr, to a maximum of 32 mg/day.

Special Populations. *Pediatric Dosage.* Inhal for asthma (metered-dose inhaler) (<12 yr) 90–180 µg (1–2 puffs) q 4–6 hr using spacer; (≥12 yr) same as adult dosage; (inhalation solution) (<12 yr) 0.05–0.15 mg/kg q 4–6 hr prn, or (<20 kg) 0.25 mL of 0.5% solution; (>20 kg) 0.5 mL of 0.5% solution to a maximum of

1 mL diluted in 2–3 mL NS q 4–6 hr prn (q 1–2 hr for severe bronchospasm under medical supervision); (≥12 yr) same as adult dosage. **PO for asthma** (2–6 yr) 100–200 μg/kg/dose q 8 hr, to a maximum of 4 mg q 8 hr; (6–12 yr) 2 mg q 6–8 hr, to a maximum of 24 mg/day; (>12 yr) same as adult dosage. **SR Tab** (<12 yr) dosage not established; (>12 yr) same as adult dosage.

Geriatric Dosage. **Inhal for asthma** same as adult dosage. **PO** 2 mg tid–qid initially, increasing prn to a maximum of 8 mg tid–qid.

Dosage Forms. **Inhal** (metered-dose) 90 μg/puff (200 puffs/inhaler); **Inhal** (metered-dose, HFA, does not contain chlorofluorocarbons as a propellant) (Proventil HFA, Ventolin HFA) 90 μg/puff (200 puffs/inhaler); **Inhal Soln** 0.5% (5 mg/mL), 0.083% (unit dose solution, 3 mL); **Inhal Cap** (Rotacap) 200 μg for use with powder inhaler; **Tab** 2, 4 mg; **Syrup** 0.4 mg/mL; **SR Tab** 4, 8 mg. **Inhal** 90 μg plus ipratropium bromide 18 μg/puff (Combivent); **Inhal Soln** 3 mg plus ipratropium bromide 0.5 mg/3 mL (DuoNeb).

Patient Instructions. (*See* Class Instructions: Antiasthmatic Inhalers.)

Pharmacokinetics. *Onset and Duration.* (Inhal) onset within 15 min, peak 60–90 min or less; (PO) onset 30–60 min, peak 2–3 hr. Duration 4–6 hr, depending on the dose, dosage form, and clinical condition. (*See* Sympathomimetic Bronchodilators Comparison Chart.)

Fate. Peak serum level after 0.15 mg/kg by inhalation is 5.6 μg/L (23 nmol/L). Oral bioavailability is 50% because of hepatic first-pass metabolism; peak after 4 mg tablet is 10 μg/L (42 nmol/L); 50% is excreted in urine as an inactive sulfate conjugate. The drug does not appear to be metabolized in the lung.[2]

t½. (IV) 2–3 hr; apparent half-life is 5–6 hr after oral and up to 7 hr after inhalation because of prolonged absorption.[2]

Adverse Reactions. Dose-related reflex tachycardia from peripheral vasodilation and direct stimulation of cardiac β_2-receptors. Tremor, palpitations, and nausea are other dose-related effects that are markedly reduced with aerosol administration. All β_2-agonists lower serum potassium concentrations.

Precautions. Pregnancy; cardiac disorders including coronary insufficiency and hypertension; diabetes. Excessive or prolonged use may lead to tolerance.

Drug Interactions. Concurrent β-blockers may antagonize effects.

Parameters to Monitor. Inhalation technique, asthma symptoms, frequency of use, pulmonary function, and heart rate.

Notes. A relationship between regular (ie, not prn) use of inhaled β_2-agonists and death from asthma has been a concern.[3,4] Regardless of whether β_2-agonists are directly responsible or simply a marker for more severe asthma, heavy use (>1 canister/month or 12 puffs/day) of these agents should alert clinicians that it is necessary to re-evaluate the patient's condition. Proventil HFA inhalers use a nonchlorofluorocarbon propellant; drug delivery is similar, but not identical, to Ventolin and Proventil. **Levalbuterol** (Xopenex) is the active L-isomer of albuterol. It is available as solution for inhalation 0.63 mg and 1.25 mg/3 mL.

CROMOLYN SODIUM
Gastrocrom, Intal, Nasalcrom, Opticrom, Various

Pharmacology. Cromolyn stabilizes the membranes of mast cells and other inflammatory cells (eg, eosinophils), thereby inhibiting release and production of soluble mediators (eg, histamine, leukotrienes) that produce inflammation and bronchospasm. The mechanism appears to be the inhibition of calcium ion influx through the cell membrane. Cromolyn inhibits the early and late responses to specific allergen and exercise challenges. It also prevents the increase in nonspecific bronchial hyperreactivity that occurs during a specific allergen season in atopic asthmatics.[5]

Administration and Adult Dosage. Inhal for asthma 20 mg qid at regular intervals in nebulizer (1 ampule inhalant solution) or 0.8–1.6 mg qid via a pressurized metered-dose inhaler. Initiate therapy in conjunction with an aerosolized β_2-agonist. (*See* Notes.) **Inhal for prevention of exercise-induced bronchospasm** single dose (as above) just before exercise. **Intranasal for prophylaxis of allergic rhinitis** 5.2 mg/nostril 3–6 times/day at regular intervals. **Ophth for allergic ocular disorders** 1–2 drops (1.6–3.2 mg) in each eye 4–6 times/day at regular intervals. For chronic conditions, the drug must be used continuously to be effective. **PO for mastocytosis** 200 mg qid, 30 min before meals and hs.

Special Populations. *Pediatric Dosage.* **Inhal** (<2 yr) dosage not established; (≥2 yr) same as adult dosage. **Intranasal or Ophth** same as adult dosage. **PO for mastocytosis** (term infants–2 yr) 20 mg/kg/day in 4 divided doses, to a maximum of 30 mg/kg/day; (2–12 yr) 100 mg qid, 30 min before meals and hs, increasing, if necessary, to a maximum of 40 mg/kg/day.

Geriatric Dosage. Same as adult dosage.

Other Conditions. The therapeutic effect is dose dependent, and patients with more severe disease may require more frequent administration initially. After a patient becomes symptom free, the frequency of administration may be reduced to bid–tid.

Dosage Forms. Inhal Soln 10 mg/mL; **Inhal** 800 μg/puff (112, 200 doses/inhaler); **Nasal Inhal** 5.2 mg/spray (100, 200 doses/inhaler); **Ophth Drp** 4% (40 mg/mL, 250 drops/container); **PO Soln** 20 mg/mL.

Patient Instructions. (*See* Class Instructions.) (Asthma) this medication must be used regularly and continuously to be effective. Do not stop therapy abruptly, except on medical advice. Carefully follow directions for inhaler use included with the device. You may mix the nebulizer solution with any bronchodilator inhalant solution that does not contain benzalkonium chloride. (Mastocytosis) dissolve oral capsules in one-half glass (4 fluid ounces) of hot water, add an equal amount of cold water, and drink the entire amount. Do not mix with fruit juice, milk, or foods.

Missed Doses. Take this drug at regular intervals. If you miss a dose, take it as soon as you remember. If it is about time for the next dose, take that dose only. Do not double the dose or take extra.

Pharmacokinetics. *Onset and Duration.* (Asthma) onset within 1 min for prevention of allergen-induced mast cell degranulation; duration dose dependent,

2–5 hr.[5] It may require 4–6 weeks to achieve maximal response, although most asthmatics respond within 2 weeks.[6]

Fate. Oral bioavailability is 0.5–1%. Amount absorbed after inhalation depends on the delivery system; about 10% of the dosage for a Spinhaler and <2% with the nebulizer solution.[5] Peak serum levels occur 15–20 min after inhalation. V_d is 0.2 ± 0.04 L/kg; Cl is 0.35 ± 0.1 L/hr/kg. Rapidly excreted unchanged in equal portions in the bile and urine.[5]

$t_{1/2}$. 22.5 ± 1.6 min.[5]

Adverse Reactions. Mild burning or stinging can occur with ophthalmic solution. Occasionally, headache and diarrhea occur with oral capsules.

Precautions. Use with caution in patients with lactose sensitivity (capsules only). Watch for worsening of asthma in patients discontinuing the drug. The ophthalmic solution contains 0.01% benzalkonium chloride; therefore, do not wear soft contact lenses during therapy.

Drug Interactions. None known.

Parameters to Monitor. Monitor relief of asthmatic symptoms and the proper dosage and inhalation technique. Patient noncompliance or inappropriate inhalation technique often contributes to treatment failure. The measurement of peak expiratory flow rate with a peak flow meter is useful in severe chronic asthma. Periodic standard pulmonary function tests are indicated q 1–6 months.

Notes. Comparative studies have shown cromolyn and **theophylline** to be equally effective for the prophylaxis of chronic asthma, although cromolyn produces fewer side effects.[5,6] The inhalant solution is stable with all β_2-agonist and anticholinergic solutions for nebulization, although benzalkonium chloride–free solutions are preferred.[5,7] The nasal spray is most effective if started 1 week before the allergen season; however, patients receive benefit even if treatment is begun after symptoms occur.[6] Oral cromolyn has been used in the management of GI conditions such as food allergy and irritable bowel syndrome.[8] Cromolyn solution is incompatible with benzalkonium chloride.[7]

IPRATROPIUM BROMIDE   Atrovent, Various

Pharmacology. Ipratropium is a competitive antagonist of acetylcholine at peripheral, but not central, muscarinic receptors because of its quaternary structure.[9] It is used primarily as a bronchodilator in COPD, emphysema, and bronchitis.

Administration and Adult Dosage. **Inhal for bronchospasm of COPD (including chronic bronchitis)** 36–72 μg (2–4 puffs) qid by metered-dose inhaler, to a maximum of 288 μg (16 puffs)/day.[9,10] **Inhal for acute, severe asthma** 500 μg tid–qid by nebulizer. Combivent or extemporaneous ipratropium/albuterol mixtures have the same dosage as above. **Nasal spray for rhinorrhea of perennial rhinitis** 2 sprays (84 μg)/nostril of 0.03% solution bid–tid; **Nasal spray for rhinorrhea of the common cold** 2 sprays (84 μg)/nostril tid–qid for up to 4 days.

Special Populations. *Pediatric Dosage.* (<12 yr) safety and efficacy not established. **Inhal** (<2 yr) 125 μg/dose by nebulizer,[11] (>2 yr) 18–36 μg (1–2 puffs) q 6–8 hr by metered-dose inhaler, or 250 μg q 6–8 hr by nebulizer has been used.[10,12] **Nasal spray for rhinorrhea of perennial rhinitis** (<6 yr) safety and efficacy not established; (6–11 yr) 1 spray (42 μg)/nostril of 0.03% solution bid–tid; (≥12 yr) same as adult dosage.

Geriatric Dosage. Same as adult dosage.

Dosage Forms. **Inhal** 18 μg/puff (200 doses/inhaler); **Inhal Soln** 200 μg/mL (500 μg/vial); **Nasal Spray** 0.03, 0.06%. **Inhal** 18 μg plus 90 μg albuterol/puff (Combivent); 500 μg plus albuterol 3 mg/3 mL (DuoNeb).

Patient Instructions. (*See* Class Instructions: Antiasthmatic Inhalers.) Temporary blurring of vision can occur if the drug is sprayed into eyes.

Pharmacokinetics. *Onset and Duration.* Onset 3 min; peak 1–2 hr;[10] duration 4–6 hr, depending on intensity of response.[13]

Fate. Only ≤32% is orally absorbed and <1% of inhaled dose is absorbed.[10] Metabolized to eight metabolites, which are excreted in urine and bile.

$t_{1/2}$. 1.5–4 hr.[10]

Adverse Reactions. Dryness of the mouth. Because of the quaternary nature of the molecule, typical systemic anticholinergic side effects are absent.[10,13] With the nasal spray, epistaxis, nasal dryness, dry mouth, or throat and nasal congestion occur in 1–10% of patients. During long-term use, headache, nausea, and upper respiratory tract infections also occur frequently.

Contraindications. (Aerosol inhaler) hypersensitivity to soy lecithin, soybeans, or related products.

Precautions. Use with caution in narrow-angle glaucoma, prostatic hypertrophy, or bladder neck obstruction.

Drug Interactions. None known.

Parameters to Monitor. Inhalation technique, asthma symptoms, frequency of use, pulmonary function, and anticholinergic symptoms.

Notes. Anticholinergics appear to be as potent bronchodilators as β_2-adrenergic drugs in bronchitis and emphysema but less potent in asthma.[9,10] Anticholinergics produce an additive bronchodilation with β_2-adrenergic agents in severe asthma.[10,12] Ipratropium and albuterol nebulizer solutions can be mixed if the mixture is used within 1 hr. **Tiotropium bromide** (Spiriva—Boehringer-Ingelheim) is similar to ipratropium and is being studied in COPD.

MONTELUKAST SODIUM   Singulair

Pharmacology. Montelukast sodium is a selective and orally active leukotriene-receptor antagonist that inhibits the cysteinyl leukotriene $CysLT_1$ receptor.[14,15]

Administration and Adult Dosage. **PO for mild persistent asthma** 10 mg/day in the evening.

Special Populations. *Pediatric Dosage.* **PO for mild persistent asthma** (<2 yr) safety and efficacy not established; (2–5 yr) 4 mg chewable tablet every evening; (6–14 yr) 5 mg chewable tablet every evening; (≥15 yr) same as adult dosage.

Geriatric Dosage. Same as adult dosage.

Dosage Forms. Chew Tab 4, 5 mg; Tab 10 mg.

Patient Instructions. This drug is used for long-term control and prevention of mild persistent asthma symptoms. Take this medication daily, even when you are having no symptoms, and during periods of worsening asthma. This medication is not for the treatment of acute asthma attack management of exercise-induced bronchospasm. You should have appropriate short-acting β_2-agonist medication available to treat acute symptoms. Seek medical attention if short-acting inhaled bronchodilators are needed more often than usual, or if the maximum number of inhalations of short-acting bronchodilator treatment prescribed for a 24-hour period is needed.

Missed Doses. Take a missed dose as soon as possible. If it is almost time to take the next dose, skip the missed dose and go back to your regular dosage schedule. Do not double doses.

Pharmacokinetics. *Onset and Duration.* Duration is 24 hr.[14,15]

Fate. Montelukast is rapidly absorbed after oral administration. Mean oral bioavailabilities are 64% for the film-coated tablet and 73% for the chewable tablet in the fasted state, and 63% with a standard morning meal. Peak concentrations occur 3–4 hr after administration of a 10 mg film-coated tablet and 2–2.5 hr after the 5 mg chewable tablet in fasted adults. Montelukast is >99% protein bound; V_{dss} is 8–11 L; Cl is 2.7 L/hr. CYP3A4 and 2C9 are involved in the metabolism of montelukast. Montelukast and its metabolites are excreted almost exclusively via the bile.

$t_{1/2}$. 2.7–5.5 hr in healthy young adults.

Adverse Reactions. Generally well tolerated. Adverse events that occur with a frequency of $\geq 2\%$ and more frequently in patients on montelukast than on placebo are diarrhea, laryngitis, pharyngitis, nausea, otitis, sinusitis, and viral infection.

Contraindications. Patients with known aspirin sensitivity should continue to avoid aspirin or other NSAIDs while taking montelukast. Inform phenylketonurics that the chewable tablets contain phenylalanine (a component of aspartame) 0.824 mg/tablet.

Precautions. (*See* Patient Instructions.) Reduction in systemic corticosteroid dosage in patients on a leukotriene modifier has been followed rarely by eosinophilia, vasculitic rash, worsening pulmonary symptoms, cardiac complications, and/or neuropathy, sometimes presenting as Churg-Strauss syndrome. A causal relationship with leukotriene-receptor antagonists is not established.

Parameters to Monitor. Clinical symptoms of asthma. Appropriate monitoring recommended when systemic corticosteroid reduction is considered.

Notes. **Zafirlukast** (Accolate) is similar to montelukast but has the disadvantages of twice-daily administration, the need to take on an empty stomach, cases of severe lever damage and several drug–drug interactions; the anticoagulant effect of warfarin is increased by zafirlukast; erythromycin and theophylline decrease zafirlukast serum concentrations, whereas aspirin increases zafirlukast serum concentrations. Interactions with other drugs are not well studied. (*See* Precautions.) The dosages of zafirlukast are 10 mg bid on a empty stomach in patients 7–11 yr and

20 mg bid on on empty stomach in those ≥12 yr; it is available as 10 and 20 mg tablets.

NEDOCROMIL SODIUM Tilade

Pharmacology. Nedocromil sodium is the disodium salt of a pyranoquinolone dicarboxylic acid that is chemically dissimilar, but pharmacologically similar, to cromolyn sodium. Like cromolyn, nedocromil inhibits the activation of and mediator release from inflammatory cells important in asthma and allergy. Nedocromil appears to have more potent in vitro activity against allergic response than cromolyn.[16,17]

Adult Dosage. Inhal for asthma 2 metered-dose actuations qid. In patients under good control with qid administration (ie, patients requiring inhaled or oral β-agonists not more than twice a week), a lower dosage can be tried. First reduce to a tid regimen, then, after several weeks of continued good control, attempt to reduce to a bid regimen. **Ophth for allergic conjunctivitis** 1–2 drops into each eye bid.

Pediatric Dosage. (>12 yr) same as adult dosage.

Dosage Forms. Inhal 16.2 g, containing at least 104 actuations of 2 mg doses (1.75 mg reaches the patient); **Ophth Soln** 2%.

Pharmacokinetics. Oral bioavailability is only 2–3%. After inhalation, bioavailability is 5%, with peak serum concentrations occurring in 20–40 min; concentrations fall monoexponentially, with a half-life of 1.5–2.3 hr, reflecting absorption from lungs.

Adverse Reactions. Bronchospasm, headache, distinctive taste, nausea, and vomiting occur frequently. In a limited number of trials, nedocromil was effective for long-term prophylaxis of asthma. Like cromolyn, it can decrease bronchial hyperreactivity but is only partly effective in steroid-dependent asthmatics. Nedocromil sodium is intended for regular maintenance treatment and should not be used in acute asthma attacks.

SALMETEROL XINAFOATE Serevent

Pharmacology. Salmeterol is a β2-agonist structurally and pharmacologically similar to albuterol. Salmeterol is intended for regular treatment of reversible airway obstruction and not for immediate symptomatic relief. The place of salmeterol in asthma therapy is being debated, in part because patients in need of regular β2-agonist therapy should be regarded as candidates for an inhaled corticosteroid to treat underlying inflammation.[18] (*See* Sympathomimetic Bronchodilators Comparison Chart.)

Administration and Adult Dosage. Inhal for asthma prophylaxis or COPD 42 μg (2 puffs) q 12 hr by metered-dose inhaler or 1 dry powder blister inhaled q 12 hr. **Inhal to prevent exercise-induced bronchospasm** 2 puffs 30–60 min before exercise. (*See also* Inhaled Corticosteroid Comparison Chart for combination product dosages.)

Pediatric Dosage. Inhal (Aerosol) (<12 yr) safety and efficacy not established; (≥12 yr) same as adult dosage. (Dry powder) (≥4 yr) same as adult dosage.

Dosage Forms. Inhal 21 μg/metered-dose puff, in 6.5 g (60 actuations) and 13 g (120 actuations) canisters; **Dry Pwdr Inhal** 50 μg/blister. **Dry Pwdr Inhal** 50 μg plus fluticasone 100, 250, or 500 μg/blister.

Patient Instructions. Shake metered-dose canister well before using. For asthma, use this medication regularly every 12 hours. If asthma symptoms occur between doses, use a short-acting inhaler to treat symptoms. If you regularly need more than 4 inhalations of the short-acting inhaler, see your health care provider.

Pharmacokinetics. Onset of effective bronchodilation is achieved in 20–30 min; peak effect occurs within 3–4 hr. Bronchodilation lasts for at least 12 hr after inhalation of a single dose of 50 μg. After inhalation, salmeterol is extensively metabolized by hydroxylation, with the majority of a dose being eliminated within 72 hr. About 23% of administered radioactivity was recovered in the urine and 57% in the feces over 168 hr.

Adverse Reactions. (*See* Albuterol.)

Notes. Formoterol (Foradil—Novartis) is a long-acting β_2-adrenergic agonist that is similar to salmeterol in duration but with a more rapid onset. Dosage (≥12 yr) is 12 μg bid for maintenance or 15 min before exercise. It is available as a dry powder for inhalation. A fixed-dose combination with budesonide (Symbicort—Astra Zeneca) is being investigated.

SYMPATHOMIMETIC BRONCHODILATORS COMPARISON CHART

DRUG	DOSAGE FORMS	DOSAGE Adult	DOSAGE Pediatric[a]	RECEPTOR SELECTIVITY[b] β_1	RECEPTOR SELECTIVITY[b] β_2	RELATIVE β_2 POTENCY[c]	DURATION OF ACTION BY INHALATION (HR)[d]
SINGLE-INGREDIENT PRODUCTS							
Albuterol AccuNeb Proventil Ventolin Volmax Various	Inhal (soln) 0.5%; (unit dose) 0.021%, 0.042%, 0.083%, (metered-dose) 90 µg/puff; (Rotacaps) 200 µg/cap SR Tab 4, 8 mg Syrup 0.4 mg/mL Tab 2, 4 mg.	Inhal (soln) 2.5–5 mg in 2–3 mL NS q 4–6 hr prn by nebulizer; may use q 1–2 hr prn status asthmaticus under medical supervision; (metered-dose) 1–2 puffs q 4–6 hr prn and before exercise; 1 Rotacap is equivalent to 2 metered-dose puffs PO 2–4 mg q 6–8 hr, to a maximum of 32 mg/day SR Tab 4–8 mg q 12 hr, to a maximum of 32 mg/day.	Inhal (soln) 0.05–0.15 mg/kg in 2–3 mL NS q 4–6 hr prn by nebulizer, may use q 1–2 hr prn or 0.5 mg/kg/hr continuously nebulized for status asthmaticus under medical supervision; (metered-dose) 1–2 puffs q 4–6 hr prn and before exercise PO 0.1–0.2 mg/kg q 6–8 hr, to a maximum of 24 mg/day.	+	++++	5	4–6

(continued)

777

SYMPATHOMIMETIC BRONCHODILATORS COMPARISON CHART *(continued)*

DRUG	DOSAGE FORMS	DOSAGE Adult	DOSAGE Pediatric[a]	RECEPTOR SELECTIVITY[b] β_1	RECEPTOR SELECTIVITY[b] β_2	RELATIVE POTENCY[c]	DURATION OF ACTION BY INHALATION (HR)[d]
Bitolterol[e] Tornalate	Inhal (metered-dose) 0.37 mg/puff; (soln) 0.2%.	Inhal (metered-dose) 1–3 puffs q 4–6 hr prn.	Inhal (metered-dose) 1–2 puffs q 4–6 hr prn.	+	++++	2.5	4–8
Epinephrine Adrenalin Various	Inhal (soln) 2.25% (racemic); Inj 0.1, 1 mg/mL.	SC 0.2–0.5 mg q 20 min–4 hr prn. Inhal not recommended.	SC 0.01 mL/kg of 1:1000 q 15–20 min for 2 doses, then q 4 hr prn. Inhal not recommended for asthma.	+++	+++	5	0.5–2
Formoterol Foradil	Inhal (dry pwdr) 12 µg.	Inhal 12 µg bid, or 15 min before exercise prn.	(≥5 yr) same as adult dosage.	+	++++	70	12
Isoetharine Various	Inhal (soln)1%.	Inhal (soln) 2.5–10 mg diluted 1:3 in NS q 2–4 hr prn.	Inhal (soln) 0.1–0.2 mg/kg q 2–4 hr prn.	++	+++	1.7	0.5–2
Isoproterenol Isuprel Various	Inhal (soln) 0.5, 1%; (metered-dose) 80, 103 µg/puff Inj 0.02, 0.2 mg/mL.	Not recommended because of short duration and lack of selectivity.	Not recommended because of short duration and lack of selectivity.	++++	++++	10	0.5–2

(continued)

SYMPATHOMIMETIC BRONCHODILATORS COMPARISON CHART *(continued)*

DRUG	DOSAGE FORMS	DOSAGE Adult	DOSAGE Pediatric[a]	RECEPTOR SELECTIVITY[b] β_1	RECEPTOR SELECTIVITY[b] β_2	RELATIVE POTENCY[c]	DURATION OF ACTION BY INHALATION (HR)[d]
Metaproterenol Alupent Various	Inhal (soln) 0.4% (unit dose 10 mg), 0.6% (unit dose 15 mg), 5%; (metered-dose) 0.65 mg/puff Syrup 2 mg/mL Tab 10, 20 mg.	Inhal (soln) 5–15 mg q 2–4 hr prn (q 1–2 hr under medical supervision); (metered-dose) 1–3 puffs q 4–6 hr prn and before exercise; PO 20 mg 3–4 times/day.	Inhal (soln) 0.25–0.5 mg/kg up to 15 mg q 2–4 hr prn; (metered-dose) 1–2 puffs prn and before exercise; PO 0.5 mg/kg q 4–6 hr, increase by 0.25 mg/kg as tolerated.	++	++	1	3–4
Pirbuterol Maxair	Inhal (metered-dose) 0.2 mg/puff.	Inhal 1–2 puffs q 4–6 hr and before exercise.	Inhal 1–2 puffs q 4–6 hr prn and before exercise.	+	++++	2.5	4–8
Salmeterol Serevent	Inhal (metered-dose) 21 µg/puff Inhal (dry pwdr) 50 µg/blister.	Inhal (metered-dose) 2 puffs q 12 hr Inhal (dry pwdr) 1 blister q 12 hr.	Inhal (aerosol) (<12 yr) not established; (≥12 yr) same as adult dosage; (dry powder) (≥4 yr) same as adult dosage.	+	++++	20	12

(continued)

SYMPATHOMIMETIC BRONCHODILATORS COMPARISON CHART (*continued*)

		DOSAGE		RECEPTOR SELECTIVITY[b]		DURATION OF RELATIVE POTENCY[c]	ACTION BY INHALATION (HR)[d]
DRUG	DOSAGE FORMS	Adult	Pediatric[a]	β_1	β_2		
Terbutaline	Inhal (metered-dose)	Inhal 1–3 puffs	Inhal 1–2 puffs	+	++++	2.5	4–8
Brethaire	0.2 mg/puff	q 4–6 hr prn; 5–7	q 4–6 hr prn;				
Brethine	Inj 1 mg/mL	mg undiluted by	0.1–0.3 mg/kg				
Bricanyl	Tab 2.5, 5 mg.	nebulizer q 4–6	q 4–6 hr prn				
		hr prn[g]	(q 1–2 hr				
		SC 0.25–0.5 mg q	under medical				
		2–6 hr prn	supervision)[g]				
		PO 5 mg q 6–8 hr.	SC 0.01 mg/kg up				
			to 0.25 mg q				
			2–6 hr prn				
			PO 0.075 mg/kg				
			q 6–8 hr.				

COMBINATION PRODUCTS

		DOSAGE		RECEPTOR SELECTIVITY[b]		DURATION OF RELATIVE POTENCY[c]	ACTION BY INHALATION (HR)[d]
DRUG	DOSAGE FORMS	Adult	Pediatric[a]	β_1	β_2		
Albuterol and Ipratropium	Inhal (metered-dose) albuterol 90 µg plus	Inhal 2 puffs qid to a maximum of	—			—	—
Combivent	ipratropium 18 µg/puff.	12 puffs/day.					
DuoNeb	Inhal Soln albuterol						
	3 mg plus ipratropium						
	0.5 mg/3 mL.						

(continued)

SYMPATHOMIMETIC BRONCHODILATORS COMPARISON CHART (*continued*)

| DRUG | DOSAGE FORMS | DOSAGE | | RECEPTOR SELECTIVITY[b] | | DURATION OF RELATIVE POTENCY[c] | ACTION BY INHALATION (HR)[d] |
		Adult	Pediatric[a]	β_1	β_2		
Salmeterol and Fluticasone Advair Diskus	Inhal (dry pwdr) salmeterol 50 mg plus fluticasone 100, 250 or 500 µg/inhal.	Inhal 1 inhal bid.	(≥12 yr) Same as adult dosage.	—	—	—	—

+ = Minimal effect; ++++ = Pronounced effect.

[a]Isoproterenol and isoetharine are the only metered-dose aerosols labeled for use in children <12 yr.

[b]β_2-selectivity does not equate to bronchoselectivity; β_2-stimulation produces reflex tachycardia from vasodilation as well as stimulation of cardiac β_2-receptors.

[c]Molar potency relative to metaproterenol; large numbers indicate more potent compounds.

[d]Onset and duration data apply to aerosol therapy only. Duration of bronchodilation only applies to otherwise stable asthmatics and is not applicable to acute severe asthma or protection from severe provocation (eg, allergen, exercise, ozone). Duration may be shorter during acute exacerbation or with long-term therapy because of downregulation of β-receptors (tolerance). Oral tablets (especially SR tablets) and syrups are slower in onset but may be slightly longer acting than aerosols.

[e]Bitolterol is a prodrug converted in the body to **colterol,** the active drug, which is more potent than isoproterenol; the relative potency value because of incomplete conversion.

[f]For prophylaxis only; acute attacks must be treated with a short-acting agent.

[g]Use injectable solution; not a labeled indication.

THEOPHYLLINE
Theo-Dur, Slo-bid, Various

Pharmacology. Theophylline directly relaxes smooth muscles of bronchial airways and pulmonary blood vessels to act as a bronchodilator and pulmonary vasodilator. It is also a diuretic, coronary vasodilator, cardiac stimulant, and cerebral stimulant; it improves diaphragmatic contractility; and it lessens diaphragmatic fatigue. The exact cellular mechanism of smooth muscle relaxation is unknown, but intracellular calcium sequestration, inhibition of specific phosphodiesterase isozymes, adenosine-receptor antagonism, and stimulation of endogenous catecholamine release have been postulated to play a role.[19] **Aminophylline** is the ethylenediamine salt of theophylline.

Administration and Adult Dosage. **PO** (theophylline) or **IV** (aminophylline) **for acute asthma symptoms in the emergency department or in the hospital** no longer recommended because it appears to provide no additional benefit over optimal inhaled β_2-agonist therapy and might increase adverse effects; addition of IV theophylline to other therapies in hospitalized adults remains controversial.[20] The following dosages have been used: 5 mg/kg (6 mg/kg aminophylline), if patient has taken no theophylline in previous 24 hr. In emergencies, 2.5 mg/kg (3 mg/kg aminophylline) may be given if an immediate serum level cannot be obtained. Each 1 mg/kg (1.25 mg/kg aminophylline) results in about a 2 mg/L increase in serum theophylline. Infuse IV aminophylline no faster than 25 mg/min. **Maintenance dosage** (*see* Theophylline Dosage Adjustment Chart.) **PO for chronic asthma (theophylline)** (*see* Theophylline Dosage Adjustment Chart.) Adjust dosage to achieve serum concentration of 5–15 mg/L.[21,22] **IM, PR Supp** not recommended.

Special Populations. All dosage recommendations are based on the average theophylline clearance for a given population group. There is a wide interpatient variability (often >2-fold) within all patient groups. Therefore, it is essential that serum concentrations be monitored in all patients. If no doses have been missed or extra doses have been taken during the previous 48 hr, and if peak serum concentrations have been obtained (1–2 hr after liquid or plain uncoated tablet and 4–6 hr after most SR products), adjust dosage using the Theophylline Dosage Adjustment Chart.

Pediatric Dosage. **PO or IV for acute symptoms** not recommended for children hospitalized for severe asthma. **PO for chronic asthma** (theophylline) (<1 yr) 0.2 × (age in weeks) + 5 = dosage in mg/kg/day.[20] **IM, PR Supp** not recommended.

Geriatric Dosage. Not established, but the elderly as a group have slower hepatic clearance. Therefore, use lower initial doses and monitor closely for response and adverse reactions.

Other Conditions. Many factors can alter theophylline dosage requirements. (*See* Precautions and Factors Affecting Serum Theophylline Concentrations Chart.) Use IBW for dosage calculations in obese patients.

THEOPHYLLINE DOSAGE ADJUSTMENT CHART[a]

EVENT	DOSAGE	ACTION
Initial dosage	10 mg/kg/day to a maximum of 300 mg/day.	If initial dosage is tolerated, increase dosage no sooner than 3 days to the first increment.
First increment	13 mg/kg/day to a maximum of 450 mg/day.	If the first incremental increase is tolerated, increase dosage no sooner than 3 days to the second increment.
Second increment	16 mg/kg/day to a maximum of 600 mg/day.	If the second incremental increase is tolerated, measure an estimate of the peak serum concentration after at least 3 days.

SERUM THEOPHYLLINE CONCENTRATION

<10 mg/L	—	Increase dosage by about 25%.
10–15.9 mg/L	—	Maintain dosage if tolerated.
16–19.9 mg/L	—	Consider a 10% dosage reduction.
20–25 mg/L	—	Hold next dose, then resume first incremental dosage.
>25 mg/L	—	Hold next 2 doses, then resume initial dosage.

[a]For children >1 yr and adults with no risk factors for decreased clearance. These recommendations acknowledge interpatient variability in dosage requirements and are based on the principle of not exceeding two-thirds of mean dosage requirements initially and not reaching or exceeding mean dosage requirements without measurement of the serum theophylline concentration. The initial low dosage and spaced increases provide time for the tolerance to caffeine-like effects to occur.
From references 22 and 23.

Dosage Forms. (*See* Theophylline Products Comparison Chart.}

Patient Instructions. Do not chew or crush sustained-release tablets or capsules. Take at equally spaced intervals around the clock. Report any nausea, vomiting, gastrointestinal pain, headache, or restlessness. Contents of sustained-release bead-filled capsules may be mixed with a vehicle (applesauce or jam) and swallowed without chewing for patients who have difficulty swallowing capsules. Take Theo-24 and Uniphyl products at least 1 hour before meals to avoid too rapid absorption of the drug.

Missed Doses. Take the missed dose as soon as possible. However, if it is almost time to take the next dose, skip the missed dose and go back to the regular dosage schedule. Do not double doses. Do not have your theophylline levels measured until you have missed no doses for 3 days.

Pharmacokinetics. *Onset and Duration.* IV onset within 15 min with loading dose.

Serum Levels. Well correlated with clinical effects: therapeutic is 10–15 mg/L (56–83 μmol/L); however, improvement in respiratory function can be observed with serum concentrations of 5 mg/L (28 μmol/L).[21,24] A serum concentration of 5–10 mg/L is often adequate for treatment of neonatal apnea. Toxicity increases at levels >20 mg/L. (*See* Adverse Reactions.)

Fate. Plain uncoated tablets and solution are well absorbed orally; enteric-coated tablets and some SR dosage forms might be unreliably absorbed. Food can affect the rate and extent of absorption of some SR formulations but has minimal effects on rapid-release forms. Food can increase the rate of absorption (Theo-24, Uniphyl), producing dose dumping, or impair absorption (Theo-Dur Sprinkle).[25] Rectal suppository absorption is slow and erratic, and suppositories (including aminophylline) are not recommended under any circumstances. Rectal solutions might result in serum concentrations comparable to oral solution. About 60% is plasma protein bound (less in neonates); V_d is 0.5 ± 0.1 L/kg (greater in neonates). There can be marked intrapatient variability in clearance over time.[22] Cl also is affected by many factors. (*See* Precautions.) Smoking increases theophylline metabolism; this effect can last for 3 months–2 yr after cessation of smoking. Clearance progressively increases in infants during the first year of life. Dose-dependent pharmacokinetics in the therapeutic range occur often in children and rarely in adults.[22] In the elderly, clearance declines with age to about 35 mL/hr/kg.[26] Extensively metabolized in the liver to several inactive metabolites; 10% excreted unchanged in the urine.

t½. 8 ± 2 hr in adult nonsmokers, 4.4 ± 1 hr in adult smokers (1–2 packs per day); 3.7 ± 1.1 hr in children 1–9 yr. In newborn infants, older patients with COPD or cor pulmonale, and patients with CHF or liver disease, the drug can have a half-life >24 hr.

Adverse Reactions. Local GI irritation can occur. Reactions occur more frequently at serum concentrations >20 mg/L and include anorexia, nausea, vomiting, epigastric pain, diarrhea, restlessness, irritability, insomnia, and headache. Serious arrhythmias and convulsions (frequently leading to death or permanent brain damage) usually occur at levels >35 mg/L but have occurred at lower concentrations and might *not* be preceded by less serious toxicity; cardiovascular reactions include sinus tachycardia and life-threatening ventricular arrhythmias with PVCs. Rapid IV administration can cause hypotension, syncope, cardiac arrest (particularly if administered directly into central line), and death.[27] IM administration is painful and offers no advantage.

Contraindications. Active peptic ulcer disease; untreated seizure disorder. (Aminophylline) hypersensitivity to ethylenediamine.

Precautions. Use with caution in severe cardiac disease, hypoxemia, hepatic disease, acute myocardial injury, cor pulmonale, CHF, fever, viral illness, underlying seizure disorder, migraine, hepatic cirrhosis, and neonates. Do not give with other xanthine preparations. The alcohol in some oral liquid preparations might cause side effects in infants.

Drug Interactions. Numerous drugs and conditions can alter theophylline clearance and serum levels. Factors that can decrease serum levels are carbamazepine, charcoal-broiled beef, high-protein/low-carbohydrate diet, isoproterenol (IV), phenytoin, rifampin, and smoking. Factors that can increase serum levels are allopurinol (>600 mg/day), cimetidine, ciprofloxacin, cor pulmonale, macrolides (eg, erythromycin, troleandomycin), oral contraceptives, and propranolol. (*See* Factors Affecting Serum Theophylline Concentrations Chart.)

Parameters to Monitor. (Inpatients) obtain serum theophylline concentrations before starting therapy (if patient previously took theophylline) and 1, 6, and 24 hr after start of infusion; monitor daily during continuous infusion. (Outpatients) monitor serum concentrations q 6 months, 3–5 days after any dosage change, and whenever there are symptoms of toxicity.[21,22]

Notes. The oral theophylline preparations of choice for long-term use, to achieve sustained therapeutic concentrations and improved compliance, are completely and slowly absorbed SR formulations that are minimally affected by food and pH.[25] (*See* Theophylline Products Comparison Chart.) Combination products containing **ephedrine** increase CNS toxicity and have no therapeutic advantage over adequate serum concentrations of theophylline alone. **Diphylline** is chemically related to, but not a salt of, theophylline; the amount of diphylline equivalent to theophylline is unknown. Because its potency is less than that of theophylline and it has a short half-life (2 hr), its dosage is greater than that of theophylline and it must be given more frequently.

FACTORS AFFECTING SERUM THEOPHYLLINE CONCENTRATIONS CHART[a]

FACTOR	DECREASES IN THEOPHYLLINE CONCENTRATIONS	INCREASES IN THEOPHYLLINE CONCENTRATIONS	ACTION
Age	↑ metabolism (1–9 yr)	↓ metabolism (<6 months, elderly)	Adjust dosage according to serum concentration.
Diet	↑ metabolism (high protein)	↓ metabolism (high carbohydrate)	Inform patient that major changes in diet are not recommended while taking theophylline.
Food	↓ or delays absorption of some SR preparations	↑ rate of absorption (fatty food)	Select theophylline product that is not affected by food.
Hypoxia, cor pulmonale, decompensated CHF, cirrhosis	—	↓ metabolism	Decrease dosage according to serum concentration.
Cimetidine	—	↓ metabolism	Use alternative H₂ blocker (eg, famotidine, nizatadine, ranitidine).
Macrolides: troleando-mycin, erythromycin, clarithromycin	—	↓ metabolism	Use alternative antibiotic or decrease theophylline dosage.
Phenobarbital, phenytoin, carbamazepine	↑ metabolism	—	Increase dosage according to serum concentration.

(continued)

FACTORS AFFECTING SERUM THEOPHYLLINE CONCENTRATIONS CHART[a] (*continued*)

FACTOR	DECREASES IN THEOPHYLLINE CONCENTRATIONS	INCREASES IN THEOPHYLLINE CONCENTRATIONS	ACTION
Quinolones: ciprofloxacin, enoxacin	—	↓ metabolism	Use alternative antibiotic or adjust theophylline dosage. Circumvent with levofloxacin if quinolone therapy is required.
Rifampin	↑ metabolism	—	Increase dosage according to serum concentration.
Smoking	↑ metabolism	—	Advise patient to stop smoking; increase dosage according to serum concentration.
Ticlopidine	—	↓ metabolism	Decrease dosage according to serum concentration.
Viral illness, systemic febrile (eg, influenza)	—	↓ metabolism	Decrease theophylline dosage according to serum concentration. Decrease dosage by 50% if serum concentration is not available.

[a]This chart is not all inclusive; for other factors, see Cytochrome P450 Interactions and product information.
From reference 20.

THEOPHYLLINE PRODUCTS COMPARISON CHART[a]

PRODUCT	ANHYDROUS THEOPHYLLINE CONTENT	MEASURABLE DOSE INCREMENT[b] (MG)	COMMENTS
RAPIDLY ABSORBED			
Plain Uncoated Tablets			
Various	Tab 100 mg scored.	50	Serum level fluctuations are 459%/117%.[c]
	Tab 125 mg scored.	62.5	
	Tab 200 mg scored.	100	
	Tab 250 mg scored.	125	
	Tab 300 mg scored.	150	
Oral Liquids (Alcohol-Free)			
Aerolate	10 mg/mL.	5	Sugar free.
Slo-Phyllin 80 Syrup	5.3 mg/mL.	5	Sugar free.
Intravenous Solution			
Aminophylline[d]	20 mg/mL.	5	Use rubber-stoppered vials to avoid glass particles from the breaking of ampules.
Theophylline	0.4, 0.8, 1.6, 2, 3.2, 4 mg/mL.	—	Available in large volume solutions only.

(continued)

THEOPHYLLINE PRODUCTS COMPARISON CHART[a] (continued)

PRODUCT	ANHYDROUS THEOPHYLLINE CONTENT	MEASURABLE DOSE INCREMENT[b] (MG)	COMMENTS
SLOW-RELEASE PRODUCTS[e]			
Slo-bid Gyrocaps	Cap 50 mg. Cap 75 mg. Cap 100 mg. Cap 125 mg. Cap 200 mg. Cap 300 mg.	25	Excellent bioavailability in young infants; beads can be sprinkled on small amount of food; serum level fluctuations are 43%/18%.[c]
Theo-Dur	Tab 100 mg scored. Tab 200 mg scored. Tab 300 mg scored. Tab 450 mg scored.	25 100 150 225	Serum level fluctuations are 38%/16% for 200, 300, and 450 mg, and 87%/34% for 100 mg tablets;[c] some rapid metabolizers may require 8-hr dosage intervals to avoid breakthrough of symptoms.
Uni-Dur	Tab 400 mg scored. Tab 600 mg scored.	200 300	The extent of absorption of Uni-Dur does not appear to be affected by food; however, large serum level fluctuations (78% in adults) may render this agent unreliable for once-daily administration.[28,29]

[a]Only products with documented bioavailability that are minimally affected by food and with dosage forms that permit incremental changes in dose are listed.

[b]Accuracy of measurement decreases below 0.5 mL with suspensions and syrups because of viscosity; smaller amounts cannot be accurately measured; measure all liquid dosage forms with a syringe.

[c]Predicted child/adult fluctuation between peak and trough (%) for 12-hr dosage interval; average child $t_{1/2}$ = 3.7 hr, average adult $t_{1/2}$ = 8.2 hr.[25]

[d]The ethylenediamine portion of aminophylline may cause urticaria or exfoliative dermatitis rarely.

[e]Only Slo-bid Gyrocaps and Theo-Dur tablets have sufficiently slow and complete absorption to allow 12-hr dosage intervals with minimal serum concentration fluocuations in most patients. Many products advertised for bid dosage do not maintain serum concentrations within the therapeutic range in many patients, especially children.[25] Some once-daily dosage products (eg, Uniphyl) are affected by food and may be unreliable.[21,22]

ZILEUTON
Zyflo

Pharmacology. Zileuton is an inhibitor of leukotriene synthesis. It has anti-inflammatory activity and inhibits the antigen-induced contraction of the trachea and bronchospasm that occurs in asthma.

Adult Dosage. PO for asthma prophylaxis 600 mg qid; dosage reduction may be necessary in hepatic dysfunction.

Pediatric Dosage. PO (<12 yr) safety and efficacy not established; (≥12 yr) same as adult dosage.

Dosage Forms. Tab 600 mg.

Pharmacokinetics. Zileuton is orally absorbed; food has no important effect on absorption. It is 93% plasma protein bound; V_d is about 1.2 L/kg. It is metabolized by CYP1A2, 2C9, and 3A4 and has a half-life of 2.5 hr.

Adverse Reactions. It is generally well tolerated, with headache reported in about 10% of patients in clinical trials. GI effects such as nausea and dyspepsia occur occasionally. Hepatic enzyme abnormalities have been reported. It is contraindicated in patients with active hepatic disease. Low WBC counts occur at rates greater than those in placebo-treated patients.

Drug Interactions. Zileuton markedly increases the effects of propranolol, theophylline, and warfarin.

Parameters to Monitor. Obtain ALT at baseline and monthly for 3 months, then q 2–3 months for the remainder of the first year, then periodically.

Antihistamines

Class Instructions. Antihistamines. This drug (with the exceptions of fexofenadine and loratadine) can cause drowsiness, dry mouth, or occasional dizziness. Until the extent of drowsiness is known, use caution when driving, operating machinery, or performing other tasks requiring mental alertness or motor coordination. Avoid excessive concurrent use of alcohol and other central nervous system depressants that cause drowsiness. This drug effectively suppresses seasonal allergic rhinitis only when taken continuously.

Missed Doses. Missed doses should be taken as soon as possible. However, if it is almost time for the next dose, skip the missed dose and go back to the regular dosage schedule. Do not double doses.

CETIRIZINE
Zyrtec

Pharmacology. Cetirizine is a low-sedating, long-acting H_1-receptor antagonist that is a metabolite of hydroxyzine. Cetirizine competitively inhibits the interaction of histamine with H_1 receptors, thereby preventing the allergic response.

Administration and Adult Dosage. PO for allergic rhinitis or urticaria 5–10 mg/day depending on symptom severity.

Special Populations. *Pediatric Dosage.* **PO for allergic rhinitis or urticaria** (2–5 yr) 2.5–5 mg/day; (≥6 yr) same as adult dosage.

Geriatric Dosage. **PO** Same as adult dosage. Reducing dosage in geriatric patients might be necessary because of a 50% increase in cetirizine's half-life and a 40% decrease in clearance.

Other Conditions. In patients with Cl_{cr} of 11–31 mL/min, those on hemodialysis, and in hepatically impaired patients, give 5 mg/day.

Dosage Forms. **Tab** 5, 10 mg; **Syrup** 1 mg/mL.

Patient Instructions. (*See* Class Instructions: Antihistamines.)

Pharmacokinetics. *Onset and Duration.* Onset is within 1 hr; duration is 24 hr.

Fate. Cetirizine is rapidly absorbed after oral administration. Peak serum levels are reached within 1 hr. Food does not affect the amount absorbed but might decrease the absorption rate. Protein binding averages 93%. Cl in normal adults is 0.04–0.05 L/kg/hr. Cetirizine is oxidized to a small extent to inactive metabolites. After a 10 mg dose, 70% of the drug is excreted unchanged in the urine within 72 hr and 10% is excreted in feces. Cetirizine is not appreciably dialyzable.[30–34]

$t_{1/2}$. (Adults) 7–10 hr; (children) 6–7 hr; (elderly/renal insufficiency) 18–21 hr.[30–34]

Adverse Reactions. The most frequent side effects are sedation, headache, dry mouth, fatigue, and nausea. Cetirizine 10 mg/day produces more sedation than loratadine 10 mg/day or placebo. Cetirizine has not been implicated in cardiac adverse events. Higher-than-recommended doses of cetirizine (up to 60 mg daily) did not prolong the QT interval in 25 healthy volunteers.

Contraindications. Hypersensitivity to hydroxyzine or cetirizine.

Precautions. Sedative effects may be dose dependent.

Drug Interactions. Exercise caution when cetirizine is combined with anticholinergic agents, alcohol, or other CNS depressants. Because most of cetirizine is eliminated renally, cytochrome P450 interactions are not likely. Clinically important drug interactions have not been found with cetirizine and azithromycin, pseudoephedrine, ketoconazole, or erythromycin. Clearance of cetirizine was reduced slightly by a 400 mg dose of theophylline, but this reduction was not clinically important; however, larger doses might have a greater effect. Therefore, it seems appropriate to monitor patients for increased sedation or other CNS-related side effects when administering theophylline concomitantly with cetirizine.

Parameters to Monitor. (Allergic rhinitis) observe for sneezing, rhinorrhea, itchy nose, and conjunctivitis. Monitor for side effects such as sedation.

Notes. Cetirizine and **loratadine** have the advantages of noncardiotoxicity, once-daily administration, and availability of liquid dosage forms. (*See* Antihistamines Comparison Chart.)

CHLORPHENIRAMINE MALEATE
Chlor-Trimeton, Various

Pharmacology. Chlorpheniramine is a competitive antagonist of histamine at the H_1-histamine receptor. It also has anticholinergic and transient sedative effects when used intermittently.

Administration and Adult Dosage. **PO for seasonal allergic rhinitis** (effectiveness is maximized if given continuously, starting just before the pollen season)

4 mg hs initially, increasing gradually over 10 days as tolerated to 24 mg/day in 1–2 divided doses until the end of the season. **PO for acute allergic reactions** 12 mg in 1–2 divided doses. **SR** (*see* Notes.)

Special Populations. *Pediatric Dosage.* **PO for seasonal allergic rhinitis** (2–6 yr) 1 mg q 4–6 hr up to 4 mg/day; (6–12 yr) 2 mg hs initially, increasing gradually over 10 days as tolerated to 12 mg/day in 1–2 divided doses until the end of the season.[35] **SR** not recommended. (*See* Notes.)

Geriatric Dosage. **PO** (≥60 yr) 4 mg daily–bid.

Dosage Forms. **Chew Tab** 2 mg; **Tab** 4 mg; **Syrup** 0.4 mg/mL; **SR Cap** 8, 12 mg (*see* Notes); **SR Tab** 8, 12 mg (*see* Notes); **Cap** 4, 10 mg with pseudoephedrine HCl 60 and 65 mg, respectively (various), and 8, 12 mg with pseudoephedrine HCl 120 mg (various).

Patient Instructions. (*See* Class Instructions: Antihistamines.)

Pharmacokinetics. *Onset and Duration.* Onset is 0.5–1 hr; duration of suppression of wheal and flare response (IgE mediated) to skin tests with allergenic extract is 2 days.[36] Fast metabolizers have an earlier, greater, and more prolonged antihistaminic response than slow metabolizers because of rapid conversion to active metabolite.[37] In the elderly, duration of action can be ≥36 hr, even when serum concentrations are low.[38]

Serum Levels. Serum chlorpheniramine levels do not correlate with histamine antagonist activity because of an unidentified active metabolite.[37] (Children) 2.3–12 μg/L (6–31 nmol/L) suppress allergic rhinitis symptoms; (children) 4–10 μg/L (11–26 nmol/L) suppress histamine-induced wheal and flare.[35]

Fate. Oral bioavailability is about 34%; 72% is plasma protein bound.[38] V_d is (adults) 3.2 ± 0.3 L/kg; (children) 7 ± 2.8 L/kg; Cl is (adults) 0.1 ± 0.006 L/hr/kg; (children) 0.43 ± 0.19 L/hr/kg.[35,39] Rapidly and extensively metabolized by CYP2D6 to mono- and didesmethylchlorpheniramine and unidentified metabolites, one or more of which are active. Metabolites and a small amount of parent drug are excreted in urine.[36,40]

$t_{1/2}$. (Adults) 20 ± 5 hr; (children) 13 ± 6 hr; (chronic renal failure) 280–330 hr.[35,39,40]

Adverse Reactions. Frequent drowsiness, dry mouth, dizziness, and irritability occur with intermittent therapy; however, most patients develop tolerance to these side effects during continuous therapy, particularly if the dosage is increased slowly.

Contraindications. Lactation; premature and newborn infants.

Precautions. Use chlorpheniramine with caution in patients ≥60 yr. It might cause paradoxical CNS stimulation in children. OTC labeling states to avoid in patients with narrow-angle glaucoma, symptomatic prostatic hypertrophy, asthma, emphysema, chronic pulmonary disease, shortness of breath, or breathing difficulties except under physician supervision; however, many studies have shown some bronchodilator effect of H_1-receptor antagonists.[37]

Drug Interactions. MAOIs prolong and intensify the anticholinergic effects of antihistamines.[41] Alcohol or sedative-hypnotics can increase CNS depressant effects.

Parameters to Monitor. In seasonal allergic rhinitis, observe for sneezing, rhinorrhea, itchy nose, and conjunctivitis.

Notes. Not effective for nasal stuffiness. SR formulations offer no advantage over syrup or plain, uncoated tablets because the drug has an inherently long duration of action. (*See* Antihistamines Comparison Chart.)

DIPHENHYDRAMINE HYDROCHLORIDE   Benadryl, Various

Pharmacology. (*See* Chlorpheniramine.) Diphenhydramine has strong sedating and anticholinergic properties.

Administration and Adult Dosage. **PO as an antihistamine or for parkinsonism** 25–50 mg tid–qid. **PO for motion sickness** 50 mg 30 min before exposure, then ac and hs. **PO as a nighttime sleep aid** 25–50 mg hs. **PO as an antitussive** 25 mg q 4–6 hr. **Deep IM or IV as an antihistamine, or for allergic reactions to blood or plasma, motion sickness, adjunctive treatment of anaphylaxis, or parkinsonism** 10–50 mg/dose, 100 mg if required, to a maximum of 400 mg/day.

Special Populations. *Pediatric Dosage.* **PO as an antihistamine** 5 mg/kg/day, or (≤9 kg) 6.25–12.5 mg tid–qid; (>9 kg) 12.5–25 mg tid–qid, to a maximum of 300 mg/day. **PO as an antitussive** (2–6 yr) 6.25 mg q 4 hr, to a maximum of 25 mg/day; (6–12 yr) 12.5 mg q 4 hr, to a maximum of 75 mg/day. **Deep IM or IV** 5 mg/kg/day in 4 divided doses, to a maximum of 300 mg/day.

Geriatric Dosage. **PO as an antihistamine** 25 mg bid–tid initially, then increase as needed.[42] (*See* Notes.)

Other Conditions. In renal impairment, increase dosage interval as follows: (Cl_{cr} 10–50 mL/min), increase to 6–12 hr; (Cl_{cr} <10 mL/min), increase to 12–18 hr.[42]

Dosage Forms. **Cap** 25, 50 mg; **Chew Tab** 12.5 mg; **Elxr** 2.5 mg/mL; **Syrup** 1.25, 2.5 mg/mL; **Tab** 25, 50 mg; **Inj** 50 mg/mL.

Patient Instructions. (*See* Class Instructions: Antihistamines.)

Pharmacokinetics. *Onset and Duration.* Onset is 15 min after single oral dose; duration of suppression of wheal and flare is up to 2 days.[37,43] Duration of effect does not appear to be related to serum levels.

Serum Levels. (Antihistaminic effect) >25 µg/L (0.09 µmol/L); (sedation) 30–50 µg/L (0.1–0.17 µmol/L); (mental impairment) >60 µg/L (0.2 µmol/L).[39,43]

Fate. As a result of first-pass metabolism, oral bioavailability is variable, 61 ± 25%.[39,44] A single 50 mg oral dose in adults usually produces serum concentrations of 25–50 µg/L.[43] About 85% is plasma protein bound and lower in Asians and those with cirrhosis.[45,46] V_d is 17.4 ± 4.8 L/kg in adults and larger in Asians and those with cirrhosis. Cl is 1.4 ± 0.6 L/hr/kg in adults and higher in Asians and 0.7 ± 0.2 L/hr/kg in the elderly.[39,42,44,45] Metabolized to *N*-dealkylated and acidic metabolites.[44,47] Less than 4% is excreted unchanged in urine.[48]

$t_{1/2}$. (Adults) 9.2 ± 2.5 hr; (elderly >65 yr) 13.5 ± 4.2 hr; (children 8–12 yr) 5.4 ± 1.8 hr;[39,44] (cirrhosis) 15 hr.[46]

Adverse Reactions. (*See* Chlorpheniramine.)

Contraindications. (*See* Chlorpheniramine.)

Precautions. (*See* Chlorpheniramine.)

Drug Interactions. (*See* Chlorpheniramine.)

Parameters to Monitor. (*See* Chlorpheniramine.)

Notes. Because of its low degree of efficacy for pruritus, weak suppression of IgE-mediated skin tests, and high sedative potential, diphenhydramine is not the antihistamine of choice for most conditions. In the elderly, diphenhydramine is discouraged as a nighttime sleep aid because of its high anticholinergic potential. **Dimenhydrinate** (Dramamine), used for motion sickness, is the 8-chlorotheophyllinate salt of diphenhydramine; 100 mg dimenhydrinate is about equal to 50 mg diphenhydramine.

FEXOFENADINE   Allegra

Pharmacology. Fexofenadine is a histamine H_1-receptor antagonist that is a metabolite of terfenadine. It causes little sedation and has little anticholinergic activity. (*See* Antihistamines Comparison Chart.)

Adult Dosage. **PO for allergic rhinitis** 180 mg once daily or 60 mg bid; **PO for chronic idiopathic urticaria** 60 mg bid. In renal impairment, reduce initial dosage to 60 mg/day.

Pediatric Dosage. **PO** (<6 yr) safety and efficacy not established; (6–11 yr) 30 mg bid; (≥12 yr) same as adult dosage.

Dosage Forms. **Cap** 60 mg; **Tab** 30, 60, 180 mg; **Tab** 60 mg with pseudoephedrine 120 mg (Allegra-D).

Pharmacokinetics. *Onset and Duration.* Onset is rapid; peak serum levels occur at 2.6 hr. Food decreases oral absorption. It is 60–70% plasma protein bound and excreted unchanged in urine and feces. Its half-life is about 14 hr in normal renal function and increases to about 19 hr in severe renal impairment.

Adverse Reactions. Drowsiness or fatigue occur in <2% of patients; GI effects occur in about 1.5% and headache in >1%. Pharyngitis and menstrual disturbances have been reported.

HYDROXYZINE HYDROCHLORIDE   Atarax, Vistaril, Various
HYDROXYZINE PAMOATE   Vistaril, Various

Pharmacology. Hydroxyzine is a competitive antagonist of histamine at the H_1-histamine receptor. It also has antiemetic and sedative effects, thought to be a result of CNS subcortical suppression. Claims of long-term antianxiety properties have not been substantiated by well-designed studies.

Administration and Adult Dosage. **PO for pruritus** 25 mg tid–qid. **PO for seasonal allergic rhinitis** (effectiveness is maximized if given continuously just before the pollen season) 25 mg initially q hs until no sedation in the morning, then increase dosage q 2–3 days, to a maximum of 150 mg/day in 1–2 divided doses and maintain until the end of the season. Reduce dosage by one-third or more if sedation persists. Dosage may be increased, if tolerated, for symptoms during the peak of pollen season.[49] **IM for sedation before and after general anesthesia** 50–100 mg. **IM for nausea and vomiting and pre- and postoperative adjunctive medication** 25–100 mg. Preferred IM injection site is upper outer quadrant of gluteus maximus or midlateral thigh. **Not for SC or intra-arterial use.**

Special Populations. *Pediatric Dosage.* **PO for pruritus** (<6 yr) 50 mg/day in 2–3 divided doses; (≥6 yr) 50–100 mg/day in divided doses. **PO for seasonal allergic rhinitis** 10 mg initially q hs until no sedation in the morning, then increase dosage q 2–3 days, to a maximum of 75 mg/day in 1–2 divided doses and maintain until the end of the season. Reduce dosage by one-third or more if sedation persists. Dosage may be increased, if tolerated, for symptoms during the peak of pollen season.[49] **IM for pre- and postoperative sedation** 0.7 mg/kg. **IM for nausea and vomiting and pre- and postoperative adjunctive medication** 1.1 mg/kg. Preferred site in children is midlateral muscles of the thigh.

Geriatric Dosage. **PO for pruritus** 10 mg tid–qid, increasing to 25 mg tid–qid if necessary.[51]

Dosage Forms. **Cap** (as pamoate equivalent of HCl salt) 25, 50, 100 mg; **Susp** (as pamoate equivalent of HCl salt) 5 mg/mL; **Syrup** (as HCl) 2 mg/mL; **Tab** (as HCl) 10, 25, 50, 100 mg; **Inj** (as HCl) 25, 50 mg/mL (IM only).

Patient Instructions. (*See* Class Instructions: Antihistamines.)

Pharmacokinetics. *Onset and Duration.* Onset 15–30 min after oral administration. Duration of suppression of wheal and flare response to allergenic extract skin test is 4 days.[37,50]

Serum Levels. (Pruritus) 6–42 μg/L (14–102 nmol/L) suppress pruritus in children.[52]

Fate. Peak serum level of 73 ± 11 μg/L occurs 2 ± 0.4 hr after a 0.7 mg/kg dose in healthy adults, 117 ± 61 μg/L at 2.3 ± 0.7 hr in primary biliary cirrhosis (mean dose 44 mg).[53,54] V_d is (healthy adults) 16 ± 3 L/kg,[53] (elderly) 23 ± 6 L/kg, (children) 19 ± 9 L/kg,[52] and (primary biliary cirrhosis) 23 ± 13 L/kg.[54] Cl is (healthy young and elderly adults) 0.6 ± 0.2 L/hr/kg,[51,53] (children) 1.9 L/hr/kg,[52] (primary biliary cirrhosis) 0.5 ± 0.4 L/hr/kg.[54]

$t_{1/2}$. (Healthy adults) 20 ± 4 hr;[53] (elderly) 29 ± 10 hr;[51] (children) 7 hr, increasing with age;[53] (primary biliary cirrhosis) 37 ± 13 hr.[54]

Adverse Reactions. Transient drowsiness and dry mouth occur frequently when the drug is taken intermittently. Most patients develop tolerance to these effects when the drug is taken continuously, particularly if the dosage is slowly increased over 7–10 days. IM injection can be painful and has caused sterile abscess. Hemolysis has been associated with IV administration and tissue necrosis with SC or intra-arterial administration.

Contraindications. Early pregnancy; SC or intra-arterial use of injectable solution.

Precautions. Use with caution in the elderly.

Drug Interactions. MAOIs prolong and intensify the anticholinergic effects of antihistamines. Alcohol or sedative-hypnotics can increase CNS depressant effects.

Parameters to Monitor. In seasonal allergic rhinitis, observe for sneezing, rhinorrhea, itchy nose, and conjunctivitis.

Notes. Hydroxyzine suppresses wheal and flare response to the greatest degree and for the longest duration of all antihistamines,[37] including the newer nonsedating antihistamines.[50]

LORATADINE
Claritin

Pharmacology. Loratadine is a long-acting piperadine antihistamine that is structurally similar to azatadine, with little or no action at α-adrenergic or cholinergic receptors.[55] (*See* Antihistamines Comparison Chart.)

Adult Dosage. PO for allergic rhinitis or urticaria 10 mg/day on an empty stomach. In patients with hepatic impairment, begin with 10 mg every other day. The dosage of Claritin-D is 1 tablet bid on an empty stomach; Claritin-D 24-hr is given once daily.

Pediatric Dosage. **PO** (<2 yr) safety and efficacy not established; (2–6 yr) 5 mg/day; (>6 yr) same as adult dosage.

Dosage Forms. Tab 10 mg (conventional and rapidly dissolving); **Syrup** 1 mg/mL; **Tab** 5 mg with pseudoephedrine 120 mg (Claritin-D); **Tab** 10 mg with pseudoephedrine 240 mg (Claritin-D 24-hr).

Pharmacokinetics. The drug is rapidly absorbed; bioavailability and peak serum levels are increased by about 50% in the elderly (66–78 yr) or when taken with food. It is 97% bound to plasma proteins and extensively metabolized to an active metabolite, descarboethoxyloratadine. Approximately 80% of a dose is excreted equally in urine and feces as metabolites after 10 days. The half-lives in healthy adults are 8.4 hr (range 3–20) for loratadine and 28 hr (range 8.8–92) for descarboethoxyloratadine.[55,56]

Adverse Reactions. Headache and mild, dose-related drowsiness or fatigue occur occasionally.

Notes. Desloratadine (Clarinex) is the active metabolite of loratadine given in a dose of 5 mg once daily. It might have some advantages such as fewer adverse reactions and drug interactions.

ANTIHISTAMINES COMPARISON CHART

DRUG	DOSAGE FORMS	ADULT DOSAGE	PEDIATRIC DOSAGE	HALF-LIFE (HR)	SIDE EFFECTS	
					Sedation[a]	Anticholinergic
Acrivastine	Tab 8 mg with pseudoephedrine 60 mg (Semprex-D).	PO 1 tab q 4–6 hr, to a maximum of 4/day.	PO (>12 yr) same as adult dosage.	1.5–3	+	±
Azatadine Maleate Optimine	Tab 1 mg.	PO 1–2 mg bid.	(<12 yr) safety and efficacy not established.	12	++	++
Azelastine HCl Astelin	Nasal spray 125 µg/spray.	2 sprays/nostril bid.	(5–11 yr) 1 spray/nostril bid; (≥12 yr) same as adult dosage.	22 (metabolite: 54)	++	++
Brompheniramine Maleate Dimetapp Allergy Various	Cap 4 mg Inj 10 mg/mL.	PO 4 mg q 4–6 hr, to a maximum of 24 mg/day SC, IM, or slow IV 5–20 mg q 12 hr, to a maximum of 40 mg/day.	PO (<12 yr) 0.5 mg/kg/day in 3–4 doses SC, IM, or slow IV 0.5 mg/kg/day in 3–4 divided doses.	25	+	++

(continued)

ANTIHISTAMINES COMPARISON CHART (*continued*)

DRUG	DOSAGE FORMS	ADULT DOSAGE	PEDIATRIC DOSAGE	HALF-LIFE (HR)	Sedation[a]	Anticholinergic
Carbinoxamine Maleate	Drp 2 mg with pseudoephedrine 25 mg/mL Soln 0.4 mg/mL Syrup 0.4, 0.8 mg with pseudoephedrine 6, 12 mg/mL, respectively Tab 4 mg with pseudoephedrine 60 mg Carbodec, Rondec). SR Tab 8 mg with pseudoephedrine 90 mg (Palgic-D).	PO 1 tab qid.	PO 0.2–0.4 mg/kg/day; (1–3 yr) 2 mg tid-qid; (3–6 yr) 2–4 mg tid-qid; (>6 yr) 4–6 mg tid-qid (dosage refers to carbinox-amine component).	10–20	++	+++
Cetirizine HCl Zyrtec	Tab 5, 10 mg Syrup 1 mg/mL.	PO 5–10 mg/day.	PO (2–5 yr) 2.5–5 mg/day; (6–11 yr) 5–10 mg/day.	7–10	+	±
Chlorpheniramine Maleate Chlor-Trimeton Various	Syrup 0.4 mg/mL Chew Tab 2 mg Tab 4 mg SR Tab 8, 12 mg Inj 10, 100 mg/mL.	PO (acute allergic reactions) 12 mg/day in 1–2 divided doses; PO (seasonal allergic rhinitis) 24 mg/day in 1–2 divided doses; IV (acute allergic reactions) 5–40 mg.	PO (seasonal allergic rhinitis) (2–6 yr) 1 mg tid up to 4 mg/day, SR not recommended; (6–12 yr) 2 mg tid up to 12 mg/day; SR not recommended.	15–25	+	++

(continued)

ANTIHISTAMINES COMPARISON CHART (*continued*)

DRUG	DOSAGE FORMS	ADULT DOSAGE	PEDIATRIC DOSAGE	HALF-LIFE (HR)	SIDE EFFECTS Sedation[a]	SIDE EFFECTS Anticholinergic
Clemastine Fumarate Tavist Various	Syrup 0.13 mg (equivalent to 0.1 mg clemastine)/mL Tab 1.34, 2.68 mg (equivalent to 1 and 2 mg clemastine, respectively.	PO 1.34 mg bid–2.68 mg tid, to a maximum of 8.04 mg/day.	PO (6–12 yr) 0.67–1.34 mg bid, to a maximum of 4.02 mg/day.	21	++	+++
Cyproheptadine HCl Periactin Various	Tab 4 mg Syrup 0.4 mg/mL.	PO 4–20 mg/day, usually 4 mg tid–qid, to a maximum of 0.5 mg/kg/day.	PO (2–6 yr) 2 mg bid–tid, to a maximum of 12 mg/day; (7–14 yr) 4 mg bid–tid, to a maximum of 16 mg/day.	—	+	++
Desloratadine Clarinex	Tab 5 mg.	PO 5 mg/day.	—	28	±	±
Dexchlorphenir-amine Maleate Polaramine Various	Syrup 0.4 mg/mL Tab 2 mg SR Tab 4, 6 mg.	PO 2 mg q 4–6 hr, to a maximum of 12 mg/day or SR 4–6 mg hs or q 8–10 hr during the day.	PO (2–5 yr) 0.5 mg q 4–6 hr, to a maximum of 3 mg/day, SR not recommended; (6–12 yr) 1 mg q 4–6 hr or SR 4 mg hs.	15–25	+	++

(continued)

799

ANTIHISTAMINES COMPARISON CHART (continued)

					SIDE EFFECTS	
DRUG	DOSAGE FORMS	ADULT DOSAGE	PEDIATRIC DOSAGE	HALF-LIFE (HR)	Sedation[a]	Anticholinergic
Diphenhydramine HCl Benadryl Various	Cap 25, 50 mg Chew Tab 12.5 mg Elxr 2.5 mg/mL Syrup 1.25, 2.5 mg/mL Tab 25, 50 mg Inj 50 mg/mL.	PO (antihistamine) 25–50 mg tid–qid PO (motion sickness) 50 mg 30 min before exposure, ac and hs PO (antitussive) 25 mg q 4–6 hr PO (nighttime sleep aid) 25–50 mg hs IM, IV 10–50 mg, to a maximum of 400 mg/day.	PO (>9 kg) 5 mg/kg/day, usually 12.5–25 mg tid–qid, to a maximum of 300 mg/day PO (antitussive) (6–12 yr) 12.5 mg q 4 hr, to a maximum of 75 mg/day IM, IV 5 mg/kg, to a maximum of 300 mg/day.	9	+++	+++
Ebastine Kestine (Investigational—RPR)	—	PO 10–20 mg/day.	—	15 (metabolite)	±	±
Fexofenadine HCl Allegra	Cap 60 mg Tab 30, 60, 180 mg	PO 60 mg bid or 180 mg once daily.	PO (>12 yr) same as adult dosage.	14	±	±

(continued)

ANTIHISTAMINES COMPARISON CHART (*continued*)

DRUG	DOSAGE FORMS	ADULT DOSAGE	PEDIATRIC DOSAGE	HALF-LIFE (HR)	Sedation[a]	Anticholinergic
Hydroxyzine HCl/ Pamoate Atarax Vistaril Various	Cap (as pamoate equivalent of HCl salt) 25, 50, 100 mg Susp (as pamoate equivalent of HCl salt) 5 mg/mL Syrup (as HCl) 2 mg/mL Tab (as HCl) 10, 25, 50, 100 mg Inj (as HCl) 25, 50 mg/mL.	PO (pruritus) 25 mg tid-qid; (seasonal allergic rhinitis) titrate up to 150 mg/ day in 1–2 divided doses IM 25–100 mg.	PO (pruritus) (<6 yr) 50 mg/day in 2–3 divided doses; (≥6 yr) 50–100 mg/day in divided doses; (seasonal allergic rhinitis) 25–75 mg/day in 1–2 divided doses IM (perioperative sedation) 0.7 mg/kg/dose; (nausea, vomiting, perioperative adjunctive medication) 1 mg/kg.	16–24	++	++
Levocabastine HCl Livostin	Ophth Susp 0.05% Nasal Spray (Investigational)	Ophth 1 drop qid.	(>12 yr) same as adult dosage.	35–40	+	+
Loratadine Claritin	Tab 10 mg Syrup 1 mg/mL.	PO 10 mg/day.	PO (2–6 yr) 5 mg/day; (>6 yr) 10 mg/day.	8 (metabolite: 28)	±	±
Phenindamine Tartrate Nolahist	Tab 25 mg.	PO 25 mg q 4–6 hr, to a maximum of 150 mg/day.	PO (6–11 yr) 12.5 mg q 4–6 hr, to a maximum of 75 mg/day.	—	+	++

(*continued*)

801

ANTIHISTAMINES COMPARISON CHART (continued)

DRUG	DOSAGE FORMS	ADULT DOSAGE	PEDIATRIC DOSAGE	HALF-LIFE (HR)	SIDE EFFECTS	
					Sedation[a]	Anticholinergic
Promethazine HCl Phenergan Various	Syrup 1.25, 5 mg/mL Tab 12.5, 25, 50 mg Inj 25, 50 mg/mL Supp 12.5, 25, 50 mg.	PO (allergy) 25 mg hs or 12.5 mg ac and hs; (nausea and vomiting) 25 mg initial dose, then 12.5–25 mg q 4–6 hr prn; (adjunctive preoperative use) 25–50 mg/dose IM, IV (IV maximum concentration 25 mg/mL, maximum rate 25 mg/min) or PR (allergy) 25 mg, may repeat in 2 hr; (nausea and vomiting) 12.5–25 mg q 4 hr prn; (ad- junctive pre- and postoperative use) 25–50 mg/dose.	PO (allergy) 6.25–12.5 mg qid; (motion sickness or sedation) 12.5–25 mg/bid; IM, IV, or PR (PR not recommended <2 yr); (allergy) 0.5 mg/kg/day in 4 divided doses; (adjunctive preoperative use) 1 mg/kg/dose, maximum dosage not to exceed one-half of adult dosage.	12	++++	++++

(continued)

ANTIHISTAMINES COMPARISON CHART (continued)

DRUG	DOSAGE FORMS	ADULT DOSAGE	PEDIATRIC DOSAGE	HALF-LIFE (HR)	SIDE EFFECTS	
					Sedation[a]	Anticholinergic
Tripelennamine HCl PBZ Various	Tab 25, 50 mg SR Tab 100 mg.	PO 25–50 mg q 4–6 hr, to a maximum of 600 mg/day.	PO 5 mg/kg/day in 4–6 divided doses, to a maximum of 300 mg/day; SR not recommended.	2–4	++	±
Triprolidine HCl	Syrup 0.25 mg with pseudoephedrine 6 mg/mL Tab 2.5 mg with pseudoephedrine 60 mg (Actifed).	PO 2.5 mg q 4–6 hr, to a maximum of 10 mg/day.	PO (4 months–2 yr) 0.3 mg tid–qid; (2–5 yr) 0.625 mg tid–qid; (6–12 yr) 1.25 mg q 4–6 hr, to a maximum of 4 doses/day.	3	++	++

++++ = very high; +++ = high; ++ = moderate; + = low; ± = low to none; — = not known
[a]Tolerance usually develops during long-term therapy.
From references 55, and 56–60 and product information.

Corticosteroids

BECLOMETHASONE DIPROPIONATE   Beconase, Beclovent, QVAR,
Vancenase, Vanceril

Pharmacology. Potent topical glucocorticoid with little systemic activity because of low systemic bioavailability.

Administration and Adult Dosage. Inhal for asthma (Beclovent, Vanceril) 168-840 μg bid; (QVAR) 80–320 μg bid. (*See* Notes.) **Intranasal for nasal congestion** 42–84 μg/nostril bid–qid (168–336 μg/day total dosage) for several days, then decrease dosage (if symptoms do not recur) to minimum amount necessary to control stuffiness.

Special Populations. *Pediatric Dosage.* Titrate dosage to the lowest effective dosage. **Inhal for asthma** (Beclovent, Vanceril) (6–12 yr) 42–336 μg bid; (>12 yr) same as adult dosage. **Intranasal for nasal congestion** (<6 yr) not recommended; (6–12 yr) 42 μg/nostril bid or tid.[61]

Geriatric Dosage. Same as adult dosage.

Other Conditions. During a severe asthma attack, patients require supplementary treatment with systemic steroids.

Dosage Forms. Inhal (Beclovent, Vanceril) 42, 84 μg/puff (80 and 200 doses/inhaler, and 40 and 120 doses/inhaler, respectively); (QVAR) 40, 80 μg/puff (*see* Notes); **Nasal Inhal** (Beconase, Vancenase) 42 μg/spray (80, 200 doses/inhaler); **Aq Susp** (Beconase AQ, Vancenase AQ) 42, 84 μg/spray (200 and 120 doses/bottle, respectively).

Patient Instructions. Metered-dose Oral Inhaler. (Aerosols) Remove inhaler cap and hold inhaler upright. Shake inhaler. Tilt your head back and breathe out slowly. To position the inhaler, open your mouth with the inhaler 1–2 inches away or in your mouth. (For young children and corticosteroid inhalers, use a spacer or holding chamber.) Press down on the inhaler to release medication as you start to breathe slowly. Breathe slowly for 3 to 5 seconds. Hold your breath for 10 seconds to allow the medication to reach deep into the lungs. Repeat as directed. (Dry Powder) close your mouth tightly around the mouthpiece and inhale rapidly. Hold the device horizontally (parallel to the ground) after it has been activated. Do not exhale into the device. Rinsing your mouth and gargling with water or mouthwash after administration may be beneficial. This medication is for preventive therapy and should not be used to treat acute asthma attacks. **Nasal Inhaler.** Blow your nose before use. Shake the container well. Remove the protective cap and hold the inhaler between your thumb and forefinger. Tilt your head back slightly and insert the end of the inhaler into one nostril. While holding the other nostril closed with one finger, press down once to release 1 dose and, at the same time, inhale gently. Hold your breath for a few seconds and then breathe out slowly through your mouth. Repeat the process in the other nostril. Avoid blowing your nose for the next 15 minutes.

Missed Doses. Take the missed dose as soon as possible. If it is almost time for the next dose, skip the missed dose and go back to regular dosage schedule. Do not double doses.

Pharmacokinetics. *Onset and Duration.* Effect is usually evident within a few days but might take 2–4 weeks for maximum improvement.[62]

Fate. Only ≤10% of an inhaled dose is deposited in the lung; 80% is deposited in the mouth and swallowed. Oral absorption is slow and incomplete (61–90%), and the drug undergoes extensive first-pass metabolism, resulting in oral bioavailability of less than 5%.[63] Well absorbed from the lung and extensively metabolized, with 65% excreted in the bile and <10% of unchanged drug and metabolites excreted in urine.[63]

t½. 15 hr.

Adverse Reactions. After oral use, localized growth of *Candida* in the mouth occurs frequently, but clinically apparent infections occur only occasionally. Hoarseness and dry mouth occur occasionally; minimal to no suppression of the pituitary–adrenal axis occurs at the recommended dosage; however, dose-dependent suppression occurs at higher dosages.[62,64–67] After intranasal use, irritation and burning of the nasal mucosa and sneezing occur occasionally; intranasal and pharyngeal *Candida* infections, nasal ulceration, and epistaxis occur rarely. Cases of growth suppression unrelated to suppression of the pituitary–adrenal axis have been reported after use of intranasally or orally inhaled corticosteroids in children. With oral inhalation, the mean reduction in growth velocity is 1 cm/yr (range 0.3–1.8 cm/yr). The long-term implications for ultimate adult height are unknown.

Contraindications. Status asthmaticus or other acute episodes of asthma in which intensive measures are required; beclomethasone-exacerbated symptoms.

Precautions. During stress or severe asthmatic attacks, patients withdrawn from systemic corticosteroid should contact their physician immediately. Use the lowest effective dosage possible in children. The potential growth effects of inhaled corticosteroids in children should be weighed against the clinical benefits of the corticosteroids and the availability of nonsteroid alternatives.

Drug Interactions. None known.

Parameters to Monitor. For treatment of asthma, frequency of daytime asthmatic symptoms, and nocturnal use of prn sympathomimetic inhaler. For nasal congestion, relief of symptoms. Routinely monitor the growth of children receiving inhaled corticosteroids (eg, via stadiometry).

Notes. Patients needing long-term use of an orally inhaled corticosteroid should be continued on therapeutic doses of a bronchodilator. Before use, a patient should be as free of symptoms as possible, which can be achieved with a 1-week course of oral **prednisone.** The nasal inhalation provides effective, prompt relief of nasal congestion when the maximally tolerated dosage of oral sympathomimetics is inadequate. (*See also* Inhaled Corticosteroids Comparison Chart.)

INHALED CORTICOSTEROIDS COMPARISON CHART

| DRUG | DOSAGE FORMS[b] | DAILY DOSAGE[a] | | | | RECEPTOR BINDING HALF-LIFE | TOPICAL POTENCY[c] | ORAL BIOAVAILABILITY[d] |
		Low (Step 2)	Medium (Step 3)	High (Step 4)			
SINGLE-INGREDIENT PRODUCTS							
Beclomethasone Dipropionate Beclovent Vanceril	MDI: 42, 84 μg/puff.	Adult: 168–504 μg Child: 84–336 μg	504–840 μg 336–672 μg	>840 μg >672 μg	7.5 hr	600	20%
Beclomethasone Dipropionate HFA QVAR	MDI: 40, 80 μg/puff.	Adult: 80–160 μg	160–320 mg	>320 μg	7.5 hr	600	20%
Budesonide Pulmicort	DPI: 200 μg/inhal Neb Susp: 125, 250 μg/mL.	Adult: 200–400 μg Child: 100–200 μg	400–600 μg 200–400 μg	>600 μg >400 μg	5.1 hr	980	11%
Flunisolide AeroBid AeroBid-M	MDI: 250 μg/puff.	Adult: 500–1000 μg Child: 500–750 μg	1000–2000 μg 750–1250 μg	>2000 μg >1250 μg	3.5 hr	330	21%
Fluticasone Propionate Flovent	MDI: 44, 110, 220 μg/puff. DPI: 50, 100, 250 μg/inhal.	Adult: 88–264 μg Child: 88–176 μg	264–660 μg 176–440 μg	>660 μg >440 μg	10.5 hr	1200	1%

(continued)

INHALED CORTICOSTEROIDS COMPARISON CHART (*continued*)

| DRUG | DOSAGE FORMS[b] | DAILY DOSAGE[a] | | | RECEPTOR BINDING HALF-LIFE | TOPICAL POTENCY[c] | ORAL BIOAVAILABILITY[d] |
		Low (Step 2)	Medium (Step 3)	High (Step 4)			
Triamcinolone Acetonide Azmacort	MDI: 100 μg/puff.	Adult: 400–1000 μg Child: 400–800 μg	1000–2000 μg 800–1200 μg	>2000 μg >1200 μg	3.9 hr	330	11%
COMBINATION PRODUCTS							
Fluticasone Propionate and Salmeterol Advair Diskus	DPI: Fluticasone 100 μg, salmeterol 50 μg/inhal; Fluticasone 250 μg, salmeterol 50 μg/inhal; Fluticasone 500 μg, salmeterol 50 μg/inhal.	Adult: 100–50 bid	250–50 bid	500–50 bid	—	—	—

DPI = dry powder inhaler; MDI = metered-dose inhaler; Neb = nebulizer.

[a]Dosage ranges correspond to recommended treatment intensities for steps 2–4 of the NIH guidelines for diagnosis and management of asthma: step 1 = mild intermittent; step 2 = mild persistent; step 3 = moderate persistent; step 4 = severe persistent.[20] The most important determinant of appropriate dosage is the clinician's judgment of the patient's response to therapy; the clinician must monitor the patient's response on several clinical parameters and adjust the dosage accordingly. The stepwise approach to therapy emphasizes that once control of symptoms is achieved, the dosage of medication should be carefully titrated to the minimum dosage required to maintain control, thereby reducing the potential for adverse effects.

[b]MDI dosages are expressed as the actuator dose (the amount of drug leaving the actuator and delivered to the patient), which is the labeling required in the United States. This is different from the dosage expressed as the valve dose (the amount of drug leaving the valve, not all of which is available to the patient), which is used in many European countries and in some of the scientific literature. DPI doses are expressed as the amount of drug in the inhaler following activation.

[c]Potency determined from skin blanching; dexamethasone is the reference drug and has a value of 1 in this assay.

[d]Oral bioavailability of the swallowed portion of the dose received by the patient. About 80% of the dose from an MDI without a spacer is swallowed. Nearly all of the drug delivered to the lungs is bioavailable. From 10–30% of an MDI dose is delivered to the lungs, depending on the product and device. Both the relative potency and the total bioavailability (inhaled + swallowed) determine the systemic activity of the product.

From references 20 and 68–70.

INTRANASAL CORTICOSTEROIDS COMPARISON CHART

DRUG	DOSAGE FORMS	ADULT DOSAGE	PEDIATRIC DOSAGE[a]
Beclomethasone Dipropionate Beconase Vancenase	Aerosol, Metered-Dose 42 µg/spray Spray, Aqueous 42, 84 µg/spray.	1–2 sprays into each nostril bid-qid.	1 spray into each nostril bid-tid.
Budesonide Rhinocort	Aerosol, Metered-Dose 32 µg/spray.	2 sprays into each nostril bid or 4 sprays into each nostril q AM, to a maximum of 800 µg/day.	2 sprays into each nostril bid or 4 sprays into each nostril q AM, to a maximum of 400 µg/day.
Flunisolide Nasalide Nasarel	Spray, Aqueous 25 µg/spray.	2 sprays into each nostril bid, to a maximum of 8 sprays/day into each nostril.	1 spray into each nostril tid-qid.
Fluticasone Propionate Flonase	Spray, Aqueous 50 µg/spray.	2 sprays into each nostril daily or 1 spray into each nostril bid; maintenance 1 spray into each nostril daily, to a maximum of 200 µg/day.	(≥4 yr) 1 spray in each nostril daily (100 µg/day); for nonresponders, 2 sprays in each nostril daily or 1 spray in each nostril bid, decrease to 100 µg/day once a response is achieved.
Mometasone Furoate Nasonex	Spray, Aqueous 50 µg/spray.	2 sprays into each nostril once daily.	(<12 yr) not established.
Triamcinolone Acetonide Nasacort Nasarel	Spray, Aqueous 55 µg/spray.	2 sprays into each nostril daily; adjust to a maximum of 4 sprays/day in 1–4 divided doses; maintenance as low as 1 spray/day.	Same as adult dosage.

[a]Unless otherwise stated, pediatric dosage is for patients 6–12 yr; dosages for patients <6 yr have generally not been established.
From references 68–70.

Cough and Cold

DEXTROMETHORPHAN HYDROBROMIDE   Various

Pharmacology. Dextromethorphan is the nonanalgesic, nonaddictive D-isomer of the codeine analogue of levorphanol. With usual antitussive doses, the cough threshold is elevated centrally with little effect on the respiratory, cardiovascular, or GI systems.

Administration and Adult Dosage. PO as cough suppressant 10–30 mg q 4–8 hr, to a maximum of 120 mg/day; **SR** 60 mg q 12 hr.

Special Populations. *Pediatric Dosage.* **PO as cough suppressant** (<2 yr) not recommended; (2–6 yr) 2.5–7.5 mg q 4–8 hr, to a maximum of 30 mg/day (as syrup); (6–12 yr) 5–10 mg q 4 hr or 15 mg q 6–8 hr, to a maximum of 60 mg/day; (>12 yr) same as adult dosage. **SR** (2–5 yr) 15 mg q 12 hr; (6–12 yr) 30 mg q 12 hr. (*See* Notes.)

Geriatric Dosage. Same as adult dosage.

Dosage Forms. Cap 30 mg; **Lozenge** 2.5, 5, 7.5, 15 mg; **Syrup** 0.66, 0.7, 1, 1.5, 2, 3 mg/mL; **SR Susp** 6 mg/mL; (available in many combination products in different concentrations).

Patient Instructions. Do not use this drug to suppress productive cough or chronic cough that occurs with smoking, asthma, or emphysema. Report if your cough persists.

Pharmacokinetics. *Onset and Duration.* PO onset 1–2 hr; duration up to 6–8 hr with non-SR, 12 hr for SR suspension.[71]

Fate. Extensively metabolized, including appreciable first-pass effect, mainly to the active metabolite dextrorphan. Genetically determined polymorphic metabolism primarily by CYP2D6 with extensive (93%) and poor (7%) metabolizers.[72] (*See* Notes.)

t½. (Extensive metabolizers) <4 to about 9 hr; (poor metabolizers) 17–138 hr.[73]

Adverse Reactions. Occasional mild drowsiness and GI upset. Intoxication, bizarre behavior, CNS depression, and respiratory depression can occur with extremely high dosages. Naloxone might be effective in reversing these effects.[74–77] Reports of dextromethorphan abuse have increased, especially among teenagers.[78,79]

Contraindications. MAOI therapy.[80]

Precautions. Generally, do not use in patients with chronic cough or cough associated with excessive secretions.

Drug Interactions. Concurrent MAOIs can cause hypotension, hyperpyrexia, nausea, and coma. Drugs that inhibit CYP2D6 can inhibit dextromethorphan metabolism, but serious effects are not reported.

Parameters to Monitor. Observe for relief of cough and CNS side effects.

Notes. Approximately equipotent with **codeine** in antitussive effectiveness in adults.[71,74] One trial of dextromethorphan and codeine for night cough in children found neither superior to placebo, and their efficacies have been questioned for this or any other use in children.[75,81] Used commonly for CYP2D6 phenotyping.[82] Dextromethorphan is currently being investigated for its analgesic-sparing effect.[83] (*See also* Codeine Salts.)

GUAIFENESIN
2/G, Robitussin, Organidin NR, Various

Pharmacology. Guaifenesin is proposed to have an expectorant action through an increased output of respiratory tract fluid, enhancing the flow of less viscid secretions, promoting ciliary action, and facilitating the removal of inspissated mucus. Evidence of the effectiveness of guaifenesin is largely subjective and not well established clinically.[74,84–87]

Administration and Adult Dosage. PO as an expectorant 100–400 mg q 4 hr; SR 600–1200 mg q 12 hr, to a maximum of 2.4 g/day.[85]

Special Populations. *Pediatric Dosage.* PO as an expectorant (2–6 yr) 50–100 mg q 4 hr, to a maximum of 600 mg/day; (6–12 yr) 100–200 mg q 4 hr, to a maximum of 1200 mg/day; (≥12 yr) same as adult dosage. SR (2–6 yr) 300 mg q 12 hr; (6–12 yr) 600 mg q 12 hr.

Geriatric Dosage. Same as adult dosage.

Dosage Forms. Cap 200 mg; Syrup 20, 40 mg/mL; Tab 100, 200, 1200 mg; SR Cap 300 mg; SR Tab 600, 1200 mg. SR Tab 600 mg with pseudoephedrine 120 mg (Entex PSE, various).

Patient Instructions. Take this drug with a large quantity of fluid to ensure proper drug action. Report if your cough persists for more than 1 week, recurs, or is accompanied by a high fever, rash, or persistent headache. Excessive dosage can cause nausea and vomiting.

Adverse Reactions. Occasional nausea and vomiting, especially with excessive dosage; dizziness; headache.

Precautions. Generally, do not use in patients with chronic cough or cough associated with excessive secretions.

Drug Interactions. None known.

Notes. May interfere with certain laboratory determinations of 5-hydroxyindoleacetic acid and vanillylmandelic acid but does not cause a positive stool guaiac reaction in normal subjects.[86]

PSEUDOEPHEDRINE HYDROCHLORIDE
Efidac/24, Sudafed, Various

Pharmacology. Pseudoephedrine is an indirect-acting agent that stimulates α-, β_1-, and β_2-adrenergic receptors via release of endogenous adrenergic amines. It is used primarily for decongestion of nasal mucosa.

Administration and Adult Dosage. PO as a decongestant 60 mg q 4–6 hr, to a maximum of 240 mg/day. PO SR Cap/Tab 120 mg q 12 hr; (Efidac/24) 240 mg once daily.

Special Populations. *Pediatric Dosage.* PO (3–12 months) 3 drops/kg q 4–6 hr, to a maximum of 4 doses/day; (1–2 yr) 7 drops (0.2 mL)/kg q 4–6 hr, to a maximum of 4 doses/day; (2–5 yr) 15 mg (as syrup) q 4–6 hr prn, to a maximum of

60 mg/day; (6–12 yr) 30 mg q 4–6 hr prn, to a maximum of 120 mg/day; (>12 yr) same as adult dosage. Do not give SR Cap/Tab 120 or 240 mg to patients <12 yr.

Geriatric Dosage. Demonstrate safe use of short-acting formulation before using an SR product.

Dosage Forms. **Cap** 60 mg; **Drp** 9.4 mg/mL; **Syrup** 3, 6 mg/mL; **Tab** 30, 60 mg; **SR Tab** (12-hr) 120 mg; (24-hr) 240 mg (Efidac/24). **Tab** 60 mg with triprolidine HCl 2.5 mg (Actifed, various). **SR Cap** 120 mg with chlorpheniramine maleate 8 mg (Deconamine SR, various).

Patient Instructions. Avoid taking the last dose of the day near bedtime if you have difficulty sleeping. Do not crush or chew sustained-release preparations.

Pharmacokinetics. *Onset and Duration.* Onset within 30 min on an empty stomach, within 1 hr for SR forms; duration $\geq$3 hr, 8–12 hr for most SR forms, 24 hr for Efidac/24.[88,89]

Fate. Solution and immediate-release tablets are rapidly and completely absorbed orally. SR dosage forms attain peak serum levels in (12-hr product) 4–6 hr or (24-hr product) 12 hr. Food appears to delay absorption of non-SR forms, but not the SR forms.[90,91] V_d is 2.7 $\pm$ 0.2 L/kg; Cl averages 0.44 L/hr/kg. Partly metabolized to inactive metabolite(s), and 6% metabolized to active metabolite, norpseudoephedrine; 45–90% excreted unchanged in urine depending on urinary pH and flow.[92,93]

$t_{1/2}$. Urinary flow and pH dependent; 13 $\pm$ 3 hr at pH 8; 6.9 $\pm$ 1.2 hr at pH 5.5–6; 4.7 $\pm$ 1.4 hr at pH 5.[92,93]

Adverse Reactions. Frequent mild transient nervousness, insomnia, irritability, or headache. Usually negligible pressor effect in normotensive patients.[94,95]

Contraindications. Severe hypertension; coronary artery disease; MAOI therapy.

Precautions. Use with caution in patients with renal failure,[96] hypertension, diabetes mellitus, ischemic heart disease, increased intraocular pressure, prostatic hypertrophy, urinary retention, or thyroid disease. Elderly patients might be particularly sensitive to CNS effects. If use is necessary in infants with phenylketonuria, reduce dosage to avoid possible increased agitation.[97]

Drug Interactions. Concurrent MAOIs can increase pressor response. Urinary alkalinizers can decrease pseudoephedrine clearance.

Parameters to Monitor. Nasal stuffiness, CNS stimulation, blood pressure in hypertensive patients.

Notes. Combination with an antihistamine can provide additive benefit in seasonal allergic rhinitis because antihistamines do not relieve nasal stuffiness.[98,99] Neither these combinations nor decongestants alone provide consistent long-term benefit for reduction of middle ear effusion in children with otitis media and are not recommended for this use.[100,101]

REFERENCES

1. Tashkin DP, Jenne JW. Beta adrenergic agonists. In, Weiss EB et al., eds. *Bronchial asthma: mechanisms and therapeutics.* 3rd ed. Boston: Little, Brown; 1993:700–48.

2. Hochhaus G, Möllmann H. Pharmacokinetic/pharmacodynamic characteristics of the β_2-agonists terbutaline, salbutamol and fenoterol. *Int J Clin Pharmacol Ther Toxicol* 1992;30:342–62.

3. Spitzer OW et al. The use of β-agonists and the risk of death and near death from asthma. *N Engl J Med* 1992; 326:501–6.

4. Mullen M et al. The association between β-agonist use and death from asthma. A meta-analytic integration of case-control studies. *JAMA* 1993;270:1842–5.

5. Murphy S, Kelly HW. Cromolyn sodium: a review of its mechanisms and clinical use in asthma. *Drug Intell Clin Pharm* 1987;21:22–35.

6. Berman BA. Cromolyn: past, present, and future. *Pediatr Clin North Am* 1983;30:915–30.

7. Joseph JC. Compatibility of nebulized admixtures. *Ann Pharmacother* 1997;31:487–9.

8. Edwards AM. Oral sodium cromoglycate: its use in the management of food allergy. *Clin Exp Allergy* 1995; 25(suppl 1):31–3.

9. Trujillo MH, Bellorin-Font E. Drugs commonly administered by intravenous infusion in intensive care units: a practical guide. *Crit Care Med* 1990;18:232–8.

10. Gross NJ, Skorodin MS. Anticholinergic agents. In, Jenne JW, Murphy S, eds. *Drug therapy for asthma: research and clinical practice.* New York: Marcel Dekker; 1987:615–68.

11. Milner AD. Ipratropium bromide in airways obstruction in childhood. *Postgrad Med J* 1987;63(suppl 1):53–6.

12. Shuk S et al. Efficacy of frequent nebulized ipratropium bromide added to frequent high-dose albuterol therapy in severe childhood asthma. *J Pediatr* 1995;126:639–45.

13. Gross NJ. Ipratropium bromide. *N Engl J Med* 1988;319:486–94.

14. Chung KF. Leukotriene receptor antagonists and biosynthesis inhibitors: potential breakthrough in asthma therapy. *Eur Respir J* 1995;8:1203–13.

15. Larsen JS et al. Antileukotriene therapy for asthma. *Am J Health Syst Pharm* 1996;53:2821–30.

16. Wasserman SI. A review of some recent clinical studies with nedocromil sodium. *J Allergy Clin Immunol* 1993;92:210–5.

17. Brogden RN, Sorkin EM. Nedocromil sodium. An updated review of its pharmacological properties and therapeutic efficacy in asthma. *Drugs* 1993;45:693–715.

18. Brogden RN, Faulds D. Salmeterol xinafoate. A review of its pharmacological properties and therapeutic potential in reversible obstructive airway disease. *Drugs* 1991;42:895–912.

19. Jenne JW. Physiology and pharmacodynamics of the xanthines. In, Jenne JW, Murphy S, eds. *Drug therapy for asthma: research and clinical practice.* New York: Marcel Dekker; 1987:297–334.

20. *Expert Panel Report 2: guidelines for the diagnosis and management of asthma.* Publication No. 97-4051. Bethesda, MD: National Heart, Lung, and Blood Institute, National Asthma Education and Prevention Program; U.S. Department of Health and Human Services; 1997.

21. Weinberger MM et al. Theophylline in asthma. *N Engl J Med* 1996;334:1380–8.

22. Weinberger MM, Hendeles L. Theophylline. In, Middleton E et al., eds. *Allergy: principles and practice.* St. Louis: Mosby; 1993:816–55.

23. Asmus MJ et al. Pharmacokinetics and drug disposition: apparent decrease in population clearance of theophylline: implications for dosage. *Clin Pharmacol Ther* 1997;62:483–9.

24. Self TH et al. Reassessing the therapeutic range for theophylline on laboratory report forms: the importance of 5–15 μg/ml. *Pharmacotherapy* 1993;13:590–4.

25. Hendeles L, Weinberger M. Selection of a slow-release theophylline product. *J Allergy Clin Immunol* 1986;78:743–51.

26. Morris JF. Geriatric considerations. In, Weiss EB et al., eds. *Bronchial asthma: mechanisms and therapeutics.* 3rd ed. Boston: Little, Brown; 1993:1017–22.

27. Kelly HW. Theophylline toxicity. In, Jenne JW, Murphy S, eds. *Drug therapy for asthma: research and clinical practice.* New York: Marcel Dekker; 1987:925–51.

28. González MA et al. Pharmacokinetic comparison of a once-daily and twice-daily theophylline delivery system. *Clin Ther* 1994;16:686–92.

29. González MA, Straughn AB. Effect of meals and dosage-form modification on theophylline bioavailability from a 24-hour sustained-release delivery system. *Clin Ther* 1994;16:804–14.

30. Campoli-Richards DM et al. Cetirizine. A review of its pharmacological properties and clinical potential in allergic rhinitis, pollen-induced asthma, and chronic urticaria. *Drugs* 1990;40:762–81.

31. Mansmann HC et al. Efficacy and safety of cetirizine in perennial allergic rhinitis. *Ann Allergy* 1992;68:348–53.

32. Spencer CM et al. Cetirizine. A reappraisal of its pharmacological properties and therapeutic use in selected allergic disorders. *Drugs* 1993;46:1055–80.

33. Barnes CL et al. Cetirizine: a new, nonsedating antihistamine. *Ann Pharmacother* 1993;27:464–70.

34. Sheffer AL et al. Cetirizine: antiallergic therapy beyond traditional H_1 antihistamines. *J Allergy Clin Immunol* 1990;86:1040–6.

35. Simons FER et al. Pharmacokinetics and efficacy of chlorpheniramine in children. *J Allergy Clin Immunol* 1982;69:376–81.
36. Cook TJ et al. Degree and duration of skin test suppression and side effects with antihistamines. *J Allergy Clin Immunol* 1973;51:71–7.
37. Usdin Yasuda S et al. Chlorpheniramine plasma concentration and histamine H_1-receptor occupancy. *Clin Pharmacol Ther* 1995;58:210–20.
38. Huang SM et al. Pharmacokinetics of chlorpheniramine after intravenous and oral administration in normal adults. *Eur J Clin Pharmacol* 1982;22:359–65.
39. Benet LZ et al. Design and optimization of dosage regimens; pharmacokinetic data. In, Hardman JG et al., eds. *Goodman and Gilman's the pharmacological basis of therapeutics.* 9th ed. New York: McGraw-Hill; 1996:1707–92.
40. Paton DM, Webster DR. Clinical pharmacokinetics of H_1-receptor antagonists (the antihistamines). *Clin Pharmacokinet* 1985;10:477–97.
41. Simons FER. H_1-receptor antagonists: clinical pharmacology and therapeutics. *J Allergy Clin Immunol* 1989;84:845–61.
42. Simons KJ et al. Diphenhydramine: pharmacokinetics and pharmacodynamics in elderly adults, young adults, and children. *J Clin Pharmacol* 1990;30:665–71.
43. Carruthers SG et al. Correlation between plasma diphenhydramine level and sedative and antihistamine effects. *Clin Pharmacol Ther* 1978;23:375–82.
44. Blyden GT et al. Pharmacokinetics of diphenhydramine and a demethylated metabolite following intravenous and oral administration. *J Clin Pharmacol* 1986;26:529–33.
45. Spector R et al. Diphenhydramine in Orientals and Caucasians. *Clin Pharmacol Ther* 1980;28:229–34.
46. Meredith CG et al. Diphenhydramine disposition in chronic liver disease. *Clin Pharmacol Ther* 1984;35:474–9.
47. Glazko AJ et al. Metabolic disposition of diphenhydramine. *Clin Pharmacol Ther* 1974;16:1066–76.
48. Albert KS et al. Pharmacokinetics of diphenhydramine in man. *J Pharmacokinet Biopharm* 1975;3:159–70.
49. Schaaf L et al. Suppression of seasonal allergic rhinitis symptoms with daily hydroxyzine. *J Allergy Clin Immunol* 1979;63:129–33.
50. Gendreau-Reid L et al. Comparison of the suppressive effect of astemizole, terfenadine, and hydroxyzine on histamine-induced wheals and flares in humans. *J Allergy Clin Immunol* 1986;77:335–40.
51. Simons KJ et al. Pharmacokinetic and pharmacodynamic studies of the H_1-receptor antagonist hydroxyzine in the elderly. *Clin Pharmacol Ther* 1989;45:9–14.
52. Simons FER et al. Pharmacokinetics and antipruritic effects of hydroxyzine in children with atopic dermatitis. *J Pediatr* 1984;104:123–7.
53. Simons FE et al. The pharmacokinetics and antihistaminic of the H_1 receptor antagonist hydroxyzine. *J Allergy Clin Immunol* 1984;73(1 pt 1):69–75.
54. Simons FER et al. The pharmacokinetics and pharmacodynamics of hydroxyzine in patients with primary biliary cirrhosis. *J Clin Pharmacol* 1989;29:809–15.
55. Simons FER, Simons KJ. Antihistamines. In, Middleton E et al., eds. *Allergy. Principles and practice.* St. Louis: Mosby; 1993:856–79.
56. Gonzalez MA, Estes KS. Pharmacokinetic overview of oral second-generation H_1 antihistamines. *Int J Clin Pharmacol Ther* 1998;36:292–300.
57. Corey JP. Advances in the pharmacotherapy of allergic rhinitis: second-generation H_1-receptor antagonists. *Otolaryngol Head Neck Surg* 1993;109:584–92.
58. Krause HF. Antihistamines and decongestants. *Otolaryngol Head Neck Surg* 1992;107:835–40.
59. Korenblat PE, Wedner HJ. *Allergy. Theory and practice.* 2nd ed. Philadelphia: WB Saunders; 1992:300–3.
60. Desager J-P, Horsmans Y. Pharmacokinetic-pharmacodynamic relationships of H_1-antihistamines. *Clin Pharmacokinet* 1995;28:419–32.
61. Kobayaski RH et al. Beclomethasone dipropionate aqueous nasal spray for seasonal allergic rhinitis in children. *Ann Allergy* 1989;62:205–8.
62. Fauci AS et al. Glucocorticoid therapy: mechanisms of action and clinical considerations. *Ann Intern Med* 1976;84:304–15.
63. Azarnoff DL, ed. *Steroid therapy.* Philadelphia: WB Saunders; 1975.
64. Barnes PJ. Inhaled glucocorticoids for asthma. *N Engl J Med* 1995;332:868–75.
65. Barnes PJ, Pederson S. Efficacy and safety of inhaled corticosteroid in asthma. *Am Rev Respir Dis* 1993;149:S1–26.
66. Szefler SJ. A comparison of aerosol glucocorticoids in the treatment of chronic bronchial asthma. *Pediatr Asthma Allergy Immunol* 1991;5:227–35.
67. Kamada AK. Therapeutic controversies in the treatment of asthma. *Ann Pharmacother* 1994;28:904–14.

814   RESPIRATORY DRUGS

68. Toogood JH et al. Aerosol corticosteroid. In, Weiss EB et al., eds. *Bronchial asthma: mechanisms and therapeutics.* 3rd ed. Boston: Little, Brown; 1993:818–41.
69. McCubbin MM et al. A bioassay for topical and systemic effect of three inhaled steroids. *Clin Pharmacol Ther* 1995;57:455–60.
70. Holliday SM et al. Inhaled fluticasone propionate. A review of its pharmacodynamic and pharmacokinetic properties, and therapeutic use in asthma. *Drugs* 1994;47:318–31.
71. Matthys H et al. Dextromethorphan and codeine: objective assessment of antitussive activity in patients with chronic cough. *J Int Med Res* 1983;11:92–100.
72. Jacqz-Aigrain E et al. CYP2D6- and CYP3A-dependent metabolism of dextromethorphan in humans. *Pharmacogenetics* 1993;3:197–204.
73. Woodworth JR et al. The polymorphic metabolism of dextromethorphan. *J Clin Pharmacol* 1987;27:139–43.
74. Bryant BG, Lombardi TP. Cold, cough, and allergy products. In, Covington TR, ed. *Handbook of nonprescription drugs.* 10th ed. Washington, DC: American Pharmaceutical Association; 1993:89–115.
75. American Academy of Pediatrics. Committee on Drugs. Use of codeine- and dextromethorphan-containing cough syrups in pediatrics. *Pediatrics* 1997;99:918–20.
76. Shaul WL et al. Dextromethorphan toxicity: reversal by naloxone. *Pediatrics* 1977;59:117–9.
77. Katona B, Wason S. Dextromethorphan danger. *N Engl J Med* 1986;314:993. Letter.
78. Bem JL, Peck R. Dextromethorphan. An overview of safety issues. *Drug Safety* 1992;190–9.
79. Cranston JW, Yoast R. Abuse of dextromethorphan. *Arch Fam Med* 1999;8:99–100.
80. Nierenberg DW, Semprebon M. The central nervous system serotonin syndrome. *Clin Pharmacol Ther* 1993;53:84–8.
81. Taylor JA et al. Efficacy of cough suppressants in children. *J Pediatr* 1993;122:799–802.
82. Streetman DS et al. Dose dependency of dextromethorphan for cytochrome P450 2D6 (CYP2D6) phenotyping. *Clin Pharmacol Ther* 1999;66:535–41.
83. Henderson DJ et al. Perioperative dextromethorphan reduces postoperative pain after hysterectomy. *Anesth Analg* 1999;89:399–402.
84. Anon. Guaiphenesin and iodide. *Drug Ther Bull* 1985;23:62–4.
85. Anon. Cold, cough, allergy, bronchodilator, and antiasthmatic drug products for over-the-counter human use; expectorant drug products for over-the-counter human use; final monograph. *Fed Regist* 1989;54:8494–509.
86. Ziment I. Drugs modifying the sol-layer and the hydration of mucus. In, Braga PC, Allegra L, eds. *Drugs in bronchial mucology.* New York: Raven Press; 1989:293–322.
87. Sisson JH et al. Effects of guaifenesin on nasal mucociliary clearance and ciliary beat frequency in healthy volunteers. *Chest* 1995;107:747–51.
88. Roth RP et al. Nasal decongestant activity of pseudoephedrine. *Ann Otol Rhinol Laryngol* 1977;86:235–42.
89. Hamilton LH et al. A study of sustained action pseudoephedrine in allergic rhinitis. *Ann Allergy* 1982;48:87–92.
90. Hwang SS et al. In vitro and in vivo evaluation of a once-daily controlled-release pseudoephedrine product. *J Clin Pharmacol* 1995;35:259–67.
91. Kanfer I et al. Pharmacokinetics of oral decongestants. *Pharmacotherapy* 1993;13(6 pt 2):116S–28.
92. Brater DC et al. Renal excretion of pseudoephedrine. *Clin Pharmacol Ther* 1980;28:690–4.
93. Kuntzman RG et al. The influence of urinary pH on the plasma half-life of pseudoephedrine in man and dog and a sensitive assay for its determination in human plasma. *Clin Pharmacol Ther* 1971;12:62–7.
94. Chua SS, Benrimoj SI. Non-prescription sympathomimetic agents and hypertension. *Med Toxicol* 1988;3:387–417.
95. Beck RA et al. Cardiovascular effects of pseudoephedrine in medically controlled hypertensive patients. *Arch Intern Med* 1992;152:1242–5.
96. Sica DA, Comstock TJ. Case report: pseudoephedrine accumulation in renal failure. *Am J Med Sci* 1989;298:261–3.
97. Spielberg SP, Schulman JD. A possible reaction to pseudoephedrine in a patient with phenylketonuria. *J Pediatr* 1977;90:1026.
98. Hendeles L. Selecting a decongestant. *Pharmacotherapy* 1993;13(6 pt 2):129S–34.
99. Bryant BG, Lombardi TP. Cold, cough, and allergy products. In, Covington TR, ed. *Handbook of nonprescription drugs.* 10th ed. Washington, DC: American Pharmaceutical Association; 1993:89–115.
100. Thoene DE, Johnson CE. Pharmacotherapy of otitis media. *Pharmacotherapy* 1991;11:212–21.
101. Bahal N, Nahata MC. Recent advances in the treatment of otitis media. *J Clin Pharm Ther* 1992;17:201–15.

PART II

Clinical Information

Principal Editor: William G. Troutman, PharmD

- Drug-Induced Diseases
- Drug Use in Special Populations
- Immunization
- Medical Emergencies
- Drug Interactions and Interferences
- Nutrition Support

Drug-Induced Diseases

William G. Troutman

Drug-Induced Blood Dyscrasias

This table does not include all drugs capable of causing the specified dyscrasias and excludes cancer chemotherapeutic agents, which are known for producing dose-related bone marrow suppression. Five major types of blood dyscrasias have been selected for inclusion in this table; the following abbreviations indicate specific blood dyscrasias:

AA   — Aplastic Anemia
AGN — Agranulocytosis, Granulocytopenia, or Neutropenia
HA   — Hemolytic Anemia
MA   — Macrocytic Anemia
Th   — Thrombocytopenia

DRUG AND DYSCRASIA	NATURE OF DYSCRASIA
Abciximab	
Th	The combination of abciximab and heparin presents twice the risk of mild and severe thrombocytopenia as the combination of placebo and heparin. (*See also* Heparin.)[1]
Acetaminophen	
Th	Scattered reports only; observed in 6 of 174 overdose patients in one report; might be an immune reaction.[2,3]
Alcohol	
HA	Most commonly encountered in chronic alcoholism.[4]
MA	Results from malnutrition and decreased folate absorption and/or utilization. Responds rapidly to folic acid administration.[4]
Th	Transient in many drinkers; persistent thrombocytopenia can accompany advanced alcoholic liver disease.[4]

(*continued*)

DRUG AND DYSCRASIA	NATURE OF DYSCRASIA
Amphotericin B	
AGN	Scattered reports only.[4,5]
Th	Scattered reports only.[5,6]
Antidepressants, Heterocyclic	
AGN	Idiosyncratic reaction, probably resulting from a direct toxic effect rather than allergy. Most commonly occurs between the 2nd and 8th weeks of therapy.[4,10,11]
Ascorbic Acid	
HA	In G-6-PD deficiency with large doses.[4]
Aspirin	
HA	Almost always encountered in patients with G-6-PD deficiency, usually in conjunction with infection or other complicating factors.[4,12]
Th	Can occur in addition to the drug's effects on platelet adhesiveness. Some evidence for an immune reaction.[2,4,13]
Azathioprine	
AGN	WBC counts <2500/μL occur in about 3% of rheumatoid arthritis patients treated with azathioprine; an additional 15% develop some lesser degree of leukopenia.[14]
Captopril	
AGN	Prevalence estimated at 1/5000 patients. The prevalence increases greatly in patients with reduced renal function or collagen–vascular diseases and reaches 7% in patients with renal impairment and a collagen–vascular disease. Most common during the first 3 weeks of therapy.[15]
Carbamazepine	
AA	27 cases reported from 1964–1988; onset can be delayed until weeks or months after the initiation of therapy.[4,16]
AGN	Transient leukopenia occurs in about 10% of patients, usually during the first month of therapy. Recovery usually occurs within a week of drug withdrawal. Persistent leukopenia occurs in 2%.[16,17]
Th	Prevalence estimated at 2%.[16,18]
Cephalosporins	
AGN	Rare; possibly the result of an immune reaction but occurs most often with high dosages and parenteral therapy lasting >2 weeks.[4,19,20]
HA	Positive direct Coombs' test occurs frequently and can persist for up to 2 months after discontinuation of therapy. Hemolysis is rare.[4,19]
Th	Rare; possibly the result of an immune reaction. Usually occurs late in the course of therapy.[4,19]

(*continued*)

DRUG AND DYSCRASIA	NATURE OF DYSCRASIA
Chloramphenicol	
AA	Prevalence estimated at 1/12,000 to 1/50,000 patients. Most cases develop with oral administration and after discontinuation of therapy, suggesting the development of a toxic metabolite. An association between the ophthalmic use of chloramphenicol and the development of aplastic anemia is weak, if it exists at all. Blacks might be more susceptible than whites. Do not confuse with the dose-related anemia seen with chloramphenicol. (Note: One case report suggests that a patient's dose-related anemia might have progressed to aplastic anemia, but most sources separate the two dyscrasias.)[4,21–24]
AGN	Rare when compared with the prevalence of aplastic anemia.[4,21]
HA	In G-6-PD deficiency.[4]
Chloroquine	
AGN	Scattered reports only; might be dose related.[4]
HA	Only a few cases have been reported; some association with G-6-PD deficiency is suspected.[4]
Cimetidine	
AA	Scattered reports only; however, at least two fatalities reported (one fatality also was receiving chloramphenicol).[25]
AGN	Usually occurs in patients with systemic disease or other drug therapy that might have contributed to the dyscrasia.[25]
Clopidogrel	
Th	At least 11 cases of clopidogrel-associated thrombotic thrombocytopenic purpura have been reported. Most cases occurred during the first 2 weeks of treatment.[26]
Clozapine	
AGN	Frequency of granulocytopenia is calculated to be 0.4–0.8% in closely monitored patients. Mild to moderate neutropenia occurs in 3–20%. Most cases occur in the first 4 months. Asians are more than twice as susceptible as whites. Recovery usually occurs 2–3 weeks after drug withdrawal. Frequent WBC counts are mandated.[27–29]
Cocaine	
Th	Reported with IV and inhalational use.[30]
Contraceptives, Oral	
MA	Results from impaired folate absorption and/or activity; of consequence only if the patient's folate status is markedly impaired.[4]
Dapsone	
AGN	Many cases have occurred during combination therapy, so it is difficult to determine if dapsone alone is the causative agent.[4,31]
HA	In G-6-PD deficiency; might have other mechanism(s). Might be dose related; uncommon at 100 mg/day but frequent at 200–300 mg/day.[4]

(*continued*)

DRUG AND DYSCRASIA	NATURE OF DYSCRASIA
Digoxin	
Th	Scattered reports only; evidence of an immune mechanism.[2,32,33]
Dimercaprol	
HA	In G-6-PD deficiency.[4]
Dipyridamole	
Th	Relative risk of thrombocytopenia calculated to be 14 times higher than in untreated individuals, but needs confirmation.[34]
Diuretics, Thiazide	
HA	Exact mechanism is unclear; might be an immune reaction.[4,35]
Th	Mild thrombocytopenia occurs frequently, but severe cases are rare. Might be caused by an immune reaction.[2,4,36]
Eflornithine	
AA	Deaths caused by aplastic anemia have been reported.[37]
AGN	Leukopenia is reported in 18–37% of patients.[37]
MA	Megaloblastic anemia is frequently reported.[37]
Th	Thrombocytopenia is frequently reported.[37]
Etanercept	
AA	Although the causal relationship is unclear, some cases of aplastic anemia, including fatalities, have been associated with etanercept.[113]
Felbamate	
AA	More than 30 cases were reported shortly after the introduction of felbamate, resulting in the manufacturer and FDA urging withdrawal of patients from therapy. When a strict definition of aplastic anemia is applied and confounding factors are accounted for, the risk of aplastic anemia from felbamate might not be markedly different from the risk posed by carbamazepine. Most cases developed 2–6 months after initiation of therapy. Monitoring has not been effective for early identification of cases.[38,39]
Fluconazole	
Th	Scattered reports only.[40]
Flucytosine	
AGN	Dose-related; usually requires plasma concentrations ≥125 mg/L.[41]
Th	Dose-related; usually requires plasma concentrations ≥125 mg/L.[41]
Foscarnet	
AGN	Neutropenia occurs in 14% of patients treated for cytomegalovirus retinitis.[42]
Furosemide	
Th	Uncommon, mild, and asymptomatic.[3]

(*continued*)

DRUG AND DYSCRASIA	NATURE OF DYSCRASIA
Ganciclovir	
AGN	Granulocytopenia occurs in about 40% of patients; it is usually reversible with drug discontinuation, but irreversible neutropenia and deaths have occurred.[42,43]
Th	Thrombocytopenia occurs in about 20% of patients.[43]
Gold Salts	
AA	Not dose-dependent; although this reaction is not common, numerous fatalities have been reported.[14,44]
AGN	Often brief and self-limiting; usually responds to withdrawal of therapy.[45,46]
Th	Not dose- or duration-dependent; prevalence estimated at 1–3%; onset usually during the loading phase (first 1000 mg) but can be delayed until after the drug has been discontinued. Mechanism is unclear, but it often appears to be immunologically mediated. Up to 85% of patients with gold-induced thrombocytopenia have HLA-DR3 phenotype compared with 30% of all rheumatoid arthritis patients.[2,4,47,48]
Heparin	
Th	Many patients demonstrate a mild to moderate transient decrease in platelets after only a few days of heparin therapy. Up to 3% experience immune-mediated, persistent thrombocytopenia, which is associated with increased thrombin generation and development of serious thrombotic complications in 30–60%. Intermittent, continuous infusion and "minidose" regimens have been implicated; this is uncommon with SC administration. Prompt cessation of heparin minimizes serious complications; platelet count usually returns to normal within 7–10 days. Low-molecular-weight heparins (eg, **dalteparin, enoxaparin, tinzaparin**) are much less likely than unfractionated heparin to stimulate the formation of immune complexes, leading to thrombocytopenia. Low-molecular-weight heparins offer very little protection from thrombocytopenia in patients who have already formed heparin-associated antibodies.[49–52]
Immune Globulin	
AGN	Transient neutropenia frequently accompanies IV use.[53]
HA	Acute Coombs' positive hemolysis has been reported in patients receiving high-dose therapy.[53]
Inamrinone	
Th	18.6% prevalence in one study of oral therapy (oral form not marketed in the United States); the prevalence during parenteral therapy has been estimated at 2.4%, although 8 of 16 children receiving parenteral inamrinone developed thrombocytopenia in one report. Thrombocytopenia might be caused by nonimmune peripheral platelet destruction.[7–9]
Indomethacin	
AA	Although rare, indomethacin has been associated with a risk 12.7 times higher than in untreated individuals, especially when used regularly and for a long duration.[54]
AGN	Although rare, risk can be 8.9 times higher than in untreated individuals.[54]

(continued)

DRUG AND DYSCRASIA	NATURE OF DYSCRASIA
Interferon Alfa	
Th	Scattered reports only.[55]
Isoniazid	
AGN	Scattered reports only; some evidence of an immune reaction.[4,56]
Th	Scattered reports only; some evidence of an immune reaction.[2,4,56]
Lamotrigine	
AGN	Scattered reports only; too early to establish a pattern of risk.[57]
Levamisole	
AGN	Might be the result of an autoimmune reaction, with a prevalence of ≥4% in some series. Presence of the HLA-B27 phenotype in seropositive rheumatoid arthritis might be an important predisposing factor.[10,54,58]
Th	Scattered reports only.[2,59]
Levodopa	
HA	Autoimmune reaction; positive direct and indirect Coombs' tests are frequent, but hemolysis is rare. **Carbidopa–levodopa** combinations also have produced hemolysis.[4]
Mefenamic Acid	
HA	Thought to be autoimmune.[4,12]
Methimazole	
AA	Scattered reports only, but some increased risk is present. Most cases occur during the first 3 months of therapy.[60,61]
AGN	Prevalence estimated at 0.31%. Encountered overwhelmingly in women and appears to increase with age. Most cases occur in the first 3 months of therapy; monitoring during this time might detect agranulocytosis before it is clinically apparent.[4,60,62,63]
Methyldopa	
HA	Autoimmune reaction; positive direct Coombs' test occurs in 5–25% of patients, depending on dosage; hemolysis occurs in <1%, and its onset is gradual after ≥4 months of therapy. Recovery is rapid after discontinuation of the drug.[4,12,64]
Th	Rare; might be caused by an immune reaction.[4,12,65]
Methylene Blue	
HA	In G-6-PD deficiency.[4]
Nalidixic Acid	
HA	In G-6-PD deficiency; might have other mechanisms.[4]
Th	Scattered reports only; possibly associated with renal impairment in one series.[66]
Nitrofurantoin	
HA	In G-6-PD deficiency; also encountered with enolase deficiency (mechanism unknown).[4]

(continued)

DRUG AND DYSCRASIA	NATURE OF DYSCRASIA
Penicillamine	
AA	Rare; develops after several months of therapy; due to direct marrow toxicity.[67,68]
AGN	Rare; most cases occur during the first month of therapy.[4,68]
HA	Scattered reports only; might be caused by G-6-PD deficiency or fluctuations in copper levels during therapy of Wilson's disease.[68,69]
Th	Prevalence estimated at 10%; some decrease in platelet counts occurs in 75% of penicillamine-treated patients. Might be the result of an immune reaction; most commonly occurs during the first 6 months of therapy.[4,68,70]
Penicillins	
AA	Prevalence very low when extent of use is considered.[4]
AGN	Uncommon with most penicillins but frequent with methicillin; in one report, neutropenia developed in 23 of 68 methicillin-treated patients; resolution occurred within 3–7 days after drug withdrawal. The risk of penicillin-induced neutropenia is increased with parenteral treatment lasting >2 weeks.[4,10,20,71]
HA	Positive direct Coombs' test occurs with large IV doses; hemolysis is rare.[4,12]
Phenazopyridine	
HA	Prevalence and mechanism unknown; renal insufficiency and overdose might be contributing factors. Often accompanied by methemoglobinemia.[4,72]
Phenobarbital	
MA	More than 100 cases reported; usually responds to folic acid.[4]
Phenothiazines	
AGN	Most common during the first 2 months of therapy and in older patients (>85% are >40 yr). Rapid onset and general lack of dose dependence suggest an idiosyncratic mechanism. Prevalence estimated as high as 1/1200.[4,10,73,74]
Phenytoin	
AA	Fewer than 25 reported cases, but the association with phenytoin is strong.[4]
AGN	Scattered reports only; onset after days to years of therapy.[4,10]
MA	Caused by impaired absorption and/or utilization of folate and responds to folic acid therapy (although folate replacement can lower phenytoin levels). Mild macrocytosis is very common (>25%); onset is unpredictable but usually appears after >6 months of therapy.[4]
Th	Scattered reports only; might be the result of an immune reaction.[2,4,75]
Primaquine	
HA	In G-6-PD deficiency.[4]
Primidone	
MA	Similar to phenobarbital, but prevalence might be lower; onset is unpredictable and can be delayed for several years during therapy. Some cases have responded to folic acid.[4]

(*continued*)

DRUG AND DYSCRASIA	NATURE OF DYSCRASIA
Procainamide	
AGN	Prevalence usually estimated at <1%, but with a 25% fatal outcome. Occurs with conventional and sustained-release products; usually occurs within the first 90 days of use. No relationship with daily or total dosage.[4,10,76–78]
Propylthiouracil	
AA	Scattered reports only, but some increased risk is present. Most cases occur within the first 3 months of therapy.[60,61]
AGN	Prevalence estimated at 0.55%. Occurs overwhelmingly in women and appears to increase with age. Most cases occur in the first 3 months of therapy, and monitoring during this time might detect agranulocytosis before it becomes clinically apparent. Some evidence for an immune reaction.[4,10,60–63,79]
Quinacrine	
AA	About one-half of reported cases were preceded by a rash or lichenoid eruption; prevalence estimated at 3/100,000.[4,80]
HA	In G-6-PD deficiency; usually requires concurrent infection or other complicating factors.[4]
Quinidine	
AGN	Scattered reports only; an immune mechanism has been described.[10,81]
HA	In G-6-PD deficiency (but not in blacks). A rapid onset immune mechanism has also been described.[4,10,12,82]
Th	Caused by quinidine-specific antibodies; little or no cross-reactivity with quinine. Accounts for a large portion of drug-induced thrombocytopenia.[2,4,34,75,83]
Quinine	
AGN	Scattered reports only.[4]
HA	In G-6-PD deficiency (but not in blacks). An immune mechanism is also suspected because quinine-dependent antibodies to RBCs have been demonstrated in cases of quinine-induced hemolytic-uremic syndrome.[4,84]
Th	Caused by quinine-specific antibodies; little or no cross-reactivity with quinidine. Fatalities have been reported. It has occurred in people drinking quinine-containing tonic water.[2,4,34,85–87]
Rifabutin	
AGN	In a study of the pharmacokinetic interactions between rifabutin and azithromycin or clarithromycin, rifabutin, alone or in combination with either of those drugs, produced neutropenia in most of the patients. Neutropenia was not seen when either of the other drugs was used without rifabutin.[88]
Rifampin	
HA	Rare but many patients develop a positive Coombs' test; onset in hours in some sensitized patients.[4,56,89]
Th	Peripheral destruction of platelets appears to result from an immune reaction; difficult to separate rifampin contribution from that of other drugs because it is usually used in combination therapy.[2,4,56]

(continued)

DRUG AND DYSCRASIA	NATURE OF DYSCRASIA
Sulfasalazine	
AGN	Leukopenia reported in 5.6% of patients receiving the drug for rheumatoid arthritis and agranulocytosis/neutropenia in 4/1000 patients; prevalence of agranulocytosis/neutropenia among inflammatory bowel disease patients is considerably lower (0.3/1000 patients). Onset is usually during the first 3 months of therapy; recovery takes 2 weeks after drug discontinuation.[14,90,91]
HA	In G-6-PD deficiency but also occurs in nondeficient patients. Hemolysis might be more common in slow acetylators.[4,91–93]
MA	One series of 130 arthritis patients reported macrocytosis in 21% and macrocytic anemia in 3%.[94]
Sulfonamides	
AA	Historically an important cause of aplastic anemia, but most cases were reported after use of older sulfonamides; rarely occurs with products currently in use.[4]
AGN	Occurs mostly with older products; rarely occurs with products currently in use. Most current cases are in combined use with **trimethoprim;** also reported with **silver sulfadiazine.** Onset is usually rapid.[4,12,95,96]
HA	In G-6-PD deficiency but also occurs in nondeficient patients.[4,97]
Th	Scattered reports only; probably an immune reaction. (*See also* Trimethoprim.)[2,34,75]
Ticlopidine	
AA	The growing number of cases of aplastic anemia associated with ticlopidine is disturbing; the incidence cannot be estimated.[98]
AGN	Incidence of neutropenia estimated at 2.4% of treated patients with severe neutropenia or agranulocytosis in 0.85%. Obtain CBC every 2 weeks during the first 3 months of treatment. Discontinue ticlopidine if the ANC is <1200/μL.[98]
Th	Thrombotic thrombocytopenia purpura occurs in 1 of every 1600–5000 exposed. Mean time to onset is 22 days. Plasmapheresis reduces the death rate from 60% to 21%.[99,100]
Tocainide	
AGN	Prevalence estimated at 0.07–0.18% of patients.[101,102]
Triamterene	
MA	Few cases reported, but it is a potent inhibitor of dihydrofolate reductase; greatest risk in those with folate deficiency before therapy (eg, alcoholics).[4]
Trimethoprim	
AGN	Rare; occurs when used alone and in combination with **sulfonamides,** with the latter numerically more common.[4,96,103]
MA	Most cases occur after 1–2 weeks of therapy; this drug can have weak antifolate action in humans that becomes important only in those with folate deficiency before therapy (eg, alcoholics).[4]
Th	Thrombocytopenia is common, but severe cases are rare. Most commonly occurs in combination therapy with sulfonamides. Relative risk calculated at 124 times that of untreated individuals.[2,4,34]

(continued)

DRUG AND DYSCRASIA	NATURE OF DYSCRASIA
Vaccines	
Th	A study of 9 million doses of measles, rubella, and mumps vaccines administered to children determined that the prevalence of thrombocytopenia was 0.17 cases/100,000 doses for measles vaccine and 0.23, 0.87, and 0.95 cases/100,000 doses for rubella, measles–rubella, and mumps–measles–rubella vaccines, respectively. These rates are similar to the rates of thrombocytopenia after the natural courses of the disease in unvaccinated children. Most of the cases had platelet counts >10,000/μL.[104]
Valproic Acid	
MA	Macrocytosis occurred in 11 of 60 patients in one report.[105]
Th	Thrombocytopenia occurred in 12 of 60 patients in one report. Immune and dose-dependent mechanisms have been suggested.[2,105]
Vancomycin	
AGN	Scattered reports only, but prevalence might be as high as 2%; mechanism unknown.[3,106,107]
Vesnarinone	
AGN	Reversible neutropenia occurs in about 3%, mostly in the first 16–24 weeks of treatment. Absolute granulocyte count $<1 \times 10^9$/L occur in 0.85%, with counts $<0.1 \times 10^9$/L in 0.25%.[108,109]
Vitamin K	
HA	In G-6-PD deficiency; usually requires concurrent infection or other complicating factors. Hemolysis from high doses can contribute to jaundice in neonates; rarely toxic in older children and adults.[4]
Zidovudine	
AGN	Most patients experience at least a 25% reduction in neutrophil count; ANC of <500/μL occurs in 16% of patients. Usual onset is during the first 3 months of therapy.[110,111]
MA	Macrocytosis develops in most patients, usually beginning during the first few weeks of therapy. Zidovudine is the leading cause of drug-induced macrocytosis.[110–112]

■ REFERENCES

1. Dasgupta H et al. Thrombocytopenia complicating treatment with intravenous glycoprotein IIb/IIIa receptor inhibitors: a pooled analysis. *Am Heart J* 2000;140:206–11.
2. Hackett T et al. Drug-induced platelet destruction. *Semin Thromb Hemost* 1982;8:116–37.
3. Fischereder M, Jaffe JP. Thrombocytopenia following acute acetaminophen overdose. *Am J Hematol* 1994; 45:258–9.
4. Swanson M, Cook R. *Drugs chemicals and blood dyscrasias.* Hamilton, IL: Drug Intelligence Publications; 1977.
5. Wilson R, Feldman S. Toxicity of amphotericin B in children with cancer. *Am J Dis Child* 1979;133:731–4.
6. Chan CSP et al. Amphotericin-B–induced thrombocytopenia. *Ann Intern Med* 1982;96:332–3.
7. Ansell J et al. Amrinone-induced thrombocytopenia. *Arch Intern Med* 1984;144:949–52.
8. Treadway G. Clinical safety of intravenous amrinone—a review. *Am J Cardiol* 1985;56:39B–40B.

9. Ross MP et al. Amrinone-associated thrombocytopenia: pharmacokinetic analysis. *Clin Pharmacol Ther* 1993;53:661–7.

10. Heimpel H. Drug-induced agranulocytosis. *Med Toxicol Adverse Drug Exp* 1988;3:449–62.

11. Levin GM, DeVane CL. A review of cyclic antidepressant-induced blood dyscrasias. *Ann Pharmacother* 1992;26:378–83.

12. Sanford-Driscoll M, Knodel LC. Induction of hemolytic anemia by nonsteroidal anti-inflammatory drugs. *Drug Intell Clin Pharm* 1986;20:925–34.

13. Garg SK, Sarker CR. Aspirin-induced thrombocytopenia on an immune basis. *Am J Med Sci* 1974;267:129–32.

14. George CS, Lichtin AE. Hematologic complications of rheumatic disease therapies. *Rheum Dis Clin North Am* 1997;23:425–37.

15. Cooper RA. Captopril-associated neutropenia. Who is at risk? *Arch Intern Med* 1983;143:659–60. Editorial.

16. Sobotka JL et al. A review of carbamazepine's hematologic reactions and monitoring recommendations. *DICP* 1990;24:1214–9.

17. Tohen M et al. Blood dyscrasias with carbamazepine and valproate: a pharmacoepidemiological study of 2,228 patients at risk. *Am J Psychiatry* 1995;152:413–8.

18. Bradley JM et al. Carbamazepine-induced thrombocytopenia in a young child. *Clin Pharm* 1985;4:221–3.

19. Thompson JW, Jacobs RF. Adverse effects of newer cephalosporins. An update. *Drug Saf* 1993;9:132–42.

20. Olaison L et al. Incidence of β-lactam–induced delayed hypersensitivity and neutropenia during treatment of infective endocarditis. *Arch Intern Med* 1999;159:607–15.

21. Chaplin S. Bone marrow depression due to mianserin, phenylbutazone, oxyphenbutazone, and chloramphenicol—part I. *Adverse Drug React Acute Poison Rev* 1986;2:97–136.

22. Chaplin S. Bone marrow depression due to mianserin, phenylbutazone, oxyphenbutazone, and chloramphenicol—part II. *Adverse Drug React Acute Poison Rev* 1986;3:181–96.

23. Laporte J-R et al. Possible association between ocular chloramphenicol and aplastic anaemia—the absolute risk is very low. *Br J Clin Pharmacol* 1998;46:181–4.

24. Flegg P et al. Chloramphenicol. Are concerns about aplastic anemia justified? *Drug Saf* 1992;7:167–9.

25. Aymard J-P et al. Haematological adverse effects of histamine H₂-receptor antagonists. *Med Toxicol Adverse Drug Exp* 1988;3:430–48.

26. Bennett CL et al. Thrombotic thrombocytopenic purpura associated with clopidogrel. *N Engl J Med* 2000;342:1773–7.

27. Atkin K et al. Neutropenia and agranulocytosis in patients receiving clozapine in the UK and Ireland. *Br J Psychiatry* 1996;169:483–8.

28. Honigfeld G. Effects of the Clozapine National Registry System on incidence of deaths related to agranulocytosis. *Psychiatr Serv* 1996;47:52–6.

29. Munro J et al. Active monitoring of 12 760 clozapine recipients in the UK and Ireland. Beyond pharmacovigilance. *Br J Psychiatry* 1999;175:576–80.

30. Leissinger CA. Severe thrombocytopenia associated with cocaine use. *Ann Intern Med* 1990;112:708–10.

31. Cockburn EM et al. Dapsone-induced agranulocytosis: spontaneous reporting data. *Br J Dermatol* 1993; 128:702–3. Letter.

32. Young RC et al. Thrombocytopenia due to digitoxin. Demonstration of antibody and mechanisms of action. *Am J Med* 1966;41:605–14.

33. Pirovino M et al. Digoxin-associated thrombocytopaenia. *Eur J Clin Pharmacol* 1981;19:205–7.

34. Kaufman DW et al. Acute thrombocytopenic purpura in relation to the use of drugs. *Blood* 1993;82:2714–8.

35. Beck ML et al. Fatal intravascular immune hemolysis induced by hydrochlorothiazide. *Am J Clin Pathol* 1984;81:791–4.

36. Okafor KC et al. Hydrochlorothiazide-induced thrombocytopenic purpura. *Drug Intell Clin Pharm* 1986; 20:60–1.

37. Sahai J, Berry AJ. Eflornithine for the treatment of *Pneumocystis carinii* pneumonia in patients with the acquired immunodeficiency syndrome: a preliminary review. *Pharmacotherapy* 1989;9:29–33.

38. Pennell PB et al. Aplastic anemia in a patient receiving felbamate for complex partial seizures. *Neurology* 1995;45:456–60.

39. Kaufman DW et al. Aplastic anemia among users of felbamate. *Pharmacoepidemiol Drug Saf* 1996;5(suppl): S106. Abstract.

40. Mercurio MG et al. Thrombocytopenia caused by fluconazole therapy. *J Am Acad Dermatol* 1995;32:525–6.

41. Kauffman CA, Frame PT. Bone marrow toxicity associated with 5-fluorocytosine therapy. *Antimicrob Agents Chemother* 1977;11:244–7.

42. Morbidity and toxic effects associated with ganciclovir or foscarnet therapy in a randomized cytomegalovirus retinitis trial. Studies of Ocular Complications of AIDS Research Group, in collaboration with the AIDS Clinical Trials Group. *Intern Med* 1995;155:65–74.

43. Cytovene product information. Palo Alto, CA: Syntex Laboratories; 1994.

44. Gibson J et al. Aplastic anemia in association with gold therapy for rheumatoid arthritis. *Aust N Z J Med* 1983;13:130–4.

45. Gibbons RB. Complications of chrysotherapy. A review of recent studies. *Arch Intern Med* 1979;139:343–6.

46. Gottlieb NL et al. The course of severe gold-associated granulocytopenia. *Clin Res* 1982;30:659A. Abstract.

47. Coblyn JS et al. Gold-induced thrombocytopenia. A clinical and immunogenetic study of twenty-three patients. *Ann Intern Med* 1981;95:178–81.

48. Adachi JD et al. Gold induced thrombocytopenia: platelet associated IgG and HLA typing in three patients. *J Rheumatol* 1984;11:355–7.

49. Warkentin TE et al. Heparin-induced thrombocytopenia in patients treated with low-molecular-weight heparin or unfractionated heparin. *N Engl J Med* 1995;332:1330–5.

50. Warkentin TE. Heparin-induced thrombocytopenia. *Drug Saf* 1997;17:325–41.

51. Schmitt BP, Adelman B. Heparin-associated thrombocytopenia: a critical review and pooled analysis. *Am J Med Sci* 1993;305:208–15.

52. Raible MD. Hematologic complications of heparin-induced thrombocytopenia. *Semin Thromb Hemost* 1999;25(suppl 1):17–21.

53. Misbah SA, Chapel HM. Adverse effects of intravenous immunoglobulin. *Drug Saf* 1993;9:254–62.

54. Risks of agranulocytosis and aplastic anemia. A first report of their relation to drug use with special reference to analgesics. The International Agranulocytosis and Aplastic Anemia Study. *JAMA* 1986;256:1749–57.

55. Murakami CS et al. Idiopathic thrombocytopenic purpura during interferon-α_{2a} treatment for chronic hepatitis. *Am J Gastroenterol* 1994;89:2244–5.

56. Holdiness MR. A review of blood dyscrasias induced by the antituberculosis drugs. *Tubercle* 1987;68:301–9.

57. Nicholson RJ et al. Leucopenia associated with lamotrigine. *BMJ* 1995;310:504.

58. Mielants H, Veys EM. A study of the hematological side effects of levamisole in rheumatoid arthritis with recommendations. *J Rheumatol* 1978;5(suppl 4):77–83.

59. El-Ghobarey AF, Capell HA. Levamisole-induced thrombocytopenia. *Br Med J* 1977;2:555–6.

60. Risk of agranulocytosis and aplastic anemia in relation to use of antithyroid drugs. International Agranulocytosis and Aplastic Anaemia Study. *BMJ* 1988;297:262–5.

61. Biswas N et al. Case report: aplastic anemia associated with antithyroid drugs. *Am J Med Sci* 1991;301:190–4.

62. Tajiri J et al. Antithyroid drug-induced agranulocytosis. The usefulness of routine white blood cell count monitoring. *Arch Intern Med* 1990;150:621–4.

63. Meyer-Gebner M et al. Antithyroid drug-induced agranulocytosis: clinical experience with ten patients treated at one institution and review of the literature. *J Endocrinol Invest* 1994;17:29–36.

64. Kelton JG. Impaired reticuloendothelial function in patients treated with methyldopa. *N Engl J Med* 1985;313:596–600.

65. Manohitharajah SM et al. Methyldopa and associated thrombocytopenia. *Br Med J* 1971;1:494.

66. Meyboom RHB. Thrombocytopenia induced by nalidixic acid. *Br Med J* 1984;289:962.

67. Kay AGL. Myelotoxicity of D-penicillamine. *Ann Rheum Dis* 1979;38:232–6.

68. Camp AV. Hematologic toxicity from penicillamine in rheumatoid arthritis. *J Rheumatol* 1981;8(suppl 7):164–5.

69. Lyle WH. D-penicillamine and haemolytic anaemia. *Lancet* 1976;1:428. Letter.

70. Thomas D et al. A study of D-penicillamine induced thrombocytopenia in rheumatoid arthritis with Cr^{51}-labelled autologous platelets. *Aust N Z J Med* 1981;11:722. Abstract.

71. Mallouh AA. Methicillin-induced neutropenia. *Pediatr Infect Dis J* 1985;4:262–4.

72. Jeffery WH et al. Acquired methemoglobinemia and hemolytic anemia after usual doses of phenazopyridine. *Drug Intell Clin Pharm* 1982;16:157–9.

73. Hollister LE. Allergic reactions to tranquilizing drugs. *Ann Intern Med* 1958;49:17–29.

74. Pisciotta AV et al. Agranulocytosis following administration of phenothiazine derivatives. *Am J Med* 1958;25:210–23.

75. Cimo PL et al. Detection of drug-dependent antibodies by the ^{51}Cr platelet lysis test: documentation of immune thrombocytopenia induced by diphenylhydantoin diazepam, and sulfisoxazole. *Am J Hematol* 1977; 2:65–72.

76. Meyers DG et al. Severe neutropenia associated with procainamide: comparison of sustained release and conventional preparations. *Am Heart J* 1985;109:1393–5.

77. Thompson JF et al. Procainamide agranulocytosis: a case report and review of the literature. *Curr Ther Res* 1988;44:872–81.

78. Danielly J et al. Procainamide-associated blood dyscrasias. *Am J Cardiol* 1994;74:1179–80.

79. Fibbe WE et al. Agranulocytosis induced by propylthiouracil: evidence of a drug dependent antibody reacting with granulocytes, monocytes and haematopoietic progenitor cells. *Br J Haematol* 1986;64:363–73.

80. Custer RP. Aplastic anemia in soldiers treated with atabrine (quinacrine). *Am J Med Sci* 1946;212:211–24.

81. Ascensao JL et al. Quinidine-induced neutropenia: report of a case with drug-dependent inhibition of granulocyte colony generation. *Acta Haematol* 1984;72:349–54.

82. Geltner D et al. Quinidine hypersensitivity and liver involvement. A survey of 32 patients. *Gastroenterology* 1976;70:650–2.

83. Reid DM, Shulman NR. Drug purpura due to surreptitious quinidine intake. *Ann Intern Med* 1988;108:206–8.

84. Webb RF et al. Acute intravascular haemolysis due to quinine. *N Z Med J* 1980;91:14–6.

85. McDonald SP et al. Quinine-induced hemolytic uremic syndrome. *Clin Nephrol* 1977;47:397–400.

86. Murray JA et al. Bitter lemon purpura. *Br Med J* 1979;2:1551–2.

87. Freiman JP. Fatal quinine-induced thrombocytopenia. *Ann Intern Med* 1990;112:308–9. Letter.

88. Apseloff G et al. Severe neutropenia caused by recommended prophylactic doses of rifabutin. *Lancet* 1996;348:685. Letter.

89. Tahan SR et al. Acute hemolysis and renal failure with rifampicin-dependent antibodies after discontinuous administration. *Transfusion* 1985;25:124–7.

90. Marabani M et al. Leucopenia during sulfasalazine treatment for rheumatoid arthritis. *Ann Rheum Dis* 1989;48:505–7.

91. Jick H et al. The risk of sulfasalazine- and mesalazine-associated blood disorders. *Pharmacotherapy* 1995; 15:176–81.

92. Cohen SM et al. Ulcerative colitis and erythrocyte G6PD deficiency. Salicylazosulfapyridine-provoked hemolysis. *JAMA* 1968;205:528–30.

93. Das KM et al. Adverse reactions during salicylazosulfapyridine therapy and the relation with drug metabolism and acetylator phenotype. *N Engl J Med* 1973;289:491–5.

94. Hopkinson ND et al. Haematological side-effects of sulphasalazine in inflammatory arthritis. *Br J Rheumatol* 1989;28:414–7.

95. Jarrett F et al. Acute leukopenia during topical burn therapy with silver sulfadiazine. *Am J Surg* 1978;135:818–9.

96. Anti-infective drug use in relation to the risk of agranulocytosis and aplastic anemia. The International Agranulocytosis and Aplastic Anemia Study. *Arch Intern Med* 1989;149:1036–40.

97. Zinkham WH. Unstable hemoglobins and the selective hemolytic action of sulfonamides. The International Agranulocytosis and Aplastic Anemia Study. *Arch Intern Med* 1977;137:1365–6. Editorial.

98. Love BB et al. Adverse haematological effects of ticlopidine. Prevention, recognition and management. *Drug Saf* 1998;19:89–98.

99. Steinhubl SR et al. Incidence and clinical course of thrombotic thrombocytopenic purpura due to ticlopidine following coronary stenting. *JAMA* 1999;281:806–10.

100. Bennett CL et al. Thrombotic thrombocytopenic purpura associated with ticlopidine in the setting of coronary stents and stroke prevention. *Arch Intern Med* 1999;159:2524–8.

101. Volosin K et al. Tocainide associated agranulocytosis. *Am Heart J* 1985;109:1392–3.

102. Roden DM, Woosley RL. Tocainide. *N Engl J Med* 1986;315:41–5.

103. Hawkins T et al. Severe trimethoprim induced neutropenia and thrombocytopenia. *N Z Med J* 1993; 106: 251–2.

104. Jonville-Béra AP et al. Thrombocytopenic purpura after measles, mumps and rubella vaccination: a retrospective survey by the French Regional Pharmacovigilance Centres and Pasteur-Mérieux Sérums et Vaccins. *Pediatr Infect Dis J* 1996;15:44–8.

105. May RB, Sunder TR. Hematologic manifestations of long-term valproate therapy. *Epilepsia* 1993; 34:1098–101.

106. Mackett RL, Guay DRP. Vancomycin-induced neutropenia. *Can Med Assoc J* 1985;132:39–40.

107. Sacho H, Moore PJ. Vancomycin-induced neutropenia. *S Afr Med J* 1989;76:701. Letter.

108. Bertolet BD et al. Neutropenia occurring during treatment with vesnarinone (OPC-8212). *Am J Cardiol* 1994;74:968–70.

109. Furusawa S et al. Vesnarinone-induced granulocytopenia: incidence in Japan and recommendations for safety. *J Clin Pharmacol* 1996;36:477–81.

110. Richman DD et al. The toxicity of azidothymidine (AZT) in the treatment of patients with AIDS and AIDS-related complex. A double-blind, placebo-controlled trial. *N Engl J Med* 1987;317:192–7.

111. Rachlis A, Fanning MM. Zidovudine toxicity. Clinical features and management. *Drug Saf* 1993;8:312–20.

112. Snower DP, Weil SC. Changing etiology of macrocytosis. Zidovudine as a frequent causative factor. *Am J Clin Pathol* 1993;99:57–60.

113. Food and Drug Administration. Important drug warning. http://www.fda.gov/medwatch/safety/2000/enbrel2.htm (accessed Oct 12, 2000).

Drug-Induced Hepatotoxicity

This table includes only those drugs with well-established records of hepatotoxicity. A drug not listed in the table does not mean it cannot produce liver damage because virtually all drugs have been reported to elevate serum liver enzymes. Combining drugs that have hepatotoxic potential commonly results in greater than additive liver damage. In general, drug-induced hepatotoxicity is most prevalent in older patients, women, and those with pre-existing hepatic impairment.

ACE Inhibitors

Hepatic injury occurs occasionally with ACE inhibitors. **Captopril** and **enalapril** are implicated in most reported cases, but other ACE inhibitors likely have similar hepatotoxic potential. Most cases show cholestatic injury, but mixed and hepatocellular damage also are reported.[1,2]

Acetaminophen

Centrilobular hepatic necrosis can follow acute overdose with ≥140 mg/kg in children or ≥6 g in adults. These doses saturate the normal metabolic pathways, producing large quantities of a hepatotoxic metabolite. Children appear to have a lower risk than adults of developing acetaminophen-induced hepatitis. Laboratory evidence of hepatotoxicity peaks 3–4 days after the acute exposure. Therapy with **acetylcysteine** to bind the metabolite is indicated when the 4-hr postingestion serum acetaminophen level is >150 mg/L. Even without acetylcysteine, fatalities are uncommon after acetaminophen overdose. Nonfatal cases usually recover fully in a few weeks. Chronic **alcohol** ingestion increases acetaminophen toxicity, as does recent fasting. Acute alcohol ingestion is thought by some to have a protective action. Less destructive, but still detectable, hepatitis is reported in patients taking large acetaminophen doses for therapeutic purposes.[1,3–5]

Alcohol

Fatty infiltration of the liver occurs in 70–100% of alcoholics. Fatty liver is generally without clinical manifestation, but 30% of alcoholics develop alcoholic hepatitis and about 10% develop cirrhosis. Malnutrition can potentiate alcoholic liver disease, and alcohol can enhance the hepatotoxicity of other drugs.[1]

Aldesleukin

Increases in serum bilirubin, alkaline phosphatase, and transaminases occur frequently. These primarily cholestatic changes are rapidly reversible after drug discontinuation.[1,6]

Allopurinol

Hepatic granulomas, hepatitis and hepatic necrosis can accompany other symptoms (especially rash, fever, eosinophilia, and vasculitis) of allopurinol hypersensitivity. Damage is usually focal, but widespread damage also is reported. This reaction is rare but serious when it occurs. Onset is usually after 3–6 weeks of treatment. Renal impairment might be a predisposing factor for allopurinol-induced hepatitis. Cholestasis also has been attributed to allopurinol.[1,7]

Aminoglutethimide

Laboratory evidence of cholestasis is common, but clinical evidence is rare.[1,8]

Aminosalicylic Acid

Up to 5% of patients develop a generalized hypersensitivity reaction. About 25% of these patients have evidence of mixed cholestatic and hepatocellular injuries as part of their hypersensitivity reactions. Fatalities have been reported.[1,9]

(continued)

Amiodarone

Mild increases in transaminases and LDH levels occur in up to one-half of patients, whereas phospholipidosis occurs in virtually all; normal values often return despite continued therapy. Symptoms (eg, jaundice, nausea and vomiting, hepatomegaly, or weight loss) occur in 1–4% of patients. Onset is typically after 2–4 months of therapy but can be delayed for ≥1 yr. Recovery after drug discontinuation can take from several months to ≥1 yr. The dose-related hepatotoxicity of amiodarone is reminiscent of alcoholic hepatitis. Cirrhosis and fatalities are also reported.[1,10–12]

Amoxicillin and Clavulanic Acid

Based on an extensive review of medical records, the frequency of acute hepatic injury with amoxicillin and clavulanic acid is 1.7 cases/10,000 prescriptions (compared with 0.3 for amoxicillin alone). In most cases, the hepatic injury is cholestatic. The risk of hepatic injury is increased by repeated prescriptions for amoxicillin and clavulanic acid and by advancing age.[2,13]

Androgens

(*See* Steroids, C-17-α-Alkyl.)

Antidepressants, Heterocyclic

The prevalence of hepatic injury is estimated at about 1%, with most of the cases presenting as cholestasis. This idiosyncratic reaction resembles the cholestasis associated with phenothiazines.[1]

Asparaginase

Slowly reversible steatosis occurs in 50–90% of patients, apparently due to the drug's influence on protein synthesis. Daily administration might be more hepatotoxic than weekly administration.[1,14–16]

Azathioprine

This drug is less hepatotoxic than its metabolite, mercaptopurine. Azathioprine's hepatotoxicity is predominantly cholestatic rather than hepatocellular. Vascular lesions, including venous occlusion and peliosis hepatis, have been reported, but their prevalence is unknown. Nodular regenerative hyperplasia has followed use of this drug in kidney and liver transplantations.[1,14,17]

Busulfan

Use in bone marrow transplant patients is associated with apparently dose-related veno-occlusive disease of the liver. Although the exact contribution of the drug is difficult to discern, this syndrome occurs in 20% of adults and 5% of children with total doses ≥16 mg/kg.[1,14,18,19]

Carbamazepine

Mild changes in liver function tests occur frequently. Hepatic necrosis, granulomas, and cholestasis have occurred, with some cases showing signs of hypersensitivity. Onset is most often in the first 4 weeks of therapy. Fatalities have been reported.[1,20]

Carmustine

Changes in liver function tests in 20–30% of patients, from a few days to several weeks after drug administration. Changes are usually mild and resolve quickly with drug discontinuation.[1,14]

Cephalosporins

Transient minor increases in AST, ALT, and alkaline phosphatase occur frequently. **Ceftriaxone** use is associated with development of "gallbladder sludge" in up to 25% of patients.[1,21]

Chlorpropamide

Most hepatotoxic reactions are cholestatic and probably are caused by an immune mechanism. Prevalence is estimated at 0.5–1.5%, with onset usually within the first 2 months of therapy.[1]

(*continued*)

Chlorzoxazone

Idiosyncratic hepatocellular damage occurs rarely, but fatalities have been reported. Discontinue the drug if elevated levels of transaminases or bilirubin are detected.[1,23]

Cisplatin

Transient, dose-related elevations of hepatic enzymes occur frequently.[1,14]

Clozapine

Transient elevations of hepatic enzymes occur frequently during the first 3 months of clozapine use. Although several cases of fulminant hepatitis have been reported, the risk of serious clozapine-induced hepatotoxicity remains small and some investigators recommend against routine testing.[1,24,25]

Cocaine

Hepatic necrosis has been reported in cases of cocaine abuse, including at least one fatality. The prevalence of this reaction is not known.[1,10,26]

Contraceptives, Oral

Data from two large, long-term cohort studies (about 33,000 users) did not detect any association between oral contraceptive use and serious liver disease. One study detected an increase in the frequency of mild liver disease among users of older, high-estrogen (>50 μg) products. Older combination oral contraceptives were associated with an increase in the annual incidence of hepatic adenomas (3.4/100,000 vs 1.3/100,000 in nonusers), especially after ≥5 yr of use. The frequency of gallbladder disease also was increased by older oral contraceptives.[1,27,28]

Cyclosporine

Elevated serum levels of alkaline phosphatase and conjugated bilirubin consistent with cholestasis occur in 50–60% of patients. These changes are usually mild and pose little threat.[1,29,30]

Dantrolene

At least 1.8% of patients develop laboratory evidence of hepatic dysfunction, with symptomatic hepatitis in about 0.6%; the fatality rate among jaundiced patients is about 25%. Predisposing factors seem to include dosage (>300 mg/day), sex (women more than men), age (>30 yr), and duration of therapy (≥2 months).[1,31,32]

Dapsone

Hepatitis can occur as part of the "dapsone syndrome," a generalized hypersensitivity reaction that includes rash, fever, and lymphadenopathy. The true prevalence is unknown but might be as high as 5%. The onset is usually during the first 2 months of therapy. Although most dapsone-associated liver injury is hepatocellular, some cases of cholestasis have occurred.[1,33–35]

Disulfiram

Small increases in serum transaminase levels occur frequently. Hepatitis is reported occasionally, which can be caused by hypersensitivity. Most cases develop during the first few months of treatment. The best estimate of the incidence of fatal hepatitis is about 1/30,000 users/year.[1,36]

Erythromycin

Erythromycin was thought to be a frequent cause of jaundice, but recent studies indicate that jaundice occurs only occasionally. Cholestasis apparently results from hypersensitivity (60% have eosinophilia and 50% have fever), appearing after 10–14 days of initial therapy or after 1–2 days in patients with a history of erythromycin exposure. Despite extensive use in children, most cases are reported in adults. Rapid reversal of symptoms follows drug discontinuation, but laboratory

(continued)

changes can persist for up to 6 months. Although most cases involve the estolate salt, hepatotoxicity has occurred with the ethylsuccinate, stearate, and propionate salts and with erythromycin base.[1,37–39]

Ethionamide

Hepatitis can occur in 3–5% of patients, and serum enzyme elevations can occur in ≥30%. Onset of hepatitis is usually after several months of therapy.[1,40]

Felbamate

Although the prevalence of hepatocellular destruction is unclear, it is of sufficient concern to limit the use of felbamate to carefully selected patients. At least 6 cases of fatal felbamate-induced hepatic necrosis have been reported.[1,42]

Ferrous Salts

Hepatic necrosis can appear within 1–3 days of an acute overdose. The fatality rate is high if the patient is not treated promptly.[1]

Floxuridine

Hepatic arterial infusion of floxuridine results in 9% sclerosing cholangitis at 9 months and 26% after 1 yr. Elevations of liver enzyme levels are common but not predictive of greater hepatotoxicity.[2,16,43]

Flutamide

Through 1994, there were as least 20 reported deaths reasonably attributed to flutamide-induced hepatotoxicity. Those deaths, typically the result of massive hepatic necrosis, occurred between 5 days and 9 months (mean 3 months) after initiation of flutamide therapy. Further, the hospitalization rate for noninfectious liver disease in flutamide-treated patients was 10 times the expected rate. Monthly liver function testing is recommended for the first 4 months.[1,44,45]

Gold Salts

Cholestasis occurs occasionally with normal doses of parenteral gold salts; hypersensitivity is the suspected mechanism. Onset is commonly within the first few weeks of therapy, and recovery usually occurs within 3 months after drug discontinuation. Lipogranulomas are frequently found in liver biopsies of parenteral gold-treated patients. These can persist long after drug withdrawal but do not seem to impair liver function. Hepatic necrosis can result from overdose.[1,46,47]

Halothane

As many as 30% of patients have increased serum transaminases or other evidence of mild hepatic impairment. Despite extensive publicity, the actual frequency of severe halothane hepatitis is low, ranging from 1/3500 to 1/35,000, with reported case fatality rates of 14–67%. Susceptibility is greatest in adults, women, obese patients, and especially in patients with prior exposure to halothane. The mechanism of hepatitis is poorly understood, but hypersensitivity is most likely. Fever precedes jaundice in most patients. The onset of jaundice is usually 5–8.5 days after exposure but can occur 1–26 days after exposure; shorter latent periods are associated with prior halothane exposure. **Methoxyflurane** and **enflurane** produce similar hepatotoxic reactions, although less frequently.[1,48,49]

Histamine H₂-Receptor Antagonists

Cimetidine and **ranitidine** are associated with increased liver enzymes. The risk of acute liver injury with cimetidine is about 1/5000, with most cases occurring during the first 2 months of use.[1,50]

(continued)

Isoniazid

Elevated serum transaminase levels occur frequently, are presumed to be associated with sub-clinical hepatitis, resolve rapidly after drug discontinuation, and can resolve despite continued isoniazid therapy. A syndrome resembling viral hepatitis occurs in 1–2% of patients, with the onset usually during the first 20 weeks of therapy. The fatality rate from isoniazid hepatitis has fallen steadily over the past 2 decades, probably in response to more aggressive monitoring, and is now estimated to be 1–1.7/100,000 patients starting isoniazid and 1.5–2.9/100,000 patients completing a course of therapy. Most fatalities occur in women. Despite the widespread assumption that patients <35 yr are unlikely to develop isoniazid-induced fatal hepatotoxicity, reported deaths indicate otherwise. **Alcohol** consumption increases the risk of hepatotoxicity; the contribution of concomitant **rifampin** is poorly defined. The role of acetylator phenotype remains unclear, but a case-control study found that patients admitted to the hospital for suspected isoniazid-induced hepatotoxicity were significantly more likely to be slow acetylators than those who completed their courses of therapy without hepatotoxicity.[1,10,51–53]

Itraconazole

The FDA has received reports of liver failure and death apparently associated with itraconazole use, included some cases without predisposing risk factors.[98]

Ketoconazole

Elevated hepatic enzyme levels occur in about 20% of ketoconazole-treated patients, with overt hepatitis in 3%. The typical onset for overt hepatitis is 30–60 days after initiation of ketoconazole therapy. There have been a few deaths attributed to ketoconazole hepatotoxicity.[1,54]

Lamotrigine

At least 9 cases of lamotrigine-associated hepatotoxicity have been published, including at least 1 case of severe hepatic failure. Most of these cases were complicated by multiple-drug therapy.[55]

Mercaptopurine

Jaundice associated with cholestasis, hepatic necrosis, and mixed reactions occurs in 6–40% of patients, with the highest prevalence associated with doses ≥2 mg/kg/day. Onset is usually during the first 2 months of therapy.[1,56]

Methotrexate

Hepatic injury (macrovesicular steatosis, necrosis, and bridging fibrosis) occurs frequently, depends on dose and duration of therapy, and can progress to cirrhosis if the drug is not stopped. Intermittent high doses pose less risk than daily low doses. Cirrhosis is reported in up to 24% of patients receiving long-term daily doses; other contributing factors are alcoholism and pre-existing liver or kidney disease. Hepatic fibrosis is not detected by standard liver function tests and is best detected by biopsy. Biopsy has been recommended at intervals of up to 36 months, after every 1.5 g of methotrexate, if 6 of 12 monthly transaminase levels are elevated, or if the serum albumin level drops below normal. Isolated elevations of transaminase levels do not preclude continued methotrexate therapy.[1,14,57–60]

Methyldopa

Mild changes in liver function tests occur in up to 35% of patients taking methyldopa, but the prevalence of clinical hepatitis is probably <1%. Most cases occur during the first 3 months of therapy. Hepatitis is more common in women, and most patients have rapid recovery after drug discontinuation. The fatality rate is <10% among patients who develop hepatitis. There is evidence to support a hypersensitivity mechanism in some patients.[1,61]

(continued)

Minocycline

The long-term use of minocycline for acne or arthritis has resulted in at least 65 reported cases of minocycline-induced hepatitis. Autoimmune hepatitis associated with lupus-like symptoms occurs with a median onset of 1 yr, and an apparent hypersensitivity mechanism is responsible for other cases occurring during the first month of minocycline therapy.[62,63]

Nevirapine

Severe, life-threatening hepatotoxicity has been reported in patients taking nevirapine for HIV infection and health care workers taking the drug for postexposure prophylaxis. Fatalities have occurred in HIV-infected patients.[64]

Niacin

Elevations of hepatic enzyme and bilirubin levels occur in 30–50% of patients taking sustained-release niacin in therapeutic doses, with jaundice in 3% of patients taking 3 g/day for >1 yr. Symptomatic hepatic dysfunction occurs frequently and limits the use of the sustained-release product. Immediate-release niacin also is hepatotoxic but to a lesser extent than sustained-release.[1,65]

Nitrofurantoin

Hepatic damage occurs occasionally, usually during the first month of therapy. Cholestasis is the most common presentation; hepatic necrosis also is reported. Hypersensitivity is the suspected mechanism, and the onset is frequently associated with fever, rash, and eosinophilia. Several late-developing cases of chronic active hepatitis have been reported; almost all are in women and after >6 months of therapy.[1,66]

Nonsteroidal Anti-inflammatory Drugs

The incidence of clinically apparent hepatic injury from nonsalicylate NSAIDs is estimated to be about 1/10,000 patient–years. The incidence for **sulindac** may be 5–10 times higher than for the other nonsalicylate NSAIDs. Half of the reactions to sulindac are cholestatic and 25% are hepatocellular. Despite previous reports to the contrary, current data analysis does not support a higher incidence of hepatotoxicity with **diclofenac**.[1,5,67]

Octreotide

Most patients on long-term therapy develop cholelithiasis and/or gallbladder sludge; some require cholecystectomy. The prevalence and speed of onset of symptoms might be dosage related.[68]

Papaverine

Numerous reports of hepatocellular injury and elevated liver enzymes in 27–43% of patients indicate a marked hepatotoxic potential.[1,69]

Pemoline

Pemoline occasionally causes elevated liver enzymes. The prescribing information for pemoline includes a boxed warning describing 15 cases of acute hepatic failure reported to the FDA between 1975 and 1998; 12 cases resulted in death or required liver transplantation. The earliest onset of hepatic abnormalities in these cases occurred 6 months after the start of pemoline therapy. The few published reports of possible pemoline-induced fulminant hepatic failure do not hold up well under close scrutiny.[1,70,71]

Penicillamine

Cholestasis resulting from a hypersensitivity reaction occurs occasionally.[1,72]

Penicillins

Cloxacillin and **flucloxacillin** are rarely associated with cholestatic hepatitis. The effect is reversible but can persist for months after drug discontinuation.[1,73–75]

(continued)

Phenothiazines

Most reports of liver damage involve **chlorpromazine**. The prevalence of hepatic enzyme elevation with this drug has been estimated to be as high as 42%, although 10% is probably more realistic. Similarly, cholestatic jaundice has been projected to occur in up to 5% of patients receiving chlorpromazine, but the actual prevalence is closer to 1%. The onset of cholestasis is generally in the first month of therapy and usually follows a prodrome of GI or influenza-like symptoms. About 70% of affected patients show signs of hypersensitivity, most frequently fever and eosinophilia, and only 5% have rash. Cholestasis usually follows a benign course, and most patients recover 1–2 months after drug discontinuation. A syndrome resembling primary biliary cirrhosis occasionally can occur. Despite the dominance of chlorpromazine in the reported cases, other phenothiazines can produce similar hepatic damage.[1,76]

Phenytoin

Hepatocellular necrosis is occasionally associated with phenytoin therapy, usually accompanied by other signs of hypersensitivity (eg, eosinophilia, fever, rash, and lymphadenopathy). Onset is usually during the first 6 weeks of therapy. Reported fatality rates have been as high as 30%. Increasing age is an apparent risk factor, with <5% of cases occurring in patients <10 yr old.[1,10,77,78]

Plicamycin

Laboratory evidence of dose-related hepatotoxicity occurs in virtually all patients. A common lesion is perivenous necrosis.[1,79]

Progestins

(*See* Steroids, C-17-α-Alkyl.)

Propoxyphene

A small number of cases of propoxyphene-induced cholestasis have been reported; these are thought to be the result of hypersensitivity.[1,80]

Propylthiouracil

Increased ALT levels occur in up to 30% of patients. Onset is usually within the first 2 months of therapy, and ALT levels commonly return to normal with dosage reduction. Clinical hepatitis occurs rarely.[1,81]

Pyrazinamide

Pyrazinamide-induced hepatitis depends on dose and duration of therapy. Daily administration appears to present a greater risk than weekly administration.[1,82,83]

Riluzole

Elevated hepatic enzymes occur frequently; the prevalence appears to be dosage related.[84]

Ritonavir

Elevations of serum AST and ALT greater than 3.6 times base line occur in 30% of patients treated with ritonavir.[85]

Quinidine

Hepatic damage is rare and usually accompanied by other signs of hypersensitivity, especially fever. Most reactions occur in the first month of therapy. The pathology is usually a mixture of hepatocellular necrosis and cholestasis; granulomas also have been reported.[1,86]

(*continued*)

Salicylates

Up to 50% of patients taking antiarthritic dosages have laboratory evidence of liver damage. The risk of liver damage is greatest in patients with connective tissue disorders such as SLE or juvenile rheumatoid arthritis. Clinically apparent salicylate-induced hepatitis is uncommon, usually mild, and readily reversible. Hepatotoxicity most often occurs at serum salicylate concentrations >250 mg/L, and only 7% of cases have serum salicylate levels <150 mg/L. Salicylates can cause microvesicular steatosis after intentional overdose.[1,5]

Steroids, C-17-α-Alkyl

Canalicular cholestasis occurs with a minimal amount of hepatic inflammation. The prevalence appears to be dose related; although laboratory changes are common (occurring in almost all patients taking anabolic steroids), jaundice is not. Jaundice may or may not be preceded by other clinical signs and usually follows 1–6 months of therapy. Peliosis hepatis also has been associated with these compounds, especially the anabolic steroids. Examples are **methyltestosterone, norethandrolone, methandrostenolone, fluoxymesterone, oxandrolone, oxymetholone,** and **stanozolol.** C-17-α-ethinyl steroids such as **ethinyl estradiol, mestranol, norethindrone,** and **norethynodrel** can produce similar reactions. An association between C-17-α-alkyl steroids and an increase in the prevalence of hepatocellular carcinoma is unclear.[1,87]

Sulfasalazine

A small number of cases of sulfasalazine-associated hepatic damage, including fatalities, have been reported in children and adults. Hepatic necrosis is apparently part of a generalized hypersensitivity reaction that includes rash, fever, and lymphadenopathy. Onset is usually within the first 4 weeks of therapy.[1,88]

Sulfonamides, Antibacterial

The sulfonamides currently in use have a lower prevalence of hepatitis than their predecessors, with most reported cases appearing before 1947. Most cases of hepatotoxicity develop during the first 2 weeks of therapy and many are accompanied by other signs of hypersensitivity.[1,39,89] (*See also* Trimethoprim-Sulfamethoxazole.)

Tacrine

In a study of 2446 patients receiving tacrine, 25% had serum ALT levels at least 3 times greater than the upper limit of normal (ULN), 6% had levels at least 10 times greater than the ULN, and 2% had levels at least 25 times greater than the ULN. Most increases were detected in the first week of therapy. Most patients' ALT levels returned to no more than twice the ULN within 1 month after drug discontinuation, and no patients developed jaundice. Only 33% developed ALT levels more than 3 times the ULN on rechallenge.[1,90]

Terbinafine

The FDA has received reports of liver failure and death apparently associated with oral terbinafine use, including some cases without predisposing risk factors.[98]

Tetracycline

Microvesicular steatosis can occur in patients receiving large doses of tetracycline IV, usually >1.5 g/day. Contributing factors include pregnancy, malnutrition, and impaired renal function, but hepatotoxicity has been reported in patients with none of these factors. Onset is usually during the first 10 days of therapy. Most cases of overt liver disease have resulted in death. Oral therapy also can produce signs of hepatotoxicity, although far less frequently.[1,39]

(*continued*)

Tolcapone

ALT levels increase to >3 times the upper limit of normal in about 8% of tolcapone-treated patients. These elevations usually develop 6–12 weeks after the start of tolcapone use and can resolve despite continued therapy. At least 3 deaths from fulminant hepatic failure have been reported.[91,92]

Trimethoprim-Sulfamethoxazole

"Clinically important" liver disease occurs in at least 5.2/100,000 patients (3.8/100,000 with trimethoprim alone). Patients with AIDS are much more susceptible to hepatic injury. The available evidence supports hypersensitivity as the mechanism and cholestasis as the predominant form of injury. Fulminant hepatic failure has been reported.[1,39,93]

Troleandomycin

From 30 to 50% of patients receiving the drug show some laboratory evidence of abnormal liver function, and up to 4% develop jaundice.[1]

Valproic Acid

Hepatic enzyme elevations occur in 7–44% of patients, with clinically apparent liver disease in 0.05–1%. Fatal hepatotoxicity occurs most often in children ≤2 yr old on polydrug therapy (1/600) and 3–10 yr old on monotherapy (1/16,000) or polytherapy (1/8300). The diffuse hepatocellular injury, microvesicular steatosis, and hepatic necrosis do not appear to be dose related and most commonly occur in the first 2–3 months of therapy. Serial liver function tests in asymptomatic patients do not predict patients at risk but are commonly recommended because immediate discontinuation might reverse the condition.[1,78,94,95]

Vitamin A

Hepatomegaly, portal hypertension, and mild increases in liver enzyme levels are common features of chronic vitamin A toxicity. Central vein sclerosis and perisinusoidal fibrosis, which can progress to cirrhosis, have been reported in cases of chronic intoxication. These effects are associated with doses >50,000 IU/day (sometimes with doses as low as 25,000 IU/day). Hepatotoxicity also is possible with acute doses >600,000 IU.[1,96]

Zafirlukast

Asymptomatic hepatic enzyme elevations occur frequently. At least three cases of severe hepatitis have been reported including one that resulted in liver transplantation.[97]

■ REFERENCES

1. Zimmerman HJ. *Hepatotoxicity: the adverse effects of drugs and other chemicals on the liver.* 2nd ed. Philadelphia: Lippincott Williams & Wilkins; 1999.
2. Hagley MT et al. Hepatotoxicity associated with angiotensin-converting enzyme inhibitors. *Ann Pharmacother* 1993;27:228–31.
3. Whitcomb DC, Block GD. Association of acetaminophen hepatotoxicity with fasting and ethanol use. *JAMA* 1994;272:1845–50.
4. Heubi JE et al. Therapeutic misadventures with acetaminophen: hepatotoxicity after multiple doses in children. *J Pediatr* 1998;132:22–7.
5. Tolman KG. Hepatotoxicity of non-narcotic analgesics. *Am J Med* 1998;105(1B):13S–19S.
6. Fisher B et al. Interleukin-2 induces profound reversible cholestasis: a detailed analysis in treated cancer patients. *J Clin Oncol* 1989;7:1852–62.
7. Arellano F, Sacristán JA. Allopurinol hypersensitivity syndrome: a review. *Ann Pharmacother* 1993;27:337–43.
8. Nagel GA et al. Phase II study of aminoglutethimide and medroxyprogesterone acetate in the treatment of patients with advanced breast cancer. *Cancer Res* 1982;42(suppl):3442S–4S.
9. Simpson DG, Walker JH. Hypersensitivity to para-aminosalicylic acid. *Am J Med* 1960;29:297–306.
10. Lee WM. Drug-induced hepatotoxicity. *N Engl J Med* 1995;333:1118–27.

11. Guigui B et al. Amiodarone-induced hepatic phospholipidosis: a morphological alteration independent of pseudoalcoholic liver disease. *Hepatology* 1988;8:1063–8.

12. Richer M, Robert S. Fatal hepatotoxicity following oral administration of amiodarone. *Ann Pharmacother* 1995;29:582–6.

13. Garcia Rodriguez LA et al. Risk of acute liver injury associated with combination of amoxicillin and clavulanic acid. *Arch Intern Med* 1996;156:1327–32.

14. Perry MC. Chemotherapeutic agents and hepatotoxicity. *Semin Oncol* 1992;19:551–65.

15. Pratt CB et al. Comparison of daily versus weekly L-asparaginase for the treatment of childhood acute leukemia. *J Pediatr* 1970;77:474–83.

16. Pratt CB, Johnson WW. Duration and severity of fatty metamorphosis of the liver following L-asparaginase therapy. *Cancer* 1971;28:361–4.

17. Gane E et al. Nodular regenerative hyperplasia of the liver graft after liver transplantation. *Hepatology* 1994; 20:88–94.

18. Grochow LB et al. Pharmacokinetics of busulfan: correlation with veno-occlusive disease in patients undergoing bone marrow transplantation. *Cancer Chemother Pharmacol* 1989;25:55–61.

19. Vassal G et al. Busulfan and veno-occlusive disease of the liver. *Ann Intern Med* 1990;112:881. Letter.

20. Horowitz S et al. Hepatotoxic reactions associated with carbamazepine therapy. *Epilepsia* 1988;29:149–54.

21. Thompson JW, Jacobs RF. Adverse effects of newer cephalosporins. An update. *Drug Saf* 1993;9:132–42.

22. Schoenfield LJ et al. Chenodiol (chenodeoxycholic acid) for dissolution of gallstones: the National Cooperative Gallstone Study. A controlled trial of efficacy and safety. *Ann Intern Med* 1981;95:257–82.

23. Labeling change. *FDA Med Bull* 1996;26(1):3.

24. MacFarlane B et al. Fatal fulminant liver failure due to clozapine: a case report and review of clozapine-induced hepatotoxicity. *Gastroenterology* 1997;112:1707–9.

25. Hummer M et al. Hepatotoxicity of clozapine. *J Clin Psychopharmacol* 1997;17:314–7.

26. Wanless IR et al. Histopathology of cocaine hepatotoxicity. Report of four patients. *Gastroenterology* 1990;98:497–501.

27. Lindberg MC. Hepatobiliary complications of oral contraceptives. *J Gen Intern Med* 1992;7:199–209.

28. Hannaford PC et al. Combined oral contraceptives and liver disease. *Contraception* 1997;55:145–51.

29. Atkinson K et al. Cyclosporine-associated hepatotoxicity after allogeneic marrow transplantation in man: differentiation from other causes of posttransplant liver disease. *Transplant Proc* 1983;15(suppl 1):2761–7.

30. Kassianides C et al. Liver injury from cyclosporine A. *Dig Dis Sci* 1990;35:693–7.

31. Utili R et al. Dantrolene-associated hepatic injury. Incidence and character. *Gastroenterology* 1977;72:610–6.

32. Ward A et al. Dantrolene. A review of its pharmacodynamic and pharmacokinetic properties and therapeutic use in malignant hyperthermia, the neuroleptic malignant syndrome and an update of its use in muscle spasticity. *Drugs* 1986;32:130–68.

33. Tomecki KJ, Catalano CJ. Dapsone hypersensitivity. The sulfone syndrome revisited. *Arch Dermatol* 1981; 117:38–9.

34. Kromann NP et al. The dapsone syndrome. *Arch Dermatol* 1982;118:531–2.

35. Mohle-Boetani J et al. The sulfone syndrome in a patient receiving dapsone prophylaxis for *Pneumocystis carinii* pneumonia. *West J Med* 1992;156:303–6.

36. Chick J. Safety issues concerning the use of disulfiram in treating alcohol dependence. *Drug Saf* 1999;20:427–35.

37. Inman WHW, Rawson NSB. Erythromycin estolate and jaundice. *Br Med J* 1983;286:1954–5.

38. Derby LE et al. Erythromycin-associated cholestatic hepatitis. *Med J Aust* 1993;158:600–2.

39. Carson JL et al. Acute liver disease associated with erythromycins, sulfonamides, and tetracyclines. *Ann Intern Med* 1993;119:576–83.

40. Conn HO et al. Ethionamide-induced hepatitis. A review with a report of an additional case. *Am Rev Resp Dis* 1964;90:542–52.

41. Sanchez MR et al. Retinoid hepatitis. *J Am Acad Dermatol* 1993;28:853–8.

42. O'Neil MG et al. Felbamate associated fatal acute hepatic necrosis. *Neurology* 1996;46:1457–9.

43. Rougier P et al. Hepatic arterial infusion of floxuridine in patients with liver metastases from colorectal carcinoma: long-term results of a prospective randomized trial. *J Clin Oncol* 1992;10:1112–8.

44. Wysowski DK, Fourcroy JL. Flutamide hepatotoxicity. *J Urol* 1996;155:209–12.

45. Food and Drug Administration. Important prescribing information. http://www.fda.gov/medwatch/safety/1999/eulexi.htm (accessed 1999 Oct 29).

46. Howrie DL, Gartner JC. Gold-induced hepatotoxicity: case report and review of the literature. *J Rheumatol* 1982;9:727–9.

47. Landas SK et al. Lipogranulomas and gold in the liver in rheumatoid arthritis. *Am J Surg Pathol* 1992;16:171–4.

48. Neuberger JM. Halothane and hepatitis. Incidence, predisposing factors and exposure guidelines. *Drug Saf* 1990;5:28–38.

49. Elliott RH, Strunin L. Hepatotoxicity of volatile anaesthetics. *Br J Anaesth* 1993;70:339–48.
50. Garcia Rodriguez LA et al. The risk of acute liver injury associated with cimetidine and other acid-suppressing anti-ulcer drugs. *Br J Clin Pharmacol* 1997;43:183–8.
51. Millard PS et al. Isoniazid-related fatal hepatitis. *West J Med* 1996;164:486–91.
52. Pande JN et al. Risk factors for hepatotoxicity from antituberculosis drugs: a case-control study. *Thorax* 1996;51:132–6.
53. Nolan CM et al. Hepatotoxicity associated with isoniazid preventive therapy. A 7-year survey from a public health tuberculosis clinic. *JAMA* 1999;281:1014–8.
54. Chien R-N et al. Hepatic injury during ketoconazole therapy in patients with onychomycosis: a controlled cohort study. *Hepatology* 1997;25:103–7.
55. Fayad M et al. Potential hepatotoxicity of lamotrigine. *Pediatr Neurol* 2000;22:49–52.
56. Einhorn M, Davidsohn I. Hepatotoxicity of mercaptopurine. *JAMA* 1964;188:802–6.
57. Kremer JM et al. Methotrexate for rheumatoid arthritis. Suggested guidelines for monitoring liver toxicity. *Arthritis Rheum* 1994;37:316–28.
58. Farrow AC et al. Serum aminotransferase elevation during and following treatment of childhood acute lymphoblastic leukemia. *J Clin Oncol* 1997;15:1560–6.
59. Ahern MJ et al. Methotrexate hepatotoxicity: what is the evidence? *Inflamm Res* 1998;47:148–51.
60. Zachariae H. Liver biopsies and methotrexate: a time for reconsideration? *J Am Acad Dermatol* 2000;42:531–4.
61. Rodman JS et al. Methyldopa hepatitis. A report of six cases and review of the literature. *Am J Med* 1976; 60:941–8.
62. Lawrenson RA et al. Liver damage associated with minocycline use in acne. A systematic review of the published literature and pharmacovigilance data. *Drug Saf* 2000;23:333–49.
63. Gough A et al. Minocycline induced autoimmune hepatitis and systemic lupus erythematosis-like syndrome. *BMJ* 1996;312:169–72.
64. Serious adverse events attributed to nevirapine regimens for postexposure prophylaxis after HIV exposures—worldwide, 1997–2000. *MMWR* 2001;49:1153–6.
65. McKenney JM et al. A comparison of the efficacy and toxic effects of sustained- vs immediate-release niacin in hypercholesterolemic patients. *JAMA* 1994;271:672–7.
66. Stricker BH et al. Hepatic injury associated with the use of nitrofurans: a clinicopathological study of 52 reported cases. *Hepatology* 1988;8:599–606.
67. Walker AM. Quantitative studies of the risk of serious hepatic injury in persons using nonsteroidal antiinflammatory drugs. *Arthritis Rheum* 1997;40:201–8.
68. Trendle MC et al. Incidence and morbidity of cholestasis in patients receiving chronic octreotide for metastatic carcinoid and malignant islet cell tumors. *Cancer* 1997;79:830–4.
69. Pathy MS, Reynolds AJ. Papaverine and hepatotoxicity. *Postgrad Med J* 1980;56:488–90.
70. Shevell M, Schreiber R. Pemoline-associated hepatic failure: a critical analysis of the literature. *Pediatr Neurol* 1997;16:14–6.
71. Food and Drug Administration. http:www.fda.gov/medwatch/safety/1999/cylert.htm (accessed 1999 Jun 18).
72. Seibold JR et al. Cholestasis associated with D-penicillamine therapy: case report and review of the literature. *Arthritis Rheum* 1981;24:554–6.
73. Olsson R et al. Liver damage from flucloxacillin, cloxacillin, and dicloxacillin. *J Hepatol* 1992;15:154–61.
74. Derby LE et al. Cholestatic hepatitis associated with flucloxacillin. *Med J Aust* 1993;158:596–600.
75. Presti ME et al. Nafcillin-associated hepatotoxicity. Report of a case and review of the literature. *Dig Dis Sci* 1996;41:180–4.
76. Regal RE et al. Phenothiazine-induced cholestatic jaundice. *Clin Pharm* 1987;6:787–94.
77. Smythe MA, Umstead GS. Phenytoin hepatotoxicity: a review of the literature. *DICP* 1989;23:13–8.
78. Wyllie E, Wyllie R. Routine laboratory monitoring for serious adverse effects of antiepileptic medications: the controversy. *Epilepsia* 1991;32(suppl 5):S74–9.
79. Green L, Donehower RC. Hepatic toxicity of low doses of mithramycin in hypercalcemia. *Cancer Treat Rep* 1984;68:1379–81.
80. Bassendine MF et al. Dextropropoxyphene induced hepatotoxicity mimicking biliary tract disease. *Gut* 1986;27:444–9.
81. Liaw Y-F et al. Hepatic injury during propylthiouracil therapy in patients with hyperthyroidism. A cohort study. *Ann Intern Med* 1993;118:424–8.
82. Hong Kong Chest Service/British Medical Research Council. Controlled trial of four thrice-weekly regimens and a daily regimen all given for 6 months for pulmonary tuberculosis. *Lancet* 1981;1:171–4.
83. Cohen CD et al. Hepatic complications of antituberculosis therapy revisited. *S Afr Med J* 1983;63:960–3.

84. Miller RG et al. Clinical trials of riluzole in patients with ALS. ALS/Riluzole Study Group—II. *Neurology* 1996;47(suppl 2):S86–92.

85. Sulkowski MS et al. Hepatotoxicity associated with antiretroviral therapy in adults infected with human immunodeficiency virus and the role of hepatitis C or B virus infection. *JAMA* 2000;283:74–80.

86. Geltner D et al. Quinidine hypersensitivity and liver involvement. A survey of 32 patients. *Gastroenterology* 1976;70:650–2.

87. Haupt HA, Rovere GD. Anabolic steroids: a review of the literature. *Am J Sports Med* 1984;12:469–84.

88. Boyer DL et al. Sulfasalazine-induced hepatotoxicity in children with inflammatory bowel disease. *J Pediatr Gastroenterol Nutr* 1989;8:528–32.

89. Dujovne CA et al. Sulfonamide hepatic injury. Review of the literature and report of a case due to sulfamethoxazole. *N Engl J Med* 1967;277:785–8.

90. Watkins PB et al. Hepatotoxic effects of tacrine administration in patients with Alzheimer's disease. *JAMA* 1994;271:992–8.

91. Waters CH et al. Tolcapone in stable Parkinson's disease: efficacy and safety of long-term treatment. The Tolcapone Stable Study Group. *Neurology* 1997;49:665–71.

92. Food and Drug Administration. New warnings for Parkinson's drug, Tasmar. http://www.fda.gov/bbs/topics/ANSWERS/AN00924.html (accessed 1998 Nov 17).

93. Jick H, Derby LE. A large population-based follow-up study of trimethoprim-sulfamethoxazole, trimethoprim, and cephalexin for uncommon serious drug toxicity. *Pharmacotherapy* 1995;15:428–32.

94. Siemes H et al. Valproate (VPA) metabolites in various clinical conditions of probable VPA-associated hepatotoxicity. *Epilepsia* 1993;34:332–46.

95. Bryant AE, Dreifuss FE. Valproic acid hepatic fatalities. III. U.S. experience since 1986. *Neurology* 1996;46:465–9.

96. Kowalski TE et al. Vitamin A hepatotoxicity: a cautionary note regarding 25,000 IU supplements. *Am J Med* 1994;97:523–8.

97. Reinus JF et al. Severe liver injury after treatment with the leukotriene receptor antagonist zafirlukast. *Ann Intern Med* 2000;133:964–8.

98. Food and Drug Administration. FDA issues health advisory regarding the safety of Sporanox® products and Lamisil® tablets to treat fungal nail infections. http://www.fda.gov/bbs/topics/answers/2001/ans01083.html (accessed 2001 May 19).

Drug-Induced Nephrotoxicity

This table includes agents that are associated with drug-induced nephrotoxicity but excludes drugs that produce nephrotoxicity as a result of damage to tissues other than the kidney (eg, liver or skeletal muscle). The following abbreviations are used in the table:

Cl_{cr} — Creatinine Clearance
Cr_s — Serum Creatinine
GFR — Glomerular Filtration Rate
mOsm — Milliosmole

Acetaminophen

Tubular necrosis has been reported, usually in association with hepatotoxicity from acute overdose. Whether nephrotoxicity is a direct effect of acetaminophen or the result of liver damage is the subject of controversy. There is a possible association between prolonged acetaminophen use (1–5 kg cumulative dosage) and the development of chronic renal failure. There is insufficient evidence to associate acetaminophen use alone with analgesic nephropathy. (*See* Analgesics.)[1–8]

ACE Inhibitors

ACE inhibitors are frequently associated with proteinuria and renal insufficiency. The prevalence of proteinuria in **captopril-**treated patients is estimated at 1%. The risks of renal insufficiency are greater with long-acting ACE inhibitors such as **enalapril** or **lisinopril** than with captopril. Immune complex glomerulopathy is a major contributor to ACE inhibitor nephrotoxicity. Hyponatremia, diuretic therapy (and other causes of hypovolemia), pre-existing renal impairment, CHF, and diabetes mellitus contribute to an increased risk of nephrotoxicity. Recovery of renal function usually follows ACE inhibitor discontinuation.[1,2,9–12]

Acetazolamide

Glaucoma therapy with acetazolamide is associated with a 10-fold increase in the risk of renal stone formation. Calcium phosphate and calcium oxalate stones have been identified.[13,14]

Acyclovir

Acyclovir is concentrated in the urine, and its precipitation in the collecting tubules with subsequent obstructive nephropathy frequently accompanies high-dose (500 mg/m^2) IV use; oral therapy is apparently free from this problem. Aggressive hydration (100–150 mL urine/hr) and administration over 1–2 hr should minimize the risk. Normal renal function usually returns within 6 weeks after drug withdrawal.[2,9,15,16]

Aldesleukin

Almost all patients receiving aldesleukin develop acute renal impairment marked by decreased Cl$_{cr}$, oliguria or anuria, and fluid retention. Most patients recover within 1 week after drug discontinuation, but some require ≥1 month.[17]

Allopurinol

Glomerulonephritis, interstitial nephritis, and interstitial fibrosis occur rarely in allopurinol-treated patients. Most cases are associated with generalized hypersensitivity reactions to allopurinol (allopurinol hypersensitivity syndrome).[18,19]

Aminoglycosides

Proximal tubular necrosis occurs in up to 30% of patients treated with aminoglycosides for >7 days. Because of slow clearance of these drugs from renal tissue, they still can be present in high concentrations in the kidney after serum levels are undetectable, but there does not appear to be a good correlation between renal tissue concentrations of individual aminoglycosides and their nephrotoxic potential. Aminoglycoside-induced acute renal failure is usually nonoliguric, which can delay its recognition. It is often first detected as an asymptomatic increase in Cr$_s$. Detectable changes in GFR usually occur at least 5 days after initiation of therapy and can progress after drug discontinuation. Aminoglycoside-induced renal damage is related to total dosage and duration of treatment. Administration of single daily doses does not markedly affect the frequency of nephrotoxicity. Recovery of some to all lost renal function can occur over several weeks after drug discontinuation. Monitoring of aminoglycoside plasma levels and serial renal function tests might be of value in recognizing nephrotoxicity. **Neomycin** has the greatest and **streptomycin** the least nephrotoxic potential of the aminoglycosides. All other currently marketed aminoglycosides have intermediate nephrotoxic potentials. Concomitant therapy with other nephrotoxic drugs should be avoided.[1,10,20–23]

(continued)

Amphotericin B

Mild or moderate renal impairment occurs in 50% of patients treated with conventional amphotericin B, with severe renal impairment in 8%. The drug causes a reduction in renal plasma flow as well as glomerular and tubular damage. Most patients experience a rapid decline in GFR, which often stabilizes at 20–60% of normal and might not return to normal until several months after drug discontinuation. Distal tubular damage can lead to loss of concentrating ability, renal tubular acidosis, and electrolyte disturbances (most commonly hypokalemia but also hyponatremia and hypomagnesemia). These effects appear to be dosage related, and many patients respond favorably to temporary drug discontinuation or reduction in dosage. The prevalence of nephrotoxicity increases as the cumulative dose increases. Some investigators suggest that the total dosage of conventional amphotericin B should be kept below 3–5 g. Nephrotoxicity is increased by the coadministration of other nephrotoxic drugs, especially cyclosporine. Sodium loading (eg, 1 L normal saline IV daily) reduces the frequency and severity of amphotericin B–induced nephrotoxicity. Newer dosage forms (eg, liposomal amphotericin B) appear to be less nephrotoxic.[1,2,9,10,24–26]

Analgesics

Analgesic nephropathy is a syndrome of papillary necrosis, interstitial nephritis, and progressive renal medullary impairment that occurs in persons with long-term consumption of large quantities of oral analgesic products, especially combination products. Most reported patients are 30–70 yr old, and women greatly outnumber men. The syndrome is characterized by proteinuria, reduced renal concentrating ability, and RBCs and WBCs in the urine. Analgesic nephropathy has been clearly associated with products containing **phenacetin,** but the removal of phenacetin from nonprescription analgesic products has not been consistently associated with a decline in analgesic nephropathy mortality. **Acetaminophen** or **salicylates** taken alone or in combination do not seem to cause analgesic nephropathy. Historically, this syndrome has been responsible for a large percentage of chronic renal failure deaths, with considerable variation in prevalence among nations (high in Australia and Germany, low in the United States), apparently reflecting analgesic abuse patterns. Mild cases are reversible, but severe cases can continue to deteriorate after the discontinuation of analgesics. The prevalence of urinary tract cancer appears higher than normal among chronic analgesic abusers.[1,2,5–8]

Azacitidine

Proximal and distal tubular dysfunction, polyuria, glucosuria, and decreases in serum bicarbonate occur occasionally during azacitidine therapy.[27]

Carboplatin

Although apparently less nephrotoxic than cisplatin, carboplatin therapy is frequently associated with reductions in GFR and increased electrolyte losses (especially calcium and magnesium). Patients with pre-existing renal impairment and those who receive inadequate hydration during drug administration are at greatest risk.[28]

Cephalosporins

The cephalosporin (and cephamycin) antibiotics are capable of producing rare interstitial nephritis similar to the penicillins. Increases in BUN and Cr_s occur occasionally. The nephrotoxicity of the newer cephalosporins is minimal compared with older drugs such as **cephalothin.**[29–31]

Cidofovir

Proteinuria occurs frequently during cidofovir therapy. **Probenecid** decreases the prevalence and magnitude of proteinuria and must be given with cidofovir.[32]

(continued)

Cisplatin

Dosage-related proximal tubular impairment is the major limiting factor in cisplatin therapy and can occur in 50–75% of patients. Cl_{cr} is typically reduced to 60–80% of baseline with repeated courses of therapy. The greatest damage occurs in the first month of therapy, and it appears to be more likely when the drug is administered repetitively at close intervals. Forced hydration and mannitol diuresis can reduce renal toxicity, at least for the first cycle of therapy. Magnesium and calcium losses are common manifestations of cisplatin-induced nephrotoxicity. Cisplatin-induced renal effects can be detected as long as 6 months after the end of therapy.[1,19,28,33]

Contrast Media, Radiopaque

Increased Cr_s occurs frequently in patients receiving iodine-containing contrast media. In unselected patients, the prevalence of Cr_s >0.5 mg/dL or >50% above pretreatment is 2–7%. Renal lesions include medullary necrosis and proximal tubular vacuolation and necrosis as well as the deposition of urate and oxalate crystals. The most common pattern is acute oliguric renal failure developing within 24 hr after the administration of the contrast agent and lasting 2–5 days; nonoliguric renal failure also has been reported. Most patients recover fully, but permanent renal impairment has been reported. Cr_s usually peaks 3–5 days after exposure and returns to baseline in 10–14 days. Patients with pre-existing renal impairment are at much greater risk and constitute 60% of those experiencing nephrotoxicity. Vigorous hydration before, during, and after drug administration with hypotonic saline reduces the risk of nephrotoxicity, but mannitol or furosemide diuresis can increase the risk. High-osmolality ionic contrast media might be more nephrotoxic than low-osmolality ionic contrast media. Nonionic contrast agents might be less nephrotoxic than ionic agents.[1,2,10,34–36]

Cyclosporine

Dose-related nephrotoxicity occurs in 30–50% of cyclosporine-treated patients and frequently limits the usefulness of the drug. Reduction in dosage usually reduces the renal toxicity. The drug produces decreased GFR, impaired tubular function, interstitial nephritis, hypertension, fluid retention, and hyperkalemia. Cyclosporine causes vasoconstriction in preglomerular arterioles, which can lead to chronic arteriopathy and tubular atrophy if the dosage is not reduced. Cyclosporine nephrotoxicity is usually reversible during the first 6 months of therapy, but the risk of permanent renal impairment increases with time. **Calcium-channel blockers** appear to reduce the prevalence of cyclosporine-induced nephrotoxicity in renal transplant patients.[1,2,9,20,37,38]

Demeclocycline

This drug can produce nephrogenic diabetes insipidus, which is usually, but not always, dosage related. For this reason, it has been used in the management of the syndrome of inappropriate antidiuretic hormone secretion.[20,39] (*See also* Tetracyclines.)

Diuretics, Thiazide

Occasional cases of interstitial nephritis have been reported, which might be the result of hypersensitivity reactions. Long-term use of diuretics might increase the risk of renal cell carcinoma, especially in women.[2,40]

Fluoroquinolones

Acute interstitial nephritis is associated with fluoroquinolone antibiotics; a hypersensitivity mechanism is suspected but remains to be confirmed. Most reported patients are >50 yr old.[41]

Foscarnet

Acute tubular necrosis occurs frequently with foscarnet. Cr_s increased during 35 of 56 courses of therapy in one retrospective study. Hydration with normal saline appears to markedly decrease the severity and frequency of nephrotoxicity.[42]

(*continued*)

Furosemide

Use of high-dose furosemide (5–10 mg/kg/day) in adults with refractory CHF is associated with a 40% decrease in Cl_{cr}. Nephrocalcinosis and nephrolithiasis occur in up to 64% of low-birthweight infants treated with furosemide. These effects usually resolve after drug discontinuation.[43,44]

Gallium Nitrate

Nephrotoxicity is the most frequent adverse effect of gallium, and elevations in BUN and Cr_s can occur after only 1 dose. At least 1 death has been associated with gallium-induced nephrotoxicity.[45,46]

Gold Salts

A lesion resembling membranous glomerulonephritis with proteinuria can occur in 3–10% of patients receiving parenteral gold therapy. Microhematuria and nephrotic syndrome are less frequent. One-half of the cases of proteinuria develop in the first 6 months of therapy. Occasionally, acute tubular necrosis and interstitial nephritis are reported. Although recovery can take up to 18 months, permanent renal impairment after drug withdrawal is uncommon. There is evidence for immune and direct toxic mechanisms for gold nephrotoxicity. Oral **auranofin** appears to be less nephrotoxic than parenteral gold products.[1,2,9,10,47,48]

Ifosamide

Reversible, subclinical nephrotoxicity occurs in almost all ifosamide-treated patients, with clinically important nephrotoxicity in many. Renal damage might correlate with total dosage, and cumulative doses >60 g/m^2 should be avoided, especially in children <5 yr old. Fanconi syndrome–like symptoms including renal loss of glucose, electrolytes, and small proteins occur in 4%.[28,49,50]

Immune Globulin

Intravenous administration of immune globulin can produce reversible acute renal failure after the first or repeated exposures. The origin of the acute renal failure is not the immune globulin but rather the large amount of sucrose used in some immune globulin products to reduce the formation of immunoglobulin aggregates. The damage is probably due to the delivery of a high-osmotic solute load to the kidneys. Maltose- and dextrose-stabilized products might have the same capacity, but there are no case reports in the literature.[51]

Indinavir

Crystalluria occurs in most indinavir-treated patients; many develop nephrolithiasis, back pain, or flank pain. The crystals contain indinavir; good hydration (2–3 L fluid/day) reduces their formation.[16,52,53]

Lithium

Lithium frequently produces nephrogenic diabetes insipidus, which is, at least in part, dosage related. This typically mild effect is usually reversible with drug withdrawal. Long-term therapy (10–15 yr) is associated with an increased prevalence of reduced Cl_{cr} and renal concentrating ability that are frequently not reversible, despite withdrawal of lithium. Interstitial nephritis and nephrotic syndrome also have been reported.[1,2,9,10,54–56]

Mannitol

High doses (>200 g/day or >400 g/2 days) are associated with acute oliguric renal failure. Although low doses act as renal vasodilators, high doses produce renal vasoconstriction. Keeping the osmolal gap to no more than 55 mOsm/kg should minimize the risk. Acute renal failure might require 7–10 days for recovery; dialysis shortens the recovery period to 1–2 days.[57,58]

(continued)

Methotrexate

This drug is directly toxic to the kidney in large doses, causing acute tubular necrosis. Acute renal impairment occurs in 30–50% of patients treated with high-dose methotrexate and leucovorin rescue. Most cases are reversible within 3 weeks. Methotrexate is eliminated primarily through the kidney, and its nephrotoxicity compounds itself by causing the serum level of the drug to rise. About 20% of deaths associated with methotrexate therapy are caused by acute renal failure. The drug and its metabolites precipitate in the distal tubule. Close monitoring of methotrexate serum concentrations and adjustment of dosage might minimize the risk of nephrotoxicity, as would vigorous hydration and alkalinization during drug administration.[2,16,59,60]

Methoxyflurane

Nephrogenic diabetes insipidus, proximal tubular damage, and interstitial nephritis are reported. The nephrotoxicity of methoxyflurane appears to be dose related and might be caused by increased circulating fluoride ion concentrations. Fluoride causes distal tubular dysfunction by inhibiting sodium and chloride transport in the ascending loop of Henle and reducing the response to antidiuretic hormone. Urinary oxalate crystallization also has been reported after methoxyflurane anesthesia.[20,61,62]

Mitomycin

Tubular necrosis occurs most frequently with daily therapy but is also reported with the intermittent therapy now recommended. Nephrotoxicity appears to be related to the total dosage administered, with the risk of renal impairment rising when the total dosage exceeds 30 mg/m^2. Onset can be delayed for many months.[63,64]

Nitrosoureas

The nitrosoureas can produce insidious nephrotoxicity in patients on long-term therapy. **Lomustine** seems to have the greatest nephrotoxic potential. Some cases of permanent renal function impairment have been reported.[65]

Nonsteroidal Anti-inflammatory Drugs

NSAIDs, including **COX-2 inhibitors,** can reduce Cl_{cr} and produce renal insufficiency as a result of renal circulatory changes caused by inhibition of prostaglandin synthesis. These effects tend to be relatively minor and usually reversible. The prevalence is usually low (0.5–1% of patients), but some patients are at increased risk; predisposing factors are advanced age, pre-existing renal impairment, and states of renal hypoperfusion (eg, sodium depletion, hypotension, diuretic use, hepatic cirrhosis, and CHF). Reversible acute interstitial nephritis and necrosis occur occasionally. It is not possible at this time to accurately categorize the prevalence associated with each NSAID. **Fenoprofen** is the NSAID most commonly associated with interstitial nephritis and nephrotic syndrome.[1,2,6–10,20,66]

Omeprazole

Interstitial nephritis occurs rarely during omeprazole therapy. At least 13 cases have been published, 10 with positive biopsies; 5 cases were rechallenged with recurrence of interstitial nephritis in all. Onset is usually after 2 weeks to 6 months of omeprazole therapy.[67]

Penicillamine

Slight to moderate proteinuria occurs in 7–30% of patients on long-term (≥6 months) therapy with penicillamine for rheumatoid arthritis. Most cases develop in the first year. Proteinuria is usually benign and slowly reversible over 6–12 months, but nephrotic syndrome is occasionally encountered. The lesions appear to be perimembranous glomerulonephritis resulting from the deposition of antigen–antibody complexes on the renal basement membrane.[1,2,10,20,68]

(continued)

Penicillins

Interstitial nephritis has been reported with most penicillins. Methicillin was by far the most frequently implicated penicillin (frequency 10–16%); the reason for its dominance in unknown. Penicillin-induced interstitial nephritis is an immune reaction that most commonly occurs during a long course of therapy. The reaction is usually accompanied by other signs of hypersensitivity such as fever, rash, and eosinophilia; hematuria also can occur. The reduction of renal function might not be oliguric, so urine volume is not a reliable parameter to monitor. Recovery usually occurs within weeks to months after drug discontinuation.[1,2,20,69]

Pentamidine

Prospective trials of IV pentamidine for the treatment of *Pneumocystis carinii* pneumonia show nephrotoxicity in 4–66% of patients. Onset is usually 8–12 days after the start of therapy.[70]

Plicamycin

High doses (50 μg/kg/day) produced renal impairment in 40% of patients, including some who died of acute renal failure. Nephrotoxicity is far less likely at the 25–30 μg/kg/day (or lower) dosage used most often.[71]

Polymyxins

Adverse reactions involving the kidney occur in about 20% of patients receiving **colistimethate** parenterally. Tubular necrosis is the most frequently described lesion, but interstitial nephritis is also reported. High dosage, long duration of therapy, and renal impairment are predisposing factors. Polymyxin-induced renal damage is usually reversible, but some patients continue to deteriorate after drug withdrawal.[72]

Rifampin

There are at least 49 published cases of rifampin-induced acute renal failure. Acute tubular necrosis is the most common lesion. This appears to be a hypersensitivity reaction and most often occurs with intermittent or interrupted dosage regimens but has accompanied continuous therapy.[73]

Streptozocin

Nephrotoxicity is the most common dosage-limiting side effect. The prevalence increases with prolonged administration until virtually all patients demonstrate renal impairment. Dosages <1.5 g/m^2/week are less toxic. The damage is glomerular and tubular. The drug should be discontinued as soon as renal damage is detected.[28,71]

Sulfonamides, Antibacterial

Early sulfonamides were poorly soluble, and urinary crystallization was a common problem. Crystalluria occurs in 8–29% of **sulfadiazine**-treated patients; symptomatic renal impairment resulting largely from nephrolithiasis occurs in 2–8%. Crystallization occurs in <0.3% of patients receiving the more soluble sulfonamides and adequate hydration. Interstitial nephritis, glomerulonephritis, and tubular necrosis are reported rarely. These reactions are probably allergic in origin.[2,9,16,74,75]

Tacrolimus

Acute nephrotoxicity occurs with a prevalence similar to that of cyclosporine. Progressive nephrotoxicity is reported with long-term (>1 yr) therapy. The risk of nephrotoxicity can be greatly limited by keeping the tacrolimus whole blood concentration <20 μg/L.[37,76,77]

(continued)

Tetracyclines

Fanconi syndrome, characterized by tubular damage with proteinuria, glycosuria, aminoaciduria, and electrolyte disturbances, was associated with the use of outdated tetracycline products. Because of changes in the manufacturing process, this syndrome is now unlikely to occur. The antianabolic effects of tetracyclines can contribute to azotemia in patients with pre-existing renal impairment.[78] (*See also* Demeclocycline.)

Topiramate

Nephrolithiasis occurs in 1.5% of topiramate-treated patients.[79]

Triamterene

Triamterene therapy is associated with an increase in urinary sediment, and the drug can be incorporated into existing renal calculi. One report suggests that 1/1500 users of the drug will develop triamterene-associated calculi during the course of 1 yr. As a precaution, the drug probably should not be used in patients with a history of renal calculi. Triamterene also might be associated with the development of interstitial nephritis.[16,80,81]

Vancomycin

Nephrotoxicity from vancomycin was commonly reported early in its history. Currently, the prevalence of vancomycin-induced renal impairment (usually mild) is 5–17%. It is usually reversible after discontinuation of the drug. Concomitant administration of **aminoglycosides** results in at least additive nephrotoxicity.[2,82–85]

■ REFERENCES

1. Koren G. The nephrotoxic potential of drugs and chemicals. Pharmacological basis and clinical relevance. *Med Toxicol Adverse Drug Exp* 1989;4:59–72.
2. Wang AYM, Lai KN. Drug-induced renal diseases. *Adverse Drug React Bull* 1994;Oct(168):635–8.
3. Blantz RC. Acetaminophen: acute and chronic effects on renal function. *Am J Kidney Dis* 1996;28(suppl 1):S3–6.
4. Barrett BJ. Acetaminophen and adverse chronic renal outcomes: an appraisal of the epidemiological evidence. *Am J Kidney Dis* 1996;28(suppl 1):S14–9.
5. De Broe ME, Elseviers MM. Analgesic nephropathy. *N Engl J Med* 1998;338:446–52.
6. Elseviers MM, De Broe ME. Analgesic nephropathy. Is it caused by multi-analgesic abuse or single substance use? *Drug Saf* 1999;20:15–24
7. Gault MH, Barrett BJ. Analgesic nephropathy. *Am J Kidney Dis* 1998;32:351–60.
8 Delzell E, Shapiro S. A review of epidemiologic studies of nonnarcotic analgesics and chronic renal disease. *Medicine* 1998;77:102–21.
9. Choudhury D, Ahmed Z. Drug-induced nephrotoxicity. *Med Clin North Am* 1997;81:705–17.
10. Hoitsma AJ et al. Drug-induced nephrotoxicity. Aetiology, clinical features and management. *Drug Saf* 1991; 61:131–47.
11. Mandal AK et al. Diuretics potentiate angiotensin converting enzyme inhibitor-induced acute renal failure. *Clin Nephrol* 1994;42:170–4.
12. Textor SC. Renal failure related to angiotensin-converting enzyme inhibitors. *Semin Nephrol* 1997;17:67–76.
13. Kass MA et al. Acetazolamide and urolithiasis. *Ophthalmology* 1981;88:261–5.
14. Tawil R et al. Acetazolamide-induced nephrolithiasis: implications for treatment of neuromuscular disorders. *Neurology* 1993;43:1105–6.
15. Sawyer MH et al. Acyclovir-induced renal failure. Clinical course and histology. *Am J Med* 1988;84:1067–71.
16. Perazella MA. Crystal-induced acute renal failure. *Am J Med* 1999;106:459–65.
17. Vial T, Descotes J. Clinical toxicity of interleukin-2. *Drug Saf* 1992;7:417–33.
18. Elasy T et al. Allopurinol hypersensitivity syndrome revisited. *West J Med* 1995;162:360–1.
19. Arellano F, Sacristán JA. Allopurinol hypersensitivity syndrome: a review. *Ann Pharmacother* 1993;27:337–43.
20. Werner M, Costa MJ. Nephrotoxicity of xenobiotics. *Clin Chim Acta* 1995;237:107–54.
21. Barclay ML, Begg EJ. Aminoglycoside toxicity and relation to dose regimen. *Adverse Drug React Toxicol Rev* 1994;13:207–34.
22. Ali MZ, Goetz MB. A meta-analysis of the relative efficacy and toxicity of single daily dosing versus multiple daily dosing of aminoglycosides. *Clin Infect Dis* 1997;24:796–809.

23. Swan SK. Aminoglycoside nephrotoxicity. *Semin Nephrol* 1997;17:27–33.

24. Anderson CM. Sodium chloride treatment of amphotericin B nephrotoxicity—standard of care? *West J Med* 1995;162:313–7.

25. Sorkine P et al. Administration of amphotericin B in lipid emulsion decreases nephrotoxicity: results of a prospective, randomized, controlled study in critically ill patients. *Crit Care Med* 1996;24:1311–5.

26. Luber AD et al. Risk factors for amphotericin B–induced nephrotoxicity. *J Antimicrob Chemother* 1999; 43:267–71.

27. Kintzel PE, Dorr RT. Anticancer drug renal toxicity and elimination: dosing guidelines for altered renal function. *Cancer Treat Rev* 1995;21:33–64.

28. Cornelison TL, Reed E. Nephrotoxicity and hydration management for cisplatin, carboplatin, and ormaplatin. *Gynecol Oncol* 1993;50:147–58.

29. Quin JD. The nephrotoxicity of cephalosporins. *Adverse Drug React Acute Poison Rev* 1989;8:63–72.

30. Zhanel GG. Cephalosporin-induced nephrotoxicity: does it exist? *DICP* 1990;24:262–5.

31. Thompson JW, Jacobs RF. Adverse effects of newer cephalosporins. An update. *Drug Saf* 1993;9:132–42.

32. Polis MA et al. Anticytomegaloviral activity and safety of cidofovir in patients with human immunodeficiency virus infection and cytomegalovirus viuria. *Antimicrob Agents Chemother* 1995;39:882–6.

33. Anand AJ, Bashey B. Newer insights into cisplatin nephrotoxicity. *Ann Pharmacother* 1993;27;1519–25.

34. Solomon R. Radiocontract-induced nephropathy. *Semin Nephrol* 1998;18:551–7.

35. Gerlach AT, Pickworth KK. Contrast medium-induced nephrotoxicity: pathophysiology and prevention. *Pharmacotherapy* 2000;20:540–8.

36. Katzberg RW. Urography into the 21st century: new contrast media, renal handling, imaging characteristics, and nephrotoxicity. *Radiology* 1997;204:297–312.

37. Andoh TF et al. Nephrotoxicity of immunosuppressive drugs: experimental and clinical observations. *Semin Nephrol* 1997;17:34–45.

38. Rossi SJ et al. Prevention and management of the adverse effects associated with immunosuppressive therapy. *Drug Saf* 1993;9:104–31.

39. Forrest JN et al. Superiority of demeclocycline over lithium in the treatment of chronic syndrome of inappropriate secretion of antidiuretic hormone. *N Engl J Med* 1978;298:173–7.

40. Grossman E et al. Does diuretic therapy increase the risk of renal cell carcinoma? *Am J Cardiol* 1999;83: 1090–3.

41. Lomaestro BM. Fluoroquinolone-induced renal failure. *Drug Saf* 2000;22:479–85.

42. Deray G et al. Foscarnet nephrotoxicity: mechanism, incidence and prevention. *Am J Nephrol* 1989;9: 316–21.

43. Alon US et al. Nephrocalcinosis and nephrolithiasis in infants with congestive heart failure treated with furosemide. *J Pediatr* 1994;125:149–51.

44. Cotter G et al. Increased toxicity of high-dose furosemide versus low-dose dopamine in the treatment of refractory congestive heart failure. *Clin Pharmacol Ther* 1997;62:187–93.

45. Samson MK et al. Phase I–II clinical trial of gallium nitrate (NSC–15200). *Cancer Clin Trials* 1980;3:131–6.

46. Warrell RP et al. Treatment of patients with advanced malignant lymphoma using gallium nitrate administered as a seven-day continuous infusion. *Cancer* 1983;51:1982–7.

47. Hall CL. Gold nephropathy. *Nephron* 1988;50:265–72.

48. Newton P et al. Proteinuria with gold therapy: when should gold be permanently stopped? *Br J Rheumatol* 1983;22:11–7.

49. Loebstein R, Koren G. Ifosamide-induced nephrotoxicity in children: critical review of predictive risk factors. *Pediatrics* 1998;101(6):E8.

50. Ho PTC et al. A prospective evaluation of ifosamide-related nephrotoxicity in children and young adults. *Cancer* 1995;76:2557–64.

51. Renal insufficiency and failure associated with immune globulin intravenous therapy—United States, 1985–1998. *MMWR* 1999;48:518–21.

52. Gagnon RF et al. Prospective study of urinalysis abnormalities in HIV-positive individuals treated with indinavir. *Am J Kidney Dis* 2000;36:507–15.

53. Saltel E et al. Increased prevalence and analysis of risk factors for indinavir nephrolithiasis. *J Urol* 2000;164: 1895–7.

54. Gitlin M. Lithium and the kidney. An updated review. *Drug Saf* 1999;20:231–43.

55. Bendz H et al. Kidney damage in long-term lithium patients: a cross-sectional study of patients with 15 years or more on lithium. *Nephrol Dial Transplant* 1994;9:1250–4.

56. Walker RG. Lithium nephrotoxicity. *Kidney Int* 1993;44(suppl 42):S93–8.

57. Dorman HR et al. Mannitol-induced acute renal failure. *Medicine* 1990;69:153–9.

58. Gadallah MF et al. Case report: mannitol nephrotoxicity syndrome: role of hemodialysis and postulate of mechanisms. *Am J Med Sci* 1995;309:219–22.

59. Condit PT et al. Renal toxicity of methotrexate. *Cancer* 1969;23:126–31.

60. Stoller RG et al. Use of plasma pharmacokinetics to predict and prevent methotrexate toxicity. *N Engl J Med* 1997;297:630–4.

61. Cousins MJ, Mazze RI. Methoxyflurane nephrotoxicity. A study of dose response in man. *JAMA* 1973;225: 1611–6.

62. Desmond JW. Methoxyflurane nephrotoxicity. *Can Anaesth Soc J* 1974;21:294–307.

63. Valavaara R, Nordman E. Renal complications of mitomycin C therapy with special reference to the total dose. *Cancer* 1985;55:47–50.

64. Verweij J et al. Mitomycin C–induced renal toxicity, a dose-dependent side effect? *Eur J Cancer Clin Oncol* 1987;23:195–9.

65. Weiss RB et al. Nephrotoxicity of semustine. *Cancer Treat Rep* 1983;67:1105–12.

66. Bennett WM et al. The renal effects of nonsteroidal anti-inflammatory drugs: summary and recommendations. *Am J Kidney Dis* 1996;28(suppl 1):S56–62.

67. Yip D et al. Omeprazole-induced interstitial nephritis. *J Clin Gastroenterol* 1997;25:450–2.

68. Hall CL et al. Natural course of penicillamine nephropathy: a long term study of 33 patients. *Br Med J* 1988; 296:1083–6.

69. Appel GB. A decade of penicillin related acute interstitial nephritis—more questions than answers. *Clin Nephrol* 1980;13:151–4.

70. O'Brien JG et al. A 5-year retrospective review of adverse drug reactions and their risk factors in human immunodeficiency virus–infected patients who are receiving intravenous pentamidine therapy for *Pneumocystis carinii* pneumonia. *Clin Infect Dis* 1997;24:854–9.

71. Ries F. Nephrotoxicity of chemotherapy. *Eur J Cancer Clin Oncol* 1988;24:951–3.

72. Koch-Weser J et al. Adverse effects of sodium colistimethate. Manifestations and specific reaction rates during 317 courses of therapy. *Ann Intern Med* 1970;72:857–68.

73. De Vriese AS et al. Rifampicin-associated acute renal failure: pathophysiologic, immunologic, and clinical features. *Am J Kidney Dis* 1998;31:108–15.

74. Appel GB, Neu HC. The nephrotoxicity of antimicrobial agents (third of three parts). *N Engl J Med* 1977;296:784–7.

75. Becker K et al. Sulfadiazine-associated nephrotoxicity in patients with the acquired immunodeficiency syndrome. *Medicine* 1996;75:185–94.

76. Porayko MK et al. Nephrotoxicity of FK 506 and cyclosporine when used as primary immunosuppression in liver transplant recipients. *Transplant Proc* 1993;25:665–8.

77. Böttiger Y et al. Tacrolimus whole blood concentrations correlate closely to side-effects in renal transplant recipients. *Br J Clin Pharmacol* 1999;48:445–8.

78. Appel GB, Neu HC. The nephrotoxicity of antimicrobial agents (second of three parts). *N Engl J Med* 1977; 296:722–8.

79. Shorvon SD. Safety of topiramate: adverse events and relationships to dosing. *Epilepsia* 1996;37(suppl 2): S18–22.

80. Ettinger B et al. Triamterene nephrolithiasis. *JAMA* 1980;244:2443–5.

81. Sica DA, Gehr TWB. Triamterene and the kidney. *Nephron* 1989;51:454–61.

82. Bailie GR, Neal D. Vancomycin ototoxicity and nephrotoxicity. A review. *Med Toxicol Adverse Drug Exp* 1988;3:376–86.

83. Eng RHK et al. Effect of intravenous vancomycin on renal function. *Chemotherapy* 1989;35:320–5.

84. Rybak MJ et al. Nephrotoxicity of vancomycin, alone and with an aminoglycoside. *J Antimicrob Chemother* 1990;25:679–87.

85. Duffull SB, Begg EJ. Vancomycin toxicity. What is the evidence for dose dependency? *Adverse Drug React Toxicol Rev* 1994;13:103–14.

Drug-Induced Oculotoxicity

Occasionally, nonspecific blurred vision occurs with almost all drugs. The agents in this table are associated with a specific pattern of drug-induced oculotoxicity when administered *systemically*.

Allopurinol

Despite the discovery of allopurinol in cataractous lenses taken from patients on long-term (>2 yr) therapy, there is no clinical evidence for an increased risk of cataracts in allopurinol-treated patients.[1–3]

(*continued*)

Amantadine

At least 9 cases of diffuse, white, subendothelial corneal opacities have been reported. These opacities usually resolved within a few weeks after amantadine discontinuation.[4]

Amiodarone

Most patients treated with amiodarone develop bilateral corneal microdeposits (75% after 1 yr of therapy). Visual symptoms occur in 6–14%. Halo vision at night is most commonly reported, but patients also might complain of photophobia and blurred vision. The deposits are apparently dose related and reversible, disappearing 3–7 months after drug discontinuation. Minute lens opacities occurred in 7 of 14 amiodarone-treated patients in one study.[5–7]

Anticholinergic Agents

Blurring of vision can result from paralysis of accommodation (cycloplegia). These drugs also dilate the pupil (mydriasis), which can produce photophobia and precipitate narrow-angle glaucoma. With systemic administration, large doses are usually required to produce mydriasis, which is most commonly associated with potent anticholinergics such as **atropine, scopolamine,** or **benztropine.** Patients being treated for narrow-angle glaucoma can usually tolerate systemic anticholinergic therapy but nevertheless should avoid these drugs unless absolutely necessary. Patients with open-angle glaucoma, particularly if treated, can receive anticholinergic medications without much risk. Patients receiving nebulized **ipratropium** by face mask are at risk for developing increased intraocular pressure and precipitation of narrow-angle glaucoma, probably from the drug escaping from beneath ill-fitting masks and directly affecting the eyes. All of the ocular effects of anticholinergics are dose related and reversible.[5,8–10]

Anticonvulsants

Diplopia and nystagmus occur frequently. Blurred vision can be caused by mydriasis (**phenytoin**) or cycloplegia (**carbamazepine**). All of these effects are dose related.[11]

Antidepressants, Heterocyclic

These drugs have anticholinergic properties and can precipitate narrow-angle glaucoma and cycloplegia at usual doses. (*See* Anticholinergic Agents.) There is a 10–30% prevalence of blurred vision resulting from cycloplegia, but it is rarely troublesome and is reversible with drug discontinuation. Blurred vision usually resolves despite continued antidepressant use as the eye becomes tolerant to the drug's effects. **SSRIs** do not seem to produce any important ocular effects.[5,12,13]

Antihistamine Drugs (H$_1$-Blockers)

With the exception of **loratadine** and **fexofenadine,** these drugs have some anticholinergic properties and can precipitate narrow-angle glaucoma and cycloplegia. (*See* Anticholinergic Agents.) These effects are minor and reversible with drug discontinuation. Antihistamines (most notably **diphenhydramine**) can reduce night vision.[5,9,14]

β-Adrenergic Blocking Agents

A reduction in tear production occurs, which can produce a hot, dry, gritty sensation in the eyes. This is rapidly reversible with drug discontinuation.

Bromocriptine

Myopia is a frequent complication of long-term bromocriptine therapy and often goes unappreciated until the patient complains of blurred vision. The cause is not fully determined but might be due to lens swelling. Myopia is reversible within 1–2 weeks after drug discontinuation.[5,15,16]

Busulfan

Long-term therapy (usually ≥1 yr) with busulfan is associated with the development of posterior subcapsular cataracts in about 10% of patients.[3,17–19]

(*continued*)

Chloramphenicol

Optic neuritis, papilledema, and visual field defects are occasionally reported. These effects can occur after weeks or years of therapy but are most common after several months of chloramphenicol use. Most cases are reported in children with cystic fibrosis, but the association with this disorder is unclear and might only reflect the types of patients who received long-term chloramphenicol therapy. Permanent visual impairment and recovery are reported after drug discontinuation. There are anecdotal reports that large doses of vitamins B_6 and B_{12} have beneficial effects on these adverse ocular effects.[5,19–22]

Chloroquine

The oculotoxicity of chloroquine limits its usefulness; two general types of ocular change occur: corneal deposits and retinopathy. About 50% of patients demonstrate corneal deposits, less than one-half of whom have visual impairment resulting from these deposits. Opacities present as punctate or whirling patterns. They can appear after 2 months and usually do not interfere with vision. They are usually reversible in 6–8 weeks after drug discontinuation. Early changes in the retina (deposition of pigment in the macula) are usually asymptomatic and reversible. More advanced damage includes hyperpigmentation of the macula surrounded by a depigmented ring and hyperpigmented retina ("bull's-eye" retinopathy). Patients complain of reading difficulty, blurred vision, visual field defects, and photophobia; some also report defective color vision and light flashes. The prevalence ranges from 3% to 45% in various reports. The drug should be discontinued if these symptoms develop. Patients receiving long-term therapy with chloroquine 3 mg/kg/day should have ophthalmologic examinations at least every 6 months initially and then annually if their vision remains stable. Those receiving >3 mg/kg/day should be examined every 6 months.[27] Daily dosage seems to be more important than the total dosage or duration of therapy for the development of retinopathy; limiting the daily dosage to 4 mg/kg up to a maximum of 250 mg in adults minimizes the risk. The prognosis of chloroquine-induced retinopathy is uncertain. Weekly use of chloroquine for malarial prophylaxis does not seem to cause retinopathy.[15,23–27]

Cidofovir

Anterior uveitis occurs in about one-third of AIDS patients receiving the drug intravenously for treatment of cytomegalovirus retinitis. The onset is usually after 4–5 days of treatment. Uveitis usually responds to topical cycloplegics and corticosteroids and does not require discontinuation of cidofovir.[28]

Cisplatin

Blurred vision and altered color perception are frequently associated with high-dose cisplatin. Blurred vision gradually improves after drug discontinuation, although altered color vision can persist. Pigmentary retinopathy is also reported.[3,18,19]

Clomiphene

Visual disturbances, most commonly blurred vision, occur frequently with clomiphene. These disturbances usually disappear after the drug is withdrawn, but one report of three patients describes prolonged afterimages, shimmering of the peripheral visual field, and photophobia.[29]

Contraceptives, Oral

A variety of retinal vascular disorders have been attributed to oral contraceptives, but the association remains unproved. It is purported that some oral contraceptive users cannot tolerate contact lenses, possibly because of ocular edema or dryness; however, a prospective study failed to show any differences in lens tolerance between oral contraceptive users and nonusers.[30,31]

(continued)

Corticosteroids

These drugs can produce a variety of ocular disorders with long-term therapy, most notably glaucoma and cataracts. Corticosteroid-induced increases in intraocular pressure occur in approximately 30% of long-term users and appear to be dose related. Glaucoma can persist for several months after drug discontinuation. Corticosteroid-induced cataracts (usually posterior subcapsular) are found in 10–40% of patients on long-term, systemic therapy and are correlated with total dosage and duration of therapy. Outcome is variable, ranging from improvement despite continued therapy to rare loss of sight. Most patients have no vision impairment. Although they most commonly occur with large oral doses, increased intraocular pressure and cataracts are reported in patients receiving corticosteroids by the topical ophthalmic, inhalation, and intranasal routes. Children develop cataracts more frequently than adults; Hispanics might be affected more often than blacks or non-Hispanic whites.[2,3,5,18,19,32–35]

Cyclophosphamide

Keratoconjunctivitis occurs in up to 50%. One report showed a 17% prevalence of transient reversible blurred vision during high-dose cyclophosphamide therapy. Recovery took from 1 hr to 14 days.[3,18,19,36]

Cyclosporine

Retinopathy occurs frequently with cyclosporine and severe visual disturbances, including cortical blindness, occur occasionally. Oculotoxicity appears to be dose related and resolves after drug discontinuation.[19,37]

Cytarabine

Keratoconjunctivitis, corneal damage, ocular pain, and photophobia are frequent, dose-related side effects of cytarabine. These symptoms usually resolve 1–2 weeks after drug discontinuation. Pretreatment with corticosteroid eye drops can be beneficial but should be used with caution in patients with corneal damage.[3,18,19,38,39]

Deferoxamine

Oculotoxicity, including blurred vision, impaired color vision, night blindness, and retinal deposits, occurs in 4–11% of patients receiving deferoxamine for chronic iron overload. These effects appear to be dose related and might be caused by the chelation of trace minerals.[40–43]

Digitalis Glycosides

The most unique ocular effect is the frosted or snowy appearance of objects or colored halos around them. These effects are most noticeable in bright light. Color vision might be affected such that objects appear yellow (green or other colors are reported, but far less frequently). With **digoxin,** color changes usually occur when the plasma level exceeds 1.5 µg/L. Digitalis glycosides also are reported to produce photophobia, blurred vision, central scotomas, and flickering or light flashes before the eyes. Reversible ocular side effects occur in up to 25% of patients with digitalis intoxication.[5,44,45]

Disopyramide

The anticholinergic effects of disopyramide frequently produce blurred vision.[46]

Disulfiram

A few cases of retrobulbar neuritis have occurred, manifested by a dramatic decline in visual acuity and impairment of color vision. In most patients, vision returns to normal after drug discontinuation.[5,47]

Doxorubicin

This drug stimulates excessive lacrimation shortly after administration in about 25% of patients. Conjunctivitis also has been reported.[18,19,48]

(continued)

Ethambutol

Retrobulbar neuritis is the primary ocular complication. Symptoms include blurred vision, scotoma, and reduction of the visual field. Color vision defects also occur, usually presenting as a reduction in green perception. Retrobulbar neuritis is dose related, occurring most frequently with dosages ≥25 mg/kg/day. Its onset is usually after 3–6 months of therapy, and it is slowly reversible after drug discontinuation. Dosages ≤15 mg/kg/day appear relatively free of ocular side effects.[5]

Fenoldopam

Treatment of hypertensive emergencies with fenoldopam results in dose-dependent, mild increases in intraocular pressure during the infusion. Increases in intraocular pressure occur in patients with and without ocular hypertension. The importance of these findings is not established.[49,50]

Fluorouracil

Adverse ocular effects occur in 25–50% of patients receiving fluorouracil systemically. Blurred vision, ocular irritation and pain, conjunctivitis, keratitis, and excessive lacrimation occur frequently. These effects resolve in 1–2 weeks after drug discontinuation. Some patients can develop eversion of the eyelid margin (cicatricial ectropion) or potentially irreversible fibrosis of the tear duct (dacryostenosis) with prolonged therapy.[3,5,18,19,51,52]

Gold Salts

Parenteral gold can produce microscopic crystalline deposits in the cornea, most commonly in the superficial layers. These deposits are dose related and rarely occur until the total dosage of parenteral gold exceeds 1 g. The deposits slowly resolve after drug discontinuation, do not appear to affect vision, and are not a reason to stop gold therapy. **Auranofin** does not seem to produce these ocular effects.[5,53,54]

Hydroxychloroquine

This drug can produce the same spectrum of ocular toxicity as **chloroquine.** (*See* Chloroquine.) Corneal deposits occur only with high daily doses. Limiting the daily dosage to 6.5 mg/kg up to a maximum of 400 mg in adults minimizes the risk of retinopathy.[5,24,25,27,55,56]

Interferon Alfa

Although the prevalence cannot be accurately determined, retinal vascular complications have been reported. Onset is usually after 2–3 months of treatment. These effects appear to be reversible after drug discontinuation.[57]

Iodine, Radioactive (^{131}I)

Ophthalmopathy, including diplopia and changes in visual acuity, occurred or worsened in 15% of patients with Graves' hyperthyroidism treated with ^{131}I after a 3–4 month course of methimazole. Patients treated with a combination of ^{131}I and prednisone or continued methimazole did not show any increased ophthalmopathy. All changes occurred during the first 6 months after ^{131}I treatment. Ophthalmic changes persisted for 2–3 months in 65% of those affected, longer in the other 35%.[58]

Isoniazid

Optic neuritis occurs occasionally, most commonly in malnourished or alcoholic patients, and often manifests itself as impaired red–green perception. It responds to **pyridoxine** therapy.[5]

Methotrexate

Adverse ocular effects associated with systemic methotrexate occur in up to 25% and include conjunctivitis, increased or decreased lacrimation, photophobia, and eye pain. Onset is during the first week of therapy, and resolution usually occurs 1–2 weeks after drug discontinuation.[13,18,19]

(*continued*)

Minocycline

Dark-blue discoloration of the sclera has been reported. Although the prevalence cannot be accurately estimated, the growing use of minocycline as an antiarthritic drug should increase the number of cases. It is not known if the discoloration is reversible.[59]

Muromonab-CD3

Conjunctivitis and photophobia occur frequently.[60]

Oprelvekin

Transient blurred vision and conjunctival injection occur frequently during oprelvekin therapy. Papilledema occurs in 1.5%.

Oxygen

Retrolental fibroplasia is an important complication of oxygen therapy in neonates, in particular premature or other low-birthweight neonates. The risk of retrolental fibroplasia in these patients increases whenever the concentration of inspired oxygen exceeds normal.[61–63]

Paclitaxel

Scintillating scotomas or photopsia occur frequently during paclitaxel infusions. The onset of these short-lived effects is usually during the last hour of the infusion. They do not always recur during subsequent infusions.[19,64,65]

Pamidronate

Reversible anterior uveitis and conjunctivitis are occasional complications of pamidronate therapy. Onset is usually 24–48 hr after IV infusion.[28,66]

Pentostatin

Conjunctivitis and keratitis frequently occur during pentostatin therapy. Whereas conjunctivitis is usually mild, keratitis can be severe.[3]

Phenothiazines

Lesions of the lens, cornea, and retina are the most important features of phenothiazine-induced oculotoxicity. White to yellow-brown deposits in the lens most frequently occur with long-term, high total-dose (>600 g) **chlorpromazine** therapy. Epithelial keratopathy, possibly resulting from a photosensitivity reaction, can occur after only a few months of high-dose therapy. It is characterized by diffuse opacification of the corneal epithelium. The consistent use of sunglasses can reduce the risk of keratopathy. Lens and corneal deposits usually do not interfere with vision, and all of these effects might be slowly reversible. **Thioridazine** is most noted for producing pigmentary retinopathy. As with most phenothiazine-induced ocular effects, pigmentary retinopathy is dose related. Patients might complain of blurred vision, decreased night vision, brown discoloration of vision, and central scotoma. Vision might improve if the drug is withdrawn soon enough; however, some cases continue to deteriorate despite drug discontinuation. Other phenothiazines can cause pigmentary retinopathy, but the supporting data are limited to case reports. Phenothiazines (especially thioridazine) have anticholinergic effects and might precipitate narrow-angle glaucoma. Corneal edema is a rare, but dangerous, complication of phenothiazine use, requiring immediate discontinuation of therapy.[12,67,68]

Psoralens

The combination of psoralens and long-wave ultraviolet light (PUVA therapy) radiation is associated with the development of conjunctivitis, photophobia, and other signs of ocular irritation. The use of UVA protective lenses during therapy greatly reduces the prevalence. An experimentally demonstrated connection between PUVA therapy and cataracts has not been confirmed clinically.[5,69,70]

(continued)

Quinine

Loss of visual acuity and reduction of the visual field to the point of blindness can occur with quinine therapy or (especially) overdose. Other reported ocular effects are impaired color vision and night blindness. These effects are usually reversible, but permanent constriction of the visual field and blindness are reported. The ocular effects of quinine might be the result of changes in the retinal vasculature.[5,71,72]

Retinoids

Blepharoconjunctivitis occurs in >50% of patients receiving **isotretinoin.** This painful condition appears to be dose related, and its onset is usually during the first 2 months of therapy. Dry eyes can occur with or without blepharoconjunctivitis. Corneal opacities, which clear in 6–7 weeks after drug discontinuation, also are reported. Similar effects were reported with etretinate. Other effects associated with retinoid therapy are papilledema and night blindness. Resolution usually occurs within a week after retinoid discontinuation.[5,19,73–76]

Rifabutin

Uveitis occurs frequently during rifabutin treatment and prophylaxis of *Mycobacterium avium* complex infection in AIDS patients. Its onset is variable (2 weeks to 7 months after starting treatment). Uveitis can be unilateral or bilateral and responds to topical corticosteroid therapy.[28,77,78]

Rifampin

Exudative conjunctivitis, ocular pain, and orange staining of tears (and consequent staining of soft contact lenses) are occasionally reported with rifampin. These effects are rapidly reversible when the drug is withdrawn.[79–81]

Sympathomimetic Agents

These drugs can dilate the pupil and precipitate narrow-angle glaucoma. Sympathomimetics with marked α-adrenergic activity (eg, **ephedrine, phenylpropanolamine, tetrahydrozoline**) should be avoided. The risk of this reaction is slight unless large doses are taken orally or the drugs are applied topically.[9]

Tamoxifen

Fine, refractile retinal opacities and retinopathy occur frequently; corneal opacities also are reported. The prevalence of retinopathy has been 1.5–11.8% in prospective studies. Although these lesions can occur with any dosage, they occur most often with daily dosages >180 mg or cumulative dosages >100 g. They can result in reduced visual acuity and are slowly reversible after drug discontinuation.[3,5,18,19,82]

Vigabatrin

Visual field loss (concentric or bilateral nasal) occurs to some degree in 29–40% of vigabatrin-treated patients and is severe in 9%. Males are more susceptible than females.[83,84]

Vinca Alkaloids

Various ocular disorders occur frequently. Most (ptosis, blurred vision, night blindness) are thought to be the result of cranial nerve impairment. Ptosis occurs in up to 50% of vincristine-treated patients. Time to onset ranges widely (2–44 weeks) as does resolution after drug discontinuation (2–24 weeks). **Vincristine** might be more oculotoxic than **vinblastine.**[3,5,18,19,85]

■ REFERENCES

1. Lerman S et al. Further studies on allopurinol therapy and human cataractogenesis. *Am J Ophthalmol* 1984; 97:205–9.
2. Clair WK et al. Allopurinol use and the risk of cataract formation. *Br J Ophthalmol* 1989;73:173–6.

3. Burns LJ. Ocular toxicities of chemotherapy. *Semin Oncol* 1992;19:492–500.

4. Fraunfelder FT, Meyer SM. Amantadine and corneal deposits. *Am J Ophthalmol* 1990;110:96–7. Letter.

5. Davidson SI, Rennie IG. Ocular toxicity from systemic drug therapy. An overview of clinically important adverse reactions. *Med Toxicol* 1986;1:217–24.

6. Flach AJ et al. Amiodarone-induced lens opacities. *Arch Ophthalmol* 1983;101:1554–6.

7. Naccarelli GV et al. Adverse effects of amiodarone. Pathogenesis, incidence and management. *Med Toxicol Adverse Drug Esp* 1989;4:246–53.

8. Hiatt RL et al. Systemically administered anticholinergic drugs and intraocular pressure. *Arch Ophthalmol* 1970;84:735–40.

9. Durkee DP, Bryant BG. Drug therapy reviews: drug therapy of glaucoma. *Am J Hosp Pharm* 1978;35: 682–90.

10. Singh J et al. Nebulized bronchodilator therapy causes acute angle closure glaucoma in predisposed individuals. *Respir Med* 1993;87:559–61. Letter.

11. Goldman MJ, Schultz-Ross RA. Adverse ocular effects of anticonvulsants. *Psychosomatics* 1993;34:154–8.

12. Oshika T. Ocular adverse effects of neuropsychiatric agents. Incidence and management. *Drug Saf* 1995;12:256–63.

13. Ritch R et al. Oral imipramine and acute angle closure glaucoma. *Arch Ophthalmol* 1994;112:67–8.

14. Luria SM et al. Effects of aspirin and dimenhydrinate (Dramamine) on visual processes. *Br J Clin Pharmacol* 1979;7:585–93.

15. Calne DB et al. Long-term treatment of Parkinsonism with bromocriptine. *Lancet* 1978;1:735–8.

16. Manor RS et al. Myopia during bromocriptine treatment. *Lancet* 1981;1:102. Letter.

17. Podos SM, Canellos GP. Lens changes in chronic granulocytic leukemia. Possible relationship to chemotherapy. *Am J Ophthalmol* 1969;68:500–4.

18. Imperia PS et al. Ocular complications of systemic cancer chemotherapy. *Surv Ophthalmol* 1989;34:209–30.

19. Al-Tweigeri T et al. Ocular toxicity and cancer chemotherapy. A review. *Cancer* 1996;78:1359–73.

20. Cocke JG et al. Optic neuritis with prolonged use of chloramphenicol. Case report and relationship to fundus changes in cystic fibrosis. *J Pediatr* 1966;68:27–31.

21. Huang NN et al. Visual disturbances in cystic fibrosis following chloramphenicol administration. *J Pediatr* 1966;68:32–44.

22. Cocke JG. Chloramphenicol optic neuritis. Apparent protective effects of very high daily doses of pyridoxine and cyanocobalamin. *Am J Dis Child* 1967;114:424–6.

23. Harley RD et al. Optic neuritis and optic atrophy following chloramphenicol in cystic fibrosis patients. *Trans Am Acad Ophthalmol Otolaryngol* 1970;74:1011–31.

24. Easterbrook M. Ocular effects and safety of antimalarial agents. *Am J Med* 1988;85(suppl 4A):23–9.

25. Kerdel F et al. Antimalarial agents and the eye. *Dermatol Clin* 1992;10:513–9.

26. Lange WR et al. No evidence for chloroquine-associated retinopathy among missionaries on long-term malaria chemoprophylaxis. *Am J Trop Med Hyg* 1994;51:389–92.

27. Easterbrook MA, Bernstein H. Ophthalmological monitoring of patients taking antimalarials: preferred practice patterns. *J Rheumatol* 1997;24:1390–2.

28. Fraunfelder FW, Rosenbaum JT. Drug-induced uveitis. Incidence, prevention and treatment. *Drug Saf* 1997;17: 197–207.

29. Purvin VA. Visual disturbance secondary to clomiphene citrate. *Arch Ophthalmol* 1995;113:482–4.

30. De Vries Reilingh A et al. Contact lens tolerance and oral contraceptives. *Ann Ophthalmol* 1978;10:947–52.

31. Petursson GJ et al. Oral contraceptives. *Ophthalmology* 1981;88:368–71.

32. Renfro L, Snow JS. Ocular effects of topical and systemic steroids. *Dermatol Clin* 1992;10:505–12.

33. Toogood JH et al. Association of ocular cataracts with inhaled and oral steroid therapy during long-term treatment of asthma. *J Allergy Clin Immunol* 1993;91:571–9.

34. Opatowsky I et al. Intraocular pressure elevation associated with inhalation and nasal corticosteroids. *Ophthalmology* 1995;102:177–9.

35. Cumming RG et al. Use of inhaled corticosteroids and the risk of cataracts. *N Engl J Med* 1997;337:8–14.

36. Kende G et al. Blurring of vision. A previously undescribed complication of cyclophosphamide therapy. *Cancer* 1979;44:69–71.

37. Memon M et al. Reversible cyclosporine-induced cortical blindness in allogenic bone marrow transplant recipients. *Bone Marrow Transplant* 1995;15:283–6.

38. Lass JH et al. Topical corticosteroid therapy for corneal toxicity from systemically administered cytarabine. *Am J Ophthalmol* 1982;94:617–21.

39. Herzig RH et al. High-dose cytosine arabinoside therapy for refractory leukemia. *Blood* 1983;62:361–9.

40. Olivieri NF et al. Visual and auditory neurotoxicity in patients receiving subcutaneous deferoxamine infusions. *N Engl J Med* 1986;314:869–73.

41. De Virgiliis S et al. Depletion of trace elements and acute ocular toxicity induced by desferrioxamine in patients with thalassemia. *Arch Dis Child* 1988;63:250–5.

42. Cases A et al. Acute visual and auditory neurotoxicity in patients with end-stage renal disease receiving desferrioxamine. *Clin Nephrol* 1988;29:176–8.

43. Cases A et al. Ocular and auditory toxicity in hemodialyzed patients receiving desferrioxamine. *Nephron* 1990;56:19–23.

44. Robertson DM et al. Ocular manifestations of digitalis toxicity. Discussion and report of three cases of central scotomas. *Arch Ophthalmol* 1966;76:640–5.

45. Aronson JK, Ford AR. The use of colour vision measurement in the diagnosis of digoxin toxicity. *Q J Med* 1980;49:273–82.

46. Bauman JL. Long-term therapy with disopyramide phosphate: side effects and effectiveness. *Am Heart J* 1986;111:654–60.

47. Norton AL, Walsh FB. Disulfiram-induced optic neuritis. *Trans Am Acad Ophthalmol Otolaryngol* 1972;76:1263–5.

48. Curran CF, Luce JK. Ocular adverse reactions associated with Adriamycin (doxorubicin). *Am J Ophthalmol* 1989;108:709–11.

49. Everitt DE et al. Effect of intravenous fenoldopam on intraocular pressure in ocular hypertension. *J Clin Pharmacol* 1997;37:312–20.

50. Elliott WJ et al. Intraocular pressure increases with fenoldopam, but not nitroprusside, in hypertensive humans. *Clin Pharmacol Ther* 1991;49:285–93.

51. Straus DJ et al. Cicatricial ectropion secondary to 5-fluorouracil therapy. *Med Pediatr Oncol* 1977;3:15–9.

52. Haidak DJ et al. Tear-duct fibrosis (dacryostenosis) due to 5-fluorouracil. *Ann Intern Med* 1978;88:657.

53. Bron AJ et al. Epithelial deposition of gold in the cornea in patients receiving systemic therapy. *Am J Ophthalmol* 1979;88:354–60.

54. Kincaid MC et al. Ocular chrysiasis. *Arch Ophthalmol* 1982;100:1791–4.

55. Easterbrook M. The ocular safety of hydroxychloroquine. *Semin Arthritis Rheum* 1993;23(suppl 1):62–7.

56. Bernstein HN. Ocular safety of hydroxychloroquine sulfate (Plaquenil). *South Med J* 1992;85:274–9.

57. Guyer DR et al. Interferon-associated retinopathy. *Arch Ophthalmol* 1993;111:350–6.

58. Bartalena L et al. Relation between therapy for hyperthyroidism and the course of Graves' ophthalmopathy. *N Engl J Med* 1998;338:73–8.

59. Fraunfelder FW, Randall JA. Minocycline-induced scleral pigmentation. *Ophthalmology* 1997;104:936–8.

60. Dukar O, Barr CC. Visual loss complicating OKT3 monoclonal antibody therapy. *Am J Ophthalmol* 1993;115:781–5.

61. Committee on Fetus and Newborn, American Academy of Pediatrics. History of oxygen therapy and retrolental fibroplasia. *Pediatrics* 1976;57(suppl):591–642.

62. Betts EK et al. Retrolental fibroplasia and oxygen administration during general anesthesia. *Anesthesiology* 1977;47:518–20.

63. Naiman J et al. Retrolental fibroplasia in hypoxic newborn. *Am J Ophthalmol* 1979;88:55–8.

64. Capri G et al. Optic nerve disturbances: a new form of paclitaxel neurotoxicity. *J Natl Cancer Inst* 1994;86:1099–101.

65. Seidman AD, Barrett S. Photopsia during 3-hour paclitaxel administration at doses ≥250 mg/m². *J Clin Oncol* 1994;12:1741–2. Letter.

66. Macarol V, Fraunfelder FT. Pamidronate disodium and possible ocular adverse drug reactions. *Am J Ophthalmol* 1994;118:220–4.

67. Bond WS, Yee GC. Ocular and cutaneous effects of chronic phenothiazine therapy. *Am J Hosp Pharm* 1980;37:74–8.

68. Ngen CC, Singh P. Long-term phenothiazine administration and the eye in 100 Malaysians. *Br J Psychiatry* 1988;152:278–80.

69. Farber EM et al. Current status of oral PUVA therapy for psoriasis. Eye protection revisions. *J Am Acad Dermatol* 1982;6:851–5.

70. Stern RS. Ocular lens findings in patients treated with PUVA. Photochemotherapy follow-up-study. *J Invest Dermatol* 1994;103:534–8.

71. Gangitano JL, Keltner JL. Abnormalities of the pupil and visual-evoked potential in quinine amblyopia. *Am J Ophthalmol* 1980;89:425–30.

72. Dyson EH et al. Death and blindness due to overdose of quinine. *Br Med J* 1985;291:31–3.

73. Fraunfelder FT et al. Adverse ocular reactions possibly associated with isotretinoin. *Am J Ophthalmol* 1985;100:534–7.

74. Lebowitz MA, Berson DS. Ocular effects of oral retinoids. *J Am Acad Dermatol* 1988;19:209–11.

75. Gold JA et al. Ocular side effects of the retinoids. *Intern J Dermatol* 1989;28:218–25.

76. Gross EG, Helfgott MA. Retinoids and the eye. *Dermatol Clin* 1992;10:521–31.

77. Saran BR et al. Hypopyon uveitis in patients with acquired immunodeficiency syndrome treated for systemic *Mycobacterium avium* complex infection with rifabutin. *Arch Ophthalmol* 1994;112:1159–65.

78. Karbassi M, Nikou S. Acute uveitis in patients with acquired immunodeficiency syndrome receiving prophylactic rifabutin. *Arch Ophthalmol* 1995;113:699–701.
79. Cayley FE, Majumdar SK. Ocular toxicity due to rifampicin. *Br Med J* 1976;1:199–200.
80. Lyons RW. Orange contact lenses from rifampin. *N Engl J Med* 1979;300:372–3. Letter.
81. Harris J, Jenkins P. Discoloration of soft contact lenses by rifampin. *Lancet* 1985;2:1133. Letter.
82. Nayfield SG, Gorin MB. Tamoxifen-associated eye disease: a review. *J Clin Oncol* 1996;14:1018–26.
83. Wild JM et al. Characteristics of a unique visual field defect attributed to vigabatrin. *Epilepsia* 1999;40:1784–94.
84. Kälviäinen R et al. Vigabatrin, a gabaergic antiepileptic drug, causes concentric visual field defects. *Neurology* 1999;53:922–6.
85. Albert DM et al. Ocular complications of vincristine therapy. *Arch Ophthalmol* 1967;78:709–13.

Drug-Induced Ototoxicity

Drug-induced ototoxicity can affect hearing (auditory or cochlear function), balance (vestibular function), or both, depending on the drug. Drugs of almost every class have been reported to produce tinnitus, as have placebos. The agents in this table are associated with measurable changes in hearing or vestibular defect when administered *systemically*.

Aminoglycosides

Aminoglycoside antibiotics can cause cochlear and vestibular toxicities. Cochlear toxicity presents as progressive hearing loss, starting with the highest tones and advancing to lower tones. Thus, considerable damage can occur before the patient is cognizant of it. Vestibular damage presents as dizziness, vertigo, or ataxia. Both forms of ototoxicity are usually bilateral and potentially reversible, but permanent damage is common and can progress after aminoglycoside discontinuation. Estimates of the prevalence of aminoglycoside-induced ototoxicity vary widely depending on the criteria applied. Clinically detectable ototoxicity probably occurs in as many as 5% of patients, with a much higher percentage demonstrating audiometrically detectable damage. Most aminoglycoside-induced ototoxicity is associated with parenteral therapy, but it has followed topical, oral, and irrigation use of these drugs, especially **neomycin.** A patient should receive dosages by these routes that are no greater than the dosages given by injection. Possible predisposing factors for ototoxicity are decreased renal function, long duration of therapy, large total dosage, plasma levels exceeding the therapeutic range, previous aminoglycoside use, concurrent use of other ototoxic drugs, dehydration, and old age. There is some evidence of an inherited susceptibility to aminoglycoside-induced ototoxicity. Hearing impairment is less common in neonates and children. Two meta-analyses found no difference in the effects on hearing of single daily dosing and multiple daily dosing of aminoglycosides. The comparative effects on vestibular function have not been adequately investigated. Serial audiometry might be useful in early detection of ototoxicity. Each aminoglycoside has a slightly different spectrum of ototoxicity; the table below serves as a general guide to their relative ototoxic potentials.[1–10]

RELATIVE OTOTOXIC POTENTIAL

DRUG	COCHLEAR	VESTIBULAR
Amikacin	+++	++
Gentamicin	++	+++

RELATIVE OTOTOXIC POTENTIAL (*continued*)

DRUG	COCHLEAR	VESTIBULAR
Kanamycin	+++	++
Neomycin	++++	++
Netilmicin	+	+
Streptomycin	++	++++
Tobramycin	++	++

Antidepressants, Heterocyclic

The prevalence of **tricyclic antidepressant**–associated tinnitus is estimated to be 1%. Tinnitus can subside despite continued therapy.[2,4,11]

Azithromycin

In elderly patients or patients with AIDS treated with 600 mg/day for *Mycobacterium avium* complex or toxoplasmosis, hearing loss occurs in 15–25%. Hearing loss occurs at all frequencies, but lower frequencies, including the speech range, are affected most often. Drug withdrawal or reduction of the dose to 300 mg/day resolves the hearing loss. Tinnitus and vestibular disturbances also occur frequently.[12–14]

Carboplatin

Although carboplatin is generally considered to be far less ototoxic than **cisplatin**, it can contribute to hearing loss when used in consolidation-phase treatment after cisplatin-containing induction. IV injection of 16–20 g/m^2 of **sodium thiosulfate** 2 hr after IV carboplatin showed significant protection against hearing loss in patients with CNS malignancies.[4,15–17]

Chloroquine

Nerve deafness is a rare but consistent feature of chloroquine therapy. Its onset is usually delayed and thought of as irreversible and accompanying long-term therapy. A partly reversible case and a case resulting from only 1 g of chloroquine have been reported.[2–4,18]

Cisplatin

Tinnitus occurs frequently and usually subsides within 1 week of drug discontinuation. It cannot be relied on to predict further ototoxicity. Hearing loss occurs frequently in patients receiving cisplatin and can be dose limiting. Audiometric abnormalities can be detected in most patients and appear within a few days after the drug is started, although a delay of several months is common. High frequencies are lost first. If therapy continues despite early hearing loss, most patients experience hearing loss in the speech frequencies. Effects are cumulative, dose related, and probably irreversible. Prolonged, low-dose therapy might produce less ototoxicity than short-term, high-dose treatment. Ototoxicity occurs more frequently in children and the elderly, and those with pre-existing hearing loss appear to be at increased risk.[1–5,16,19–23]

Deferoxamine

Dosage-related hearing impairment occurs during long-term deferoxamine therapy. The prevalence reported varies among studies from 6% to 57%. High-frequency hearing is affected first; reversible and irreversible hearing losses have been reported.[4,24–26]

(*continued*)

Diuretics, Loop

Rapid-onset hearing loss is a frequent feature of high-dose, rapid IV administration of **furosemide.** The onset might be more gradual with **ethacrynic acid.** Renal failure is usually listed as a predisposing factor, but only renal failure patients are likely to receive large IV doses. Co-administration with **aminoglycoside antibiotics** is often said to result in increased ototoxicity, but one study did not confirm this. The hearing loss is usually transient, but permanent loss has been reported, more often with ethacrynic acid than with furosemide. Hearing loss and vestibular toxicity after oral therapy have been reported. **Bumetanide** or **torsemide** produce less ototoxicity than ethacrynic acid or furosemide.[1–5,27,28]

Eflornithine

High- and low-frequency hearing impairments are reported frequently and dizziness occurs occasionally.[23]

Erythromycin

Hearing loss has occasionally followed high-dose (>4 g/day) parenteral or oral therapy and does not seem to be caused by any particular salt form. Impaired hepatic or renal function and advanced age can increase the risk. The loss occurs at speech frequencies and is usually reversible, but irreversible hearing loss has been reported. Recovery usually begins within 24 hr of drug discontinuation.[1,3–5,29,30]

Interferons

Tinnitus and hearing loss occur frequently during parenteral interferon therapy. These effects usually resolve 1–2 weeks after drug discontinuation. Interferon beta is more ototoxic than interferon alfa.[4,31]

Minocycline

Reversible vestibular toxicity, manifested primarily by dizziness, loss of balance, and lightheadedness, is a frequent occurrence. This adverse effect was noted in an average of 76% of patients in 6 studies and required 12–52% of affected patients to discontinue the drug or to stop working. Other studies have found lower, but still large, percentages of patients with vestibular toxicity. Women are more susceptible than men. Onset is often during the first 2 days of therapy, and recovery begins soon after minocycline discontinuation.[1,4,32–34]

Nonsteroidal Anti-inflammatory Drugs

Although not as common as with salicylates, NSAIDs have been associated with hearing impairment and deafness, including some cases of permanent damage. Tinnitus and vestibular dysfunction also have been reported.[1–4,35]

Quinine

Tinnitus and high-frequency hearing impairment occur frequently. Although these effects are usually reversible, permanent hearing impairment has occurred with long-term therapy. Vestibular effects also have been described.[1,4,5,35]

Salicylates

Tinnitus, high-frequency hearing loss, and occasional vertigo are common features of salicylate intoxication. Hearing loss appears to be related to the unbound plasma salicylate level, explaining the marked interpatient variability in the total salicylate serum level at which it is first detected. Most patients demonstrating ototoxicity from salicylates are receiving long-term, high-dose therapy, such as for rheumatoid arthritis. Salicylate ototoxicity, even if severe, is almost always reversible in 48–72 hr, but permanent hearing loss has been reported.[1–5,35,36]

(*continued*)

Vancomycin

Transient and permanent hearing loss, tinnitus, and dizziness have occurred. Hearing impairment is rare with plasma levels <30 mg/L (21 µmol/L). In many of the reported cases, the patients also had been exposed to other ototoxic drugs, especially **aminoglycoside antibiotics.** The prevalence of purely vancomycin-induced ototoxicity is unknown but probably low, especially with the current, highly purified vancomycin products.[1,4,5,37–39]

Zidovudine

Audiometry determined that hearing loss occurred in 29% of 99 patients receiving antiretroviral drugs, with most cases associated with zidovudine. The prevalence of hearing loss was marked for patients >35 yr.[40]

■ REFERENCES

1. Huang MY, Schacht J. Drug-induced ototoxicity. Pathogenesis and prevention. *Med Toxicol Adverse Drug Exp* 1989;4:452–67.
2. Griffin JP. Drug-induced ototoxicity. *Br J Audiol* 1988;22:195–210.
3. Norris CH. Drugs affecting the inner ear. A review of their clinical efficacy, mechanisms of action, toxicity, and place in therapy. *Drugs* 1988;36:754–72.
4. Seligmann H et al. Drug-induced tinnitus and other hearing disorders. *Drug Saf* 1996;14:198–212.
5. Tange RA. Ototoxicity. *Adverse Drug React Toxicol Rev* 1998;17:75–89.
6. Brummett RE, Fox KE. Aminoglycoside-induced hearing loss in humans. *Antimicrob Agents Chemother* 1989;33:797–800.
7. Garrison MW et al. Aminoglycosides: another perspective. *DICP* 1990;24:267–72.
8. Matz GJ. Aminoglycoside cochlear ototoxicity. *Otolaryngol Clin North Am* 1993;26:705–12.
9. Bailey TC et al. A meta-analysis of extended-interval dosing versus multiple daily dosing of aminoglycosides. *Clin Infect Dis* 1997;24:786–95.
10. Ali MZ et al. A meta-analysis of the relative efficacy and toxicity of single daily dosing versus multiple daily dosing of aminoglycosides. *Clin Infect Dis* 1997;24:798–809.
11. Tandon R et al. Imipramine and tinnitus. *J Clin Psychiatry* 1987;48:109–11.
12. Tseng AL et al. Azithromycin-related ototoxicity in patients infected with human immunodeficiency virus. *Clin Infect Dis* 1997;24:76–7.
13. Brown BA et al. Relationship of adverse events to serum drug levels in patients receiving high-dose azithromycin for mycobacterial lung disease. *Clin Infect Dis* 1997;24:958–64.
14. Lo SE et al. Azithromycin-induced hearing loss. *Am J Health Syst Pharm* 1999;56:380–3.
15. Freilich RJ et al. Hearing loss in children with brain tumors treated with cisplatin and carboplatin-based high-dose chemotherapy with autologous bone marrow rescue. *Med Pediatr Oncol* 1996;26:95–100.
16. van der Hulst RJAM et al. High frequency audiometry in prospective clinical research of ototoxicity due to platinum derivatives. *Ann Otol Rhinol Laryngol* 1988;97:133–7.
17. Neuwelt EA et al. First evidence of otoprotection against carboplatin-induced hearing loss with a two-compartment system in patients with central nervous system malignancy using sodium thiosulfate. *J Pharmacol Exp Ther* 1998;286:77–84.
18. Mukherjee DK. Chloroquine ototoxicity—a reversible phenomenon? *J Laryngol Otol* 1979;93:809–15.
19. Blakley BW, Myers SF. Patterns of hearing loss resulting from *cis*-platinum therapy. *Otolaryngol Head Neck Surg* 1993;109:385–91.
20. Berg AL et al. Ototoxic impact of cisplatin in pediatric oncology patients. *Laryngoscope* 1999;109:1806-14.
21. Bokemeyer C et al. Analysis of risk factors for cisplatin-induced ototoxicity in patients with testicular cancer. *Br J Cancer* 1998;77:1355–62.
22. Ilveskoski I et al. Ototoxicity in children with malignant brain tumors treated with the "8 in 1" chemotherapy protocol. *Med Pediatr Oncol* 1996;27:26–31.
23. Schweitzer VG. Ototoxicity of chemotherapeutic agents. *Otolaryngol Clin North Am* 1993;26:759–89.
24. Gallant T et al. Serial studies of auditory neurotoxicity in patients receiving deferoxamine therapy. *Am J Med* 1987;83:1085–90.
25. Cases A et al. Ocular and auditory toxicity in hemodialyzed patients receiving desferrioxamine. *Nephron* 1990;56:19–23.

26. Chiodo AA et al. Desferrioxamine ototoxicity in an adult transfusion-dependent population. *J Otolaryngol* 1997;26:116–22.
27. Rybak LP. Ototoxicity of loop diuretics. *Otolaryngol Clin North Am* 1993;26:829–44.
28. Smith CR, Lietman PS. Effect of furosemide on aminoglycoside-induced nephrotoxicity and auditory toxicity in humans. *Antimicrob Agents Chemother* 1983;23:133–7.
29. Brummett RE. Ototoxic liability of erythromycin and analogues. *Otolaryngol Clin North Am* 1993;26:811–9.
30. Sacristán JA et al. Erythromycin-induced hypoacusis: 11 new cases and literature review. *Ann Pharmacother* 1993;27:950–5.
31. Kanda Y et al. Sudden hearing loss associated with interferon. *Lancet* 1994;343:1134–5.
32. Schofield CBS, Masterton G. Vestibular reactions to minocycline. *MMWR* 1976;25:31.
33. Gump DW et al. Side effects of minocycline: different dosage regimens. *Antimicrob Agents Chemother* 1977;12:642–6.
34. Greco TP et al. Minocycline toxicity: experience with an altered dosage regimen. *Curr Ther Res* 1979;25:193–201.
35. Jung TTK et al. ototoxicity of salicylate, nonsteroidal anti-inflammatory drugs, and quinine. *Otolaryngol Clin North Am* 1993;26:791–810.
36. Brien J. ototoxicity associated with salicylates. A brief review. *Drug Saf* 1993;9:143–8.
37. Brummett RE. Ototoxicity of vancomycin and analogues. *Otolaryngol Clin North Am* 1993;26:821–8.
38. Duffull SB, Begg EJ. Vancomycin toxicity. What is the evidence for dose dependency? *Adverse Drug React Toxicol Rev* 1994;13:103–14.
39. Gendeh BS et al. Vancomycin administration in continuous ambulatory peritoneal dialysis: the risk of ototoxicity. *Otolaryngol Head Neck Surg* 1998;118:551–8.
40. Marra CM et al. Hearing loss and antiretroviral therapy in patients infected with HIV-1. *Arch Neurol* 1997;54:407–10.

Drug-Induced Pancreatitis

Pancreatitis can be acute or chronic, and most drug-induced cases are acute. The diagnosis of acute drug-induced pancreatitis requires laboratory (elevated serum amylase and lipase levels) and clinical (abdominal pain) evidence. The strongest associations are made when readministration of the drug results in a recurrence of pancreatitis (ie, a positive rechallenge). Pancreatitis has occurred during therapy with many drugs; the drugs included in this table are those that present sufficient evidence to establish themselves as probable causes of pancreatitis.

ACE Inhibitors

There are numerous cases of ACE inhibitor–induced pancreatitis in the literature and the files of manufacturers. **Captopril, enalapril,** and **lisinopril** have been implicated. It is not possible to estimate a prevalence. A few cases have been confirmed by rechallenge.[1,3–5]

Alcohol

Alcohol is the greatest cause of drug-induced pancreatitis, easily exceeding the number of cases caused by all other drugs. Acute pancreatitis occurs in about 5% of alcoholics and usually develops after several years of alcohol abuse. It probably represents an acute flare of chronic pancreatitis.[6]

Asparaginase

The estimated prevalence of asparaginase-induced acute pancreatitis is 1–26%, with fatalities in 1.8–4.6% of cases. Many patients who develop pancreatitis during asparaginase therapy are in poor condition and receiving other chemotherapeutic agents. Asparaginase inhibits amylase and lipase production, complicating the diagnosis and evaluation of asparaginase-induced pancreatitis.[1,2,7–9]

(continued)

Azathioprine

There are many published cases of azathioprine-induced pancreatitis including at least 11 with positive rechallenge. Most cases occur in transplant recipients who are receiving other drugs implicated in causing pancreatitis.[1,2]

Calcium Salts

Pancreatitis is associated with hypercalcemia from pathologic causes, and it is likely that hypercalcemia resulting from the administration of exogenous calcium also can produce pancreatitis. There are at least 6 published cases of pancreatitis from parenteral nutrition–induced hypercalcemia.[1,10]

Contrast Media

Up to 11% of patients receiving contrast media through endoscopic retrograde cholangiopancreatography develop pancreatitis. Use of lower-osmolarity agents reduces the prevalence of pancreatitis.[2,11]

Corticosteroids

Although corticosteroids are commonly implicated as causes of pancreatitis, most of the reported cases involve disease states that predispose to pancreatitis. The weak evidence against corticosteroids is further complicated by data supporting the use of corticosteroids in the treatment of acute pancreatitis.[1,2,12]

Cyclosporine

Cyclosporine-induced pancreatitis was identified in 5 of 143 heart and heart–lung transplant recipients in one study. In another, 4 of 105 cyclosporine-treated renal transplant recipients developed pancreatitis, compared with only 2 of 180 **azathioprine**-treated patients. All cases occurred within 4 months of the start of cyclosporine therapy.[1,2,13,14]

Didanosine

Estimates of the prevalence of pancreatitis in didanosine-treated patients are 3–26%. A published report of didanosine treatment of 51 adult males with AIDS (10–12 mg/kg/day) found clinical pancreatitis in 12 (24%) and asymptomatic elevations of amylase and lipase levels in 10 others. Two patients died from fulminant pancreatitis. Pancreatitis might be dose related because in one study pancreatitis developed in 7 of 60 HIV-infected children receiving doses $\geq$360 mg/m^2/day but not in any of the 35 patients receiving $\leq$270 mg/m^2/day.[1,2,15,16]

Diuretics, Thiazide

Although there are at least 25 published case reports of thiazide-associated pancreatitis, the quality of the evidence is poor. Some of the cases are complicated by hypercalcemia, a known risk factor for pancreatitis.[1,2]

Estrogens

Estrogen therapy increases the risk of pancreatitis in patients with pre-existing hyperlipidemia, especially hypertriglyceridemia. Hypertriglyceridemia is a known cause of pancreatitis, and estrogen therapy raises serum triglyceride levels. In one report, 4 of 7 women with serum triglycerides >1500 mg/dL (17 mmol/L) while receiving postmenopausal estrogen replacement therapy (ERT) developed pancreatitis. Cases also have been reported in younger patients taking **oral contraceptives.** ERT is relatively contraindicated when serum triglycerides are >350 mg/dL (4 mmol/L) and absolutely contraindicated at >750 mg/dL (8.5 mmol/L).[1,2,17,18]

Furosemide

There are few published cases of furosemide-associated pancreatitis. The dosage range for these cases is 40–160 mg/day and most cases occurred during the first few weeks of treatment. The evidence for furosemide-associated pancreatitis is weakened by the small number of positive rechallenges.[1,2,19]

(*continued*)

Interferon Alfa

Although few cases have been reported, the association with the administration of interferon alfa is strong.[20]

Mercaptopurine

Inflammatory bowel disease is associated with pancreatitis. In one study of 400 patients with inflammatory bowel disease, 13 (4.25%) developed pancreatitis while receiving mercaptopurine (50–100 mg/day). Seven of the 13 were rechallenged and all developed recurrent pancreatitis, thereby establishing a strong cause-and-effect relationship. Pancreatitis developed during the first month of initial treatment in all patients and within 24 hr for 4 of the 7 rechallenges.[1,2,21]

Mesalamine Derivatives

Inflammatory bowel disease is associated with pancreatitis, but **mesalamine, sulfasalazine,** and **olsalazine** have been implicated in cases of acute pancreatitis confirmed by rechallenge. Positive rechallenge can occur after rectal administration.[1,2,22,23]

Metronidazole

Pancreatitis occurs occasionally with metronidazole. One study of 6485 HMO patients found a rate of pancreatitis requiring hospitalization of 3.9–4.6/10,000 in patients receiving metronidazole. The study did not report on nonhospitalized cases.[1,2,24]

Nonsteroidal Anti-inflammatory Drugs

There are isolated case reports of pancreatitis associated with most NSAIDs, but **sulindac** is clearly the most commonly reported. Many cases have positive rechallenges. The onset of symptoms is from 2 weeks to 9 months after initiation of therapy.[1,2]

Octreotide

When placebo or 100 μg doses of octreotide were administered before and immediately after endoscopic retrograde cholangiopancreatography in 84 patients, the frequencies of pancreatitis within the first 24 hr after the procedure were 11% in the placebo group and 35% in the octreotide group. Despite the higher frequency of pancreatitis, the octreotide patients were NPO for fewer days.[1,2,25]

Pegaspargase

The risk of pancreatitis with pegaspargase is similar to or greater than that of asparaginase. Onset is usually within a few days to 2 weeks after the start of therapy but has occurred up to 6 weeks after the start of therapy.[26] (*See also* Asparaginase.)

Pentamidine

Injected and aerosolized pentamidine have been implicated in causing pancreatitis; a few fatalities have been reported. Most of the patients had AIDS, which might have contributed to their pancreatitis.[2]

Propofol

At least 25 cases of pancreatitis associated with propofol have been reported. Many, but not all, of the cases were patients who developed hypertriglyceridemia that was attributed to the lipid-containing vehicle for injectable propofol.[27,28]

Valproic Acid

Five of 72 valproate-treated, mentally retarded patients in one series developed pancreatitis. There are at least 50 other published cases, including some fatalities. The prevalence of asymptomatic elevations of serum amylase might be as high as 20%. There is no obvious connection with dosage or duration of therapy, although one-half of the cases occur in the first 3 months of therapy and two-thirds occur during the first year. When detected, pancreatitis is rapidly reversible after drug withdrawal.[1,2,29–31]

(*continued*)

Vinca Alkaloids

Pancreatitis with vinca alkaloid (ie, **vincristine**) therapy occurs primarily in patients receiving multiple-drug therapy, making the establishment of a cause-and-effect association difficult. Animal data show that vinca alkaloids can severely disrupt pancreatic architecture.[1]

■ REFERENCES

1. Wilmink T, Frick TW. Drug-induced pancreatitis. *Drug Saf* 1996;14:406–23.
2. Underwood TW, Frye CB. Drug-induced pancreatitis. *Clin Pharm* 1993;12:440–8.
3. Maringhini A et al. Enalapril-associated acute pancreatitis: recurrence after rechallenge. *Am J Gastroenterol* 1997;92:166–7.
4. Jeandidier N et al. Captopril-induced acute pancreatitis. *Diabetes Care* 1995;18:410–1.
5. Dabaghi S. ACE inhibitors and pancreatitis. *Ann Intern Med* 1991;115:330–1. Letter.
6. Steinberg W, Tenner S. Acute pancreatitis. *N Engl J Med* 1994;330:1198–210.
7. Haskell CM et al. L-Asparaginase. Therapeutic and toxic effects in patients with neoplastic disease. *N Engl J Med* 1969;281:1028–34.
8. Nguyen DL et al. Serial sonograms to detect pancreatitis in children receiving L-asparaginase. *South Med J* 1987;80:1133–6.
9. Sadoff J et al. Surgical pancreatic complications induced by L-asparaginase. *J Pediatr Surg* 1997;32:860–3.
10. Izsak EM et al. Pancreatitis in association with hypercalcemia in patients receiving total parenteral nutrition. *Gastroenterology* 1980;79:555–8.
11. Banerjee AK et al. Trial of low versus high osmolar contrast media in endoscopic retrograde cholangiopancreatography. *Br J Clin Pract* 1990;44:445–7.
12. Steinberg WM, Lewis JH. Steroid-induced pancreatitis: does it really exist? *Gastroenterology* 1981;81:799–808.
13. Steed DL et al. General surgical complications in heart and heart–lung transplantation. *Surgery* 1985;98:739–45.
14. Yoshimura N et al. Effect of cyclosporine on the endocrine and exocrine pancreas in kidney transplant recipients. *Am J Kidney Dis* 1988;12:11–7.
15. Maxson CJ et al. Acute pancreatitis as a common complication of 2′, 3′-dideoxyinosine therapy in the acquired immunodeficiency syndrome. *Am J Gastroenterol* 1992;87:708–13.
16. Butler KM et al. Pancreatitis in human immunodeficiency virus-infected children receiving dideoxyinosine. *Pediatrics* 1993;91:747–51.
17. Parker WA. Estrogen-induced pancreatitis. *Clin Pharm* 1983;2:75–9.
18. Glueck CJ et al. Severe hypertriglyceridemia and pancreatitis when estrogen replacement therapy is given to hypertriglyceridemic women. *J Lab Clin Med* 1994;123:59–64.
19. Banerjee AK et al. Drug-induced pancreatitis. A critical review. *Med Toxicol Adv Drug Exp* 1989;4:186–98.
20. Eland IA et al. Acute pancreatitis attributed to the use of interferon alfa-2b. *Gastroenterology* 2000;119:230–3.
21. Haber CJ et al. Nature and course of pancreatitis caused by 6-mercaptopurine in the treatment of inflammatory bowel disease. *Gastroenterology* 1986;91:982–6.
22. Fernández J et al. Acute pancreatitis after long-term 5-aminosalicylic acid therapy. *Am J Gastroenterol* 1997;92:2302–3.
23. Isaacs KL, Murphy D. Pancreatitis after rectal administration of 5-aminosalicylic acid. *J Clin Gastroenterol* 1990;12:198–9.
24. Friedman GD, Selby JV. How often does metronidazole induce pancreatitis? *Gastroenterology* 1990;98:1702–3.
25. Sternlieb JM et al. A multicenter, randomized, controlled trial to evaluate the effect of prophylactic octreotide on ERCP-induced pancreatitis. *Am J Gastroenterol* 1992;87:1561–6.
26. Alvarez OA, Zimmerman G. Pegaspargase-induced pancreatitis. *Med Pediatr Oncol* 2000;34:200–5.
27. Leisure GS et al. Propofol and postoperative pancreatitis. *Anesthesiology* 1996;84:224–7.
28. Kumar AN et al. Propofol-induced pancreatitis: recurrence of pancreatitis after rechallenge. *Chest* 1999;115:1198–9.
29. Binek J et al. Valproic-acid–induced pancreatitis. Case report and review of the literature. *J Clin Gastroenterol* 1991;13:690–3.
30. Asconapé JJ et al. Valproate-associated pancreatitis. *Epilepsia* 1993;34:177–83.
31. Buzan RD et al. Valproate-associated pancreatitis and cholecystitis in six mentally retarded adults. *J Clin Psychiatry* 1995;56:529–32.

Drug-Induced Sexual Dysfunction

The large subjective component of human sexual response makes the evaluation of drug-induced sexual dysfunction difficult. Variations in study design have produced widely divergent reported rates of sexual dysfunction in the "normal" or control populations. Common drug-induced sexual dysfunctions are decreased libido or sexual drive, impotence (failure to achieve or maintain an erection in men), priapism (persistent and often painful erection), delayed ejaculation or failure of ejaculation, retrograde ejaculation (into the urinary bladder), and, in women, failure to achieve orgasm and decreased vaginal lubrication. Gynecomastia (enlargement of the male breast) has been included in this table. Although not life-threatening, drug-induced sexual dysfunction has a negative effect on quality of life and is an important contributor to noncompliance with prescribed drug regimens.

Alcohol

Low doses result in behavioral disinhibition. With higher doses, sexual response is impaired, frequently resulting in failure of erection in men and reduced vaginal vasodilation and delayed orgasm in women. In chronic alcoholics, sexual dysfunction frequently persists long after alcohol withdrawal and is permanent in some. The long-term effects are probably neurologic and endocrine in origin; alcohol reduces testosterone levels and increases luteinizing hormone levels. Long-term effects are independent of liver disease.[1–8]

Alprostadil

Intracavernous injection of alprostadil produces penile pain in 44% of patients, prolonged erection in 8%, and priapism in 1%. Fibrotic nodules or scarring occur frequently. Intraurethral administration does not appear to cause priapism or fibrosis, but 36% experience penile pain.[9–11]

Aminocaproic Acid

This drug can inhibit ejaculation without affecting libido and has produced "dry" ejaculation. Effects are rapidly reversible with drug discontinuation.[1,2,12,13]

Amphetamines

Low doses can increase libido and delay male orgasm. High doses have been associated with failure to achieve an erection in men and loss of orgasm in both sexes.[2,14–16]

Anabolic Steroids

Impotence and gynecomastia occur frequently in men and might be the result of reduction in the circulating levels of natural testosterone.[1,3,17]

Anticonvulsants

Female and male libido can be reduced. Self-reported sexual dysfunction has been described in a widely varying percentage of patients. Social and psychological aspects of epilepsy probably play important roles in these findings. Some effects might be caused by a reduction in the level of free testosterone, resulting from hepatic enzyme induction and higher concentrations of sex hormone–binding globulins.[1,4,18–20]

Antidepressants, Heterocyclic

Impotence, delayed ejaculation, and painful ejaculation have been reported in men. Women and men have reported delayed orgasm and anorgasmia. **Clomipramine** is the worst offender. Increased and, more commonly, decreased libido have been reported in men and women. The frequency of these effects varies considerably among published reports, perhaps reflecting the influence of the underlying depressive illness.[1–4,16,21–24] (*See also* Selective Serotonin Reuptake Inhibitors and Trazodone.)

(*continued*)

β-Adrenergic Blocking Agents

These drugs are associated with a variety of sexual problems, most commonly impotence. In a study of 46 men taking **propranolol,** 7 experienced "complete" impotence, 13 noted reduced potency, and 2 complained of reduced libido. In a larger trial, the frequencies of impotence during propranolol therapy were 13.8% and 13.2% after 12 weeks and 2 years, respectively. However, these figures did not differ significantly from placebo. Most of the published reports implicate propranolol; other more cardioselective β-blockers are less frequently associated with complaints of adverse sexual effects. There have been at least 25 reported patients who complained of sexual dysfunction (18 impotence, 9 decreased libido) while receiving topical ophthalmic treatment with **timolol.** Some of these patients were rechallenged, with positive results.[1,4,12,25–31]

Calcium-Channel Blockers

Although these drugs are generally thought to be free of adverse effects on sexual function, they are associated with gynecomastia. **Verapamil** is the most commonly implicated calcium-channel blocker, but **nifedipine** and **diltiazem** also can produce gynecomastia. Other calcium-channel blockers seem less likely to cause gynecomastia.[1,32]

Carbonic Anhydrase Inhibitors

Many patients receiving carbonic anhydrase inhibitors (eg, **acetazolamide, methazolamide**) develop a syndrome of malaise, fatigue, weight loss, and depression that often includes loss of libido. These patients appear to be more acidotic than those without the syndrome and some respond to therapy with sodium bicarbonate. Decreased libido has occurred in men and women and usually requires 2 weeks of carbonic anhydrase inhibitor therapy to develop.[1,2]

Cimetidine

In a group of 22 men treated with high dosages of cimetidine for hypersecretory states, 11 developed gynecomastia and 9 experienced impotence. These effects appear to be dose related and readily reversible and are not an important problem at dosages used for peptic ulcers. Cimetidine has some antiandrogenic effects, possibly the result of hyperprolactinemia, which are thought to be responsible for sexual dysfunction. Displacement of androgens from breast androgen receptors might contribute to the development of gynecomastia. **Ranitidine** does not appear to be associated with as high a prevalence of sexual dysfunction, and **famotidine** is not antiandrogenic.[1–4,12,17,32,33]

Clofibrate

In large multicenter trials, impotence has been reported more frequently than with placebo.[1–4,12,34,35]

Clonidine

Although some reports have indicated no sexual problems, others have indicated problems in up to 24% of patients. Impotence is the most frequently noted effect, but delayed or retrograde ejaculation in men and failure of arousal and orgasm in women have been described.[1–4,12,18,36,37]

Cocaine

Although cocaine is often perceived as a sexual stimulant, its use is associated with difficulty in establishing an erection and delayed ejaculation.[2,16,38,39]

Cyproterone

Gynecomastia results from the antiandrogen effects of cyproterone.[17]

Danazol

Most women treated with danazol for endometriosis experience reversible decreased libido.[40]

(continued)

Digoxin

Digitalis glycosides have some estrogen-like activity, and digoxin has been associated with decreased libido, impotence, and gynecomastia in men. In one study, digoxin use was associated with a 60% decrease in testosterone and a similar increase in estrogen in men.[1–4,12,41]

Diuretics, Thiazide

In one large study, the prevalence of impotence was reported to be significantly higher with **bendroflumethiazide** than with placebo (23% after 2 yr compared with 10% for placebo), and in another, **hydrochlorothiazide** was reported to produce more impotence and loss of libido than **propranolol**. In a well-designed study, 14% of men taking **chlorthiazide** complained of impotence, as did 14% of placebo-treated men. In three studies, **chlorthalidone** therapy resulted in more impotence than placebo (17% vs 8% in one).[1–4,12,27–29,36,42–44]

Estrogens

Impotence and gynecomastia occur frequently in men taking estrogens for prostate cancer. Estrogens have been used to reduce libido and sexual activity of male sex offenders.[1–4,45]

Finasteride

Gynecomastia occurs in 0.4% of finasteride-treated men. Onset is usually delayed until after 5–6 months of treatment.[46]

Flutamide

Gynecomastia might result from the antiandrogen effects of flutamide.[17]

Gonadotropin-Releasing Hormone Analogues

Most men and women treated with **goserelin** experience reversible decreased libido. **Leuprolide**-treated patients likely react similarly.[40]

Growth Hormone

(*See* Somatropin.)

Guanethidine

Up to 54% of men have reported impotence and up to 71% have reported ejaculatory impairment. Guanethidine does not affect parasympathetic function and would not be expected to produce impotence, leading some to suggest that the impotence is secondary to the inhibition of ejaculation. Retrograde ejaculation occurs as a result of the failure of the internal urethral sphincter to close; this action is sympathetically mediated. Although not well characterized, decreased libido in women taking guanethidine has been reported. Guanethidine effects are reversible with drug discontinuation and can be alleviated by a reduction in dosage.[1–4,12,36]

HMG-CoA Reductase Inhibitors

At least 47 cases of **simvastatin**-associated impotence have been reported, including some with positive rechallenge. There are scattered reports of impotence with **lovastatin** and **pravastatin**.[47,48]

Ketoconazole

Gynecomastia has been reported, apparently the result of the inhibition of testosterone synthesis.[1,17,32]

Marijuana

Positive and negative effects on sexual function are possible. Low doses can have a disinhibiting effect, whereas large doses have been associated with decreased libido and impotence. Long-term use also can result in gynecomastia.[2,32,49]

(*continued*)

Methyldopa

Impotence and ejaculatory failure in men and reduced libido in both sexes have been described. The frequency of sexual dysfunction varies from quite low in some reports to >50% in response to direct questioning. These effects are dose related and reversible. They might be the result of drug-induced sympathetic inhibition and mild CNS depression. Gynecomastia in men and painful breast enlargement in women have occurred.[1–4,12,29,36]

Metoclopramide

Gynecomastia and galactorrhea have been reported in adults and children receiving metoclopramide. These effects are probably due to metoclopramide-induced hyperprolactinemia.[50]

Monoamine Oxidase Inhibitors

Reported adverse sexual effects of MAOIs are highly variable. Impotence, spontaneous erections, and ejaculatory delay in men and orgasmic failure in men and women have been described. The true prevalence of these effects cannot be determined from available data, but MAOIs might be associated with more sexual dysfunction than heterocyclic antidepressants.[1,2,4,16]

Narcotics

Long-term narcotic use (especially abuse) is frequently associated with decreased libido and orgasmic failure in both sexes and impotence in men. These effects are dose related, with the highest frequency of impotence reported in narcotic addicts (80–90% in some series), and are reversible with drug discontinuation.[2,51–53]

Nitrates and Nitrites

These vasodilators have been used (primarily by inhalation) to enhance the perception of orgasm. When they are used too soon before orgasm, however, the vasodilation rapidly produces loss of erection. This effect has been used therapeutically to reduce spontaneous erections in men undergoing urologic procedures.[2,54,55]

Omeprazole

Although the prevalence is unclear, impotence and gynecomastia in men and breast enlargement in women have been described.[1,56]

Papaverine

Intracavernous injection of papaverine resulted in priapism (defined as an erection lasting >3 hr) in 17% of 400 patients. Those with psychogenic or neurogenic impotence were more likely to experience priapism than those with vasculogenic impotence.[9,57]

Phenothiazines

These drugs have been implicated in producing a wide variety of adverse sexual effects such as impotence and priapism, absent and spontaneous ejaculation, painful ejaculation, retrograde ejaculation, menstrual irregularities, and decreased libido. These effects result from the complex actions of the drugs on the patient's hormonal balance and central sympathetic and parasympathetic pathways. With the exception of priapism, these effects are usually benign and respond to drug discontinuation. **Thioridazine** is the most commonly implicated drug. The possible contribution of the underlying disease state cannot be overlooked.[1–4,16,25,58]

Phenoxybenzamine

This α-adrenergic blocker is associated with dosage-related failure of ejaculation but not interference with orgasm. This effect was present in all 19 patients in one study and reversed 24–48 hr after drug discontinuation.[1–3,59]

(continued)

Progestins

Impotence has been reported in 25–70% of men receiving progestins for prostatic hypertrophy. Progestins have been used to reduce libido and sexual activity of male sex offenders.[2,44,60]

Reserpine

Impotence (33%) and failure of ejaculation (14%) in men and reduced libido in both sexes occur frequently.[1,2,4,12,36]

Sedative-Hypnotics

In a manner similar to alcohol, low doses can produce some disinhibition, whereas large doses can reduce sexual performance.[1–4]

Selective Serotonin Reuptake Inhibitors

Anorgasmia and delay of orgasm are frequent adverse effects of SSRIs, affecting the majority of patients in some studies. These effects have been confirmed in patients without depression. **Fluvoxamine, fluoxetine, paroxetine,** and **sertraline** are the most frequently mentioned. Some patients have benefited from dosage reduction. **Bupropion, mirtazapine,** and **nefazodone** have limited, if any, adverse effects on sexual function and should be considered in patients with SSRI-induced dysfunction.[1,3,24,61–63]

Somatropin

Benign gynecomastia can occur in prepubertal and adult males receiving somatropin. Onset might not occur until after months or years of treatment.[64]

Spironolactone

Gynecomastia in men and painful breast enlargement or menstrual irregularities in women are frequent with large dosages. Less frequently reported effects are impotence, inhibition of vaginal lubrication, and loss of libido. The structural similarity of the drug to estrogens and progestins is thought to be a key factor in the genesis of adverse sexual effects. Spironolactone might inhibit the formation of testosterone and its breast receptor binding. It also might increase the metabolic clearance of testosterone and its rate of peripheral conversion to estradiol. These effects appear to be dosage related.[1,2,4,12,17,32,36]

Tamoxifen

Use of tamoxifen increases the prevalence of vaginal dryness and painful intercourse.[65]

Trazodone

Numerous cases of priapism have been reported, usually during the first month of therapy.[1,4,12,57,66]

■ REFERENCES

1. Forman R et al. *Drug-induced infertility and sexual dysfunction.* Cambridge: Cambridge University; 1996.
2. Buffum J. Pharmacosexology: the effects of drugs on sexual function. A review. *J Psychoact Drugs* 1982; 14:5–44.
3. Brock GB, Lue TF. Drug-induced male sexual dysfunction. An update. *Drug Saf* 1993;8:414–26.
4. McWaine DE, Procci WR. Drug-induced sexual dysfunction. *Med Toxicol Adverse Drug Exp* 1988;3:289–306.
5. Lemere F, Smith JW. Alcohol-induced sexual impotence. *Am J Psychiatry* 1973;130:212–3.
6. Wilson GT, Lawson DM. Effects of alcohol on sexual arousal in women. *J Abnorm Psychol* 1976;85:489–97.
7. Gordon GG et al. Effect of alcohol (ethanol) administration on sex-hormone metabolism in normal men. *N Engl J Med* 1976;295:793–7.
8. Dudek FA, Turner DS. Alcoholism and sexual functioning. *J Psychoact Drugs* 1982;14:47–54.
9. The long-term safety of alprostadil (prostaglandin-E$_1$) in patients with erectile dysfunction. The European Alprostadil Study Group. *Br J Urol* 1998;82:538–43.

(continued)

10. Chen RN et al. Penile scarring with intracavernous injection therapy using prostaglandin E1: a risk factor analysis. *J Urol* 1996;155:138–40.

11. Padma-Nathan H et al. Treatment of men with erectile dysfunction with transurethral alprostadil. *N Engl J Med* 1997;336:1–7.

12. Buffum J. Pharmacosexology update: prescription drugs and sexual function. *J Psychoact Drugs* 1986; 18:97–106.

13. Evans BE, Aledort LM. Inhibition of ejaculation due to epsilon aminocaproic acid. *N Engl J Med* 1978; 298:166–7. Letter.

14. Greaves G. Sexual disturbances among chronic amphetamine users. *J Nerv Ment Dis* 1972;155:363–5.

15. Smith DE et al. Amphetamine abuse and sexual dysfunction: clinical and research considerations. In, Smith DE et al, eds. *Amphetamine use, misuse, and abuse: proceedings of the National Amphetamine Conference, 1978.* Boston: GK Hall; 1979:228–48.

16. Segraves RT. Effects of psychotropic drugs on human erection and ejaculation. *Arch Gen Psychiatry* 1989; 46:275–84.

17. Braunstein GD. Gynecomastia. *N Engl J Med* 1993;328:490–5.

18. Toone BK et al. Sex hormone changes in male epileptics. *Clin Endocrinol* 1980;12:391–5.

19. Dana-Haeri J et al. Reduction of free testosterone by antiepileptic drugs. *Br Med J* 1982;284:85–6.

20. Morrell MJ. Sexual dysfunction in epilepsy. *Epilepsia* 1991;32(suppl 6):S38–45.

21. Harrison WM et al. Effects of antidepressant medication on sexual function: a controlled study. *J Clin Psychopharmacol* 1986;6:144–9.

22. Shen WW, Sata LS. Inhibited female orgasm resulting from psychotropic drugs. A five-year, updated, clinical review. *J Reprod Med* 1990;35:11–4.

23. Balon R et al. Sexual dysfunction during antidepressant treatment. *J Clin Psychiatry* 1993;54:209–12.

24. Segraves RT. Antidepressant-induced sexual dysfunction. *J Clin Psychiatry* 1998;59(suppl 4):48–54.

25. Pollack MH et al. Genitourinary and sexual adverse effects of psychotropic medication. *Int J Psychiatry Med* 1992;22:305–27.

26. Fraunfelder FT, Meyer SM. Sexual dysfunction secondary to topical ophthalmic timolol. *JAMA* 1985; 253: 3092–3. Letter.

27. Medical Research Council Working Party on Mild to Moderate Hypertension. Adverse reactions to bendrofluazide and propranolol for the treatment of mild hypertension. *Lancet* 1981;2:539–42.

28. Veterans Administration Cooperative Study Group on Antihypertensive Agents. Comparison of propranolol and hydrochlorothiazide for the initial treatment of hypertension. II. Results of long-term therapy. *JAMA* 1982; 248:2004–11.

29. Bansal S. Sexual dysfunction in hypertensive men. A critical review of the literature. *Hypertension* 1988; 12:1–10.

30. Prisant LM et al. Sexual dysfunction with antihypertensive drugs. *Arch Intern Med* 1994;154:730–6.

31. Grimm RH Jr et al. Long-term effects on sexual function of five antihypertensive drugs and nutritional hygienic treatment in hypertensive men and women. Treatment of Mild Hypertension Study (TOMHS). *Hypertension* 1997;29:8–14.

32. Thompson DF, Carter JR. Drug-induced gynecomastia. *Pharmacotherapy* 1993;13:37–45.

33. Jensen RT et al. Cimetidine-induced impotence and breast changes in patients with gastric hypersecretory states. *N Engl J Med* 1983;308:883–7.

34. The Coronary Drug Project Research Group. Clofibrate and niacin in coronary heart disease. *JAMA* 1975;231: 360–81.

35. Oliver MF et al. A co-operative trial in the primary prevention of ischaemic heart disease using clofibrate. Report from the Committee of Principal Investigators. *Br Heart J* 1978;40:1069–118.

36. Duncan L, Bateman DN. Sexual function in women. Do antihypertensive drugs have an impact? *Drug Saf* 1993;8:225–34.

37. Meston CM. Inhibition of subjective and physiological sexual arousal in women by clonidine. *Psychosom Med* 1997;59:399–407.

38. Siegel RK. Cocaine and sexual dysfunction: the curse of mama coca. *J Psychoact Drugs* 1982;14:71–4.

39. Wesson DR. Cocaine use by masseuses. *J Psychoact Drugs* 1982;14:75–6.

40. Shaw RW. An open randomized comparative study of the effect of goserelin depot and danazol in the treatment of endometriosis. Zoladex Endometriosis Study Team. *Fertil Steril* 1992;58:265–72.

41. Neri A et al. Subjective assessment of sexual dysfunction of patients on long-term administration of digoxin. *Arch Sex Behav* 1980;9:343–7.

42. Wassertheil-Smoller S et al. Effect of antihypertensives on sexual function and quality of life: the TAIM study. *Ann Intern Med* 1991;114:613–20.

43. Chang SW et al. The impact of diuretic therapy on reported sexual function. *Arch Intern Med* 1991;151:2402–8.

44. Grimm RH et al. Long-term effects on sexual function of five antihypertensive drugs and nutritional hygienic treatment in hypertensive men and women. Treatment of Mild Hypertension Study (TOMHS). *Hypertension* 1997;29:8–14.

45. Bancroft J et al. The control of deviant sexual behavior by drugs: I. Behavioural changes following oestrogens and anti-androgens. *Br J Psychiatry* 1974;125:310–5.

46. Wilton L et al. The safety of finasteride used in benign prostatic hypertrophy: a non-interventional observational cohort study in 14,772 patients. *Br J Urol* 1996;78:379–84.

47. Boyd IW. HMG-CoA reductase inhibitor-induced impotence. *Ann Pharmacother* 1996;30:1199. Letter.

48. Jackson G. Simvastatin and impotence. *BMJ* 1997;315:31.

49. Halikas J et al. Effects of regular marijuana use on sexual performance. *J Psychoact Drugs* 1982;14:59–70.

50. Madani S, Tolia V. Gynecomastia with metoclopramide use in pediatric patients. *J Clin Gastroenterol* 1997;24:79–81.

51. Cushman P. Sexual behavior in heroin addiction and methadone maintenance. Correlation with plasma luteinizing hormone. *N Y State J Med* 1972;72:1261–5.

52. Langrod J et al. Methadone treatment and physical complaints: a clinical analysis. *Int J Addict* 1981;16:947–52.

53. Rosenbaum M. When drugs come into the picture, love flies out the window: women addicts' love relationships. *Int J Addict* 1981;16:1197–206.

54. Sigell LT et al. Popping and snorting volatile nitrites: a current fad for getting high. *Am J Psychiatry* 1978;135:1216–8.

55. Welti RS, Brodsky JB. Treatment of intraoperative penile tumescence. *J Urol* 1980;124:925–6.

56. Lindquist M, Edwards IR. Endocrine adverse effects of omeprazole. *BMJ* 1992;305:451–2.

57. Lomas GM, Jarow JP. Risk factors for papaverine-induced priapism. *J Urol* 1992;147:1280–1.

58. Thompson JW et al. Psychotropic medication and priapism: a comprehensive review. *J Clin Psychiatry* 1990;51:430–3.

59. Kedia KR, Persky L. Effect of phenoxybenzamine (dibenzyline) on sexual function in man. *Urology* 1981;18:620–2.

60. Meiraz D et al. Treatment of benign prostatic hyperplasia with hydroxyprogesterone-caproate: placebo-controlled study. *Urology* 1977;9:144–8.

61. Piazza LA et al. Sexual functioning in chronically depressed patients treated with SSRI antidepressants: a pilot study. *Am J Psychiatry* 1997;154:1757–9.

62. Modell JG et al. Comparative sexual side effects of bupropion, fluoxetine, paroxetine, and sertraline. *Clin Pharmacol Ther* 1997;61:476–87.

63. Nafziger AN et al. Incidence of sexual dysfunction in healthy volunteers on fluvoxamine therapy. *J Clin Psychiatry* 1999;60:187–90.

64. Malozowski S, Stadel BV. Prepubertal gynecomastia during growth hormone therapy. *J Pediatrics* 1995;126:659–61.

65. Mortimer JE et al. Effect of tamoxifen on sexual functioning in patients with breast cancer. *J Clin Oncol* 1999;17:1488–92.

66. Warner MD et al. Trazodone and priapism. *J Clin Psychiatry* 1987;48:244–5.

Drug-Induced Skin Disorders

Most drugs occasionally have been associated with rashes or other dermatologic reactions. The difficulty of determining a correct diagnosis of a skin disorder and the complexity of establishing a causal relationship with drug therapy make estimating the frequency of occurrence of these reactions virtually impossible. Only skin disorders resulting from *systemic* administration of drugs are represented in this table. Drugs believed to be among the most common causes of a particular drug-induced skin disorder are designated by "XX" in the table. Stevens–Johnson syndrome and toxic epidermal necrolysis have been combined into a single column because of their similarity in histopathology and because they are usually caused by the same drugs. The following abbreviations are used to indicate specific skin disorders:

AE — Acneiforms Eruptions
AL — Alopecia
ED — Exfoliative Dermatitis

FE — Fixed Eruptions
LE — Lupus Erythematosus-Like Reactions
Ph — Photosensitivity and Phototoxicity Reactions
SJ/TN — Stevens–Johnson Syndrome/Toxic Epidermal Necrolysis

DRUG	AE	AL	ED	FE	LE	Ph	SJ/TN	REFERENCES
Acetaminophen		X		X			X	1–3
Allopurinol				X			XX	1–6
Amantadine		X				X		1
Aminosalicylic Acid			X					5
Amiodarone		X				X		1,4,7
Amphetamines		X						2
Androgens	XX	X						1,2,4,5
Antidepressants, Heterocyclic	X					X		1,4,7
Auranofin		X						1
Azathioprine		X						1
Barbiturates	X			X			XX	1–6,8
Bleomycin		XX						1,2
Bromocriptine		X						1,2,4
Captopril		X	X					1
Carbamazepine			X	X			X	1–3,5,8
Carboplatin		X						1
Chloral Hydrate	X			X				1,2
Chlordiazepoxide				X				1
Chloroquine				X		X	X	2,4,7
Cimetidine							X	2,4
Clofibrate		X						2,5
Colchicine		XX					X	1–3,5
Contraceptives, Oral	X	X		X	X	X		1,2,4,5,7
Corticosteroids	XX							1,2,4,5
Cyclophosphamide		XX					X	1,2
Cyclosporine	X	X						1
Cytarabine		XX						1
Dacarbazine						X		1,2,7
Dactinomycin	XX						X	1,2,5
Danazol	XX							1,2
Dapsone				X		X	X	1,2,7
Daunorubicin		X						1,2

(continued)

DRUG	AE	AL	ED	FE	LE	Ph	SJ/TN	REFERENCES
Disulfiram	X							1
Diuretics, Thiazide						XX		1,2,4,5,7
Doxorubicin		XX						1
Ethionamide	X							1
Etoposide		XX						1
Fluoroquinolones						XX	X	1,7,8
Fluorouracil		XX				X		1,2,4,7
Gold Salts		X	XX	X		X	X	1,2,5,7
Griseofulvin				X		X		2,4,7
Heparin		X						1,2
Hydralazine					XX			1,2,5,9
Ifosfamide		XX						1
Interferon Alfa (2a, 2b)		XX						1,2
Isoniazid	X	X	X	X	X	X	X	1,2,4,5,9
Isotretinoin		XX				X		1,2,4,7
Ketoconazole		X						1
Lamotrigine							XX	10
Levodopa		X						2,5
Lithium	XX	X	X					1,2,4,5
Meprobamate				X				1
Methotrexate		XX				X	X	1,2,4,7
Methyldopa				X				1,5,9
Methysergide		X						1
Metronidazole				X				1,2
Minocycline					X	X		7,11
Mitomycin		X						1
Nalidixic Acid						X		2,7
Nitrofurantoin		X		X			X	2,4
NSAIDs		X		X		X	X	1–4,7
Paclitaxel		XX						1
Penicillamine		X		X	X			1,2,4,9
Penicillins			XX	X			X	1–6,8
Phenolphthalein				X			X	1,2,4,5
Phenothiazines			X	X	X	XX		1,2,4,5,7,9
Phenytoin	X		X	X	X		X	1,2,4,5,8,9

(*continued*)

DRUG	AE	AL	ED	FE	LE	Ph	SJ/TN	REFERENCES
Plicamycin							X	2,4
Procainamide					XX			1,5,9
Propranolol		X		X				4,5
Propylthiouracil		X			X			1,2,5
Psoralens	X				X	XX		1,2
Quinacrine		X						2,5
Quinidine	X		X	X	X	X		2,5,7,9
Quinine	X			X		X		1,2
Rifampin	X						X	1,8
Salicylates					X		X	1–4
Streptomycin			XX	X			X	1,2,4
Sulfonamides			XX	X	X	XX	XX	1–9
Sulfonylureas						X	X	1,2,4–7
Tamoxifen		X						1
Tetracyclines				X		XX		1,2,4–7
Tretinoin						X		1,7
Trimethadione	X	X			X			1,2,5
Valproic Acid		X						1,2,5,6
Vinblastine		XX				X		1,2,4,7
Vincristine		XX						1
Vitamin A		X						1,2,4,5
Warfarin		X						1,2,4,5

■ REFERENCES

1. Zürcher K, Krebs A. *Cutaneous drug reactions,* 2nd ed. Basel: S Karger; 1992.
2. Bork K. *Cutaneous side effects of drugs.* Philadelphia: WB Saunders; 1988.
3. Roujeau J-C et al. Toxic epidermal necrolysis (Lyell syndrome). Incidence and drug etiology in France, 1981–1985. *Arch Dermatol* 1990;126:37–42.
4. Blacker KL et al. Cutaneous reactions to drugs. In Fitzpatrick TB et al, eds. *Dermatology in general medicine,* 4th ed. New York: McGraw-Hill; 1993:1783–806.
5. Millikan LE. Drug eruptions (dermatitis medicamentosa). In Moschella SL, Hurley HJ, eds. *Dermatology,* 3rd ed. Philadelphia: WB Saunders; 1992:535–73.
6. Chan H-L et al. The incidence of erythema multiforme, Stevens–Johnson syndrome, and toxic epidermal necrolysis. A population-based study with particular reference to reactions caused by drugs among outpatients. *Arch Dermatol* 1990;126:43–7.
7. Drugs that cause photosensitivity. *Med Lett Drugs Ther* 1995;37:35–6.
8. Roujeau JC, Stern RS. Severe adverse cutaneous reactions to drugs. *N Engl J Med* 1994;331:1272–85.
9. Price EJ, Venables PJW. Drug-induced lupus. *Drug Saf* 1995;12:283–90.
10. Mackay FJ et al. Safety of long-term lamotrigine in epilepsy. *Epilepsia* 1997;38:881–6.
11. Shapiro LE et al. Comparative safety of tetracycline, minocycline, and doxycycline. *Arch Dermatol* 1997;133: 1224–30.

Drug Use in Special Populations

2

Drugs and Pregnancy

Anna Taddio

In the United States, fetal malformations occur in 3 to 6% of pregnancies. These include major and minor malformations from any cause, be it drug, infection, maternal disease state, genetic defect, or pollutant.[1,2] Drug use during pregnancy can be associated with risk to the developing fetus and the pregnant woman. Drugs are probably responsible for only about 1 to 5% of fetal malformations; 60 to 70% of malformations have unknown causes.[2-4]

The genetic makeups of the fetus and the mother influence the extent to which an agent affects the developing fetus. For example, the rates of absorption, metabolism, and elimination of an agent by the mother, its rate of placental transfer, or the way it interacts with cells and tissues of the embryo are genetically determined factors. Thus, human teratogenicity cannot be predicted based only on animal data or extrapolated from one pregnancy to another.

■ PHYSIOLOGIC AND DEVELOPMENTAL FACTORS

Teratogenic substances rarely cause a single defect. Most often, a spectrum of defects occurs that corresponds with the systems undergoing major development at the time of exposure. Major malformations are usually the result of first-trimester exposure during critical periods of organogenesis. Exposures during the second and third trimesters can result in alterations or damage in fine structure and function. Intrauterine growth retardation is perhaps the most reliable indicator that a teratogen was present during the second and third trimesters of fetal development. Several organs and systems continue to develop after birth. Therefore, exposure to agents late in pregnancy carries some risk and can result in debilitating alterations in development such as mental retardation. Figure 2–1 shows the stages of human structural development in relation to teratogenic potential.[5]

■ DRUG FACTORS

Most chemicals in the maternal bloodstream cross the placenta. Movement of compounds across the placenta is generally bidirectional, although the net transfer occurs from mother to fetus in most instances.[6,7] Although active and facilitated transport of some substances across the placenta have been demonstrated, the

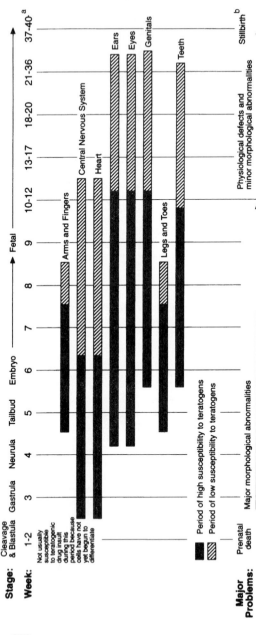

Figure 2–1. Variation in teratogenic susceptibility of organ systems during stages of human intrauterine development. (Reproduced with permission from Pagliaro LA, Pagliaro AM. *Problems in pediatric drug therapy.* 3rd ed. Hamilton, IL: Drug Intelligence Publications; 1995.)

[a]Average time for fertilization to parturition is 38 weeks.

[b]Drugs administered during this period can cause neonatal depression at birth (or other effects directly related to the pharmacologic effect of the administered drug).

transplacental passage of most agents occurs primarily by simple diffusion.[6,8,9] Only the unbound (free) fraction of a drug is subject to placental transfer; therefore, the greater the degree of protein binding of a drug, the less will be transferred to the fetus.[6,8,9] Early in pregnancy, the placental membrane is relatively thick, and this characteristic tends to reduce permeability.[6] The thickness of the trophoblastic epithelium decreases and surface area increases in the last trimester. The passage of drugs is increased during this stage of pregnancy.[6,10]

The rate-limiting factors in placental transfer of drugs are the same as those that govern membrane diffusion by molecules in general. Thus, the rate of diffusion across the placental barrier is directly proportional to the maternal–fetal concentration gradient and the surface area of the placenta.[6,8,9] Higher concentrations are generally attained in fetal serum and amniotic fluid after bolus injection than after continuous infusion of drug into the mother and by multiple-dose rather than single-dose therapy.[6] Certain physicochemical properties of drugs or chemicals favor transport to the fetus, including low molecular weight, lipid solubility, and nonionization at pH 7.4.[7,9,10]

Each drug has a threshold above which fetal defects can occur and below which no effects are discernible. Whether an agent reaches a "threshold concentration" in the fetus depends on maternal factors (eg, rates of absorption and clearance) and the chemical nature of the agent.

Administration of drugs near term poses another potential threat to the fetus. Before birth, the fetus relies on maternal systems for drug elimination. After birth, the infant must rely on its own metabolic and excretory capabilities, which have not yet fully developed. Drugs given near term or during birth, especially those with long half-lives, can have an even more prolonged action in the neonate. Drugs that cause maternal addiction also are known to cause fetal addiction. Neonatal withdrawal symptoms can occur when mothers have been addicted to drugs during pregnancy or when they have taken addicting drugs near term, even though the mothers themselves are not addicted.

■ EFFECTS OF PREGNANCY ON THE MOTHER

Maternal physiology changes as pregnancy progresses and can have an effect on drug disposition and clearance. Maternal plasma volume increases by about 20% at midgestation and 50% at term[9] and then falls toward prepregnancy levels postpartum. The volume of distribution for many drugs increases as the fetal compartment enlarges, causing changes in maternal serum drug concentrations. Drugs with narrow therapeutic ranges require careful monitoring during pregnancy and possibly dosage increases. As postpartum maternal plasma volume returns to normal, dosages of many drugs require reduction. Changes in plasma protein concentrations during pregnancy can affect the degree of binding and thus the amount of unbound drug.[8,9] Despite an increase in production of serum albumin, the increased intracellular and intravascular volumes cause serum albumin concentrations to decline.[11] A decrease in total plasma protein concentrations of about 10 g/L occurs during pregnancy.[8] Body fat increases by 3–4 kg during pregnancy and can act as a depot for fat-soluble drugs, thereby increasing their volume of distribution.[9] Renal blood flow and glomerular filtration rate increase by almost 50%

during pregnancy because of increased cardiac output. Renally excreted drugs therefore can have increased rates of clearance.[9]

■ INTERPRETATION OF STUDIES

There are few controlled, prospective studies of drug use in pregnancy. Most of the available information comes from case reports or case-control studies. Cause-and-effect relationships between drugs and teratogenicity are difficult to establish retrospectively because of the numerous variables in each report. These include maternal drug dosage, time of ingestion relative to the date of conception, duration of therapy, concomitant exposure to other potential teratogens, and questionable study design or methodology. Because studies cannot disprove that a slight teratogenic risk might occur with in utero exposure to drugs, drugs should be used during pregnancy only when absolutely necessary. The following table provides information concerning the effects of drugs used during pregnancy on the pregnant woman and on pregnancy outcome. For a more thorough discussion of the principles of teratology, the reader should consult reference 1.

The following abbreviation is used in the table:

IUGR—intrauterine growth retardation, less than the 10th percentile (of an appropriate standard) birth weight for gestational age.[12]

DRUGS AND PREGNANCY

ANALGESIC AND ANTI-INFLAMMATORY DRUGS

ANTIMIGRAINE DRUGS

Ergotamine

Ergotamine can stimulate uterine contraction and potentially cause abortion.[13]

Sumatriptan

Evidence collected through the Swedish Medical Birth Registry indicates no increased risk of birth defects in 658 pregnancies with drug exposure.[14] A prospective study of 86 women showed no increased risk of birth defects.[15] Sumatriptan does not have the oxytocic effect of the ergot alkaloids.

NONSTEROIDAL ANTI-INFLAMMATORY DRUGS

Acetaminophen

Acetaminophen does not cause congenital malformations and is the analgesic-antipyretic of choice for use near term because it does not affect platelet function or peripheral prostaglandin synthesis.[16,17] In maternal acetaminophen overdose, most infants are normal at birth,[18–21] but there have been a few cases of neonatal liver toxicity.[18,22] Acetaminophen might prevent fetal distress in laboring women with chorioamnionitis and fever.[23]

(continued)

ANALGESIC AND ANTI-INFLAMMATORY DRUGS

Nonsteroidal Anti-inflammatory Drugs

Early case reports implicating **indomethacin** as a cause of prenatal closure of the ductus arteriosus are inconclusive.[24–27] Indomethacin might cause oligohydramnios because of decreased fetal urine output, which places the fetus at risk for pulmonary hypoplasia and umbilical cord compromise.[13,26–29] Indomethacin inhibits uterine contractions and has been used as a tocolytic agent. Echocardiographic surveillance of the fetus might be indicated to monitor effects on the ductus arteriosus.

A large prospective study of more than 50,000 pregnancies did not show an increased risk of birth defects, altered birth weight, or perinatal deaths associated with exposure to **aspirin.**[30] First-trimester aspirin use does not increase the risk of congenital heart defects compared with other structural malformations.[31] Repeated third-trimester administration of aspirin 325 mg can result in prolonged constriction of the ductus arteriosus and pulmonary hypertension.[32] Maternal ingestion of aspirin 325 mg during the third trimester can interfere with uterine contractility and prolong gestation and labor.[32] Maternal and neonatal platelet function can be affected, resulting in increased maternal blood loss at delivery and abnormal platelet function tests and clinical bleeding in newborns, including intracranial hemorrhage.[13,33] Second- or third-trimester use of low-dose (20–100 mg/day) aspirin in mothers at risk of developing pregnancy-related hypertension decreases the frequency of this disorder and its complications.[34,35] A study of more than 9000 women found that 60 mg/day was not protective.[36] A follow-up 18 months after delivery of infants exposed in utero to aspirin 50 mg/day showed no increase in malformations and normal physical and neurologic development.[37] Newborns exposed to low-dose aspirin have not been found to have bleeding abnormalities.[35] Systematic evaluations of other commonly used NSAIDs have not been conducted in humans, but no substantive reports of NSAID teratogenicity exist.[24,38] However, caution is warranted because of their similarity to indomethacin and aspirin. **Ibuprofen** can cause mild oligohydramnios and mild constriction of the fetal ductus arteriosus.[13,38] Similar effects are likely with **naproxen.**[13] Persistent pulmonary hypertension occurred in a neonate whose mother had ingested 5 g naproxen 8 hr before delivery.[24] There are no reports of adverse effects of **ketorolac;** it is usually avoided during pregnancy.[13]

OPIOIDS

Narcotics

Narcotic analgesics do not cause fetal malformations, but narcotic abuse during pregnancy or use near term can lead to fetal tolerance and neonatal withdrawal. Meconium might be present in the amniotic fluid, caused most likely by increased bowel activity during periods of fetal withdrawal and/or hypoxia, putting the fetus at risk for meconium aspiration.[39] (*See* Heroin.) Withdrawal symptoms such as irritability, increased muscle tone, sleep disturbances, vague autonomic nervous system symptoms, tremulousness, high-pitched crying, frantic and uncoordinated sucking, and seizures can occur in neonates born to narcotic-addicted women and nonaddicted women using narcotics near term. Neonatal respiratory depression can occur when narcotic analgesics are given during labor and is dependent on the drug, dose, dosing interval, and route of administration (IV > IM).[40] Epidural **alfentanil** can cause neonatal hypotonus.[41,42] **Meperidine** crosses the placenta rapidly and can cause a sinusoidal fetal heart rate pattern. It is eliminated by the fetus at a rate much slower than the mother's; its metabolite, normeperidine, is long acting.[43] Meperidine given during delivery can interfere with the early establishment of breastfeeding because of infant sedation.[44,45] Meperidine by patient-controlled analgesia (PCA) for postcesarean pain causes a much greater decrease in neonatal alertness and sucking than an equivalent dosage of PCA **morphine.** Infants born to narcotic-dependent women maintained on **methadone** during

(*continued*)

ANALGESIC AND ANTI-INFLAMMATORY DRUGS

pregnancy are reported to have lower birth weights, jaundice, thrombocytosis, and withdrawal. Divided doses of methadone better stabilize the fetal activity pattern (which might indicate fetal withdrawal) before and after drug administration than do single daily doses.[46] It is not known if opioids can cause alterations in the neurobehavioral function of infants exposed in utero.

Narcotic Partial Agonists

All narcotics can cause respiratory depression and possibly some behavioral abnormalities in the newborn if used at the time of delivery. **Buprenorphine** used by a pregnant woman daily near term resulted in a mild narcotic-like withdrawal syndrome in her newborn.[47] **Butorphanol**[48] and **nalbuphine**[49] during labor can cause a sinusoidal fetal heart rate pattern. Nalbuphine offers no advantage over pure narcotics and can cause more abnormal Apgar scores (<7) at 1 min.[13,46] Nalbuphine with **pentazocine** use throughout pregnancy has caused infant withdrawal symptoms similar to those reported in offspring of heroin and methadone addicts.[13,40] Small-for-gestational-age infants, prematurity, and fetal distress also have been observed.[50] **Tramadol** withdrawal has been reported in a neonate exposed in utero throughout pregnancy.[51]

OTHER ANTI-INFLAMMATORY DRUGS

Gold Salts

Although teratogenic in animals, reports have described normal children born to women using gold salts during pregnancy. A few cases of musculoskeletal problems and one case of IUGR occurred among 128 infants exposed to parenterally administered gold during pregnancy.[24,52] Six women given **auranofin** during pregnancy delivered normal infants.[52]

Penicillamine

Data on the teratogenicity of penicillamine are contradictory. Most pregnant women taking penicillamine deliver normal healthy babies, even at the high dosages used in treating Wilson's disease.[24,52] However, there have been cases of fetal connective tissue abnormalities.[24,52] Penicillamine is best avoided during pregnancy.[52]

ANTIMICROBIAL DRUGS

AMINOGLYCOSIDES

There is no evidence that aminoglycosides are teratogenic. **Streptomycin** can cause congenital hearing loss, ranging from minor high-frequency loss to total deafness, when given to pregnant women for the treatment of tuberculosis. Prevalence is low, especially with careful dosage calculation and limited duration of therapy.[6,40,53,54] There is a theoretical risk of nephrotoxicity and ototoxicity for all aminoglycosides.[6,40,55]

ANTIMYCOBACTERIAL DRUGS

Antituberculars

The treatment of choice for tuberculosis during pregnancy is **isoniazid** and **rifampin** with **ethambutol** added if isoniazid resistance is suspected.[56] Isoniazid is the safest and most effective antitubercular during pregnancy,[6] although there can be an increased risk of hepatotoxicity in pregnant women. Of the reported isoniazid exposures during pregnancy, only 1% demonstrated any malformations. No pattern of malformation was shown, but several abnormalities involved the CNS.[6,40,53,54] Exposures were confounded by concomitant ethambutol therapy. Rifampin safety during pregnancy is less well established; however, it has not been associated with an increased risk of fetal malfor-

(continued)

ANTIMICROBIAL DRUGS

mations. In most reports, rifampin was taken with isoniazid or ethambutol. Neonatal hypoprothrombinemia has been reported and raises some concern about the use of rifampin, especially near term.[6,40,53,54] If rifampin is given during pregnancy, maternal oral prophylaxis with vitamin K 20 mg/day for 2 weeks before delivery is recommended.[6,40,53] Infants should receive 0.5–1 mg of vitamin K IM or SC immediately after delivery and again 6–8 hr later.[40] Ethambutol does not appear to cause malformations, but several anomalies involving the CNS occurred in 655 reported exposures.[6,40,53,54]

Sulfones

Dapsone does not appear to increase the risk of fetal abnormalities.[57] There are, however, some reports of hemolytic anemia in mothers and their infants after dapsone use.[58] Because dapsone is similar to sulfonamides, it might displace bilirubin from albumin binding sites and increase the risk of kernicterus in the infant due to hyperbilirubinemia. This risk is minimized if the drug is discontinued 1 month before the expected date of delivery.[6,53,59] (*See* Sulfonamides.)

Thalidomide

Thalidomide causes bilateral limb reduction defects, facial hemangioma, esophageal or duodenal atresia, and anomalies of the kidneys, heart, and external ears. The time of greatest risk is between gestational days 22 and 32. If exposure occurs between days 27 and 30, the arms are most often affected; with exposure between days 30 and 33, the legs and arms are affected.[2]

ANTIPARASITIC DRUGS

Antimalarials

Chloroquine is the drug of choice for prophylaxis and treatment of malaria during pregnancy.[60] Chloroquine or **hydroxychloroquine** malaria prophylaxis does not cause adverse fetal effects; however, larger anti-inflammatory doses have resulted in spontaneous abortion and fetal retinal and vestibular damage.[6,52,53,61] These drugs are best avoided in anti-inflammatory dosages during pregnancy. There is a risk of hemolysis in fetuses that are G-6-PD deficient. There are no reports of **primaquine** teratogenicity. It might induce hemolysis in neonates by the same mechanism as in adults.[40] **Pyrimethamine** is a microbial folate antagonist and should be used cautiously because the mammalian folate antagonist methotrexate is teratogenic; folic acid supplementation might be warranted during treatment.[6,40,52,53,62] In a study of 210 women exposed during pregnancy, however, no increased risk of birth defects was observed.[63] **Quinine** has been used as a folk medicine abortifacient, despite its poor efficacy. Maternal deaths have been reported. Fetal anomalies include blindness, optic nerve hypoplasia, deafness, and hearing impairment.[6,40,52,53]

ANTIVIRAL DRUGS

Acyclovir

Maternal acyclovir has not been shown to cause malformations[53,64–72] and is recommended for various infections during pregnancy.

Zidovudine

Use of zidovudine in pregnant women has not been shown to cause an increased rate of birth defects.[73–75] Concentrations of zidovudine are 2.5–7 times higher in amniotic fluid than in cord blood; concentrations in cord blood are higher (113 to 140%) than those in maternal blood.[76,77] Transmission of HIV from mother to fetus is substantially reduced with zidovudine treatment, and treatment is recommended for HIV-infected pregnant women.[74,78,79] In a long-term study of almost 200 children prenatally exposed to zidovudine, no adverse effects were observed on lymphocyte function, height, weight, or malignancy.[80] (*continued*)

ANTIMICROBIAL DRUGS

β-LACTAMS

Cephalosporins and penicillins are thought to be without teratogenic risk.[6,8,53,55,81] Treatment of early syphilis with penicillin (or other drugs) during pregnancy might produce the Jarisch–Herxheimer reaction, resulting in uterine cramping, decreased fetal movement, and, in some cases, fetal death.[82]

MACROLIDES

There is no evidence that erythromycin is harmful to the fetus.[6,40,53,81] About 10–15% of women treated with erythromycin estolate in the second trimester develop elevated serum AST levels that normalize when therapy is discontinued;[40] other derivatives might be preferred. Preliminary studies of women exposed to clarithromycin during pregnancy show no increased risk of anomalies.[83,84] Clarithromycin currently is not recommended during pregnancy because of limited data.

QUINOLONES

Nalidixic acid use during pregnancy can cause increased intracranial pressure, papilledema, and bulging fontanelles in the newborn. Avoid first-trimester use.[6,53,55] Fluoroquinolones (eg, ciprofloxacin, norfloxacin, ofloxacin) cause arthropathy in immature animals,[53] but preliminary data have not shown this effect in humans.[85,86]

SULFONAMIDES

There are occasional reports of abnormalities, but no malformation pattern has emerged. Evidence associating sulfonamide use near term with neonatal kernicterus is lacking, despite sulfonamide displacement of bilirubin from albumin binding sites.[6,53,55,81,87–89] There is a theoretical risk for hemolysis in the fetus or neonate because of its relative deficiencies in G-6-PD and glutathione.[6,53]

TETRACYCLINES

Tetracyclines can cause depression of fetal bone growth and permanent staining of the teeth when taken after the 12th week of pregnancy. Rebound bone growth can follow tetracycline discontinuation.[90] The risk of enamel discoloration increases with dose, duration of therapy, and advancing pregnancy; one-third to one-half of third-trimester exposures can be affected.[6,53,55,81] Pregnant women with pyelonephritis or underlying renal disease or after an overdose are at risk for developing acute fatty necrosis of the liver and azotemia.[6,53,55,81] Doxycycline might be less likely to discolor enamel.

MISCELLANEOUS ANTIMICROBIALS

Chloramphenicol

Although reports of fetal abnormality or toxicity from maternal chloramphenicol are lacking, there is a theoretical risk of blood dyscrasias. Particular caution should be exercised near term because of the "gray baby" syndrome, the result of toxic accumulation of chloramphenicol in neonates caused by their slow elimination of the drug.[6,53,55]

Metronidazole

Twenty years' experience and several studies demonstrate no association of metronidazole with congenital malformations, abortions, or stillbirths.[91–94] However, a few cases of facial clefting have been reported.[95] Metronidazole has not been demonstrated to be carcinogenic in humans.[96,97]

(continued)

ANTIMICROBIAL DRUGS

Nitrofurantoin

No fetal abnormalities or neonatal hemolytic anemia have been observed with nitrofurantoin use during pregnancy.[6,55,98–100] A theoretical risk for the development of hemolysis in neonates exists if the drug is taken by mothers near term because of infants' relative G-6-PD and glutathione deficiencies.[100]

Trimethoprim

Because it is a folate antagonist, caution is advised in pregnancy.[6,64] (*See* Methotrexate and Pyrimethamine.) However, data suggest a lack of teratogenicity.[6,55,81,88,89,100,101–103] Neither single-dose trimethoprim 600 mg nor the usual 5-day course (300 mg/day) for asymptomatic bacteriuria caused any detrimental effects on pregnancy outcome when given between the 16th and 30th weeks of gestation.[103]

Vancomycin

There is a theoretical risk for auditory and renal toxicity in the fetus.[6,53] However, in one small prospective trial, IV vancomycin during the second or third trimester produced no cases of fetal renal toxicity or hearing impairment.[104]

ANTINEOPLASTICS AND IMMUNOSUPPRESSANTS

ANTINEOPLASTICS

Antineoplastic agents have teratogenic and mutagenic potential, and reports of infertility and congenital defects exist. Nevertheless, several studies indicate that fertility is preserved, with normal pregnancy outcome, among women and men treated for cancer before conception. Although aggressive treatment of malignancy is necessary on occasion, avoidance or minimum use of these drugs, especially during the first trimester, is recommended because of reports of teratogenicity and spontaneous abortion. However, normal pregnancy outcome has occurred, particularly if exposure is early in gestation (first 2 weeks after conception).[105] Chemotherapy generally produces a decrease in birth weight but not IUGR.[106] Use of antineoplastics near delivery might cause neonatal bone marrow suppression[107] because the drugs might not have been eliminated before delivery. Chemotherapy should be avoided within 3 weeks of delivery, if possible.[105] Chemotherapy-induced tumors in the infant are a theoretical possibility.

ALKYLATING AGENTS

Busulfan

Use during pregnancy has been associated with IUGR and multiple malformations, although no specific pattern is evident.

Chlorambucil

Treatment in the first and second trimesters can cause spontaneous abortion, cleft palate, renal aplasia, or skeletal abnormalities.[105] There also have been reports of normal pregnancy.[108]

Cyclophosphamide

Use in the first trimester has resulted in fetal malformations, particularly of the toes; syndactyly; cleft palate; facial anomalies; IUGR; and possible developmental delay. The overall risk of malformation is estimated to be 16–22%. No malformations have been reported with second- or third-trimester use, but pancytopenia occurred in neonates exposed late in pregnancy. A report of malignancies in a child that occurred 10 and 14 yr after exposure in utero raises the question of

(*continued*)

ANTINEOPLASTICS AND IMMUNOSUPPRESSANTS

whether intrauterine exposure to cyclophosphamide can cause iatrogenic or secondary cancers.[109] Cyclophosphamide should be avoided in pregnancy.

Procarbazine

Use in pregnancy is limited, but several fetal abnormalities have occurred, all with first-trimester exposure.[40]

ANTIMETABOLITES

Fluorouracil

Use can cause malformations consistent with inhibition of cell division and cell growth.[40] Inadvertent first-trimester topical administration of 5% fluorouracil to the lower genital tract did not result in abnormal-appearing infants in 10 pregnancies.[110,111]

Methotrexate

Use in the first trimester causes spontaneous abortion and congenital abnormalities such as cranial anomalies, cleft palate, syndactyly, growth retardation, and developmental abnormalities.[2] One study of 10 pregnancies in 8 women taking methotrexate 7.5–10 mg/week during the first trimester for arthritis resulted in three spontaneous abortions, two elective abortions, and the birth of five full-term normal infants who had no medical illnesses or learning disabilities. Normal pregnancy outcome has occurred after use in the second and third trimesters.[2,112] It is recommended that methotrexate be discontinued for at least three menstrual cycles before conception and that the mother be taking folic acid.

Thioguanine

Use in the first and second trimesters has been associated with abnormalities.[40,113]

DNA INTERCALATING DRUGS

Daunorubicin and **doxorubicin** have been given without resultant fetal malformation, although some spontaneous abortions have occurred.[105] Premature delivery and transient bone marrow suppression have been reported.[114]

MITOTIC INHIBITORS

Most reports of **vinblastine** and **vincristine** use during pregnancy describe a lack of congenital malformations.[105]

IMMUNOSUPPRESSANTS

Azathioprine

Normal pregnancy outcome has occurred with azathioprine taken for renal transplantation, SLE, or acute or chronic leukemias.[115] However, IUGR, neonatal lymphopenia, hypogammaglobulinemia, thymic hypoplasia, fetal bone marrow suppression, leukopenia, and thrombocytopenia have occurred.[116] Azathioprine for inflammatory bowel disease with or without a corticosteroid plus sulfasalazine resulted in no congenital anomalies or developmental problems.[116] Older studies showed some chromosomal aberrations; however, there is no evidence of permanent genomal or gonadal damage.

Cyclosporine

Use of cyclosporine throughout pregnancy after renal or hepatic transplant does not appear to cause malformations, although experience is limited.[52] IUGR occurred in 11 of 20 infants, and

(continued)

ANTINEOPLASTICS AND IMMUNOSUPPRESSANTS

6 had severe IUGR (below the 3rd percentile). However, normal-size-for-gestational-age infants are often delivered. No neonatal distress or increased mortality has been reported.[117,118]

Mycophenolate

There are no data on the safety of mycophenolate taken during pregnancy.

Tacrolimus

Use in pregnancy after liver transplant resulted in preterm deliveries of 27 infants of 21 mothers.[119] However, prenatal and postnatal growth were appropriate for age. One infant was born with unilateral polycystic kidney disease.

CARDIOVASCULAR DRUGS

ANTIARRHYTHMIC DRUGS

Amiodarone

Neonatal hypothyroidism with and without goiter and hyperthyroidism have occurred with amiodarone use.[120] A child with transient congenital hypothyroidism showed some delay in motor development and impaired speech performance at age 5 yr.[120]

Digoxin

Digoxin is not a teratogen. It may be given to pregnant women to treat fetal CHF and supraventricular tachycardia. Maternal digitalis toxicity has caused fetal toxicity and miscarriage in one case and neonatal ECG changes with subsequent infant death in another. As pregnancy progresses, renal clearance of digoxin increases and its bioavailability can increase. Therefore, maternal serum concentrations might decrease or increase and should be monitored.[121,122]

Disopyramide

Use during pregnancy has not been well studied, but in one report, uterine contractions precipitated by disopyramide subsided when the drug was discontinued.[121]

Procainamide

Limited data indicate that procainamide use during pregnancy is probably safe. However, because of the potential for SLE, caution is advised.[121]

Quinidine

Quinidine is not teratogenic.[40,121] Neonatal thrombocytopenia has occurred after maternal use of quinidine.[40]

ANTIHYPERTENSIVE DRUGS

ACE Inhibitors

Several cases of IUGR and prolonged neonatal anuria and hypotension with resultant renal failure have occurred after maternal **captopril** or **enalapril** use.[123–126] Oligohydramnios or anhydramnios was present in 7 of 9 cases (not recorded in the other 2 cases) and led to pulmonary hypoplasia and death in some. Respiratory problems occurred in several neonates. Some infants had altered or absent skull formation with dysmorphic facial features, microcephaly, and occipital encephalocele. One infant exposed during the second and third trimesters had prolonged anuria and hypotension requiring dialysis, and one infant exposed throughout pregnancy had hypoglycemia; others have had persistent ductus arteriosus (this might have been caused by low birth weight).[125–127]

(continued)

CARDIOVASCULAR DRUGS

There might be an increased frequency of fetal loss with ACE inhibitors.[126] The FDA warns against their use in the second and third trimesters.

Diazoxide

When given by rapid IV bolus, diazoxide can cause excessive maternal hypotension and fetal distress. Slow IV infusion or minibolus administration might prevent these effects. Other reported effects are inhibition of labor, neonatal hyperglycemia when exposure preceded delivery, alopecia, hypertrichosis lanuginosa, and decreased bone age after exposure in the last 19–70 days of gestation. Other investigators report no problems after long-term oral administration of diazoxide.[121,128,129]

Hydralazine

Hydralazine is not associated with congenital anomalies. Use in pregnancy can cause reduced uteroplacental blood flow, fetal heart rate changes after acute administration, and neonatal hypothermia and thrombocytopenia.[121,128,129]

Methyldopa

Methyldopa in pregnancy has been studied more extensively than any other antihypertensive. Available data show no teratogenicity. Transient reduction in neonatal blood pressure can occur after maternal methyldopa ingestion. There is a questionable association of IUGR and maternal treatment with methyldopa. One study suggested IUGR was caused by chronic hypertension rather than by methyldopa.[121,128,129]

Reserpine

When given to mothers within 24 hr of delivery, reserpine produces edema of the neonatal nasal mucosa. This effect is especially important because newborns are obligate nose breathers. Lethargy, hypothermia, and bradycardia also have been reported in infants whose mothers received antenatal reserpine.[128,130]

β-ADRENERGIC BLOCKING DRUGS

β-Blockers such as **atenolol, pindolol, metoprolol,** and **propranolol** are not associated with congenital anomalies and are generally safe in pregnancy. Maternal hypertension can cause IUGR, decreased placental size, neonatal respiratory depression, and hypoglycemia. IUGR and neonatal hypoglycemia and hypotension have occurred after taking β-blockers. Whether these effects are caused by the drugs or maternal disease has not been established. Neonatal bradycardia might be caused by these agents; it is usually mild but was severe after an intravenous infusion in one case.[131] β-Blockers can adversely affect fetal adaptation to intrauterine hypoxia such as that associated with umbilical cord compression.[121,123,128,132–136] Although generally regarded as safe during pregnancy, **labetalol** given intravenously to control severe hypertension has caused neonatal bradycardia, weak femoral pulses, inadequate breathing, hypotonia, hypotension, and hypoglycemia.[128,129,136,137]

CALCIUM-CHANNEL BLOCKING DRUGS

No malformations have been associated with the use of calcium-channel blocking agents during pregnancy.[138–140] Bolus doses of IV **isradipine** during labor decrease maternal blood pressure and increase fetal heart rate.[138] **Nifedipine** does not appear to alter uterine arterial resistance when given at 17–22 weeks or 26–35 weeks of gestational age.[139,140]

(continued)

CARDIOVASCULAR DRUGS

INOTROPIC DRUGS

The treatment of hypotension during pregnancy with sympathomimetic agents (eg, **dopamine, dobutamine, norepinephrine**) is complicated by the fact that the uterine vasculature is supplied solely with α-adrenergic receptors and maximally dilated under basal conditions. Pure α-adrenergic agents markedly constrict uterine vessels and decrease blood flow, thereby compromising the fetus. β-Adrenergic agents cause peripheral vasodilation and tend to shunt blood away from the uterus and also can cause fetal compromise. Volume-expanding agents seem to be the most prudent treatment for sudden hypotension in pregnancy.

CENTRAL NERVOUS SYSTEM DRUGS

ANTICONVULSANTS

Many congenital malformations have been reported in children of epileptic mothers, and all anticonvulsants for which data are adequate have been implicated as possible causes of malformations. Epileptic mothers have increased frequencies of fetal malformation compared with nonepileptic mothers, and anticonvulsant drugs appear to increase these frequencies.[141] Major malformations seem to be more common after combination therapy than with monotherapy.[141] Fetal deficiency of epoxide hydrolase, a major enzyme in the metabolic pathway of many anticonvulsants (eg, **carbamazepine, phenytoin, and valproic acid**) that helps eliminate toxic intermediates, might mediate teratogenic effects. Deficient function of this enzyme might be inherited as an autosomal recessive trait.[142–146] Total concentrations of carbamazepine, phenytoin, phenobarbital, and valproic acid decline as pregnancy progresses, caused mainly by changes in plasma protein binding.[141] However, free or unbound drug concentrations fall appreciably only for phenobarbital. Free concentrations of valproic acid increase. Measurement of free anticonvulsant drug concentrations allows for appropriate dosage adjustment.[141] Decreased fetal **folic acid** concentrations have been reported with several anticonvulsants (eg, carbamazepine, phenobarbital, phenytoin, and valproic acid). Folic acid supplementation during pregnancy might decrease the risk of abnormal offspring.[147]

Carbamazepine

Carbamazepine is associated with a 1% risk of spina bifida.[141,147,148] Malformations similar to those ascribed to other anticonvulsants also have been reported: specific facial features, nail hypoplasia, and small head circumference. Data concerning developmental delay or impairment require substantiation.[141,149] Higher serum concentrations of carbamazepine were found in mothers of abnormal offspring than in mothers of normal offspring.[150] Mothers receiving carbamazepine should receive supplemental folic acid.[147]

Gabapentin

There is little information about gabapentin in pregnancy. Of 9 exposed women reported to the manufacturer, 4 had elective abortions, 4 had normal infants, and 1 infant had pyloric stenosis and an inguinal hernia.

Lamotrigine

There are no studies of the safety of lamotrigine in pregnancy. The manufacturer maintains a pregnancy registry with birth outcomes reported. As of 1994, no constellation of defects was observed.

Oxazolidinediones

Long-term use of **trimethadione** or **paramethadione** during pregnancy has resulted in children with abnormalities such as mental deficiency, prominent forehead with V-shaped eyebrows, epi-

(continued)

CENTRAL NERVOUS SYSTEM DRUGS

canthal folds, microcephaly, low-set ears with anteriorly folded helices, short stature, and hypospadias. This syndrome of abnormalities is called fetal trimethadione syndrome. The frequency of spontaneous abortion also might be increased.[2,40,141]

Phenobarbital

Abnormalities have been reported with phenobarbital alone and in combination, but causality is not established. Malformations similar to those of phenytoin and alcohol have been reported with phenobarbital and might be related to the folate deficiency that each of these can cause.[141] These effects might be more likely when maternal serum concentrations exceed usual therapeutic concentrations. Barbiturates can cause a decrease in vitamin K-dependent clotting factors, leading to bleeding in the newborn.[40,141] Neonatal withdrawal can occur after phenobarbital use during pregnancy.

Phenytoin

Phenytoin is a teratogen that causes a number of anomalies such as heart defects and facial clefts. It also can cause a cluster of anomalies called the fetal hydantoin syndrome (FHS), the principal features of which are craniofacial anomalies (eg, bowed upper lip, ocular hypertelorism, broad nasal bridge, short nose, epicanthal folds), digital hypoplasia with small or absent nails, and pre- and postnatal growth deficiency.[2,141,151] The risk of developing the full-blown FHS is about 5 to 10% when phenytoin is taken throughout pregnancy; the risk of a less serious effect is 30%.[152] Serum anticonvulsant concentrations were higher in mothers of malformed infants than in mothers of normal infants in some studies.[149] Maternal phenytoin use also can result in developmental delay and intellectual impairment.[149] Phenytoin can cause a decrease in vitamin K-dependent clotting factors, leading to bleeding in the newborn.[40,141] Phenytoin serum concentrations often decrease during pregnancy because of increased plasma clearance. Adjustment of phenytoin dosage to maintain serum free drug concentrations seems to improve seizure control.[153]

Primidone

The teratogenicity of primidone alone is difficult to assess because few cases have been reported and primidone is often taken with other anticonvulsants, primarily phenytoin. Although no specific pattern is established, reported malformations include craniofacial alterations, hirsute forehead, cardiac defects, pre- and postnatal growth retardation, digital hypoplasia with small or flat nails, inguinal hernias, and hypospadias.[40,141] Some cases of developmental delay also have been reported. These effects might be more likely when maternal serum concentrations exceed usual therapeutic concentrations. Phenobarbital is one metabolite of primidone. (See Phenobarbital.)

Valproic Acid

Neural tube defects (eg, spina bifida) occur in 1 to 2% of valproic acid–exposed fetuses compared with 0.4% in fetuses exposed to other anticonvulsants.[141,152] The risk for neural tube defects might be 5- to 10-fold higher with valproic acid compared with the background frequency.[142] The rate of spina bifida appears to be related to valproate serum concentration. Serum concentrations should be kept as low as possible during pregnancy and the mother should be given supplemental folic acid.[141] External ear anomalies, congenital heart defects, hypospadias, craniofacial anomalies, low birth weight, and small head circumference have been reported.[141,150,152,154–156] Cases of limb reduction defects, radial ray aplasia, talipes equinovarus, developmental delay, neurologic abnormality, and brain atrophy have been reported.[152,154] Congenital liver damage has been described.[157]

(continued)

CENTRAL NERVOUS SYSTEM DRUGS

ANTIDEPRESSANTS

Selective Serotonin Reuptake Inhibitors

Prospective follow-up of exposed pregnancies, including first-trimester exposure and spontaneous reports to the manufacturer, do not implicate **fluoxetine** as a teratogen.[158] However, a prospective study found increased risks of multiple minor malformations, prematurity, large-for-gestational-age size, admission to a special care nursery, and poor neonatal adaptation.[158] Several case reports of neonatal withdrawal after maternal fluoxetine or **sertraline** use during the third trimester have been reported.[158,159] Symptoms are restlessness, irritability, crying, tremors, increased muscle tone, poor feeding, and sleep disturbance. Neurodevelopmental assessments in offspring exposed to fluoxetine did not substantiate behavioral teratogenicity.[160]

Tricyclic Antidepressants

Although there are several case reports of different fetal anomalies after maternal use of tricyclic antidepressants (TCAs) during pregnancy, no consistent pattern of malformation has been observed and they are not considered to pose a teratogenic risk. Maternal use of TCAs during pregnancy occasionally has produced neonatal symptoms of breathlessness, respiratory distress, hypertonia with tremor, clonus, spasm, cyanosis, tachypnea, irritability, and feeding difficulties. In one case, neonatal urinary retention occurred after maternal **nortriptyline** use.[161] Neurodevelopmental assessments of offspring exposed in utero did not show abnormalities.[160]

ANTIPSYCHOTIC DRUGS

There is some evidence that women with psychoses have twice the rate of fetal malformation as the general population.[162] Most data do not implicate **phenothiazines, haloperidol,** or **clozapine** as teratogens.[162] Phenothiazine use near term can result in extrapyramidal effects and withdrawal reactions in the neonate.[162,163] If drug therapy is necessary during pregnancy, high-potency agents (eg, **haloperidol, fluphenazine**) are preferred to low-potency agents (eg, **chlorpromazine, thioridazine**) because the latter can cause maternal hypotension.[162]

ANXIOLYTICS, SEDATIVES, AND HYPNOTICS

High dosages of any sedative-hypnotic close to or during delivery can result in neonatal CNS and respiratory depression.

Anesthetics, General

Single exposures to general anesthesia in early pregnancy have not been associated with an increased risk of birth defects.[164] There is, however, a possible association between general anesthesia for surgery performed between gestational weeks 4 and 5 and neural tube defects,[165] and first-trimester exposure to general anesthesia is associated with hydrocephalus and eye defects.[166] However, not all patients in these studies received the same preoperative medications or inhalation anesthetics, although **nitrous oxide** was received by >98% in one study and a causal relationship between other factors (eg, underlying disease) could not be ruled out.[167] Although a 2- to 4-fold increase in the rate of spontaneous abortion in pregnant women with long-term exposure to inhalation anesthetics (eg, operating room and dental personnel) has been suggested, poor study design makes these conclusions suspect.[167,168] CNS and respiratory depression in the neonate can occur after inhalation anesthetic use during labor. During labor, **halothane** is not recommended because of its low analgesic activity. Nitrous oxide, **methoxyflurane,** and **enflurane** are commonly used.[169] Halogenated anesthetics can cause uterine relaxation and, theoretically, increase maternal blood loss. Neonatal EEG recordings have documented that **thiopental**

(continued)

CENTRAL NERVOUS SYSTEM DRUGS

general anesthesia has more neonatal depressant effects than 0.5% **bupivacaine** epidural anesthesia when used for cesarean section.[170]

Barbiturates

Long-term use of barbiturates during pregnancy for control of seizures might be associated with an increased risk of birth defects. First-trimester use of thiopental or **pentobarbital** has not been associated with defects.[171] Barbiturate addiction during pregnancy can result in neonatal withdrawal. Symptoms include tremors, irritability, restlessness, high-pitched crying, increased tone, hyperphagia, and overreaction to stimuli, which can persist for up to 6 months.[40] (*See* Anticonvulsants and Phenobarbital.)

Benzodiazepines

Recent data do not support a previously reported association between **diazepam** or **chlordiazepoxide** and oral clefting.[12,40,161,172–174] Infants of mothers using benzodiazepines near term might exhibit withdrawal symptoms (including tremors, irritability, and hypertonicity) and cardiovascular, respiratory, and CNS effects consistent with benzodiazepine pharmacology. Many exhibit the "floppy baby syndrome" characterized by muscular relaxation, poor sucking, disturbances in thermoregulation, and regurgitation.[13,40,169,172,175–177] **Oxazepam, lorazepam,** and **temazepam** are short acting and predominantly metabolized into inactive glucuronides and subsequently excreted by the kidneys; therefore, they might be preferred to diazepam, although irritability, feeding difficulties, and muscle tone disorders lasting 2 months were reported in two infants of mothers who used lorazepam 2–3 mg/day throughout pregnancy.[176,178] It is not known if benzodiazepines cause behavioral abnormalities after prolonged intrauterine exposure.

Meprobamate

In one study, meprobamate ingestion during the first 42 days of pregnancy resulted in 8 of 66 exposed children having abnormalities, 5 of whom had cardiovascular malformations. Other large-scale investigations have not confirmed these findings.[40] Alternative agents are advised, especially during the first trimester.

LITHIUM

Lithium use during the first trimester of pregnancy, particularly from the 3rd to 8th weeks, might increase the risk of cardiovascular abnormalities, including Ebstein's anomaly.[179–183] Anomalies of the external ear, ureters, CNS, and endocrine system, as well as macrosomia also have been reported.[181,182] A case of polyhydramnios possibly caused by lithium-induced fetal polyuria has occurred.[184] Of lithium-exposed pregnancies followed by the Lithium Registry, 39% delivered prematurely, 36% had macrosomia (>90th percentile body weight for gestational age), and there was an 8.3% perinatal mortality rate. Symptoms of lithium toxicity, including lethargy, hypotonia, poor sucking reflex, respiratory distress, cyanosis, arrhythmias, and thyroid depression with goiter and hypothermia, have been reported in newborns of women on long-term lithium therapy. Newborn blood concentrations were 0.6–1 mEq/L. Monitor maternal serum concentrations frequently during pregnancy because lithium clearance changes as pregnancy progresses.[161,179–181]

GASTROINTESTINAL DRUGS

ACID-PEPTIC THERAPY

Antacids

Available data do not suggest teratogenicity for commonly used antacids (aluminum, magnesium, calcium salts).[185–187] Long-term administration, however, is not recommended because of the potential toxicity.[188]

(continued)

GASTROINTESTINAL DRUGS

Histamine H_2-Receptor Antagonists

No reports link **cimetidine** or **ranitidine** to adverse pregnancy outcome.[189,190] Manufacturer data on cimetidine use in 50 pregnant women showed no increased risk to the developing fetus, although time of exposure was not noted. No reported adverse effects on the course of delivery or on the neonate have been reported following the use of H_2-antagonists as preanesthetic agents to prevent aspiration of acidic stomach contents.[87,191,192]

Sucralfate

No adequate studies exist on the use of sucralfate in pregnant women. Because little drug is absorbed, little risk is expected.[87]

ANTIEMETICS

Studies of women with hyperemesis gravidarum treated with **metoclopramide, prochlorperazine,** or placebo found no malformations or neonatal problems.[171,193,194] However, a reanalysis of some early data questions the initial negative findings and suggests an increased risk of malformations with antinauseant phenothiazine use during the 4th to 10th weeks of gestation.[163] Antihistamines used for pregnancy-induced emesis (**dimenhydrinate, diphenhydramine, doxylamine, meclizine**) are not considered teratogens.[195,196] (*See* Antihistamines.)

GASTROINTESTINAL MOTILITY

Metoclopramide

There are no reports of adverse fetal outcome with use of metoclopramide during pregnancy; however, the drug has not been used widely in this setting.[87,193] The use of metoclopramide during labor, anesthesia, or cesarean section to prevent acid aspiration has not resulted in adverse maternal, fetal, or neonatal outcomes.[87,193]

MISCELLANEOUS GASTROINTESTINAL DRUGS

Mesalamine Derivatives

Mesalamine derivatives including **sulfasalazine** have not been associated with teratogenic risk. It is not clear, however, if the drugs or the disease for which they are used (eg, Crohn's disease) contribute adverse effects such as low birth weight.[52,87,197–202] (*See also* Antimicrobial Drugs, Sulfonamides.)

HEMATOLOGIC DRUGS

COAGULANTS AND ANTICOAGULANTS

Heparin

Heparin has not been associated with an increased risk for structural or functional defects or with IUGR. Its large molecular size prevents it from crossing into the fetal circulation. Maternal thrombocytopenia and hemorrhage can occur.[203–206]

Low-Molecular-Weight Heparins

Low-molecular-weight heparins do not cross the placenta. Limited data do not suggest a teratogenic risk.[207,208]

Warfarin

Warfarin and related anticoagulants can produce the fetal warfarin syndrome or warfarin embryopathy. The critical period of risk appears to be between 6 and 12 weeks of gestation. Features include nasal hypoplasia, neonatal respiratory distress from upper airway obstruction, stippled

(*continued*)

HEMATOLOGIC DRUGS

epiphyses, IUGR, and different degrees of hypoplasia of the extremities. Eye abnormalities, including blindness, have also been reported. About one-third of exposed cases result in adverse pregnancy outcomes. One-half of these are spontaneous abortions or stillbirths, and the other half exhibit some type of congenital abnormality.[2,152,203–206,209–212] A few cases of diaphragmatic malformation have been reported when warfarin was used early in pregnancy.[213] CNS defects occur in about 3% of those exposed and appear to occur independent of the fetal warfarin syndrome. Critical periods of risk for CNS effects appear to be during the second and third trimesters.[212] Warfarin also increases the risk for fetal and maternal hemorrhage, especially when used near term.[203,209]

HORMONAL DRUGS

ADRENAL HORMONES

Corticosteroid use during pregnancy can increase the risk for maternal gestational diabetes, hypertension, and excessive weight gain.[118] Although corticosteroids do not represent a major teratogenic risk, there might be a small increased risk of oral clefts, which is consistent with animal studies.[214] Large prospective investigations and cases of pregnant women with inflammatory bowel disease, asthma, or rheumatoid arthritis do not show an increase in spontaneous abortions or congenital defects in infants exposed prenatally. Some studies show decreased birth weight and increased rates of prematurity, although these effects might have been due to underlying maternal disease.[118,215] Women who had status asthmaticus during pregnancy were more likely to have infants with low birth weight or IUGR.[215] A placental enzyme (11-β-OH-dehydrogenase) inactivates certain corticosteroids, leading to low fetal concentrations. This inactivation is greater with **hydrocortisone, prednisone,** or **prednisolone** than with **betamethasone** or **beclomethasone.** The fetal liver is relatively ineffective in converting prednisone into the active prednisolone, even at term. Therefore, prednisone or hydrocortisone might be preferred during pregnancy. When appropriate, corticosteroids can be administered by aerosol inhalation or intrasynovial injection to minimize systemic availability.[215] Neonates born to women taking long-term corticosteroids should be monitored for adrenal insufficiency, although this rarely occurs. Maternal betamethasone therapy is used to prevent respiratory distress in infants born between 28 and 34 weeks of gestation, with no apparent adverse effects.[216,217] No differences in psychological or physical development, pulmonary function, ophthalmologic findings, or neurologic function were noted between exposed and nonexposed children 10 to 12 yr old.[218] However, there was a significantly increased frequency of hospitalizations for infections during early childhood in the exposed group.

ANDROGENS

Androgen (eg, **testosterone, methyltestosterone,** and **danazol**) exposure during the first week of gestation can cause masculinization of the female embryo. Clitoromegaly, with or without fusion of the labia minora, can occur. In some cases, a urogenital sinus opening at the base of the clitoris has been observed. The extent of the defect is correlated with the time of exposure and dosage.[2,219,220] Although danazol dosages <400 mg/day can carry a lower risk, virilization was observed with 200 mg/day in one case.[220] Because differentiation of external genitalia occurs 8–12 weeks postconception, exposure beyond the 12th week of gestation is expected to produce only clitoral hypertrophy. If danazol is discontinued by the 8th week of gestation, the risk is substantially lower. Internal genitalia are unaffected because they are not androgen responsive. Male fetuses do not appear to be adversely affected.

(continued)

HORMONAL DRUGS

ANTIDIABETIC DRUGS

Maternal diabetes increases the rate of malformations and perinatal mortality.[221,222] Pregnancy in 20 women exposed to an oral hypoglycemic (16 to a sulfonylurea, 3 to a biguanide, 1 unknown) during organogenesis resulted in a higher proportion of major and minor malformations than a similar, unexposed control group.[222] A retrospective case review did not find a similar increase in malformations.[223] Malformations reported included auricular, vertebral, cardiac, neural tube, and limb defects.[222–224] Complicating the issue is a study that shows **glyburide** does not cross the human placenta ex vivo in appreciable amounts.[225] Sulfonylureas (eg, **chlorpropamide, glyburide,** and **glipizide**) and biguanides (eg, **metformin**) can cause prolonged hypoglycemia or hyperinsulinism in the newborn.[2,40,152,222,226] Pregnant diabetics should be treated with **insulin.**

FEMALE SEX HORMONES

Clomiphene

Clomiphene-induced ovulation results in an increased frequency of multiple ovulations (primarily twinning), delayed follicular rupture, ectopic pregnancy, and female fetuses. There also is an increase in abnormal karyotypes in oocytes and abortuses. The high proportion of abnormal karyotypes might be related to the increase in spontaneous abortions and low pregnancy rate noted after ovulation induction and in vitro fertilization.[227,228] The rate of birth defects reported after ovulation induction in most studies has been within the expected range.[227,229,230] A pooled analysis of available studies concluded that, if clomiphene causes neural tube defects, the elevated risk is no greater than twice the baseline rate.[231]

Diethylstilbestrol (DES)

Daughters of DES-exposed mothers have an increased frequency of vaginal adenosis; structural defects of the cervix, vagina, uterus, and fallopian tubes; and reproductive complications such as infertility, spontaneous abortion, ectopic pregnancy, premature deliveries, and perinatal deaths.[2,232–235] Two large cohort studies do not confirm the relation of DES to clear cell carcinoma. Early studies showing such an association were retrospective and had serious methodologic flaws.[236] If an association exists, the risk of developing this cancer in exposed females is very low. Data on DES-exposed males suggest an increased risk for infertility, various urogenital abnormalities, and testicular cancer.[237]

Progestins

High doses of progestins (eg, **medroxyprogesterone, norethindrone,** and **norethynodrel**) during pregnancy can cause masculinization of female external genitalia (clitoral hypertrophy or labioscrotal fusion). Hypospadias has occurred in males.[238,239] This most likely occurs during the period of external genitalia development (8–12 weeks postconception).[2,40,240–242] Doses used in oral or implantable contraceptives do not appear to carry these risks.[243]

THYROID AND ANTITHYROID DRUGS

Propylthiouracil and **methimazole** are not considered major human teratogens.[244] However, both drugs were associated with neonatal goiter in early reports, possibly because of the use of iodine in addition to unnecessarily high dosages of antithyroid medication. However, even conservative management does not completely eliminate the risk of congenital goiter. Transient neonatal hypothyroidism and neonatal thyrotoxicosis can occur. Hypothyroidism can be prevented by discontinuing the drug 4–6 weeks before delivery if the mother has remained euthyroid. Monitor in-

(continued)

HORMONAL DRUGS

fants for thyrotoxicosis because it can be masked by the antithyroid agent. Cases of infants with ulcer-like midline scalp defects have been associated with maternal methimazole. Another report, however, did not confirm an association of methimazole with skin defects.[245] Mothers with moderate to severe hyperthyroidism not receiving treatment have an increased risk of complications including toxemia, small-for-gestational-age babies, and neonatal morbidity.[246–249] Excessive **iodine** use during pregnancy can cause congenital goiter and hypothyroidism. Goiters might be large enough to cause tracheal compression and interfere with delivery. Severe maternal iodine deficiency produces hypothyroidism and cretinism.[246,247]

No adverse effects have been reported after inadvertent exposure to ^{131}I before 10 weeks of gestation. After 10 weeks of gestation, the fetal thyroid actively concentrates iodine; any radioactive iodine ingested by the mother will cross the placenta and destroy fetal thyroid tissue.[2,246]

Thyroid hormones (**levothyroxine, liothyronine**) may be used during pregnancy for the treatment of hypothyroidism.[171]

MISCELLANEOUS HORMONAL AGENTS

Oxytocin

Oxytocin given for induction of labor can cause tetanic uterine contractions, resulting in decreased uterine blood flow and fetal distress. The risk of neonatal hyperbilirubinemia is increased 1.6-fold after oxytocin-induced labor compared with spontaneous labor, and neonatal jaundice has occurred.[249]

Prostaglandins

Misoprostol has uterotonic effects and should not be used during pregnancy. In 56 pregnant women who requested first-trimester abortions, 1 or 2 oral doses of misoprostol 400 g resulted in spontaneous fetal expulsions.[250] Twenty-five women had uterine bleeding. High doses of misoprostol in early pregnancy, such as those used to induce abortion, cause defects. Anomalies reported include paralysis of cranial nerves VI and VII and limb, orofacial, and musculoskeletal defects.[251–254] **Dinoprostone,** when administered as vaginal tablets to mildly hypertensive women at term to induce labor, produces significant decreases in the percentage of time occupied by fetal body and breathing movements 3–4 hr later.[255] Fetal outcome is normal. Dinoprostone might shorten labor more than oxytocin.[256,257]

RENAL AND ELECTROLYTES

DIURETICS

Diuretics should be used with great caution during pregnancy because they can decrease maternal intravascular volume and consequently diminish uteroplacental perfusion, thereby compromising fetal oxygenation. This effect is most rapid and severe with loop diuretics (eg, **bumetanide, furosemide,** and **torsemide**). IV furosemide administration to the pregnant woman has enabled ultrasonic imaging of the fetal bladder because of increased fetal urine output. **Thiazide diuretic** use is not associated with birth defects; however, use during late pregnancy can produce neonatal hypoglycemia, hyponatremia, hypokalemia, and thrombocytopenia.[121,128,129,258]

ELECTROLYTES

Long-term infusion of **magnesium sulfate** during the second trimester occasionally causes bone abnormalities and dental enamel hypoplasia.[259,260] However, infusions between 24 and 34 weeks of gestation in women with preterm labor generally do not cause adverse neonatal outcomes.[261]

(*continued*)

RENAL AND ELECTROLYTES

Use of magnesium sulfate as a tocolytic agent near term can cause dosage-related neonatal hypotonia, hyporeflexia, respiratory distress, hypocalcemia, and hypermagnesemia.[259,262] Magnesium also is used for prophylaxis of seizures due to eclampsia.[263] Serial serum magnesium concentrations should be used to guide therapy.

RESPIRATORY DRUGS

ANTIALLERGICS

Cromolyn sodium use during pregnancy is not known to have any teratogenic effects. A prescription event monitoring study of **nedocromil** in the United Kingdom identified 79 exposed pregnancies.[264] Routine follow-up showed no abnormalities among the 33 infants with first-trimester exposure.

ANTIASTHMATICS

β-Adrenergic Agonists

Aerosol inhalation of **metaproterenol, albuterol, isoetharine,** or **terbutaline** is considered safe during pregnancy. Less is known about the oral use of these products, but experience suggests no adverse outcome. In one series, **salmeterol** was taken during the first trimester during 64 pregnancies and only during the second and third trimesters in 3 pregnancies.[265] The 67 pregnancies resulted in 50 live births, 6 spontaneous abortions, 2 ectopic pregnancies, 4 elective terminations, and 5 unknown outcomes. The small number of fetuses exposed to salmeterol during this study precludes any definitive conclusions about its safety. Albuterol, terbutaline, and **ritodrine** have been given in large IV or PO doses for their tocolytic effects in the third trimester without permanent harm to the fetus, although hypertension, hypoglycemia, hypokalemia, and hypocalcemia have been reported.[262] **Ephedrine** use during labor can alter neonatal sleep patterns.[170]

Inhaled Corticosteroids

This route is preferred during pregnancy to minimize fetal exposure. (*See* Corticosteroids.)

Theophylline

Maternal theophylline pharmacokinetics can change during the second and third trimesters, with decreased theophylline protein binding, decreased nonrenal clearance, and increased renal clearance.[266] V_d and half-life increase during the third trimester.[266] Pregnant women should have serum theophylline concentrations monitored frequently for dosage adjustments. No adverse fetal effects from long-term theophylline use during pregnancy are known.[267] Theophylline toxicity occurred in three newborns whose mothers received theophylline or **aminophylline** in late pregnancy and during labor. Symptoms included jitteriness, vomiting, and tachycardia, all of which resolved.[40]

ANTIHISTAMINES

The relative risk of malformations for first-generation antihistamines (eg, **chlorpheniramine, doxylamine**) is not statistically significant. Despite reports implicating **meclizine** and Bendectin (doxylamine and **pyridoxine** with or without **dicyclomine**) as teratogens, large-scale studies and two meta-analyses have shown no association between antihistamines and fetal malformation.[3,40,268,269] Limited data from studies of **astemizole, hydroxyzine,** and **cetirizine** have not shown a significant teratogenic risk.[269,270] **Dimenhydrinate** might have an oxytocic

(*continued*)

RESPIRATORY DRUGS

effect on the term uterus, causing shortened labor. The same concerns as with oxytocin (hyperstimulation and the possibility of uterine rupture) apply.[193] (*See* Antiemetics.)

COUGH AND COLD

Use of **sympathomimetics** (eg, **pseudoephedrine**) for treatment of nasal congestion can cause increased fetal activity and fetal tachycardia. Systemically administered sympathomimetics should be avoided in patients with hypertension or eclampsia or situations in which there is poor fetal cardiac reserve.[40,271]

MISCELLANEOUS DRUGS

ANESTHETICS, LOCAL

Maternal exposure to local anesthetics during the first 4 months of pregnancy does not cause fetal malformations.[169,170,272] However, local anesthetics have resulted in fetal and neonatal CNS and myocardial depression and fetal hyperthermia after maternal use during labor. Fetal bradycardia can occur after paracervical blocks. Epidural administration of **bupivacaine** or **lidocaine** might be the safest method for obstetric analgesia. Epidural lidocaine was shown to decrease neonatal neurobehavioral performance, but the effect was short lived and of minimal clinical consequence.[169] High-concentration (0.75%) bupivacaine is not recommended for use in obstetrics because of the profound neonatal myocardial depression and prolonged difficult resuscitation that follow accidental intravascular injection.[169,272] Lower concentrations are popular because of the high quality of analgesia with minimal degree of motor block.[169] **Mepivacaine** should not be used in obstetric anesthesia because the neonate cannot metabolize it.[169,170]

ERGOT ALKALOIDS

The use of **ergonovine** or **methylergonovine** before delivery carries the same risk of uterine stimulation as oxytocin.[13,262] (*See* Hormonal Drugs, Oxytocin.)

PODOPHYLLIN

Podophyllotoxins are antimitotic agents, and their use during pregnancy is contraindicated. Maternal oral use during the 5th through 9th weeks of gestation might be associated with congenital malformation. High doses used topically at the 34th week resulted in severe maternal toxicity and a stillborn fetus. There are several cases in which topical podophyllin use during pregnancy produced no adverse outcome.[171,273–276]

RETINOIDS

Etretinate

Etretinate is a known teratogen in humans. Fetal abnormalities include facial dysmorphia; syndactylies; absence of terminal phalanges; neural tube closure defects; malformations of the hip, ankle, and forearm; low-set ears; high palate; decreased cranial volume; and alterations of the cervical vertebrae and skull.[277] Etretinate accumulates in adipose tissue with repeated administration and has been detected in the serum of some patients up to 3 yr after discontinuing therapy. The importance of this, relative to the risk of teratogenicity, is unknown. An effective form of contraception must be used for at least 1 month before etretinate therapy, during therapy, and for an indefinite time after

(*continued*)

MISCELLANEOUS DRUGS

therapy, some say for at least 2 yr.[277–282] Unpublished data from the manufacturer indicate suspected teratogenicity in 8 of 95 fetuses reportedly exposed 1–24 months after drug discontinuation.[279]

Isotretinoin

Use during pregnancy causes defects of the CNS, heart, external ear, and thymus.[152,283–291] Other reported malformations include cleft palate, microphthalmia, micrognathia, facial dysmorphia, and limb reduction defects. Infants might exhibit hearing and visual impairments and mental retardation.[289] One report estimates the relative risk for major birth defects from isotretinoin to be 25.6.[283] Data suggest that the risk is substantial even when exposure to isotretinoin is brief or dosage is low.[290] The risk for spontaneous abortion is also increased.[284,285,290] In an analysis of cases reported to the manufacturer, 28% of exposed fetuses were malformed.[290] Exposures before day 14 of gestation resulted in the same rates of malformation and spontaneous/missed abortion as exposures between days 14 and 83.[290] An effective form of contraception must be used for at least 1 month after discontinuation of isotretinoin and before conceiving.

Tretinoin

Topical application of tretinoin results in absorption of vitamin A with equivalent activity less than that of a prenatal vitamin. Therefore, teratogenicity of this retinoid, although theoretically possible, is unlikely when used topically as directed.[292,293] Studies of first trimester use of topical retinoids and a review of cases of malformations typical of retinoids do not implicate topical retinoids in malformations.[292–294] Of note, two cases of malformations similar to those of isotretinoin have been reported after first-trimester tretinoin exposure.[295,296]

Vitamin A

Retinol or retinyl esters (but not beta-carotene) in toxic doses are teratogenic in experimental animals, producing defects in almost all organ systems. Human data on vitamin A teratogenicity consist of only a few anecdotal reports and epidemiologic studies. Epidemiologic studies show that doses of vitamin A contained in prenatal vitamin supplements (ie, ≤10,000 IU/day) do not increase the risk of fetal malformation.[297–300] However, because of methodologic flaws and incomplete data, the degree of risk with higher daily dosages of vitamin A is unclear. Defects observed when mothers ingested ≥25,000 IU/day of vitamin A during pregnancy include craniofacial, CNS, cardiac, urinary, vertebral, and other skeletal malformations.[2,301,302]

VACCINES

See Immunization, page 996, for information regarding vaccination during pregnancy.

VAGINAL SPERMICIDES

Use of vaginal spermicides was associated with major congenital anomalies in two retrospective analyses, but there were many flaws in the studies, casting doubt on the results.[303,304] Subsequent studies, including a meta-analysis of nine studies, did not implicate these agents as teratogens.[243,305–308]

VITAMIN D

Supplementation with vitamin D in pregnant women with poor dietary intake and little exposure to light is not associated with adverse outcomes. Excessive use has been associated with an idiopathic hypercalcemic syndrome including cardiovascular malformation, abnormal bone mineralization, elfin facies, mental retardation, hypercalcemia, and nephrocalcinosis. Definitive conclusions await further investigation.[2,309,310]

(continued)

MISCELLANEOUS DRUGS

DRUGS FOR NONMEDICAL USE

Alcohol

Animal studies show that alcohol and **acetaldehyde** exposure in utero results in morphologic changes in the structure and protein and endocrine content of the CNS.[311–313] As many as 5% of human congenital anomalies might be due to maternal alcohol consumption,[314] and it might be responsible for 10% of all cases of mental retardation. (Alcohol is the most frequent recognizable cause of mental retardation.)[314,315] A 2-fold increase in spontaneous abortion was noted among women who drank one to two drinks daily for the first 2 months of pregnancy; the rate was higher in those who drank more than two drinks daily. Moderate drinking (1–13 fl oz of absolute alcohol per week) results in an increase in some of the features of the "fetal alcohol syndrome" (FAS), including IUGR.[315,316] Chronic heavy alcohol consumption can cause full-blown FAS in up to 50% of children exposed in utero. Binge drinking has been associated with behavioral defects. Features of FAS include IUGR, microcephaly, postnatal growth deficiency, developmental delay, mental retardation, and craniofacial anomalies. Joint, limb, cardiac, ocular, brain, urogenital defects, and eustachian tube dysfunction also can occur. Neonates can have withdrawal symptoms similar to those of adults.[152,311–325] Alcohol-related birth defects can occur at rates higher than those of full-blown FAS, and CNS dysfunction can occur with lower alcohol exposure than that required to produce the FAS.[315] One investigator proposes that the threshold dosage for alcohol teratogenesis is 1 fl oz of absolute alcohol per day.[315] Alcohol consumption during pregnancy should be avoided because the minimum dosage that can produce adverse fetal effects has not been established.

Amphetamines

Data on the effect of prenatal amphetamines, prescribed and abused, are conflicting so no consistent pattern of abnormalities has emerged.[40,326] Most studies found no increase in severe congenital malformations, but others reported biliary atresia, congenital heart disease, and eye and CNS defects.[40,326] Reports of decreased birth weight and length, head circumference, and IUGR might reflect poor maternal nutrition, but use of other drugs and alcohol might have confounded those findings. Investigations with term neonates exposed antenatally to methamphetamine, with or without cocaine, document an increased prevalence of prematurity, IUGR, altered behavioral patterns (abnormal sleep patterns, poor feeding, tremors, and hypertonia), and the presence of cerebral injury as detected by ultrasonography.[326–328] (*See also* Cocaine.)

Caffeine

Caffeine is not suspected of causing fetal malformations. Data suggest that caffeine use before and during pregnancy increases the rate of spontaneous abortion.[329,330] A small reduction in birth weight can occur when caffeine consumption during pregnancy exceeds 300 mg/day, although cigarette smoking might contribute. There are conflicting data about whether 400–600 mg/day of caffeine increases the risk of miscarriage, stillbirth, or prematurity.[330–335] One study showed that rates of infant central and obstructive apnea positively correlated with increasing maternal caffeine consumption.[336] In one study of long-term outcome, no adverse effects were observed on the IQ of children exposed in utero to caffeine.[337]

Cocaine

Maternal cocaine use during pregnancy can cause adverse fetal and maternal outcomes. Although most data relate to use near term, preliminary findings suggest some risks from exposure early in pregnancy. Poor health care and nutrition, a high infection rate, and frequent concomitant drug (eg, narcotics, nicotine, or marijuana) and alcohol use complicate risk evaluation. A meta-analysis

(*continued*)

DRUGS FOR NONMEDICAL USE

found no significant differences in adverse fetal effects between cocaine users and polydrug users.[338] Maternal cocaine use results in an increase in the frequency of spontaneous abortion, placental hemorrhage, abruptio placentae, and stillbirth. There also is an increase in frequency of prematurity and premature rupture of the membranes. A few cases of precipitate delivery have been reported, as have cases of precipitate rupture of ectopic pregnancy. Fetal genitourinary malformations and intrauterine death have been reported when mothers used cocaine.[338–343] Cocaine most likely disrupts morphogenesis by vasoconstriction of uterine and fetal circulation. Interruption of calcium metabolism might contribute to hydronephrosis.[340,342,344,345] Infants can experience a withdrawal syndrome consisting of jitteriness, tremor, hyperreflexia, hypertonia, irritability, high-pitched crying, frantic sucking, poor feeding, tachypnea, abnormal sleep patterns, vomiting, or loose stools. Neurologic signs of toxicity, including seizures, also have been reported. Exposed infants have an increased frequency of abnormal pneumograms, respiratory distress, or other cardiorespiratory abnormalities. Some investigators feel these abnormalities can predispose infants to sudden infant death syndrome (SIDS). Retrospective population-based studies found that the risk of SIDS in cocaine-exposed infants was higher than that of infants whose mothers did not abuse any drugs; however, several confounding independent risks for SIDS were not controlled.[346,347] Several reports of neonatal or fetal cerebral infarction or intracranial hemorrhage exist.[338,339,344,348–376] Long-term behavioral abnormalities have been reported after in utero exposure to cocaine.[377]

Heroin

Poor nutrition and health care, lack of prenatal care, high infection rates, and frequent concomitant nicotine, nonmedical drug, and alcohol use complicate risk assessment. No specific pattern of fetal malformation has been noted. Some studies have associated maternal heroin use with a decrease in birth weight and length, reduced head circumference, small-for-gestational-age infants, low Apgar scores, meconium staining, neonatal respiratory distress, jaundice, and increased neonatal mortality. A narcotic withdrawal syndrome occurs frequently, usually within the first 24–48 hr after birth, although it can be delayed for as long as 6 days. The symptoms, which can persist for as long as 20 days, include irritability; feeding and sleeping problems; hyperactivity; and excessive sneezing, yawning, vomiting, mucous secretion, sweating, and face scratching. Other withdrawal symptoms such as increased muscle tone, vague autonomic nervous system symptoms, tremulousness, high-pitched crying, frantic and uncoordinated sucking, and seizures can occur in neonates born to narcotic-addicted women and nonaddicted women who use narcotics near term. The frequency of withdrawal is directly related to the daily dosage and duration of maternal heroin use. The results of studies evaluating development show conflicting results ranging from no effect to problems with behavior and perceptual and organizational abilities.[40,378] One retrospective, population-based study found that the relative risk of SIDS was 15.5 in infants of mothers who abused illicit opiates during all or part of pregnancy.[346]

Marijuana

Marijuana smoke contains carbon monoxide and can constrict uterine and placental vessels, resulting in fetal hypoxia and decreased nutrient supply (growth retardation).[374,379] Marijuana use during pregnancy did not result in any specific pattern of malformation, but exposures were confounded by nicotine and other nonmedical drug and alcohol use.[374,376,379–381]

Phencyclidine

Long-term phencyclidine use during pregnancy, especially near term, can produce neonatal withdrawal symptoms of hypertonicity, occasional darting eye movements, lethargy, and coarse flappy

(continued)

DRUGS FOR NONMEDICAL USE

tremors after stimulation. These infants have a marked increase in lability of behavioral states and poor consolability.[382,383] Long-term behavioral abnormalities have been reported in some studies but not in others.[374,382,384,385]

Tobacco

Cigarette smoke contains numerous toxins, including carbon monoxide and nicotine, that are probably responsible for reported fetal hypoxia because of decreased oxygen exchange and placental vasoconstriction.[386,387] Smoking during pregnancy increases rates of IUGR or low birth weight (5% decrease/pack smoked daily), prematurity, spontaneous abortion, neonatal and postnatal deaths, abruptio placentae, premature rupture of membranes, and placenta previa.[2,226,387–391] Women exposed to second-hand smoke also can be at risk for delivering a growth-retarded or preterm infant.[388] If a woman stops smoking by the 20th week of pregnancy, the risk of a low birth weight infant is similar to that of the general population.[386] Cigarette smoking alters the placental arterial linings and accelerates placental senescence, which might explain the placental complications of smoking.[387,390–392] One study involving 17,152 infants (15.7% of the mothers were smokers) found an increased frequency of minor malformations in infants of mothers aged ≥35 yr who smoked.[393] Some data suggest infants of smokers have increased nervous system excitation, hypertonicity, and altered breathing patterns with an increased rate of central apnea.[336,394] There also might be long-term mental and physical effects.[395] Some studies suggest an increased risk of childhood acute lymphocytic and lymphoblastic leukemias and lymphoma in those whose fathers and/or mothers smoked before or during pregnancy.[396,397] Tobacco chewing during pregnancy also greatly increases the rate of stillbirth, IUGR, and prematurity.[388]

■ REFERENCES

1. Wilson JG, Fraser RC, eds. *Handbook of teratology. Vol I. General principles and etiology.* New York: Plenum Press; 1977.
2. Beckman DA, Brent RL. Mechanism of known environmental teratogens: drugs and chemicals. *Clin Perinatol* 1986;13:649–87.
3. Brent RL. The complexities of solving the problem of human malformations. *Clin Perinatol* 1986;13: 491–503.
4. Friedman JM et al. Potential human teratogenicity of frequently prescribed drugs. *Obstet Gynecol* 1990;75: 594–9.
5. Pagliaro LA, Pagliaro AM, eds. *Problems in pediatric drug therapy.* 3rd ed. Hamilton, IL: Drug Intelligence Publications; 1995.
6. Chow AW, Jewesson PJ. Pharmacokinetics and safety of antimicrobial agents during pregnancy. *Rev Infect Dis* 1985;7:287–313.
7. Berlin CM. Effects of drugs on the fetus. *Pediatr Rev* 1991;12:282–7.
8. Landers DV et al. Antibiotic use during pregnancy and the postpartum period. *Clin Obstet Gynecol* 1983;26: 391–406.
9. Murray L, Seger D. Drug therapy during pregnancy and lactation. *Emerg Med Clin North Am* 1994;12: 129–49.
10. Pacifici GM, Nottoli R. Placental transfer of drugs administered to the mother. *Clin Pharmacokinet* 1995;28: 235–69.
11. Frey BM, O'Donnell J. Drug therapy in pregnancy and lactation. *J Pharm Pract* 1989;2:2–12.
12. Kramer MS. Intrauterine growth and gestational duration determinants. *Pediatrics* 1987;80:502–11.
13. Rathmell JP et al. Management of nonobstetric pain during pregnancy and lactation. *Anesth Analg* 1997;85: 1074–87.
14. Källén B, Lygner PE. Delivery outcome in women who used drugs for migraine during pregnancy with special reference to sumatriptan. *Headache* 2001;41:351–6.
15. Shuhaiber S et al. Pregnancy outcome following first trimester exposure to sumatriptan. *Neurology* 1998;51: 581–3.

16. Streissguth AP et al. Aspirin and acetaminophen use by pregnant women and subsequent child IQ and attention decrements. *Teratology* 1987;35:211–9.
17. Heymann MA. Non-narcotic analgesics: use in pregnancy and fetal and perinatal effects. *Drugs* 1986;32(suppl 4):164–76.
18. Ludmir J et al. Maternal acetaminophen overdose at 15 weeks of gestation. *Obstet Gynecol* 1986;67:750–1.
19. McElhatton PR et al. Paracetamol poisoning in pregnancy: an analysis of the outcomes of cases referred to the teratology information service of the national poisons information service. *Hum Exp Toxicol* 1990; 9:147–53.
20. Rosevear SK, Hope PL. Favourable neonatal outcome following maternal paracetamol overdose and severe fetal distress: case report. *Br J Obstet Gynaecol* 1989;96:491–3.
21. Robertson RG et al. Acetaminophen overdose in the second trimester of pregnancy. *J Fam Pract* 1986; 23:267–8.
22. Kurzel RB. Can acetaminophen excess result in maternal and fetal toxicity? *South Med J* 1990;83:953–5.
23. Kirshon B et al. Effect of acetaminophen on fetal acid–base balance in chorioamnionitis. *J Reprod Med* 1989; 34:955–9.
24. Brooks PM, Needs CJ. The use of antirheumatic medication during pregnancy and in the puerperium. *Rheum Dis Clin North Am* 1989;15:789–806.
25. Kirshon B et al. Influence of short-term indomethacin therapy on fetal urine output. *Obstet Gynecol* 1988; 72:51–3.
26. Morales WJ et al. Efficacy and safety of indomethacin versus ritodrine in the management of preterm labor: a randomized study. *Obstet Gynecol* 1989;74:567–72.
27. Hallak M et al. Indomethacin for preterm labor: fetal toxicity in a dizygotic twin gestation. *Obstet Gynecol* 1991;78:911–3.
28. Wurtzel D. Prenatal administration of indomethacin as a tocolytic agent: effect on neonatal renal function. *Obstet Gynecol* 1990;76:689–92.
29. Hickok DE et al. The association between decreased amniotic fluid volume and treatment with nonsteroidal anti-inflammatory agents for preterm labor. *Am J Obstet Gynecol* 1989;160:1525–31.
30. Slone D et al. Aspirin and congenital malformations. *Lancet* 1976;1:1373–5.
31. Werler MM et al. The relation of aspirin use during the first trimester of pregnancy to congenital cardiac defects. *N Engl J Med* 1989;321:1639–42.
32. Rudolph AM. Effects of aspirin and acetaminophen in pregnancy and in the newborn. *Arch Intern Med* 1981;141:358–63.
33. Benigni A et al. Effect of low-dose aspirin on fetal and maternal generation of thromboxane by platelets in women at risk for pregnancy-induced hypertension. *N Engl J Med* 1989;321:357–62.
34. Sibai BM et al. Low-dose aspirin in pregnancy. *Obstet Gynecol* 1989;74:551–7.
35. Schiff E et al. The use of aspirin to prevent pregnancy-induced hypertension and lower the ratio of thromboxane A2 to prostacyclin in relatively high risk pregnancies. *N Engl J Med* 1989;321:351–6.
36. CLASP: a randomised trial of low-dose aspirin for the prevention and treatment of pre-eclampsia among 9364 pregnant women. CLASP (Collaborative Low-dose Aspirin Study in Pregnancy) Collaborative Group. *Lancet* 1994;343:619–29.
37. Parazzini F et al. Follow-up of children in the Italian Study of Aspirin in Pregnancy. *Lancet* 1994;343:1235. Letter.
38. Barry WS et al. Ibuprofen overdose and exposure in utero: results from a postmarketing voluntary reporting system. *Am J Med* 1984;77(suppl 1a):35–9.
39. Edelin KC et al. Methadone maintenance in pregnancy: consequences to care and outcome. *Obstet Gynecol* 1988;71:399–404.
40. Briggs GG et al. *Drugs in pregnancy and lactation.* 3rd ed. Baltimore: Williams & Wilkins; 1990.
41. Curran MJA. Options for labor analgesia: techniques of epidural and spinal analgesia. *Semin Perinatol* 1991;15:348–57.
42. Wilhite AO et al. Plasma concentration profile of epidural alfentanil. Bolus followed by continuous infusion technique in the parturient: effect of epidural alfentanil and fentanyl on fetal heart rate. *Reg Anesth* 1994;19:164–8.
43. Savona-Ventura C et al. Pethidine blood concentrations at time of birth. *Int J Gynecol Obstet* 1991; 36:103–7.
44. Wittels B et al. Postcesarean analgesia with both epidural morphine and intravenous patient-controlled analgesia: neurobehavioral outcomes among nursing infants. *Anesth Analg* 1997;85:600–6.
45. Nissen E et al. Effects of routinely given pethidine during labour on infants' developing breast feeding behaviour. *Acta Paediatr* 1997;86:201–8.
46. Wittmann BK, Segal S. Comparison of the effects of single- and split-dose methadone administration on the fetus: ultrasound evaluation. *Int J Addiction* 1991;26:213–8.

47. Marquet P et al. Buprenorphine withdrawal syndrome in a newborn. *Clin Pharmacol Ther* 1997;62:569–71.
48. Hatjis CG, Meis PJ. Sinusoidal fetal heart rate pattern associated with butorphanol administration. *Obstet Gynecol* 1986;67:377–80.
49. Dan U et al. Intravenous pethidine and nalbuphine during labor: a prospective double-blind comparative study. *Gynecol Obstet Invest* 1991;32:39–43.
50. Little BB et al. Effects of T's and blues abuse on pregnancy outcome and infant health status. *Ann J Perinatol* 1990;7:359–62.
51. Meyer FP et al. Tramadol withdrawal in a neonate. *Eur J Clin Pharmacol* 1997;53:159–60.
52. Ramsey-Goldman R, Schilling E. Optimum use of disease-modifying and immunosuppressive antirheumatic agents during pregnancy and lactation. *Clin Immunother* 1996;1:40–58.
53. Anon. Safety of antimicrobial drugs in pregnancy. *Med Lett Drugs Ther* 1987;29:61–3.
54. Holdiness MR. Teratology of the antituberculosis drugs. *Early Hum Dev* 1987;15:61–74.
55. Pedler SJ, Bint AJ. Management of bacteriuria in pregnancy. *Drugs* 1987;33:413–21.
56. American Thoracic Society. Medical Section of the American Lung Association: Treatment of tuberculosis and tuberculosis infection in adults and children. *Am Rev Resp Dis* 1986;134:355–63.
57. Dapsone. In, Barnhart ER, ed. *Physicians' desk reference*. 44th ed. Oradell, NJ: Medical Economics; 1990: 1079–80.
58. Hocking DR. Neonatal haemolytic disease due to dapsone. *Med J Aust* 1968;1:1130–1.
59. Thornton YS, Bowe ET. Neonatal hyperbilirubinemia after treatment of maternal leprosy. *South Med J* 1989;82:668.
60. White NJ. The treatment of malaria. *N Engl J Med* 1996;335:800–6.
61. Levy M et al. Pregnancy outcome following first trimester exposure to chloroquine. *Am J Perinatol* 1991;8:174–8.
62. Pajor A. Pancytopenia in a patient given pyrimethamine and sulphamethoxidiazine during pregnancy. *Arch Gynecol Obstet* 1990;247:247:215–7.
63. Morley D et al. Controlled trial of pyrimethamine in pregnant women in an African village. *Br Med J* 1964; 1:667–8.
64. Landsberger EJ et al. Successful management of varicella pneumonia complicating pregnancy: a report of three cases. *J Reprod Med* 1986;31:311–4.
65. Brown ZA, Baker DA. Acyclovir therapy during pregnancy. *Obstet Gynecol* 1989;73:526–31.
66. Leen CLS et al. Acyclovir and pregnancy. *Br Med J* 1987;294:308. Letter.
67. Hankins GDV et al. Acyclovir treatment of varicella pneumonia in pregnancy. *Crit Care Med* 1987;15:336–7.
68. Boyd K, Walker E. Use of acyclovir to treat chickenpox in pregnancy. *Br Med J* 1988;296:393–4.
69. Eder SE et al. Varicella pneumonia during pregnancy: treatment of two cases with acyclovir. *Am J Perinatol* 1988;5:16–8.
70. Klein NA et al. Herpes simplex virus hepatitis in pregnancy. Two patients successfully treated with acyclovir. *Gastroenterology* 1991;100:239–44.
71. Anon. Pregnancy outcomes following systemic prenatal acyclovir exposure—June 1, 1984–June 30, 1993. *MMWR* 1993;42:806–9.
72. Andrews EB et al. Acyclovir in pregnancy registry: six years' experience. The Acyclovir in Pregnancy Registry Advisory Committee. *Obstet Gynecol* 1992;79:7–13.
73. Sperling RS et al. A survey of zidovudine use in pregnant women with human immunodeficiency virus infection. *N Engl J Med* 1992;326:857–61.
74. Anon. Birth outcomes following zidovudine therapy in pregnant women. *MMWR* 1994;43:409,415–6.
75. Kumar RM et al. Zidovudine use in pregnancy: a report on 104 cases and the occurrence of birth defects. *J Acquir Immune Defic Syndr* 1994;7:1034–9.
76. Chavanet P et al. Perinatal pharmacokinetics of zidovudine. *N Engl J Med* 1989;321:1548–9. Letter.
77. Watts DH et al. Pharmacokinetic disposition of zidovudine during pregnancy. *J Infect Dis* 1991; 163: 226–32.
78. Recommendations of the U.S. Public Health Service on the use of zidovudine to reduce perinatal transmission of human immunodeficiency virus. *MMWR* 1994;43(RR-11):1–20.
79. Public Health Service Task Force recommendations for the use of antiretroviral drugs in pregnant women infected with HIV-1 for maternal health and for reducing perinatal HIV-1 transmission in the United States. *MMWR* 1998;47(RR-2):1–30.
80. Culnane M et al. Lack of long-term effects of in utero exposure to zidovudine among uninfected children born to HIV-infected women. Pediatric AIDS Clinical Trials Group Protocol 219/076 Teams. *JAMA* 1999; 281:151–7.
81. Chapman ST. Bacterial infections in pregnancy. *Clin Obstet Gynecol* 1986;13:397–417.
82. Klein VR et al. The Jarisch–Herxheimer reaction complicating syphilotherapy in pregnancy. *Obstet Gynecol* 1990;75:375–80.

83. Einarson A et al. A prospective controlled multicentre study of clarithromycin in pregnancy. *Am J Perinatol* 1998;15:523–5.

84. Schick B et al. Pregnancy outcome following exposure to clarithromycin. *Reprod Toxicol* 1996;10:162.

85. Berkovitch M et al. Safety of the new quinolones in pregnancy. *Obstet Gynecol* 1994;84:535–8.

86. Andreou R et al. New post marketing surveillance data supports a lack of association between quinolone use in pregnancy and fetal and neonatal complications. *Reprod Toxicol* 1995:9;584.

87. Lewis JH et al. The use of gastrointestinal drugs during pregnancy and lactation. *Am J Gastroenterol* 1985;80:912–23.

88. Soper DE, Merrill-Nach S. Successful therapy of penicillinase-producing Neisseria gonorrhoeae pharyngeal infection during pregnancy. *Obstet Gynecol* 1986;68:290–1.

89. Czeizel A. A case-control analysis of the teratogenic effects of co-trimoxazole. *Reprod Toxicol* 1990; 4: 305–13.

90. Cohlan SQ et al. Effect of tetracycline on bone growth in the premature infant. *Antimicrob Agents Chemother* 1961;1:340–7.

91. Amon I. Placental transfer of metronidazole. *J Perinat Med* 1985;13:97–8. Letter.

92. Drinkwater P. Metronidazole. *Aust N Z J Obstet Gynaecol* 1987;27:228–30.

93. Roe FJC. Safety of nitroimidazoles. *Scand J Infect Dis* 1985;46(suppl):72–81.

94. Piper JM et al. Prenatal use of metronidazole and birth defects: no association. *Obstet Gynecol* 1993;82: 348–52.

95. Greenberg F. Possible metronidazole teratogenicity and clefting. *Am J Med Genetics* 1985;22:825. Letter.

96. Beard CM et al. Cancer after exposure to metronidazole. *Mayo Clin Proc* 1988;63:147–53.

97. Beard CM et al. Lack of evidence for cancer due to use of metronidazole. *N Engl J Med* 1979;301: 519–22.

98. Hailey FJ et al. Fetal safety of nitrofurantoin macrocrystals therapy during pregnancy: a retrospective analysis. *J Int Med Res* 1983;11:364–9.

99. D'Arcy PF. Nitrofurantoin. *Drug Intell Clin Pharm* 1985;19:540–7.

100. Personal communication, Carol A. Bixler, Norwich Eaton Pharmaceuticals, February 12, 1991.

101. Cruikshank DP, Warenski JC. First-trimester maternal *Listeria monocytogenes* sepsis and chorioamnionitis with normal neonatal outcome. *Obstet Gynecol* 1989;73:469–71.

102. Kelly RT, Bibbins B. Pregnancy and brucellosis. *Tex Med* 1987;83:39–41.

103. Bailey RR et al. Comparison of single dose with a five-day course of trimethoprim for asymptomatic (covert) bacteriuria of pregnancy. *N Z Med J* 1986;99:501–3.

104. Reyes MP et al. Vancomycin during pregnancy: does it cause hearing loss or nephrotoxicity in the infant? *Am J Obstet Gynecol* 1989;161:977–81.

105. Sorosky JI et al. The use of chemotherapeutic agents during pregnancy. *Obstet Gynecol Clin North Am* 1997;24:591–9.

106. Kim DS, Park MI. Maternal and fetal survival following surgery and chemotherapy of endodermal sinus tumor of the ovary during pregnancy: a case report. *Obstet Gynecol* 1989;73:503–7.

107. Raffles A et al. Transplacental effects of maternal cancer chemotherapy. Case report. *Br J Obstet Gynaecol* 1989;96;1099–100.

108. Jacobs C et al. Management of the pregnant patient with Hodgkin's disease. *Ann Intern Med* 1981;95:669–75.

109. Zemlickis D et al. Teratogenicity and carcinogenicity in a twin exposed in utero to cyclophosphamide. *Teratog Carcinog Mutagen* 1993;13:139–43.

110. Kopelman JN, Miyazawa K. Inadvertent 5-fluorouracil treatment in early pregnancy: a report of three cases. *Reprod Toxicol* 1990;4:233–5.

111. Van Le L et al. Accidental use of low-dose 5-fluorouracil in pregnancy. *J Reprod Med* 1991;36:872–4.

112. Blatt J et al. Pregnancy outcome following cancer chemotherapy. *Am J Med* 1980;69:828–32.

113. Artlich A et al. Teratogenic effects in a case of maternal treatment for acute myelocytic leukaemia—neonatal and infantile course. *Eur J Pediatr* 1994;153:488–91.

114. Colbert N et al. Acute leukaemia during pregnancy: favourable course of pregnancy in two patients treated with cytosine arabinoside and anthracyclines. *Nouv Presse Med* 1980;9:175–8.

115. Korelitz BI. Pregnancy, fertility, and inflammatory bowel disease. *Am J Gastroenterol* 1985;80:365–70.

116. Alstead EM et al. Safety of azathioprine in pregnancy in inflammatory bowel disease. *Gastroenterology* 1990; 99:443–6.

117. Pickrell MD et al. Pregnancy after renal transplantation: severe intrauterine growth retardation during treatment with cyclosporin A. *Br Med J* 1988;296:825.

118. Burrows DA et al. Successful twin pregnancy after renal transplant maintained on cyclosporine A immunosuppression. *Obstet Gynecol* 1988;72:459–61.

119. Jain A et al. Pregnancy after liver transplantation under tacrolimus. *Transplantation* 1997;64:559–65.

120. Plomp TA et al. Use of amiodarone during pregnancy. *Eur J Obstet Gynecol Reprod Biol* 1992;43:201–7.

121. Lees KR, Rubin PC. Treatment of cardiovascular diseases. *Br Med J* 1987;294:358–60.
122. Moriguchi Mitani G et al. The pharmacokinetics of antiarrhythmic agents in pregnancy and lactation. *Clin Pharmacokinet* 1987;12:253–91.
123. Kaler SG et al. Hypertrichosis and congenital anomalies associated with maternal use of minoxidil. *Pediatrics* 1987;79:434–6.
124. Rosa FW et al. Neonatal anuria with maternal angiotensin-converting enzyme inhibition. *Obstet Gynecol* 1989;74:371–4.
125. Mehta N, Modi N. ACE inhibitors in pregnancy. *Lancet* 1989;2:96. Letter.
126. Cunniff C et al. Oligohydramnios sequence and renal tubular malformation associated with maternal enalapril use. *Am J Obstet Gynecol* 1990;162:187–9.
127. Piper JM et al. Pregnancy outcome following exposure to angiotensin-converting enzyme inhibitors. *Obstet Gynecol* 1992;80:429–32.
128. Lubbe WF. Hypertension in pregnancy: pathophysiology and management. *Drugs* 1984;28:170–88.
129. Naden RP, Redman CWG. Antihypertensive drugs in pregnancy. *Clin Perinatol* 1985;12:521–38.
130. Mabie WC et al. Chronic hypertension in pregnancy. *Obstet Gynecol* 1986;67:197–205.
131. Ducey JP, Knape KG. Maternal esmolol administration resulting in fetal distress and cesarean section in a term pregnancy. *Anesthesiology* 1992;77:829–32.
132. Al Kasab SM et al. β-Adrenergic receptor blockage in the management of pregnant women with mitral stenosis. *Am J Obstet Gynecol* 1990;163:37–40.
133. Ellenbogen A et al. Metabolic effects of pindolol on both mother and fetus. *Curr Ther Res* 1988;43: 1038–41.
134. Lyons CW, Colmorgen GHC. Medical management of pheochromocytoma in pregnancy. *Obstet Gynecol* 1988;72:450–1.
135. Devoe LD et al. Metastatic pheochromocytoma in pregnancy and fetal biophysical assessment after maternal administration of alpha-adrenergic, beta-adrenergic, and dopamine antagonists. *Obstet Gynecol* 1986; 68 (suppl):15S–8.
136. Haraldsson A, Geven W. Severe adverse effects of maternal labetalol in a premature infant. *Acta Paediatr Scand* 1989;78:956–8.
137. Haraldsson A, Geven W. Half-life of maternal labetalol in a premature infant. *Pharm Weekbl Sci* 1989;11: 229–31.
138. Wide-Swensson D et al. Effects of isradipine, a new calcium antagonist, on maternal cardiovascular system and uterine activity in labour. *Br J Obstet Gynaecol* 1990;97:945–9.
139. Thaler I et al. Effect of calcium channel blocker nifedipine on uterine artery flow velocity waveforms. *J Ultrasound Med* 1991;10:301–4.
140. Moretti MM et al. The effect of nifedipine therapy on fetal and placental Doppler waveforms in preeclampsia remote from term. *Am J Obstet Gynecol* 1990;163:1844–8.
141. Yerby MS. Contraception, pregnancy and lactation in women with epilepsy. *Baillieres Clin Neurol* 1996;5: 887–908.
142. Kaneko S. Antiepileptic drug therapy and reproductive consequences: functional and morphologic effects. *Reprod Toxicol* 1991;5:179–98.
143. Sharony R, Graham JM. Identification of fetal problems associated with anticonvulsant usage and maternal epilepsy. *Obstet Gynecol Clin North Am* 1991;18:933–51.
144. Finnell RH et al. Clinical and experimental studies linking oxidative metabolism to phenytoin-induced teratogenesis. *Neurology* 1992;42(suppl 5):25–31.
145. Omtzigt JGC et al. The 10,11-epoxide-10,11-diol pathway of carbamazepine in early pregnancy in maternal serum, urine, and amniotic fluid: effect of dose, comedication, and relation to outcome of pregnancy. *Ther Drug Monit* 1993;15:1–10.
146. Van Dyke DC et al. Differences in phenytoin biotransformation and susceptibility to congenital malformations: a review. *DICP* 1991;25:987–92.
147. Eller DP et al. Maternal and fetal implications of anticonvulsive therapy. *Obstet Gynecol Clin North Am* 1997;24:523–34.
148. Rosa FW. Spina bifida in infants of women treated with carbamazepine during pregnancy. *N Engl J Med* 1991;324:674–7.
149. Scolnik D et al. Neurodevelopment of children exposed in utero to phenytoin and carbamazepine monotherapy. *JAMA* 1994;271:767–70.
150. Lindhout D et al. Antiepileptic drugs and teratogenesis in two consecutive cohorts: changes in prescription policy paralleled by changes in pattern of malformations. *Neurology* 1992;42(suppl 5):94–110.
151. Dravet C et al. Epilepsy, antiepileptic drugs, and malformations in children of women with epilepsy: a French prospective cohort study. *Neurology* 1992;42(suppl 5):75–82.
152. Cohen MM. Syndromology: an updated conceptual overview. VII. Aspects of teratogenesis. *Int J Oral Maxillofac Surg* 1990;19:26–32.

153. Dickinson RG et al. The effect of pregnancy in humans on the pharmacokinetics of stable isotope labelled phenytoin. *Br J Clin Pharmacol* 1989;28:17–27.

154. Verloes A et al. Proximal phocomelia and radial ray aplasia in fetal valproic syndrome. *Eur J Pediatr* 1990;149:266–7.

155. Hubert A et al. Aplasia cutis congenita of the scalp in an infant exposed to valproic acid in utero. *Acta Paediatr* 1994;83:789–90.

156. Sharony R et al. Preaxial ray reduction defects as part of valproic acid embryofetopathy. *Prenatal Diag* 1993;13:909–18.

157. Legius E et al. Sodium valproate, pregnancy, and infantile fatal liver failure. *Lancet* 1987;2:1518–9. Letter.

158. Baum AL, Misri S. Selective serotonin-reuptake inhibitors in pregnancy and lactation. *Harvard Rev Psychiatry* 1996;4:117–25.

159. Kent LSW, Laidlaw JDD. Suspected congenital sertraline dependence. *Br J Psychiatry* 1995;167:412–3. Letter.

160. Nulman I et al. Neurodevelopment of children exposed in utero to antidepressant drugs. *N Engl J Med* 1997;336:258–62.

161. Calabrese JR, Gulledge AD. Psychotropics during pregnancy and lactation: a review. *Psychosomatics* 1985;26:413–29.

162. Trixler M, Tényi T. Antipsychotic use in pregnancy. *Drug Saf* 1997;16:403–10.

163. Marken PA et al. Treatment of psychosis in pregnancy. *DICP* 1989;23:598–9.

164. Mazze RI, Kallen B. Reproductive outcome after anesthesia and operation during pregnancy: a registry study of 5405 cases. *Am J Obstet Gynecol* 1989;161:1178–85.

165. Kallen B, Mazze RI. Neural tube defects and first trimester operations. *Teratology* 1990;41:717–20.

166. Sylvester GC et al. First-trimester anesthesia exposure and the risk of central nervous system defects: a population-based case-control study. *Am J Public Health* 1994;84:1757–60.

167. Baeder C, Albrecht M. Embryotoxic/teratogenic potential of halothane. *Int Arch Occup Environ Health* 1990;62:263–71.

168. Tannenbaum TN, Goldberg RJ. Exposure to anesthetic gases and reproductive outcome. A review of the epidemiologic literature. *J Occup Med* 1985;27:659–68.

169. Kanto J. Obstetric analgesia: clinical pharmacokinetic considerations. *Clin Pharmacokinet* 1986;11:283–98.

170. Janowsky EC. Pharmacologic aspects of local anesthetic use. *Anesthesiol Clin North Am* 1990;8:1–25.

171. Heinonen OP et al. *Birth defects and drugs in pregnancy.* Littleton, MA: Publishing Sciences Group; 1977.

172. Shiono PH, Mills JL. Oral clefts and diazepam use during pregnancy. *N Engl J Med* 1984;311:919–20. Letter.

173. Bergman U et al. Teratogenic effects of benzodiazepine use during pregnancy. *J Pediatr* 1990;116:490–1. Letter.

174. Rivas F et al. Acentric craniofacial cleft in a newborn female prenatally exposed to a high dose of diazepam. *Teratology* 1984;30:179–80.

175. Laegreid L et al. Congenital malformations and maternal consumption of benzodiazepines: a case-control study. *Dev Med Child Neurol* 1990;32:432–41.

176. St Clair SM, Schirmer RG. First-trimester exposure to alprazolam. *Obstet Gynecol* 1992;80:843–6.

177. Laegreid L et al. The effect of benzodiazepines on the fetus and the newborn. *Neuropediatrics* 1992;23:18–23.

178. Sanchis A et al. Adverse effects of maternal lorazepam on neonates. *DICP* 1991;25:1137–8.

179. Zalzstein E et al. A case-control study on the association between first trimester exposure to lithium and Ebstein's anomaly. *Am J Cardiol* 1990;65:817–8.

180. Warkany J. Teratogen update: lithium. *Teratology* 1988;38:593–6.

181. Chapman WS. Lithium use during pregnancy. *J Fla Med Assoc* 1989;76:454–8.

182. Jacobson SJ et al. Prospective multicentre study of pregnancy outcome after lithium exposure during first trimester. *Lancet* 1992;339:530–3.

183. Cohen LS et al. A reevaluation of risk of in utero exposure to lithium. *JAMA* 1994;271:146–50.

184. Ang MS et al. Maternal lithium therapy and polyhydramnios. *Obstet Gynecol* 1990;76:517–9.

185. Nelson MM, Forfar JO. Associations between drugs administered during pregnancy and congenital abnormalities of the fetus. *Br Med J* 1971;1:523–7.

186. Dordevic M, Beric B. Our experience in the treatment of pyrosis in pregnancy with Kompensan. *Med Pregl* 1972;25:277–9.

187. Jacobs D. Maternal drug ingestion and congenital malformations. *S Afr Med J* 1975;49:2073–80.

188. Witter FR et al. The effects of chronic gastrointestinal medication on the fetus and neonate. *Obstet Gynecol* 1981;58(suppl):79S–84.

189. Koren G, Zemlickis DM. Outcome of pregnancy after first trimester exposure to H_2 receptor antagonists. *Am J Perinatol* 1991;8:37–8.

190. Magee LA et al. Safety of first trimester exposure to histamine H2 blockers. A prospective cohort study. *Dig Dis Sci* 1996;41:1145–9.

191. Qvist N et al. Cimetidine as pre-anesthetic agent for cesarean section: perinatal effects on the infant, the placental transfer of cimetidine and its elimination in the infants. *J Perinat Med* 1985;13:179–83.

192. Ikenoue T et al. Effects of ranitidine on maternal gastric juice and neonates when administered prior to caesarean section. *Aliment Pharmacol Ther* 1991;5:315–8.

193. Seto A et al. Pregnancy outcome following first trimester exposure to antihistamines: a meta-analysis. *Am J Perinatol* 1997;14:119–24.

194. Slone D et al. Antenatal exposure to the phenothiazines in relation to congenital malformations, perinatal mortality rate, birth weight, and intelligence quotient score. *Am J Obstet Gynecol* 1977;128:486–8.

195. Aselton P et al. First-trimester drug use and congenital disorders. *Obstet Gynecol* 1985;65:451–5.

196. McKeigue PM et al. Bendectin and birth defects: I. A meta-analysis of the epidemiologic studies. *Teratology* 1994;50:27–37.

197. Mogadam M et al. Pregnancy in inflammatory bowel disease: effect of sulfasalazine and corticosteroids on fetal outcome. *Gastroenterology* 1981;80:72–6.

198. Moody GA. The effects of chronic ill health and treatment with sulphasalazine on fertility amongst men and women with inflammatory bowel disease in Leicestershire. *Int J Colorectal Dis* 1997;12:220–4.

199. Diav-Citrin O et al. The safety of mesalamine in human pregnancy: a prospective controlled cohort study. *Gastroenterology* 1998;114:23–8.

200. Marteau P et al. Foetal outcome in women with inflammatory bowel disease treated during pregnancy with oral mesalazine microgranules. *Aliment Pharmacol Ther* 1998;12:1101–8.

201. Baiocco PJ, Korelitz BI. The influence of inflammatory bowel disease and its treatment on pregnancy and fetal outcome. *J Clin Gastroenterol* 1984;6:211–6.

202. Meyers S, Sacher DB. Medical management of Crohn's disease. *Hepatogastroenterology* 1990;37:42–55.

203. Hall JG et al. Maternal and fetal sequelae of anticoagulation during pregnancy. *Am J Med* 1980;68: 122–40.

204. Ginsberg JS et al. Risks to the fetus of anticoagulant therapy during pregnancy. *Thromb Haemost* 1989;61: 197–203.

205. Ginsberg JS, Hirsh J. Use of anticoagulants during pregnancy. *Chest* 1989;95(suppl):156S–60.

206. Nageotte MP et al. Anticoagulation in pregnancy. *Am J Obstet Gynecol* 1981;141:472–3.

207. Nelson-Piercy C et al. Low-molecular-weight heparin for obstetric thromboprophylaxis: experience of sixty-nine pregnancies in sixty-one women at high risk. *Am J Obstet Gynecol* 1997;176:1062–8.

208. Schneider DM et al. Retrospective evaluation of the safety and efficacy of low-molecular-weight heparin as thromboprophylaxis during pregnancy. *Am J Obstet Gynecol* 1997;177:1567–8. Letter.

209. Iturbe-Alessio I et al. Risks of anticoagulant therapy in pregnant women with artificial heart valves. *N Engl J Med* 1986;315:1390–3.

210. Born D et al. Pregnancy in patients with prosthetic heart valves: the effects of anticoagulation on mother, fetus, and neonate. *Am Heart J* 1992;124:413–7.

211. Gärtner BC et al. Phenprocoumon therapy during pregnancy: case report and comparison of the teratogenic risk of different coumarin derivatives. *Z Geburtshilfe Perinatol* 1993;197:262–5.

212. Pati S, Helmbrecht GD. Congenital schizencephaly associated with in utero warfarin exposure. *Reprod Toxicol* 1994;8:115–20.

213. Normann EK, Stray-Pedersen B. Warfarin-induced fetal diaphragmatic hernia: case report. *Br J Obstet Gynaecol* 1989;96:729–30.

214. Fraser FC, Sajoo A. Teratogenic potential of corticosteroids in humans. *Teratology* 1995;51:45–6.

215. Fitzsimons R et al. Outcome of pregnancy in women requiring corticosteroids for severe asthma. *J Allergy Clin Immunol* 1986;78:349–53.

216. Avery ME et al. Update on prenatal steroid for prevention of respiratory distress. *Am J Obstet Gynecol* 1986;155:2–5.

217. Van Marter LJ et al. Maternal glucocorticoid therapy and reduced risk of bronchopulmonary dysplasia. *Pediatrics* 1990;86:331–6.

218. Smolder-de Haas H et al. Physical development and medical history of children who were treated antenatally with corticosteroids to prevent respiratory distress syndrome: a 10- to 12-year follow-up. *Pediatrics* 1990; 85:65–70.

219. Saenger P. Abnormal sex differentiation. *J Pediatr* 1984;104:1–17.

220. Brunskill PJ. The effect of fetal exposure to danazol. *Br J Obstet Gynaecol* 1992;99:212–5.

221. Rosenn B et al. Minor congenital malformations in infants of insulin-dependent diabetic women: association with poor glycemic control. *Obstet Gynecol* 1990;70:745–9.

222. Piacquadio K et al. Effects of in-utero exposure to oral hypoglycaemic drugs. *Lancet* 1991;338:866–9.

223. Hellmuth E et al. Congenital malformations in offspring of diabetic women treated with oral hypoglycaemic agents during embryogenesis. *Diabetic Med* 1994;11:471–4.

224. Saili A, Sarna MS. Tolbutamide: teratogenic effects. *Indian Pediatr* 1991;28:936–40.

225. Elliott BD et al. Insignificant transfer of glyburide occurs across the human placenta. *Am J Obstet Gynecol* 1991;165:807–12.

226. Kramer MS et al. Determinants of fetal growth and body proportionality. *Pediatrics* 1990;86:18–26.

227. Fischer K. A rapid evolution mechanism may contribute to changes in sex ratio, multiple birth incidence, frequency of autoimmune disease and frequency of birth defects in Clomid conceptions. *Med Hypotheses* 1990;31:59–65.

228. Wramsby H et al. Chromosome analysis of human oocytes recovered from preovulatory follicles in stimulated cycles. *N Engl J Med* 1987;316:121–4.

229. Shoham Z et al. Early miscarriage and fetal malformations after induction of ovulation (by clomiphene citrate and/or human menotropins), in vitro fertilization, and gamete intrafallopian transfer. *Fertil Steril* 1991;55: 1–11.

230. Mills JL et al. Risk of neural tube defects in relation to maternal fertility and fertility drug use. *Lancet* 1990; 336:103–4.

231. Greenland S, Ackerman DL. Clomiphene citrate and neural tube defects: a pooled analysis of controlled epidemiologic studies and recommendations for future studies. *Fertil Steril* 1995;64:936–41.

232. Melnick S et al. Rates and risks of diethylstilbestrol-related clear-cell adenocarcinoma of the vagina and cervix. An update. *N Engl J Med* 1987;316:514–6.

233. Anon. Infertility among daughters exposed to diethylstilbestrol. *Drug Newslett* 1988;7:59. Abstract.

234. Adams DM et al. Intrapartum uterine rupture. *Obstet Gynecol* 1989;73:471–3.

235. Claman P, Berger MJ. Phenotypic differences in upper genital tract abnormalities and reproductive history in dizygotic twins exposed to diethylstilbestrol. *J Reprod Med* 1990;35:431–3.

236. McFarlane MJ et al. Diethylstilbestrol and clear cell vaginal carcinoma: reappraisal of the epidemiologic evidence. *Am J Med* 1986;81:855–63.

237. Leary FJ et al. Males exposed in utero to diethylstilbestrol. *JAMA* 1984;252:2984–9.

238. Harris EL. Genetic epidemiology of hypospadias. *Epidemiol Rev* 1990;12:29–40.

239. Blickstein I, Katz Z. Possible relationship of bladder exstrophy and epispadias with progestins taken during early pregnancy. *Br J Urol* 1991;68:105–6.

240. Stoll C et al. Genetic and environmental factors in hypospadias. *J Med Genet* 1990;27:559–63.

241. Progestational drug birth defects warning statement. *FDC Rep* 1987;49:T&G1–2.

242. Lammer EJ, Cordero JF. Exogenous sex hormone exposure and the risk for major malformations. *JAMA* 1986;255:3128–32.

243. Simpson JL, Phillips OP. Spermicides, hormonal contraception and congenital malformations. *Adv Contraception* 1990;6:141–67.

244. Wing DA et al. A comparison of propylthiouracil versus methimazole in the treatment of hyperthyroidism in pregnancy. *Am J Obstet Gynecol* 1994;170:90–5.

245. Van Dijke CP et al. Methimazole, carbimazole, and congenital skin defects. *Ann Intern Med* 1987;106:60–1.

246. Mestman JH. Thyroid disease in pregnancy. *Clin Perinatol* 1985;12:651–7.

247. Momotani N et al. Antithyroid drug therapy for Graves' disease during pregnancy. *N Engl J Med* 1986;315: 24–8.

248. Martinez-Frias ML et al. Methimazole in animal feed and congenital aplasia cutis. *Lancet* 1992;339:742–3. Letter.

249. Singhi S et al. Iatrogenic neonatal and maternal hyponatremia following oxytocin and aqueous glucose infusion during labour. *Br J Obstet Gynaecol* 1985;92:356–63.

250. Schönhöfer PS. Brazil: misuse of misoprostol as an abortifacient may induce malformations. *Lancet* 1991; 337;1534–5.

251. Gonzalez CH et al. Limb deficiency with or without Möbius sequence in seven Brazilian children associated with misoprostol use in the first trimester of pregnancy. *Am J Med Genet* 1993;47:59–64.

252. Pastuszak AL et al. Use of misoprostol during pregnancy and Möbius' syndrome in infants. *N Engl J Med* 1998;338:1881–5.

253. Schuller L et al. Pregnancy outcome after abortion attempt with misoprostol. *Teratology* 1997;55:36. Abstract.

254. Gonzalez CH et al. Congenital abnormalities in Brazilian children associated with misoprostol misuse in first trimester of pregnancy. *Lancet* 1998;351:1624–7.

255. Sorokin Y et al. Effects of induction of labor with prostaglandin E_2 on fetal breathing and body movements: controlled, randomized, double-blind study. *Obstet Gynecol* 1992;80:788–91.

256. Papageorgiou I et al. Labor characteristics of uncomplicated prolonged pregnancies after induction with intracervical prostaglandin E_2 gel versus intravenous oxytocin. *Gynecol Obstet Invest* 1992;34:92–6.

257. Ray DA, Garite TJ. Prostaglandin E_2 for induction of labor in patients with premature rupture of membranes at term. *Am J Obstet Gynecol* 1992;166:836–43.

258. Sibai BM et al. Effects of diuretics on plasma volume in pregnancies with long-term hypertension. *Am J Obstet Gynecol* 1984;150:831–5.

259. Lamm CI et al. Congenital rickets associated with magnesium sulfate infusion for tocolysis. *J Pediatr* 1988;113:1078–82.
260. Holcomb WL et al. Magnesium tocolysis and neonatal bone abnormalities: a controlled study. *Obstet Gynecol* 1991;78:611–4.
261. Cox SM et al. Randomized investigation of magnesium sulfate for prevention of preterm birth. *Am J Obstet Gynecol* 1990;163:767–72.
262. Doan-Wiggins L. Drug therapy for obstetric emergencies. *Emerg Med Clin North Am* 1994;12:257–3.
263. Anon. Which anticonvulsant for women with eclampsia? Evidence from the Collaborative Eclampsia Trial. *Lancet* 1995;345:1455–63.
264. Asthma. *PEM News*, no. 7. Drug Safety Research Unit, Southampton, England, August 1990.
265. Mann RD et al. Salmeterol. *PEM Report*, no. 25. Drug Safety Research Unit, Southampton, England, July 1994.
266. Frederiksen MC et al. Theophylline pharmacokinetics in pregnancy. *Clin Pharmacol Ther* 1986;40:321–8.
267. Stenius-Aarniala B et al. Slow-release theophylline in pregnant asthmatics. *Chest* 1995;107:642–7.
268. McKeigue PM et al. Bendectin and birth defects: I. A meta-analysis of the epidemiologic studies. *Teratology* 1994;50:27–37.
269. Einarson A et al. Prospective controlled study of hydroxyzine and cetirizine in pregnancy. *Ann Allergy Asthma Immunol* 1997;78:183–6.
270. Pastuszak A et al. The safety of astemizole in pregnancy. *J Allergy Clin Immunol* 1996;98:748–50.
271. Wright JW et al. Effect of tocolytic agents on fetal umbilical velocimetry. *Am J Obstet Gynecol* 1990;163:748–50.
272. Gormley DE. Cutaneous surgery and the pregnant patient. *J Am Acad Dermatol* 1990;23:269–79.
273. Chamberlain MJ et al. Toxic effect of podophyllum application in pregnancy. *Br Med J* 1972;3:391–2.
274. Ridley CM. Toxicity of podophyllum. *Br Med J* 1972;3:698. Letter.
275. Karol MD et al. Podophyllum: suspected teratogenicity from topical application. *Clin Toxicol* 1980;16:283–6.
276. Sundharam JA. Is podophyllin safe for use in pregnancy? *Arch Dermatol* 1989;125:1000–1.
277. Stamatos MN. *The most important step forward in years (etretinate)*. Nutley, NJ: Roche Laboratories; 1986. Promotional letter.
278. Etretinate approved. FDA *Drug Bull* 1986;16:16–7.
279. Vahlquist A, Rollman O. Etretinate and the risk for teratogenicity: drug monitoring in a pregnant woman for 9 months after stopping treatment. *Br J Dermatol* 1990;123:131. Letter.
280. Personal communication, Joseph B. Laudano, Roche Laboratories, January 29, 1987.
281. Anon. Etretinate for psoriasis. *Med Lett Drugs Ther* 1987;29:9–10.
282. Geiger J-M et al. Teratogenic risk with etretinate and acitretin treatment. *Dermatology* 1994;189:109–16.
283. Lammer EJ et al. Retinoic acid embryopathy. *N Engl J Med* 1985;313:837–41.
284. Holmes A, Wolfe S. When a uniquely effective drug is teratogenic: the case of isotretinoin. *N Engl J Med* 1989;321:756. Letter.
285. Faich G, Rosa F. When a uniquely effective drug is teratogenic: the case of isotretinoin. *N Engl J Med* 1989;321:756–7. Letter.
286. Rappaport EB, Knapp M. Isotretinoin embryopathy—a continuing problem. *J Clin Pharmacol* 1989;29:463–5.
287. Hansen LA, Pearl GS. Isotretinoin teratogenicity. Case report with neuropathologic findings. *Acta Neuropathol* 1985;65:335–7.
288. McBride WG. Limb reduction deformities in child exposed to isotretinoin in utero on gestation days 26–40 only. *Lancet* 1985;1:1276. Letter.
289. Anon. Birth defects caused by isotretinoin—New Jersey. *MMWR* 1988;37:171–2,177.
290. Dai WS et al. Epidemiology of isotretinoin exposure during pregnancy. *J Am Acad Dermatol* 1992;26:599–606.
291. Rizzo R et al. Limb reduction defects in humans associated with prenatal isotretinoin exposure. *Teratology* 1991;44:599–604.
292. deWals P et al. Association between holoprosencephaly and exposure to topical retinoids: results of the EUROCAT survey. *Paediatr Perinat Epidemiol* 1991;5:445–7.
293. Jick SS et al. First trimester topical tretinoin and congenital disorders. *Lancet* 1993;341:1181–2.
294. Shapiro L et al. Safety of first-trimester exposure to topical tretinoin: prospective cohort study. *Lancet* 1997;350:1143–4.
295. Camera G, Pregliasco P. Ear malformation in baby born to mother using tretinoin cream. *Lancet* 1992;339:687. Letter.
296. Lipson AH et al. Multiple congenital defects associated with maternal use of topical tretinoin. *Lancet* 1993;341:1352–3. Letter.

297. Martínez-Frías ML, Salvador J. Epidemiological aspects of prenatal exposure to high doses of vitamin A in Spain. *Eur J Epidemiol* 1990;6:118–23.

298. Werler MM et al. Maternal vitamin A supplementation in relation to selected birth defects. *Teratology* 1990;42:497–503.

299. Rothman KJ et al. Teratogenicity of high vitamin A intake. *N Engl J Med* 1995;333:1369–73.

300. Oakley GP, Erickson JD. Vitamin A and birth defects. Continuing caution is needed. *N Engl J Med* 1995;333:1414–5. Editorial.

301. Anon. Use of supplements containing high-dose vitamin A—New York State, 1983–1984. *MMWR* 1987; 36:80–2.

302. Committee on Safety of Medicines. Vitamin A and teratogenesis. *Lancet* 1985;1:319–20.

303. Shapiro S et al. Birth defects and vaginal spermicides. *JAMA* 1982;247:2381–4.

304. Jick H et al. Vaginal spermicides and congenital disorders. *JAMA* 1981;245:1329–32.

305. Louik C et al. Maternal exposure to spermicides in relation to certain birth defects. *N Engl J Med* 1987; 317:474–8.

306. Warburton D et al. Lack of association between spermicide use and trisomy. *N Engl J Med* 1987;317:478–82.

307. Einarson TR et al. Maternal spermicide use and adverse reproductive outcome: a meta-analysis. *Am J Obstet Gynecol* 1990;162:655–60.

308. Anon. Data do not support association between spermicides, birth defects. *FDA Drug Bull* 1986;16:21.

309. Martin NDT et al. Increased plasma 1,25-dihydroxyvitamin D in infants with hypercalcemia and elfin facies. *N Engl J Med* 1985;313:888–9. Letter.

310. Chesney RW et al. Increased plasma 1,25-dihydroxyvitamin D in infants with hypercalcemia and elfin facies. *N Engl J Med* 1985;313:889–90. Letter.

311. Rudeen PK, Creighton JA. Mechanisms of central nervous system alcohol-related birth defects. In, Sun G-Y et al, eds. *Molecular mechanisms of alcohol.* Clifton, NJ: Humana Press; 1989:147–65.

312. Goodwin FK. Acetaldehyde produced and transferred by human placenta. *JAMA* 1988;260:3563.

313. Blakley PM, Scott WJ. Determination of the proximate teratogen of the mouse fetal alcohol syndrome. 1. Teratogenicity of ethanol and acetaldehyde. *Toxicol Appl Pharmacol* 1984;72:355–63.

314. Little BB et al. Alcohol abuse during pregnancy: changes in frequency in a large urban hospital. *Obstet Gynecol* 1989;74:547–50.

315. Clarren SK. Fetal alcohol syndrome: diagnosis, treatment, and mechanisms of teratogenesis. In, *Transplacental disorders: perinatal detection, treatment, and management (including pediatric AIDS). Proceedings of the 1988 Albany Birth Defects Symposium XIX.* New York: Alan R. Liss; 1990:37–55.

316. Virji SK. The relationship between alcohol consumption during pregnancy and infant birthweight. An epidemiologic study. *Acta Obstet Gynecol Scand* 1991;70:303–8.

317. Kline J et al. Drinking during pregnancy and spontaneous abortion. *Lancet* 1980;2:176–80.

318. Harlap S, Shiono PH. Alcohol, smoking, and incidence of spontaneous abortions in the first and second trimester. *Lancet* 1980;2:173–6.

319. Streissguth AP et al. Natural history of the fetal alcohol syndrome: a 10-year follow-up of eleven patients. *Lancet* 1985;2:85–91.

320. Halmesmaki E et al. Low somatomedin C and high growth hormone levels in newborns: damages by maternal alcohol abuse. *Obstet Gynecol* 1989;74:366–70.

321. Strömland K. Contribution of ocular examination to the diagnosis of foetal alcohol syndrome in mentally retarded children. *J Mental Defic Res* 1990;34:429–35.

322. Froster UG, Baird PA. Congenital defects of the limbs and alcohol exposure in pregnancy: data from a population based study. *Am J Med Genet* 1992;44:782–5.

323. Ronen GM, Andrews WL. Holoprosencephaly as a possible embryonic alcohol effect. *Am J Med Genet* 1991;40:151–4.

324. Bonnemann C, Meinecke P. Holoprosencephaly as a possible embryonic alcohol effect: another observation. *Am J Med Genet* 1990;37:431–2.

325. Astley SJ et al. Analysis of facial shape in children gestationally exposed to marijuana, alcohol, and/or cocaine. *Pediatrics* 1992;89:67–77.

326. Little BB et al. Methamphetamine abuse during pregnancy: outcome and fetal effects. *Obstet Gynecol* 1988; 72:541–4.

327. Oro AS, Dixon SD. Perinatal cocaine and methamphetamine exposure: maternal and neonatal correlates. *J Pediatr* 1987;111:571–8.

328. Dixon SD, Bejar R. Echoencephalographic findings in neonates associated with maternal cocaine and methamphetamine use: incidence and clinical correlates. *J Pediatr* 1989;115:770–8.

329. Infante-Rivard C et al. Fetal loss associated with caffeine intake before and during pregnancy. *JAMA* 1993; 270:2940–3.

330. Dlugosz L, Bracken MB. Reproductive effects of caffeine: a review and theoretical analysis. *Epidemiol Rev* 1992;14:83–100.

331. Watkinson B, Fried PA. Maternal caffeine use before, during and after pregnancy and effects upon offspring. *Neurobehav Toxicol Teratol* 1985;7:9–17.

332. Cerrato PL. Caffeine: how much is too much? *RN* 1990;53:77–80.

333. Szucs Myers VA, Miwa LJ. Caffeine consumption during pregnancy. *Drug Intell Clin Pharm* 1988;22:614–6.

334. Olsen J et al. Coffee consumption, birthweight, and reproductive failures. *Epidemiology* 1991;2:370–4.

335. Narod SA et al. Coffee during pregnancy: a reproductive hazard? *Am J Obstet Gynecol* 1991;164:1109–14.

336. Toubas PL et al. Effects of maternal smoking and caffeine habits on infantile apnea: a retrospective study. *Pediatrics* 1986;78:159–63.

337. Barr HM, Streissguth AP. Caffeine use during pregnancy and child outcome: a 7-year prospective study. *Neurotoxicol Teratol* 1991;13:441–8.

338. Lutiger B et al. Relationship between gestational cocaine use and pregnancy outcome: a meta-analysis. *Teratology* 1991;44:405–14.

339. Chen C et al. Respiratory instability in neonates with in utero exposure to cocaine. *J Pediatr* 1991;119:111–3.

340. Ho J et al. Renal vascular abnormalities associated with prenatal cocaine exposure. *Clin Pediatr* 1994; 33:155–6.

341. Lezcano L et al. Crossed renal ectopia associated with maternal alkaloid cocaine abuse: a case report. *J Perinatol* 1994;14:230–3.

342. Viscarello RR et al. Limb–body wall complex associated with cocaine abuse: further evidence of cocaine's teratogenicity. *Obstet Gynecol* 1992;80:523–6.

343. Hume RF Jr et al. Ultrasound diagnosis of fetal anomalies associated with in utero cocaine exposure: further support for cocaine-induced vascular disruption teratogenesis. *Fetal Diagn Ther* 1994;9:239–45.

344. Hoyme HE et al. Prenatal cocaine exposure and fetal vascular disruption. *Pediatrics* 1990;85:743–7.

345. Greenfield SP et al. Genitourinary tract malformations and maternal cocaine abuse. *Urology* 1991;37:455–9.

346. Davidson Ward SL et al. Sudden infant death syndrome in infants of substance-abusing mothers. *J Pediatr* 1990;117:876–81.

347. Durand DJ et al. Association between prenatal cocaine exposure and sudden infant death syndrome. *J Pediatr* 1990;117:909–11.

348. Lowenstein DH et al. Acute neurologic and psychiatric complications associated with cocaine abuse. *Am J Med* 1987;83:841–6.

349. Chasnoff IJ et al. Perinatal cerebral infarction and maternal cocaine use. *J Pediatr* 1986;108:456–9.

350. Chasnoff IJ et al. Cocaine use in pregnancy. *N Engl J Med* 1985;313:666–9.

351. Oro AS, Dixon SD. Perinatal cocaine and methamphetamine exposure: maternal and neonatal correlates. *J Pediatr* 1987;111:571–8.

352. Burkett G et al. Perinatal implications of cocaine exposure. *J Reprod Med* 1990;35:35–42.

353. Collins E et al. Perinatal cocaine intoxication. *Med J Aust* 1989;150:331–4.

354. Cherukuri R et al. A cohort study of alkaloidal cocaine ("crack") in pregnancy. *Obstet Gynecol* 1988;72:147–51.

355. Kaye K et al. Birth outcomes for infants of drug abusing mothers. *NY State J Med* 1989;89:256–61.

356. Bingol N et al. Teratogenicity of cocaine in humans. *J Pediatr* 1987;110:93–6.

357. Keith LG et al. Substance abuse in pregnant women: recent experience at the Perinatal Center for Chemical Dependence of Northwestern Memorial Hospital. *Obstet Gynecol* 1989;73:715–20.

358. Roland EH, Volpe JJ. Effect of maternal cocaine use on the fetus and newborn: review of the literature. *Pediatr Neurosci* 1989;15:88–94.

359. Doering PL et al. Effects of cocaine on the human fetus: a review of clinical studies. *DICP* 1989;23:639–45.

360. Mastrogiannis DS et al. Perinatal outcome after recent cocaine usage. *Obstet Gynecol* 1990;76:8–11.

361. Cravey RH. Cocaine deaths in infants. *J Anal Toxicol* 1988;12:354–5.

362. Chouteau M et al. The effect of cocaine abuse on birth weight and gestational age. *Obstet Gynecol* 1988; 72:351–4.

363. Little BB et al. Cocaine abuse during pregnancy: maternal and fetal implications. *Obstet Gynecol* 1989;73:157–60.

364. Mercado A et al. Cocaine, pregnancy, and postpartum intracerebral hemorrhage. *Obstet Gynecol* 1989;73:467–8.

365. Ney JA et al. The prevalence of substance abuse in patients with suspected preterm labor. *Am J Obstet Gynecol* 1990;162:1562–7.

366. Thatcher SS et al. Cocaine use and acute rupture of ectopic pregnancies. *Obstet Gynecol* 1989;74:478–9.

367. Gonsoulin W et al. Rupture of unscarred uterus in primigravid woman in association with cocaine abuse. *Am J Obstet Gynecol* 1990;163:526–7.

368. Madden JD et al. Maternal cocaine abuse and effect on the newborn. *Pediatrics* 1986;77:209–11.

369. Rosenstein BJ et al. Congenital renal abnormalities in infants with in utero cocaine exposure. *J Urol* 1990; 144:110–2.

370. Chavez GF et al. Maternal cocaine use during early pregnancy as a risk factor for congenital urogenital anomalies. *JAMA* 1989;262:795–8.

371. Ward SLD et al. Abnormal sleeping ventilatory pattern in infants of substance-abusing mothers. *Am J Dis Child* 1986;140:1015–20.

372. Chasnoff IJ et al. Prenatal cocaine exposure is associated with respiratory pattern abnormalities. *Am J Dis Child* 1989;143:583–7.

373. Cregler LL, Mark H. Medical complications of cocaine abuse. *N Engl J Med* 1986;315:1495–500.

374. Braude MC et al. Perinatal effects of drugs of abuse. *Fed Proc* 1987;46:2446–53.

375. Feldman JG et al. A cohort study of the impact of perinatal drug use on prematurity in an inner-city population. *Am J Public Health* 1992;82:726–8.

376. Zuckerman B et al. Effects of maternal marijuana and cocaine use on fetal growth. *N Engl J Med* 1989; 320:762–8.

377. Nulman I et al. Neurodevelopment of adopted children exposed in utero to cocaine. *Can Med Assoc J* 1994; 151:1591–7.

378. Klenka HM. Babies born in a district general hospital to mothers taking heroin. *Br Med J* 1986;293:745–6.

379. Fried PA. Cigarettes and marijuana: are there measurable long-term neurobehavioral teratogenic effects? *Neurotoxicology* 1989;10:577–84.

380. Hatch EE, Bracken MB. Effect of marijuana use in pregnancy on fetal growth. *Am J Epidemiol* 1986;124: 986–93.

381. Tansley BW et al. Visual processing in children exposed prenatally to marijuana and nicotine: a preliminary report. *Can J Public Health* 1986;77(suppl 1):72–8.

382. Chasnoff IJ et al. Phencyclidine: effects on the fetus and neonate. *Dev Pharmacol Ther* 1983;6:404–8.

383. Golden NL et al. Phencyclidine use during pregnancy. *Am J Obstet Gynecol* 1984;148:254–9.

384. Harry GJ, Howard J. Phencyclidine: experimental studies in animals and long-term developmental effects on humans. In, Sonderegger TB, ed. *Perinatal substance abuse: research findings and clinical implications.* Baltimore: Johns Hopkins University Press; 1992:254–78.

385. Wachsman L et al. What happens to babies exposed to phencyclidine (PCP) in utero? *Am J Drug Alcohol Abuse* 1989;15:31–9.

386. Lindblad A et al. Effect of nicotine on human fetal blood flow. *Obstet Gynecol* 1988;72:371–82.

387. Pinette MG et al. Maternal smoking and accelerated placental maturation. *Obstet Gynecol* 1989;73:379–82.

388. Cole H. Studying reproductive risks, smoking. *JAMA* 1986;255:22–3.

389. Shiono PH et al. Smoking and drinking during pregnancy: their effects on preterm birth. *JAMA* 1986; 255:82–4.

390. Brown HL et al. Premature placental calcification in maternal cigarette smokers. *Obstet Gynecol* 1988;71: 914–7.

391. Newnham JP et al. Effects of maternal cigarette smoking on ultrasonic measurements of fetal growth and on Doppler flow velocity waveforms. *Early Hum Dev* 1990;24:23–6.

392. Jauniaux E, Burton GJ. The effect of smoking in pregnancy on early placental morphology. *Obstet Gynecol* 1992;79:645–8.

393. Seidman DS et al. Effect of maternal smoking and age on congenital anomalies. *Obstet Gynecol* 1990;76:1046–50.

394. Brown RW et al. Effect of maternal smoking during pregnancy on passive respiratory mechanics in early infancy. *Pediatr Pulmonol* 1995;19:23–8.

395. Fox NL et al. Prenatal exposure to tobacco: I. Effects on physical growth at age three. *Int J Epidemiol* 1990;19:66–71.

396. John EM et al. Prenatal exposure to parents' smoking and childhood cancer. *Am J Epidemiol* 1991;133:123–32.

397. Stjernfeldt M et al. Maternal smoking and irradiation during pregnancy as risk factors for child leukemia. *Cancer Detect Prev* 1992;16:129–35.

Drugs and Breastfeeding

Philip O. Anderson

With the increasing recognition of the benefits of breastfeeding, the clinician often must weigh the benefits against the risks of drug therapy in lactating women. The physicochemical, pharmacokinetic, and clinical factors involved with drug use in nursing women have been described.[1] These factors are summarized as follows.

■ PHYSICOCHEMICAL FACTORS

Small water-soluble nonelectrolytes pass into breastmilk by simple diffusion through pores in the mammary epithelial membrane that separates plasma from milk. Equilibration between the two fluids is rapid, and milk concentrations of drugs approximate plasma concentrations. For larger molecules, only the lipid-soluble, nonionized forms pass through the membrane by crossing the cell wall and diffusing across the interior of the cell to reach the milk. Because the pH of milk is generally lower than that of plasma, milk can act as an "ion trap" for basic drugs. At equilibrium, these compounds can be concentrated in milk relative to plasma. Conversely, acidic drugs are inhibited from entering milk. The pKa of weak electrolytes is an important determinant of their equilibrium concentration in milk.

Protein binding also is an important determinant because plasma proteins bind drugs much more avidly than do milk proteins. Highly protein-bound drugs do not pass into milk in high concentrations. Lipid solubility favors passage of some drugs into milk because the fat component of milk can concentrate lipid-soluble drugs. However, because milk contains only 3 to 5% fat, its capacity for concentrating drugs is limited. Active or facilitated transport of drugs into breastmilk might occur in humans, but it is rare.

■ PHARMACOKINETIC FACTORS

Because the breast is periodically emptied by the nursing infant and refilled with newly formed milk, equilibrium between plasma and milk is rarely reached. Therefore, the rate of drug passage from plasma into milk is important in determining the concentration of a drug in milk. Factors favoring rapid passage into milk are high lipid solubility and low molecular weight.

Passage of drugs between plasma and milk occurs in both directions. When the concentration of nonionized free drug is higher in milk than in plasma, net transfer of drug from milk to plasma occurs. Thus, the maneuver of pumping and discarding milk does not appreciably hasten the elimination of most drugs from milk and does not have a marked effect on overall clearance of the drug from the mother's body.

■ METHODS OF EXPRESSING THE EXTENT OF PASSAGE

The ratio of concentrations of a drug in milk and plasma (the milk/plasma, or M/P, ratio) often has been used as a measure of a drug's passage into breastmilk. However, the M/P ratio has shortcomings that make it meaningless as a measure of drug safety during nursing. There is no standard method of calculating the value, and the value is not constant, as often calculated, but changes with the time after the dose and the number of doses given. It also does not take into account the potential toxicity of the drug.

The percentage of the maternal dosage that is excreted into milk also is used to express the extent of passage. This value alone is not predictive of safety in a nursing infant but can be used to calculate the actual dosage received by the infant. Usually a weight-adjusted (ie, mg/kg) infant dosage <10% of the mother's is considered safe; of 205 drugs studied, 87% of drugs fell into this category. The likelihood of an adverse effect in the infant increases markedly in those few drugs (about 3%) that have a dosage in milk that is >25% of the maternal weight-adjusted dosage.[2]

Drug clearance can be a useful factor for identifying drugs that can accumulate in infants and thereby have a pharmacologic effect.[3] Drugs with an adult total body clearance of ≥0.3 L/hr/kg and that have no active metabolites are unlikely to have pharmacologic effects in a nursing infant because they are rapidly eliminated from the mother and infant.

All of the above methods fall short of providing a complete assessment of the safety of a drug during breastfeeding in a specific mother–infant pair. Several additional factors must be considered.

■ CLINICAL CONSIDERATIONS

Factors that should be considered when determining the advisability of using a particular drug in a nursing mother are the potential acute toxicity of the drug, dosage and duration of therapy, age of the infant (<2 months are the most susceptible), quantity of milk consumed, experience with the drug in infants, oral absorption of the drug by the infant, potential long-term effects, and possible interference with lactation.[1,4]

A stepwise approach to using medications in breastfeeding women can be followed to minimize infant exposure to medications in milk.[1] Starting from the strategies that are least disruptive to nursing and progressing to those that are most disruptive, the prescriber can consider the following steps: withhold the drug; delay drug therapy temporarily; choose drugs that pass poorly into milk; use alternative routes of administration (eg, topical, inhalation); avoid nursing at times of peak milk levels; administer the drug before the infant's longest sleep period; withhold breastfeeding temporarily; and, infrequently, discontinue breastfeeding.

Another consideration is non–dose-related adverse effects such as allergic reactions and some hemolytic anemias; however, these reactions are relatively uncommon. GI intolerance caused by antimicrobial agents in breastmilk can occur whether or not the drugs are absorbed by the infant. Antimicrobial agents are among the most commonly used maternal medications during nursing and, although serious side effects are rare, diarrhea might occur in up to 12% of infants.[5] Disruption of the infant's GI flora is uncommon but occasionally leads to thrush and rarely to pseudomembranous colitis.[6] Severe diarrhea or blood in the infant's stool during maternal antimicrobial use is an indication to stop nursing and seek medical attention.

Although the above considerations are important, follow-up of mothers who took medications while breastfeeding their infants has shown that serious side effects are uncommon.[5] Nursing seldom needs to be completely discontinued because of concern of acute toxicity from maternal drug therapy.

The following table contains information on the use of specific drugs during nursing. The risks are assessed and alternatives are presented based on the principles discussed. Information in the table is from reference 1 unless noted otherwise.

DRUGS AND BREASTFEEDING

ANALGESICS AND ANTI-INFLAMMATORY DRUGS

ANTIMIGRAINE DRUGS

Ergotamine

When given daily for 6 days postpartum, ergotamine did not affect lactation or infant weight in one study; however, the excretion of ergotamine into milk during lactation has not been studied. Avoid its use during lactation because older ergot preparations have produced toxicity in infants.

Sumatriptan

Minimally excreted in milk, sumatriptan has poor oral absorption by the infant. It poses little risk during breastfeeding.[7]

NONSTEROIDAL ANTI-INFLAMMATORY DRUGS

Acetaminophen

The amount of acetaminophen excreted into milk is small. Acetaminophen is a good analgesic choice during nursing.

Nonsteroidal Anti-inflammatory Drugs

Amounts of most NSAIDs in milk are low because they are weak acids that are extensively plasma protein bound. However, short-acting agents are preferred, particularly in the case of breastfed neonates. Some agents have active metabolites (eg, **sulindac**) or glucuronide metabolites (eg, **salicylate, fenoprofen,** and **ketoprofen**) that can add to infant intake. Because of the increased likelihood of accumulation, avoid long-acting agents such as **diflunisal, naproxen, piroxicam,** and sulindac in mothers of neonates, although amounts of piroxicam in milk are low.[1,4] Naproxen caused prolonged bleeding time, thrombocytopenia, and acute anemia in one 7-day-old infant, and possibly drowsiness and vomiting in others.[8] The more toxic NSAIDs such as **mefenamic acid** and **indomethacin** also should be avoided, although recent studies on indomethacin indicate that it might not be contraindicated.[9,10] **Ketorolac** is contraindicated during nursing. **Diclofenac** was not detected in milk after a single dose of 50 mg IM, or 100 mg/day for 1 week, and the amount of **tolmetin** in one woman's milk was low. **Ibuprofen** and **flurbiprofen** have the best documentation of safety during breastfeeding; the dose of ibuprofen that an infant receives in milk is <0.001% of the mother's dosage,[11] and flurbiprofen concentrations are low to undetectable after dosages up to 50 mg tid.[1]

Salicylates

Salicylate enters milk in a low concentration relative to that in plasma, although its glucuronide metabolite increases the overall infant dosage. Doses >1 g yield markedly higher salicylate concentrations in milk and can result in high infant serum concentrations. One case of thrombocytopenic purpura from **aspirin** in breastmilk (confirmed by rechallenge) was reported in a 5-month-old infant.[8] The risk of Reye's syndrome caused by salicylate in milk is unknown. If aspirin is taken occasionally, avoid breastfeeding for 1–2 hr after a dose to minimize antiplatelet effects. NSAIDs such as ibuprofen are preferred to aspirin for long-term therapy.

(continued)

ANALGESICS AND ANTI-INFLAMMATORY DRUGS

OTHER ANTI-INFLAMMATORY DRUGS (*See also* Antimalarials.)

Gold

During maternal administration of **aurothioglucose** and **gold sodium thiomalate,** gold was detected in the blood and urine of some nursing infants. The weight-adjusted infant dosage might be greater than the maternal dosage, but the amount of gold that infants absorb orally is not known. Sufficient amounts are absorbed, however, to potentially cause adverse effects. Gold therapy is a reason to very carefully monitor the breastfed infant and might be a reason for withholding breastfeeding.[1,12]

Penicillamine

Penicillamine was used during 3 months of breastfeeding in two women who nursed 3 infants without harm, but it is not recommended.[13,14]

OPIOIDS

Neonates are particularly susceptible to narcotics in breastmilk.[4] Postpartum maternal opioids (oral **codeine** or **propoxyphene** with or without prior IM **meperidine**) might be a causative factor in episodes of apnea, bradycardia, and cyanosis during the first week of life. Avoid maternal narcotics when the breastfed neonate has experienced such an episode. Although single analgesic doses of most narcotics are excreted into milk in small amounts, infant drowsiness caused by repeated administration of postpartum oral narcotics in milk is more prevalent than commonly thought—about 20% in one study.[5] Drowsiness is dose related and can be severe with the maximum dosage. Limiting oral dosage to 1 tablet (eg, codeine 30 mg, **hydrocodone** 5 mg, or **oxycodone** 5 mg) q 4 hr is advisable; analgesia can be supplemented with additional acetaminophen or ibuprofen.

Meperidine

Meperidine is particularly likely to interfere with infant nursing behavior when given during labor.[15,16] Furthermore, repeated postpartum meperidine doses, including patient-controlled analgesia, cause diminished alertness and orientation in breastfed neonates compared with equivalent doses of **morphine**.[1,17] Meperidine should be avoided during labor and nursing, although a single small dose for anesthesia or conscious sedation usually does not cause problems in older breastfed infants.[18]

Morphine

Morphine 10–15 mg in single parenteral doses produces only low concentrations in milk, but repeated doses can result in drug accumulation in infant serum to near therapeutic concentrations. Morphine glucuronides in milk contribute an additional 50 to 100% to the infant. Epidural administration and patient-controlled analgesia cause fewer effects in an infant than IV administration and are preferred.[4,17]

Fentanyl and Sufentanil

IV or epidural fentanyl, alfentanil, and sufentanil produce low milk levels.[19,20] In addition, these drugs have poor oral bioavailability, so they are good choices for maternal analgesia during nursing.

Narcotic Partial Agonists

IV narcotic agonist/antagonists given during labor can interfere with establishment of lactation.[15,16] Despite breastfeeding and relatively high infant serum drug levels, mild withdrawal occurred in the neonate of a mother taking **buprenorphine** during pregnancy and postpartum for heroin addiction.[21] Oral buprenorphine for narcotic abstinence appears to have little impact on the

(*continued*)

ANALGESICS AND ANTI-INFLAMMATORY DRUGS

breastfed infant.[22] **Butorphanol** and **nalbuphine** concentrations in milk are low, and oral bioavailability in the infant should be low.[8,23] Only about 0.1% of the maternal dose of **tramadol** is found in milk according to the manufacturer.[24]

ANTIMICROBIAL DRUGS

AMINOGLYCOSIDES

Systemic effects of **amikacin, gentamicin, streptomycin, tobramycin,** and other aminoglycosides are unlikely in infants because of the small amounts in milk and poor oral absorption; however, observe infants for disruptions of the GI flora such as diarrhea and thrush.

ANTIFUNGAL DRUGS

Amphotericin B and **nystatin** are virtually unabsorbed orally, and the latter is frequently used orally for treating thrush in infants; therefore, both are safe for use in nursing mothers, including topical application to the nipples. Likewise, **clotrimazole** has poor oral bioavailability and has been used orally in infants with thrush, sometimes successfully after nystatin has failed.[25] **Miconazole** has efficacy and safety similar to clotrimazole.[26] These two imidazoles are preferred for topical or vaginal application during nursing. **Fluconazole** amounts in milk are much less than the dosage prescribed for infants and can be used for recalcitrant *Candida* infections[27,28] given to the mother and infant simultaneously. **Ketoconazole** concentrations in milk are low,[29] but it is best avoided in nursing mothers orally or topically to the nipples because of its oral absorption, occasional hepatotoxicity, and the availability of safer alternatives. Other imidazole antifungals have not been studied. **Gentian violet** is potentially toxic (toxic to mucous membranes, potential tattooing of the skin, and carcinogenic and mutagenic in rodents) and is best avoided topically on the nipples or in the infant's mouth.[30]

ANTIMYCOBACTERIAL DRUGS

Clofazimine

Clofazimine is excreted into milk, reportedly coloring it bright pink.[31] Infants receive about 15 to 30% of the maternal mg/kg dose.[32] Breastfed infants can develop the typical skin discoloration.[31] The skin color returned to normal 5 months after the end of maternal therapy in one infant.

Antituberculars

Antituberculars pass into milk in small quantities. Use caution in nursing mothers because many of these drugs can cause hepatic damage. However, inadequate maternal therapy poses a much greater risk to the infant than the drugs in milk. The mother may take single daily doses of many of these drugs at bedtime and substitute a bottle for a nighttime feeding to minimize infant exposure. **Isoniazid** is excreted into milk in amounts that are less than those given to treat an infant. **Pyrazinamide** concentrations in milk in one woman were low and would give the baby less than a therapeutic dosage. **Rifampin** has not been well studied, but amounts in milk are small. **Cycloserine** is excreted in small amounts, and no adverse reactions have been reported in infants. **Ethambutol** has not been adequately studied.

Sulfones

Newborns and G-6-PD–deficient infants are particularly susceptible to **dapsone** hemolysis. Older infants might tolerate the amounts of sulfones excreted into milk.

(continued)

ANTIMICROBIAL DRUGS

ANTIPARASITIC DRUGS

Anthelmintics

Mebendazole was undetectable in milk in one woman and is poorly absorbed orally; therefore, it is unlikely to cause adverse effects in a breastfed infant. In contrast to an earlier report, it does not inhibit lactation.[33] Only small amounts of **praziquantel** and **ivermectin** reach the infant and these drugs seem safe during nursing.[1,34]

Antimalarials

Undertake breastfeeding cautiously during long-term daily therapy with **chloroquine** or **hydroxy-chloroquine** because the importance of the small amounts of drug and metabolites in milk is un-clear and accumulation can occur. Weekly prophylactic doses are probably safe because the amount of drug in milk is less than the infant prophylactic dose.[1,12] Small amounts of **quinine** in milk are unlikely to harm the infant, although allergic reactions can occur. **Pyrimethamine** ap-pears to be safe and might be excreted into milk in quantities sufficient to treat or protect infants <6 months of age against malaria; however, breastfeeding is not a reliable method of drug admin-istration. **Mefloquine** appears in milk in small amounts after a single dose but has not been stud-ied after repeated weekly administration for malaria prophylaxis.

Lindane

Lindane was excreted into milk at up to 30 times the typical background concentration (from envi-ronmental pollution) after maternal topical application of a 0.3% emulsion daily for 3 days. Milk concentrations remained elevated over background concentrations for at least 7 days. Although they have not been studied, alternative drugs (eg, **permethrin,** and **pyrethrins**) are preferred for nursing mothers because of their low toxicity.

ANTIVIRAL DRUGS

Acyclovir

Acyclovir has not been well studied, but a breastfed infant would receive about 1% of the mother's weight-adjusted oral dosage. The low dosage in milk and its poor oral bioavailability indicate that it may be well tolerated by the nursing infant, even with large IV doses.[35,36] Topical acyclovir applied to small areas of the mother's body away from the breast should pose no risk to the infant.

Amantadine

Amantadine is a dopamine agonist that decreases serum prolactin and theoretically can decrease lactation, so it is best avoided during nursing. **Rimantadine** might not have the same effect.

Antiretrovirals

Lamivudine in breastmilk adds negligibly to the neonatal treatment dose.[37] **Nevirapine** and **zidovudine** levels are also low but might offer some protection against breastmilk transmission of HIV-1.[38,39]

β-LACTAMS

Cephalosporins

Cephalosporins appear in trace amounts in milk and can lead to disruption of the GI flora or, rarely, allergic sensitization. Breastfeeding is safe with first- and second-generation agents. The risk might be greater with the third-generation cephalosporins and similar agents (eg, **aztreonam**) that are more active against GI flora. Observe infants for diarrhea, thrush, and rashes.

(*continued*)

ANTIMICROBIAL DRUGS

Penicillins

Penicillins appear in trace amounts in milk that can occasionally lead to allergic sensitization, allergic reactions in previously sensitized infants, or disruption of the GI flora, especially with the broader-spectrum agents. Unless the infant is allergic to penicillin, breastfeeding is safe. Observe infants for diarrhea, rashes, and thrush.

MACROLIDES

Erythromycin, clarithromycin, and **azithromycin** are excreted into the milk in amounts much smaller than a typical infant dosage and are usually safe.[1,40,41]

QUINOLONES

Ciprofloxacin, fleroxacin, nalidixic acid, ofloxacin, and **pefloxacin** have been detected in milk.[42,43] Ciprofloxacin seems to have caused pseudomembranous colitis in an infant via breastmilk,[6] and nalidixic acid caused hemolytic anemia in a breastfed neonate.[44] Most fluoroquinolones are best avoided during nursing. **Norfloxacin** was undetectable in milk after a 200 mg dose and might be acceptable for maternal UTI treatment because of its low milk excretion and poor oral bioavailability.

SULFONAMIDES

Some sulfonamides can cause hemolysis in G-6-PD–deficient infants; theoretically, sulfonamides increase the risk of kernicterus in neonates. **Sulfamethoxazole,** with or without trimethoprim, and **sulfisoxazole** can be used by mothers of healthy, full-term infants >2 months old.

TETRACYCLINES

Tooth staining from a tetracycline in breastmilk has not been reported. Milk calcium apparently inhibits absorption of the small amounts of **tetracycline** in milk. Infant absorption and serum concentrations have not been reported with other tetracyclines, but infants would only receive a few milligrams per day of **demeclocycline, doxycycline,** or **minocycline** with usual maternal dosages. Minocycline has caused black milk.[45] Although other drugs are preferred for most infections, tetracyclines can be used for a short time (7–14 days); avoid prolonged or repeat courses during nursing.

MISCELLANEOUS ANTIMICROBIALS

Chloramphenicol

Breastfeeding is contraindicated during maternal chloramphenicol treatment. Milk concentrations are not sufficient to induce "gray baby" syndrome but theoretically might be enough to cause the rare, idiosyncratic aplastic anemia. Adverse reactions in infants, including refusal of the breast, falling asleep during feeding, and vomiting after feeding, have occurred.

Clindamycin

Clindamycin is excreted variably in small amounts into milk. It is not certain what effects these amounts have on infants' GI flora (eg, pseudomembranous colitis), but a single case of bloody stools in an infant with normal stool flora was reported during maternal clindamycin use. Clindamycin is best avoided, if possible, but a few days of therapy with close monitoring of the infant is acceptable. Vaginal clindamycin presents less infant risk than oral or IV use.

Furazolidone

Furazolidone is poorly absorbed orally and can be used to treat maternal giardiasis if the infant is >1 month old.

(continued)

ANTIMICROBIAL DRUGS

Methenamine

The hippurate and methenamine salts of methenamine pass into milk in small quantities and seem safe to use.

Metronidazole

Metronidazole and its hydroxy metabolite are found in the serum of nursing infants in concentrations that are 10 to 20% of maternal serum concentrations. Anecdotal cases of "spitting up" (possibly from a bad taste), diarrhea, and isolation of *Candida* species in breastfed infants have been reported, but most infants do not have immediate reactions. Because of the carcinogenicity in animals, possible mutagenicity, and the relatively high infant serum concentrations achieved, metronidazole probably should be avoided in nursing mothers.[1,46] When essential to treat trichomoniasis, metronidazole may be given as a single 2 g dose, and an alternative feeding method used for the next 24 hr. After longer courses for anaerobic infections, nursing can resume 12–24 hr after the final dose.

Nitrofurantoin

Nitrofurantoin is excreted into milk in pharmacologically unimportant amounts but avoid it with infants <1 month old and those with G-6-PD deficiency because of the risk of hemolysis.

Trimethoprim

Trimethoprim is excreted into milk in amounts that are not harmful.

Vancomycin

Because it is excreted into milk in only small amounts[47] and is not orally absorbed, vancomycin is safe during nursing.

ANTINEOPLASTICS AND IMMUNOSUPPRESSANTS

Few reports exist, but breastfeeding is generally considered to be contraindicated in women receiving antineoplastics because of the potential for immunosuppression and carcinogenicity.

ALKYLATING AGENTS

Busulfan

Busulfan in a dosage of 4 mg/day for 5 weeks was taken by one woman while breastfeeding, with no apparent adverse effects on her infant's leukocytes or hemoglobin. This case is not conclusive and breastfeeding is not recommended.

Cisplatin

Platinum was not detected in the milk of one patient at any time after an IV infusion of 100 mg/m^2 of cisplatin. In another patient, milk platinum was 0.9 mg/L 19.5 hr after her third daily dose of 20 mg/m^2. Because the platinum might be in a reactive form, nursing is not recommended during cisplatin therapy.

Cyclophosphamide

Cyclophosphamide is detectable in milk and has caused bone marrow depression in infants of women who nursed while receiving the drug. Breastfeeding is contraindicated during cyclophosphamide therapy.

ANTIMETABOLITES

Methotrexate

Low amounts of methotrexate were found in milk in one patient; however, this case is not conclusive. Low weekly doses for arthritis probably pose only a slight risk to the infant.

(continued)

ANTINEOPLASTICS AND IMMUNOSUPPRESSANTS

CYTOKINES

Interferons

An IV dose of 30 million units of **interferon alfa-N3** resulted in only a slight increase over physiologic milk levels in one woman.[48]

DNA INTERCALATING DRUGS

Doxorubicin

Doxorubicin and its primary active metabolite, **doxorubicinol,** appear in milk, with their highest milk concentrations occurring 24 hr after a dose.

Mitoxantrone

Measurable levels of mitoxantrone occurred in milk for at least 28 days after 6 mg/kg was given daily for 3 days.[49]

MITOTIC INHIBITORS

Etoposide

Etoposide is undetectable in milk 24 hr after a dose.[49]

MISCELLANEOUS ANTINEOPLASTICS

Hydroxyurea

Only small amounts of hydroxyurea are found in milk, but breastfeeding is not advised.

IMMUNOSUPPRESSANTS

Three infants reportedly were breastfed safely during maternal **azathioprine** use (75–100 mg/day) after renal transplantation. Low concentrations of the azathioprine metabolite, **mercaptopurine,** were found in milk. Breastfeeding can be undertaken with close infant monitoring for infection or other signs of immunosuppression during azathioprine therapy, although there is concern over potential carcinogenicity.[1,12] Maternal **cyclosporine** therapy results in the infant receiving ≤2% of the mother's mg/kg dosage.[50,51] At least 9 infants have been breastfed safely for 4–12 months during maternal therapy with cyclosporine, prednisone, and azathioprine. Infant serum cyclosporine levels were undetectable (<30 μg/L), renal function was unaffected, and the infants grew normally.[50,51] **Tacrolimus** colostrum concentrations are about 50% of maternal serum concentrations.[52] The implications of these low concentrations for the infant are not known.

CARDIOVASCULAR DRUGS

ANTIARRHYTHMIC DRUGS

Some antiarrhythmics reach near-therapeutic serum concentrations in breastfed infants. **Amiodarone** is excreted in amounts that might pose a hazard to the infant and it should not be used during nursing.[1,53] Data on **disopyramide** indicate that infants can receive relatively large amounts of the drug and its active metabolite, with serum concentrations near the therapeutic range. Disopyramide can be used cautiously while breastfeeding older infants when other alternatives are unacceptable. Observe the infant for anticholinergic symptoms, and monitor infant serum concentrations if there is a concern. The anticholinergic activity of disopyramide might suppress lactation. (*See* Anticholinergics.) Sparse data from one patient indicate that **tocainide** should be used with caution during nursing. Because of its low oral bioavailability, maternal **bretylium** is unlikely to harm nursing infants; 400 mg q 8 hr was taken orally by one mother while nursing, with

(*continued*)

CARDIOVASCULAR DRUGS

no apparent effects on her infant. Infants receive trivial doses of **digoxin** via breastmilk. Amounts of **flecainide** in milk are small and unlikely to affect the infant. **Lidocaine** concentrations in milk during continuous IV infusion and epidural administration and in high doses as a local anesthetic are low and poorly absorbed by the infant, so it poses no hazard to the infant[54–56] Amounts of **mexiletine** in milk are too low to be detected in the serum of breastfed infants. **Procainamide** and its active metabolite, **N-acetylprocainamide,** are found in milk in fairly small concentrations; procainamide may be used with caution in nursing mothers. **Propafenone** milk concentrations are very low, but no clinical experience has been reported.[57] **Quinidine** excretion seems inconsequential.

ANTIHYPERTENSIVE DRUGS

Certain antihypertensives are less desirable than others during nursing. Breastfed infants have serum **clonidine** concentrations approaching those of the mother.[1,58] Clonidine and **guanfacine** also can decrease prolactin secretion. These drugs must be used with caution during breastfeeding and avoided if possible. Avoid **reserpine** because it can cause nasal stuffiness and increased tracheobronchial secretions in the infant. The angiotensin-converting enzyme (ACE) inhibitors, **benazepril, captopril,** and **enalapril,** are found in small amounts and no adverse effects have occurred in breastfed infants.[1,59] In addition, milk ACE activity was in the normal range after a dose of enalapril. These ACE inhibitors are good choices during lactation; others have not been studied. Limited data indicate that low-dose, short-term use of **hydralazine** (ie, a few days postpartum) is safe. There is limited information on oral **minoxidil** in milk, but amounts are small. However, use minoxidil with caution, particularly when therapy involves large dosages and long-term use. Several studies indicate that **methyldopa** is excreted in unimportant amounts.

β-ADRENERGIC BLOCKING DRUGS

The excretion of β-blockers into breastmilk has been studied extensively. The infant's dosage differs greatly among the different compounds, allowing a range of choices. The most water-soluble drugs reach the infant in the greatest amounts because of low serum protein binding. Water-soluble agents also have the longest half-lives, are renally eliminated, and therefore are more likely to accumulate in infants. Maternal therapy with **atenolol** and **acebutolol** have resulted in adverse effects (eg, bradycardia, hypotension, tachypnea, and cyanosis) in breastfed infants. These two drugs, as well as **betaxolol, nadolol, sotalol,** and **timolol,** should be avoided in mothers of newborn infants or when high dosage is required. **Oxprenolol** and **mepindolol** excretions are intermediate and should be avoided in neonates. **Propranolol, metoprolol,** and **labetalol** are excreted in low enough quantities to allow nursing even in the neonatal period.

CALCIUM-CHANNEL BLOCKING DRUGS

Case reports indicate that only small amounts of **diltiazem, nifedipine, nimodipine,** and **nitrendipine** are excreted into milk.[1,60] Several case reports indicate that the amounts of **verapamil** and **norverapamil** in milk and infant serum are low. Verapamil appears to be safe during nursing.

CENTRAL NERVOUS SYSTEM DRUGS

ANTICONVULSANTS

Breastfed infants can achieve serum anticonvulsant concentrations that produce pharmacologic effects. Mild drowsiness, irritability, and feeding difficulties are common in the infants of mothers taking sedating anticonvulsants, especially during the early neonatal period.[1,61] Breastfeeding can

(continued)

CENTRAL NERVOUS SYSTEM DRUGS

mitigate withdrawal symptoms in infants whose mothers took sedating anticonvulsants during pregnancy, and withdrawal symptoms have been observed after abrupt weaning. Serum concentration monitoring in breastfed infants might be indicated, particularly in infants who are excessively drowsy, feed poorly, or gain weight inadequately. Long-term effects of exposure are not well studied. Infants of mothers taking anticonvulsants might have more difficulty nursing and breastfed for a shorter duration, possibly because of negative or equivocal safety advice given by health professionals.[62–64]

No data are available for some of the newer anticonvulsants such as **felbamate, gabapentin, levetiracetam, oxcarbazepine, tiagabine,** and **topiramate.** Breastfeeding is not recommended during felbamate use.[65–67]

Carbamazepine

Carbamazepine and its major active metabolite are excreted into milk and can be detected in nursing infants' serum; concentrations are usually low but near the therapeutic range in some infants. Two cases of hepatic dysfunction in breastfed neonates have been reported. Poor feeding also has been reported. Carbamazepine can be used during lactation, but close observation of the infant for jaundice and other signs of possible adverse idiosyncratic effects is advisable.[67] Measurement of infant serum concentration might be indicated if symptoms occur.

Clonazepam

Serum concentrations of clonazepam were low in two nursing infants, and no effects were noted.[1] In another infant, breastfeeding increased serum concentrations over those present at birth.[68] Clonazepam has been detected in the serum of a breastfed neonate whose mother was receiving the drug before and after delivery but was undetectable in 4 others.[69] Observation of the infant for drowsiness and monitoring of the infant's serum concentration might be indicated.

Ethosuximide

Breastfed infants can attain ethosuximide serum concentrations near the therapeutic range, and some infants might become drowsy or fussy. Breastfeed with caution and keep the mother's serum concentrations as low as possible while remaining in the therapeutic range. Infant serum drug concentration monitoring is indicated.

Lamotrigine

Lamotrigine concentrations in infants breastfed during maternal lamotrigine therapy have ranged from 22 to 85% of the maternal serum concentration, but no adverse effects have been reported with these relatively high levels.[67,70,71] Infants can be allowed to nurse, but close monitoring for side effects such as rash (which can be life-threatening), drowsiness, or poor sucking is essential. Obtain an infant serum concentration if adverse effects are suspected and discontinue breastfeeding if rash occurs.

Phenobarbital

The effect of phenobarbital is unpredictable: drowsiness leading to feeding difficulties can occur; breastfeeding can prevent withdrawal symptoms in infants whose mothers took phenobarbital during pregnancy; and withdrawal symptoms have been observed after abrupt weaning. Phenobarbital can be used in low to moderate dosages but monitor infant behavior, weight gain, and, if there is concern, serum concentrations. Sometimes breastfeeding must be discontinued because of excessive drowsiness and poor weight gain.

Phenytoin

Only small amounts of phenytoin are excreted into milk. Rarely, infants might experience idiosyncratic reactions such as cyanosis and methemoglobinemia, but infants generally tolerate phenytoin in milk well.

(continued)

CENTRAL NERVOUS SYSTEM DRUGS

Primidone

Primidone and its metabolites (phenylethylmalonamide, **phenobarbital**, and parahydroxypheno-barbital) appear in milk in large amounts. Considerations are the same as those for phenobarbital. (*See* Phenobarbital.)

Valproic Acid

Milk concentrations of valproate are low, and usually no effects occur in infants. One case of probable infant thrombocytopenic purpura from valproate in milk has been reported.[72] Observe infants for rare idiosyncratic effects such as thrombocytopenia and hepatotoxicity.[67]

Vigabatrin

Limited data from two mothers indicate that a breastfed infant would receive <4% of the mother's mg/kg dose of vigabatrin.[73]

Zonisamide

Peak milk concentrations were 9–10 mg/L with a maternal dose of 300 mg/day in one mother. No data are available on effects in breastfed infants.[74]

ANTIDEPRESSANTS

Heterocyclic Antidepressants

Most of these drugs have not been well studied during lactation. Some investigators recommend against the use of antidepressants because of theoretical (but undemonstrated) long-term effects on infants' neurologic development; others consider **tricyclic antidepressants** to be acceptable. Follow-up for 1–3 yr in a small group of breastfed infants indicates no adverse effects on growth and development.[75] Another study found that breastfed infants of mothers taking **dothiepin** had cognitive development equal to controls at 3 yr of age.[76] Sedating TCAs and those with active metabolites (eg, **amitriptyline, doxepin,** and **imipramine**) might be less desirable than other TCAs. Respiratory depression was reported in one breastfed infant whose mother was taking doxepin 25 mg tid, but an infant whose mother was taking 150 mg at night had no problems. Another report found poor sucking and swallowing, muscle hypotonia, and vomiting in a 9-day-old whose mother was taking doxepin 35 mg/day.[77] Maternal dosages of amitriptyline up to 150 mg/day, **clomipramine** 150 mg/day, **desipramine** 300 mg/day, imipramine 200 mg/day, or **nortriptyline** 125 mg/day have not caused observable effects in the infants studied. In several infants, nortriptyline serum concentrations were undetectable with maternal nortriptyline dosages of up to 125 mg/day or amitriptyline 175 mg/day.[69,78,79] One nortriptyline metabolite has been detected in low levels in the serum of breastfed infants without adverse consequences.[78,80] Nortriptyline (and probably the other secondary amine, desipramine) is the TCA of choice during breastfeeding. Doxepin should be avoided. Giving the drug as a single dose at bedtime and skipping nighttime feeding(s) can further minimize infant exposure. A dose of 250 mg/day of **amoxapine** or 100–150 mg/day of **maprotiline** produces low drug concentrations in milk, but effects of these drugs on infants have not been well studied.

Selective Serotonin Reuptake Inhibitors

Although the average daily dosages of **fluoxetine** and **norfluoxetine** in milk are about 7% of the mother's weight-adjusted dosages, some mothers excrete as much as 12% of a dosage and the drugs' half-lives are very long.[81] One case of colic (increased crying, decreased sleep, watery stools, and vomiting) and unexplained high serum concentrations were reported in a breastfed 6-week-old infant. The infant improved after switching to formula and colic reappeared with rechallenge. Other case reports include seizure-like activity, irritability, hyperglycemia and

(*continued*)

CENTRAL NERVOUS SYSTEM DRUGS

glycosuria, and withdrawal symptoms.[81] Norfluoxetine is often detectable in infants' serum.[69,81,82] Fluoxetine in breastmilk had no effect on neurologic development in 4 infants,[83] but a larger retrospective study found that fluoxetine can reduce the growth rate of infants who are exposed via breastmilk from birth.[84] Fluoxetine should be avoided during breastfeeding if possible, although older infants might be less susceptible to fluoxetine's effects than newborns. Monitor infants carefully for behavioral symptoms and adequate weight gain. **Citalopram** reaches the infant in dosages of about 5% of the mother's mg/kg dosage.[85–87] The manufacturer states that drowsiness and weight loss in breastfed infants have occurred, and uneasy sleep occurred in the infant of a mother taking citalopram.[88] Citalopram is not a good choice while breastfeeding a newborn. Infants receive a dose <1% of the maternal **fluvoxamine** dose. Several infants grew and developed normally with maternal fluvoxamine use.[89,90] With **paroxetine,** infants receive about 1.5% of the maternal dosage. Of 23 infants studied, only 1 had detectable serum concentrations of paroxetine. No adverse behavioral or growth effects have been observed in studies, but one case of infant agitation and feeding difficulties has been reported.[91–93] **Sertraline** dosage to the breastfed infant is <2% of the maternal dosage; concentrations in infant serum are usually low to undetectable, platelet serotonin is unaffected, and no adverse effects on growth have been seen in controlled follow-up.[94–97] One case of infant agitation and one of somnolence and developmental difficulties have been reported spontaneously to Australian authorities.[97] Sertraline and paroxetine are considered the SSRIs of choice during breastfeeding, especially with a neonate.

Monoamine Oxidase Inhibitors

There are no data on the amounts of older nonselective MAOIs excreted into milk. Because of their potential for toxicity and lactation inhibition, avoid MAOIs during nursing. With **moclobemide,** a reversible MAO-A inhibitor not available in the United States, infants receive a dose <1% of the mother's dose and no side effects have been reported in a small number of infants studied.[98,99]

Other Antidepressants

Bupropion and its metabolites were undetectable in one 14-month-old infant whose mother was taking 300 mg/day and nursing twice daily.[99,100] **Nefazodone** and **trazodone** dosages in the infant are <1% of the mother's mg/kg dosage, but only a few cases have been reported.[1,101] One case of drowsiness, lethargy, poor feeding, and inability to maintain normal body temperature was reported in a small preterm breastfed infant whose mother was taking nefazodone 300 mg/day.[102] Infants receive **venlafaxine** doses of up to 9.2% of the mother's mg/kg dosage and the active metabolite is detectable in the infant's serum. Although adverse effects were not seen in 3 breastfed infants, caution should be used with venlafaxine until more experience is gained.[99]

ANTIPSYCHOTIC DRUGS

Data on the use of antipsychotics during lactation are sparse.[103–105] **Phenothiazines** and **thioxanthenes** pass into milk somewhat unpredictably but usually in small amounts. Drowsiness can occur with the more sedating agents, such as **chlorpromazine.** Other effects, such as extrapyramidal symptoms, are possible but have not been reported. Limited follow-up, ranging from 15 months to 6 yr, indicates no long-term effects on infant development in most infants. However, 3 infants whose mothers were taking large dosages of chlorpromazine (200–600 mg/day) and **haloperidol** (20–40 mg/day) in combination showed deterioration of mental and psychomotor developmental scores over the first 12–18 months of life.[106] Nine other infants whose mothers were taking lower dosages of a single antipsychotic (including haloperidol up to 20 mg/day) showed normal development. It appears that maternal phenothiazines, thioxanthenes, and haloperidol

(*continued*)

CENTRAL NERVOUS SYSTEM DRUGS

cause no problems for nursing infants unless dosages are at the high end of the range or combinations of drugs are used.[104,105] Breastfeeding during **clozapine** use in 4 infants resulted in sedation in 1 and agranulocytosis in another, which resolved with discontinuation; nursing is not recommended during clozapine use.[100,107] Exposure of 2 infants to **olanzapine** in breastmilk for a few days each caused no untoward events, but more experience is needed.[108] One mother taking **risperidone** excreted about 4% of her mg/kg dosage into breastmilk; no infant side effects were noted.[109]

ANXIOLYTICS, SEDATIVES, AND HYPNOTICS

Many sedatives and hypnotics pass into breastmilk in measurable and potentially important amounts. Minimize sedative and hypnotic intake during lactation.

Anesthetics, General

Compared with epidural anesthesia, general anesthesia used during cesarean delivery can decrease the frequency and duration of breastfeeding.[19] Excretion of most inhalation anesthetics in breastmilk has not been well studied. Blood levels of anesthetic gases such as **desflurane, enflurane, halothane, isoflurane, nitrous oxide,** and **sevoflurane** drop rapidly after termination of anesthesia, are predicted to pass poorly into milk, and are probably poorly absorbed by the infant.[19,20] **Etomidate** milk levels drop rapidly after a dose and should pose little risk to the infant.[110] Amounts of **propofol** in milk are small and do not have good oral bioavailability in the infant. Typical IV doses of **methohexital** or **thiopental** for induction of anesthesia produce low concentrations in milk that do not cause effects in the infant.[1,18,110] Current opinion suggests that breastfeeding can be resumed as soon as the mother has recovered sufficiently from general anesthesia to nurse.[19,20]

Barbiturates

These drugs can stimulate metabolism of endogenous compounds in the infant when small amounts pass into milk. Short-acting agents are preferable to long-acting agents because smaller amounts are excreted into milk. Large single doses might have more potential for causing infant drowsiness than multiple small doses. (*See also* Anesthetics, General; Anticonvulsants.)

Benzodiazepines

Long-acting benzodiazepines and those with active metabolites (eg, **diazepam**) can accumulate and cause adverse effects in infants, especially with repeated doses, and in neonates because of their immature excretory mechanisms. **Bromazepam** taken by the mother might have contributed to the death of her 4-week-old breastfed infant with a 5-day history of apneic episodes.[111] A single dose of diazepam for short dental, surgical, or diagnostic procedures is not likely to cause sedation in infants past the neonatal period.[18] Milk **alprazolam** concentrations are low,[112] but infant drowsiness and withdrawal symptoms have been reported with alprazolam use during nursing.[1,5] When oral therapy is essential, the short-acting agents, **oxazepam** or **lorazepam,** are preferred; **temazepam** also might be acceptable.[103,113] **Midazolam** concentrations in milk are low and unlikely to affect the infant after a single dose or short course of therapy.[19,114]

Chloral Hydrate

Chloral hydrate and its active metabolite, **trichloroethanol,** appear in milk in dosages that approximate an infant sedative dosage and are detectable for up to 24 hr after a single dose. Using another hypnotic is advisable during nursing.

(*continued*)

GASTROINTESTINAL DRUGS

Zaleplon

The dose in milk is very small and the drug disappears from breastmilk rapidly.[115]

Zolpidem

Zolpidem milk concentrations are low for 3 hr after a dose and undetectable thereafter.[116]

LITHIUM

Lithium in milk can adversely affect the infant when its elimination is impaired, as in dehydration or in neonates or premature infants. Neonates also can have transplacentally acquired serum lithium levels. The long-term effects of lithium on infants are not known; many investigators consider lithium therapy a contraindication to breastfeeding, but others do not. Lithium may be used cautiously in mothers who are carefully selected for their ability to monitor their full-term infants. Discontinue breastfeeding immediately if the infant appears restless or looks ill. Measurement of serum lithium concentrations in the infant can help rule out lithium toxicity.[1,67,80]

PARKINSONISM DRUGS

Dopamine Agonists

Some ergot alkaloids have dopaminergic activity that can suppress prolactin release and lactation. **Bromocriptine** was used therapeutically for this purpose but has lost this indication in the United States because of potentially serious maternal toxicity (ie, stroke, death).

Levodopa

Levodopa decreases serum prolactin in non-nursing women with hyperprolactinemia and galactorrhea in a dose-dependent fashion and inhibits lactation in animals at high dosages.[1] One mother taking sustained-release levodopa/carbidopa 200 mg/50 mg qid successfully breastfed her infant whose development was normal at age 2 yr.[117]

GASTROINTESTINAL DRUGS

ACID-PEPTIC THERAPY

Antacids

Although **aluminum, calcium,** and **magnesium** antacids are partially absorbed, they are unlikely to appreciably increase concentrations of these ions in milk and are safe to use.

Histamine H_2-Blockers

Cimetidine is concentrated in milk because of ion trapping and possibly active secretion;[118] **ranitidine** doses in milk are lower. **Famotidine** and **nizatidine** have the lowest concentrations in milk and are preferred during nursing.

Proton Pump Inhibitors

Omeprazole and **lansoprazole** have not been adequately studied. In one mother, omeprazole milk levels were low and her newborn infant was breastfed without harm.[119]

Sucralfate

Because sucralfate is virtually nonabsorbable, it might be preferable to H_2-receptor antagonists.

GASTROINTESTINAL MOTILITY

Antidiarrheals

Nonabsorbable products such as **kaolin-pectin** are preferred in nursing mothers. The **loperamide** prodrug loperamide oxide results in only small amounts of loperamide in breastmilk.

(continued)

GASTROINTESTINAL DRUGS

Diphenoxylate excretion into milk has not been studied. One or two small doses of loperamide or diphenoxylate daily should pose little risk to the nursing infant. Avoid **bismuth subsalicylate** because salicylate is absorbable.

Cathartics and Laxatives

Some **anthraquinone** derivatives, such as **aloe** and **cascara,** and other stimulant cathartics (eg, **phenolphthalein**) should be avoided during nursing because of a laxative effect in breastfed infants. Laxatives that are nonabsorbable or poorly absorbed, such as bulk-forming (eg, **psyllium**), osmotic (eg, **magnesium** or **phosphate salts**), or stool-softening (eg, **docusate**) types, are preferred during lactation. **Senna** in moderate dosages is acceptable if other measures fail. **Bisacodyl** is virtually unabsorbed from the GI tract and should be safe.

Gastrokinetic Agents

Metoclopramide elevates serum prolactin via central dopaminergic antagonism and results in increased milk production and a more rapid transition from colostrum to mature milk. It can be used therapeutically in mothers who are producing insufficient quantities of milk, such as the mothers of premature or sick infants or adoptive mothers. Although infant dosages of metoclopramide from milk are low, the infant's serum prolactin concentrations can become elevated. Metoclopramide can induce depression, so caution is warranted. Limiting the duration of metoclopramide therapy to 14 days is essential, and it should not be used in mothers with a history of depression. **Domperidone** (not available in the U.S.) also has been used to increase milk supply and results in lower milk drug levels than metoclopramide.[120,121]

MISCELLANEOUS GASTROINTESTINAL DRUGS

Mesalamine Derivatives

Small amounts of **sulfasalazine** and **sulfapyridine** have been found in milk and infants' sera after oral sulfasalazine use. The small amount of sulfapyridine released should cause no bilirubin displacement. **Olsalazine** is not detectable in milk, but its metabolite, *N*-acetyl-5-ASA, is found in small amounts.[122] Small amounts of **mesalamine** and larger amounts of its metabolite are found in milk after oral administration.[123] Diarrhea has been reported in infants of mothers using mesalamine derivatives, but a controlled study found the frequency of diarrhea to be no greater than that in infants of untreated mothers.[124] Sulfasalazine and mesalamine and its derivatives may be used during nursing.

Ursodiol

Ursodiol was undetectable in the milk of 1 lactating mother, and her nursing infant developed normally during therapy.[125] Maternal ursodiol therapy decreased the bile acid concentration in colostrum and was found in trivial amounts in breastmilk in 16 mothers with intrahepatic cholestasis of pregnancy.[126] Their infants showed no adverse effects.

HEMATOLOGIC DRUGS

COAGULANTS AND ANTICOAGULANTS

Coumarins

Amounts of **warfarin** in milk are of no clinical consequence with a maternal dosage of ≤12 mg/day because of extensive protein binding. Higher dosages have not been studied. Other coumarin derivatives (eg, **acenocoumarol, dicumarol,** and **phenprocoumon**) also appear to be safe.[127]

(continued)

HEMATOLOGIC DRUGS

Heparins

Although minimal documentation exists, it is unlikely that **heparin** or low-molecular-weight heparins (eg, **enoxaparin, dalteparin**) pass into milk or are absorbed orally by the infant; anticoagulant activity was undetectable in 1 breastfed infant whose mother received 20–40 mg/day of enoxaparin.[128] **Hirudin** was not detectable in milk.[129]

Indandiones

Anisindione and **phenindione** are contraindicated because infant hemorrhage has occurred.[127]

HORMONES AND SYNTHETIC SUBSTITUTES

ADRENAL HORMONES

Corticosteroids

Prednisone and **prednisolone** excretions into milk are minimal even with large oral doses.[130] The infant dosage can be reduced even further by using prednisolone rather than prednisone and avoiding nursing for 3–4 hr after a dose. Three infants have been breastfed during long-term maternal use of **methylprednisolone** 6–8 mg/day with apparent safety. Large IV doses of corticosteroids or use of long-acting agents such as **dexamethasone** have not been studied, and caution is warranted. Depot injections, inhaled corticosteroids (eg, **beclomethasone, fluticasone**), or topical corticosteroids should present little or no risk to the infant because of low maternal serum concentrations. However, topical application to the nipple has caused adverse effects in the infant because of direct ingestion.[131]

ANTIDIABETIC DRUGS

Insulin

Diabetic mothers using insulin may nurse their infants. However, it has been found empirically that the mother might need to reduce her insulin dosage to 55–75% of the prepregnancy dosage. Close monitoring is required postpartum because the return to prepregnancy insulin dosage has been variably reported to take 1–6 weeks.[132,133]

Sulfonylureas

Tolbutamide is excreted in milk in small amounts that should cause no harm. The manufacturer reports that **chlorpropamide** concentrations in milk are low, but no published clinical data are available on this or other sulfonylureas.

CONTRACEPTIVES

Estrogen–Progestin Combinations

Although present in milk in small amounts, estrogens and progestins are readily metabolized by nursing infants. Rare case reports of breast enlargement in infants have been attributed to estrogen-containing oral contraceptives. These effects occur primarily with products containing >50 μg of estrogen. These high-estrogen contraceptives also markedly suppress lactation, especially when administered immediately postpartum. When currently available low-dose estrogen–progestin combination contraceptives are begun ≥6 weeks postpartum, a dramatic immediate effect on milk supply is usually not seen, but long-term negative effects on milk yield lead to early feeding supplementation and discontinuation of breastfeeding and decreased infant growth. An 8-year follow-up of breastfed infants of mothers taking contraceptives containing **ethinyl estradiol** 50 μg found no adverse effects on the infants' development or behavior. Progestin-only contraceptives are preferred during lactation.

(continued)

HORMONES AND SYNTHETIC SUBSTITUTES

Progestin Only

No immediate effects have been reported with progestin-only contraceptives such as **levo-norgestrel** implants, depot **medroxyprogesterone** acetate, or oral **norethindrone** or **norgestrel**. Progestin-only contraceptives generally have no effect on, or enhance, milk supply and might extend the duration of lactation. Although infant growth might undergo a slight, transient depression after insertion of levonorgestrel implants, large multicenter studies have found no effect of progestin-only contraceptives on growth and development of infants and children up to puberty.[134–137] Early (ie, immediately postpartum) initiation of these agents is controversial. Because physiologic postpartum progesterone withdrawal is a primary stimulus for lactation, it appears best to wait for at least 3 days postpartum before starting a progestin-only contraceptive.[138] One small study found no adverse effects on lactation or infant growth when depot medroxyprogesterone was given immediately postpartum,[139] but anecdotal reports of lactation suppression with immediate postpartum administration exist. Progestin-only contraceptives started 6 weeks postpartum are the preferred hormonal contraceptives during lactation.[140,141] (*See also* Progesterone.)

FEMALE SEX HORMONES

Progesterone

Contraceptive use via implants (investigationally) or intrauterine devices transfers little progesterone to the breastfed infant, and any drug in milk is minimally absorbed by the infant.[1,140,141] Milk progesterone concentrations have not been measured after higher doses used to treat premenstrual syndrome.

THYROID AND ANTITHYROID DRUGS

Iodides

Inorganic iodide is contraindicated during breastfeeding because of possible thyroid suppression and rash. Topical and vaginal **povidone–iodine** in nursing mothers results in elevated milk iodine concentrations and occasional thyroid suppression in nursing infants. Avoid povidone–iodine preparations while nursing and minimize their use during delivery.

Thioamides

Propylthiouracil is the antithyroid drug of choice during lactation; little passes into milk and infant thyroid suppression does not occur. Dosages as high as 750 mg/day have been given to nursing mothers with no adverse effects in their infants.[142] **Methimazole** 20 mg/day or **carbimazole** (a methimazole prodrug) 15 mg/day also can be used, but these drugs pass into milk in greater quantities and have longer half-lives than propylthiouracil.[143] Infants of mothers who took 20 mg/day of methimazole while nursing had no decrease in intellectual or physical development at age 1 yr.[144] A potential for idiosyncratic reactions (eg, agranulocytosis) and hypothyroidism exists, and measurement of the infant's serum thyroxine and TSH concentrations at 2–4-week intervals might be prudent during maternal antithyroid drug use.

Thyroid Hormones

Normal lactation requires thyroid hormones. **Levothyroxine** (T_4) passes into milk poorly, although **liothyronine** (T_3) might pass in more physiologically relevant amounts. Milk concentrations of thyroid hormones have not been measured after exogenous administration, but a physiologic replacement dosage of levothyroxine to a breastfeeding mother is not expected to result in excessive thyroid administration to the infant. Replacement therapy with liothyronine or supraphysiologic maternal levothyroxine dosage might transfer larger amounts of liothyronine to the infant.

(*continued*)

HORMONES AND SYNTHETIC SUBSTITUTES

Protirelin

Protirelin (thyrotropin-releasing hormone [TRH]) causes an increase in prolactin secretion and can enhance milk yield.[145]

MISCELLANEOUS HORMONAL AGENTS

Ergot Alkaloids

Ergonovine can lower postpartum serum prolactin concentrations, but **methylergonovine** apparently does not. Methylergonovine is not found in milk in important quantities. Short-term, low-dose regimens of these agents immediately postpartum pose no hazard to the infant, but methylergonovine is preferred because it does not inhibit lactation. Courses of these drugs given several days postpartum can expose the infant to greater risk of ergot side effects because of the larger amount of milk consumed at this age.

Calcitriol

Calcitriol requirements in hypoparathyroid women decrease during lactation. Failure to substantially decrease (by up to two-thirds) the calcitriol dosage results in maternal hypercalcemia.[146,147]

Desmopressin

Desmopressin is excreted in negligible amounts into milk and is poorly absorbed orally by the infant, so it appears safe to use.

Human Growth Hormone

Somatropin can increase milk production in mothers with an insufficient milk supply.[148,149]

RENAL AND ELECTROLYTES

DIURETICS

Large dosages of short-acting thiazide-type diuretics (eg, **hydrochlorothiazide**), usual dosages of loop diuretics (eg, **furosemide**), or long-acting thiazide-type diuretics (eg, **chlorthalidone** and **bendroflumethiazide**) can suppress lactation and should be avoided. Long-acting agents also can accumulate in infants' serum. Low dosages of short-acting thiazide-type diuretics should pose no problems to the infant or suppress lactation. **Acetazolamide** appears in milk in small amounts that are unlikely to harm the infant. The amounts of **spironolactone** and its metabolites in milk are inconsequential.

ELECTROLYTES

Bisphosphonates

Pamidronate was used successfully in one patient to treat bone loss associated with reflex sympathetic dystrophy. The drug was undetectable in breastmilk.[150]

Fluoride

Fluoride supplementation is not recommended during the first 6 months after birth; from 6 months to 3 yr of age, fluoride supplementation of the breastfed infant is recommended only if the mother's water supply contains <0.3 ppm fluoride.[151]

Magnesium Sulfate

When given IV, magnesium sulfate increases milk magnesium concentrations only slightly. Oral absorption of magnesium is poor, so maternal magnesium therapy is not a contraindication to breastfeeding.

(continued)

RENAL AND ELECTROLYTES

ANTIGOUT AGENTS

Allopurinol

This drug and its active metabolite, **oxypurinol**, are excreted into milk in nearly therapeutic amounts, and oxypurinol is detectable in the nursing infant's serum in near-therapeutic levels.[152] Although one infant breastfed without harm during maternal allopurinol therapy, observe infants for side effects, especially hypersensitivity reactions. If possible, give allopurinol to the mother in a single dose after the last nursing of the day.

Colchicine

Several infants have been breast-fed safely during long-term, low-dose administration of colchicine to the mother for familial Mediterranean fever.[153,154] The amount excreted in milk indicates that toxicity might occur with higher dosages.[153] Colchicine decreases milk production and alters milk composition in animals when infused into the udder. Use it with great caution and in low dosages when breastfeeding, especially with a neonate.

RESPIRATORY DRUGS

ANTIASTHMATICS

Anticholinergics

Excretion of anticholinergics into milk has not been studied. Theoretical hazards of the orally absorbable compounds include anticholinergic effects such as drying of secretions, temperature elevations, and CNS disturbances in the infant. Anticholinergics might inhibit lactation by inhibiting growth hormone and oxytocin secretion.[1,155] Observe infants carefully for anticholinergic symptoms and signs of decreased lactation (eg, insatiety, poor weight gain) when anticholinergics are given to the mother. It is unlikely that inhaled **ipratropium** affects the infant or milk production.

Terbutaline

Oral administration results in low milk terbutaline concentrations, causes no symptoms in breastfed infants, and is not expected to decrease milk supply. Other β_2-receptor agonists (eg, **albuterol**) appear safe to use orally, but inhaler products should transfer less drug to the infant and are preferred.

Theophylline

Maternal theophylline use occasionally can cause irritability and fretful sleep in infants. Newborn infants are most likely to be affected because of their slow elimination and low serum protein binding of theophylline. There is no need to avoid theophylline products; however, keep maternal serum concentrations in the lower part of the therapeutic range and measure infant serum concentrations if side effects occur. The related drug **dyphylline** is excreted into milk in greater amounts and is best avoided.

ANTIHISTAMINES

There are few studies on antihistamine use during lactation. One study found drowsiness or irritability in 12% of breastfed infants whose mothers took antihistamines.[5] Older sedating (and more anticholinergic) antihistamines are more problematic because they can affect the infant and might suppress lactation. (*See* Anticholinergics.) Nonsedating antihistamines are preferred agents for long-term therapy. However, single bedtime doses of a sedating antihistamine after the last feeding of the day might be adequate and minimize the amount the infant receives. Avoid sedating antihistamines in high dosages, in SR formulations, or in combinations with sympathomimetic agents.

(continued)

RESPIRATORY DRUGS

Cetirizine

Cetirizine has not been studied and is not a preferred agent because of its sedative and anticholinergic effects.

Cyproheptadine

Cyproheptadine lowers maternal serum prolactin and should be avoided during lactation.

Fexofenadine

Based on terfenadine experience, fexofenadine is likely to be well tolerated by breastfed infants.[5,156]

Loratadine

Loratadine is excreted into milk in seemingly unimportant amounts.

Triprolidine

Only small amounts of triprolidine are found in breastmilk.

COUGH AND COLD

α-Adrenergic **sympathomimetics** decrease milk flow in animals by central inhibition of secretion and release of oxytocin and by peripheral vasoconstriction, which limits the access of oxytocin to myoepithelial cells in the mammary glands. **Norepinephrine** also might decrease prolactin release. Although these effects are not well documented in humans, lactation inhibition seems to occur with oral decongestant (eg, **pseudoephedrine**) use; therefore, sympathomimetic nasal sprays (eg, **oxymetazoline**) are recommended over oral decongestant products. Pseudoephedrine also can cause irritability in some infants.[5]

MISCELLANEOUS DRUGS

CHOLINERGIC DRUGS

Six infants of mothers treated with **neostigmine** for myasthenia gravis were reportedly breastfed successfully. Neostigmine was not found in milk, but 1 infant appeared to have abdominal cramps after each breastfeeding. **Pyridostigmine** has been used safely during breastfeeding in 3 patients with myasthenia gravis.

Baclofen

Only small amounts of baclofen appear in milk, and it may be used in nursing mothers with caution.

Bupivacaine

Bupivacaine appears in milk in small amounts when administered to the mother by intrapleural or epidural routes but has no effect on the infant.[55] Epidural analgesia with bupivacaine postcesarean section improved breastfeeding performance in one study.[157] (*See also* Lidocaine in Antiarrhythmics.)

Dantrolene

Several dantrolene doses totaling 720 mg IV over 2 days to a postpartum mother yielded peak milk levels of 12 mg/L. Dantrolene half-life in milk was 9.2 hr.[158]

Pyridoxine

In high doses (200–600 mg/day), pyridoxine has been used therapeutically to suppress lactation, although it is often not effective. With usual dosages found in foods and low-dose vitamin supplements, pyridoxine has no effect on prolactin or lactation.

(*continued*)

MISCELLANEOUS DRUGS

Radiopharmaceuticals

Exposure of the infant to excessive amounts of radioactivity is usually the primary concern raised by administration of radiopharmaceuticals to nursing mothers, rather than any pharmacologic toxicity of the agent. Some, but not all, radiopharmaceuticals require discontinuation of breastfeeding, at least temporarily, after administration to a nursing mother. **Radioactive iodine** compounds are the most dangerous and might require complete cessation of breastfeeding. The period needed for milk radioactivity to decline (by means of radioactive decay and maternal excretion) to a safe exposure level depends on several factors: dosage, biological half-life, radionuclide half-life, and "contamination" with other isotopes. The age of the infant, potential for oral absorption of the radionuclide from the infant's GI tract, and threshold level that is considered safe are also important factors. Measurement of milk radioactivity can aid in determining when breastfeeding can resume. Consult specialty sources for more detailed information.[159,160]

Retinoids

Acitretin passes into breastmilk in a quantity sufficient to merit avoidance of nursing while taking it. Although there is no information on use during lactation, the manufacturers of oral **isotretinoin** and topical **tretinoin** state that they are not compatible with nursing. Based on the systemic bioavailability of tretinoin applied topically to a small area such as the face, it is unlikely that harmful amounts reach the infant via breastmilk. Avoid contact of the infant's skin with treated areas of the mother's skin.

Vaccines

Breastfeeding is not a contraindication to the use of any vaccine (live or inactivated) in the nursing mother.[161]

DIAGNOSTIC AGENTS

Iodinated Contrast Media

Iopanoic acid contains free iodide that can be detected in milk. (*See* Iodides.) **Diatrizoate, iodamide, iohexol, metrizoate,** and **metrizamide** are detectable in milk after IV administration. Although no adverse effects have been reported in infants, breastfeeding probably should be withheld for a period after administration of most iodinated contrast media, the period depending on its rate of elimination. A few hours is probably adequate after an IV pyelogram. Large amounts of iodine are excreted into milk for weeks after lymphangiography with **ethiodized oil,** and nursing should be discontinued after this procedure.

Fluorescein

Fluorescein is detectable in milk after IV or topical administration. After IV administration, it had a milk half-life of 62 hr in one mother. The drug might present a risk to neonates who are undergoing phototherapy. Temporarily withholding nursing after fluorescein use (especially IV) seems appropriate in this situation.

Gadolinium

Gadodiamide and **gadopentetate**, used in magnetic resonance imaging, are detectable in milk but have poor oral absorption and are rapidly excreted renally. Suspension of breastfeeding is not necessary after use of these agents.[162]

(*continued*)

DRUGS FOR NONMEDICAL USE

Alcohol

Alcohol equilibrates rapidly between blood and milk, resulting in milk concentrations equivalent to simultaneous blood concentrations. Peak maternal serum alcohol levels occur later (1 hr after the drink) in nursing mothers than in non-nursing women;[163] alteration in milk odor parallels milk alcohol levels.[164,165] Potential effects on infants depend on the pattern of use. Drunkenness (deep, unarousable sleep with snoring, deep respiration, no reaction to pain, inability to suck, excessive perspiration, and a feeble pulse) was reported after maternal binge drinking. Pseudo-Cushing syndrome was reported in the infant of a chronic alcoholic mother. One prospective study suggests that as little as 1 drink daily can cause slight impairment of the infant's motor development; the impairment increases in a dose-dependent fashion.[166] Infants suck more but consume less milk after maternal alcohol ingestion.[164] Alcohol also affects lactation; it inhibits the milk ejection reflex in a dose-dependent fashion, with single doses >2 g/kg completely blocking suckling-induced oxytocin release. Animal studies show that alcohol consumption results in a reduced suckling-induced prolactin release and reduced milk yield. An unknown substance in beer increases maternal serum prolactin; this effect also occurs with nonalcoholic beer.[1,167] Use alcohol in moderation during lactation and withhold nursing temporarily after alcohol consumption, with the duration dependent on the amount consumed—at least 2 hr per drink is suggested.[168]

Amphetamine

In a mother taking amphetamine 20 mg/day therapeutically, amphetamine concentrations in milk were less than those in serum and no adverse effects on the infant were noted. However, there is likely to be substantial intersubject variation in excretion, and concentrations in milk have not been measured during high-dose abuse of amphetamines. Anecdotally, infants breastfed by amphetamine abusers seem to experience drug-induced behavioral abnormalities such as agitation and crying. Amphetamine also inhibits prolactin release and, in high dosages, can interfere with lactation.

Caffeine

Anecdotal reports of infant jitteriness and difficulty sleeping have been reported with very high maternal intake of caffeine, but infant serum caffeine concentrations were not measured. Systematic studies have indicated that caffeine and its metabolites are excreted into milk in relatively small amounts with usual maternal intake and infants are usually not affected, even with high maternal intake.[1,169,170] Effects are more likely in premature and newborn infants because of their greatly diminished ability to metabolize caffeine.

Cocaine

Although not well studied in humans, the chemical nature of cocaine and results from animal studies indicate that it probably appears in milk in amounts that affect the infant. Cocaine was detectable in milk for 24–36 hr after use. In addition, serum cholinesterase, which is needed to metabolize the drug, is low in newborns. Cocaine and its toxic metabolite can be detected in milk and can cause adverse effects (vomiting, diarrhea, irritability, and dilated pupils) in breastfed infants. Convulsions occurred in an infant whose mother used topical cocaine to treat sore nipples. Breastfeeding is not recommended when the mother is a chronic cocaine user, and even occasional use of cocaine is discouraged during breastfeeding. Withhold breastfeeding for at least 24 hr after occasional cocaine use.[1,171]

Heroin

Abuse can result in high enough concentrations in milk to cause addiction or alleviate withdrawal symptoms in infants; however, breastfeeding is not a reliable method of preventing withdrawal.

(continued)

DRUGS FOR NONMEDICAL USE

Most authorities consider breastfeeding safe during **methadone** maintenance in doses up to 80 mg/day.[1,172]

Marijuana

Marijuana excretion into milk is not well studied, but **dronabinol** (tetrahydrocannabinol) can reach high concentrations in milk and be detected in the infant, particularly with heavy maternal use. Short-term effects in infants have not been reported, but a decrement in motor development at age 1 yr in the infants of marijuana-smoking mothers was reported in one study. Marijuana lowers serum prolactin slightly in nonlactating women and oxytocin release in rodents. One survey indicated that women who smoke marijuana breastfed for a shorter duration than nonusers and that the effect appears to be dose related.[173] Avoid breastfeeding in heavy marijuana users and during therapeutic dronabinol use. Withhold breastfeeding for several hours after occasional marijuana use and use caution to avoid exposing the infant to marijuana smoke.

Phencyclidine

Phencyclidine is concentrated in milk and remains detectable in milk for weeks after heavy use. Avoid breastfeeding after phencyclidine use; a sufficient duration of abstinence has not been defined.

Tobacco

Nicotine and its metabolite, **cotinine**, are excreted into breastmilk in amounts proportional to the number of cigarettes smoked by the mother.[1,174] The milk of smokers contains higher concentrations of cadmium than the milk of nonsmokers; other toxins from smoke have not been measured. Smokers also produce lower milk volumes, have lower milkfat content, use formula supplements more often, and wean their infants from breastfeeding earlier than nonsmokers, in part because nicotine lowers maternal basal prolactin concentrations.[175,176] Infants of smoking mothers have increased infantile colic, large postnursing decreases in respiratory rate and oxygen saturation, and more respiratory infections.[174] However, among infants of smokers, breastfeeding reduces the risk of respiratory illness by half that of formula-fed infants.[177] In nonsmokers, breastfeeding reduces the risk of sudden infant death syndrome compared with formula feeding, but smoking negates this advantage.[178] Advise nursing mothers to (1) stop or decrease smoking to the greatest degree possible, (2) not breastfeed right after smoking, and (3) not smoke in the same room with the infant.[179] The use of nicotine chewing gum, topical patches, or nasal spray has not been studied during lactation. Although they are not recommended by the manufacturer during nursing, these products are likely to be less hazardous to the nursing infant than maternal smoking.

■ REFERENCES

1. Anderson PO. Drug use during breast-feeding. *Clin Pharm* 1991;10:594–624.
2. Bennett PN, Notarianni LJ. Risk from drugs in breast milk: an analysis by relative dose. *Br J Clin Pharmacol* 1996;42:P673–4. Abstract.
3. Ito S, Koren G. A novel index for expressing exposure to the infant to drugs in breast milk. *Br J Clin Pharmacol* 1994;38:99–102.
4. Anderson PO. Medication use while breast-feeding a neonate. *Neonatal Pharmacol Q* 1993;2:3–14.
5. Ito S et al. Prospective follow-up of adverse reactions in breast-fed infants exposed to maternal medication. *Am J Obstet Gynecol* 1993;168:1393–9.
6. Harmon T et al. Perforated pseudomembranous colitis in the breast-fed infant. *J Pediatr Surg* 1992;27:744–6.
7. Wojnar-Horton RE et al. Distribution and excretion of sumatriptan in human milk. *Br J Clin Pharmacol* 1996;41:217–21.
8. Spigset O, Hägg S. Analgesics and breast-feeding: safety considerations. *Pediatr Drugs* 2000;2:223–8.

938 Drug Use in Special Populations

9. Beaulac-Baillargeon L, Allard G. Distribution of indomethacin in human milk and estimation of its milk to plasma ratio in vitro. *Br J Clin Pharmacol* 1993;36:413–6.
10. Lebedevs TH et al. Excretion of indomethacin in breast milk. *Br J Clin Pharmacol* 1991;32:751–4.
11. Walter K, Dilger C. Ibuprofen in human milk. *Br J Clin Pharmacol* 1997;44:211–2.
12. Janssen NM, Genta MS. The effects of immunosuppressive and anti-inflammatory medications on fertility, pregnancy and lactation. *Arch Intern Med* 2000;160:610–9.
13. Ramsey-Goldman R, Schilling E. Optimum use of disease-modifying and immunosuppressive antirheumatic agents during pregnancy and lactation. *Clin Immunother* 1996;5:40–58.
14. Messner U et al. Morbus Wilson und schwangerschaft. Literaturübersicht und kausuistische mitteilung. *Z Geburtsh Neonatol* 1998;202:77–9.
15. Rajan L. The impact of obstetric procedures and analgesia/anaesthesia during labour and delivery on breast-feeding. *Midwifery* 1994;10:87–103.
16. Nissen E et al. Effects of routinely given pethidine during labour on infants' developing breastfeeding behaviour. Effects of dose-delivery time interval and various concentrations of pethidine/norpethidine in cord plasma. *Acta Paediatr* 1997;86:201–8.
17. Wittels B et al. Postcesarean analgesia with both epidural morphine and intravenous patient-controlled analgesia: neurobehavioral outcomes among nursing neonates. *Anesth Analg* 1997;85:600–6.
18. Borgatta L et al. Clinical significance of methohexital, meperidine, and diazepam in breast milk. *J Clin Pharmacol* 1997;37:186–92.
19. Lee JJ, Rubin AP. Breast-feeding and anaesthesia. *Anaesthesia* 1993;48:616–25.
20. Hale TW. Anesthetic medications in breastfeeding mothers. *J Hum Lact* 1999;15:185–94.
21. Marquet P et al. Buprenorphine withdrawal syndrome in a newborn. *Clin Pharmacol Ther* 1997;62:569–71.
22. Jernite M et al. Buprenorphine excretion in breast milk. *Anesthesiology* 1999;91:A1095. Abstract.
23. Wischnik A et al. Elimination von nalbuphin in die muttermilch. *Arzneimittelforschung* 1988;38:1496–8.
24. Lee CR et al. Tramadol. A preliminary review of its pharmacodynamic and pharmacokinetic properties, and therapeutic potential in acute and chronic pain states. *Drugs* 1993;46:313–40.
25. Johnstone HA, Marcinak JF. Candidiasis in the breastfeeding mother and infant. *J Obstet Gynecol Neonatal Nurs* 1990;19:171–3.
26. Amir LH, Pakula S. Nipple pain, mastalgia and candidiasis in the lactating breast. *Aust N Z J Obstet Gynaecol* 1991;31:378–80.
27. Schilling CG et al. Excretion of fluconazole in human breast milk. *Pharmacotherapy* 1993;13:287. Abstract.
28. Force RW. Fluconazole concentrations in breast milk. *Pediatr Infect Dis J* 1995;14:235–6.
29. Moretti ME et al. Disposition of maternal ketoconazole in breast milk. *Am J Obstet Gynecol* 1995;173: 1625–6.
30. Utter AR. Gentian violet treatment for thrush: can its use cause breastfeeding problems? *J Hum Lact* 1990; 6:178–80. Letter.
31. Waters MFR. G 30 320 or B 663—Lampren (Geigy). A working party held at the Royal Garden Hotel London, September 1968. *Lepr Rev* 1969;40:21–47.
32. Venkatesan K et al. Excretion of clofazimine in human milk in leprosy patients. *Lepr Rev* 1997;68:242–6.
33. Kurzel RB et al. Mebendazole and postpartum lactation. *N Z Med J* 1994;107:439. Letter.
34. Ogbuokiri JE et al. Ivermectin levels in human breast milk. *Eur J Clin Pharmacol* 1994;46:89–90. Letter.
35. Taddio A et al. Acyclovir excretion in human breast-milk. *Ann Pharmacother* 1994;28:585–7.
36. Bork K, Benes P. Concentration and kinetic studies of intravenous acyclovir in serum and breast milk of a patient with eczema herpeticum. *J Am Acad Dermatol* 1995;32:1053–5.
37. Moodley J et al. Pharmacokinetics and antiretroviral activity of lamivudine alone or when coadministered with zidovudine in human immunodeficiency virus type 1–infected pregnant women and their offspring. *J Infect Dis* 1998;178:1327–33.
38. Musoke P et al. A phase I/II study of the safety and pharmacokinetics of nevirapine in HIV-1–infected pregnant Ugandan women and their neonates (HIVNET 006). *AIDS* 1999;13:479–86.
39. Ruff A et al. Excretion of zidovudine (ZDV) in human breast milk. 34th Interscience Conference on Antimicrobial Agents and Chemotherapy. October 4–7, 1995. Abstract I11.
40. Sedlmayr T et al. Clarithromycin, ein neues macrolid-antibiotikum. Wirksamkeit bei puerperalen infektionen und übertritt in die muttermilch. *Geburtshilfe Frauenheilkd* 1993;53:488–91.
41. Kelsey JJ et al. Presence of azithromycin breast milk concentrations: a case report. *Am J Obstet Gynecol* 1994;170:1375–6.
42. Dan M et al. Penetration of fleroxacin into breast milk and pharmacokinetics in lactating women. *Antimicrob Agents Chemother* 1993;37:293–6.
43. Gardner DK et al. Simultaneous concentrations of ciprofloxacin in breast milk and in serum in mother and breast-fed infant. *Clin Pharm* 1992;11:352–4.
44. Belton EM, Jones RV. Haemolytic anaemia due to nalidixic acid. *Lancet* 1965;2:691. Letter.

45. Hunt MJ et al. Black breast milk due to minocycline therapy. *Br J Dermatol* 1996;134:943–44.

46. Dobias L et al. Genotoxicity and carcinogenicity of metronidazole. *Mutat Res* 1994;317:177–94.

47. Reyes MP et al. Vancomycin during pregnancy: does it cause hearing loss or nephrotoxicity in the infant? *Am J Obstet Gynecol* 1989;161:977–81.

48. Kumar AR et al. Transfer of interferon alfa into human breast milk. *J Human Lactation* 2000;16:226-8.

49. Azuno Y et al. Mitoxantrone and etoposide in breast milk. *Am J Hematol* 1995;48:131–2. Letter.

50. Thiagarajan KD et al. Breast-feeding by cyclosporine-treated mother. *Obstet Gynecol* 2001;97:816–8.

51. Nyberg G et al. Breast-feeding during treatment with cyclosporine. *Transplantation* 1998;65:253–5.

52. Jain A et al. Pregnancy after liver transplantation under tacrolimus. *Transplantation* 1997;64:559–65.

53. Plomp TA et al. Use of amiodarone during pregnancy. *Eur J Obstet Gynecol Reprod Biol* 1992;43:201–7.

54. Zeisler JA et al. Lidocaine excretion in breast milk. *Drug Intell Clin Pharm* 1986;20:691–3.

55. Ortega D et al. Excretion of lidocaine and bupivacaine in breast milk following epidural anesthesia for cesarean delivery. *Acta Anesthesiol Scand* 1999;43:394–7.

56. Dryden RM, Lo MW. Breast milk lidocaine levels in tumescent liposuction. *Plast Reconstr Surg* 2000;105: 2267–8. Letter.

57. Libardoni M et al. Transfer of propafenone and 5-OH-propafenone to foetal plasma and maternal milk. *Br J Clin Pharmacol* 1991;32:527–8.

58. Bunjes R et al. Clonidine and breast-feeding. *Clin Pharm* 1993;12:178–9. Letter.

59. Kaiser G et al. Benazepril and benazeprilat in human plasma and breast milk. *Eur J Clin Pharmacol* 1989; 36(suppl):A303. Abstract.

60. Carcas AJ et al. Nimodipine transfer into human breast milk and cerebrospinal fluid. *Ann Pharmacother* 1996; 30:148–50.

61. Yerby MS. Contraception, pregnancy and lactation in women with epilepsy. *Bailliere Clin Neurol* 1996;5: 887–908.

62. Hartmann AM et al. Stillen, gewichtszunahme und verhalten bei neugeborenen epileptischer frauen. [Breast feeding, weight gain and behaviour in newborns of epileptic women.]. *Monatsschr Kinderheilkd* 1994;142:505–12.

63. Ito S et al. Initiation and duration of breast-feeding in women receiving antiepileptics. *Am J Obstet Gynecol* 1995;172:881–6.

64. Lee A et al. Physicians' advice as an influential factor on the decision to breastfeed in a cohort of women on carbamazepine. *Pediatr Res* 2000;47:472A. Abstract.

65. Bar-Oz B et al. Anticonvulsants and breastfeeding. A critical review. *Pediatr Drugs* 2000;2:113–26.

66. Hägg S, Spigset O. Anticonvulsant use during lactation. *Drug Saf* 2000;22:425–40.

67. Chaudron LH, Jefferson JW. Mood stabilizers during breastfeeding: a review. *J Clin Psychiatry* 2000; 61:79–90.

68. Bossi L, et al. Pharmacokinetics and clinical effects of antiepileptic drugs in newborns of chronically treated epileptic mothers. In: Janz D et al, eds. *Epilepsy, pregnancy and the child*. New York: Raven Press; 1982:373–81.

69. Birnbaum CS et al. Serum concentrations of antidepressants and benzodiazepines in nursing infants: a case series. *Pediatrics* 1999;104:e11

70. Ohman I et al. Lamotrigine in pregnancy: pharmacokinetics during delivery, in the neonate, and during lactation. *Epilepsia* 2000;41:709–13.

71. Berry DJ. The disposition of lamotrigine throughout pregnancy. *Ther Drug Monit* 1999;21:450. Abstract 90.

72. Stahl MMS et al. Thrombocytopenic purpura and anemia in a breast-fed infant whose mother was treated with valproic acid. *J Pediatr* 1997;130:1001–3.

73. Tran A et al. Vigabatrin: placental transfer in vivo and excretion into breast milk of the enantiomers. *Br J Clin Pharmacol* 1998;45:409–11.

74. Shimoyama R et al. Monitoring of zonisamide in human breast milk and maternal plasma by solid-phase extraction HPLC method. *Biomed Chromatography* 1999;13:370–2.

75. Misri S, Sivertz K. Tricyclic drugs in pregnancy and lactation: a preliminary report. *Int J Psychiatry Med* 1991;21:157–71.

76. Buist A, Janson H. Effect of exposure to dothiepin and northiaden in breast milk on child development. *Br J Psychiatry* 1995;167:370–3.

77. Frey OR et al. Adverse effects in a newborn infant breast-fed by a mother treated with doxepin. *Ann Pharmacother* 1999;33:690–3.

78. Wisner KL et al. Nortriptyline and its hydroxymetabolites in breastfeeding mothers and newborns. *Psychopharmacol Bull* 1997;33:249–51.

79. Yoshida K et al. Investigation of pharmacokinetics and possible adverse effects in infants exposed to tricyclic antidepressants in breast-milk. *J Affect Disord* 1997;43:225–37.

80. Mammen O et al. Antidepressants and breast-feeding. *Am J Psychiatr* 1997;154:1174–5. Letter.

81. Kristensen JH et al. Distribution and excretion of fluoxetine and norfluoxetine in human milk. *Br J. Clin Pharmacol* 1999;48:521–7.

82. Isenberg KE. Excretion of fluoxetine in human breast milk. *J Clin Psychiatry* 1990;51;169. Letter.
83. Yoshida K et al. Fluoxetine in breast-milk and developmental outcome of breastfed infants. *Br J Psychiatry* 1998;172:175–9.
84. Chambers CD et al. Weight gain in infants breastfed by mothers who take fluoxetine. *Pediatrics* 1999; 104:e61.
85. Jensen PN et al. Citalopram and desmethylcitalopram concentrations in breast milk and in serum of mother and infant. *Ther Drug Monit* 1997;19:236–9.
86. Spigset O et al. Excretion of citalopram in breast milk. *Br J Clin Pharmacol* 1997;44:295–8.
87. Rampono J et al. Citalopram and demethylcitalopram in human milk; distribution, excretion and effects in breast fed infants. *Br J Clin Pharmacol* 2000;50:263–8.
88. Schmidt K et al. Citalopram and breast-feeding: serum concentration and side effects in the infant. *Biol Psychiatry* 2000;47:164–5.
89. Hägg S et al. Excretion of fluvoxamine into breast milk. *Br J Clin Pharmacol* 2000;49:286–7. Letter.
90. Piontek CM et al. Serum fluvoxamine levels in breastfed infants. *J Clin Psychiatry* 2001;62:111–3.
91. Öhman R et al. Excretion of paroxetine into breast milk. *J Clin Psychiatry* 1999;60:519–23.
92. Begg EJ et al. Paroxetine in human milk. *Br J Clin Pharmacol* 1999;48:142–7.
93. Stowe ZN et al. Paroxetine in human breast milk and nursing infants. *Am J Psychiatr* 2000;157:185–9.
94. Altshuler LL et al. Breastfeeding and sertraline: a 24-hour analysis. *J Clin Psychiatry* 1995;56:243–5.
95. Mammen OK et al. Sertraline and norsertraline levels in three breastfed infants. *J Clin Psychiatr* 1997;58:100–3.
96. Wisner KL et al. Serum sertraline and N-desmethylsertraline levels in breast-feeding mother–infant pairs. *Am J Psychiatry* 1998;155:690–2.
97. Dodd S et al. Sertraline in paired blood plasma and breast-milk samples from nursing mothers. *Hum Psychopharmacol Clin Exp* 2000;15:261–4.
98. Buist A et al. Plasma and human milk concentrations of moclobemide in nursing mothers. *Hum Psychopharmacol Clin Exp* 1998;13:579–82.
99. Dodd S et al. Antidepressants and breast-feeding. A review of the literature. *Paediatr Drugs* 2000;2:183–92.
100. Spigset O, Hägg S. Excretion of psychotropic drugs into breast milk. Pharmacokinetic overview and therapeutic implications. *CNS Drugs* 1998;9:111–34.
101. Dodd S et al. Nefazodone in the breast milk of nursing mothers: a report of two patients. *J Clin Psychopharmacol* 2000;20:717–8. Letter.
102. Yapp P et al. Drowsiness and poor feeding in a breast-fed infant: association with nefazodone and its metabolites. *Ann Pharmacother* 2000;34:1269–72.
103. Pons G et al. Excretion of psychoactive drugs into breast milk. Pharmacokinetic principles and recommendations. *Clin Pharmacokinet* 1994;27:270–89.
104. Yoshida K et al. Psychotropic drugs in mothers' milk: a comprehensive review of assay methods, pharmacokinetics and safety of breast-feeding. *J Psychopharmacol* 1999;13:64–80.
105. Tényi T et al. Antipsychotics and breast-feeding. A review of the literature. *Paediatr Drugs* 2000;2:23–8.
106. Yoshida K et al. Neuroleptic drugs in breast-milk: a study of pharmacokinetics and of possible adverse effects in breast-fed infants. *Psychol Med* 1998;28:81–91.
107. Dev VJ, Krupp P. Adverse event profile and safety of clozapine. *Rev Contemp Pharmacother* 1995;6: 197–208.
108. Goldstein DJ et al. Olanzapine-exposed pregnancies and lactation: early experience. *J Clin Psychopharmacol* 2000;20:399–403.
109. Hill RC et al. Risperidone distribution and excretion into human milk: case report and estimated infant exposure during breast-feeding. *J Clin Psychopharmacol* 2000;20:285–6. Letter.
110. Esener Z et al. Thiopentone and etomidate concentrations in maternal and umbilical plasma, and in colostrum. *Br J Anaesth* 1992;69:586–8.
111. Martens PR. A sudden infant death like syndrome possibly induced by a benzodiazepine in breast-feeding. *Eur J Emerg Med* 1994;1:86–7.
112. Oo CY et al. Pharmacokinetics in lactating women: prediction of alprazolam transfer into milk. *Br J Clin Pharmacol* 1995;40:231–6.
113. Lebedevs TH et al. Excretion of temazepam in breast milk. *Br J Clin Pharmacol* 1992;33:204–6. Letter.
114. Spigset O. Anaesthetic agents and excretion in breast milk. *Acta Anaesthesiol Scand* 1994;38:94–103.
115. Darwish M et al. Rapid disappearance of zaleplon from breast milk after oral administration to lactating women. *J Clin Pharmacol* 1999;39:670–4.
116. Pons G et al. Zolpidem excretion in breast-milk. *Eur J Clin Pharmacol* 1989;37:245–8.
117. Thulin PC et al. Levodopa in human breast milk: clinical implications. *Neurology* 1998;50:1920–1.
118. Oo CY et al. Active transport of cimetidine into human milk. *Clin Pharmacol Ther* 1995;58:548–55.

119. Marshall JK et al. Omeprazole for refractory gastroesophageal reflux disease during pregnancy and lactation. *Can J Gastroenterol* 1998;12:225–7.

120. Hofmeyr GJ et al. Domperidone: secretion in breast milk and effect on puerperal prolactin levels. *Br J Obstet Gynecol* 1985;92:141–4.

121. da Silva OP et al. Effect of domperidone on milk production in mothers of premature newborns: a randomized, double-blind, placebo-controlled trial. *CMAJ* 2001;164:17-21.

122. Miller LG et al. Disposition of olsalazine and metabolites in breast milk. *J Clin Pharmacol* 1993;33:703–6.

123. Klotz U, Harings-Kaim A. Negligible excretion of 5-aminosalicylic acid in breast milk. *Lancet* 1993;342: 618–9. Letter.

124. Moretti ME et al. Prospective follow-up of infants exposed to 5-aminosalicylic acid containing drugs through maternal milk. *J Clin Pharmacol* 1998;38:867. Abstract.

125. Rudi J et al. Therapie mit ursodeoxycholsäure bei primär biliärer zirrhose während der schwangerschaft. *Z Gastroenterol* 1996;34:188–91.

126. Brites D, Rodrigues CMP. Elevated levels of bile acids in colostrum of patients with cholestasis of pregnancy are decreased following ursodeoxycholic acid therapy. *J Hepatol* 1998;29:743–51.

127. Clark SL et al. Coumarin derivatives and breast-feeding. *Obstet Gynecol* 2000;95:938–40.

128. Guillonneau M et al. L'allaitement est possible en cas de traitement maternal par l'enoxaprine. *Arch Pediatr* 1996;4:513–4.

129. Lindhoff-Last E et al. Hirudin treatment in a breastfeeding woman. *Lancet* 2000;355:467–8.

130. Greenberger PA. Pharmacokinetics of prednisolone transfer to breast milk. *Clin Pharmacol Ther* 1993;53: 324–8.

131. De Stefano B et al. Factitious hypertension with mineralocorticoid excess in an infant. *Helv Paediatr Acta* 1983;38:185–9.

132. Alban Davies H et al. Insulin requirements of diabetic women who breast feed. *BMJ* 1989;298:1357–8.

133. Murtaugh MA et al. Energy intake and glycemia in lactating women with type 1 diabetes. *J Am Diet Assoc* 1998;98:642–8.

134. Pardthaisong T et al. The long-term growth and development of children exposed to Depo-Provera during pregnancy or lactation. *Contraception* 1992;45:313–24.

135. Dunson TR et al. A multicenter clinical trial of a progestin-only oral contraceptive in lactating women. *Contraception* 1993;47:23–35.

136. World Health Organization Task Force for Epidemiological Research on Reproductive Health. Progestogen-only contraceptives during lactation: I. Infant growth. *Contraception* 1994;50:35–53.

137. World Health Organization Task Force for Epidemiological Research on Reproductive Health et al. Progestogen-only contraceptives during lactation: II. Infant development. *Contraception* 1994;50:55–68.

138. Kennedy KI et al. Premature introduction of progestin-only contraceptive methods during lactation. *Contraception* 1997;55:347–50.

139. Hannon PR et al. The influence of medroxyprogesterone on the duration of breast-feeding in mothers in an urban community. *Arch Pediatr Adolesc Med* 1997;151:490–6.

140. Chi I-C et al. The progestin-only oral contraceptive—its place in postpartum contraception. *Adv Contracept* 1992;8:93–103.

141. Díaz S, Croxatto HB. Contraception in lactating women. *Curr Opin Obstet Gynecol* 1993;5:815–22.

142. Momotani N et al. Thyroid function in wholly breast-feeding infants whose mothers take high doses of propylthiouracil. *Clin Endocrinol* 2000;53:177–81.

143. Azizi F. Effect of methimazole treatment of maternal thyrotoxicosis on thyroid function in breast-feeding infants. *J Pediatr* 1996;128:855–8.

144. Azizi F et al. Thyroid function and intellectual development of infants nursed by mothers taking methimazole. *J Clin Endocrinol Metab* 2000;85:3233–8.

145. Hanew K et al. Simultaneous administration of TRH and sulpiride caused additive but not synergistic PRL responses in normal subjects. *Endocrinol Jpn* 1992;39:465–8.

146. Caplan RH, Wickus GG. Reduced calcitriol requirements for treating hypoparathyroidism during lactation. A case report. *J Reprod Med* 1993;38:914–8.

147. Cathébras P et al. Hypercalcémie induite par la lactation chez deux patientes hypoparathyroïdiennes traitees. *Rev Med Interne* 1996;17:675–6.

148. Gunn AJ et al. Growth hormone increases breast milk volumes in mothers of preterm infants. *Pediatrics* 1996;98:279–82.

149. Milsom SR et al. Potential role for growth hormone in human lactation insufficiency. *Horm Res* 1998;50: 147–50.

150. Siminoski K et al. Intravenous pamidronate for treatment of reflux sympathetic dystrophy during breastfeeding. *J Bone Mineral Res* 2000;15:2052–5.

151. American Academy of Pediatrics. Committee on Nutrition. Fluoride supplementation. *Pediatrics* 1986;77: 758–61.

152. Kamilli I et al. Allopurinol in breast milk. *Adv Exp Biol Med* 1991;309A:143–5.
153. Guillonneau M et al. Colchicine is excreted at high concentrations in human breast milk. *Eur J Obstet Gynecol Reprod Biol* 1995;61:177–8. Letter.
154. Ben-Cherit E et al. Colchicine in breast milk of patients with familial Mediterranean fever. *Arthritis Rheum* 1996;39:1213–7.
155. Daniel JA et al. Methscopolamine bromide blocks hypothalamic-stimulated release of growth hormone in ewes. *J Anim Sci* 1997;75:1359–62.
156. Lucas BD Jr et al. Terfenadine pharmacokinetics in breast milk in lactating women. *Clin Pharmacol Ther* 1995;57:398–402.
157. Hirose M et al. The effect of postoperative analgesia with continuous epidural bupivacaine after cesarean section on the amount of breast-feeding and infant weight gain. *Anesth Analg* 1996;82:1166–9.
158. Fricker RM et al. Secretion of dantrolene into breast milk after acute therapy of a suspected malignant hyperthermia crisis during Cesarean section. *Anesthesiology* 1998;89:1023–5.
159. US Nuclear Regulatory Commission. Regulatory guide 8.39. Release of patients administered radioactive materials. 1997. (http://198.213.116.218/lact/html/radioactive.html)
160. Stabin MG, Breitz HB. Breast milk excretion of radiopharmaceuticals: mechanisms, findings, and radiation dosimetry. *J Nucl Med* 2000;41:663–73.
161. Gizurason S. Optimal delivery of vaccines. *Clin Pharmacokinet* 1996;30:1–15.
162. Kubik-Huch RA et al. Gadopentetate dimeglumine excretion into human breast milk during lactation. *Radiology* 2000;216:555–8.
163. da-Silva VA et al. Ethanol pharmacokinetics in lactating women. *Braz J Med Biol Res* 1993;26:1097–103.
164. Mennella JA, Beauchamp GK. The transfer of alcohol to human milk. Effects on flavor and the infant's behavior. *N Engl J Med* 1991;325:981–5.
165. Mennella JA, Beauchamp GK. Effects of beer on breast-fed infants. *JAMA* 1993;269:1637–8. Letter.
166. Little RE et al. Maternal alcohol use during breast-feeding and infant mental and motor development at one year. *N Engl J Med* 1989;321:425–30.
167. Mennella JA, Beauchamp GK. Beer, breast feeding, and folklore. *Dev Psychobiol* 1993;26:459–66.
168. Anderson PO. Alcohol and breastfeeding. *J Hum Lact* 1995;11:321–3.
169. Blanchard J et al. Methylxanthine levels in breast milk of lactating women of different ethnic and socioeconomic classes. *Biopharm Drug Dispos* 1992;13:187–96.
170. Oo CY et al. Pharmacokinetics of caffeine and its demethylated metabolites in lactation: predictions of milk to serum concentration ratios. *Pharm Res* 1995;12:313–6.
171. Dickson PH et al. The routine analysis of breast milk for drugs of abuse in a clinical toxicology laboratory. *J Forensic Sci* 1994;39:207–14.
172. Wojnar-Horton RE et al. Methadone distribution and excretion into breast milk of clients in a methadone maintenance programme. *Br J Clin Pharmacol* 1997;44:543–7.
173. Astley SJ, Little RE. Maternal marijuana use during lactation and infant development at one year. *Neurotoxicol Teratol* 1990;12:161–8.
174. Stepans MB, Wilkerson N. Physiologic effects of maternal smoking on breast-feeding infants. *J Am Acad Nurse Pract* 1993;5:105–13.
175. Mansbach IK et al. Onset and duration of breast feeding among Israeli mothers: relationships with smoking and type of delivery. *Soc Sci Med* 1991;33:1391–7.
176. Hopkinson JM et al. Milk production by mothers of premature infants: influence of cigarette smoking. *Pediatrics* 1992;90:934–8.
177. Jin C, Rossignol AM. Effects of passive smoking on respiratory illness from birth to age eighteen months, in Shanghai, People's Republic of China. *J Pediatr* 1993;123:553–8.
178. Klonoff-Cohen HS et al. The effect of passive smoking and tobacco exposure through breast milk on sudden infant death syndrome. *JAMA* 1995;273:795–8.
179. Håkansson A, Cars H. Maternal cigarette smoking, breast-feeding, and respiratory tract infections. A matched-pair study. *Scand J Prim Health Care* 1991;9:115–9.

Pediatric Drug Therapy

William E. Murray

Pediatric drug therapy presents a challenge to the practitioner in many respects. The pediatric population is comprised of a range of patient weights and organ maturity. Often there are no pediatric-specific data in the literature from which to derive appropriate dosage regimens. At times, medications must be used for which data are extrapolated on the basis of limited pharmacokinetic knowledge about the pediatric population. It must be remembered that children should not be treated as "little adults" when designing dosage regimens. Dosage administration nomograms derived from adult data should not be used in the pediatric population. Pharmacodynamic responses for the majority of medications used in children are even less well known. Children often react much differently from adults to certain medications. Examples are the use of stimulants such as methylphenidate to control hyperactivity common with attention deficit disorders and paradoxical hyperactivity, which can be observed in children taking phenobarbital. With therapeutically monitored medications, the standard adult therapeutic range is typically used because age-specific, concentration-effect information is scarce. Because of protein binding differences, infants might respond to lower total drug concentrations than those used in adults for certain medications (eg, phenytoin, theophylline).

One of the problems facing the clinician and caregiver of small children is the administration of medications. Dosage forms are usually designed with the adult population in mind, and the dosage cannot easily be individualized in small patients. This is especially true for most sustained-release products. Most young children cannot swallow tablets and capsules; thus, liquid preparations are generally preferred in this age group. For many drugs, liquid forms are not commercially available and must be extemporaneously compounded. Stability of these preparations is often unknown or of limited duration. Even when appropriate dosage forms suitable for young children are available, palatability, resistance to taking medications, and compliance issues can hinder optimal therapy.

■ PHARMACOKINETICS

ABSORPTION

At birth, gastric pH is neutral but falls to values of 1–3 in the first day of life. Subsequently, gastric pH returns toward neutrality because gastric acid secretion is low in the first several weeks to months. Adult values are usually achieved after the age of 2 yr.[1,2] Medications that require gastric acidity for absorption can have poor bioavailability in this age group, rendering them ineffective or requiring much higher doses than normal for therapeutic serum concentrations to be reached. Examples of medications in this group are phenytoin, ketoconazole, and itraconazole.[1,3] Alternative agents might have to be used if adequate serum levels cannot be documented when these drugs are administered orally. Certain medications that are acid labile actually might have increased bioavailability in infants, and these are antibiotics such as penicillin G and ampicillin.[4]

Gastric emptying time can be delayed in infants, especially premature infants.[1,3,5] Peak drug concentrations can occur much later in infants than in older children and adults. Other factors that can influence overall bioavailability of a particular medication in infants are the relatively high frequencies of gastroesophageal reflux, which can cause the dose to be spit up or vomited, and acute gastroenteritis (diarrhea), which can considerably shorten intestinal transit time. The oral route must be used with caution in these instances, especially in critically ill patients.

Other routes of administration can pose difficulties in the pediatric population. Overall muscle mass is decreased, and intramuscular administration might not be practical and certainly is not appreciated by most children. Most adults still remember their first injections in the doctor's office when they were children. Also, the dose of drug to be administered might require multiple injections.

Rectal administration may be used in situations where the oral route is not practical or available; however, absorption might be incomplete and/or erratic. Topical administration of medications can lead to undesired systemic absorption, especially in infants in whom the skin thickness is less and the total skin surface area is proportionally greater than in adults.[1,2,4]

DISTRIBUTION

Rapid changes in body composition can dramatically alter the V_d for many medications during the first several months of life. Newborns have a higher percentage of total body water and extracellular fluid than older children and adults.[1,3,6] Hydrophilic drugs such as the aminoglycosides have a much larger V_d in newborns; this gradually decreases over the first year of life to approach adult values.

Total body fat in newborns (especially premature infants) is much lower than in older children and adults.[6] Medications that are lipophilic might have a lower weight-adjusted V_d in the very young.

Protein binding is an important determinant of the V_d for drugs that are bound by albumin and other plasma proteins. In the neonatal period, the binding affinity of albumin is decreased compared with that in older children and adults (because of the persistence of fetal albumin).[1–3] Highly protein-bound drugs such as phenytoin have higher free fractions in neonates, and there might be an increased pharmacodynamic response at lower concentrations of total drug. The V_d of these drugs is inversely related to the degree of protein binding.

In addition, the clinician must be aware of the potential for highly protein-bound substances to displace bilirubin from binding sites on albumin, particularly in the newborn.[1–3,7] The blood–brain barrier in newborns is more permeable than in older patients, and free bilirubin can readily cross into the CNS and cause kernicterus.

Tissue binding for many medications is unknown but can differ dramatically from that in adults. One example is digoxin, which binds to erythrocytes in pediatric patients to a much greater extent than in adult patients.[2,4] Digoxin has a much larger V_d in pediatric patients, and recommended loading doses in this age group are much larger on a mg/kg basis than in adult patients. In general, drug distribution volumes are larger in neonates and gradually approach adult values (in L/kg) by the first year of life.

METABOLISM

Metabolic processes show dramatic changes in the first weeks to months of life. At birth, most hepatic enzymes are immature and drug metabolizing capacity is greatly reduced. Phase I reactions (ie, oxidation) are controlled largely by the mixed-function oxidase system, of which the cytochrome P450 enzymes are the major determinant. These enzymes are largely undeveloped in newborns, especially premature infants, but maturation can take place quickly in the first weeks to months of life. Phase II reactions (ie, conjugation) include glucuronidation, sulfation, and acetylation. These reactions also are immature at birth, and drug toxicity has resulted (eg, with chloramphenicol) because of the absence of knowledge about reduced dosage requirements in newborns.[1–3,6]

The liver size relative to body weight in newborns is much larger than that in adults.[1] Rapid weight gain, with subsequent increases in liver size and metabolic capacity, might require many dosage adjustments to prevent newborns from growing out of their dosages for many medications. When full metabolic capacity is reached in the pediatric patient, the hepatic clearance can greatly exceed that observed in adult patients on a weight-adjusted basis. Pediatric dosages of many medications on a mg/kg basis are often much greater than adult dosages. Figure 2–2 illustrates the change in clearance with age for theophylline.[6] Most medications have similar curves but can be shifted to the left or have different relative peaks compared with adult values. A decrease in hepatic clearance relative to body weight typically begins after a child weighs approximately 30 kg.[8] Thereafter, the increase in total body weight in proportion to liver size becomes greater. Thus, in adolescence, drug dosages typically begin to approach adult values. Drug toxicity can be observed in the adolescent patient if drug dosages on a mg/kg basis (designed for younger patients) are used.

RENAL ELIMINATION

The kidneys are the major route of drug elimination for many drugs. The kidneys are functionally immature at birth with regard to glomerular filtration and tubular secretion. Glomerular filtration at birth adjusted for body surface area is only

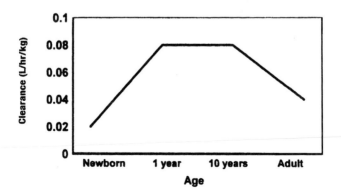

Figure 2–2. Maturation of theophylline metabolism.

30 to 40% of values in older infants and healthy young adults.[1–3] Premature infants often have even lower values during the first few weeks of life. Dosages of many medications (eg, aminoglycosides, vancomycin) that are eliminated largely by glomerular filtration must be decreased on the basis of the relative immaturity of the kidneys at birth. Maturation of glomerular filtration occurs over the first several weeks to months of life. The dosages of most medications are similar to those in older children by age 4–6 months. Although the frequency of renal disease in children is much lower than in the adult population, factors that can alter renal function, such as shock, nonsteroidal anti-inflammatory drugs, or hypoxia, must be considered when evaluating dosage regimens. Serum creatinine, the usual marker for renal function, is usually lower in young children than in adults because of children's lower muscle mass. Thus, a serum creatinine that indicates normal renal function in an adult might indicate renal impairment in a young child.

Tubular secretion also is diminished in the newborn. Drugs that have a component of tubular secretion (eg, penicillin) are typically administered at reduced dosages in the newborn. Maturation of tubular secretion occurs somewhat more slowly than glomerular filtration, but approaches adult values by age 8–12 months.[1–3]

EVALUATING DRUG DATA IN CHILDREN

With the numerous maturational changes observed in children from birth through adolescence, results of pediatric drug studies must be used with caution in children whose ages differ from those in the study. Dosages extrapolated only on a weight basis have the potential to underdose or overdose other age groups, depending on the population studied. Body surface area might correlate better than body weight with total body water and extracellular water and can be useful in certain instances in calculating dosage regimens. With the exception of cancer chemotherapeutic agents, information on drug dosage is more widely available in mg/kg than by body surface area.[5] Medications with narrow therapeutic ranges should have serum concentrations measured to aid in individualizing drug therapy, especially in critically ill children or those with known decreased renal or hepatic function.

Pharmacodynamic changes are poorly studied in the pediatric population, and responses to specific drug concentrations might be much different from those in the adult population. Diseases of childhood often differ from those in adults. Medications tolerated by adult patients might be inappropriate for the pediatric population (eg, aspirin for fever).

Caution must be used in the interpretation of drug levels because there might be much greater fluctuation in serum concentrations because of shorter drug half-lives in children than in adults. Further, the total volume of blood needed for drug level monitoring in small children can limit monitoring.

Detailed information on specific drugs can be found in the Pediatric Dosage sections of the individual drug monographs.

■ REFERENCES

1. Stewart CF, Hampton EM. Effect of maturation on drug disposition in pediatric patients. *Clin Pharm* 1987;6:548–64.

2. Besunder JB et al. Principles of drug biodisposition in the neonate. A critical evaluation of the pharmacokinetic-pharmacodynamic interface (part I). *Clin Pharmacokinet* 1988;14:189–216.

3. Milsap RL et al. Special pharmacokinetic considerations in children. In, Evans WE et al, eds. *Applied pharmacokinetics. Principles of therapeutic drug monitoring.* 3rd ed. Vancouver, WA: Applied Therapeutics; 1992:10-1–32.

4. Morselli PL et al. Clinical pharmacokinetics in newborns and infants. Age-related differences and therapeutic implications. In, Gibaldi M, Prescott LF, eds. *Handbook of clinical pharmacokinetics.* Section II. Balgowlah, NSW, Australia: ADIS Health Science Press; 1983:98–141.

5. Maxwell GM. Paediatric drug dosing. Bodyweight versus surface area. *Drugs* 1989;37:113–5.

6. McLeod HL, Evans WE. Pediatric pharmacokinetics and therapeutic drug monitoring. *Pediatr Rev* 1992;13:413–21.

7. Morselli PL. Clinical pharmacokinetics in neonates. In, Gibaldi M, Prescott LF, eds. *Handbook of clinical pharmacokinetics.* Section II. Balgowlah, NSW, Australia: ADIS Health Science Press; 1983:79–97.

8. Rane A, Wilson JT. Clinical pharmacokinetics in infants and children. In, Gibaldi M, Prescott LF, eds. *Handbook of clinical pharmacokinetics.* Section II. Balgowlah, NSW, Australia: ADIS Health Science Press; 1983:142–68.

Geriatric Drug Therapy

Dianne E. Tobias

Geriatric drug therapy is an important area of therapeutics and research, because of the growing elderly population, their disproportionately high use of medications, and their increased risk of drug misadventures. Although they represent approximately 12% of the U.S. population, the elderly consume more than 30% of all medications.[1] Trends include increasing numbers of the extreme elderly (over age 80) and elderly with functional disabilities. It is estimated that the number of elderly who are dependent in their activities of daily living will triple from 1985 to 2060. Ethical considerations, such as a patient's right to exercise decisions regarding treatment, are particularly relevant to the elderly population.[2,3] As the number of elderly increases and health care resources diminish, cost–benefit considerations will become increasingly important.[4]

The elderly are the most physiologically heterogeneous category of the adult population. The rate of normal aging varies considerably, and comparing data from persons of chronologically similar age can be misleading; health status is probably as important as age. Optimization of drug therapy in the elderly requires an understanding of how aging and concomitant pathology affect the pharmacokinetics and pharmacodynamics of drugs, the need to assess elderly patients individually, and elderly patients' expectations of therapy.[5]

Compliance issues leading to misuse and medication errors can be important in the elderly.[6] The cost of medications, physical difficulty in opening medication containers, swallowing large tablets, reading the prescription label, and the presence of depression or cognitive impairment can contribute to compliance problems.[7–9]

Adverse drug reactions are more common in the elderly,[10–13] although the correlation with age alone is debatable.[1,14] Increased medication use, especially medications with greater potential for toxicity, and chronic pathology with intermittent acute exacerbations are thought to contribute to the higher frequency and severity of adverse drug reactions. Most reactions in the elderly are dose related rather than idiosyncratic as a result of changes in pharmacokinetics and/or pharmacodynamics. Given the wide physiologic variability in the elderly population, the contribution of pharmacokinetic and pharmacodynamic changes can vary considerably. Additionally, the elderly are more sensitive to specific adverse reactions. For example, they have an increased sensitivity to anticholinergic side effects, especially central effects such as disorientation and memory impairment. These effects can be additive because many drugs commonly taken by the elderly are centrally active.[15–17] Varying degrees of cognitive impairment or even delirium can be induced by drugs in several classes including benzodiazepines, centrally acting antihypertensive agents, and antidepressants.[15,18] The onset can be insidious and mistakenly attributed solely to the aging process.

■ PHARMACOKINETICS

ABSORPTION

With aging there is some decrease in gastric secretions, acidity, gastric emptying, peristalsis, absorptive surface area, and splanchnic blood flow,[9,19] although the effect on gastric pH may not be as pronounced as once believed.[20,21] Taken together, the changes predict an altered extent or rate of absorption of orally administered drugs, yet most formal studies show no difference in oral bioavailability. Some factors might counterbalance each other (eg, acidity and gastric emptying; decreased absorptive surface and longer transit time). Some drugs (eg, digoxin) have shown a clinically unimportant slowed rate of absorption with equivalent quantities absorbed. Drugs with high extraction ratios may have increased bioavailability in the elderly compared with young patients, because of a decreased first-pass effect secondary to reduced hepatic blood flow. Decreased first-pass metabolism in the elderly has been shown for labetalol, propranolol, lidocaine, and verapamil.[22] It is known that the elderly have drier skin with lower lipid content, which is expected to be less permeable to hydrophilic compounds. Although neither conclusively nor well studied, percutaneous drug absorption appears to decrease with age.[23]

DISTRIBUTION

Body weight generally decreases, but more important, body composition changes with age. Total body water and lean body mass decrease, while body fat increases in proportion to total body weight. The percentage of body weight contributed by fat changes from 18% and 33% in young men and women, respectively, to 36% and 45% in their elderly counterparts.[24] These factors can alter the V_d of drugs in the elderly, although other aspects of drug disposition (binding, metabolism, elimination) can be additive or negate the effect. The V_d changes are most marked for highly lipophilic and hydrophilic drugs, and elderly patients are particularly susceptible to overdosage from drugs whose doses should be based on ideal body weight or lean body weight.[25] Theoretically, highly lipidsoluble drugs (eg, long-acting benzodiazepines, lidocaine) may have an increased V_d and a prolonged effect if drug clearance remains constant. Conversely, watersoluble drugs (eg, gentamicin) may have a decreased V_d, and at least transiently increased serum levels, leading to possible toxicity if initial doses are not conservative.[9] Although cardiac output does not appear to decrease with age,[26] some chronic diseases affecting the elderly do contribute to a decrease in cardiac output and regional blood flow. There is some evidence that blood is preferentially shunted away from the liver and kidneys to the brain, heart, and muscles.[15,27] These changes could explain the slowed elimination of some drugs and the heightened sensitivity to others.

PROTEIN BINDING

The proportion of albumin among total plasma proteins decreases with frailty, catabolic disease states, and immobility seen in many elderly,[28] but it is no longer believed that serum albumin decreases with age alone.[23] Serum albumin determinations should be performed to aid monitoring and dosage adjustment of drugs that are highly protein bound in the chronically immobile or ill elderly. A decrease in serum albumin can increase the percentage of free drug available for pharmacologic effect and elimination. Changes in albumin binding are more important with highly bound (greater than 90%) acidic drugs such as salicylates, phenytoin, and warfarin.[9] Conversely, basic drugs, including lidocaine, propranolol, and meperidine, have affinity for α_1-acid-glycoprotein, which may increase with age, especially when associated with conditions such as inflammatory diseases and malignancies.[9] Protein binding theoretically may be increased and result in less free drug available, although the clinical relevance of this is unclear.[23] With both types of binding, the net effect on clearance varies, depending on metabolism and elimination. Although not always available, free drug concentration measurements are often desirable in the elderly. There is also some evidence that the elderly may have a greater potential for protein displacement drug interactions.[29,30]

METABOLISM

Liver size and hepatic blood flow decrease with age and especially with disease. Studies show hepatic blood flow decreases by 35%, and liver volume by 44% and 28% in elderly women and men, respectively, when compared to younger counterparts.[13] Such a decrease in hepatic blood flow can limit the first-pass effect of drugs with high extraction ratios and markedly reduce their systemic clearance. Studies on phase I drug metabolism (ie, oxidation) do not consistently show a correlation with age,[23] although most show that the elderly, especially men, have prolonged elimination. Differences may be explained by environmental factors such as smoking habits and genetics. Phase II metabolism (ie, conjugation) does not appear to be influenced as much by age, although there has been less study in this area.[9,13,23] The effect of aging on drug acetylation is inconsistent and the importance unclear.[9,23] There does not appear to be any age difference in the degree of inhibition or induction of cytochrome P450 isozymes.[13,31] Monitoring and management of interactions with drugs such as cimetidine should be handled in the same manner as in younger patients. The changes described in liver size and metabolic function help to explain why certain drugs may have prolonged elimination; however, the variability of data cautions against generalizing about the effect of age alone. The initial dosage of metabolized drugs should be conservative and subsequent dosage adjustments based on careful monitoring of therapeutic and toxic parameters.

RENAL ELIMINATION

The effect of aging on the renal elimination of drugs is probably the most completely understood and important aspect affecting geriatric drug therapy. Glomerular filtration, tubular secretion, and renal blood flow all decrease with age. Creatinine clearance decreases approximately 1% per year after age 40,[32] the effect is variable, and volume depletion, CHF, and renal disease can further decrease organ function. Because creatinine production also decreases with age, serum creatinine may be normal despite a substantial decrease in renal function. It is therefore recommended that Cl_{cr} be measured or estimated using a method that incorporates age and weight.[33,34] The dosage of renally excreted drugs with low therapeutic indices should be conservative initially, with subsequent dosage titrated by close clinical and serum drug level monitoring, if applicable.

■ PHARMACODYNAMICS

Heightened drug effects that cannot be explained by altered pharmacokinetic variables alone have been hypothesized to be caused by changes in compensatory homeostasis, drug receptor sensitivity, or complications of chronic diseases that occur in the elderly. There is a gradual decrease in homeostatic reserve with aging. Postural control and orthostatic circulatory response are examples of compensatory mechanisms that are slowed in aging. Adequate postural blood pressure control relies on several factors, including central coordination, muscle tone, and proprioception, all of which can be blunted in the elderly.[15] As a result, side effects that are minimal or absent in a young patient with normal compensatory response can be marked in the elderly. The administration of long-acting anxiolytics, hypnotics, or antipsychotics can further alter these mechanisms and lead to an increased risk of falls in the elderly.[9,35] Similarly, symptomatic postural hypotension can result from the administration of a variety of antihypertensive agents (especially calcium-channel blockers and ACE inhibitors) and other drugs (eg, antipsychotics, antidepressants) that affect vasomotor tone. Physiologic mechanisms such as vasoconstriction and tachycardia cannot fully compensate for postural hypotension in the elderly.[15] Temperature regulation and intestinal motility are other homeostatic mechanisms that change with aging and can explain heightened effects of certain drugs.

The number and characteristics of drug receptors can change with aging and produce altered, often heightened, drug response. Research has shown age-related decreases in several autonomic receptors. There is some evidence of increased sensitivity to oral anticoagulants and digoxin, apart from the alterations in pharmacokinetics, which might contribute to the higher frequency of adverse reactions to these two agents in the elderly.[15]

Preliminary data indicate a possible increase in brain sensitivity to certain drugs with aging. It is unknown whether this effect is caused by changes in blood-brain permeability or tissue receptor sensitivity.[9] More research into drug pharmacodynamics in the elderly is needed, especially the interrelationship with pharmacokinetic alterations. The presence and impact of multiple concurrent pathologies and their treatments cannot be overemphasized in their contribution to the various drug effects seen in the elderly.

■ OTHER FACTORS

Cigarette smoking can cause clinically important induction of the metabolism of some drugs to a similar degree in both the elderly and the young.[23,36] This, and the fact that many published studies do not indicate smoking history, could explain some interpatient variability of pharmacokinetic data.

Nutritional intake is sometimes diminished in the elderly and can lead to nutritional and vitamin deficiencies. Nutritional status of the elderly can impact the outcome of drug therapy, and, conversely, drug therapy can affect nutritional status.[19,36,37]

■ EVALUATING DRUG DATA FOR THE ELDERLY

Because of age-related changes that may impact the outcome of drug therapy as outlined in this chapter, the results of drug studies using young subjects cannot always be extrapolated accurately to the elderly. Studies on diseases and drugs in the elderly do not always include sufficient numbers of elderly, especially extremely aged subjects, to draw appropriate conclusions.[38] Studies that include the elderly do not always separate results by decade of age and health status, two criteria that are helpful in assessing applicability of data in this heterogeneous population. Many studies also do not mention data on nutrition, alcohol, and smoking, which might explain some variability of results.[19] Although single-dose studies in healthy volunteers can be useful, long-term studies in afflicted elderly patients often yield data more applicable to therapeutics. Drugs are often not studied over a wide dosage range, so a minimal effective dosage in the elderly cannot be determined.[39]

When reviewing studies that include the elderly, one should consider the following potential problems: numbers of subjects must be sufficient to allow for high attrition rates and the typically wide variation in this population; study lengths must be sufficient for a chronic disease; concomitant diseases and medications must be acknowledged and their impact assessed; and "normal" values can be different from those of a younger population.[40–42]

■ CONCLUSION

The effects of aging as related to drug therapy illustrate the challenges in caring for the elderly. Clinical practice guidelines that have been developed for conditions commonly afflicting the elderly, such as those published by the Agency for Health Care Research and Quality, can be a helpful guide.[43] Conservative dosage, especially initially, with close clinical monitoring for dose-dependent effects is critical and should be emphasized by all health care practitioners caring for the elderly. For detailed information on specific drugs in the elderly, refer to the Geriatric Dosage section of the individual drug monographs.

■ REFERENCES

1. Gerety MB et al. Adverse events related to drugs and drug withdrawal in nursing home residents. *J Am Geriatr Soc* 1993;41:1326–32.
2. Faden R, German PS. Quality of life. Considerations in geriatrics. *Clin Geriatr Med* 1994;10:541–55.
3. Goldstein MK. Ethical considerations in pharmacotherapy of the aged. *Drugs Aging* 1991;1:91–7.
4. Livesley B. Cost-benefit considerations in the treatment of elderly people. *Drugs Aging* 1991;1:249–53.
5. Tobias DE. Ensuring and documenting the quality of drug therapy in the elderly. *Generations* 1994;18:40–2.
6. Burns JMA et al. Elderly patients and their medication: a post-discharge follow-up study. *Age Aging* 1992;21: 178–81.

7. Honig PK, Cantilena LR. Polypharmacy. Pharmacokinetic perspectives. *Clin Pharmacokinet* 1994;26:85–90.
8. Botelho RJ, Dudrak R. Home assessment of adherence to long-term medication in the elderly. *J Fam Pract* 1992;35:61–5.
9. Tregaskis BF, Stevenson IH. Pharmacokinetics in old age. *Br Med Bull* 1990;46:9–21.
10. Denham MJ. Adverse drug reactions. *Br Med Bull* 1990;46:53–62.
11. Beard K. Adverse reactions as a cause of hospital admission in the aged. *Drugs Aging* 1992;2:356–67.
12. Owens NJ et al. Distinguishing between the fit and frail elderly, and optimising pharmacotherapy. *Drugs Aging* 1994;4:47–55.
13. Woodhouse KW, James OFW. Hepatic drug metabolism and ageing. *Br Med Bull* 1990;46:22–35.
14. Walker J, Wynne H. Review: the frequency and severity of adverse drug reactions in elderly people. *Age Ageing* 1994;23:255–9.
15. Hämmerlein A et al. Pharmacokinetic and pharmacodynamic changes in the elderly. Clinical implications. *Clin Pharmacokinet* 1998;35:49–64.
16. Feinberg M. The problems of anticholinergic adverse effects in older patients. *Drugs Aging* 1993;3:335–48.
17. Nolan L, O'Malley K. Adverse effects of antidepressants in the elderly. *Drugs Aging* 1992;2:450–8.
18. Bowen JD, Larson EB. Drug-induced cognitive impairment. Defining the problem and finding solutions. *Drugs Aging* 1993;3:349–57.
19. Iber FL et al. Age-related changes in the gastrointestinal system. Effects on drug therapy. *Drugs Aging* 1994;5:34–48.
20. Gainsborough N et al. The association of age with gastric emptying. *Age Aging* 1993;22:37–40.
21. Russell TL et al. Upper gastrointestinal pH in seventy-nine healthy, elderly, North American men and women. *Pharm Res* 1993;10:187–96.
22. Durnas C et al. Hepatic drug metabolism and aging. *Clin Pharmacokinet* 1990;19:359–89.
23. Roskos KV, Maibach HI. Percutaneous absorption and age. Implications for therapy. *Drugs Aging* 1992;2:432–49.
24. Novak LP. Aging, total body potassium, fat-free mass, and cell mass in males and females between ages 18 and 85 years. *J Gerontol* 1972;27:438–43.
25. Morgan DJ, Bray KM. Lean body mass as a predictor of drug dosage. Implications for drug therapy. *Clin Pharmacokinet* 1994;26:292–307.
26. Rodeheffer RJ et al. Exercise cardiac output is maintained with advancing age in healthy human subjects: cardiac dilatation and increased stroke volume compensate for a diminished heart rate. *Circulation* 1984; 69:208–13.
27. Schumacher GE. Using pharmacokinetics in drug therapy. VII: pharmacokinetic factors influencing drug therapy in the aged. *Am J Hosp Pharm* 1980;37:559–62.
28. Woo J et al. Effect of age and disease on two drug binding proteins: albumin and α-1-acid glycoprotein. *Clin Biochem* 1994;27:289–92.
29. Wallace S et al. Factors affecting drug binding in plasma of elderly patients. *Br J Clin Pharmacol* 1976;3:327–30.
30. Ritschel WA. Drug disposition in the elderly: gerontokinetics. *Methods Find Exp Clin Pharmacol* 1992;14:555–72.
31. Vestal RE et al. Aging and the response to inhibition and induction of theophylline metabolism. *Exp Gerontol* 1993;28:421–33.
32. Lindeman RD. Changes in renal function with aging. Implications for treatment. *Drugs Aging* 1992;2:423–31.
33. Siersbaek-Nielsen K et al. Rapid evaluation of creatinine clearance. *Lancet* 1971;1:1133–4.
34. Cockcroft DW, Gault MH. Prediction of creatinine clearance from serum creatinine. *Nephron* 1976;16:31–41.
35. Campbell AJ. Drug treatment as a cause of falls in old age. A review of the offending agents. *Drugs Aging* 1991;1:289–302.
36. O'Mahony MS, Woodhouse KW. Age, environmental factors and drug metabolism. *Pharmacol Ther* 1994;61:279–87.
37. Roe DA. Medications and nutrition in the elderly. *Prim Care* 1994;21:135–47.
38. Gurwitz JH et al. The exclusion of the elderly and women from clinical trials in acute myocardial infarction. *JAMA* 1992;268:1417–22.
39. Kitler ME. Clinical trials and clinical practice in the elderly. A focus on hypertension. *Drugs Aging* 1992;2:86–94.
40. Zimmer AW et al. Conducting clinical research in geriatric populations. *Ann Intern Med* 1985;103:276–83.
41. Butler RN. The importance of basic research in gerontology. *Age Aging* 1993;22:S53–4.
42. Fraser CG. Age-related changes in laboratory test results. Clinical implications. *Drugs Aging* 1993;3:246–57.
43. Agency for Health Care Policy and Research. Guidelines for pressure ulcer prevention: improving practice and a stimulus for research. *J Gerontol* 1993;48:M3–5.

Renal Disease

Gary R. Matzke

■ DOSAGE REGIMEN OPTIMIZATION FOR PATIENTS WITH RENAL INSUFFICIENCY

Eleven million Americans have early renal insufficiency, defined as a Cr_s ≥ 1.5 mg/dL or Cl_{cr} <70 mL/min; approximately 1 million have concentrations >2 mg/dL.[1] The number of individuals with end-stage renal disease (ESRD) has been increasing at a rate of about 7–9% annually during the past decade.[2]

Reduced renal function can be associated with drug effects, age, or chronic disease states.[3–5] Medical problems can contribute to the development of a patient's initial renal injury, enhance the rate of their progressive decline in renal function, or develop as sequelae of chronic renal disease.[6] Hypertension, diabetes mellitus, infection, bone disease, neurological dysfunction, GI disturbances, and bleeding abnormalities are but a few of the medical conditions frequently encountered in renal failure patients.[7] These patients are often given medications early in the course of their disease in an attempt to slow the rate of decline in renal function and prevent cardiovascular complications. Surveys of dialysis patients have found that they average more than eight scheduled prescription drugs and two or more "prn" drugs.[8–10] Thus, patients with early renal insufficiency and those with ESRD are at increased risk for adverse reactions because of the number of drugs received, concurrent medical problems, and impaired drug excretion.[11–12]

Renal insufficiency in any patient requires that the clinician understand the aspects of drug disposition that are altered and the appropriate methods to individualize drug therapy.[3,5] Complications of drug administration can be minimized by the application of pharmacokinetic and pharmacodynamic principles.[13] The advent of specific and sensitive methods for measuring drug concentrations in biological fluids has resulted in a voluminous literature on drug disposition in renal disease and evaluations of the effects of dialysis.[14–17]

This section provides a conceptual discussion of how renal disease alters drug disposition with selected literature examples. It also describes an approach for determining the individual dosage adjustment necessary to achieve the optimal therapeutic effect with minimal toxicity for a patient with a given degree of renal function. The subsequent section, Dialysis of Drugs, presents the concepts of drug removal by hemodialysis, peritoneal dialysis, and continuous renal replacement therapies that are now frequently used in critically ill patients. Data on the amount of drug removed by dialysis are tabulated and dosage modification schemes for a number of drugs during dialysis are presented.

FOUR BASIC QUESTIONS

A practical approach to drug therapy in patients with renal insufficiency can be arrived at if one considers the following questions:

1. What is the patient's renal function status?
2. What is the degree of alteration in the pharmacokinetics or pharmacodynamics of the patient's drug(s) in the presence of renal insufficiency?
3. What approaches to dosage modification are useful for a specific drug?
4. What is the impact of dialysis on drug disposition, and is dosage modification or supplementation necessary?

QUANTIFYING RENAL FUNCTION

Several common laboratory tests provide an assessment of a patient's renal function: blood urea nitrogen (BUN), serum creatinine (Cr_s), the ratio of BUN to Cr_s, and creatinine clearance (Cl_{cr}).[18] The BUN concentration can change because of many factors in addition to changes in renal function. Urea is filtered and reabsorbed by the nephron, and its renal excretion is a function of urine flow. Diuretic use, dehydration, and bleeding can increase the BUN concentration without a decline in renal function.[18] These conditions usually result in an increased BUN/Cr_s ratio to values above the normal range of 10–15. Creatinine production and elimination in adults are usually constant at approximately 20 mg/kg/day under steady-state conditions.[18] Creatinine is filtered predominantly by the glomerulus with little renal tubular secretion (about 10%) in those with normal renal function. However, secretion becomes an important excretory pathway for patients with a Cl_{cr} <50 mL/min. In these individuals, accurate measurement of Cl_{cr} can be obtained by giving cimetidine before initiating the urine collection because cimetidine inhibits the tubular secretion of creatinine.[19,20]

Because the nonrenal factors that can affect BUN do not alter serum or urine creatinine concentrations, Cr_s and Cl_{cr} serve as better markers of changing renal function. The relationship between Cr_s and Cl_{cr} is a hyperbolic one, as is shown in Figure 2–3. Small increases in Cr_s represent a larger absolute decrease in renal function in subjects with normal renal function than do similar increases in Cr_s in individuals with moderate to severe renal insufficiency. For example, doubling the Cr_s is associated with a halving in Cl_{cr} (ie, as Cr_s changes from 1 to 2 mg/dL, the Cl_{cr} declines from 120 to 60 mL/min, whereas an increase from 2 to 4 mg/dL represents a decrease in Cl_{cr} of 60 to 30 mL/min).

Although Cr_s is easy to determine, requiring collection of only a single blood sample, measurement of Cl_{cr} is more difficult. The standard method consists of a continuous 24-hr urine collection for urine creatinine with a single blood sample for Cr_s at approximately the middle of the urine collection period. The most difficult problem from a practical standpoint is obtaining a complete urine collection. Almost invariably, the urine collection is incomplete and consequently the Cl_{cr} is underestimated. However, the accuracy of the Cl_{cr} and urine collection can be assessed by determining the daily creatinine excretion rate—the amount of creatinine (in mg/day) excreted in the urine during the 24-hr collection period. This can be compared with the expected amount of creatinine to be excreted, which is approximately 20–25 mg/day/kg ideal body weight in males and 15–20 mg/day/kg in females who are age 18–50 yr. Urinary creatinine excretion declines in males and females who are >50 yr.[21] For example, in a 70-kg man, the expected creatinine production and excretion in the urine is approximately 1.4 g/day. If his total creatinine excretion is less than this value, it is likely he did not collect all his urine and

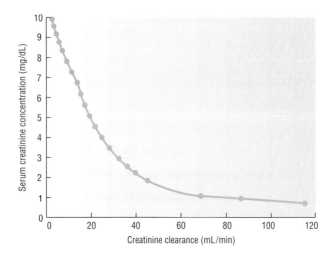

Figure 2–3. Relationship between serum creatinine concentration and creatinine clearance. (Reproduced with permission from DiPiro J et al, eds. *Pharmacotherapy: a pathophysiologic approach,* 4th ed. New York: McGraw-Hill; 1999.)

the calculated Cl_{cr} is an underestimate. The use of this approach is valid only under steady-state conditions when creatinine production and excretion are equivalent.

If it is impractical to measure a patient's Cl_{cr}, it can be estimated from equations based on the patient's age, height, and weight.[18] The most frequently used equation for adults with stable renal function was derived by Cockcroft and Gault.[21] Equations are given for men, women, and children in Appendix 2, Anthropometrics. These equations assume steady-state serum creatinine values and do not provide valid Cl_{cr} estimates in patients with fluctuating renal function or those receiving dialysis of any type. The advantages and disadvantages of the several methods for Cl_{cr} estimation in patients with changing renal function have been reviewed recently.[18]

■ PHARMACOKINETIC/PHARMACODYNAMIC ALTERATIONS OF DRUGS IN RENAL FAILURE

Decreased renal function can alter the absorption, distribution, protein binding, metabolism, or excretion of drugs.[3,22] Furthermore, the pharmacodynamic effects of a drug can be different in patients with renal insufficiency because of biochemical or pathophysiologic changes associated with renal disease. The bioavailability of drugs can be altered in symptomatic (uremic) patients because of GI disturbances such as nausea, vomiting, and diarrhea, increased gastric pH because of the ingestion of histamine H_2-receptor antagonists, or increased salivary urea concentration as a result of markedly increased BUN (>100–120 mg/dL).[23] This can decrease the absorption of ferrous sulfate and other drugs that are best absorbed from an acidic environment. In addition, patients who routinely take aluminum or calcium antacids might have reduced bioavailability of some drugs because of complexation in the GI tract. Propoxyphene, dihydrocodeine, and some β-blockers might have increased bioavailability because of reduced first-pass metabolism.[24–26]

The plasma protein binding of some drugs is altered in patients with severe renal insufficiency. This might be secondary to hypoalbuminemia; accumulation of acidic byproducts of uremia resulting in competitive displacement of drugs from binding sites; or changes in the structure of albumin resulting in a decreased number of effective binding sites.[3,22,27] Most weak organic acid drugs, such as cefazolin, phenytoin, salicylate, valproic acid, and warfarin, exhibit decreased plasma protein binding (increased free fraction). Weak organic basic drugs might have decreased or unchanged binding. The protein binding of carbamazepine, dapsone, diazepam, and morphine is decreased, whereas the binding of propranolol, quinidine, verapamil, and trimethoprim is unchanged. Propranolol and lidocaine are bound primarily to α_1-acid glycoprotein from which little displacement occurs in renal disease or hypoalbuminemia. If the protein binding of a drug is decreased, the patient can experience an increased pharmacodynamic effect, an increased V_d, and increased or unchanged total body clearance depending on whether it is a high or low extraction ratio drug.

Phenytoin has altered protein binding and disposition in ESRD patients that results in important differences in dosage.[28] The percentage of unbound phenytoin in plasma is normally 10% but increases to 20 to 35% in ESRD patients. This results in an increase in the V_d from 0.65 L/kg in those with normal kidney function to 1–1.8 L/kg in ESRD patients. Further, the terminal half-life is decreased from 11–16 hr to 6–10 hr and the apparent plasma clearance increases from 28–41 mL/hr/kg to 64–225 mL/hr/kg in ESRD patients compared with those with normal renal function. These changes in the pharmacokinetics of phenytoin result in a change in its therapeutic concentration range. In patients with normal kidney function, the usual therapeutic plasma concentration range for total phenytoin (unbound plus bound) is 10–20 mg/L; in those with ESRD, the range is approximately 4–8 mg/L. Both ranges of total drug represent the same concentration of unbound drug, 1–2 mg/L.

The V_d of drugs can be increased, decreased, or unchanged in renal failure patients.[3,22,27] An increase in V_d could be due to decreased protein binding, fluid overload secondary to reduced renal excretion, or increased tissue binding. A decrease in V_d could be due to decreased tissue binding or increased protein binding. Examples of drugs with increased V_d are cefazolin, furosemide, gentamicin, naproxen, phenytoin, and vancomycin. Digoxin exhibits a decreased V_d in renal impairment, whereas minoxidil and procainamide are drugs whose V_d does not change markedly in ESRD.

Drugs are eliminated from the body by two primary pathways: renal and nonrenal elimination (predominantly hepatic metabolism).[29] The degree of reduction in renal clearance depends on the percentage of drug excreted unchanged by the kidney. The influence of renal function is very important for aminoglycosides, cephalosporins, penicillins, vancomycin, acyclovir, lithium, and ranitidine, all of which are extensively (>80%) eliminated unchanged renally. For many of these drugs, linear correlations have been established between the drug's plasma and renal clearance and Cl_{cr}.[17,27] These correlations can be used as guides to project the drug dosage requirement for those with a given degree of renal insufficiency. For example, the linear correlation between gentamicin plasma clearance and Cl_{cr} demonstrates that the clearance of gentamicin can change from 120 mL/min with normal renal function to as little as 2 mL/min in ESRD. The half-life of gentamicin in ESRD is markedly prolonged (range 40–60 hr) compared with the 1–2 hr values of patients with normal renal function. This relationship then can be used to determine the desired maintenance dosage of gentamicin in patients with different degrees of renal insufficiency, as outlined later in this chapter.

Drug metabolism typically involves enzymatic conversion of drugs to more water-soluble compounds. These metabolites are formed through the processes of oxidation, reduction, synthesis (eg, conjugation), or hydrolysis. Once formed, these metabolites often are excreted predominantly by the kidney.[27,29] Most metabolites are inactive or have minimal pharmacologic activity. However, some active metabolites might accumulate, especially in ESRD patients, and lead to exaggerated pharmacodynamic responses that warrant dosage reduction. Active metabolites that are excreted by the kidney include oxypurinol from allopurinol, which is an active inhibitor of xanthine oxidase; desacetylcefotaxime from cefotaxime, which is microbiologically active; normeperidine from meperidine, which can cause seizures; and N-acetylprocainamide from procainamide, which has its own unique antiarrhythmic properties.[27]

Renal insufficiency also can lead to alterations in drug metabolism.[30,31] Animal experiments indicate that the activity of many drug metabolic pathways is reduced in the presence of renal insufficiency by up to 70%.[32,33] The decrement in enzyme activity is larger in the animals with the most severe renal dysfunction. The nonrenal clearance of several drugs is decreased in ESRD.[3,27] For example, the antiviral agent acyclovir and the antihypertensive agent captopril demonstrate 50% decreases in nonrenal clearance in patients with ESRD.[34,35] As a consequence, the elimination half-life for both drugs is increased 6-fold in the presence of renal failure. This shows that predictions of the disposition of drugs in renal failure based on general principles and nomograms are subject to considerable error if one assumes that nonrenal clearance is unaffected by renal disease.

The pharmacodynamics of a drug also can be altered in ESRD and result in the pharmacologic effects being different from those one would expect in patients with normal renal function. One well-defined example is that of nifedipine, where marked differences in E_{max} (maximal change in diastolic blood pressure) were observed. The average E_{max} values were 12 and 29% in healthy controls and ESRD patients, respectively.[36,37] Thus, at the same plasma concentration of unbound nifedipine, a greater blood pressure reduction occurs in patients with renal insufficiency.

■ DOSAGE ADJUSTMENT APPROACHES THAT ARE USEFUL AND PRACTICAL FOR SPECIFIC DRUGS

The general approaches for dosage adjustments of drugs in renal insufficiency are to (1) decrease the dose and maintain the usual dosage interval, (2) lengthen the dosage interval and maintain the usual dose, or (3) modify the dose and interval. The primary goal of these approaches is to provide average steady-state plasma concentrations or AUCs in renal insufficiency similar to those in normal kidney function. The choice of approach depends on the type of drug and the desirability, from a therapeutic or toxic standpoint, of having small or large peak-to-trough fluctuations.[38,39] Other considerations are that the dosage regimen adjustment should be practical and the reduced dose or prolonged dosage interval should be relatively easy to implement.[14,27]

When presented with a patient with renal insufficiency for whom drug dosage regimen decisions must be made, the most practical and efficient approach is to first consult published tables or guidelines that provide a quick reference source for drug dosage in renal failure.[14] Additional sources are the appendices of *Handbook of Drug Therapy in Liver and Kidney Disease*[29] and "Use of Drugs in Renal Failure" in *Diseases of the Kidney*,[40] which describe specific pharmacokinetic alterations of drugs in kidney disease, recommended dosage regimens, and tabulate the effects of dialysis. The reader also is advised to refer to specific drug monographs in this book and in *AHFS Drug Information*,[41] which briefly describe the effect of renal failure on drug disposition and provide initial dosage recommendations. These sources allow the user to determine whether dosage adjustments are necessary and if there are any important toxicities or precautions in using a particular drug. These sources, however, provide only general guidelines.

For drugs requiring marked dosage adjustment in renal insufficiency or for which the achievement of specific therapeutic plasma concentrations is critical, the reader should consult the original publications, which provide specific data on individual drugs. Consulting the original publications or authoritative reviews will provide details regarding the relationship of renal function to drug elimination and can provide a dosage nomogram or specific dosage recommendations and precautions for the use of the drug in patients with various degrees of renal insufficiency.[17]

If drug-specific data or guidelines are not available, one can use general dosage equations such as those developed by Rowland and Tozer.[42] Only basic pharmacokinetic information about the drug is needed—primarily the fraction of the available dose that is normally excreted unchanged in the urine, f_e. The fraction of normal renal function (KF) in a given patient is determined as the ratio of the patient's Cl_{cr} to the accepted normal value of 120 mL/min. The patient's Cl_{cr} can be determined from Cr_s values at steady state with the method of Cockcroft and Gault.[21]

The following equation, which takes into consideration the renal clearance and extrarenal clearance of unbound drug, can be used to determine the dosage adjustment factor, Q:[42]

$$Q = \frac{[(KF \times f_e) + [1 - f_e] \times [(140 - age) \times weight\ in\ kg^{0.7}]}{1660}$$

Q is analogous to the ratio of the unbound drug clearance of the patient to that observed in those with a $Cl_{cr} \geq 120$ mL/min, or $[Cl_u$ (failure)/Cl_u (normal)]. If a drug is minimally protein bound (<25%) and not extensively metabolized ($f_e \geq 70\%$), this equation can be simplified to:[5]

$$Q = 1 - [f_e(1 - KF)]$$

Once the value of Q is obtained, the dosage regimen adjustment can be made with the following equations and scenarios:

$$D_{RI} = Q \times D_N$$

where D_{RI} is the maintenance dose in the renally insufficient patient that is to be given at the normal dosage interval and D_N is the normal dose for those with Cl_{cr} ≥ 120 mL/min.

$$\tau_{RI} = \frac{\tau_N}{Q}$$

where τ_{RI} is the maintenance dosage interval for the renally insufficient patient at which the D_N is the dose to be given and τ_N is the dosage interval for those with $Cl_{cr} \geq 120$ mL/min.

The final scenario incorporates a modification of D_N and τ_N. This scenario usually is used when the calculated D_{RI} or τ_{RI} are impractical. In that situation, one chooses a clinically relevant "τ_{RI}" and calculates the D_{RI} to be given at that time.

$$D_{RI} = \frac{[D_N \times Q \times "\tau_{RI}"]}{\tau_N}$$

An example will clarify the use of this approach. An 80-kg, 45-yr-old man with a Cr_s of 5.4 mg/dL requires treatment with ceftazidime for a pseudomonal infection. This drug is 70% excreted unchanged in the urine, and the usual dosage is 1 g q 8 hr IV. With the equation of Cockcroft and Gault, the patient's Cl_{cr}, KF, and Q are calculated as follows:

$$Cl_{cr} = \frac{(140 - 45) \times 80}{(5.4 \times 72)} = 20 \text{ mL/min}$$

$$KF = \frac{20 \text{ mL/min}}{120 \text{ mL/min}} = 0.17$$

$$Q = (0.17 \times 0.7) + (1 - 0.7)$$
$$= 0.120 + 0.3$$
$$= 0.43$$

If the maintenance dose for this patient was reduced and the dosage interval maintained every 8 hr, the D_{RI} would be:

$$D_{RI} = 0.43 \times D_N$$
$$= 430 \text{ mg q 8 hr}$$

This regimen will result in reduced peak and increased trough concentrations relative to subjects with normal renal function receiving the standard dose. The average concentration would, however, be the same.

Alternatively, one might extend the dosage interval and maintain the standard dose size (D_N). This will produce the same peak and trough concentrations for the renal patient that one would expect in a patient with $Cl_{cr} \geq 120$ mL/min. Unfortunately, the use of nonstandard dosage intervals often has been associated with drug administration errors.

$$\tau_{RI} = \frac{\tau_N}{Q} = \frac{8}{0.43} = 18.6 \text{ hr}$$

In this example and many patient scenarios, the best dosage adjustment strategy might be to select a feasible prolonged dosage interval ("τ_{RI}"), eg, 12 hr, and then calculate the D_{RI}.

$$D_{RI} = \frac{[D_N \times Q \times \text{"}\tau_{RI}\text{"}]}{\tau_N} = \frac{[1000 \text{ mg} \times 0.43 \times 12]}{8} = 650 \text{ mg}$$

This general approach provides a reasonable initial method for adjusting drug dosage regimens in patients with renal insufficiency until more specific guidelines can be consulted or serum concentrations are measured. This method is based on several assumptions: (1) bioavailability is unchanged in renal failure; (2) metabolites are not therapeutically active or toxic; (3) decreased renal function does not alter metabolism of the drug; (4) metabolism or renal excretion does not exhibit concentration-dependent pharmacokinetics; (5) renal function is constant with time; and (6) the renal clearance of the drug is directly proportional to the renal clearance of the compound used to measure renal function. If any of these assumptions is invalid, the accuracy of the projected dosage regimen will be reduced.

The time to reach steady state is longer for a patient with renal insufficiency than one with normal renal function. Consequently, it is common to initiate therapy for many drugs with a loading dose (ie, at least the D_N and in some cases an even greater dose) to achieve the desired concentration in the expanded V_d and/or shorten the time to reach a therapeutic plasma concentration. The amount of the loading dose depends on the particular drug being used and the desired therapeutic objectives.

It should be noted that any dosage regimen modification for renally insufficient patients might require plasma concentration determinations of the drug, if available, and close clinical observation for assessment of toxicity and verification of achievement of the desired therapeutic serum concentrations or effects.

■ REFERENCES

1. Jones CA et al. Serum creatinine levels in the US population: Third National Health and Nutrition Examination Survey. *Am J Kidney Dis* 1998; 32:992–9.
2. US Renal Data System. *1998 Annual data report.* Bethesda: National Institutes of Diabetes and Digestive and Kidney Diseases; 1998:40.
3. Lam YW et al. Principles of drug administration in renal insufficiency. *Clin Pharmacokinet* 1997;32:30–57.
4. Sloan RW. Principles of drug therapy in geriatric patients. *Am Fam Phys* 1992;45:2709–18.

5. Matzke GR, Millikin SM. Influence of renal disease and dialysis on pharmacokinetics. In: Evans WE et al, eds. *Applied pharmacokinetics: principles of therapeutic drug monitoring.* 3rd ed. Spokane: Applied Therapeutics; 1992.

6. *NIH Publication 97.* Bethesda: National Institutes of Diabetes and Digestive and Kidney Diseases; 1997:3925.

7. St. Peter WL, Lewis MJ. Chronic renal insufficiency and end-stage renal disease. In, DiPiro J et al, eds. *Pharmacotherapy: a pathophysiologic approach.* 4th ed. Stamford, CT: Appleton & Lange; 1999:732–70.

8. Cleary DJ et al. Medication knowledge and compliance among patients receiving long-term dialysis. *Am J Health Syst Pharm* 1995;52:1895–900.

9. US Renal Data System. *1998 Annual data report.* Bethesda: National Institutes of Diabetes and Digestive and Kidney Diseases; 1998:51–62.

10. Kaplan B et al. Chronic hemodialysis patients. Part I: characterization and drug-related problems. *Ann Pharmacother* 1994;28:316–9.

11. Smith JW et al. Studies on the epidemiology of adverse drug reactions. V. Clinical factors influencing susceptibility. *Ann Intern Med* 1966;65:629–40.

12. Jick H. Adverse drug effects in relation to renal function. *Am J Med* 1977;62:514–7.

13. Matzke GR, Frye RF. Drug administration in patients with renal insufficiency: minimising renal and extrarenal toxicity. *Drug Saf* 1997;16:205–31.

14. Aronoff GR et al. *Drug prescribing in renal failure: dosing guidelines for adults.* 4ᵗʰ ed. Philadelphia: American College of Physicians; 1999.

15. Bennett WM. Guide to drug dosage in renal failure. In, Holford NHG, ed. *Drug data handbook.* 3rd ed. Auckland: ADIS International; 1998:49–119.

16. Benet LZ et al. Design and optimization of dosage regimens: pharmacokinetic data. In, Hardman JG et al, eds. *Goodman and Gilman's the pharmacological basis of therapeutics.* 9th ed. New York: McGraw-Hill; 1996:1707–9.

17. St. Peter W et al. Clinical pharmacokinetics of antibiotics in patients with impaired renal function. *Clin Pharmacokinet* 1992;22:169–210.

18. Comstock TJ. Assessment of renal function. In, DiPiro J et al, eds. *Pharmacotherapy: a pathophysiologic approach.* 4th ed. Stamford, CT: Appleton & Lange; 1999:686–705.

19. Roubenoff R et al. Oral cimetidine improves the accuracy and precision of creatinine clearance in lupus nephritis. *Ann Intern Med* 1990;113:501–6.

20. Zaltzman JS et al. Accurate measurement of impaired glomerular filtration using single-dose oral cimetidine. *Am J Kidney Dis* 1996;27:504–11.

21. Cockcroft, DW, Gault MH. Prediction of creatinine clearance from serum creatinine. *Nephron* 1976; 16:31–41.

22. Gambertoglio JG. Effects of renal disease: altered pharmacokinetics. In, Benet LZ et al, eds. *Pharmacokinetic basis for drug treatment.* New York: Raven Press; 1984:149–71.

23. Dressman JB et al. Gastrointestinal parameters that influence oral medications. *J Pharm Sci* 1993;82:857–72

24. Bianchetti G et al. Pharmacokinetics and effects of propranolol in terminal uraemic patients and in patients undergoing regular dialysis treatment. *Clin Pharmacokinet* 1976;1:373–84.

25. Gibson TP et al. Propoxyphene and norpropoxyphene plasma concentrations in the anephric patient. *Clin Pharmacol Ther* 1980;27:665–70.

26. Barnes JNet al. Dihydrocodeine in renal failure: further evidence for an important role of the kidney in the handling of opioid drugs. *Br Med J* 1985;290:740–2.

27. Frye RF, Matzke GR. Drug therapy individualization for patients with renal insufficiency. In, DiPiro J et al, eds. *Pharmacotherapy: a pathophysiologic approach.* 4th ed. Stamford, CT: Appleton & Lange; 1999:872–89.

28. Flaherty JF et al. Neuropsychiatric drugs. In, Schrier RW, Gambertoglio JG, eds. *Handbook of drug therapy in liver and kidney disease.* Boston: Little, Brown; 1991.

29. Schrier RW, Gambertoglio JG, eds. *Handbook of drug therapy in liver and kidney disease.* Boston: Little, Brown; 1991.

30. Elston AC et al. Effect of renal failure on drug metabolism by the liver. *Br J Anaesth* 1993;71:282–90.

31. Touchette MA, Slaughter RL. The effect of renal failure on hepatic drug clearance. *DICP* 1991;25:1214–24.

32. Patterson SE, Cohn VH. Hepatic drug metabolism in rats with experimental chronic renal failure. *Biochem Pharmacol* 1984;33:711–6.

33. Leblond FA, et al. Decreased in vivo metabolism of drugs in chronic renal failure. *Drug Metab Disp* 2000;28: 1317–20.

34. Laskin OL et al. Acyclovir kinetics in end-stage renal disease. *Clin Pharmacol Ther* 1982;31:594–600.

35. Duchin KL et al. Elimination kinetics of captopril in patients with renal failure. *Kidney Int* 1984;25:942–7.

36. Kleinbloesem CH et al. Nifedipine. Relationship between pharmacokinetics and pharmacodynamics. *Clin Pharmacokinet* 1987;12:12–29.

37. Kleinbloesem CH. Nifedipine: influence of renal function on pharmacokinetic/hemodynamic relationship. *Clin Pharmacol Ther* 1985;37:563–74.

38. Kays MB. Comparison of five β-lactam antibiotics against common nosocomial pathogens using the time above MIC at different creatinine clearances. *Pharmacotherapy* 1999;19:1392–9.
39. Craig WA. Pharmacokinetic/pharmacodynamic parameters: rationale for antibacterial dosing of mice and men. *Clin Infect Dis* 1998;26:1–12.
40. Gambertoglio JG et al. Use of drugs in patients with renal failure. In, Schrier RW, Gottschalk CW, eds. *Diseases of the kidney*. Boston: Little, Brown; 1993:3211–68.
41. McEvoy GK, ed. *AHFS drug information*. Bethesda: American Society of Health-System Pharmacists; 2001.
42. Rowland M, Tozer TN. *Clinical pharmacokinetics, concepts and applications*. 2nd ed. Philadelphia: Lea & Febiger; 1989. p. 238–54.

■ DIALYSIS OF DRUGS

DIALYSIS REMOVAL OF DRUGS AND DOSAGE SUPPLEMENTATION

In the United States, more than 250,000 patients with ESRD receive chronic maintenance hemodialysis or continuous ambulatory or cycling peritoneal dialysis. Further, 8000–10,000 patients each year receive a kidney transplant.[1] Therapeutic advances in immunosuppressive drugs and dialysis techniques have increased survival, and a reasonable quality of life is now possible for many patients with ESRD. These patients are managed primarily with hemodialysis, but the use of continuous ambulatory and/or continuous cycling peritoneal dialysis is now common. Although the purpose of dialysis is to remove unwanted toxic waste products from the body, it also removes many pharmacotherapeutic agents. Thus, it is important to know to what extent a drug is removed by dialysis because this can affect the patient's therapy.[2] Supplemental doses or a revised dosage regimen might be required if the dialysis procedure markedly augments the patient's clearance of the drug. Dialysis procedures, including hemoperfusion, also have been used in drug overdose situations as a means of enhancing drug removal from the body. Therefore, it is important to consider how effective these procedures are and whether they offer any substantial advantage over conventional means of treating overdoses.[3–5]

The objectives of this section are to review those drug and dialysis prescription factors that affect the efficiency of the removal of drugs by dialysis. The impact of hemodialysis on the disposition of a drug can be quantified by direct measurement of the clearance by the dialyzer.[2,6] This provides the most accurate assessment of dialyzability and requires one to assay the dialysate and/or obtain multiple blood samples. Alternatively, one can assess the clearance or half-life during dialysis just by collecting 2–3 blood samples. These pharmacokinetic data can be used to estimate the fraction of the drug removed by dialysis from the patient during the dialysis procedure.[7,8]

Peritoneal dialysis is a much less efficient means of removing waste products and drugs than hemodialysis.[9–11] The additional clearance provided by this mode of dialysis is only of clinical significance for a few agents: aminoglycosides, some antifungals, phenobarbital, theophylline, and vancomycin.[12] In contrast, the continuous renal replacement therapies, which are frequently used in critically ill patients, can dramatically alter disposition of many drugs used in the acute care setting.[13,14] These therapies are now widely used and employ hemofilters that are made of the same materials as hemodialyzers. Thus, the dialyzer filter factors, which influence drug removal, are similar. However, the patient factors are not affected as dramatically because these patients usually have some residual renal function.[15]

DETERMINANTS OF DRUG DIALYZABILITY

The Dialysis Prescription.   The literature on drug dialyzability dates back to the early 1970s. Since then there have been several marked improvements in hemodialysis therapy.[16] The blood and dialysate flow rates, two of the primary determinants of the removal of uremic waste products and drug, have increased from 200–300 and ~500 mL/min in the 1970s and much of the 1980s to 400–600 and ~700–1000 mL/min in the 1990s. As a result, the clearance of many drugs has been markedly increased. Further, in the 1990s, a major shift in the composition of dialyzer membranes occurred. Before the 1990s, >80% of ESRD patients were dialyzed with conventional dialyzers: cellulose, cuprophane, or slightly modified cellulose filters. By 2000, >75% of ESRD patients received hemodialysis with semisynthetic or synthetic dialyzers: polysulfone, polymethylmethacrylate, polyamide, or cellulose triacetate.[17] The clearance of waste products, BUN, creatinine, and all drugs evaluated to date are much higher than reported in the literature.[6,18] In fact, some drugs such as vancomycin, which was not dialyzable with conventional dialyzers, is now highly dialyzable with these new filters.[19–21] For other agents such as the aminoglycosides and cephalosporins, increases in clearance of 200 to 300% are common.[18,22]

In light of these dramatic improvements in hemodialysis, earlier data might no longer be applicable. Thus, one must accurately document what dialyzer is used, what the blood and dialysate flow rates are, and the duration of the dialysis procedure. With this information, one can begin the literature search for data on dialyzer clearance of the drugs of concern. If only older, conventional data are available, it will be necessary to extrapolate to the current situation, usually resulting in an increase in the projected impact of hemodialysis.

Pharmacokinetic Factors.   Certain drug properties can help predict drug dialyzability.[23–25] Drugs with low molecular weights, usually <500 d, cross conventional dialysis membranes readily. Large-molecular-weight drugs, such as vancomycin (MW 1449) and amphotericin B (MW 924), cross those membranes poorly and are not effectively removed by conventional hemodialysis. The use of semisynthetic and synthetic dialyzers, however, allows for removal of large-molecular-weight compounds such as vancomycin and has been associated with marked increases in the clearance of low-molecular-weight agents.

Drugs with high water solubility are removed more easily to the aqueous dialysate than more lipid-soluble compounds. In addition, the latter usually have a larger V_d than more water-soluble drugs. Drugs such as digoxin or tricyclic antidepressants, which have V_d >5–7 L/kg, are usually minimally removed by dialysis because the majority of drug is contained in tissue compartments rather than in the blood, and the drug in these tissues is not as readily accessible for removal. A large V_d and slow transport between tissue and blood also can limit the use of hemodialysis and hemoperfusion.[3,4] Although one can rapidly clear the blood compartment of a drug (shown by a dramatic decrease in plasma concentrations once the procedure has ended), plasma drug concentrations can increase (rebound) as a result of re-equilibration of drug from tissue stores.

Plasma protein binding of a drug also determines how effectively it can be dialyzed.[25] Drugs with a high degree of protein binding, such as propranolol (90–94%) and warfarin (99%), are poorly removed by dialysis because the drug–protein complex is too large to cross all dialysis membranes. This is not a limitation of hemoperfusion because the drug is removed from plasma proteins as the complex passes through the high surface area absorbent material.[4]

LITERATURE EVALUATION PITFALLS

Several problems are encountered when attempting to assess the literature on removal of drugs by dialysis.[2,26] First, for some drugs, only anecdotal reports are available. This is primarily true in the overdose setting in which the effect of dialysis on drug removal often is determined primarily by clinical response.[3,5] For example, a comatose patient awakens during or shortly after dialysis and it is assumed that dialysis removed the drug, accounting for the improved clinical status. Second, the amount of drug ingested and/or the amount of drug recovered in the dialysate often is unknown. Third, the type of dialysis system employed is frequently not specified—this is extremely important when comparing the patient's dialysis prescription with published data. Advances in dialysis technology make much of the data evaluating conventional methods inapplicable. Fourth, there often is a lack of patient data, such as weight, hematocrit, and renal and liver function. Fifth, the method used to calculate drug clearance often is unspecified. For example, was clearance determined from the amount of drug recovered in the dialysate or from differences in arterial and venous plasma concentrations across the dialyzer? The proper method for clearance calculations in hemodialysis has been described.[2,6,27]

A common error is misinterpretation of plasma drug concentrations obtained before and after dialysis. Declining plasma concentrations during dialysis often are believed to be the result of the dialysis procedure. However, a declining concentration might be due to drug elimination by metabolism or renal excretion, and the contribution of dialysis to this decline might be very small. The situation in which drug concentrations are relatively unchanged during dialysis usually means that little or no drug is being removed by dialysis. However, the drug might continue to be absorbed from the GI tract as dialysis is being carried out, as in the delayed and prolonged absorption observed in drug overdose.[3] Another problem is interpreting drug removal rate by dialysis. If 200 mg of a drug was removed in the first hour of dialysis, one might assume that 5 hr of dialysis would remove 5 times as much (ie, 1000 mg). This is incorrect because drug removal by dialysis occurs by a first-order process; as the amount of drug in the body declines, so does the amount removed per hour. Thus, the total amount removed is less than that calculated from the initial estimates.

For many drugs, there is a lack of correlation between plasma drug concentration and clinical response. Some drugs have been found to have active or toxic metabolites that correlate well with the toxic effects of the drug.[3] In attempting to collect information on dialysis removal of drugs, attention must be given to metabolites as well. In the overdose and critically ill patients, the pharmacokinetic disposition of a drug can be altered.[3] In making predictions of drug dialyzability, pharmacokinetic data are usually derived from healthy subjects receiving therapeutic dosages. However, in critically ill patients, especially those who have ingested an overdose, there might be changes in drug metabolism, V_d, or protein binding. For example, large amounts of drug in the body might saturate plasma protein binding, which in turn might alter drug distribution and metabolism.

ESTIMATION OF THE IMPACT OF DIALYSIS

The clearance of a drug by dialysis can be compared with the clearance of the drug by the body because clearance terms are additive:

$$Cl_{TD} = Cl_T + Cl_D$$

where

$$Cl_{TD} = \text{total body clearance of drug during dialysis}$$
$$Cl_T = \text{patient's residual total body clearance of drug}$$
$$Cl_D = \text{dialysis clearance of drug}$$

If dialysis clearance adds substantially to total body clearance, thereby forming a much larger total clearance, then the drug will be eliminated that much faster. For example, if the dialysis clearance of a drug is 50 mL/min and the body clearance is 50 mL/min, then the drug would be eliminated from the body twice as fast during the dialysis period. To relate clearance to drug half-life ($t_{1/2}$), the following equations are useful:

$$t_{1/2} \text{ (off dialysis)} = \frac{0.693 \times V_d}{Cl_T}$$

$$t_{1/2} \text{ (on dialysis)} = \frac{0.693 \times V_d}{Cl_T + Cl_D}$$

The more the dialysis clearance adds to the patient's residual total body clearance, the shorter the drug half-life will be on dialysis (assuming V_d remains constant). Another extension of this allows one to calculate the faction of the drug in the body that is lost during a dialysis period.

$$\text{Fraction Lost} = 1 - e^{-(Cl_T + Cl_D)(\tau_d / V_d)}$$

where τ_d is the duration of the dialysis period.

    This calculation represents the fraction of drug in the body that is lost during a dialysis period by all routes of elimination (ie, dialysis, metabolism, and renal excretion). It is necessary to acquire from literature sources (keeping in mind the limitations discussed previously) values for V_d, Cl_T, and Cl_D. If renal or liver function is diminished, this must be taken into consideration because it will result in a lower Cl_T. In addition, changes in V_d in certain disease states (eg, the decreased V_d of digoxin in renal failure) also must be taken into account.

    Clearance data are not always available in the literature. Many reports, especially those published in the 1970s and 1980s, contain only the half-lives of the drugs, on and off dialysis.[28] The following equation can be used to estimate the fraction of drug removed by dialysis alone with half-life data:[8]

$$f = \frac{\left[t_{\frac{1}{2}(\text{off})} - t_{\frac{1}{2}(\text{on})} \right] \times (1 - e^{([0.693/t_{\frac{1}{2}(\text{on})}] \times \tau)})}{t_{\frac{1}{2}(\text{off})}}$$

where

f = fraction of drug removed by dialysis

$t_{\frac{1}{2}(\text{on})}$ = half-life on dialysis

$t_{\frac{1}{2}(\text{off})}$ = half-life off dialysis

τ_d = duration of dialysis.

The assumptions made when using this equation are that all drug elimination (including dialysis removal) occurs by first-order processes, and dialysis is initiated after the completion of the absorption and distribution phases. The primary limitations of this equation are that inaccurate values of half-lives result in incorrect estimates of drug removal by dialysis and the fact that drugs might be given during dialysis. Because drug concentrations in plasma are higher in the distribution phase, especially for intravenously administered drugs, more drug can be removed by dialysis than one would predict by using this method. As an example, up to 30% of a dose of vancomycin is removed if it is given during the last hour of dialysis.[29] It is important to note the duration of dialysis in relation to the estimate of $t_{\frac{1}{2}(\text{on})}$. For example, if the $t_{\frac{1}{2}(\text{on})}$ is reported as 24 hr, but the dialysis duration is only 4 hr, the half-life value is probably not accurate. Conversely, if the $t_{\frac{1}{2}(\text{on})}$ is reported as 1 hr during a 4-hr dialysis period, the half-life value might be more reliable.

Two examples illustrate the use of pharmacokinetic data to calculate drug clearance during dialysis. Phenobarbital has a V_d of approximately 50 L, a total body clearance of 0.3 L/hr, and a conventional hemodialysis clearance of 4.2 L/hr. The half-life off dialysis is 115 hr and this will decrease to 8 hr during dialysis. Approximately 50% of the drug would be removed from the body during 8 hr of dialysis. As another example, digoxin has a V_d of about 300 L and total body clearance of 2.4 L/hr in an anephric patient. The hemodialysis clearance of digoxin is 1.2 L/hr. Therefore, in this patient, the half-lives of digoxin are 86 hr off dialysis and 58 hr on dialysis. Although this appears to be a substantial decrease in half-life, it means that the patient would have to be dialyzed continuously for 58 hr to remove one-half of the digoxin from the body. The fraction of drug lost during a routine hemodialysis period of 4 hr would be only 5%. Thus, a supplemental dose of digoxin after hemodialysis is not warranted.

USING THE TABLES

Tables 2–1 through 2–4 provide semiquantitative data on selected drugs. An additional authoritative source of information is *Drug Prescribing in Renal Failure: Dosing Guidelines for Adults.*[30] Drugs are classified on the basis of the reported range of drug removal by hemodialysis or derived by using pharmacokinetic parameters taken from the literature using the equations cited previously in the text. Drug removal is intentionally described in a semiquantitative fashion for a number of reasons. First, much of this information changes quite rapidly (eg, as new dialysis techniques are developed). Second, a given value for the amount of drug removed or the dialysis clearance determined in one study might differ from that found in another study because of differences in dialysate or blood flow during dialysis or the duration of the dialysis. The duration of dialysis has become shorter in the past 10 yr. Previously, most conventional hemodialysis runs were 4–6 hr, whereas typical dialysis procedures now lasts 2.5–3 hr. Third, the tables list comments for the clarification of certain points and selected references are provided for more specific information.

**TABLE 2–1. READILY REMOVED BY DIALYSIS
(50–100% WITHIN 1 HEMODIALYSIS SESSION)**

DRUG	TYPE OF DIALYZER[a]	% REMOVED IN N HOURS	REFERENCES
Acyclovir	CONV 1	51–60 in 4–5	32, 33
Amikacin	CONV 1	50 in 6	5
Amoxicillin	CONV 2	64 in 4	64
Cefadroxil	CONV 1	63 in 6–8	35
Cefazolin	SYN 1 and HE	40–60 in 3–4	36,37
Cefmetazole	HE	52–67 in 3	38
Ceftazidime	CONV 2	40–50 in 4	22, 39, 40
	HE	58 in 3	
	SYN2	60–75 in 3	
Cefepime	HE	68 in 3	41, 42
	SYN 1	72 in 3.5	
Cefprozil	HE	55 in 3	43
Clavulanic acid	CONV 2	65 in 4	64
Flucytosine	CONV 1	69 in 4	44
Ganciclovir	CONV 2	60 in 4	45
Gentamicin	CONV 1	30–50 in 4	46–48
	HE	40–45 in 3–4	
	SYN 1	50–60 in 3	
Isepamicin	HE	42–85 in 3	49
Imipenem/cilistatin	CONV 2	55–63 in 4	5
Lithium	CONV 2	61 in 6	50, 51
Methotrexate	SYN 1	60 in 4–6	52
Mezlocillin	CONV 1	62 in 6	53

(continued)

TABLE 2–1. READILY REMOVED BY DIALYSIS
(50–100% WITHIN 1 HEMODIALYSIS SESSION) (*continued*)

DRUG	TYPE OF DIALYZER[a]	% REMOVED IN N HOURS	REFERENCES
Netilmicin	CONV 1	50 in 4	54, 55
	SYN 3	56–62 in 4	
Phenobarbital	CONV 1	36–45 in 6–8	56
	SYN I	51 In 4	
Theophylline	CONV 1	59 in 4	57–61
Tobramycin	CONV 1	40–50 in 4	18, 45, 62
	SYN 2	60–75 in 3	

[a]CONV 1 = conventional with dialyzers that are no longer available; CONV 2 = conventional with currently available dialyzers; HE = high efficiency with cellulose acetate dialyzers CA170 and CA210; SYN 1 = synthetic; polysulfone; SYN 2 = synthetic; polysulfone, polymethylmethacrylate and cellulose triacetate; SYN 3 = synthetic; polyacrylonitrile.

TABLE 2–2. MODERATELY DIALYZABLE
(20–50% WITHIN 1 HEMODIALYSIS SESSION)

DRUG	REFERENCES	DRUG	REFERENCES
Acebutolol	65, 66	Cephradine	5
Allopurinol	5	Cyclophosphamide	84, 85
Acetaminophen	5	Didanosine	86, 87
Ampicillin/sulbactam	67	Enalapril	88
Atenolol	68–70	Ethosuximide	89
Azathioprine	71	Fluconazole	90, 91
Aztreonam	72	Foscarnet	92, 93
Bretylium	73	Lisinopril	88
Cefaclor	74	Lorazepam	94
Cefamandole	5	Methyldopa	5
Cefotaxime	75	Metronidazole	95, 96
Cefoxitin	76	Minoxidil	97
Cefpodoxime	77	Nadolol	5
Ceftizoxime	78	Ofloxacin	98–100
Ceftriaxone	79–81	Omeprazole	101
Cefuroxime	82	Penicillin G	5
Cephalexin	83	Pentoxifylline	102

(*continued*)

**TABLE 2–2. MODERATELY DIALYZABLE
(20–50% WITHIN 1 HEMODIALYSIS SESSION)** (*continued*)

DRUG	REFERENCES	DRUG	REFERENCES
Piperacillin	103–105	Sulfamethoxazole	114
Primidone	106, 107	Ticarcillin	115
Procainamide	108, 109	Tocainide	116
Pyrazinamide	110, 111	Trimethoprim	114
Sotalol	112, 113	Vancomycin	19–21

TABLE 2–3. NOT SIGNIFICANTLY REMOVED BY HEMODIALYSIS

DRUG	REFERENCES	DRUG	REFERENCES
Amantidine	5	Doxepin	131
Amiodarone	117	Doxycycline	5
Amphotericin B	5	Epoetin alfa	132
Astemizole	118	Erythromycin	133
Bleomycin	119	Esmolol	134
Captopril	120	Ethambutol	111
Carbamazepine	121	Ethchlorvynol	5
Cefonicid	5	Etodolac	135
Cefixime	122	Famotidine	136
Cefoperazone	123	Felodipine	137
Chloramphenicol	124, 125	Filgrastim	138
Chloroquine	126	Flecainide	5
Cimetidine	127	Flurbiprofen	139
Ciprofloxacin	128, 129	Furosemide	5
Clindamycin	130	Gemfibrozil	140
Clonidine	5	Glutethimide	5
Colchicine	165	Glyburide	141
Cyclosporine	5	Ibuprofen	142
Diazepam	5	Isoniazid	111
Dicloxacillin	5	Isradipine	143
Digitoxin	5	Itraconazole	144
Digoxin	5	Ketoconazole	145
Disopyramide	5	Labetalol	146

(*continued*)

TABLE 2–3. NOT SIGNIFICANTLY REMOVED BY HEMODIALYSIS (*continued*)

DRUG	REFERENCES	DRUG	REFERENCES
Lidocaine	5	Ranitidine	153
Lomefloxacin	147, 148	Rifampin	111
Meprobamate	5	Rimantadine	154
Methadone	5	Secobarbital	5
Methylprednisolone	5	Sulindac	155
Metoprolol	70	Tacrolimus	156
Miconazole	5	Temazepam	157
Nafcillin	5	Tetracycline	5
Naproxen	5	Thiabendazole	158, 159
Nifedipine	149, 150	Timolol	160
Oxacillin	151	Triazolam	161
Propoxyphene	5	Valproic acid	5
Propranolol	5	Verapamil	162, 163
Quinapril	152	Zidovudine	164
Quinidine	5		

TABLE 2–4. NO DATA

DRUG	DRUG
Alprazolam	Clorazepate
Amitriptyline[a]	Clozapine
Amlodipine	Codeine
Azithromycin[a]	Colchicine
Baclofen	Cytarabine
Betaxolol	Dapsone
Bumetanide	Desipramine
Carteolol	Diltiazem[a]
Chlorpheniramine	Dipyridamole[b]
Chlorpromazine	Dopamine
Chlorpropamide	Ethacrynic acid
Cisplatin	Felbamate
Clarithromycin	Fenoprofen[b]
Clofazimine	Fluorouracil

(*continued*)

TABLE 2–4. NO DATA (*continued*)

DRUG	DRUG
Flurazepam	Penicillamine
Glipizide	Pentamidine[c]
Griseofulvin	Pentazocine
Guanethidine	Phenothiazines
Haloperidol[a]	Phenytoin[b]
Hydralazine	Piroxicam[b]
Hydrochlorothiazide	Pravastatin
Indinavir[b]	Prazepam
Indomethacin	Prazosin
Lamivudine	Prednisone
Levodopa	Primaquine
Lovastatin	Probenecid
Melphalan	Ramipril
Meperidine	Rifabutin[c]
Methaqualone	Ritonavir[b]
Metholazone	Saquinavir[b]
Midazolam[b]	Sargramostin
Milrinone	Simvastatin
Minocycline	Spironolactone
Misoprostol	Stavudine
Morphine	Sulfisoxazole
Muromonab-CD3	Sulindac
Nelfinavir[b]	Tamoxifen
Nevirapine	Tolmetin[b]
Nitrofurantoin	Triamterene
Norfloxacin	Vinblastine[c]
Nortriptyline[a]	Vincristine[c]
Ondansetron	Warfarin[b]
Paromomycin	Zalcitabine

[a]Removal unlikely due to large V_d and high degree of protein binding.
[b]Removal unlikely due to extensive protein binding.
[c]Removal unlikely due to large V_d.

The use of multiple modes of continuous renal replacement therapy in critically ill individuals is increasing. The principles of drug removal for some of the continuous renal replacement therapies are different from those discussed in this section. Therefore, the reader is referred to selected references that provide an introduction to this topic and tabulations of literature data on drug removal.[13,14,31,32]

■ REFERENCES

1. US Renal Data System. *2000 Annual data report*. Bethesda: National Institutes of Diabetes and Digestive and Kidney Diseases; 2000.
2. Matzke GR, Millikin SM. Influence of renal disease and dialysis on pharmacokinetics. In, Evans WE et al, eds *Applied pharmacokinetics: principles of therapeutic drug monitoring*. 3rd ed. Spokane: Applied Therapeutics; 1992.
3. Rosenberg J et al. Pharmacokinetics of drug overdose *Clin Pharmacokinet* 1981;6:161–92.
4. Takki S et al. Pharmacokinetic evaluation of hemodialysis in acute drug overdose. *J Pharmacokinet Biopharm* 1978;6:427–42.
5. Aweeka FT, Gambertoglio JG. Drug overdose and pharmacologic considerations in dialysis. In, Cogan MG, Schoenfeld P, eds. *Introduction to dialysis*. 2nd ed. New York: Churchill Livingstone; 1991.
6. Frye RF, Matzke GR. Drug therapy individualization for patients with renal nsufficiency. In, DiPiro J et al, eds. *Pharmacotherapy: a pathophysiologic approach*. 4th ed. New York: McGraw Hill; 1999:872–89.
7. Gwilt PR. General equation for assessing drug removal by extracorporeal devices. *J Pharm Sci* 1981;70:345–6. Letter.
8. Lee CS. The assessment of fractional drug removal by extracorporeal dialysis. *Biopharm Drug Disp* 1982; 3:165–73.
9. Paton TW et al. Drug therapy in patients undergoing peritoneal dialysis. Clinical pharmacokinetic considerations. *Clin Pharmacokinet* 1985;10:404–25.
10. Keller E. Peritoneal kinetics of different drugs. *Clin Nephrol* 1988;30:(suppl 1):S24–8.
11. Taylor CA et al. Clinical pharmacokinetics during continuous ambulatory peritoneal dialysis. *Clin Pharmacokinet* 1996; 31:293–308.
12. Keane WF et al. Peritoneal dialysis-related peritonitis treatment recommendations. 1993 update. The ad hoc Advisory Committee on Peritonitis Management. International Society for Peritoneal Dialysis. *Perit Dial Int* 1993;13:14–28.
13. Reetze-Bonorden P et al. Drug dosage in patients during continuous renal replacement therapy. Pharmacokinetic and therapeutic considerations. *Clin Pharmacokinet* 1993;24:362–79.
14. Joy M et al. A primer on continuous renal replacement therapy for critically ill patients. *Ann Pharmacother* 1998;32:362–75.
15. Power BM et al. Pharmacokinetics of drugs used in critically ill adults. *Clin Pharmacokinet* 1998; 34:25–56.
16. Matzke GR. Pharmacotherapeutic consequences of recent advances in hemodialysis therapy. *Ann. Pharmacother* 1994;28:512–4.
17. US Renal Data System. *1999 Annual data report*. Bethesda: National Institutes of Diabetes and Digestive and Kidney Diseases; 1999.
18. Matzke GR et al. In-vitro model for tobramycin disposition during hemodialysis with conventional and high flux biocompatible membranes. American Society of Nephrology 33rd Annual Meeting. Toronto, Ontario, Canada. October 10–16, 2000. 286A.
19. Quale JM et al. Removal of vancomycin by high-flux hemodialysis membranes. *Antimicrob Agents Chemother* 1992;36:1424–6.
20. Barth RH, DeVincenzo N. Use of vancomycin in high-flux hemodialysis: experience with 130 courses of therapy. *Kidney Int* 1996;50:929–36.
21. Zoer J et al. Dosage recommendation of vancomycin during haemodialysis with highly permeable membranes. *Pharm World Sci* 1997;19:191–6.
22. Matzke GR et al. In-vitro model for ceftazidime disposition during hemodialysis with conventional and high flux biocompatible membranes. Annual Meeting of the American Association of Pharmaceutical Scientists. Indianapolis, IN. November 1, 2000.
23. Tilstone WJ et al. The use of pharmacokinetic principles in determining the effectiveness of removal of toxins from blood. *Clin Pharmacokinet* 1979;4:23–37.
24. Gibson TP, Nelson HA. Drug kinetics and artificial kidneys. *Clin Pharmacokinet* 1977;2:403–26.
25. Gwilt PR, Perrier D. Plasma protein binding and distribution characteristics of drugs as indices of their hemodialyzability. *Clin Pharmacol Ther* 1978;24:154–61.
26. Benet LZ et al. Design and optimization of dosage regimens: pharmacokinetic data. In, Hardman JG et al, eds. *Goodman and Gilman's the pharmacological basis of therapeutics*. 9th ed. New York: McGraw-Hill; 1996: 1707–9.
27. Lee CS et al. Clearance calculations in hemodialysis: application to blood, plasma, and dialysate measurements for ethambutol. *J Pharmacokinet Biopharm* 1980;8:69–82.
28. Matzke GR, Keane WF. Use of antibiotics in renal failure. In, Peterson PK, Verhoef J, eds. *The antimicrobial agents annual*. Amsterdam: Elsevier; 1986:472–88.

29. Scott MK et al. Effects of dialysis membrane on intradialytic vancomycin administration. *Pharmacotherapy* 1997;17:256–62.

30. Aronoff GR, et al. *Drug prescribing in renal failure: dosing guidelines for adults.* 4th ed. Philadelphia: American College of Physicians; 1999.

31. Kroh UF. Drug administration in critically ill patients with acute renal failure. *New Horizons* 1995; 3:748–59.

32. Bohler J et al. Pharmacokinetic principles during continuous renal replacement therapy: drugs and dosage. *Kidney Int* 1999;56(suppl 72):S24–8.

33. Almond MK et al. Avoiding acyclovir neurotoxicity in patients with chronic renal failure undergoing haemodialysis. *Nephron* 1995;69:428–32.

34. Leikin JB et al. Hemodialysis removal of acyclovir. *Vet Hum Toxicol* 1995;37:233–4.

35. Leroy A et al. Pharmacokinetics of cefadroxil in patients with impaired renal function. *J Antimicrob Chemother* 1982;10(suppl B):39–46.

36. Fogel MA et al. Cefazolin in chronic hemodialysis patients: a safe, effective alternative to vancomycin. *Am J Kidney Dis* 1998;32:401–9.

37. Marx MA et al. Cefazolin as empiric therapy in hemodialysis-related infections: efficacy and blood concentrations. *Am J Kidney Dis* 1998;32:410–4.

38. Halstenson CE et al. Disposition of cefmetazole in healthy volunteers and patients with impaired renal function. *Antimicrob Agents Chemother* 1990;34:519–23.

39. Ohkawa M et al. Pharmacokinetics of ceftazidime in patients with renal insufficiency and in those undergoing hemodialysis. *Chemother* 1985;31:410–6.

40. Matzke GR et al. Cefazolin and ceftazidime clearance during hemodialysis with low and high flux polymethylmethacrylate dialyzers. *J Am Soc Nephrol* 1999;10:193A. Abstract.

41. Barbhaiya RH et al. Pharmacokinetics of cefepime in subjects with renal insufficiency. *Clin Pharmacol Ther* 1990;48:268–76.

42. Schmaldienst S et al. Multiple-dose pharmacokinetics of cefepime in long-term hemodialysis with high-flux membranes. *Eur J Clin Pharmacol* 2000;56:61–4.

43. Shyu WC et al. Pharmacokinetics of cefprozil in healthy subjects and patients with renal impairment. *J Clin Pharmacol* 1991;31:362–71.

44. Christopher TG et al. Hemodialyzer clearances of gentamicin, kanamycin, tobramycin, amikacin, ethambutol, procainamide, and flucytosine, with a technique for planning therapy. *J Pharmacokinetic Biopharm* 1976;4: 427–41.

45. Swan SK et al. Pharmacokinetics of ganciclovir in a patient undergoing hemodialysis. *Am J Kidney Dis* 1991;17:69–72.

46. Matzke GR et al. Hemodialysis elimination rates and clearance of gentamicin and tobramycin. *Antimicrob Agents Chemother* 1984;25:128–30.

47. Agarwal R et al. Heterogeneity in gentamicin clearance between high-efficiency hemodialyzers. *Am J Kidney Dis* 1994;23:47–51.

48. Amin NB et al. Characterization of gentamicin pharmacokinetics in patients hemodialyzed by high-flux polysulfone membranes. *Am J Kidney Dis* 1999;34:222–7.

49. Halstenson CE et al. Isepamicin disposition in subjects with various degrees of renal function. *Antimicrob Agents Chemother* 1991;35:2382–7.

50. Jaeger A et al. When should dialysis be performed in lithium poisoning? A kinetic study in 14 cases of lithium poisoning. *J Toxicol Clin Toxicol* 1993;31:429–47.

51. Leblanc M et al. Lithium poisoning treated by high-performance continuous arteriovenous and venovenous hemodiafiltration. *Am J Kidney Dis* 1996;27:365–72.

52. Wall SM et al. Effective clearance of methotrexate using high-flux hemodialysis membranes. *Am J Kidney Dis* 1996;28:846–54.

53. Brogard JM et al. Pharmacokinetics of mezlocillin in patients with kidney impairment: special reference to hemodialysis and dosage adjustments in relation to renal function. *Chemotherapy* 1982;28:318–26.

54. Halstenson CE et al. Aminoglycoside redistribution phenomenon after hemodialysis: netilmicin and tobramycin. *Int J Clin Pharmacol Ther Toxicol* 1987;25:50–5.

55. Herrero A et al. Pharmacokinetics of netilmicin during hemodialysis: comparison of four artificial kidneys. *Int J Clin Pharmacol Ther Toxicol* 1988;26:605–9.

56. Palmer BF. Effectiveness of hemodialysis in the extracorporeal therapy of phenobarbital overdose. 2000; 36:640–3.

57. Anderson JR et al. Effects of hemodialysis on theophylline kinetics. *J Clin Pharmacol* 1983;23:428–32.

58. Lee CS et al. Comparative pharmacokinetics of theophylline in peritoneal dialysis and hemodialysis. *J Clin Pharmacol* 1983;23:274–80.

59. Slaughter RL et al. Hemodialysis clearance of theophylline. *Ther Drug Monit* 1982;4:191–3.

60. Blouin RA et al. Theophylline hemodialysis clearance. *Ther Drug Monit* 1980;2:221–3.

61. Shannon MW. Comparative efficacy of hemodialysis and hemoperfusion in severe theophylline intoxication. *Acad Emerg Med* 1997;4:674–8.
62. Matzke GR et al. In-vitro model for tobramycin disposition during hemodialysis with low and high flux biocompatible membranes. *J Am Soc Nephrol* 1999;10:193A. Abstract.
63. Mac-Kay MV et al. Drug dosage in end-stage renal disease (ESRD) patients undergoing haemodialysis: a predictive study based on a microcomputer program. *Clin Pharmacokinet* 1993;25:243–57.
64. Davies BE et al. Pharmacokinetics of amoxycillin and clavulanic acid in haemodialysis patients following intravenous administration of Augmentin. *Br J Clin Pharmacol* 1988;26:385–90.
65. Roux A et al. Pharmacokinetics of acebutolol after intravenous bolus administration. *Br J Clin Pharmacol* 1980;9:215–7.
66. Roux A et al. Pharmacokinetics of acebutolol in patients with all grades of renal failure. *Eur J Clin Pharmacol* 1980;17:339–48.
67. Blum RA et al. Pharmacokinetics of ampicillin (2.0 grams) and sulbactam (1.0 grams) coadministered to subjects with normal and abnormal renal function and with end-stage renal disease on hemodialysis. *Antimicrob Agents Chemother* 1989;33:1470–6.
68. Salahudeen AK et al. Atenolol pharmacokinetics in patients on continuous ambulatory peritoneal dialysis. *Br J Clin Pharmacol* 1984;18:457–60.
69. Campese VM et al. Pharmacokinetics of atenolol in patients with chronic hemodialysis or peritoneal dialysis. *J Clin Pharmacol* 1985;25:393–5.
70. Niedermayer W et al. Pharmacokinetics of antihypertensive drugs (atenolol, metoprolol, propranolol and clonidine) and their metabolites during intermittent haemodialysis in humans. *Proc Eur Dial Transplant Assoc* 1978;15:607–9.
71. Schusziarra V et al. Pharmacokinetics of azathioprine under haemodialysis. *Int J Clin Pharmacol Biopharm* 1976;14:298–302.
72. Gerig JS et al. Effect of hemodialysis and peritoneal dialysis on aztreonam pharmacokinetics. *Kidney Int* 1984;26:308–18.
73. Josselson J et al. Bretylium kinetics in renal insufficiency. *Clin Pharmacol Ther* 1983;33:144–50.
74. Spyker DA et al. Pharmacokinetics of cefaclor in renal failure: effects of multiple doses and hemodialysis. *Antimicrob Agents Chemother* 1982;21:278–81.
75. Hasegawa H et al. Pharmacokinetics of cefotaxime in patients undergoing haemodialysis and continuous ambulatory peritoneal dialysis. *J Antimicrob Chemother* 1984;14(suppl B):135–42.
76. Garcia MJ et al. Pharmacokinetics of cefoxitin in patients undergoing hemodialysis. *Int J Clin Pharmacol Biopharm* 1979;17:366–70.
77. Hoffler D et al. Cefpodoxime proxetil in patients with end stage renal failure on hemodialysis. *Infection* 1990;18:157–62.
78. Cutler RE et al. Pharmacokinetics of ceftizoxime. *J Antimicrob Chemother* 1982;10(suppl C):91–7.
79. Losno Garcia R et al. Single-dose pharmacokinetics of ceftriaxone in patients with end-stage renal disease and hemodialysis. *Chemotherapy* 1988;34:261–6.
80. Ti TY et al. Kinetic disposition of intravenous ceftriaxone in normal subjects and patients with renal failure on hemodialysis or peritoneal dialysis. *Antimicrob Agents Chemother* 1984;25:83–7.
81. Gabutti L et al. Clearance of ceftriaxone during haemodialysis using cuprophane, haemophane and polysulfone dialysers. *Eur J Clin Pharmacol* 1997;53:123–6.
82. Sanchez E et al. A new approach to pharmacokinetic parameters: estimation of cefuroxime during haemodialysis. *Biopharm Drug Dispos* 1990;11:107–20.
83. Bailey RR et al. The effect of impairment of renal function and haemodialysis on serum and urine levels of cephalexin. *Postgrad Med J* 1970;(suppl):60–4.
84. Wang LH et al. Clearance and recovery calculations in hemodialysis: application to plasma, red blood cells, and dialysate measurements for cyclophosphamide. *Clin Pharmacol Ther* 1981;29:365–72.
85. Perry JJ et al. Administration and pharmacokinetics of high-dose cyclophosphamide with hemodialysis support for allogeneic bone marrow transplantation in acute leukemia and end-stage renal disease. *Bone Marrow Transplant* 1999;23:839–42.
86. Knupp CA et al. Disposition of didanosine in HIV-seropositive patients with normal renal function or chronic renal failure: influence of hemodialysis and continuous ambulatory peritoneal dialysis. *Clin Pharmacol Ther* 1996;60:535–42.
87. Singlas E et al. Didanosine pharmacokinetics in patients with normal and impaired renal function: influence of hemodialysis. *Antimicrob Agents Chemother* 1992;36:1519–24.
88. Kelly JG et al. Pharmacokinetics of lisinopril, enalapril and enalaprilat in renal failure: effects of haemodialysis. *Br J Clin Pharmacol* 1988;26:781–6.
89. Marbury TC et al. Hemodialysis clearance of ethosuximide in patients with chronic renal disease. *Am J Hosp Pharm* 1981;38:1757–60.

90. Toon S et al. An assessment of the effects of impaired renal function and haemodialysis on the pharmacokinetics of fluconazole. *Br J Clin Pharmacol* 1990;29:221–6.

91. Berl T et al. Pharmacokinetics of fluconazole in renal failure. *J Am Soc Nephrol* 1995;6:242–7.

92. MacGregor RR et al. Successful foscarnet therapy for cytomegalovirus retinitis in an AIDS patient undergoing hemodialysis: rationale for empiric dosing and plasma level monitoring. *J Infect Dis* 1991;164:785–7.

93. Aweeka FT et al. Effect of renal disease and hemodialysis on foscarnet pharmacokinetics and dosing recommendations. *J Acquir Immune Defic Syndr Hum Retrovirol* 1999;20:350–7.

94. Morrison G et al. Effect of renal impairment and hemodialysis on lorazepam kinetics. *Clin Pharmacol Ther* 1984;35:646–52.

95. Kreeft JH et al. Metronidazole kinetics in dialysis patients. *Surgery* 1983;93(1 pt 2):149–53.

96. Lau AH et al. Hemodialysis clearance of metronidazole and its metabolites. *Antimicrob Agents Chemother* 1986;29:235–8.

97. Lowenthal DT, Affrime MB. Pharmacology and pharmacokinetics of minoxidil. *J Cardiovasc Pharmacol* 1980;2(suppl 2):S93–106.

98. Kampf D et al. Multiple dose kinetics of ofloxacin and ofloxacin metabolites in haemodialysis patients. *Eur J Clin Pharmacol* 1992;42:95–9.

99. Dorfler A et al. Pharmacokinetics of ofloxacin in patients on haemodialysis treatment. *Drugs* 1987;34(suppl 1):62–70.

100. Thalhammer F et al. Ofloxacin clearance during hemodialysis: a comparison of polysulfone and cellulose acetate hemodialyzers. *Am J Kidney Dis* 1998;32:642–5.

101. Roggo A et al. The effect of hemodialysis on omeprazole plasma concentrations in the anuric patient: a case report. *Int J Clin Pharmacol Ther Toxicol* 1990;28:115–7.

102. Silver MR, Kroboth PD. Pentoxifylline in end-stage renal disease. *Drug Intell Clin Pharm* 1987;21:976–8.

103. Giron JA et al. Pharmacokinetics of piperacillin in patients with moderate renal failure and in patients undergoing hemodialysis. *Antimicrob Agents Chemother* 1981;19:279–83.

104. Heim KL et al. The effect of hemodialysis on piperacillin pharmacokinetics. *Drug Intell Clin Pharm* 1985;19:455. Abstract.

105. Keller E et al. Single dose kinetics of piperacillin during continuous arteriovenous hemodialysis in intensive care patients. *Clin Nephrol* 1995;43(suppl 1):S20–3.

106. Lee CS et al. Pharmacokinetics of primidone elimination by uremic patients. *J Clin Pharmacol* 1982;22:301–8.

107. Streete JM et al. Clearance of phenylethylmalonamide during haemodialysis of a patient with renal failure. *Ther Drug Monit* 1990;12:281–3.

108. Gibson TP et al. Artificial kidneys and clearance calculations. *Clin Pharmacol Ther* 1976;20:720–3.

109. Low CL et al. Relative efficacy of haemoperfusion, haemodialysis and CAPD in the removal of procainamide and NAPA in a patient with severe procainamide toxicity. *Nephrol Dial Transplant* 1996;11:881–4.

110. Stamatakis G et al. Pyrazinamide and pyrazinoic acid pharmacokinetics in patients with chronic renal failure. *Clin Nephrol* 1988;30:230–4.

111. Malone RS et al. The effect of hemodialysis on isoniazid, rifampin, pyrazinamide, and ethambutol. *Am J Respir Crit Care Med* 1999;159(5 pt 1):1580–4.

112. Tjandramaga TB et al. The effect of end-stage renal failure and haemodialysis on the elimination kinetics of sotalol. *Br J Clin Pharmacol* 1976;3:259–65.

113. Singh SN et al. Sotalol-induced torsades de pointes successfully treated with hemodialysis after failure of conventional therapy. *Am Heart J* 1991;121(2 pt 1):601–2.

114. Nissenson AR et al. Pharmacokinetics of intravenous trimethoprim-sulfamethoxazole during hemodialysis. *Am J Nephrol* 1987;7:270–4.

115. Watson ID et al. Pharmacokinetics of clavulanic acid-potentiated ticarcillin in renal failure. *Ther Drug Monit* 1987;9:139–47.

116. Wiegers U et al. Pharmacokinetics of tocainide in patients with renal dysfunction and during haemodialysis. *Eur J Clin Pharmacol* 1983;24:503–7.

117. Ujhelyi MR et al. Disposition of intravenous amiodarone in subjects with normal and impaired renal function. *J Clin Pharmacol* 1996;36:122–30.

118. Zazgornik J et al. Plasma concentrations of astemizole in patients with terminal renal insufficiency, before, during, and after hemodialysis. *Int J Clin Pharmacol Ther Toxicol* 1986;24:246–8.

119. Crooke ST et al. Bleomycin serum pharmacokinetics as determined by a radioimmunoassay and a microbiologic assay in a patient with compromised renal function. *Cancer* 1977;39:1430–4.

120. Drummer OH et al. The pharmacokinetics of captopril and captopril disulfide conjugates in uraemic patients on maintenance dialysis: comparison with patients with normal renal function. *Eur J clin Pharmacol* 1987;32:267–71.

121. Kandrotas RJ et al. Carbamazepine clearance in hemodialysis and hemoperfusion. *DICP* 1989;23:137–40.

122. Guay DR et al. Pharmacokinetics of cefixime (CL284,635; FK 027) in healthy subjects and patients with renal insufficiency. *Antimicrob Agents Chemother* 1986;30:485–90.

123. Reitberg DP et al. Pharmacokinetics of cefoperazone (2.0 g) and sulbactam (1.0 g) coadministered to subjects with normal renal function, patients with decreased renal function, and patients with end-stage renal disease on hemodialysis. *Antimicrob Agents Chemother* 1988;32:503–9.

124. Blouin RA et al. Chloramphenicol hemodialysis clearance. *Ther Drug Monit* 1980;2:351–4.

125. Slaughter RL et al. Effect of hemodialysis on total body clearance of chloramphenicol. *Am J Hosp Pharm* 1980;37:1083–6.

126. Akintonwa A et al. Hemodialysis clearance of chloroquine in uremic patients. *Ther Drug Monit* 1986; 8:285–7.

127. Ziemniak JA et al. Rebound following hemodialysis of cimetidine and its metabolites. *Am J Kidney Dis* 1984; 3:430–5.

128. Singlas E et al. Pharmacokinetics of ciprofloxacin tablets in renal failure; influence of haemodialysis. *Eur J Clin Pharmacol* 1987;31:589–93.

129. Kowalsky SF et al. Pharmacokinetics of ciprofloxacin in subjects with varying degrees of renal function and undergoing hemodialysis or CAPD. *Clin Nephrol* 1993;39:53–8.

130. Roberts AP et al. Serum and plasma concentrations of clindamycin following a single intramuscular injection of clindamycin phosphate in maintenance haemodialysis patients and normal subjects. *Eur J Clin Pharmacol* 1978;14:435–9.

131. Faulkner RD et al. Hemodialysis of doxepin and desmethyldoxepin in uremic patients. *Artif Organs* 1984;8:151–5.

132. Keen ML. Epoetin alfa—focus on dialyzability. Case study of the anemic patient. *ANNA J* 1995;22:610–3.

133. Kroboth PD et al. Hearing loss and erythromycin pharmacokinetics in a patient receiving hemodialysis. *Arch Intern Med* 1983;143:1263–5.

134. Covinsky JO. Esmolol: a novel cardioselective, titratable, intravenous beta-blocker with ultrashort half-life. *Drug Intell Clin Pharm* 1987;21:316–21.

135. Brater DC. Evaluation of etodolac in subjects with renal impairment. *Eur J Rheumatol Inflamm* 1990; 10:44–55.

136. Echizen H, Ishizaki T. Clinical pharmacokinetics of famotidine. *Clin Pharmacokinet* 1991;21:178–94.

137. Buur T et al. Pharmacokinetics of felodipine in chronic hemodialysis patients. *J Clin Pharmacol* 1991;31:709–13.

138. Shishido K et al. The effects and pharmacokinetics of rhG-CSF on the treatment of neutropenia in patients with renal failure. *Nippon Jinzo Gakkai Shi* 1991;33:973–81.

139. Cefali EA et al. Pharmacokinetic comparison of flurbiprofen in end-stage renal disease subjects and subjects with normal renal function. *J Clin Pharmacol* 1991;31:808–14.

140. Knauf H et al. Gemfibrozil absorption and elimination in kidney and liver disease. *Klin Wochenschr* 1990;68:692–8.

141. Pearson JG et al. Pharmacokinetic disposition of ^{14}C-glyburide in patients with varying renal function. *Clin Pharmacol Ther* 1986;39:318–24.

142. Senekjian HO et al. Absorption and disposition of ibuprofen in hemodialyzed uremic patients. *Eur J Rheumatol Inflamm* 1983;6:155–62.

143. Schonholzer K, Marone C. Pharmacokinetics and dialysability of isradipine in chronic haemodialysis patients *Eur J Clin Pharmacol* 1992;42:231–3.

144. Boelaert J et al. Itraconazole pharmacokinetics in patients with renal dysfunction. *Antimicrob Agents Chemother* 1988;32:1595–7.

145. Daneshmend TK, Warnock DW. Clinical pharmacokinetics of ketoconazole. *Clin Pharmacokinet* 1988;14:13–34.

146. Halstenson CE et al. The disposition and dynamics of labetalol in patients on dialysis. *Clin Pharmacol Ther* 1986;40:462–8.

147. Blum RA et al. Pharmacokinetics of lomefloxacin in renally compromised patients. *Antimicrob Agents Chemother* 1990;34:2364–8.

148. Leroy A et al. Lomefloxacin pharmacokinetics in subjects with normal and impaired renal function. *Antimicrob Agents Chemother* 1990;34:17–20.

149. Martre H et al. Haemodialysis does not affect the pharmacokinetics of nifedipine. *Br J Clin Pharmacol* 1985;20:155–8.

150. Kleinbloesem CH et al. Influence of haemodialysis on the pharmacokinetics and haemodynamic effects of nifedipine during continuous intravenous infusion. *Clin Pharmacokinet* 1986;11:316–22.

151. Bulger RJ et al. Effect of uremia on methicillin and oxacillin blood levels. *JAMA* 1964;187:319–22.

152. Blum RA et al. Pharmacokinetics of quinapril and its active metabolite, quinaprilat, in patients on chronic hemodialysis. *J Clin Pharmacol* 1990;30:938–42.

153. Comstock TJ et al. Ranitidine bioavailability and disposition kinetics in patients undergoing chronic hemodialysis. *Nephron* 1989;52:15–9.

154. Capparelli EV et al. Rimantadine pharmacokinetics in healthy subjects and patients with end-stage renal failure. *Clin Pharmacol Ther* 1988;43:536–41.

155 Ravis WR et al. Pharmacokinetics and dialyzability of sulindac and metabolites in patients with end-stage renal failure. *J Clin Pharmacol* 1993;33:527–34.

156. Venkataramanan R et al. Pharmacokinetics of FK 506: preclinical and clinical studies. *Transplant Proc* 1990;22:52–6.

157. Kroboth PD et al. Effects of end-stage renal disease and aluminum hydroxide of temazepam kinetics. *Clin Pharmacol Ther* 1985;37:453–9.

158. Bauer LA et al. The pharmacokinetics of thiabendazole and its metabolites in an anephric patient undergoing hemodialysis and hemoperfusion. *J Clin Pharmacol* 1982;22:276–80.

159. Schumaker JD et al. Thiabendazole treatment of severe strongyloidiasis in a hemodialyzed patient. *Ann Intern Med* 1978;89(5 pt 1):644–5.

160. Lowenthal DT et al. Timolol kinetics in chronic renal insufficiency. *Clin Pharmacol Ther* 1978;23:606–15.

161. Kroboth PD et al. Effects of end stage renal disease and aluminum hydroxide on triazolam pharmacokinetics. *Br J Clin Pharmacol* 1985;19:839–42.

162. Shah GM, Winer RL. Verapamil kinetics during maintenance hemodialysis. *Am J Nephrol* 1985;5:338–41.

163. Hanyok JJ et al. An evaluation of the pharmacokinetics, pharmacodynamics, and dialyzability of verapamil in chronic hemodialysis patients. *J Clin Pharmacol* 1988;28:831–6.

164. Ostrop NJ et al. The use of antiretroviral agents in patients with renal insufficiency. *AIDS Patient Care STDS* 1999;13:517–26.

165. Ben-Chetrit E et al. Colchicine clearance by high-flux polysulfone dialyzers. *Arthritis Rheum* 1998;41:749–50.

■ GENERAL RECOMMENDATIONS ON IMMUNIZATION*

Recommendations for immunizing infants, children, and adults are based on characteristics of immunobiologics, principles of active and passive immunization, and judgments by public health officials and specialists in clinical and preventive medicine. Benefits and risks are associated with the use of all immunobiologics; *no* vaccine is completely safe or completely effective. Recommendations for immunization practices balance scientific evidence of benefits, costs, and risks to achieve optimal levels of protection against infectious diseases. The recommendations in this chapter describe this balance and attempt to minimize the risks by providing information regarding dose, route, and spacing of immunobiologics, and delineating situations that warrant precautions or contraindicate the use of these immunobiologics. These recommendations are for use only in the United States because vaccines and epidemiologic circumstances often differ in other countries. *Individual circumstances may warrant deviations from these recommendations.* Tables 3–1 and 3–2 list the immunobiologics available in the United States.

■ IMMUNOBIOLOGICS

The specific nature and content of immunobiologics can differ. When immunobiologics against the same infectious agent are produced by different manufacturers, active and inert ingredients in the various products are not always the same. Practitioners are urged to become familiar with the constituents of the various products.

Suspending Fluids. These may be sterile water, saline, or complex fluids containing protein or other constituents derived from the medium or biologic system in which the vaccine is produced (eg, serum proteins, egg antigens, and cell culture–derived antigens).

Preservatives, Stabilizers, Antibiotics. These components of vaccines, antitoxins, and globulins are used to inhibit or prevent bacterial growth in viral cultures

---

*Excerpted from reference 1.

TABLE 3–1. LICENSED VACCINES AND TOXOIDS AVAILABLE IN THE UNITED STATES, BY TYPE AND RECOMMENDED ROUTES OF ADMINISTRATION[a]

VACCINE	TYPE	ROUTE
Adenovirus[b]	Live virus	Oral
Anthrax	Inactivated bacteria	Subcutaneous
Bacillus of Calmette and Guérin (BCG)	Live bacteria	Intradermal/ percutaneous
Cholera	Inactivated bacteria	Subcutaneous, intramuscular, or intradermal[c]
Diphtheria-tetanus-acellular pertussis (DTaP)	Toxoids and inactivated bacterial components	Intramuscular
Diphtheria-tetanus-pertussis (DTP)	Toxoids and inactivated whole bacteria	Intramuscular
DTP–*Haemophilus influenzae* type b conjugate (DTP-Hib)	Toxoids, inactivated whole bacteria, and bacterial polysaccharide conjugated to protein	Intramuscular
Haemophilus influenzae type b conjugate (Hib)[d]	Bacterial polysaccharide conjugated to protein	Intramuscular
Hepatitis A	Inactivated virus	Intramuscular
Hepatitis B	Inactive viral antigen	Intramuscular
Influenza	Inactivated virus or viral components	Intramuscular
Lyme disease	Bacterial lipoprotein	Intramuscular
Japanese encephalitis	Inactivated virus	Subcutaneous
Measles	Live virus	Subcutaneous
Measles-mumps-rubella (MMR)	Live virus	Subcutaneous
Meningococcal	Bacterial polysaccharides of serotypes A/C/Y/W-135	Subcutaneous
Mumps	Live virus	Subcutaneous
Pertussis	Inactivated whole bacteria	Intramuscular
Plague	Inactivated bacteria	Intramuscular
Pneumococcal conjugate	Bacterial polysaccharides of 7 pneumococcal types	Intramuscular
Pneumococcal polyvalent	Bacterial polysaccharides of 23 pneumococcal types	Intramuscular or subcutaneous
Poliovirus vaccine, inactivated (IPV)	Inactivated viruses of all 3 serotypes	Subcutaneous

(*continued*)

TABLE 3–1. LICENSED VACCINES AND TOXOIDS AVAILABLE IN THE UNITED STATES, BY TYPE AND RECOMMENDED ROUTES OF ADMINISTRATION[a] (*continued*)

VACCINE	TYPE	ROUTE
Poliovirus vaccine, oral (OPV)	Live viruses of all 3 serotypes	Oral
Rabies	Inactivated virus	Intramuscular or intradermal[f]
Rubella	Live virus	Subcutaneous
Tetanus	Inactivated toxin (toxoid)	Intramuscular[f]
Tetanus-diphtheria (Td or DT)[g]	Inactivated toxins (toxoids)	Intramuscular[f]
Typhoid (parenteral)	Inactivated bacteria	Subcutaneous[h]
(Ty21a oral)	Live bacteria	Oral
(Vi CPS)	Bacterial polysaccharide	Intramuscular
Varicella	Live virus	Subcutaneous
Yellow fever	Live virus	Subcutaneous

[a]Modified from reference 1.

[b]Available only to the U.S. Armed Forces.

[c]The intradermal dose is lower than the subcutaneous dose.

[d]The recommended schedule for infants depends on the vaccine manufacturer; consult the package insert and ACIP recommendations for specific products.

[e]The intradermal dose of rabies vaccine, human diploid cell (HDCV), is lower than the intramuscular dose and is used only for pre-exposure vaccination. **Rabies vaccine, absorbed (RVA) should not be used intradermally.**

[f]Preparations with adjuvants should be administered intramuscularly.

[g]Td = tetanus and diphtheria toxoids for use among persons ≥7 years of age. Td contains the same amount of tetanus toxoid as DTP or DT, but contains a smaller dose of diphtheria toxoid. DT = tetanus and diphtheria toxoids for use among children <7 years of age.

[h]Booster doses may be administered intradermally unless vaccine that is acetone killed and dried is used.

TABLE 3–2. IMMUNE GLOBULINS AND ANTITOXINS[a] AVAILABLE IN THE UNITED STATES, BY TYPE OF ANTIBODIES AND INDICATIONS FOR USE

IMMUNOBIOLOGIC	TYPE	INDICATION(S)
Botulinum antitoxin	Specific equine antibodies	Treatment of botulism
Cytomegalovirus immune globulin, intravenous (CMV-IGIV)	Specific human antibodies	Prophylaxis for bone marrow and kidney transplant recipients
Diphtheria antitoxin	Specific equine antibodies	Treatment of respiratory diphtheria
Hepatitis B immune (HBIG)	Specific human antibodies	Hepatitis B postexposure prophylaxis
Immune globulin (IG)	Pooled human antibodies	Hepatitis A pre- and post-exposure prophylaxis; measles postexposure prophylaxis
Immune globulin, intravenous (IGIV)	Pooled human antibodies	Replacement therapy for antibody deficiency disorders; immune thrombocytopenic purpura (ITP); hypogammaglobulinemia in chronic lymphocytic leukemia; Kawasaki disease
Rabies immune globulin[b] (HRIG)	Specific human antibodies	Rabies postexposure management of persons not previously immunized with rabies vaccine
Tetanus immune globulin (TIG)	Specific human antibodies	Tetanus treatment; postexposure prophylaxis of persons not adequately immunized with tetanus toxoid
Vaccinia immune globulin (VIG)	Specific human antibodies	Treatment of eczema vaccinatum, vaccinia necrosum, and ocular vaccinia
Varicella-zoster immune globulin (VZIG)	Specific human antibodies	Postexposure prophylaxis of susceptible immunocompromised persons, certain susceptible pregnant women, and perinatally exposed newborn infants

[a]Immune globulin preparations and antitoxins are administered intramuscularly unless otherwise indicated.
[b]HRIG is administered around the wounds in addition to the intramuscular injection.

or the final product or to stabilize the antigens or antibodies. Allergic reactions can occur if the recipient is sensitive to one of these additives (eg, phenols, albumin, glycine, and neomycin).

Adjuvants.   Many antigens evoke suboptimal immunologic responses. Efforts to enhance immunogenicity include mixing antigens with a variety of substances or adjuvants (eg, aluminum adjuvants such as aluminum phosphate or aluminum hydroxide).

Storage and Handling of Immunobiologics.   Failure to adhere to recommended specifications for storage and handling of immunobiologics can make these products impotent. Recommendations included in a product's package insert should be followed closely to ensure maximum potency of vaccines. Vaccines should be stored at recommended temperatures immediately upon receipt. Certain vaccines, such as oral polio vaccine (OPV) and yellow fever vaccine, are very sensitive to increased temperature. Other vaccines are sensitive to freezing, including diphtheria and tetanus toxoids and pertussis vaccine, adsorbed (DTP); diphtheria and tetanus toxoids and acellular pertussis vaccine, adsorbed (DTaP); diphtheria and tetanus toxoids for pediatric use (DT); tetanus and diphtheria toxoids for adult use (Td); inactivated poliovirus vaccine (IPV); *Haemophilus influenzae* type b conjugate vaccine (Hib); hepatitis B vaccine; pneumococcal vaccines; and influenza vaccine. Mishandled vaccine may not be easily distinguished from potent vaccine, and, when in doubt, contact the manufacturer.

■ ADMINISTRATION OF VACCINES

General Instructions.   Persons administering vaccines should take precautions to minimize risk for spreading disease and be adequately immunized against hepatitis B, measles, mumps, rubella, and influenza. Tetanus and diphtheria toxoids are recommended for all persons. Hands should be washed between patients. Gloves are not required when administering vaccinations, unless the persons who administer the vaccine will come in contact with potentially infectious body fluids or have open lesions on their hands. Syringes and needles used for injections must be sterile and preferably disposable to minimize the risk of contamination. A separate needle and syringe should be used for each injection. Different vaccines should not be mixed in the same syringe unless specifically licensed for such use. Disposable needles and syringes should be discarded in labeled, puncture-proof containers to prevent inadvertent reuse or needlestick injury.

Routes of administration are recommended for each immunobiologic (*see* Table 3–1). Injectable immunobiologics should be administered where there is little likelihood of local, neural, vascular, or tissue injury. In general, vaccines containing adjuvants should be injected into the muscle mass; when administered subcutaneously or intradermally, they can cause local irritation, induration, skin discoloration, inflammation, and granuloma formation. Once the needle is inserted into the injection site, the syringe plunger should be pulled back. If blood appears in the needle hub, the needle should be withdrawn and a new site selected before the vaccine is expelled. The process should be repeated until no blood appears.

Subcutaneous Injections. SC injections are usually administered into the thigh of infants and into the deltoid area of older children and adults. A ⅝- to ¾-inch, 23- to 25-gauge needle should be inserted into the tissues below the dermal layer of the skin.

Intramuscular Injections. The preferred sites for IM injections are the anterolateral aspect of the upper thigh and the deltoid muscle of the upper arm. *The buttock should not be used routinely for active vaccination of infants, children, or adults because of the potential for injury to the sciatic nerve.* In addition, injection into the buttock has been associated with decreased immunogenicity of hepatitis B and rabies vaccines in adults. If the buttock is used for passive immunization when large volumes are to be injected or multiple doses are necessary (eg, large doses of immune globulin), the central region should be avoided; only the upper, outer quadrant should be used, and the needle should be directed anteriorly (ie, not inferiorly or perpendicular to the skin) to minimize the possibility of involvement with the sciatic nerve. For all IM injections, the needle should be long enough to reach the muscle mass and prevent vaccine from seeping into subcutaneous tissues, but not so long as to endanger the underlying neurovascular structures or bone.

Infants (<12 Months of Age). Among most infants, the anterolateral aspect of the thigh provides the largest muscle mass and is therefore the recommended site. However, the deltoid can also be used with the thigh, for example, when multiple vaccines must be administered on the same visit. In most cases, a ⅞- to 1-inch, 22- to 25-gauge needle is sufficient to penetrate muscle in the thigh of a 4-month-old infant. The free hand should bunch the muscle, and the needle should be directed inferiorly along the axis of the leg at an angle appropriate to reach the muscle while avoiding nearby neurovascular structures and bone.

Toddlers and Older Children. The deltoid may be used if the muscle mass is adequate. The needle size can range from 22 to 25 gauge and from ⅝ to 1¼ inches, based on the size of the muscle. As with infants, the anterolateral thigh may be used, but the needle should be longer—generally ranging from ⅞ to 1¼ inches.

Adults. The deltoid is recommended for routine intramuscular vaccination among adults, particularly for hepatitis B vaccine. The suggested needle size is 1 to 1½ inches and 20- to 25-gauge.

Intradermal Injections. Intradermal injections are generally administered on the volar surface of the forearm, except for human diploid cell rabies vaccine (HDCV), for which reactions are less severe when the vaccine is administered in the deltoid area. With the bevel facing upward, a ⅜ to ¾ inch, 25- or 27-gauge needle can be inserted into the epidermis at an angle parallel to the long axis of the forearm. The needle should be inserted so that the entire bevel penetrates the skin and the injected solution raises a small bleb. Because of the small amounts of antigen used in intradermal injections, care must be taken not to inject the vaccine subcutaneously, because it can result in a suboptimal immunologic response.

Multiple Vaccinations. If more than one vaccine preparation is administered or if live vaccine and an immune globulin preparation are administered simultaneously, it is preferable to administer each at a different anatomic site. It is also preferable to avoid administering two IM injections in the same limb, especially if DTP is one of the products administered. However, if more than one injection must be administered in a single limb, the thigh is usually the preferred site because of the greater muscle mass; the injections should be sufficiently separated (ie, 1–2 inches apart) so that any local reactions are unlikely to overlap.

Regurgitated Oral Vaccines. Infants may sometimes fail to swallow oral preparations (eg, OPV) after administration. If a substantial amount of the vaccine is spit out, regurgitated, or vomited shortly after administration (ie, within 5–10 min), another dose can be administered at the same visit. If this repeat dose is not retained, neither dose should be counted, and the vaccine should be readministered at the next visit.

■ AGE AT WHICH IMMUNOBIOLOGICS ARE ADMINISTERED

Recommendations for the age at which vaccines are administered are influenced by several factors: age-specific risks of disease, age-specific risks of complications, ability of persons of a given age to respond to the vaccine(s), and potential interference with the immune response by passively transferred by maternal antibody. In general, vaccines are recommended for the youngest age group at risk for developing disease whose members are known to develop an adequate antibody response to vaccination (*see* Tables 3–3, 3–4, and 3–5).

■ SPACING OF IMMUNOBIOLOGICS

Interval Between Multiple Doses of Same Antigen. Some products require administration of more than one dose for development of an adequate antibody response. In addition, some products require periodic reinforcement or booster doses to maintain protection (*see* Tables 3–3, 3–4, and 3–5.) Longer-than-recommended intervals between doses do not reduce final antibody concentrations. Therefore, an interruption in the immunization schedule does not require reinstitution of the entire series of an immunobiologic or the addition of extra doses. However, administering doses of a vaccine or toxoid at less-than-recommended minimum intervals may decrease the antibody response and therefore should be avoided. Doses administered at less-than-recommended minimum intervals should not be counted as part of a primary series.

Some immunobiologics produce increased rates of local or systemic reactions in certain recipients when administered too frequently (eg, adult Td, pediatric DT, tetanus toxoid, and rabies vaccine). Such reactions are thought to result from the formation of antigen-antibody complexes.

Simultaneous Administration. Many of the commonly used vaccines can safely and effectively be administered simultaneously (ie, on the same day, *not* at the same anatomic site). Simultaneous administration is important in certain situations, including imminent exposure to several infectious diseases, preparation for foreign travel, and uncertainty that the person will return for further doses of vaccine.

TABLE 3-3. RECOMMENDED CHILDHOOD IMMUNIZATION SCHEDULE[a] UNITED STATES, JANUARY–DECEMBER 2001

VACCINE	Birth	1 Mo	2 Mo	4 Mo	6 Mo	12 Mo	15 Mo	18 Mo	24 Mo	4–6 Yr	11–12 Yr	14–18 Yr
Hepatitis B[b]	Hep B-1	Hep B-1	Hep B-2			Hep B-3	Hep B-3	Hep B-3			Hep B	
Diphtheria and tetanus toxoids and pertussis[c]			DTaP	DTaP	DTaP		DTaP	DTaP		DTaP	Td	Td
Haemophilus influenzae type b[d]			Hib	Hib	Hib	Hib	Hib					
Inactivated polio[e]			IPV	IPV	IPV	IPV	IPV	IPV		IPV		
Pneumococcal conjugate[f]			PCV	PCV	PCV	PCV	PCV					

AGE

(continued)

TABLE 3–3. RECOMMENDED CHILDHOOD IMMUNIZATION SCHEDULE[a] UNITED STATES, JANUARY–DECEMBER 2001 (continued)

VACCINE	Birth	1 Mo	2 Mo	4 Mo	6 Mo	12 Mo	15 Mo	18 Mo	24 Mo	4–6 Yr	11–12 Yr	14–18 Yr
Measles-mumps-rubella[g]						MMR				MMR	MMR	
Varicella[h]						Var					Var	
Hepatitis A[i]									Hep A in selected areas			

☐ Range of recommended ages for vaccination.

⬭ Vaccines to be given if previously recommended doses were missed or given earlier than the recommended minimum age.

▬ Recommended in selected states and/or regions.

[a]From reference 2. This schedule lists the recommended ages for routine administration of currently licensed childhood vaccines as of November 1, 2000, for children up to age 18 yr. Additional vaccines might be licensed and recommended during the year. Licensed combination vaccines may be used whenever any components of the combination are indicated and the vaccine's other components are not contraindicated. Providers should consult the manufacturer's package inserts for detailed recommendations.

(continued)

TABLE 3–3. RECOMMENDED CHILDHOOD IMMUNIZATION SCHEDULE[a] UNITED STATES, JANUARY–DECEMBER 2001 (*continued*)

[b]Infants born to hepatitis B surface antigen (HBsAg)–negative mothers should receive the first dose of hepatitis B vaccine (Hep B) by age 2 months. The second dose should be administered at least 1 month after the first dose. The third dose should be administered at least 4 months after the first dose and at least 2 months after the second dose, but not before age 6 months. Infants born to HBsAg-positive mothers should receive Hep B and 0.5 mL hepatitis B immune globulin (HBIG) within 12 hr of birth at separate sites. The second dose is recommended at age 1–2 months and the third dose at age 6 months. Infants born to mothers whose HBsAG status is unknown should receive Hep B within 12 hr of birth. Maternal blood should be drawn at delivery to determine the mother's HBsAG status; if the HBsAG test is positive, the infant should receive HBIG as soon as possible (no later than age 1 week). All children and adolescents (through age 18 yr) who have not been immunized against hepatitis B should begin the series during any visit. Providers should make special efforts to immunize children who were born in or whose parents were born in areas of the world where hepatitis B virus infection is moderately or highly endemic.

[c]The fourth dose of diphtheria and tetanus toxoids and acellular pertussis vaccine (DTaP) can be administered as early as age 12 months provided 6 months have elapsed since the third dose and the child is unlikely to return at age 15–18 months. Tetanus and diphtheria toxoids (Td) is recommended at age 11–12 yr if at least 5 yr have elapsed since the last dose of Td and pertussis vaccine (DTP), DTaP, or diphtheria and tetanus (DT) toxoids. Subsequent routine Td boosters are recommended every 10 yr.

[c]Three *Haemophilus influenzae* type b (Hib) conjugate vaccines are licensed for use in infants. If Hib conjugate vaccine (PRP-OMP, Pedvax HIB or ComVax, Merck) is administered at ages 2 and 4 months, a dose at age 6 months is not required. Because clinical studies in infants have demonstrated that using some combination products can induce a lower immune response to the Hib vaccine component, DTaP/Hib combination products should not be used for primary immunization in infants at age 2, 4, or 6 months unless approved by the Food and Drug Administration for these ages.

[d]An all-inactivated polio virus vaccine (IPV) schedule is recommended for routine childhood polio vaccination in the United States. All children should receive four doses of IPV at age 2 months, age 4 months, between 6–18 months, and 4–6 yr. Oral polio virus vaccine should be used only in selected circumstances.[3]

[e]The heptavalent pneumococcal conjugate vaccine (PCV) is recommended for all children 2–23 months old. It is also recommended for certain children 24–59 months old.[4]

[f]The second dose of measles–mumps–rubella (MMR) vaccine is recommended routinely at age 4–6 yr but can be administered during any visit provided at least 4 weeks have elapsed since receipt of the first dose and both doses are administered beginning at or after age 12 months. Those who previously did not receive the second dose should complete the schedule no later than the routine visit to a heath care provider at age 11–12 yr.

[h]Varicella vaccine (Var) is recommended at any visit on or after the first birthday for susceptible children (ie, those who lack a reliable history of chickenpox as judged by a heath care provider and have not been immunized). Susceptible persons age ≥13 yr should receive two doses given at least 4 weeks apart.

[i]Hepatitis A vaccine (Hep A) is recommended for use in selected states and/or regions and for certain high-risk groups. Information is available from local public health authorities.[5]

TABLE 3–4. RECOMMENDED ACCELERATED IMMUNIZATION SCHEDULE FOR INFANTS AND CHILDREN <7 YEARS OF AGE WHO START THE SERIES LATE[a] OR WHO ARE >1 MONTH BEHIND IN THE IMMUNIZATION SCHEDULE[b] (ie, children for whom compliance with scheduled return visits cannot be assured)

TIMING	VACCINE(S)	COMMENTS
First visit (≥4 mo of age)	DTP,[c] IPV[d] or OPV, Hib,[c,e] Hepatitis B, MMR (should be given as soon as child is age 12–15 mo)	All vaccines should be administered simultaneously at the appropriate visit.
Second visit (1 mo after first visit)	DTP,[c] Hib,[c,e] Hepatitis B	
Third visit (1 mo after second visit)	DTP,[c] OPV,[d] Hib,[c,e]	
Fourth visit (6 weeks after third visit)	OPV	
Fifth visit (≥6 mo after third visit)	DTaP[c] or DTP, Hib,[c,e] Hepatitis B	
Additional visits (Age 4–6 yr)	DTaP[c] or DTP, OPV, MMR	Preferably at or before school entry.
(Age 14–16 yr)	Td	Repeat every 10 yr throughout life.

DTP, diphtheria-tetanus-pertussis; DTaP, diphtheria-tetanus-acellular pertussis; Hib, *Haemophilus influenzae* type b conjugate; MMR, measles-mumps-rubella; OPV, poliovirus vaccine, live oral, trivalent; Td, tetanus and diphtheria toxoids (for use among persons ≥7 years of age).

[a]If initiated in the first year of life, administer DTP doses 1, 2, and 3 and OPV doses 1, 2, and 3 according to this schedule; administer MMR when the child reaches 12–15 mo of age.

[b]See individual ACIP recommendations for detailed information on specific vaccines.

[c]Two DTP and Hib combination vaccines are available (DTP/HbOC [TETRAMUNE]; and PRP-T [ActHIB, OmniHIB] which can be reconstituted with DTP vaccine produced by Connaught). DTaP preparations are currently recommended only for use as the fourth and/or fifth doses of the DTP series among children 15 mo–6 yr of age (before the seventh birthday). DTP and DTaP should not be used on or after the seventh birthday.

[d]The Advisory Committee on Immunization Practices (ACIP) of the Centers for Disease Control and Prevention (CDC) recommends the use of enhanced inactivated poliomyelitis vaccine (IPV) injection for the first 2 doses of the series to minimize OPV-related paralysis.[6]

[e]The recommended schedule varies by vaccine manufacturer. For information specific to the vaccine being used, consult the package insert and ACIP recommendations. Children beginning the Hib vaccine series at age 2–6 mo should receive a primary series of three doses of HbOC, PRP-T, or a licensed DTP-Hib combination vaccine; *or* two doses of PRP-OMP. An additional booster dose of any licensed Hib conjugate vaccine should be administered at 12–15 mo of age *and* at least 2 mo after

(continued)

TABLE 3–4. RECOMMENDED ACCELERATED IMMUNIZATION SCHEDULE FOR INFANTS AND CHILDREN <7 YEARS OF AGE WHO START THE SERIES LATE[a] OR WHO ARE >1 MONTH BEHIND IN THE IMMUNIZATION SCHEDULE[b] (ie, children for whom compliance with scheduled return visits cannot be assured) (*continued*)

the previous dose. Children beginning the Hib vaccine series at 7–11 mo of age should receive a primary series of two doses of a vaccine containing HbOC, PRP-T, or PRP-OMP. An additional booster dose of any licensed Hib conjugate vaccine should be administered at 12–18 mo of age *and* at least 2 mo after the previous dose. Children beginning the Hib vaccine series at ages 12–14 mo should receive a primary series of one dose of a vaccine containing HbOC, PRP-T, or PRP-OMP. An additional booster dose of any licensed Hib conjugate vaccine should be administered 2 mo after the previous dose. Children beginning the Hib vaccine series at ages 15–59 mo should receive one dose of any licensed Hib vaccine. Hib vaccine should not be administered after the fifth birthday except for special circumstances as noted in the specific ACIP recommendations for the use of Hib vaccine.

TABLE 3–5. RECOMMENDED IMMUNIZATION SCHEDULE FOR PERSONS ≥7 YR OF AGE NOT VACCINATED AT THE RECOMMENDED TIME IN EARLY INFANCY[a]

TIMING	VACCINE(S)	COMMENTS
First visit	Td,[b] OPV,[c] MMR,[d] and Hepatitis B[e]	Primary poliovirus vaccination is not routinely recommended for persons ≥18 yr of age.
Second visit (6–8 weeks after first visit)	Td, OPV, MMR,[d,f] Hepatitis B[e]	
Third vist (6 mo after second visit)	Td, OPV, Hepatitis B[e]	
Additional visits	Td	Repeat every 10 yr throughout life.

MMR, measles-mumps-rubella; OPV, poliovirus vaccine, live oral, trivalent; Td, tetanus and diphtheria toxoids (for use among persons ≥7 yr of age).

[a]See individual ACIP recommendations for details.

[b]The DTP and DTaP doses administered to children <7 yr of age who remain incompletely vaccinated at age ≥7 yr should be counted as prior exposure to tetanus and diphtheria toxoids (eg, a child who previously received two doses of DTP needs only one dose of Td to complete a primary series for tetanus and diphtheria).

[c]When polio vaccine is administered to previously unvaccinated persons ≥18 yr of age, inactivated poliovirus vaccine (IPV) is preferred. For the immunization schedule for IPV, see specific ACIP statement on the use of polio vaccine.

[d]Persons born before 1957 can generally be considered immune to measles and mumps and need not be vaccinated. Rubella (or MMR) vaccine can be administered to persons of any age, particularly to nonpregnant women of childbearing age.

[e]Hepatitis B vaccine, recombinant. Selected high-risk groups for whom vaccination is recommended include persons with occupational risk, such as health care and public safety workers who have occupational exposure to blood, clients and staff of institutions for the developmentally disabled, hemodialysis patients, recipients of certain blood products (eg, clotting factor concentrates), household contacts and sex partners of hepatitis B virus carriers, injecting drug users, sexually active homosexual and bisexual men, certain sexually active heterosexual men and women, inmates of long-term correctional facilities, certain international travelers, and families of HBsAg-positive adoptees from countries where HBV infection is endemic. Because risk factors are often not identified directly among adolescents, universal hepatitis B vaccination of teenagers should be implemented in communities where injecting drug use, pregnancy among teenagers, and/or sexually transmitted diseases are common.

[f]The ACIP recommends a second dose of measles-containing vaccine (preferably MMR to ensure immunity to mumps and rubella) for certain groups. Children with no documentation of live measles vaccination after the first birthday should receive two doses of live measles-containing vaccine not less than 1 mo apart. In addition, the following persons born in 1957 or later should have documentation of measles immunity (ie, 2 doses of measles-containing vaccine [at least one of which being MMR], physician-diagnosed measles, or laboratory evidence of measles immunity): (a) those entering post-high school educational settings; (b) those beginning employment in health care settings who will have direct patient contact; and (c) travelers to areas with endemic measles.

Killed Vaccines.   In general, inactivated vaccines can be administered simultaneously at separate sites. However, when vaccines commonly associated with local or systemic side effects (eg, cholera, parenteral typhoid, and plague) are administered simultaneously, the side effects might be accentuated. When feasible, it is preferable to administer these vaccines on separate occasions.

Live Vaccines.   The simultaneous administration of the most widely used live and inactivated vaccines has not resulted in impaired antibody responses or increased rates of adverse reactions. Administration of combined measles, mumps, and rubella (MMR) vaccine yields results similar to administration of the individual vaccines at different sites. Concern has been raised that oral live attenuated typhoid (Ty21a) vaccine theoretically might interfere with the immune response to OPV when OPV is administered simultaneously or soon after live oral typhoid vaccine, but no published data exist to support this theory.

Routine Childhood Vaccines.   The simultaneous administration of routine childhood vaccines does not interfere with the immune response to these vaccines. When administered at the same time and at separate sites, DTP, OPV, and MMR have produced seroconversion rates and rates of side effects similar to those observed when the vaccines are administered separately. Simultaneous vaccination of infants with DTP, OPV (or IPV), and either Hib vaccine or hepatitis B vaccine has resulted in acceptable response to all antigens. Routine simultaneous administration of DTP (or DTaP), OPV (or IPV), Hib vaccine, MMR, and hepatitis B vaccine is encouraged for children who are the recommended age to receive these vaccines and for whom no specific contraindications exist at the time of the visit. Individual vaccines should not be mixed in the same syringe unless they are licensed for mixing by the U.S. Food and Drug Administration (FDA).

Other Vaccines.   The simultaneous administration of pneumococcal polysaccharide vaccine and whole-virus influenza vaccine elicits satisfactory antibody responses without increasing the frequency or severity of adverse reactions in adults. Simultaneous administration of the pneumococcal vaccine and split-virus influenza vaccine also yields satisfactory results in both children and adults.

Hepatitis B vaccine administered with yellow fever vaccine is as safe and efficacious as when these vaccines are administered separately. Measles and yellow fever vaccines have been administered together safely and with full efficacy.

The antibody response to yellow fever and cholera vaccines is decreased if administered simultaneously or within a short time of each other. If possible, separate yellow fever and cholera vaccinations by at least 3 weeks. If time constraints exist and both vaccines are necessary, the injections can be administered simultaneously or within a 3-week period with the understanding that antibody response may not be optimal. Yellow fever vaccine is required by many countries and is highly effective in protecting against a disease with substantial mortality and for which no therapy exists. The currently used cholera vaccine provides limited protection of brief duration; few indications exist for its use.

Antimalarials and Vaccination.   The antimalarial mefloquine (Lariam) could potentially affect the immune response to oral live attenuated typhoid (Ty21a) vaccine if both are taken simultaneously. To minimize this effect, it may be prudent to administer Ty21a typhoid vaccine at least 24 hours before or after a dose of mefloquine. Because chloroquine phosphate (and possibly other structurally related antimalarials, such as mefloquine) may interfere with the antibody response to human diploid cell rabies vaccine (HDCV) when HDCV is administered by the intradermal route, HDCV should be administered by the intramuscular route when chloroquine, mefloquine, or other structurally related antimalarials are used.

Nonsimultaneous Administration.   Inactivated vaccines generally do not interfere with the immune response to other inactivated vaccines or to live vaccines except in certain instances (eg, yellow fever and cholera vaccines). In general, an inactivated vaccine can be administered either simultaneously or at any time before or after a different inactivated vaccine or a live vaccine. However, limited data indicate that prior or concurrent administration of DTP vaccine may enhance anti-PRP antibody response following vaccination with certain *Haemophilus influenzae* type b conjugate vaccines (ie, PRP-T, PRP-D, and HbOC). For infants, the immunogenicity of PRP-OMP appears to be unaffected by the absence of prior or concurrent DTP vaccination.

Theoretically, the immune response to one live-virus vaccine might be impaired if administered within 30 days of another live-virus vaccine. Whenever possible, live-virus vaccines administered on different days should be administered at least 30 days apart. However, OPV and MMR vaccines can be administered at any time before, with, or after each other, if indicated. Live-virus vaccines can interfere with the response to a tuberculin test. Tuberculin testing, if otherwise indicated, can be done either on the same day the live-virus vaccines are administered or 4–6 weeks later.

IMMUNE GLOBULIN

Live Vaccines.   OPV and yellow fever vaccines can be administered at any time before, with, or after the administration of immune globulin or specific immune globulins (eg, hepatitis B immune globulin [HBIG], rabies immune globulin [RIG]). The concurrent administration of immune globulin should not interfere with the response to Ty21a typhoid vaccine. Recent evidence suggests that high doses of immune globulin can inhibit the immune response to measles vaccine for more than 3 months. Administration of immune globulin can also inhibit the response to rubella vaccine. The effect of immune globulin preparations on the response to mumps and varicella vaccines is unknown, but commercial immune globulin preparations contain antibodies to these viruses.

Blood (eg, whole blood, packed RBCs, and plasma) and other antibody-containing blood products (eg, immune globulin; specific immune globulins; and immune globulin, intravenous [IGIV]) can diminish the immune response to MMR or its individual component vaccines. Therefore, after an immune globulin preparation is received, these vaccines should not be administered before the recommended interval has passed. However, postpartum vaccination of rubella-susceptible women with rubella or MMR vaccine should not be delayed because anti-Rho(D) IG (human) or any other blood product was received during the last trimester of pregnancy or at delivery. These women should be vaccinated immediately after delivery and, if possible, tested at least 3 months later to ensure immunity to rubella and, if necessary, to measles.

If administration of an immune globulin preparation becomes necessary because of imminent exposure to disease, MMR or its component vaccines can be administered simultaneously with the immunoglobulin preparation, although vaccine-induced immunity might be compromised. The vaccine should be administered at a site remote from that chosen for the immune globulin inoculation. Unless serologic testing indicates that specific antibodies have been produced, vaccination should be repeated after the recommended interval.

If administration of an immune globulin preparation becomes necessary after MMR or its individual component vaccines have been administered, interference can occur. Usually vaccine virus replication and stimulation of immunity occurs 1–2 weeks after vaccination. Thus, if the interval between administration of any of these vaccines and subsequent administration of an immune globulin preparation is less than 14 days, vaccination should be repeated after the recommended interval unless serologic testing indicates that antibodies were produced.

Killed Vaccines. Immune globulin preparations interact less with inactivated vaccines and toxoids than with live vaccines. Therefore, administration of inactivated vaccines simultaneously with or at any interval before or after receipt of immune globulins should not substantially impair the development of a protective antibody response. The vaccine or toxoid and immune globulin preparation should be administered at different sites.

Interchangeability of Vaccines From Different Manufacturers. When at least one dose of a hepatitis B vaccine produced by one manufacturer is followed by subsequent doses from a different manufacturer, the immune response has been shown to be comparable with that resulting from a full course of vaccination with a single vaccine.

Both HDCV and rabies vaccine, adsorbed (RVA) are considered equally efficacious and safe. When used as licensed and recommended, they are considered interchangeable during the vaccine series. *RVA should not be used intradermally.* The full 1 mL dose of either product, administered by IM injection, can be used for both pre-exposure and postexposure prophylaxis.

When administered according to their licensed indications, different diphtheria and tetanus toxoids and pertussis vaccines as single antigens or various combinations, as well as the live and inactivated polio vaccines, also can be used interchangeably.

Currently licensed *Haemophilus influenzae* type b conjugate vaccines (ie, PRP-OMP, PRP-T, HbOC, and combination DTP-Hib vaccines) have been shown to induce different temporal patterns of immunologic response in infants. Data suggest that infants who receive sequential doses of different vaccines produce a satisfactory antibody response after a complete series. The primary vaccine series should be completed with the same Hib vaccine, if feasible. However, if different vaccines are administered, a total of 3 doses of Hib vaccine is considered adequate for the primary series among infants, and any combination of Hib conjugate vaccines licensed for use among infants may be used. Any of the licensed conjugate vaccines can be used for the recommended booster dose at 12–18 months of age.

■ HYPERSENSITIVITY TO VACCINE COMPONENTS

Vaccine components can cause allergic reactions in some recipients. These reactions can be local or systemic, and can include mild to severe anaphylaxis or anaphylactoid responses (eg, generalized urticaria or hives, wheezing, swelling of the mouth and throat, difficulty breathing, hypotension, and shock). The responsible vaccine components can derive from vaccine antigen, animal protein, antibiotics, preservatives, and stabilizers.

Egg Allergy.   The most common animal protein allergen is egg protein found in vaccines prepared using embryonated chicken eggs (eg, influenza and yellow fever vaccines) or chicken embryo cell cultures (eg, measles and mumps vaccines). Ordinarily, persons who are able to eat eggs or egg products safely can receive these vaccines; persons with histories of anaphylactic or anaphylactoid allergy to eggs or egg proteins should not. Asking persons whether they can eat eggs without adverse effects is a reasonable way to determine who might be at risk for allergic reactions. Protocols for testing and vaccinating those persons with anaphylactic reactions to egg ingestion or vaccinating children with egg hypersensitivity and severe asthma have been developed. Rubella vaccine is grown in human diploid cell cultures and can be safely administered to persons with histories of severe allergy to eggs or egg proteins.

Antibiotic Allergy.   Some vaccines contain trace amounts of antibiotics to which patients may be hypersensitive. The information provided in the vaccine package insert should be carefully reviewed before deciding if the uncommon patient with such hypersensitivity should receive the vaccine(s). No currently recommended vaccine contains penicillin or penicillin derivatives. MMR and its individual component vaccines contain trace amounts of neomycin and, although the amount present is less than would usually be used for a skin test to determine hypersensitivity, persons who have experienced anaphylactic reactions to neomycin should not receive these vaccines. Most often, neomycin allergy is a contact dermatitis—a manifestation of a delayed-type (cell-mediated) immune response—rather than anaphylaxis. A history of delayed-type reactions to neomycin is not a contraindication for these vaccines.

Thimerosal Allergy.   Exposure to vaccines containing the preservative thimerosal (eg, DTP, DTaP, DT, Td, Hib, hepatitis B, influenza, and Japanese encephalitis) can lead to induction of hypersensitivity. However, most patients do not develop reactions to thimerosal given as a component of vaccines even when patch or intradermal tests for thimerosal indicate hypersensitivity, which usually consists of local delayed-type hypersensitivity reactions. Manufacturers are removing thimerosal from many products.

Vaccine Allergy.   Certain parenteral bacterial vaccines (ie, cholera, DTP, plague, and typhoid) are frequently associated with local or systemic adverse effects, such as redness, soreness, and fever. These reactions are difficult to link with a specific sensitivity to vaccine components and appear to be toxic rather than hypersensitive. Urticarial or anaphylactic reactions in DTP, DT, or Td or tetanus toxoid recipients have been reported rarely. When these reactions are reported, appropriate skin tests should be performed to determine sensitivity to tetanus toxoid before its use is discontinued. Alternatively, serologic testing to determine immunity to tetanus can be performed to evaluate the need for a booster dose of tetanus toxoid.

■ VACCINATION IN SPECIAL POPULATIONS

Preterm Infants.   Infants born prematurely, regardless of birth weight, should be vaccinated at the same chronologic age and according to the same schedule and precautions as full-term infants and children. Birthweight and size generally are not factors in deciding whether to postpone routine vaccination of a clinically stable premature infant. The full recommended dose of each vaccine should be used. To prevent the theoretical risk of poliovirus transmission in the hospital, the administration of OPV should be deferred until discharge.

Any premature infant born to a hepatitis B surface antigen (HBsAg)-positive mother should receive immunoprophylaxis with hepatitis B vaccine and HBIG beginning at or shortly after birth. For premature infants of HBsAg-negative mothers, the optimal timing of hepatitis B vaccination has not been determined. Some studies suggest that decreased conversion rates might occur in some premature infants with low birthweights (ie, <2000 g) following administration of hepatitis B vaccine at birth. Such low-birthweight premature infants of HBsAg-negative mothers should receive the hepatitis B vaccine series, which can be initiated at discharge from the nursery if the infant weighs at least 2000 g or at 2 months of age along with DTP, OPV, and Hib vaccine.

Breastfeeding and Vaccination.   Neither killed nor live vaccines affect the safety of breastfeeding for mothers of infants. Breastfeeding does not adversely affect immunization and is not a contraindication for any vaccine. Breast-fed infants should be vaccinated according to routine recommended schedules.

Inactivated or killed vaccines do not multiply within the body. Therefore, they should pose no special risk for mothers who are breastfeeding or for their infants. Although live vaccines do multiply within the mother's body, most are not excreted in breastmilk. Although rubella vaccine virus may be transmitted in breastmilk, the virus usually does not infect the infant, and, if it does, the infection is well tolerated. There is no contraindication for vaccinating breastfeeding mothers with yellow fever vaccine. Breastfeeding mothers can receive OPV without any interruption in feeding schedule.

Vaccination During Pregnancy.   Risk from vaccination during pregnancy is largely theoretical. The benefit of vaccination among pregnant women usually outweighs the potential risk when the risk for disease is high, infection would pose a special risk to the mother or fetus, and the vaccine is unlikely to cause harm.

Combined tetanus and diphtheria toxoids are the only immunobiologic agents routinely indicated for susceptible pregnant women. Previously vaccinated pregnant women who have not received a Td vaccination within the past 10 years should receive a booster dose. Pregnant women who are unimmunized or only partially immunized against tetanus should complete the primary series. Depending on when a woman seeks prenatal care and the required interval between doses, one or two doses of Td can be administered before delivery. Women for whom the vaccine is indicated but who have not completed the required three-dose series during pregnancy should be followed up after delivery to ensure they receive the doses necessary for protection.

There is no convincing evidence of risk from immunizing pregnant women with other inactivated virus or bacteria vaccines or toxoids. Hepatitis B vaccine is recommended for women at risk for hepatitis B infection, and influenza and pneumococcal vaccines are recommended for women at risk for infection and for complications of influenza and pneumococcal disease.

OPV can be administered to pregnant women who are at substantial risk of exposure to natural infection. Although OPV is preferred, IPV may be considered if the complete vaccination series can be administered before the anticipated exposure. Pregnant women who must travel to areas where the risk of yellow fever is high should receive yellow fever vaccine. In these circumstances, the small theoretical risk from vaccination is far outweighed by the risk of yellow fever infection. Known pregnancy is a contraindication for rubella, measles, and mumps vaccines. Although a theoretical concern, no cases of congenital rubella syndrome or abnormalities attributable to rubella vaccine virus infection have been observed in infants born to susceptible mothers who received rubella vaccine during pregnancy.

Persons who receive measles, mumps, or rubella vaccines can shed these viruses, but generally do not transmit them. These vaccines can be administered safely to the children of pregnant women. Although live poliovirus is shed by persons recently immunized with OPV (particularly after the first dose), this vaccine can also be administered to the children of pregnant women because experience has not revealed any risk of polio vaccine virus to the fetus.

All pregnant women should be evaluated for immunity to rubella and tested for the presence of HBsAg. Women susceptible to rubella should be immunized immediately after delivery. A woman infected with hepatitis B virus should be followed carefully to ensure that the infant receives HBIG and begins the hepatitis B vaccine series shortly after delivery.

There is no known risk to the fetus from passive immunization of pregnant women with immune globulin. Further information regarding immunization of pregnant women is available in the American College of Obstetricians and Gynecologists Technical Bulletin Number 160, October 1991.[7]

Altered Immunocompetence.   This section is a summary of the more extensive recommendations on vaccines and immune globulin preparations for immunocompromised persons. Additional information can be found in references 8 and 9.

Severe immunosuppression can be the result of congenital immunodeficiency. HIV infection, leukemia, lymphoma, generalized malignancy, or therapy with alkylating agents, antimetabolites, radiation, or large amounts of corticosteroids. Severe complications have followed vaccination of immunocompromised patients with live, attenuated-virus vaccines and with live-bacteria vaccines. In general, these patients should not receive live vaccines except in certain circumstances that are noted below. In addition, OPV should *not* be administered to any household contact of a severely immunocompromised person. If polio immunization is indicated for immunosuppressed patients, their household members, or other close contacts, IPV should be administered. MMR is not contraindicated in close contacts of immunocompromised patients.

Killed or inactivated vaccines can be administered to all immunocompromised patients, although response to such vaccines may be suboptimal. All such childhood vaccines are recommended for immunocompromised persons in usual doses and schedules. Certain vaccines such as pneumococcal vaccine or Hib vaccine are recommended specifically for certain groups of immunocompromised patients, including those with functional or anatomic asplenia.

HIV Infection.   Limited studies of MMR vaccination in HIV-infected patients have not documented serious or unusual adverse events. Because measles may cause severe illness in persons with HIV infection, MMR vaccine is recommended for all asymptomatic HIV-infected persons and should be considered for all symptomatic HIV-infected persons. HIV-infected persons on regular IGIV therapy may not respond to MMR or its individual component vaccines because of the continued presence of passively acquired antibody. However, because of the potential benefit, measles vaccination should be considered approximately 2 weeks before the next monthly dose of IGIV (if not otherwise contraindicated), although an optimal immune response is unlikely to occur. Unless serologic testing indicates that specific antibodies have been produced, vaccination should be repeated (if not otherwise contraindicated) after the recommended interval. An additional dose of IGIV should be considered for persons on routine IGIV therapy who are exposed to measles 3 or more weeks after administration of a standard dose (100–400 mg/kg) of IGIV.

Chemotherapy or Radiation Therapy.   Vaccination during chemotherapy or radiation therapy should be avoided because antibody response is poor. Patients vaccinated while on immunosuppressive therapy or in the 2 weeks before starting therapy should be considered unimmunized and should be revaccinated at least 3 months after therapy is discontinued. Patients with leukemia in remission whose chemotherapy has been terminated for 3 months may receive live-virus vaccines.

Corticosteroid Therapy.   The exact amount of systemically absorbed corticosteroids and the duration of administration needed to suppress the immune system of an otherwise healthy child are not well defined. Most experts agree that corticosteroid therapy usually does not contraindicate administration of live-virus vaccine when it is short term (ie, <2 weeks); low to moderate dose; long-term, alternate-day treatment with short-acting preparations; maintenance physiologic doses (replacement therapy); or administered topically (skin or eyes), by aerosol, or by intra-articular, bursal, or tendon injection. Although of recent theoretical concern, no evidence of increased severe reactions to live vaccines has been reported among persons receiving corticosteroid therapy by aerosol, and such therapy is not in itself a reason to delay vaccination. The immunosuppressive effects of corticosteroid treatment vary, but many clinicians consider a dose equivalent to a total of 20 mg/day of prednisone in adults as sufficiently immunosuppressive to raise concern about the safety of vaccination with live-virus vaccines. Corticosteroids used in greater than physiologic doses can also reduce the immune response to vaccines. Physicians should wait at least 3 months after discontinuation of therapy before administering a live-virus vaccine to patients who have received high systemically absorbed doses of corticosteroids for 2 or more weeks.

Vaccination of Persons with Hemophilia. Persons with bleeding disorders such as hemophilia have an increased risk of acquiring hepatitis B and at least the same risk as the general population of acquiring vaccine-preventable diseases. However, because of the risk of hematomas, intramuscular injections are often avoided among persons with bleeding disorders by using the subcutaneous or intradermal routes for vaccines that are normally administered by the intramuscular route. Hepatitis B vaccine administered intramuscularly to hemophiliacs using a 23-gauge needle, followed by steady pressure at the site for 1 to 2 minutes has resulted in a 4% bruising rate with no patients requiring clotting factor supplementation. Whether an antigen that produces more local reactions, such as pertussis, would produce an equally low rate of bruising is unknown.

When hepatitis B or any other intramuscular vaccine is indicated for a patient with a bleeding disorder, it should be administered intramuscularly if, in the opinion of a physician familiar with the patient's bleeding risk, the vaccine can be administered with reasonable safety by this route. If the patient received antihemophilic or other similar therapy, intramuscular vaccination can be scheduled for shortly after such therapy is administered. A fine needle (≤ 23 gauge) can be used for the vaccination and firm pressure applied to the site (without rubbing) for at least 2 minutes. The patient or family should be instructed concerning the risk of hematoma from the injections.

■ REFERENCES

1. General recommendations on immunization. Recommendations of the Advisory Committee on Immunization Practices (ACIP). *MMWR* 1994;43(RR-1):1–38.
2. Recommended childhood immunization schedule—United States, 2001. *MMWR* 2001;50:1–4.
3. Poliomyelitis prevention in the United States: updated recommendations of the Advisory Committee on Immunization Practices (ACIP). *MMWR* 2000;49(RR-5).
4. Preventing pneumococcal disease among infants and young children: recommendations of the Advisory Committee on Immunization Practices (ACIP). *MMWR* 2000;49(RR-9).
5. Prevention of hepatitis A through active or passive imunization recommendations of the Advisory Committee on Immunization Practices (ACIP). *MMWR* 1999;48(RR-12).
6. Marwick C. Switch to inactivated polio vaccine recommended. *JAMA* 1996;276:89. News.
7. Immunization during pregnancy. ACOG technical bulletin number 160—October 1991. *Int J Gynaecol Obstet* 1993;40:69–79. Also available from the American College of Obstetricians and Gynecologists. Attention: Resource Center, 409 12th Street SW, Washington, DC 20024–2188.
8. Recommendations of the Advisory Committee on Immunization Practices (ACIP): use of vaccines and immune globulins for persons with altered immunocompetence. *MMWR* 1993;42(RR-4):1–18.
9. Gardner P et al. Update: adult immunizations. *Ann Intern Med* 1996;12(1 pt 1):35–40.

Medical Emergencies: Anaphylaxis, Cardiac Arrest, Poisoning, Status Epilepticus

4

The clinical management of medical emergencies is an area in which there continues to be some variability in treatment philosophy. Thus, the therapeutic approaches, drugs, and adult dosages given here are based on somewhat divergent and conflicting sources of information. In addition, some recommendations have been made based on the authors' experience and suggestions from specialists and researchers in the field. As a result, the therapeutic concepts and dosages contained herein, although conforming to medical standards, may differ from those advocated by specific practitioners and institutions.

Anaphylaxis

William G. Troutman

Anaphylaxis is a systemic response to exposure to an allergen caused by rapid, IgE-mediated release of histamine and other mediators from tissue mast cells and circulating basophils. Symptoms usually occur within a few seconds or minutes of exposure but can be delayed or recur many hours after apparent resolution. The treament of anaphylaxis is directed toward its three major presentations: skin manifestations (angioedema, urticaria), respiratory distress (wheezing, stridor and dyspnea from laryngeal edema, laryngospasm and bronchospasm), and hypotension. Upper airway obstruction and cardiovasuclar collapse are the most common causes of death in anaphylaxis. All specific treatment measures should be accompanied by basic resuscitative measures including clear airway, supplemental oxygen and IV access.

■ GENERAL THERAPY AND SKIN MANIFESTATIONS

1. **Epinephrine HCl, IM or SC, 0.3–0.5 mg** (0.3–0.5 mL of 1:1000 soln), may repeat q 10–15 min. In children, 10 µg/kg up to 500 µg/dose (0.5 mL of 1:1000 soln).

2. **Diphenhydramine, IV or IM, 1–2 mg/kg (up to 50 mg) over 5–10 min.**
3. **Cimetidine, IV, 300 mg over 5 min** for urticaria or if hypotension does not respond to fluid replacement and pressors. In children, 3–5 mg/kg IV.
4. Although controversial, corticosteroids such as **hydrocortisone phosphate** or **succinate, IV, 200 mg** or **methylprednisolone, IV, 1–2 mg/kg** might reduce the risk of recurrent or prolonged anaphylaxis.

■ RESPIRATORY DISTRESS

1. Assure adequate oxygenation with supplemental **oxygen by mask** titrated to an oxygen saturation above 90%.
2. In addition to the general therapy described above, add **albuterol, by nebulization, 2.5–5 mg q 20 min.** In children, 0.15 mg/kg by nebulization q 20 min.
3. If response is inadequate after 3–4 doses of intermittent albuterol, consider **albuterol, by continuous nebulization, 10–15 mg/hr.** In children, 0.5 mg/kg/hr by continuous nebulization.

■ HYPOTENSION

1. If response to the general therapy described above is inadequate, give **NS or lactated Ringer's injection, IV, 500–1000 mL** initially and continue at high flow rate. In children, 10–20 mL/kg IV initially.
2. **Epinephrine HCl, IV continuous infusion, 1 μg/min** (as a 1:10,000 or 1:100,000 soln), up to 10 μg/min.
3. **Dopamine HCl, IV, 2–5 μg/kg/min,** titrate to desired effect.
4. Patients taking **β-adrenergic blockers** may not respond adequately to epinephrine and fluid replacement and can be adversely affected by unopposed α-adrenergic stimulation from epinephrine. **Glucagon, IV, 5–10 mg** followed by 1–5 mg/hr by continuous infusion can increase myocardial contractility independent of β-receptors.

■ REFERENCES

1. deShazo RD, Kemp SF. Allergic reactions to drugs and biologic agents. *JAMA* 1997;278:1895–906.
2. Anon. The diagnosis and management of anaphylaxis. Joint Task Force on Practice Parameters, American Academy of Allergy, Asthma and Immunology, American College of Allergy, Asthma and Immunology, and Joint Council of Allergy, Asthma and Immunology. *J Allergy Clin Immunol* 1998;101(6 Pt 2):S465–528.
3. Lucke W. Anaphylaxis (Disease and Trauma Monograph for Acute Care). In: Klasco R, ed. EMERGINDEX® System. Greenwood Village, CO: MICROMEDEX (edition expires June 30, 2001).

Cardiac Arrest

Robert J. DiDomenico
Allison E. Einhorn

Cardiac arrest is a medical emergency requiring a systematic approach. Early recognition must be followed by prompt, effective application of Basic Life Support (BLS) techniques to sustain the patient until Advanced Cardiac Life Support (ACLS) capabilities are available. The management of cardiac arrest is a four-step approach:

- **Recognition and Assessment**
- **Basic Life Support (BLS)**
- **Advanced Cardiovascular Life Support (ACLS)**
- **Postresuscitation Care**

■ RECOGNITION AND ASSESSMENT

Verify that respiration and circulation have ceased:

1. Loss of consciousness.
2. Loss of functional ventilation (respiratory arrest or inadequate respiratory effort).
3. Loss of functional perfusion (no pulse).

■ BASIC LIFE SUPPORT (BLS)

The findings listed above are sufficient to justify the immediate application of BLS techniques. The goal in cardiac arrest is the restoration of spontaneous circulation (ROSC). The first step toward achieving ROSC is prompt initiation of BLS, where the goal is to rapidly and effectively perfuse the tissues with oxygenated blood. A delay in initiating BLS or providing ineffective BLS can result in irreversible hypoxic brain injury.

1. Summon help and resuscitation equipment.
2. Establish an adequate airway.
3. Provide rescue breathing by delivering two slow, deep breaths. Ventilate by mouth-to mouth, mouth-to-mask, or bag-valve-mask techniques.
4. Check for pulse and other signs of circulation. Lay persons are not expected to perform a pulse check. Rather, they are instructed to look for other signs of circulation such as normal breathing, coughing, or movement. When available, assess heart rhythm with an automated external defibrillator or monophasic/biphasic defibrillator.
   - If ventricular tachycardia or ventricular fibrillation are documented, defibrillate with 200 joules of direct current shock.

- If the first shock fails to terminate the dysrhythmia, a second shock with 200–300 joules should be attempted. If the first two shocks fail, shock again with 360 joules.
5. Reassess cardiac rhythm and check for a pulse. If no pulse or other signs of circulation are present, initiate rescue breathing and chest compressions.
   - For rescue breathing:
     —Give each breath slowly over 2 sec.
     —Deliver 10–12 breaths per minute or 1 breath q 4–5 sec.
   - For external chest compressions:
     —Position patient supine on a firm surface.
     —Ensure proper placement of hands on sternum.
     —Depress sternum at a rate of 80–100 cycles per min (50% of cycle should be compression).
     —For every 15 chest compressions, give 2 breaths.

■ ADVANCED CARDIOVASCULAR LIFE SUPPORT (ACLS)

Note: Only adult dosages are given in this section.

Trained personnel should attempt to maintain a patent airway, establish intravenous access for administration of fluids and drugs, establish an electrocardiographic diagnosis, and apply specific treatments to correct any recognized electrical and/or mechanical abnormalities.

DRUG THERAPY IN ACLS

Ventricular Tachyarrhythmias. In this category, and treated the same way, are unstable ventricular flutter and ventricular tachycardia (pulseless VT), and ventricular fibrillation (VF). All are associated with decreased cardiac output and hypotension.

1. **Electrical defibrillation** with 200 joules. If tachyarrhythmias persist, deliver subsequent shocks with 200, 300 and 360 joules, respectively. Any further shocks should be with 360 joules.
   - Class recommendation: I (excellent supporting evidence)
   - Defibrillation is the only treatment proven to decrease mortality in pulseless VT/VF. The objective is to shock soon and shock often. When drug administration is initiated, the sequence is CPR–drug–shock–repeat or CPR–drug–shock–shock–shock–repeat.
2. For pulseless VT/VF refractory to initial defibrillation, administration of medications should follow the sequence below:
   - **Epinephrine HCl, 1 mg IV push** (10 mL of 1:10,000 solution) q 3–5 min until the ROSC *or* **vasopressin 40 units** (2 mL of 20 units/mL vial) IV, *one* dose only. If after 5–10 min there is no response to vasopressin, administer epinephrine as instructed.
   - If IV access has not been established or has been lost, consider administering **epinephrine HCl via endotracheal tube** (2–2.5 times the intravenous dose; *see* Special Considerations), followed by 3 or 4 rapid

ventilations to aerosolize the drug. There is no evidence to support administration of vasopressin via endotracheal tube.

—Class recommendation: Indeterminate for epinephrine and vasopressin (insufficient data to support class recommendation).

—Epinephrine is used not as an aid to defibrillation but rather to increase perfusion and sustain blood pressure. Epinephrine stimulates α- and β-adrenergic receptors. Stimulation of α-receptors causes vasoconstriction, increasing systemic vascular resistance (SVR) and blood pressure. However, the β-agonist activity of epinephrine increases heart rate and contractility, increasing myocardial oxygen demand in resuscitated patients, and might precipitate or worsen myocardial ischemia.

—Vasopressin is an alternative to epinephrine (at least initially). It is an endogenous antidiuretic hormone that, at high doses (ie, ACLS doses), possesses considerable vasoconstrictor activity. Unlike epinephrine, vasopressin has no β-agonist activity and does not increase myocardial oxygen demand.

3. If pulseless VT/VF persists, the next step is to initiate antiarrhythmic drug therapy. Management has changed in that the initial antiarrhythmic of choice is now:

- **Amiodarone, 300 mg IV push** (6 mL of 50 mg/mL ampule diluted to 20–30 mL of NS or D5W). If pulseless VT/VF persists, give an additional 150 mg IV push. If ROSC occurs, initiate intravenous infusion (450 mg in 250 mL NS, 1.8 mg/mL) at 1 mg/min for 6 hr and then decrease to 0.5 mg/min. Maximum dose is 2.2 g in 24 hr.

  —Class recommendation: IIb (Fair to good supporting evidence).

  —Amiodarone, in addition to its sodium, potassium, and calcium channel blocking activity, possesses α- and β-antagonistic properties. The short-term side effects of amiodarone are bradycardia, hypotension, and QT prolongation. Hypotension, likely secondary to the polysorbate 80 diluent of the injectable formulation, can be prevented by slowing the rate of drug infusion. A polysorbate 80–free formulation of amiodarone is currently under investigation. Bradycardia and QT prolongation might respond to a dose reduction.

  —IV infusions of amiodarone should be admixed in glass bottles because drug adsorption to plastic containers is likely with prolonged exposure. This phenomenon was taken into account during clinical trials, so traditional PVC tubing for administration is acceptable.

4. If amiodarone fails to control the arrhythmia, consider:

- **Lidocaine HCl, 1.0-1.5 mg/kg IV push** (2.5–5 mL of 2% solution or 5–10 mL of 1% solution), may repeat in 3–5 min to a cumulative dose of 3 mg/kg. If the arrhythmia is controlled, initiate an intravenous infusion (1 g/250 mL D5W, 4 mg/mL) at 1–4 mg/min.

- If IV access has not been established or has been lost, consider administering **lidocaine HCl via endotracheal tube** (2–2.5 times the intravenous dose; *see* Special Considerations), followed by 3 or 4 rapid ventilations to aerosolize the drug.

—Class recommendation: Indeterminate (insufficient data to support class recommendation).

—Lidocaine is a class Ib antiarrhythmic agent that blocks cellular sodium ion channels and increases the electrical stipulation threshold of the heart. Lidocaine inhibits its own hepatic metabolism after 24–48 hr of therapy; therefore, it should be used with caution in the elderly and in patients with hepatic dysfunction. Signs of toxicity are mental status changes, muscle twitching, seizures, and bradycardia. If prolonged administration is likely, monitoring of serum concentrations might be helpful.

5. If amiodarone- and lidocaine-resistant dysrhythmias persist, consider the administration of:

   • **Procainamide HCl, 30 mg/min IV infusion,** (1 g/250 NS, 4 mg/mL or 2 g/250 mL NS, 8 mg/mL) to a maximum dose of 17 mg/kg. If the arrhythmia terminates with procainamide, initiate an IV infusion at 1–4 mg/min.

     —Class recommendation: IIb for intermittent/recurrent VT/VF (Fair to good supporting evidence).

     —Procainamide is a class Ia antiarrhythmic agent that blocks the sodium ion channels of the heart. Avoid rapid administration (>30 mg/min) because this can lead to hypotension. Because procainamide must be administered slowly, it is not a first-line antiarrhythmic agent in the management of VT/VF. Serum concentrations of procainamide and its active metabolite N-acetylprocainamide, should be monitored and doses should be decreased in the presence of renal dysfunction. Procainamide also can prolong the QT interval; therefore, it should be avoided in patients with pre-existing QT prolongation and torsades de pointes.

6. If the rhythm is documented polymorphic VT (torsades de pointes) or secondary to hypomagnesemia, administer:

   • **Magnesium sulfate, 1–2 g IV infusion** over 15–30 min. Rapid IV push administration can lead to hypotension, bradycardia, and asystole; therefore, it is not recommended. Consider a maintenance infusion of 0.5–1 g/hr if arrhythmia successfully terminates with magnesium.

     —Class recommendation: IIb (Fair to good supporting evidence).

7. Administering sodium bicarbonate during cardiac arrest has traditionally been a controversial issue. Its use in VT/VF arrests should be considered only after other accepted interventions (eg, defibrillation, intubation/ventilation, chest compressions, and vasopressors) have been ineffective. If desired, administer:

   • **Sodium bicarbonate, 1 mEq/kg slow IV push** (50 mL of 8.4% solution, 1 mEq/mL).

8. Bretylium is no longer recommended by the American Heart Association because of a shortage of natural resources, limited product availability, high occurrence of side effects, and the availability of safer and at least as efficacious agents. It is not featured on the VT/VF algorithm but is still an appropriate choice for treatment *after attempting lidocaine.*

- **Bretylium tosylate, 5 mg/kg slow IV push,** may repeat with 10 mg/kg q 5 min to a maximum dose of 30–35 mg/kg. If a response to the loading dose occurs, initiate an intravenous infusion (500 mg/250 mL D5W, 2 mg/mL) at 1–2 mg/min.
  —Class recommendation: IIb (Fair to good supporting evidence).
  —Bretylium is a class III antiarrhythmic that inhibits the potassium channel, prolonging action potential duration and refractoriness of the myocardium. Bretylium also causes a release of catecholamines shortly after administration but subsequently exhibits postganglionic adrenergic receptor blockade, frequently leading to the development of hypotension. Prolongation of the QT interval also can occur.

Pulseless Electrical Activity (PEA). PEA was previously known as electromechanical dissociation and is characterized by ineffective cardiac output (hypotension) in the face of ECG evidence of electrical myocardial activity. Etiologies of PEA can be remembered by the 5 Hs and 5 Ts:

Hypovolemia	**T**ablets (drugs)
Hypoxia	**T**amponade (cardiac)
Hydrogen ions (acidosis)	**T**ension pneumothorax
Hypo/hyperkalemia	**T**hrombosis, coronary
Hypothermia	**T**hrombosis, pulmonary (embolism)

The most effective way to treat PEA is to correct the underlying cause. The methods discussed below are temporizing measures until the causative etiology is found and remedied.

1. Nonspecific treatment measures include administration of:
   - **Epinephrine HCl, 1 mg IV push** (10 mL of 1:10,000 solution) q 3–5 min.
   - If bradycardic, give **atropine sulfate, 1 mg IV push** (10 mL of 0.1 mg/mL solution) every 3–5 min to a maximum dose of 3 mg or 0.04 mg/kg. Atropine may be given via endotracheal tube at 2–2.5 times the intravenous dose (2–2.5 mg; *see* Special Considerations) followed by 3 or 4 rapid ventilations to aerosolize the drug.
2. The use of buffering agents is controversial. When clinical situations arise where alkalinization is necessary (*see* Class Recommendations, below), administer:
   - **Sodium bicarbonate, 1 mEq/kg slow IV push** (50 mL of 8.4% solution, 1 mEq/mL).
     —Class recommendation: I (Excellent supporting evidence) for documented hyperkalemia.
       - In addition to sodium bicarbonate, calcium is indicated for hyperkalemia with ECG changes. Calcium acts as a cardioprotectant and offsets the arrhythmogenic potential of excessive potassium. Administer **calcium chloride, 0.5–1 g slow IV push** (5–10 mL of

10% solution = 6.8–13.6 mEq) *or* **calcium gluconate 1–2 g slow IV push** (10–20 mL of 10% solution = 4.7–9.4 mEq).

—Class recommendation: IIa (Good to very good supporting evidence) for bicarbonate-sensitive acidosis, tricyclic antidepressant overdose, or for urine alkalinization in aspirin and other drug overdoses.

—Class recommendation: IIb (Fair to good supporting evidence) following ROSC in mechanically ventilated patients after a prolonged arrest.

—Sodium bicarbonate can be harmful in hypercarbic acidosis; therefore, administration should be limited to those situations described above.

3. Hypovolemia is the most common underlying cause of PEA; therefore, rapid assessment of fluid status is crucial. In hypovolemic patients, fluid resuscitation using crystalloid (NS or lactated Ringer's solution) or colloid (hetastarch or human albumin) products should be initiated immediately.

4. If volume is adequate and there is no evidence of cardiac tamponade, consider vasopressors for vasoconstrictor and inotropic/chronotropic effects.

   • **Dopamine HCl, start at 5 μg/kg/min IV infusion** (400 mg/500 mL D5W, 800 μg/mL or 800 mg/500 mL D5W, 1600 μg/mL) and titrate to effect (BP and heart rate). Maximum dosage is 20 μg/kg/min. Dosages >20 μg/kg/min have no increased effect on BP and increase the risk for drug-induced tachyarrhythmias.

   —Dopamine possesses dopaminergic and α- and β-adrenergic activity. At dosages <5 μg/kg/min, dopaminergic receptor activation causes an increase in renal and mesenteric blood flow. At dosages of 5–10 μg/kg/min, β-adrenergic receptor stimulation ($\beta_1 > \beta_2$) occurs, increasing heart rate and contractility. At dosages >10 μg/kg/min, α-receptor stimulation leads to an increase in SVR and elevation in BP.

   • **Norepinephrine bitartrate, start at 0.5–1 μg/min IV infusion** (4 mg/250 mL D5W, 16 μg/mL, or 8 mg/250 mL D5W, 32 μg/mL) and titrate to effect (BP and heart rate). No maximum dose is noted.

   —Norepinephrine stimulates α- and β-adrenergic receptors, increasing BP (secondary to increased SVR), heart rate, and contractility.

   —Because increased doses of norepinephrine enhance β-agonist activity (especially in patients with prior cardiac disease), patients are at increased risk for drug-induced tachyarrhythmias.

Asystole. Asystole is characterized by cessation of cardiac muscular and electrical activities. It is important to note that true asystole, unless as a result of excessive vagal tone (bradyasystolic event), is frequently associated with irreversible cardiac damage. Like PEA, the most effective management of the asystolic patient is identifying and treating the underlying causes (*see* PEA management). However, many times a cause cannot be determined.

1. Initial management of asystole starts with transcutaneous or transvenous pacing, when the capability is available.
2. In conjunction with pacing, medications for managing asystole include:
   - **Epinephrine HCl, 1 mg IV push** (10 mL of 1:10,000 solution) q 3–5 min and **atropine sulfate, 1 mg IV push** (10 mL of 0.1 mg/mL solution) q 3–5 min to a maximum dose 3 mg or 0.04 mg/kg.

If asystole persists, the potential for a successful resuscitation should be evaluated and a decision made to continue or cease resuscitation efforts.

Bradyarrhythmias. Considered in this category, and treated the same way, are complete heart block, slow ventricular focus, sinus bradycardia, and agonal rhythm. In dealing with any of these symptomatic arrhythmias, transvenous pacing is the best long-term approach but is often not readily accessible. Therefore, drugs are used to enhance or initiate cardiac activity, at least until transcutaneous or transvenous pacing capabilities are available.

1. If symptomatic bradycardia occurs, initiate management with:
   - **Atropine sulfate, 1 mg IV push** (10 mL of 0.1 mg/mL solution) every 3–5 min to a maximum dose of 3 mg or 0.04 mg/kg.
     —Patients with denervated transplanted hearts will not respond to atropine; therefore, proceed immediately to transcutaneous pacing, administration of catecholamines, or both.
2. If capabilities are available, attempt:
   - *Transcutaneous* **pacing** to capture the slow rhythm and increase heart rate to a level at which symptoms disappear. If continued pacing is necessary, continue transcutaneous pacing until a transvenous pacer can be placed.

SUPPORTIVE THERAPY

Management of Acidosis. Severe acidosis can develop within 5 min after cardiac arrest and will continue unless BLS is provided. Acidosis can be respiratory and/or (to a lesser extent) metabolic in etiology.

1. Respiratory Acidosis
   - Secondary to hypoventilation and an accumulation of CO_2.
   - Treat by providing adequate ventilation. There is no role for sodium bicarbonate in this situation.
2. Metabolic Acidosis
   - Due to tissue hypoxia and subsequent anaerobic metabolism that results in the slow accumulation of lactic acid.
   - Treat by adequate tissue perfusion and return to aerobic metabolism. Sodium bicarbonate administration is not indicated unless there is evidence of pre-existing acidosis, hyperkalemia, or TCA overdose. There is no evidence supporting routine use of bicarbonate and it should be limited to specific clinical situations.

- If sodium bicarbonate is to be given, the following guidelines should be followed:
  —If an arterial blood gas (ABG) is *not* available, empirically administer **sodium bicarbonate, 1 mEq/kg slow IV push** (50 mL of 8.4% solution, 1 mEq/mL).
  —If an ABG *is* available, the sodium bicarbonate dose can be calculated from the base deficit with the following equation:

$$\text{NaHCO}_3 \text{ dose in mEq} = \text{base deficit (mEq/L)} \times 0.2 \times \text{body weight (kg)}$$

■ POSTRESUSCITATION CARE

With the ROSC after cardiac arrest, cardiovascular and hemodynamic compromise is often considerable and can be manifested as different types of shock (hypovolemic, cardiogenic, and vasodilatory associated with systemic inflammatory response syndrome). If the patient is not already in an intensive care setting, transport to an intensive care unit should occur as soon as possible. Continuous monitoring, resuscitation equipment, and skilled nursing care are needed. Health care providers should be diligent in identifying the underlying causes and correcting them, if possible. The goal of postresuscitation care is to restore functional ventilation and maintain adequate tissue perfusion.

■ SPECIAL CONSIDERATIONS

- Time to Drug Effect
  —Systemic circulation times are grossly prolonged during external chest compressions. Remember to allow *at least* 2 min between the time of peripheral injection and anticipated response. To enhance the onset and activity of peripherally administered medications, give as a rapid bolus injection, followed by a 10–20 mL NS flush and, if possible, elevate the extremity.
- High-dose Epinephrine
  —It was once believed that high-dose epinephrine was more effective than standard ACLS doses. However, recent studies have found no advantage using high-dose over standard-dose epinephrine. There is some also preliminary evidence that higher doses of epinephrine can be harmful in resuscitated patients.
- Endotracheal Administration
  —Administration of epinephrine, lidocaine, and atropine can be done via endotracheal tube if IV access has not been established or has been lost. Doses are 2–2.5 times the IV dose. Undiluted drug (eg, epinephrine 1:1000) can be given, but it must be diluted to 10 mL with NS or followed by a 10-mL NS or sterile water flush. After administration of medications via the endotracheal route, 3 to 4 rapid ventilations should be performed to aerosolize the drug and maximize absorption. This route of administration may not be as effective as IV.

- Intraosseous Administration
  —Epinephrine, atropine, sodium bicarbonate, lidocaine, vasopressors, or calcium via the distal tibia can be used in situations in which IV access and endotracheal intubation have not been established. This route of administration is often reserved for pediatric patients but may be attempted in adults in rare situations.
- Intracardiac Administration
  —Administration of mediation directly into the myocardium has *no role* in the modern management of cardiac arrest. Drugs do not work within the chambers of the heart but rather at the cellular level after delivery via the coronary circulation. Stopping BLS to attempt intracardiac injections only serves to interrupt vital CNS perfusion.
- Physical Incompatibilities
  —With many medications being given during a cardiac arrest (often through the same IV access site), it is important to recognize the likelihood of physical incompatibilities. Sodium bicarbonate inactivates catecholamines and can form a precipitate when mixed with calcium-containing solutions. Concomitant administration should be avoided, if possible. If sodium bicarbonate is administered through the same vascular access site, the line must be flushed before and after bicarbonate administration.

■ REFERENCES

1. American Heart Association in collaboration with the International Liaison Committee on Resuscitation (ILCOR). Guidelines 2000 for cardiopulmonary resuscitation and emergency cardiovascular care: an international consensus on science. *Circulation* 2000;102(suppl I):I1–291.
2. Lindner KH et al. Vasopressin administration in refractory cardiac arrest. *Ann Intern Med* 1996;124:1061–4.
3. Kudenchuk PJ et al. Amiodarone for resuscitation after out-of-hospital cardiac arrest due to ventricular fibrillation. *N Eng J Med* 1999;341:871–8.
4. Raehl CL. Endotracheal drug therapy in cardiopulmonary resuscitation. *Clin Pharm* 1986;5:572–9.
5. Iserson KV. Intraosseous infusions in adults. *J Emerg Med* 1989;7:587–91.

Poisoning

Blaine E. Benson

Management of the poisoned patient involves procedures designed to prevent the absorption, minimize the toxicity, and hasten the elimination of the suspected toxin. The prompt employment of appropriate emergency management procedures often can prevent unnecessary morbidity and mortality.

A regional poison center is a practitioner's best source of definitive treatment information and should be consulted in all poisonings, regardless of the apparent simplicity of the case. Contact the regional poison center in your area to learn of its staffing, resources, and capabilities before a need for its services arises. Well-qualified regional centers are certified by the American Association of Poison Control Centers.

In all cases, every attempt should be made to accurately identify the toxin, estimate the quantity involved, and determine the time that has passed since the exposure. These data, plus patient-specific parameters such as age, weight, sex, and underlying medical conditions or drug use, will assist you and the regional poison center in designing an appropriate therapeutic plan for the patient.

The techniques described below are intended for the initial management of the poisoned patient with the use of materials that should be readily available.

■ TOPICAL EXPOSURES

1. *Immediately* irrigate affected areas with a copious amount of water; use soap only if a stubborn, oily substance is the contaminant. Skin should be gently washed, not scrubbed, and special attention should be given to the hair, skin folds, umbilicus, and other areas where the contaminant might be trapped.
2. If the patient's clothes have been contaminated, remove them during the irrigation and clean them before they are worn again or destroy them. Clothing can interfere with the irrigation process and serve as a reservoir of toxic material.
3. Do not attempt to "neutralize" the contaminant with another chemical (eg, acids and alkalis). Attempts at neutralization waste valuable time, are of no benefit, and might be harmful.
4. Do not cover the affected area with emollients. These can trap unremoved contaminant against the skin. Severely damaged skin may be temporarily covered with a light, dry dressing.
5. Protect yourself from contamination. Gloves, aprons, or a change of clothes might be necessary.
6. After the irrigation is complete, contact a regional poison center for definitive treatment information.

■ EYE EXPOSURES

1. *Immediately* irrigate the eye; damage can occur within seconds. The stream of water from the tap or a pitcher should strike the patient on the forehead, temple, or bridge of the nose and then flow into the eye.
2. The eyelids should be open, with frequent blinking during the irrigation.
3. The irrigation should continue for at least 15 min (by the clock) to ensure adequate removal of the contaminant and normalization of the conjunctival pH. Body temperature water or saline may be substituted for tap water as the irrigation proceeds, but only if these can be obtained without interrupting the irrigation.
4. After the irrigation is complete, contact a regional poison center for definitive treatment information.

■ INHALATION EXPOSURES

1. Remove the patient from the suspected contaminated area, regardless of its apparent safety. Carbon monoxide, a common inhaled toxin, cannot be detected by sight, smell, or taste.
2. Institute artificial ventilation, if necessary, and provide supplementary humidified oxygen, if available and needed.
3. Protect yourself from contamination at all times.
4. Contact a regional poison center for definitive treatment information.

■ INGESTIONS

1. Remove any remaining contaminant from inside and around the mouth of the patient.
2. Give a small amount of water to clear the mouth and esophagus.
3. Contact a regional poison center for definitive treatment information.
4. In many cases, it will not be necessary to take additional steps. The following information can be used if additional care is recommended by the regional poison center.

■ GASTROINTESTINAL DECONTAMINATION

Gastrointestinal (GI) decontamination can be accomplished by the administration of activated charcoal, gastric lavage, ipecac-induced emesis, or whole-bowel irrigation. Indications for GI decontamination are ingestion of a known toxic dose, ingestion of an unknown dose of a known toxic substance, and ingestion of a substance of unknown toxicity. For all methods of GI decontamination, the value of the procedure diminishes rapidly with time. Some investigators now question the usefulness of gastric lavage or ipecac-induced emesis more than 1 hr after ingestion. None of these techniques should be presumed to provide complete removal or binding of the ingested toxin(s). Comparative experimental studies have shown only limited success with these techniques, and there is considerable interpatient variability in the results. In general, activated charcoal is the most useful agent for preventing absorption of ingested toxic substances. Other methods of GI decontamination may be considered if the ingested contaminant is not adsorbed by activated charcoal or if circumstances do not permit its prompt administration.

ACTIVATED CHARCOAL

Activated charcoal is a nonspecific absorbent that binds unabsorbed toxins within the GI tract. There is limited experience using activated charcoal in the home setting. Activated charcoal is not effective for absorbing strong acids and alkalis, cyanide, ethanol, methanol, ethylene glycol, iron, or lithium.

1. Activated charcoal is administered orally or by gastric tube in doses that range from 30 to 120 g.
2. Activated charcoal is commercially supplied as a slurry in water or a concentrated solution of sorbitol. The water-based products are preferred because the large amount of sorbitol that accompanies a typical dose of activated charcoal can result in excessive sorbitol-induced catharsis, producing fluid and electrolyte imbalance. Gentle encouragement may be needed to make children swallow the charcoal. Having the child take the liquid through a drinking straw from an opaque container is sometimes helpful.
3. Activated charcoal administration is commonly followed by the administration of a cathartic (eg, sorbitol, magnesium citrate, or magnesium sulfate) to hasten the elimination of the activated charcoal–toxin complex. There is no evidence to support cathartic use.
4. Alert the patient that charcoal will cause the stools to turn black.
5. Repeated oral doses of activated charcoal (eg, 25 g q 2 hr) have been used to enhance the elimination of some drugs, most notably carbamazepine, dapsone, phenobarbital, quinine, or theophylline. Multiple-dose activated charcoal is suitable only for patients with active bowel sounds. Co-administration of a cathartic is not recommended during multiple-dose activated charcoal therapy.

GASTRIC LAVAGE

Gastric lavage can be used to remove toxic substances poorly adsorbed by activated charcoal. Lavage is contraindicated for patients who have ingested corrosives or aliphatic hydrocarbons (ie, gasoline) and for patients at risk for esophageal or gastric perforation due to underlying medical conditions (eg, esophageal varices).

1. If the patient's gag reflex is weak or absent, the airway must be protected by the use of a cuffed endotracheal tube.
2. The largest possible orogastric tube should be used (26–28 F for children and 34–42 F for adults): the larger the tube diameter, the more efficient the lavage. The tube should be introduced through the mouth with the aid of a water-soluble lubricant. Nasogastric passage is not recommended.
3. Gastric lavage may be done with water, but a solution such as 0.45% NaCl may be used to minimize the risk of dilutional hyponatremia, especially in children. Aliquots of fluid up to 100 mL in children and 200 mL

in adults are introduced through the tube and then removed by gravity or suction-assisted drainage. The lavage should be continued for several cycles after the returning fluid is clear. Warming the lavage fluid reduces the risk of hypothermia.

INDUCTION OF EMESIS

Do not induce emesis if the patient is experiencing or is at risk for CNS depression, seizures, or loss of gag reflex, or if the patient has ingested a caustic substance or a hydrocarbon with high aspiration potential (eg, gasoline).

1. Induce emesis only with **syrup of ipecac.** Salt water, mustard water, other "home remedies," or gagging have no place in the management of the poisoned patient. These techniques are ineffective and can be dangerous.
2. The usual initial dose of syrup of ipecac is 30 mL in persons older than 12 yr, 15 mL in children 1–12 yr old, and 10 mL in children between 6 months and 1 yr.
3. Give the patient additional water to drink: 125–250 mL (4–8 fluid ounces) in children, 250–500 mL (8–16 fluid ounces) in adults. Activated charcoal should not be given until after ipecac-induced emesis has occurred.
4. Emesis usually occurs within 15–20 min. If 30 min have passed without emesis, administer an additional dose of syrup of ipecac and more water.
5. Have the patient vomit into a bowl or other container so that the vomitus can be inspected for the presence of the ingested toxin.

WHOLE-BOWEL IRRIGATION

Whole-bowel irrigation with an orally administered **polyethylene glycol electrolyte solution** (eg, GoLYTELY or CoLyte) is commonly used before bowel procedures. It has drawn attention as an alternative to other methods of GI decontamination in the management of acute poisoning. Results of studies are promising and the technique may have value in cases of ingestion of iron, enteric-coated or sustained-release products, foreign bodies, and drug-smuggling packets. Instillation rates have ranged from 500 mL/hr in children to 2 L/hr in adults. Typically, 4–6 L of fluid is administered. The endpoint is clearing of the rectal effluent. Contraindications to whole-bowel irrigation are persistent vomiting, adynamic ileus, bowel obstruction or perforation, and GI hemorrhage.

■ REFERENCES

1. Shannon M. Ingestion of toxic substances by children. *N Engl J Med* 2000;342:186–91.
2. AACT/EAPCCT position statement on gastrointestinal decontamination. *J Toxicol Clin Toxicol* 1997;35:695–762.
3. AACT/EAPCCT position statement and practice guidelines on the use of multi-dose activated charcoal in the treatment of acute poisoning. *J Toxicol Clin Toxicol* 1999;37:731–51.
4. Manoguerra AS. Gastrointestinal decontamination after poisoning: where is the science? *Crit Care Clin* 1997;709–25.

Status Epilepticus

Brian K. Alldredge

Status epilepticus is a medical emergency in which prompt recognition and effective medical intervention are required to reduce the risk of permanent sequelae and death. Status epilepticus is defined as continuous seizures lasting at least 5 min, or two or more sequential seizures without full recovery of consciousness between seizures.

Status epilepticus can be categorized into two major types: convulsive and nonconvulsive. Convulsive status epilepticus is associated with the highest risk of morbidity and mortality, so this section focuses on the clinical features and management of this form of status epilepticus.

In about one-half of patients, status epilepticus is the first manifestation of seizures. The causes of status epilepticus are similar to those for new-onset seizures and include CNS infection, cerebral tumor, trauma, stroke, metabolic disorders, cardiopulmonary arrest, and drug toxicity. In the remainder of patients, status occurs in the setting of a pre-existing seizure disorder. Among persons with a history of epilepsy, antiepileptic drug withdrawal (usually noncompliance with prescribed therapy) is the most common cause of status epilepticus.

The primary determinant of patient outcome after status epilepticus is the underlying cause of the episode. In general, patients with status caused by an acute or progressive neurologic insult (eg, cardiopulmonary arrest, stroke) have poorer outcomes than patients in whom status epilepticus occurs in the setting of a more chronic or stable underlying condition (eg, antiepileptic drug withdrawal or medically refractory epilepsy). Nonetheless, aggressive medical intervention and administration of effective antiepileptic drug therapy are important to reduce status-related morbidity and mortality, regardless of the etiology.

Status epilepticus should be managed in an emergency department or an environment where continuous skilled medical and nursing support are available. The emergency management of status epilepticus should include the following:

- Ensure airway patency and adequate oxygenation.
- Obtain blood specimens for baseline laboratory measurements, including CBC, serum electrolytes (including calcium and magnesium), screen, and anticonvulsant serum levels.
- Establish IV access.
- Administer IV glucose (100 mg thiamine followed by 50 mL of 50% glucose in adults).
- Administer IV antiepileptic drugs.
- Monitor BP, respiratory rate and temperature. Treat hyperthermia with passive cooling.
- Obtain other diagnostic studies as needed.
- Treat precipitating factors.

■ DRUG THERAPY OF STATUS EPILEPTICUS

Adult doses only are given in this section.

If a treatable cause of status epilepticus can be identified rapidly, then drug therapy to terminate seizures might be unnecessary. In these situations, treatment of the underlying cause might be sufficient to stop status. Examples are status caused by an acute metabolic derangement (where correction of the underlying abnormality often stops seizures) or status after isoniazid overdose (where IV pyridoxine is usually effective). However, when a treatable cause is not known, drug therapy should begin immediately. The goal of drug treatment is to terminate seizures as rapidly as possible. Evidence from animal and human studies indicate that 60–120 min of status epilepticus is associated with neurologic sequelae and that the risk increases as status continues. Thus, it is important to have a clear, stepwise plan for the administration of effective drug therapy. Figure 4–1 shows an example of a status epilepticus treatment protocol. In addition, adequate support should be available to manage cardiac and respiratory complications that might occur during drug administration.

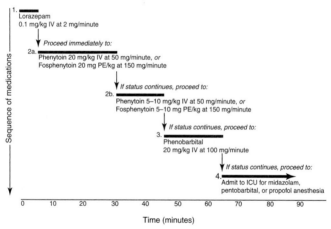

Figure 4–1. Timeline for administration of drug therapy for convulsive status epilepticus. Heavy bars (━) indicate duration (in minutes) of intravenous drug administration. PE = phenytoin equivalents.

1. For rapid termination of seizures:
   - **Lorazepam, IV, 0.1 mg/kg (4–8 mg) at rate of 2 mg/min;** may repeat in 10 min if seizures continue (to maximum of 0.2 mg/kg). Lorazepam has a longer duration of anticonvulsant effect than diazepam and is often preferred for this reason.

   or

- **Diazepam, IV, 0.2 mg/kg (5–10 mg) at rate of 5 mg/min;** may repeat in 10 min if seizures continue (to maximum of 20 mg). Diazepam has a short duration of anticonvulsant effect (15–60 min) and must be immediately followed by a long-acting agent (eg, phenytoin).

2a. After benzodiazepine administration, give:
- **Phenytoin, IV infusion, 20 mg/kg at rate of 50 mg/min** or **fosphenytoin 20 mg/kg phenytoin equivalents IV at a rate of 150 mg/min.** Monitor BP and ECG during administration of phenytoin or fosphenytoin loading dose. Elderly and severely ill patients are predisposed to phenytoin-related hypotension.

2b. If status persists, *then:*
- **Phenytoin or fosphenytoin, IV,** up to 2 additional doses of 5 mg/kg, to a total dosage of 30 mg/kg.

2c. If status is terminated, then begin maintenance phenytoin or fosphenytoin therapy.

3. If seizures are not terminated after administration of phenytoin or fosphenytoin 30 mg/kg, *then:*
- **Phenobarbital, IV, 20 mg/kg at rate of 100 mg/min.** The risk of hypoventilation is increased markedly when phenobarbital is administered after a benzodiazepine; respiratory support is often required.

4. For patients who continue in status epilepticus despite the above recommendations, anesthetic doses of a benzodiazepine, barbiturate, or propofol are often required to suppress seizure activity. Ventilatory assistance and vasopressor drug therapy are often required; therefore, the patient should be admitted to the ICU and the following therapies considered:

4a. **Midazolam, IV slow push, 200 μg/kg,** *then maintenance:*
- **Midazolam, IV infusion, 0.75–10 μg/kg/min.** High-dose midazolam is probably associated with a lower risk of hypotension than high-dose pentobarbital; however, there is less experience with its use.

4b. **Propofol, IV slow push, 1 mg/kg,** *then maintenance:*
- **Propofol, IV infusion 2–4 mg/kg/hr.** Reduce dosage by one-half in elderly or hemodynamically unstable patients.

The EEG should be monitored continuously during the first 1–2 hr of therapy, and infusion rates should be adjusted until suppression of electrographic seizures is evident. After seizures are terminated, the rate of the maintenance infusion can be slowed periodically to determine if status has remitted.

4c. **Pentobarbital, IV infusion, 1–2 mg/kg/hr.** Hypotension is a frequent complication of high-dose pentobarbital therapy; a vasopressor (eg, dopamine) may be required.

■ REFERENCES

1. Working Group on Status Epilepticus. Treatment of convulsive status epilepticus. Recommendations of the Epilepsy Foundation of America's working group on status epilepticus. *JAMA* 1993;270:854–9.
2. Treiman DM et al. A comparison of four treatments for generalized convulsive status epilepticus. *N Engl J Med* 1998;339:792–8.

3. Lowenstein DH et al. Barbiturate anesthesia in the treatment of status epilepticus: clinical experience with 14 patients. *Neurology* 1988;38:395–400.
4. Parent JM, Lowenstein DH. Treatment of refractory generalized status epilepticus with continuous infusion of midazolam. *Neurology* 1994;44:1837–40.
5. Shorvon SD. *Status epilepticus: its clinical features and treatment in children and adults.* New York: Cambridge University Press; 1994.
6. Stecker MM et al. Treatment of refractory status epilepticus with propofol: clinical and pharmacokinetic findings. *Epilepsia* 1998;39:18–26.
7. Lowenstein DH, Alldredge BK. Current concepts: status epilepticus. *N Engl J Med* 1998;338:970–6.

Drug Interactions and Interferences

5

Cytochrome P450 Enzyme Interactions

Philip D. Hansten

Cytochrome P450 enzymes are found throughout the body and play an important role in the metabolism of many drugs by catalyzing α-hydroxylation, N-demethylation, ring oxidation, and more.[1,2] Most substrates are metabolized by a specific enzyme, whereas each cytochrome P450 enzyme is generally capable of metabolizing many different compounds.[2,3] Induction or inhibition of these enzymes can dramatically affect the outcome of drug therapy.

Cytochrome P450 enzymes are identified by the prefix "CYP" followed by an Arabic number identifying the family, although Roman numerals are still sometimes used. The three important enzyme families in humans are CYP1, CYP2, and CYP3. Subfamilies are given letters (eg, CYP2B, CYP2C) that are followed by numbers identifying the specific enzyme.

Although most concentrated in the liver, cytochrome P450 enzymes exist in all tissues of the human body.[2,3] Intestinal mucosal cytochrome P450 enzymes appear to be primarily from the CYP3A family, probably CYP3A4 in humans.[3] These enzymes affect the bioavailability of some drugs.

■ INDUCTION AND INHIBITION

When the amount of enzyme present in the body is increased by a drug or chemical, the enzyme is said to be "induced." Although most inducers are P450 substrates, this is not always the case. Induction can increase the rate of clearance of a drug, decreasing its efficacy. It also can increase the rate of formation of an active or toxic metabolite, resulting in exaggeration of therapeutic effect or increased toxicity.

Theoretically, all substrates metabolized by the same enzyme can compete for the same binding site, causing competitive inhibition. However, the clinical relevance depends on the concentrations, relative affinities, and other elimination pathways of each substrate. Like inducers, not all inhibitors are enzyme substrates. Some drugs or their metabolites can form an inactive complex with a cytochrome P450 enzyme or its heme group. Inhibition can lead to increased toxic

1019

effects by causing drug accumulation, or it can lower toxic or therapeutic effects by decreasing the amount of toxic or active metabolite(s).

■ DRUG INTERACTIONS

Knowing which drugs are metabolized by each cytochrome P450 enzyme and the drugs that influence those enzymes can help in predicting drug–drug interactions. However, there are additional points to consider when predicting drug interactions.

The effect of inhibition on drug elimination depends partly on whether a substrate has alternate elimination pathways. Inhibition of an enzyme might not be clinically important if there are alternative metabolic pathways. However, phenytoin, which is metabolized by CYP2C9 and CYP2C19, can interact with CYP2C9 and CYP2C19 inhibitors, resulting in phenytoin toxicity.

Therapeutic range also is important. If a drug has a wide therapeutic range, factors such as induction or inhibition might be clinically unimportant. The opposite is true for drugs with a narrow therapeutic range, such as tricyclic antidepressants and antiarrhythmics.[4,5]

Last, consider metabolites. Not only does inhibition and induction of cytochrome P450 enzymes influence the formation of active metabolites, the formation of active metabolites can enhance inhibition or induction. Fluoxetine, an inhibitor of CYP2D6, has an active metabolite norfluoxetine, which also inhibits CYP2D6.[6,7]

The following table is meant to serve as an aid in the prediction of drug–drug interactions. However, it is also important to consider many other parameters: whether the patient is a poor or extensive metabolizer, the affinity of the drug for the binding site, the concentration of drug in the liver, the presence of alternate elimination pathways, and the therapeutic range. Because research on P450 metabolism is currently being published at a rapid rate, the table is not complete. The absence of a drug from the table does not necessarily imply that it is not metabolized by one of the P450 enzymes. When using the table, consider the following principles:

- Inhibition of drug metabolism tends to be substrate independent. That is, a potent inhibitor of CYP2D6 is likely to inhibit the metabolism of any drug metabolized by CYP2D6.
- The magnitude of cytochrome P450 enzyme inhibition is usually dose related over the dosage range of the inhibitor. For example, fluconazole 100 mg/day is usually a modest inhibitor of CYP3A4, but at 400 mg/day it can substantially inhibit the isozyme.
- Some cytochrome P450 inhibitors affect more than one enzyme. For example, ritonavir inhibits both CYP2D6 and CYP3A4.
- Drug enantiomers can be metabolized by different cytochrome P450 isozymes. For example, (R)-warfarin is metabolized by CYP1A2 and CYP3A4, and the more potent (S)-warfarin is metabolized primarily by CYP2C9. Thus, CYP1A2 or CYP3A4 inhibitors tend to produce only small increases in the hypoprothrombinemic response to warfarin, and CYP2C9 inhibitors produce large increases in warfarin effect.

COMMON DRUGS THAT INTERACT WITH P450 ENZYMES

	SUBFAMILY SUBSTRATES	INDUCERS	INHIBITORS
1A2	acetaminophen, amitriptyline, antipyrine, caffeine, clomipramine, clozapine, imipramine, olanzapine, propranolol, tacrine, theophylline, (R)-warfarin, zileuton	charcoal-broiled food, omeprazole, smoking	ciprofloxacin, enoxacin, fluvoxamine, macrolides,[a] mexietine, tacrine, zileuton
2B6	cyclophosphamide, ifosfamide	phenobarbital, phenytoin	
2C8	benzphetamine, cerivastatin, diazepam, diclofenac, (R)-mephenytoin, paclitaxel, pioglitazone, rosiglitazone, tolbutamide		
2C9/10	celecoxib, diclofenac, dronabinol, flubiprofen, hexobarbital, ibuprofen, losartan, (R)-mephenytoin, montelukast, naproxen, phenytoin, piroxicam, tolbutamide, torsemide, (S)-warfarin	barbiturates, carbamazepine, phenytoin, primidone, rifampin	amiodarone, clopidogrel, disulfiram, efavirenz, fluconazole, fluoxetine, fluvastatin, metronidazole, miconazole (IV), ritonavir, sulfamethoxazole, sulfaphenazole, sulfinpyrazone, zafirlukast
2C18	cimetidine, (S)-mephenytoin, propranolol, retinoic acid	omeprazole, piroxicam	
2C19	amitriptyline, clomipramine, diazepam, hexobarbital, imipramine, lansoprazole, mephenytoin, mephobarbital, omeprazole, pantoprazole, phenytoin, propranolol, rabeprazole	rifampin	efavirenz, felbamate, fluoxetine, fluvoxamine, omeprazole, ritonavir, ticlopidine
2D6	chlorpheniramine, codeine, debrisoquine, dextromethorphan, flecainide, fluoxetine, galantamine, haloperidol, hydrocodone, loratadine, metoprolol, mexiletine, paroxetine, perphenazine, propafenone, propranolol, risperidone, thioridazine, timolol, tramadol, trazodone, tricyclic antidepressants, venlafaxine, voriconazole		amiodarone, chloroquine, cimetidine, diphenhydramine, fluoxetine, haloperidol, paroxetine, perphenazine, propoxyphene, quinidine, ritonavir, SSRIs,[b] terbinafine, thioridazine

(continued)

COMMON DRUGS THAT INTERACT WITH P450 ENZYMES (continued)

	SUBFAMILY SUBSTRATES	INDUCERS	INHIBITORS
2E1	acetaminophen, alcohol, chlorzoxazone, dapsone, halothane, isoflurane, methoxy-flurane, sevoflurane	alcohol (chronic), isoniazid	alcohol (acute intoxication), disulfiram
3A3/4	alfentanil, alprazolam, amiodarone,[c] amitriptyline, amlodipine, androgens, astemizole, atorvastatin, benzphetamine, bepridil, bromocriptine, buspirone, carbamazepine, cilostazol, cisapride, clomipramine, clonazepam, cocaine, corticosteroids, cyclosporine,[c,d] dapsone, dexamethasone,[d] diazepam, diltiazem,[c,d] disopyramide, doxorubicin,[d] ergotamine, erythromycin,[c] ethinyl estradiol, ethosuximide, etoposide,[d] felodipine,[c] fentanyl, fexofenadine, finasteride, galantamine, hydrocortisone,[c,d] ifosfamide, imatinib, imipramine, indinavir, isradipine, itraconazole,[c] ketoconazole,[c] lidocaine,[c] losartan, lovastatin, miconazole, midazolam, mifepristone,[c] montelukast, nefazodone, nelfinavir,[c,d] nicardipine,[c,d] nifedipine,[c] nimodipine, nisoldipine, nitrendipine,[c] omeprazole, paclitaxel,[d] pimozide, pioglitazone, progesterone, propafenone, quinidine,[c] quinine, rifabutin, ritonavir,[c,d] saquinavir,[c,d] sertraline, sibutramine, sildenafil, simvastatin, sirolimus,[d] tacrolimus,[c,d] tamoxifen, teniposide, testosterone,[c] theophylline, triazolam, troleandomycin, verapamil,[c,d] vinca alkaloids,[d] voriconazole, (R)-warfarin, zolpidem	aminoglutethimide, barbiturates, carbamazepine, corticosteroids,[d] efavirenz, griseofulvin, phenytoin, primidone, rifabutin, rifampin, sulfinpyrazone	cyclophosphamide, cyclosporine,[c,d] delavirdine, diltiazem,[c,d] fluconazole, fluvoxamine, grapefruit juice, ifosfamide, indinavir,[c,d] itraconazole,[c] ketoconazole,[c] macrolides,[a] metronidazole, miconazole (IV), nefazodone, nelfinavir,[c,d] nicardipine,[c,d] nifedipine,[c] quinidine,[c] ritonavir,[c,d] verapamil,[c,d] zafirlukast

[a]CYP3A4 enzyme inhibition by macrolide antibiotics varies by drug: troleandomycin > erythromycin > clarithromycin > azithromycin = dirithromycin = 0.
[b]CYP2D6 enzyme inhibition by SSRI varies by drug: paroxetine = fluoxetine >> sertraline > ctalopram > fluvoxamine.
[c]Also an inhibitor of p-glycoprotein.[36]
[d]Also a substrate of p-glycoprotein.[36]
Compiled from references 3, 8–36.

■ REFERENCES

1. Almira M. Drug biotransformation. In, Katzung BG, ed. *Basic and clinical pharmacology*. Norwalk, CT: Appleton & Lange; 1992:49–59.
2. Watkins PB. Role of cytochromes P450 in drug metabolism and hepatotoxicity. *Semin Liver Dis* 1990; 10:235–50.
3. Watkins PB. Drug metabolism by cytochromes P450 in the liver and small bowel. *Gastroenterol Clin North Am* 1992;21:511–26.
4. DeVane CL. Pharmacogenetics and drug metabolism of newer antidepressant agents. *J Clin Psychiatry* 1994;55(suppl):38–4–5.
5. Lennard M. Genetically determined adverse drug reactions involving metabolism. *Drug Saf* 1993;9:60–77.
6. Crewe HK et al. The effect of selective serotonin reuptake inhibitors on cytochrome P4502D6 (CYP2D6) activity in human liver microsomes. *Br J Clin Pharmacol* 1992;34:262–5.
7. Otton SV et al. Inhibition by fluoxetine of cytochrome P4502D6 activity. *Clin Pharmacol Ther* 1993;53:401–9.
8. Spinler SA et al. Possible inhibition of hepatic metabolism of quinidine by erythromycin. *Clin Pharmacol Ther* 1995;57:89–94.
9. Ereshefsky L et al. Antidepressant drug interactions and the cytochrome P450 system, the role of cytochrome P4502D6. *Clin Pharmacokinet* 1995;29(suppl):10–9.
10. von Moltke LL et al. Metabolism of drugs by cytochrome P450 3A isoforms. *Clin Pharmacokinet* 1995; 29(suppl):33–44.
11. Flockhart DA. Drug interactions and the cytochrome P450 system. *Clin Pharmacokinet* 1995;29(suppl):45–52.
12. Slaughter RL, Edwards DJ. Recent advances: the cytochrome P450 enzymes. *Ann Pharmacother* 1995;29:619–24.
13. Pollock BG. Recent developments in drug metabolism of relevance to psychiatrists. *Harvard Rev Psychiatry* 1994;2:204–13.
14. Gonzalez FJ. Human cytochromes P450: problems and prospects. *Trends Pharmacol Sci* 1992;13:346–52.
15. Tatro DS, ed. *Drug interactions facts*. St. Louis: Facts and Comparisons; 2000.
16. Riesenman C. Antidepressant drug interactions and the cytochrome P450 system: a critical appraisal. *Pharmacotherapy* 1995;6(pt 2):84S–99S.
17. Kivisto KT et al. The role of human cytochrome P450 enzymes in the metabolism of anticancer agents: implications for drug interactions. *Br J Clin Pharmacol* 1995;40:523–30.
18. Schein JR. Cigarette smoking and clinically significant drug interactions. *Ann Pharmacother* 1995;29:1139–48.
19. Mitra AK et al. Metabolism of dapsone to its hydroxylamine by CYP2E1 in vitro and in vivo. *Clin Pharmacol Ther* 1995;58:556–66.
20. Transon C et al. In vivo inhibition profile of cytochrome P450TB (CYP2C9) by (+/–)-fluvastatin. *Clin Pharmacol Ther* 1995;58:412–7.
21. Periti P et al. Pharmacokinetic drug interactions of macrolides. *Clin Pharmacokinet* 1992;23:106–31.
22. Crewe HK et al. The effect of selective serotonin re-uptake inhibitors on cytochrome P4502D6 (CYP2D6) activity in human liver microsomes. *Br J Clin Pharmacol* 1992;34:262–5.
23. Manufacturer's Product Information.
24. Ketter TA et al. The emerging role of cytochrome P4503A in psychopharmacology. *J Clin Psychopharmacol* 1995;15:387–98.
25. Bertz RJ, Granneman GR. Use of in vitro and in vivo data to estimate the likelihood of metabolic pharmacokinetic interactions. *Clin Pharmacokinet* 1997;32:210–58.
26. Rendic S, Di Carlo FJ. Human cytochrome P450 enzymes: a status report summarizing their reactions, substrates, inducers and inhibitors. *Drug Metab Rev* 1997;29:413–580.
27. Michalets EL. Update: clinically significant cytochrome P-450 drug interactions. *Pharmacotherapy* 1998; 18:84–112.
28. Suri A et al. Effects of CYP3A inhibition on the metabolism of cilostazol. *Clin Pharmacokinet* 1999;37(suppl 2):61–8.
29. Moody DE et al. The involvement of cytochrome P450 3A4 in the N-demethylation of L-alpha-acetylmethadol (LAAM), norLAAM, and methadone. *Drug Metab Dispos* 1997;25:1347–53.
30. Libersa CC et al. Dramatic inhibition of amiodarone metabolism induced by grapefruit juice. *Br J Clin Pharmacol* 2000;49:373–8.
31. Karol MD et al. Lack of interaction between lansoprazole and propranolol, a pharmacokinetic and safety assessment. *J Clin Pharmacol* 2000;40:301–8.
32. Song JC, White CM. Pharmacologic, pharmacokinetic, and therapeutic differences among angiotensin II receptor antagonists. *Pharmacotherapy* 2000;20:130–9.
33. Vickers AE et al. Multiple cytochrome P-450s involved in the metabolism of terbinafine suggest a limited potential for drug–drug interactions. *Drug Metab Dispos* 1999;27:1029–38.

34. Cagnoni PJ et al. Modification of the pharmacokinetics of high-dose cyclophosphamide and cisplatin by antiemetics. *Bone Marrow Transplant* 1999;24:1–4.

35. Hansten PD, Horn JR. *Drug interactions analysis and management.* St. Louis: Facts and Comparisons; 2000.

36. Zhang Y, Benet LZ. The gut as a barrier to drug absorption. *Clin Pharmacokinet* 2001;40:159–68.

Drug-Induced Discoloration of Feces and Urine

The drugs and drug classes in the following tables have been associated with the discoloration of feces or urine. Drugs and drug classes are listed generically.

DRUGS THAT CAN DISCOLOR FECES	
DRUG/DRUG CLASS	**COLOR PRODUCED**
Antacids, Aluminum Hydroxide Types	Whitish or speckling
Anthraquinones	Brownish staining of rectal mucosa
Antibiotics, Oral	Greenish gray
Anticoagulants	Pink to red or black[a]
Bismuth Salts	Greenish black
Charcoal	Black
Clofazimine	Red to brownish black
Ferrous Salts	Black
Heparin	Pink to red or black[a]
Indocyanine Green	Green
Indomethacin	Green because of biliverdinemia
NSAIDs	Pink to red or black[a]
Omeprazole	Discoloration
Phenazopyridine	Orange-red
Pyrvinium Pamoate	Red
Rifampin	Red-orange
Risperidone	Discoloration
Salicylates (especially Aspirin)	Pink to red or black[a]

[a]These colors can indicate intestinal bleeding.

DRUGS THAT CAN DISCOLOR URINE	
DRUG/DRUG CLASS	**COLOR PRODUCED**
Aminopyrine	Red
Aminosalicylic Acid	Discoloration; red in hypochlorite solution[a]

(continued)

DRUGS THAT CAN DISCOLOR URINE (*continued*)

DRUG/DRUG CLASS	COLOR PRODUCED
Amitriptyline	Blue-green
Anthraquinones	Yellow-brown in acid urine; yellow-pink-red in alkaline urine
Antipyrine	Red-brown
Azuresin	Blue or green
Chloroquine	Rust yellow to brown
Chlorzoxazone	Orange or purplish red
Cimetidine (injection)	Green[b]
Clofazimine	Red to brownish black
Daunorubicin	Red
Deferoxamine	Reddish
Doxorubicin	Red
Entacapone	Brownish-orange
Ethoxazene	Orange to orange-brown
Ferrous Salts	Black
Flutamide	Amber or yellow-green
Furazolidone	Brown
Idarubicin	Red
Indandiones	Orange-red in alkaline urine
Indomethacin	Green because of biliverdinemia
Iron Sorbitex	Brown-black
Levodopa	Red-brown; dark on standing in hypochlorite solution[a]
Loratadine	Discoloration
Methocarbamol	Dark to brown, black or green on standing
Methyldopa	Dark on standing in hypochlorite solution[b]
Methylene Blue	Blue or green
Metronidazole	Dark, brown
Mitoxantrone	Blue-green
Niacin	Dark
Nitrofurantoin	Rust yellow to brown
Pamaquine	Rust yellow to brown
Phenacetin	Dark brown to black on standing
Phenazopyridine	Orange to red
Phenolphthalein	Pink to purplish red in alkaline urine
Phenothiazines	Pink to red or red-brown

(*continued*)

DRUGS THAT MIGHT DISCOLOR URINE (*continued*)

DRUG/DRUG CLASS	COLOR PRODUCED
Phensuximide	Pink to red or red-brown
Phenytoin	Pink to red or red-brown
Primaquine	Rust yellow to brown
Promethazine (injection)	Green[b]
Propofol (injection)	Green, white, pink, brown, or red-brown
Quinacrine	Deep yellow in acidic urine
Quinine	Brown to black
Resorcinol	Dark green
Riboflavin	Yellow fluorescence
Rifabutin	Discoloration
Rifampin	Red-orange
Sulfasalazine	Orange-yellow in alkaline urine
Sulfonamides, Antibacterial	Rust yellow to brown
Sulindac	Discoloration
Tolcapone	Bright yellow
Tolonium	Blue-green
Triamterene	Pale blue fluorescence
Warfarin	Orange

[a]Hypochlorite solution in toilet bowl from prior use of chlorine bleach.
[b]Caused by phenol as a preservative in the injectable formulation.

■ REFERENCES

1. *Physicians' desk reference*. 49th ed. Montvale, NJ: Medical Economics Data Production; 1995.
2. Baran RB, Rowles B. Factors affecting coloration of urine and feces. *J Am Pharm Assoc* 1973;NS13:139–42.
3. Bodenham A et al. Propofol infusion and green urine. *Lancet* 1987;2:740. Letter.
4. Bowling P et al. Intravenous medications and green urine. *JAMA* 1981;246:216. Letter.
5. Devereaux MW, Mancall EL. Brown urine, bleach, and L-DOPA. *N Engl J Med* 1974;291:1142. Letter.
6. Michaels RM, ed. Discolored urine. *Phys Drug Alert* 1981;2(9):71.
7. Nates J et al. Appearance of white urine during propofol anesthesia. *Anesth Analg* 1995;81:204–13. Letter.
8. Raymond JR, Yarger WE. Abnormal urine color: differential diagnosis. *South Med J* 1988;81:837–41.
9. Wallach J. *Interpretation of diagnostic tests*. 6th ed. Boston: Little, Brown; 1996:867–8, 879.
10. Blakey SA, Hixson-Wallace JA. Clinical significance of rare and benign side effects: propofol and green urine. *Pharmacotherapy* 2000;20:1120-2.

Nutrition Support | 6

Fred Shatsky

Nutrition status is a major determinant of patients' morbidity and mortality. Morbidity increases with malnutrition, as manifested by depressed immunocompetence and impaired wound healing.[1] Conditions that indicate a possible need for nutrition support are inadequate oral nutrition for longer than 7 days, recent body weight loss >10%, an illness lasting longer than 3 weeks, recent major surgery, a lymphocyte count <1.2 × 10^3/μL, serum albumin <3 g/dL, serum transferrin <150 mg/dL, and serum prealbumin <15 mg/dL. Sepsis, trauma, and other factors that induce hypermetabolism might intensify the need.

The term "nutrition support" can be applied to any nutrition regimen that is provided for conditions that preclude the use of regular foods. There are two broad categories of nutrition support, enteral and parenteral, determined by their route of administration. Enteral nutrition applies to regimens provided via any portion of the GI tract. Parenteral nutrition (PN), although implying all routes other than the GI tract, refers primarily to regimens that are provided directly by the intravenous route of administration. Less frequently used modes of PN such as intradialytic parenteral nutrition and intraperitoneal nutrition are not discussed in this chapter.

Whenever possible, maintenance rather than repletion should be the primary objective of nutrition support. Early provision of nutrition requirements without exceeding energy balance promotes the synthesis of lean body mass rather than adipose tissue.[2]

■ NUTRITION ASSESSMENT

Nutrition assessment of the patient can aid in diagnosing malnutrition and determining its degree of severity, so that a proper nutrition support regimen can be formulated. The patient's physical and dietary history should be obtained to establish baseline data. Clinical parameters for assessing the patient's nutrition status can be evaluated through the use of an assessment form (Table 6–1). Because a patient's nutrition status is best reflected by body protein, nutrition assessment should focus on the protein compartments. Protein compartments are classified into two types: somatic (muscle protein) and visceral (all other protein).

TABLE 6–1. NUTRITION ASSESSMENT[a]

NAME: AGE: HT (CM): DATE: SEX: WT (KG):	STANDARD	DEPLETION		
		MILD	*MODERATE*	*SEVERE*
TSF (mm)	M 12.5	11.3	11.3–7.5	<7.5
	F 16.5	14.9	14.9–9.9	<9.9
Ideal Body Weight: $\frac{ABW}{IBW} \times 100 =$	100%	90%	90–60%	<60%
MUAC (cm)	M 29.3	26.4	26.4–17.6	<17.6
	F 28.5	25.7	25.7–17.1	<17.1
MUAMC: MUAC (cm) − (0.314 × TSF [mm]) =	M 25.3	22.8	22.8–15.2	<15.2
	F 23.2	21.0	21.0–13.9	<13.9
Creatinine/Height Index: $\frac{Cr_u}{ICr_u \text{ for height}} \times 100 =$	100%	90%	90–60%	<60%
Serum Albumin (g/dL)	3.5–5.0	3.5–3.0	3.0–2.1	<2.1
Serum Prealbumin (mg/dL)	>20	20–15	15–10	<10
Serum Transferrin (mg/dL)	200–400	200–150	150–100	<100
Total Lymphocytes/μL: $\frac{WBC/\mu L \times \% \text{ Lymphocytes}}{100}$	1800–3000	1800–1200	1200–800	<800

[a]The standards specified represent those of healthy persons. Measurements in patients can be affected by nonnutritional and nutritional factors.
ABW, actual body weight; Cr_u, urinary creatinine; IBW, ideal body weight; ICr_u, ideal urinary creatinine; MUAC, mid–upper arm circumference; MUAMC, mid-upper arm muscle circumference; TSF, triceps skinfold.

SOMATIC PROTEIN ASSESSMENT PARAMETERS

Percentage Ideal Body Weight.   A simple initial measurement of a patient's nutrition status is body weight expressed as a percentage of ideal body weight. (*See* Appendix 2, Anthropometrics.)

$$\text{Percentage Ideal Body Weight} = \frac{\text{Actual Body Weight}}{\text{Ideal Body Weight}} \times 100$$

Creatinine/Height Index.   Creatinine/height index (CHI), when accurately obtained, is a more sensitive indicator of somatic protein and nutrition status than is percentage of ideal body weight. Creatinine, a product of muscle metabolism, is normally excreted in urine at a constant rate proportional to the amount of skeletal muscle and lean body mass catabolized. CHI is calculated from a 24-hr urinary creatinine measurement, and the ideal urinary creatinine value found in Table 6–2, using the following formula:

$$CHI = \frac{\text{Actual Urinary Creatinine}}{\text{Ideal Urinary Creatinine for Height}} \times 100$$

It is important that the urine sample be an aliquot drawn from a 24-hr collection of urine rather than a random sample.

TABLE 6–2. IDEAL URINARY CREATININE

MALES[a]		FEMALES[b]	
Height (cm)	Ideal Creatinine (mg/24 hr)	Height (cm)	Ideal Creatinine (mg/24 hr)
157.5	1288	147.3	830
160.0	1325	149.9	851
162.6	1359	152.4	875
165.1	1386	154.9	900
167.6	1426	157.5	925
170.2	1467	160.0	949
172.7	1513	162.6	977
175.3	1555	165.1	1006
177.8	1596	167.6	1044
180.3	1642	170.2	1076
182.9	1691	172.7	1109
185.4	1739	175.3	1141
188.0	1785	177.8	1174
190.5	1831	180.3	1206
193.0	1891	182.9	1240

[a]Creatinine coefficient (men) = 23 mg/kg of ideal body weight.
[b]Creatinine coefficient (women) = 18 mg/kg of ideal body weight.
From Blackburn GL et al. Nutritional and metabolic assessment of the hospitalized patient. JPEN 1977;1:11–22, reproduced with permission.

There are limitations in using CHI as an indicator of malnutrition. Patients sometimes excrete amounts of creatinine and nitrogen that change with diet, medications, degree of renal function, conditions of illness, or stress. Certain drugs interfere with urine creatinine determinations. (*See* Drug–Laboratory Test Interferences, page 1070.)

Anthropometric Measurements.   Anthropometric measurements can be of questionable value because of slow changes over time and interobserver variability. If used, the triceps skinfold (TSF) and mid–upper arm circumference (MUAC) should be measured on the mid–upper portion of the nondominant arm by trained personnel. Detailed procedures and methods of measurement are available.[3,4] TSF measurement with calipers is compared with the standards in Table 6–1 to give a reasonable estimate of subcutaneous fat reserves. TSF and MUAC, obtained with a tape measure, can be used to derive the mid upper arm muscle circumference MUAMC by the formula:

$$MUAMC = MUAC \text{ (cm)} - (0.314 \times TSF \text{ [mm]})$$

VISCERAL PROTEIN ASSESSMENT PARAMETERS

The status of visceral protein reflects the patient's ability to respond to stress by means such as immunocompetence and wound healing. Visceral protein status can be determined by measurements of serum albumin, serum thyroxine–binding pre-albumin (also referred to as transthyretin or prealbumin), and serum transferrin. These visceral protein indicators usually decrease after trauma or surgical proce-dures; however, consistently low levels for at least 1 week might indicate a degree of malnutrition.[4] Serum albumin is unreliable as an assessment parameter in cer-tain patients. Serum albumin can be elevated as a result of dehydration, shock, hemoconcentration, or administration of anabolic hormones or IV albumin. De-creased albumin levels can result from chronic illness, malabsorption, pregnancy, nephrotic syndrome, hepatic insufficiency, protein-losing enteropathy, overhydra-tion, or severe burns.[5,6]

Prealbumin and transferrin are visceral proteins with a more rapid turnover than albumin; they are effective assessment parameters with half-lives of approxi-mately 2 and 8 days, respectively.

Visceral protein levels and nitrogen balance are expected to decline postop-eratively. In a comparison between postoperative prealbumin and transferrin serum levels, the decline in prealbumin was much greater, and changes in trans-ferrin were more closely correlated with changes in nitrogen balance.[7] Transferrin levels can be elevated in patients who are iron deficient, pregnant, or taking estro-gens or oral contraceptives. Serum albumin, prealbumin, and transferrin values in-dicative of different degrees of depletion are given in Table 6–1.

■ PERIODIC REASSESSMENT

An initial assessment can be made before beginning a nutrition support regimen. Periodic reassessment of the patient, using some or all of the previously men-tioned parameters, can provide a means of objectively evaluating the efficacy of nutrition support. Additional parameters to consider during this stage of assess-ment are nitrogen balance and body weight.

NITROGEN BALANCE

Nitrogen balance determinations indicate the extent to which exogenous protein is being used and can serve as a method for evaluating the efficacy of nutrition sup-port. Because nitrogen balance data are subject to errors of collection and other variables, they should be used only as a relative index of daily change and not an absolute measure of depletion or improvement. Nitrogen balance is calculated for a 24-hr period with the following formula:[4]

$$\text{Nitrogen Balance} = \text{Total Nitrogen In} - \text{Total Nitrogen Out}$$

Urinary urea nitrogen (UUN), although a less sensitive indicator of nitrogen output than total urea nitrogen, is a simpler laboratory procedure and is therefore a more frequently used measurement to estimate nitrogen balance. Nitrogen balance is calculated as follows:

$$\text{Nitrogen Balance} = \frac{\text{Protein Intake (in g)}}{6.25} - (\text{UNN [in g]} + 4)$$

UUN is usually reported in mg/dL; therefore, to derive the amount in grams for use in the above formula, the value must be multiplied by the total 24-hr volume of urine output. The urine sample sent to the laboratory should be an aliquot drawn from an accurate 24-hr urine collection. The factor 4 is added as an empirical number to account for nonurinary nitrogen such as that excreted in feces, sweat, and other normal losses. Excessive nitrogen losses that cannot be measured, such as nitrogen lost in exudates from severe burns or other fluid losses, render nitrogen balance data less reliable.

Positive nitrogen balance can indicate a retention of nitrogen as newly synthesized body protein tissue and nitrogen retained in body fluids. A positive nitrogen balance of 4–6 g/day is the maximum that should be expected;[8] greater amounts are not considered efficient. Because only synthesized protein is of therapeutic interest, increments in BUN above baseline (in grams) should be subtracted from total nitrogen balance. This calculation is summarized as follows:

$$\text{Corrected Nitrogen Balance} = \text{Nitrogen Balance} - \text{BUN Increment (g)}$$

To derive the BUN increment above baseline in grams, the total body water volume of the patient must be considered. Body water can be estimated to be 55% of total body weight (0.55 L/kg).[8] A BUN of 10 mg/dL above baseline in a 70-kg patient represents a BUN increment of 3.85 g (70 kg × 0.55 L/kg × 100 mg/L = 3850 mg).

BODY WEIGHT

The weight difference between body water and tissue is indistinguishable unless water balance is measured. Body weight gain alone is therefore not a reliable maintenance assessment parameter. It is known, however, that weight gain in excess of 200 g/day is undesirable because patients cannot synthesize lean body tissue at a greater rate.[8] Despite its shortcomings as a monitoring parameter, body weight should be measured throughout the support regimen at the same time each day, and intake and output should be considered in the interpretation of body weight changes.

NUTRIENT REQUIREMENTS

The nutrients required for enteral and parenteral nutrition are virtually the same. Either mode of nutrition support must consist of the basic components of a normal diet: water, carbohydrate, fat, protein, electrolytes, vitamins, and trace elements.

CALORIC REQUIREMENTS

Accurate estimation of caloric requirements is essential, particularly for the severely stressed or depleted patient, to avoid problems associated with overfeeding and underfeeding.[9] Requirements can be calculated accurately by indirect calorimetry using instruments that measure respiratory gas exchange. When this is not possible, requirements can be estimated as a multiple of the patient's basal energy expenditure (BEE). BEE is the amount of energy required to maintain basic metabolic functions in the resting state and can be derived from the Harris-Benedict equations:[9]

$$\text{BEE (Men): } 66 + (13.8 \times \text{wt in kg}) + (5 \times \text{ht in cm}) - (6.8 \times \text{age in yr})$$

$$\text{BEE (Women): } 655 + (9.6 \times \text{wt in kg}) + (1.8 \times \text{ht in cm}) - (4.7 \times \text{age in yr})$$

Mechanically ventilated nonsurgical patients without stress or sepsis should receive a total caloric intake no greater than the calculated BEE.[9] Trauma and sepsis increase energy and protein requirements, and the nutrition support regimen should be adjusted accordingly. One means of determining the severity of catabolism in stress conditions is by measurement of UUN excreted per 24 hr. Caloric requirements can then be estimated as a multiple of BEE, as shown in Table 6–3.[10]

TABLE 6–3. CALORIC REQUIREMENTS DURING CATABOLISM

24-HR UUN	DEGREE OF NET CATABOLISM	CALORIC REQUIREMENTS
0–5 g	1° (normal)	1 × BEE
5–10 g	2° (mild)	1.5 × BEE
10–15 g	3° (moderate)	1.75 × BEE
>15 g	4° (severe)	2 × BEE

BEE, basal energy expenditure; UUN, urinary urea nitrogen.

In estimating the calories to be provided by each substrate, yields may be considered as follows: dextrose, 3.4 kcal/g; fat, 9 kcal/g; and protein, 4 kcal/g. Although protein is considered a calorigenic substrate, it is not usually included in estimating caloric goals because the main role of protein is the preservation or synthesis of lean body mass.

PROTEIN REQUIREMENTS

The minimum requirement for protein is about 0.8 g/kg/day of a balanced mixture of amino acids (AAs), and can be as high as 2.5 g/kg/day in severely stressed or traumatized patients. For optimal synthesis of protein, concurrent provision of nonprotein calories must be sufficient. To calculate the nonprotein calorie–to–nitrogen ratio, assume that the nitrogen content is 1 g/6.25 g of AAs. The optimal ratio of nonprotein calories to nitrogen for efficient nitrogen retention and nitrogen balance is not definite, but differs with the metabolic state of the patient. Nonprotein calorie-to-nitrogen ratios of standard enteral nutrition and PN formulas are typically about 150:1. Lower ratios are indicated for stress or trauma and higher ratios for nonstressed patients and those with impaired protein metabolism.

ENTERAL NUTRITION

For physiologic and economic reasons, the enteral route should be used whenever possible, but adequacy of the GI tract must be established before enteral nutrition is provided. The IV route should be strictly reserved for patients who cannot be adequately nourished by the enteral route.

Formulas for enteral nutrition are available for supplemental oral feeding or enteral feeding through different types of tubes. When the oral route is not feasible, transnasal passage of a feeding tube into the stomach (nasogastric) or intestine (nasoduodenal or nasojejunal) is the feeding route generally employed. Feeding ostomies, most commonly the gastrostomy, jejunostomy, or combination gastrostomy–jejunostomy, are generally indicated when insertion through the nares is not feasible or when long-term feeding is anticipated.

FORMULA SELECTION

The abundance of products and lack of an ideal system of categorization can cause confusion in selecting the most appropriate enteral formula for a patient. It is not within the scope of this chapter to fully describe criteria for formula selection or provide a complete list of formulas.

Some nutritionally complete, ready-to-use liquid enteral formulas that are suitable for a variety of patients are presented in Table 6–4. Carbohydrate, fat, and protein sources differ with products and can be important criteria for selecting a product. Because patients with abnormal intestinal function are usually lactose intolerant, only lactose-free products are included. Disease-specific formulas, such as those with high content of branched-chain amino acids (BCAAs) for liver disease or essential AAs for renal disease, might be nutritionally incomplete and are not included because of inadequate evidence of their superiority.

ADMINISTRATION

One of two types of feeding schedules can be employed, continuous or intermittent. Continuous drip infusion is the preferred method of administration, particularly for patients who have not eaten for a long time. Large 24-hr volumes may be given by infusion without challenging the GI tract, thereby allowing readaptation of the starved gut. Although gravity can be used, an infusion pump is recommended when initiating therapy. For most patients, it is recommended that the first day's feeding be infused at a rate of 50 mL/hr using a lactose-free, nutrient-intact, isotonic formula of 1 kcal/mL. Many protocols recommend diluting the initial formula to one-half strength; however, this practice has been questioned.[11]

TABLE 6–4. REPRESENTATIVE ENTERAL FORMULAS

PRODUCT	CALORIES (per mL)	PROTEIN (g/L)	FAT (g/L)	CARBOHYDRATE (g/L)	NONPROTEIN CALORIES:N (cal/g nitrogen)	SODIUM (mEq/L)	POTASSIUM (mEq/L)	CALCIUM (mg/L)	PHOSPHORUS (mg/L)	OSMOLARITY (mOsm/L)
Compleat Modified	1.07	43	37	140	135	44	36	670	930	300
Criticare HN	1.06	38	5	220	152	27	34	530	530	650
Ensure Plus	1.5	54	53	197	146	45	49	705	705	690
Ensure Plus HN	1.5	62	49	197	125	51	46	1057	1057	650
Impact	1.0	56	28	130	86	48	33	800	800	375
Isocal	1.06	34	44	135	172	23	34	630	530	270
Isocal HCN	2.0	75	102	200	143	35	43	1000	1000	640
Isosource HN	1.2	53	41	160	119	48	44	670	670	330
Jevity	1.06	44	35	151	130	40	40	910	760	300
Magnacal	2.0	70	80	250	154	43	32	1000	1000	590
Nitrolan	1.24	60	40	160	104	30	30	800	800	310
Osmolite	1.06	37	37	143	153	27	26	528	528	300
Osmolite HN	1.06	44	35	140	124	40	40	758	758	300
Pulmocare	1.5	62	92	104	125	56	44	1060	1060	475
Reabilan HN	1.3	58	52	158	119	44	42	500	500	490
Suplena	2.0	30	92	253	389	34	28	1386	728	600
Sustacal	1.0	61	23	138	78	40	52	1010	930	620
Sustacal Plus	1.5	61	53	200	131	55	53	850	850	600
TraumaCal	1.5	83	69	195	105	52	36	750	750	490
Ultracal	1.06	44	45	123	127	40	41	850	850	310

Incremental advances in rate and strength can be attempted daily until the desired rate of a full-strength formula is achieved. To minimize the risk of aspiration, proper placement of the tube must be confirmed, and the patient's head and shoulders must be kept at a 30–45° angle during and for 1 hr after feeding. The stomach should be checked periodically for residual volumes during gastric feedings.

Once a patient has been stabilized on maintenance therapy, intermittent infusions can be used, allowing the patient to rest from feedings at selected hours. A volume of 250–400 mL may be administered 5–8 times/day. This method is preferred for ambulatory patients because it permits more freedom of movement than does continuous feeding.

Formulas should be given at room temperature and kept no longer than 12 hr after the time of preparation and 6 hr from the start of administration to avoid excessive bacterial growth. The delivery system, including bag and tubing, should be changed q 24 hr.

COMPLICATIONS

Mechanical and GI complications known to occur with tube feedings are summarized in Table 6–5. Metabolic complications that occur with enteral nutrition are similar to those with PN and are included in Table 6–12.

To prevent metabolic complications, monitoring of the patient as suggested in Table 6–13 is recommended.

TABLE 6–5. TUBE FEEDING COMPLICATIONS AND MANAGEMENT

COMPLICATION	PREVENTION OR MANAGEMENT
Mechanical	
Clogged Tube	Flush with water, replace tube if necessary. Avoid passing crushed tablets through small-bore feeding tubes.
Nasal, Pharyngeal, Esophageal Irritation	Use small-lumen flexible tube. Provide daily care of nose and mouth.
Aspiration	Ensure proper tube placement and verify location. Maintain patient's head and shoulders at 30–45° in the upright position during and for 1 hr after feeding. Monitor for gastric reflux and abdominal distention. Stop infusion if vomiting occurs. Check residual gastric volume before and q 2–4 hr during infusion. Hold if the residual exceeds the hourly volume or 150 mL.
Dislocated Tube	Verify tube location and mark tube at insertion site.
Gastrointestinal	
Diarrhea and Cramps	Reduce flow rate, dilute formula, or consider alternative formula. Rule out alternative causes. If persistent, add antidiarrheal agent.
Vomiting or Bloating	Check stool output and measure residual formula in gut q 2–4 hr if necessary, stop or reduce flow.
Constipation	Consider different formula or a laxative.

■ PARENTERAL NUTRITION

PN may be administered by one of two routes of access: peripheral veins or larger central veins. The peripheral route is indicated for those patients who require only short-term supplementation or supplementation in addition to enteral support or for those in whom the risks of central venous administration are too great. Peripheral veins are susceptible to thrombophlebitis, particularly when the osmolarity of the solution exceeds 600 mOsm/L. Therefore, it is recommended that formulas for peripheral administration not exceed final concentrations of 10% dextrose and

4.5% AAs plus electrolyte and vitamin additives. Many techniques to prevent or delay onset of peripheral vein thrombophlebitis have been reported.[12] Addition of small amounts of hydrocortisone (5 mg/L) and heparin (1000 units/L) to PN formulas, as well as the topical use of agents such as nitroglycerin, have demonstrated success. Concurrent administration of IV fat emulsion, which is a concentrated, iso-osmotic calorie source, is vital because it increases the caloric content of a peripheral regimen and minimizes the risk of thrombophlebitis.

The complete nutrition needs of the malnourished or hypermetabolic patient are difficult to provide through peripheral vein for long periods. The concentrated, hyperosmolar solutions required by such patients for PN *must* be administered into a large central vein, such as the superior vena cava, where rapid dilution occurs.

ADMINISTRATION

Initiation of PN should be gradual, particularly in the malnourished patient, to avoid glucose intolerance and the dangers of refeeding syndrome.[13] With high concentrations of dextrose and AAs intended for central vein administration, an initial rate of 40 mL/hr for the first 24 hr is suggested. Infusion rates may then be increased daily in accordance with assessment goals. Less concentrated formulas that are suited for peripheral vein administration do not warrant such slow initial rates of infusion.

Different catheters exist for infusion of PN formulas by central or peripheral vein. Use of an in-line filter is recommended to minimize adverse consequences in case precipitation occurs in the PN solution.[14]

PARENTERAL NUTRIENTS

Each of the following nutrient substrate groups are required in formulas for effective PN.

Water. The average healthy adult can tolerate a fluid infusion volume of about 5 L/day. The patient who is fluid restricted might be limited to an intake of ≤ 2 L/day. This might be the deciding factor in selecting a hypertonic concentrated solution for infusion through a large central vein rather than a more dilute solution for peripheral administration.

Carbohydrate. The presently preferred carbohydrate substrate for PN is dextrose. The concentration of dextrose should be determined by the osmotic limitation of the administration route and the nonprotein calorie requirement of the patient. The concentrations of available dextrose solutions with their corresponding caloric concentrations and osmolarities are shown in Table 6–6.

Dextrose remains the primary source of calories for PN through central vein, and the rate of infusion should be limited to its maximum rate of oxidation, which is 5 mg/kg/min or 7.2 g/kg/day.[15] On a calorie-for-calorie basis, carbohydrate is more efficient than fat in sparing body protein during hypocaloric feedings.[16] The inclusion of dextrose and fat is recommended in PN regimens, but the optimal proportion of each has not been established.

Fat. Fat is an important parenteral substrate for three major reasons: (1) it is a concentrated source of calories in an isotonic medium, which makes it useful for

TABLE 6–6. IV DEXTROSE SOLUTIONS

CONCENTRATION	kcal/L	mOsm/L
5%	170	252
10%	340	505
20%	680	1010
40%	1360	2020
50%	1700	2520
60%	2040	3030
70%	2380	3530

peripheral administration; (2) it is a source of essential fatty acids (EFAs) required for prevention or treatment of EFA deficiency, which can develop during prolonged fat-free PN;[17] and (3) it is a useful substitute for carbohydrate when dextrose calories must be limited because of glucose intolerance or diminished ventilatory capacity. When a patient's ventilatory effort is hampered, it is important to avoid excessive calories of any type. In comparison with dextrose, the metabolism of fat increases heat production, decreases respiratory quotient (RQ), and increases oxygen consumption. Because it has a lower RQ, fat produces less CO_2 for a given number of calories, thereby minimizing the ventilatory effort required to eliminate CO_2. The RQ of fat is 0.7 compared with 1 for carbohydrate. An RQ in excess of 1 indicates net lipogenesis and is undesirable.[18]

Fat is available as emulsions of 10, 20, or 30% soybean oil or 10 or 20% soybean–safflower oil mixtures. Clinical studies have not shown any major advantages of one lipid source over the other. The major differences between these products are their fatty acid contents, which are summarized in Table 6–7. The 20 and 30% emulsions are more readily cleared than the 10% one because of the lower proportion of phospholipid to triglyceride.[19]

Fat emulsions that are currently marketed in the United States contain only long-chain triglycerides (LCTs); however, the use of fat emulsions that contain LCTs and medium-chain triglycerides (MCTs) is being investigated. MCTs are reported to be more rapidly cleared from the blood and more ketogenic than

TABLE 6–7. IV FAT EMULSIONS

FATTY ACID	SOYBEAN OIL	SOYBEAN OIL/SAFFLOWER OIL
Linoleic Acid	54%	65.8%
Linolenic Acid	8%	4.2%
Oleic Acid	26%	17.7%
Palmitic Acid	9%	8.8%
Stearic Acid	2.5%	3.4%

LCTs, and emulsions containing MCTs and LCTs have greater protein-conserving properties than pure LCT emulsions.[20] LCTs are required for their EFA content, however.

The caloric density of 10% fat emulsions is 1.1 kcal/mL, of which 1 kcal is supplied by lipid and 0.1 kcal by glycerol (carbohydrate); the 20% and 30% emulsions have caloric densities of 2 and 3 kcal/mL, respectively, of which 0.1 kcal/mL is glycerol. The average particle size (0.5 μ) is the same in all concentrations, and all are nearly iso-osmotic.

Fat emulsion can be infused concurrently with AA/dextrose solution through peripheral or central veins. The 10% or 20% emulsion may be infused separately or combined with AAs and dextrose in a single container to form a total nutrient ("3-in-1") admixture (TNA).[21] The 30% concentration is intended only for compounding TNA. Because lipid emulsion is iso-osmolar, it reduces the thrombophlebitic effect of hyperosmolar AA/dextrose solutions on the endothelium of peripheral veins when they are infused concurrently.[22] For this reason and its potential adverse effect on the immune system, fat emulsion should be infused as slowly as possible.[23] The use of IV fat emulsion in patients with pancreatitis is often questionable because it is harmful if lipid is not adequately cleared from the blood. IV fat emulsion can be used safely if serum triglyceride levels are monitored and remain below 400 mg/dL (4.5 mmol/L).[24] Product literature suggests that fat be provided in quantities no greater than 3 g/kg or 60% of total calories. For further information on dosage, administration, and precautions of fat emulsion, the product literature should be consulted.

Protein.   Various brands and concentrations of AA solutions are available as sources of protein for parenteral use. The AA profile differs in each; therefore, their nitrogen contents are not equivalent. A comparison of formulations is summarized in Table 6–8. AA solutions >3.5% concentration should be diluted to a lower final concentration with dextrose and other additives.

SPECIAL AMINO ACID SOLUTIONS

Special AA solutions are available for specific metabolic or disease states. Discretion is recommended in the use of these solutions because they are expensive and clinical benefit is not proved.

Protein Sparing.   A low concentration of AAs infused with or without concurrent nonprotein calories conserves endogenous nitrogen more efficiently than the traditional 5% dextrose infusion alone.[25] For a limited infusion of no more than 1 week's duration in patients who are not severely catabolic, low-concentration AA formulas merit consideration. Low-concentration AA formulas are available with or without electrolytes and with or without a nonprotein calorie source (*see* Table 6–8).

Renal Failure.   The objective of PN in patients with renal failure is to provide sufficient AAs and calories for protein synthesis without exceeding the renal capacity for excretion of fluid and metabolic wastes. Four parenteral products that contain primarily essential AAs have been developed for this purpose (*see* Table 6–8), but controversy exists regarding their use. Patients who undergo renal re-

TABLE 6–8. AMINO ACID SOLUTIONS COMPARISON CHART

AA SOLUTION AND OSMOLARITY CONCENTRATION	TOTAL BCAAs (g/dL)	TOTAL ESSENTIAL AAs (g/dL)	TOTAL N (g/dL)	ELECTROLYTES (mEq/L)						OSMOLARITY (mOsm/L)
				Na+	K+	Mg++	Cl−	Ac−	PO₄ (mmol/L)	
FOR GENERAL PURPOSE										
Aminosyn 3.5%[a]	0.86	1.65	0.55	7	—	—	—	46	—	357
Aminosyn 5%[a]	1.23	2.35	0.79	—	5.4	—	—	86	—	500
Travasol 5.5%	0.86	2.15	0.93	—	—	—	22	48	—	575
(with electrolytes)				70	60	10	70	102	30	850
Aminosyn 7%[a]	1.73	3.32	1.1	—	5.4	—	—	105	—	700
(with electrolytes)				76	66	10	96	124	30	1013
Aminosyn 8.5%[a]	2.11	4.06	1.34	—	5.4	—	35	90	—	850
(with electrolytes)				70	66	10	86	142	30	1160
Travasol 8.5%	1.32	3.34	1.43	—	—	—	34	72	—	890
(with electrolytes)				70	60	10	70	141	30	1160
FreAmine III 8.5%	1.92	3.94	1.43	10	—	—	<3	72	10	810
(with electrolytes)				60	60	10	60	125	20	1045
Aminosyn 10%	2.46	4.7	1.57	—	5.4	—	—	148	—	1000
Aminosyn II 10%	2.16	4.3	1.53	45	—	10	—	72	—	873
FreAmine III 10%	2.26	4.63	1.53	10	—	—	<3	89	10	950
Travasol 10%	1.91	4.05	1.65	—	—	—	40	87	—	1000
Novamine	2.09	5.11	1.8	—	—	—	—	114	—	1057

(continued)

TABLE 6–8. AMINO ACID SOLUTIONS COMPARISON CHART (continued)

AA SOLUTION AND OSMOLARITY CONCENTRATION	TOTAL BCAAs (g/dL)	TOTAL ESSENTIAL AAs (g/dL)	TOTAL N (g/dL)	ELECTROLYTES (mEq/L)						OSMOLARITY (mOsm/L)
				Na+	K+	Mg++	Cl-	Ac-	PO4 (mmol/L)	
Aminosyn II 15%	3.24	6.42	2.3	63	—	—	—	108	—	1300
Novamine 15%	2.75	6.72	2.37	—	—	—	—	151	—	1388
FOR PROTEIN SPARING										
ProcalAmine 3%[b]	0.68	1.4	0.46	35	24	5	41	47	3.5	735
FreAmine III 3% (with electrolytes)	0.68	1.4	0.46	35	24.5	5	41	44	3.5	405
Aminosyn 3.5% M[a]	0.86	1.65	0.55	47	13	3	40	58	3.5	477
3.5% Travasol (with electrolytes)	0.55	1.38	0.59	25	15	5	25	52	7.5	450
FOR RENAL FAILURE										
Aminess 5.2%	1.95	5.18	0.66	—	—	—	—	50	—	416
Aminosyn RF 5.2%	1.72	4.83	0.79	—	5.4	—	—	105	—	475
NephrAmine 5.4%	2.08	5.33	0.65	5	—	—	<3	44	—	435
RenAmin 6.5%	1.92	4.32	1.0	—	—	—	31	60	—	600
FOR TRAUMA										
BranchAmin 4%[c,d]	4.0	4.0[d]	0.44	—	—	—	—	—	—	316
FreAmine HBC 6.9%[c]	3.01	4.28	0.97	10	—	—	<3	57	—	620
Aminosyn HBC 7%[c]	3.15	4.21	1.12	7	40	—	—	72	—	665

(continued)

TABLE 6–8. AMINO ACID SOLUTIONS COMPARISON CHART (continued)

AA SOLUTION AND OSMOLARITY CONCENTRATION	TOTAL BCAAs (g/dL)	TOTAL ESSENTIAL AAs (g/dL)	TOTAL N (g/dL)	ELECTROLYTES (mEq/L)						PO$_4$ (mmol/L)	OSMOLARITY (mOsm/L)
				Na$^+$	K$^+$	Mg^{++}	Cl$^-$	Ac$^-$			
FOR LIVER DISEASE											
HepatAmine^c	2.84	4.17	1.2	10	—	—	<3	62		10	785
FOR PEDIATRICS											
Aminosyn-PF 7%	1.82	3.2	1.07	3.4	—	—	—	33		—	586
Aminosyn-PF 10%	2.63	4.61	1.52	3.4	—	—	—	46		—	834
TrophAmine 6%	1.8	4.28	0.93	5	—	—	<3	56		—	525
TrophAmine 10%	3.0	7.2	1.55	5	—	—	<3	97		—	875

^{a}Also available as Aminosyn II which contains glutamic and aspartic acids, and differs slightly in content of other amino acids, acetate, and chloride.
^{b}Contains glycerol as a nonprotein calorie source.
^{c}BCAA-enriched products. Each of these products has distinct indications for use and should not be interchanged.
^{d}Contains only BCAA. Other essential AA are not included.
AA, amino acid; BCAA, branched-chain amino acid.

placement therapy such as peritoneal or hemodialysis require essential and nonessential AAs and should receive standard AA solutions.

Hepatic Failure.   Patients with hepatic failure, in whom muscle breakdown and an altered serum and CNS AA profile might contribute to hepatic encephalopathy, can benefit from a special AA formula. This formula has relatively greater amounts of BCAAs (ie, leucine, isoleucine, valine) and smaller amounts of the aromatic acids (ie, phenylalanine, tyrosine, tryptophan) and methionine.[26] One parenteral formula, HepatAmine, is currently available specifically for therapeutic and nutrition support of patients with liver disease (*see* Table 6–8).

Stress and Trauma.   The hypermetabolism that occurs in response to stress and trauma presents difficulty in providing nutrition support. BCAAs, in addition to their useful effect in metabolic support of the patient with liver disease, are reported to be useful for patients with stress and trauma.[27,28] Three BCAA-enriched products are available (*see* Table 6–8). FreAmine HBC and Aminosyn HBC are solutions of nonessential and essential AAs enriched with BCAAs. BranchAmin 4% is a solution of only BCAAs intended for use as a supplement to be admixed with a complete AA and a nonprotein caloric source. These products are indicated only for stress and trauma and should not be confused with the BCAA-enriched product that is indicated for hepatic encephalopathy.

Pediatrics.   It is beyond the scope of this chapter to describe procedures for nutrition support of pediatric patients except for this brief mention of parenteral AA products. Crystalline AA solutions marketed for infants are based on the essentiality of certain AAs in these patients (*see* Table 6–8).[29] Compared with adult AA formulations, these products contain taurine and glutamic and aspartic acids. Increased amounts of tyrosine and histidine and lower amounts of phenylalanine, methionine, and glycine are included. Although cysteine is also assumed to be essential for infants, adequate amounts cannot be included in AA formulas because of its limited solubility. A cysteine solution (50 mg/mL) is available separately for admixture to the formula before administration.

■ ELECTROLYTES

Formulas also are available with standard electrolyte compositions that might be suitable for most patients, after the addition of certain additives. Electrolyte provision, however, should be based on close monitoring of patients' laboratory values. Average daily requirements are summarized in Table 6–9.

VITAMINS

Vitamin requirements for PN have been suggested in a report by an advisory group to the American Medical Association (AMA).[30] Multiple vitamins are available in adult and pediatric formulations for once-daily IV administration (*see* Table 6–10). The usual daily dosage of the adult formulation is 10 mL to provide the amounts of vitamins specified in Table 6–10. The daily dosage of the pediatric formulation for infants who weigh <1 kg is 1.5 mL. For infants weighing 1–3 kg, the daily dosage is 3 mL. For infants and children weighing ≥3 kg up to 11 yr of

TABLE 6–9. ELECTROLYTES AND REQUIREMENTS

ELECTROLYTES	AVERAGE DAILY REQUIREMENT	DOSAGE FORMS	COMMENTS
CATIONS			
Sodium	60–150 mEq	Sodium chloride concentrate (4 mEq/mL) Sodium acetate (2 mEq/mL) Sodium phosphate (4 mEq Na+/mL)	Requirements during parenteral nutrition should not differ from normal fluid therapy requirements unless there is excessive sodium loss. Lactate and bicarbonate salts of sodium should not be used.
Potassium	40–240 mEq	Potassium chloride (2 mEq/mL) Potassium acetate (2 mEq/mL) Potassium phosphate (4.4 mEq K+/mL)	Requirements are related to glucose metabolism and therefore increase with higher concentrations of dextrose infused.
Magnesium	10–45 mEq	Magnesium sulfate (4 mEq/mL)	Requirements increase with anabolism but with less variation than with potassium.
Calcium	5–30 mEq	Calcium gluconate 10% (4.5 mEq/10 mL) Calcium chloride 10% (13 mEq/10 mL)	Requirements increase only slightly during parenteral nutrition. Limited amounts of calcium and phosphate, as determined by compatibility references, may be combined in solutions that contain amino acids.
ANIONS			
Phosphate	10 mmol/1000 kcal	Potassium phosphate (3 mmol P/mL, Abbott) Sodium phosphate (3 mmol P/mL, Abbott) (other concentrations may vary according to manufacturer)	Requirements increase with anabolism. Safe empirical dosage guidelines should be developed, taking into account the sodium or potassium content of the phosphate solution.
Acetate and Chloride	The amounts of acetate and chloride contained in each amino acid solution vary. (See Table 6–8.) Acetate is metabolized to bicarbonate. Bicarbonate salts should not be added to PN solutions because of incompatibility.		

age, the daily dosage is 5 mL. Vitamin K is included in the pediatric product only. Phytonadione 5 mg may be given to adults weekly in the PN formula, or by IM or SC administration, if needed.[30]

Fat emulsion contains vitamin K. Intralipid 10% contains about 0.31 mg/L and Liposyn II contains 0.13 mg/L; 20% products contain twice as much. Intralipid 20% 500 mL provides about 300 μg of vitamin K, an amount that exceeds maintenance recommendations and interferes with oral anticoagulant therapy.[30]

TABLE 6–10. IV MULTIVITAMINS

	AMOUNT	
TYPICAL FORMULA	Adult (per vial)	Pediatric (5 mL)
Ascorbic Acid (C)	100 mg	80 mg
Vitamin A	3300 IU	2300 IU
Vitamin D	200 IU	400 IU
Vitamin E	10 IU	7 IU
Thiamine (B$_1$)	3 mg	1.2 mg
Riboflavin (B$_2$)	3.6 mg	1.4 mg
Niacinamide (B$_3$)	40 mg	17 mg
Pantothenic Acid (B$_5$)	15 mg	5 mg
Pyridoxine (B$_6$)	4 mg	1 mg
Biotin	60 μg	20 μg
Folic Acid	400 μg	140 μg
Cyanocobalamin (B$_{12}$)	5 μg	1 μg
Phytonadione (K$_1$)	0	200 μg

TRACE ELEMENTS

Solutions of individual trace elements are available in several concentrations from different manufacturers. Solutions of multiple trace elements also are commercially available in products containing 4, 5, 6, or 7 elements and in concentrations suitable for adult or pediatric use. Guidelines for the use of trace elements in PN have been reported in an AMA statement[31] and the recommended daily dosages appear in Table 6–11. Although a need for molybdenum and iodine in long-term PN has been described, there are no officially recommended requirements for these elements.[32–34]

IRON

Iron deficiency can occur in patients deprived of iron during long-term PN. Iron dextran is sometimes added to PN solutions, but the advisability of its routine use

TABLE 6–11. SUGGESTED DAILY IV DOSAGE OF TRACE ELEMENTS

TRACE ELEMENT	PEDIATRIC PATIENTS (μG/kg)[a]	STABLE ADULT	ADULT IN ACUTE CATABOLIC STATE[b]	STABLE ADULT WITH INTESTINAL LOSSES[b]
Zinc	400 (preterm)[c] 250 (<3 months)[d] 100 (>3 months–1 yr)[d] 50 (>1 yr)[d]	2.5–4 mg	Additional 2 mg	Add 12.2 mg/L of small-bowel fluid lost; 17.1 mg/kg of stool or ileostomy output.[e]
Copper	20	0.5–1.5 mg	—	—
Chromium	0.14–0.2	10–15 μg	—	20 μg[f]
Manganese	1	0.15–0.8 mg	—	—
Selenium	2	20–60 μg	—	—

[a]Limited data are available for infants weighing <1500 g. Their requirements might be more than the recommendations because of their low body reserves and increased requirements for growth.
[b]Frequent monitoring of plasma levels in these patients is essential to provide proper dosage.
[c]Premature infants (weight <1500 g) up to 3 kg of body weight. Thereafter, the recommendations for full-term infants apply.
[d]Full-term infants and children ≤5 yr old. Thereafter, the recommendations for adults apply, up to a maximum dosage of 4 mg/day.
[e]Values derived by mathematical fitting of balance data from a 71 patient-week study in 24 patients.
[f]Mean from balance study.
Modified from references 31 and 35.

and its compatibility with fat emulsion are questionable. Dosage recommendations by this route are 1–12.5 mg/day of iron.[36]

INSULIN

Many patients who receive PN become hyperglycemic. When feasible, the cause should be investigated and controlled by means other than insulin before insulin is employed (*see* Table 6–12). Although the efficacy of PN is reportedly enhanced by insulin,[37] it should be used cautiously to avoid hypoglycemia and because it promotes deposition of fatty acids in body fat stores, making them less available for important biochemical pathways.[38] When it is required, insulin may be provided separately by SC or IV administration or added to the PN formula. Until a patient is stabilized on a consistent dosage of insulin, it is more cost effective to provide insulin separately to avoid wasting of PN formulations that might be discarded if the insulin dosage needs to be changed.[39] Human insulin is the least immunogenic and is therefore the insulin of choice. Guidelines for dosage are empirical; one-half to two-thirds of the previous day's sliding scale requirements may be added as regular human insulin to the daily PN formula. Standardized admixture procedures should be used to minimize variations of insulin activity caused by adsorption loss.

TABLE 6–12. NUTRITION SUPPORT: METABOLIC COMPLICATIONS AND MANAGEMENT

COMPLICATION	FREQUENT CAUSES	MANAGEMENT
Hyponatremia	Excessive GI or urinary sodium losses, or inadequate sodium intake.	Increase sodium provision.
	Excessive water intake.	Limit free water.
Hypokalemia	Excessive GI or urinary potassium losses; deficit of potassium; or large glucose infusion.	Increase potassium provision.
Hypocalcemia	Insufficient calcium.	Increase calcium provision.
	Magnesium deficit.	Increase magnesium provision.
Hypomagnesemia	Insufficient magnesium; or excessive GI or urinary losses.	Increase magnesium provision.
Hypophosphatemia	Inadequate phosphate.	Increase phosphate provision.
	Refeeding syndrome.	Refeed gradually.
Hypoglycemia	Abrupt interruption of formula infusion.	Begin dextrose infusion and monitor blood glucose and potassium.
	Excessive insulin.	Decrease insulin.
Hyperglycemia	Deficit of potassium or phosphorus.	Increase potassium or phosphate provision.
	Insufficient insulin.	Give insulin.
	Corticosteriod use.	Reduce rate of glucose infusion.
	Sepsis.	Sepsis workup and treatment.
Hypertriglyceridemia	Impaired clearance.	Hold IV lipid if serum triglycerides >400 mg/dL (4.5 mmol/L).
Elevated BUN	Dehydration.	Correct dehydration.
	Renal dysfunction; or calorie: nitrogen ratio imbalance.	Increase nonprotein calorie:nitrogen ratio.
Elevated Liver Function Tests	Underlying disease; lack of GI use; or GI bacterial overgrowth.	Attempt enteral feeding.
	Essential fatty acid deficiency.	Provide lipid.
	Excessive nutrients.	Decrease PN.
Metabolic Acidosis	Excessive GI or urinary losses of base.	Increase acetate provision.
	Inadequate amount of base-producing substance in formula.	Decrease chloride in formula or increase acetate provision.
Osmotic Diuresis	Failure to recognize initial hyperglycemia and increased glucose in urine.	Reduce infusion rate.
		Give insulin to correct hyperglycemia.

(continued)

TABLE 6–12. NUTRITION SUPPORT: METABOLIC COMPLICATIONS AND MANAGEMENT (*continued*)

COMPLICATION	FREQUENT CAUSES	MANAGEMENT
		Give 5% dextrose and 0.2% or 0.45% NaCl rather than PN solution to correct dehydration. Continue to monitor blood glucose, sodium, and potassium.
Essential Fatty Acid Deficiency	Insufficient provision of fat during PN.	Provide lipid.

ALBUMIN

Albumin is compatible when admixed with PN formulas; however, its supply is too limited and its cost is too prohibitive for casual use. Although inclusion of albumin in PN is reported to rapidly increase serum albumin levels[40] and enhance tolerance of enteral feedings,[41] the clinical benefits of such treatment are not proved. For synthesis of endogenous protein, albumin is inferior to crystalline AAs as a parenteral source of nitrogen. If administration of albumin is necessary, it should not be included in the PN formula.

CARNITINE

Carnitine is a micronutrient that is vital to energy metabolism because of its role in transporting long-chain fatty acids across the mitochondrial membrane. Certain patients, such as those with chronic renal failure on dialysis and premature neonates, are at increased risk of developing carnitine deficiency, especially if they are receiving long-term PN.[42,43] L-carnitine, the physiologically active form, is available for IV administration as a 1 g/5 mL solution that is stable when added to PN formulas.[44] Consult the carnitine product information for detailed usage information.

MEDICATIONS

There may be advantages to the admixture of certain medications such as antibiotics, chemotherapeutic agents, and H_2-receptor antagonists to PN, if there is compatibility reported with all components of the formula. Consult other sources for information regarding the stability and compatibility of medication/PN admixtures.

■ MONITORING THE PATIENT

Metabolic complications known to occur with enteral or parenteral nutrition are summarized in Table 6–12. Most of these can be avoided by proper precautions and close monitoring of the patient. Laboratory parameters for patient monitoring are summarized in Table 6–13.

TABLE 6–13. ROUTINE PATIENT MONITORING PARAMETERS

PARAMETER	FREQUENCY[a]
Urinary glucose and specific gravity.	Every voided specimen until stable, then daily.
Finger stick glucose.	Every 6 hr until stable.
Vital signs, weight, intake, and output.	Daily.
Serum glucose, electrolytes, creatinine, and BUN	Daily until stable, then twice weekly.
Magnesium, calcium, and phosphorus.	Daily until stable, then once weekly.
CBC, hemoglobin, WBC, platelets, and prothrombin time.	Baseline, then weekly.
Serum protein, albumin, prealbumin, and liver functions.	Baseline, then weekly.
Serum cholesterol and triglycerides.	Baseline, then weekly.
Blood ammonia.	Baseline, then weekly in renal and hepatic patients.

[a]Frequency should be increased in critically ill patients.

■ FUTURE DEVELOPMENTS

Technologic advancements in nutrition formulas and the means of preparing, providing, and monitoring their effects on patients continue to be made. These modifications enable safer and more cost-effective nutrition support of patients in the hospital or at home.

Body composition research is presenting innovative approaches to metabolic and nutrition assessments.[45] Formulas with specialized AA mixtures continue to be investigated. The benefits of using BCAA-enriched formulas are reported for patients with hepatic encephalopathy[46] or hypermetabolism[47] but remain unproved in terms of morbidity and mortality. Recombinant human growth factors,[48] arginine,[49] and glutamine[50] offer promise for their beneficial influences on protein synthesis rates, immunocompetence, and intestinal mucosal barrier protection, respectively.

In vitro and animal studies report an improvement in tissue protein synthesis and reduction in hypermetabolic response with the enteral use of structured lipids containing MCTs and omega-3 fish oil.[51,52] Because of difficulties reported with the IV use of currently available LCT emulsions such as hepatic and pulmonary complications and immunosuppression, alternate shorter-chain lipid preparations have been investigated.[53] MCTs continue to be explored for IV use as an obligate fuel and an important component of PN.[54] Animal studies with short-chain triglycerides such as triacetin show potential for better protein-sparing properties than MCTs, with less toxicity.[53] Short-chain fatty acids also have been shown to be beneficial in inhibiting small-bowel mucosal atrophy when infused IV or intra-colonically.[55]

New insights into the relationship between nutrition and immune function are emerging through advances with recombinant monokines and new discoveries concerning the involvement of interleukin-1 and tumor necrosis factor in energy metabolism.[52,56] Although all of these are promising areas of research, they are not considered standard therapy in nutrition support.

■ REFERENCES

1. Albina JE. Nutrition and wound healing. *JPEN* 1994;18:367–76.
2. Elwyn DH. Nutritional requirements of adult surgical patients. *Crit Care Med* 1980;8:9–19.
3. Grant JP et al. Current techniques of nutritional assessment. *Surg Clin North Am* 1981;61:437–63.
4. Blackburn GL et al. Nutritional and metabolic assessment of the hospitalized patient. *JPEN* 1977;1:11–22.
5. Traub SL, ed. *Basic skills in interpreting laboratory data.* Bethesda, MD: American Society of Hospital Pharmacists; 1992.
6. Vanlandingham S et al. Prealbumin: a parameter of visceral protein levels during albumin infusion. *JPEN* 1982; 6:230–1.
7. Fletcher JP et al. A comparison of serum transferrin and serum prealbumin as nutritional parameters. *JPEN* 1987;11:144–7.
8. Bistrian BR. Recent advances in parenteral and enteral nutrition: a personal perspective. *JPEN* 1990;14:329–34.
9. Liggett SB, Renfro AD. Energy expenditures of mechanically ventilated nonsurgical patients. *Chest* 1990;98: 682–6.
10. Rutten P et al. Determination of optimal hyperalimentation infusion rate. *J Surg Res* 1975;18:477–83.
11. Rees RGP et al. Elemental diet administered nasogastrically without starter regimens to patients with inflammatory bowel disease. *JPEN* 1986;10:258–62.
12. Payne-James JJ, Khawaja HT. First choice for total parenteral nutrition: the peripheral route. *JPEN* 1993;17: 468–78.
13. Solomon SM, Kirby DF. The refeeding syndrome: a review. *JPEN* 1990;14:90–7.
14. Food and Drug Administration. Safety alert: hazards of precipitation associated with parenteral nutrition. *Am J Hosp Pharm* 1994;51:1427–8.
15. Barton RG. Nutrition support in critical illness. *Nutr Clin Pract* 1994;9:127–39.
16. Shizgal HM, Forse RA. Protein and calorie requirements with total parenteral nutrition. *Ann Surg* 1980; 192:562–9.
17. Barr LH et al. Essential fatty acid deficiency during total parenteral nutrition. *Ann Surg* 1981;193:304–11.
18. Mattox TW, Teasley-Strausberg KM. Overview of biochemical markers used for nutrition support. *DICP* 1991; 25:265–71.
19. Roulet M et al. Effects of intravenously infused egg phospholipids on lipid and lipoprotein metabolism in postoperative trauma. *JPEN* 1993;17:107–12.
20. Crowe PJ et al. A new intravenous emulsion containing medium-chain triglyceride: studies of its metabolic effects in the perioperative period compared with a conventional long-chain triglyceride emulsion. *JPEN* 1985;9:720–4.
21. Driscoll DF et al. Practical considerations regarding the use of total nutrient admixtures. *Am J Hosp Pharm* 1986;43:416–9.
22. Pineault M et al. Beneficial effect of coinfusing a lipid emulsion on venous patency. *JPEN* 1989;13:637–40.
23. Hardin TC. Intravenous lipids—depression of the immune function: fact or fantasy? *Hosp Pharm* 1994;29: 182,185–6.
24. Guidelines for the use of parenteral and enteral nutrition in adult and pediatric patients. American Society for Parenteral and Enteral Nutrition. *JPEN* 1993;17(4 suppl):1SA–52SA.
25. Humbestone DA et al. Relative importance of amino acid infusion as a means of sparing protein in surgical patients. *JPEN* 1989;13:223–7.
26. Freund H et al. Infusion of branched-chain enriched amino acid solution in patients with hepatic encephalopathy. *Ann Surg* 1982;196:209–20.
27. Freund H et al. Infusion of the branched-chain amino acids in postoperative patients: anticatabolic properties. *Ann Surg* 1979;190:18–23.

28. Cerra FB et al. Branched-chains support postoperative protein synthesis. *Surgery* 1982;92:192–9.

29. Heird WC et al. Pediatric parenteral amino acid mixture in low birth weight infants. *Pediatrics* 1988;81:41–50.

30. Baumgartner T, ed. *Clinical guide to parenteral nutrition*. 3rd ed. Deerfield, IL: Fujisawa, Inc; 1997.

31. American Medical Association Department of Foods and Nutrition. Guidelines for essential trace element preparations for parenteral use: a statement by an expert panel. *JAMA* 1979;241:2051–4.

32. Lane HW et al. The effect of selenium supplementation on selenium status of patients receiving chronic total parenteral nutrition. *JPEN* 1987;11:177–82.

33. Abumrad NN et al. Amino acid intolerance during prolonged total parenteral nutrition reversed by molybdate therapy. *Am J Clin Nutr* 1981;34:2551–9.

34. Shils ME, Jacobs DH. Plasma iodide levels and thyroid function studies in long term home TPN patients. *Am J Clin Nutr* 1983;37:731. Abstract.

35. Greene HL et al. Guidelines for the use of vitamins, trace elements, calcium, magnesium, and phosphorus in infants and children receiving total parenteral nutrition: report of the Subcommittee on Pediatric Parenteral Nutrient Requirements from the Committee on Clinical Practice Issues of the American Society for Clinical Nutrition. *Am J Clin Nutr* 1988;48:1324–42.

36. Norton JA et al. Iron supplementation of total parenteral nutrition: a prospective study. *JPEN* 1983;7:457–61.

37. Shizgal HM, Posner B. Insulin and the efficacy of total parenteral nutrition. *Am J Clin Nutr* 1989;50:1355–63.

38. Rothkopf MM et al. Nutritional support in respiratory failure. *Nutr Clin Pract* 1989;4:166–72.

39. Sajbel TA et al. Use of separate insulin infusions with total parenteral nutrition. *JPEN* 1987;11:97–9.

40. Brown RO et al. Response of serum albumin concentrations to albumin supplementation during central total parenteral nutrition. *Clin Pharm* 1987;6:222–6.

41. Andrassy RJ, Durr ED. Albumin: use in nutrition and support. *Nutr Clin Pract* 1988;3:226–9.

42. Wolk R. Micronutrition in dialysis. *Nutr Clin Pract* 1993;8:267–76.

43. Bonner CM et al. Effects of parenteral L-carnitine supplementation on fat metabolism and nutrition in premature neonates. *J Pediatr* 1995;126:287–92.

44. Borum PR. Is L-carnitine stable in parenteral nutrition solutions prepared for preterm neonates? *Neonatal Intens Care* 1993;Sept/Oct:30–2.

45. Heymsfield SB, Matthews D. Body composition: research and clinical advances—1993 ASPEN research workshop. *JPEN* 1994;18:91–103.

46. Alexander WF et al. The usefulness of branched chain amino acids in patients with acute or chronic hepatic encephalopathy. *Am J Gastroenterol* 1989;84:91–6.

47. Teasley KM, Buss RL. Do parenteral nutrition solutions with high concentrations of branched-chain amino acids offer significant benefits to stressed patients? *DICP* 1989;23:411–6.

48. Hatton J et al. Growth factors in nutritional support. *Pharmacotherapy* 1993;13:17–27.

49. Daly JM et al. Immune and metabolic effects of arginine in the surgical patient. *Ann Surg* 1998;208:512–23.

50. Li J et al. Glycyl-L-glutamine–enriched total parenteral nutrition maintains small intestine gut-associated lymphoid tissue and upper respiratory tract immunity. *JPEN* 1998;22:31–6.

51. Teo TC et al. Administration of structured lipid composed of MCT and fish oil reduces net protein catabolism in enterally fed burned rats. *Ann Surg* 1989;210:100–6.

52. Endres S. The effect of dietary supplementation with n-3 polyunsaturated fatty acids on the synthesis of interleukin-1 and tumor necrosis factor by mononuclear cells. *N Engl J Med* 1989;320:265–71.

53. Bailey JW et al. Triacetin: a potential parenteral nutrient. *JPEN* 1991;15:32–6.

54. Mascioli EA et al. Thermogenesis from intravenous medium-chain triglycerides. *JPEN* 1991;15:27–31.

55. Koruda MJ et al. Parenteral nutrition supplemented with short-chain fatty acids: effect on the small-bowel mucosa in normal rats. *Am J Clin Nutr* 1990;51:685–9.

56. Pomposelli JJ et al. Role of biochemical mediators in clinical nutrition and surgical metabolism. *JPEN* 1988;12:212–8.

PART 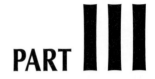 III

Appendices

Principal Editor: William G. Troutman, PharmD

- Conversion Factors
- Anthropometrics
- Laboratory Indices
- Drug–Laboratory Test Interferences
- Pharmacokinetic Equations

Conversion Factors

1

■ SI UNITS

SI units (*le Système International d'Unités*) are being introduced in the United States to express clinical laboratory and serum drug concentration data. Instead of employing units of mass (such as micrograms), the SI system uses moles (mol) to represent the amount of a substance. A molar solution contains 1 mole (the molecular weight of the substance in grams) of the solute in 1 liter of solution. The following formula is used to convert units of mass to moles (μg/mL to μmol/L or, by substitution of terms, mg/mL to mmol/L or ng/mL to nmol/L).

Micromoles per Liter (μmol/L)

$$\mu mol/L = \frac{\text{Drug concentration } (\mu g/mL) \times 1000}{\text{Molecular weight of drug } (g/mol)}$$

■ MILLIEQUIVALENTS

An equivalent weight of a substance is that weight which will combine with or replace 1 g of hydrogen; a milliequivalent is 1/1000 of an equivalent weight.

Milliequivalents per Liter (mEq/L)

$$mEq/L = \frac{\text{Weight of salt } (g) \times \text{Valence of ion} \times 1000}{\text{Molecular weight of salt}}$$

$$\text{Weight of salt } (g) = \frac{mEq/L \times \text{Molecular weight of salt}}{\text{Valence of ion} \times 1000}$$

APPROXIMATE MILLIEQUIVALENTS—WEIGHTS OF SELECTED IONS

SALT	mEq/g SALT	mg SALT/mEq
Calcium Carbonate ($CaCO_3$)	20.0	50.0
Calcium Chloride ($CaCl_2 \cdot 2H_2O$)	13.6	73.5
Calcium Gluceptate ($Ca[C_7H_{13}O_8]_2$)	4.1	245.2
Calcium Gluconate ($Ca[C_6H_{11}O_7]_2 \cdot H_2O$)	4.5	224.1
Calcium Lactate ($Ca[C_3H_5O_3]_2 \cdot 5H_2O$)	6.5	154.1
Magnesium Gluconate ($Mg[C_6H_{11}O_7]_2 \cdot H_2O$)	4.6	216.3
Magnesium Oxide (MgO)	49.6	20.2

(continued)

APPROXIMATE MILLIEQUIVALENTS—WEIGHTS OF SELECTED IONS (*continued*)

SALT	mEq/g SALT	mg SALT/mEq
Magnesium Sulfate ($MgSO_4$)	16.6	60.2
Magnesium Sulfate ($MgSO_4 \cdot 7H_2O$)	8.1	123.2
Potassium Acetate ($K[C_2H_3O_2]$)	10.2	98.1
Potassium Chloride (KCl)	13.4	74.6
Potassium Citrate ($K_3[C_6H_5O_7] \cdot H_2O$)	9.2	108.1
Potassium Iodide (KI)	6.0	166.0
Sodium Acetate ($Na[C_2H_3O_2]$)	12.2	82.0
Sodium Acetate ($Na[C_2H_3O_2] \cdot 3H_2O$)	7.3	136.1
Sodium Bicarbonate ($NaHCO_3$)	11.9	84.0
Sodium Chloride (NaCl)	17.1	58.4
Sodium Citrate ($Na_3[C_6H_5O_7] \cdot 2H_2O$)	10.2	98.0
Sodium Iodide (NaI)	6.7	149.9
Sodium Lactate ($Na[C_3H_5O_3]$)	8.9	112.1
Zinc Sulfate ($ZnSO_4 \cdot 7H_2O$)	7.0	143.8

VALENCES AND ATOMIC WEIGHTS OF SELECTED IONS

SUBSTANCE	ELECTROLYTE	VALENCE	MOLECULAR WEIGHT
Calcium	Ca^{++}	2	40.1
Chloride	Cl^-	1	35.5
Magnesium	Mg^{++}	2	24.3
Phosphate	$HPO_4^=$ (80%)	1.8	96.0[*]
(pH = 7.4)	$H_2PO_4^-$ (20%)		
Potassium	K^+	1	39.1
Sodium	Na^+	1	23.0
Sulfate	$SO_4^=$	2	96.0[*]

[*]The molecular weight of phosphorus only is 31; that of sulfur only is 32.1.

■ ANION GAP

The anion gap is the concentration of plasma anions not routinely measured by laboratory screening. It is useful in the evaluation of acid–base disorders. The anion gap is greater with increased plasma concentrations of endogenous (eg, phosphate, sulfate, lactate, ketoacids) or exogenous (eg, salicylate, penicillin, ethylene glycol, ethanol, methanol) species. The formulas for calculating the anion gap follow:

(A) Anion Gap = $(Na^+ + K^+) - (Cl^- + HCO_3^-)$

or

(B) Anion Gap = $Na^+ - (Cl^- + HCO_3^-)$

where

the expected normal value for A is 11–20 mmol/L;
the expected normal value for B is 7–16 mmol/L.*

*Note that there is variation at the upper and lower limits of the normal range.

■ TEMPERATURE

Fahrenheit to Centigrade: $(°F - 32) \times 5/9 = °C$
Centigrade to Fahrenheit: $(°C \times 9/5) + 32 = °F$
Centigrade to Kelvin: $°C + 273 = °K$

■ WEIGHTS AND MEASURES

Metric Weight Equivalents
1 kilogram (kg) = 1000 grams
1 gram (g) = 1000 milligrams
1 milligram (mg) = 0.001 gram
1 microgram (mcg, μg) = 0.001 milligram
1 nanogram (ng) = 0.001 microgram
1 picogram (pg) = 0.001 nanogram
1 femtogram (fg) = 0.001 picogram

Metric Volume Equivalents
1 liter (L) = 1000 milliliters
1 deciliter (dL) = 100 milliliters
1 milliliter (mL) = 0.001 liter
1 microliter (μL) = 0.001 milliliter
1 nanoliter (nL) = 0.001 microliter
1 picoliter (pL) = 0.001 nanoliter
1 femtoliter (fL) = 0.001 picoliter

Apothecary Weight Equivalents
1 scruple (℈) = 20 grains (gr)
60 grains (gr) = 1 dram (ℨ)
8 drams (ℨ) = 1 ounce (℥)
1 ounce (℥) = 480 grains
12 ounces (℥) = 1 pound (lb)

Apothecary Volume Equivalents
60 minims (m) = 1 fluidram (fl ʒ)
8 fluidrams (fl ʒ) = 1 fluid ounce (fl ʒ)
1 fluid ounce (fl ʒ) = 480 minims
16 fluid ounces (fl ʒ) = 1 pint (pt)

Avoirdupois Equivalents
1 ounce (oz) = 437.5 grains
16 ounces (oz) = 1 pound (lb)

Weight/Volume Equivalents
1 mg/dL = 10 μg/mL
1 mg/dL = 1 mg%
1 ppm = 1 mg/L

Conversion Equivalents
1 gram (g) = 15.43 grains
1 grain (gr) = 64.8 milligrams
1 ounce (ʒ) = 31.1 grams
1 ounce (oz) = 28.35 grams
1 pound (lb) = 453.6 grams
1 kilogram (kg) = 2.2 pounds
1 milliliter (mL) = 16.23 minims
1 minim (m) = 0.06 milliliter
1 fluid ounce (fl oz) = 29.57 mL
1 pint (pt) = 473.2 mL
0.1 mg = 1/600 gr
0.12 mg = 1/500 gr
0.15 mg = 1/400 gr
0.2 mg = 1/300 gr
0.3 mg = 1/200 gr
0.4 mg = 1/150 gr
0.5 mg = 1/120 gr
0.6 mg = 1/100 gr
0.8 mg = 1/80 gr
1 mg = 1/65 gr

Anthropometrics 2

CREATININE CLEARANCE FORMULAS

FORMULAS FOR ESTIMATING CREATININE CLEARANCE IN PATIENTS WITH STABLE RENAL FUNCTION

Adults [Age 18 Years and Older][1]

$$Cl_{cr} \text{ (Males)} = \frac{(140 - Age) \times (Weight)}{Cr_s \times 72}$$

$$Cl_{cr} \text{ (Females)} = 0.85 \times \text{Above value*}$$

where

Cl_{cr} = creatinine clearance in mL/min
Cr_s = serum creatinine in mg/dL
Age is in years
Weight is in kg.

*Some studies suggest that the predictive accuracy of this formula for women is better *without* the correction factor of 0.85.

Children [Age 1–18 Years][2]

$$Cl_{cr} = \frac{0.48 \times (Height) \times (BSA)}{Cr_s \times 1.73}$$

where

BSA = body surface area in m^2
Cl_{cr} = creatinine clearance in mL/min
Cr_s = serum creatinine in mg/dL
Height is in cm.

FORMULA FOR ESTIMATING CREATININE CLEARANCE FROM A MEASURED URINE COLLECTION

$$Cl_{cr} \text{ (mL/min)} = \frac{U \times V*}{P \times t}$$

where

U = concentration of creatinine in a urine specimen (in same units as P)
V = volume of urine in mL

P = concentration of creatinine in serum at the midpoint of the urine collection period (in same units as U)

t = time of the urine collection period in minutes (eg, 6 hr = 360 min; 24 hr = 1440 min).

*The product of U × V equals the production of creatinine during the collection period and, at steady state, should equal 20–25 mg/kg/day ideal body weight (IBW) in males and 15–20 mg/kg/day IBW in females. If it is less than this, inadequate urine collection may have occurred and Cl_{cr} will be under-estimated.

■ IDEAL BODY WEIGHT

IBW is the weight expected for a nonobese person of a given height. The IBW formulas below and various life insurance tables can be used to estimate IBW. Most dosing methods described in the literature use IBW as a method in dosing obese patients.

Adults [Age 18 years and Older][3]

$$IBW \text{ (Males)} = 50 + (2.3 \times \text{Height in inches over 5 feet})$$

$$IBW \text{ (Females)} = 45.5 + (2.3 \times \text{Height in inches over 5 feet})$$

where IBW is in kg.

Children [Age 1–18 Years][2]
Under 5 Feet Tall:

$$IBW = \frac{(\text{Height}^2 \times 1.65)}{1000}$$

where

IBW is in kg;
Height is in cm.

5 Feet or Taller:

$$IBW \text{ (Males)} = 39 + (2.27 \times \text{Height in inches over 5 feet})$$
$$IBW \text{ (Females)} = 42.2 + (2.27 \times \text{Height in inches over 5 feet})$$

where IBW is in kg;

■ SURFACE AREA NOMOGRAMS

Nomograms represent the relationship between height, weight, and body surface area in infants and adults. To use a nomogram, a ruler is aligned with the height and weight on the two lateral axes. The point at which the centerline is intersected provides the corresponding value for body surface area.

NOMOGRAM FOR DETERMINATION OF BODY SURFACE AREA
FROM HEIGHT AND WEIGHT (INFANTS)[4]

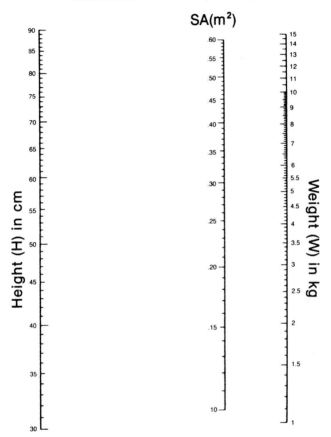

$$SA = W^{0.5378} \times H^{0.3964} \times 0.024265$$

where

SA is in m^2
Height (H) is in cm
Weight (W) is in kg.

Reproduced from reference 4, with permission.

NOMOGRAM FOR DETERMINATION OF BODY SURFACE AREA
FROM HEIGHT AND WEIGHT (ADULTS)[5]

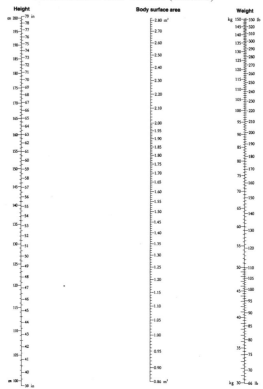

$$SA = W^{0.425} \times H^{0.725} \times 71.84$$

where

SA is in m^2
Height (H) is in cm
Weight (W) is in kg.

Reproduced from reference 5, with permission.

REFERENCES

1. Cockcroft DW, Gault MH. Prediction of creatinine clearance from serum creatinine. *Nephron* 1976;16:31–41.
2. Traub SL, Johnson CE. Comparison of methods of estimating creatinine clearance in children. *Am J Hosp Pharm* 1980;37:195–201.
3. Devine BJ. Gentamicin therapy. *Drug Intell Clin Pharm* 1974;8:650–5.
4. Haycock GB et al. Geometric method for measuring body surface area: a height–weight formula validated in infants, children, and adults. *J Pediatr* 1978;93:62–6.
5. DuBois and DuBois. *Arch Intern Med* 1916;17:863.

Laboratory Indices

Blood, Serum, Plasma Chemistry; Urine, Renal Function Tests; Hematology

William G. Troutman

The following table lists typical reference ranges for clinical laboratory tests in common use. Reference ranges for laboratory tests can vary widely among testing facilities, often as a result of methodologic differences. It is therefore always advisable to obtain reference ranges from the laboratory performing the analyses. Laboratory test results should never be accepted without correct identification of the units of measurement because most tests can be reported in several systems of measurement. The table presents conventional and international (usually the same as *Système International,* or SI) units.

The following abbreviations are used to identify the specimen:

(P)   — Plasma
(S)   — Serum
(U)   — Urine
(WB)   — Whole Blood
(WB, art) — Whole Blood, Arterial

The table begins on page 1062.

BLOOD, SERUM, PLASMA CHEMISTRY

| TEST/SPECIMEN | AGE GROUP OR OTHER FACTOR | REFERENCE RANGE | |
		Conventional	International Units
Acid Phosphatase (S)		0.11–0.60 units/L	0.11–0.60 units/L
Alanine Aminotransferase (S)		*units/L*	*units/L*
(ALT, SGPT)	Adult	8–20	8–20
	>60 yr, M	7–24	7–24
	>60 yr, F	7–16	7–16
Alkaline Phosphatase (S)		*units/L*	*units/L*
	Child	20–150	20–150
	Adult	20–70	20–70
	>60 yr	30–75	30–75
Ammonia Nitrogen (S,P)	Adult	15–45 mg/dL	11–32 μmol/L
Amylase (S)		*units/L*	*units/L*
	Adult	25–125	25–125
	>70 yr	20–160	20–160
Anion Gap (Na$^+$ 2 [Cl$^-$ + HCO$_3^-$]) (P)		7–16 mEq/L	7–16 mmol/L
Aspartate Aminotransferase (S)		*units/L*	*units/L*
(AST, SGOT)	Adult	8–20	8–20
	>60 yr, M	11–26	11–26
	>60 yr, F	10–20	10–20
Bicarbonate (S)		*mEq/L*	*mmol/L*
	Arterial	21–28	21–28
	Venous	22–29	22–29
(WB, art)	Adult	18–23	18–23
Bilirubin (S)		*mg/dL*	*mmol/L*
Total	Child, Adult	0.2–1.0	3.4–17.1
Conjugated (direct)	Child, Adult	0–0.2	0–3.4
Calcium (S)		*mg/dL*	*mmol/L*
Ionized	Adult	4.48–4.92	1.12–1.23
Total	Child	8.8–10.8	2.20–2.70
	Adult	8.4–10.2	2.10–2.55
Carbon Dioxide, Partial Pressure (WB, art)		*mm Hg*	*kPa*
(pCO$_2$)	Adult, M	35–48	4.66–6.38
	Adult, F	32–45	4.26–5.99
Chloride (S,P)		98–107 mEq/L	98–107 mmol/L

(continued)

BLOOD, SERUM, PLASMA CHEMISTRY (*continued*)

TEST/SPECIMEN	AGE GROUP OR OTHER FACTOR	REFERENCE RANGE			
		Conventional		*International Units*	
Cholesterol, Total (S,P)		*mg/dL*		*mmol/L*	
	Child	120–200		3.11–5.18	
	Adolescent	120–210		3.11–5.44	
	Adult	140–310		3.63–8.03	
	Desired, Adult	<200		<2.6	
Cortisol (S,P)		*µg/dL*		*nmol/L*	
	08:00 hr	5–23		138–635	
	16:00 hr	3–15		83–414	
	20:00 hr	≤50% of 08:00 hr		≤50% of 08:00 hr	
Creatine Kinase (CK) (S)		*units/L*		*units/L*	
	Adult, M	38–174		38–174	
	Adult, F	26–140		26–140	
Creatinine (S,P)		*mg/dL*		*µmol/L*	
	Child	0.3–0.7		27–62	
	Adolescent	0.5–1.0		44–88	
	Adult, M	0.7–1.3		62–115	
	Adult, F	0.6–1.1		53–97	
(γ)-Glutamyltransferase (S) (GGT)		*units/L*		*units/L*	
	Adult, M	9–50		9–50	
	Adult, F	8–40		8–40	
Glucose, 2-hr Postprandial (S)		<120 mg/dL		<6.7 mmol/L	
Glucose Tolerance Test (S) (Oral)		*mg/dL*		*mmol/L*	
		Normal	*Diabetic*	*Normal*	*Diabetic*
	Fasting	70–105	>140	3.9–5.8	>7.8
	60 min	120–170	≥200	6.7–9.4	≥11.1
	90 min	100–140	≥200	5.6–7.8	≥11.1
	120 min	70–120	≥140	3.9–6.7	≥7.8
HDL-Cholesterol (S,P)		*mg/dL*		*mmol/L*	
	15–19 yr, M	30–65		0.78–1.68	
	15–19 yr, F	30–70		0.78–1.81	
	20–29 yr, M	30–70		0.78–1.81	
	20–29 yr, F	30–75		0.78–1.94	
	30–39 yr, M	30–70		0.78–1.81	
	30–39 yr, F	30–80		0.78–2.07	

(*continued*)

BLOOD, SERUM, PLASMA CHEMISTRY (*continued*)

TEST/SPECIMEN	AGE GROUP OR OTHER FACTOR	REFERENCE RANGE	
		Conventional	*International Units*
	>40 yr, M	30–70	0.78–1.81
	>40 yr, F	30–85	0.78–2.20
Iron (S)		*µg/dL*	*mmol/L*
	Child	50–120	8.95–21.48
	Adult, M	65–170	11.64–30.43
	Adult, F	50–170	8.95–30.43
Iron-Binding Capacity, Total (S) (TIBC)		250–450 µg/dL	44.75–80.55 µmol/L
Isocitrate Dehydrogenase (S)		1.2–7.0 units/L	1.2–7.0 units/L
Lactate Dehydrogenase (S)		*units/L*	*units/L*
	Child	60–170	60–170
	Adult	100–190	100–190
	>60 yr	110–210	110–210
Isozymes (S)		*% of Total*	*Fraction of Total*
	Fraction 1	14–26	0.14–0.26
	Fraction 2	29–39	0.29–0.39
	Fraction 3	20–26	0.20–0.26
	Fraction 4	8–16	0.08–0.16
	Fraction 5	6–16	0.06–0.16
Lead (WB)		*µg/dL*	*µmol/L*
	Child	<15	<0.72
	Adult	<30	<1.45
Lipase (S)		*units/L*	*units/L*
	Adult	10–150	10–150
	>60 yr	18–180	18–180
β-Lipoprotein (LDL) (S)		28–53% of total lipoproteins.	0.28–0.53
Magnesium (S)		*mEq/L*	*mmol/L*
	6–12 yr	1.7–2.1	0.70–0.86
	12–20 yr	1.7–2.2	0.70–0.91
	Adult	1.6–2.6	0.66–1.07
Osmolality (S)		*mOsmol/kg*	*mOsmol/kg*
	Child, Adult	275–295	275–295
	>60 yr	280–301	280–301

(*continued*)

BLOOD, SERUM, PLASMA CHEMISTRY (*continued*)

TEST/SPECIMEN	AGE GROUP OR OTHER FACTOR	REFERENCE RANGE	
		Conventional	*International Units*
Osmolal Gap		≤10	≤10
Measured Osmolality − Calculated Osmolality			
Calculated Osmolality = $2(Na^+)$ + (Glucose/18) + (BUN/2.8)			
Oxygen, Partial Pressure (WB, art) (pO_2) (Decreases with age and altitude)		83–108 mm Hg	11.04–14.36 kPa
pH (WB, art)		7.35–7.45	7.35–7.45
Phosphorus, Inorganic (S)		*mg/dL*	*mmol/L*
	Child	4.5–5.5	1.45–1.78
	Adult	2.7–4.5	0.87–1.45
	>60 yr, M	2.3–3.7	0.74–1.20
	>60 yr, F	2.8–4.1	0.90–1.32
Potassium (S,P)		*mEq/L*	*mmol/L*
	Child	3.4–4.7	3.4–4.7
	Adult	3.5–5.1	3.5–5.1
Protein, Total (S)		*g/dL*	*g/L*
	Adult		
	Ambulatory	6.4–8.3	64–83
	Recumbent	6.0–7.8	60–78
	>60 yr	lower by 0.2	lower by 2
Albumin	Adult	3.5–5.0	35–50
	>60 yr	3.7–4.7	37–47
Globulins	Adult	2.3–3.5	23–35
Prealbumin	Adult	10–40 mg/dL	100–400 mg/L
Sodium (S,P)		*mEq/L*	*mmol/L*
	Child	138–145	138–145
	Adult	136–146	136–146
Thyroid-Stimulating Hormone (S,P) (TSH)		*μunits/mL*	*munits/L*
	Child	4.5 ± 3.6	4.5 ± 3.6
	Adult	<10	<10
	>60 yr, M	2–7.3	2–7.3
	>60 yr, F	2–16.8	2–16.8

(*continued*)

BLOOD, SERUM, PLASMA CHEMISTRY (*continued*)

TEST/SPECIMEN	AGE GROUP OR OTHER FACTOR	REFERENCE RANGE	
		Conventional	International Units
Thyroxine, Total (S)		µg/dL	nmol/L
(T₄)	5–10 yr	6.4–13.3	83–172
	Adult	5–12	65–155
	>60 yr, M	5–10	65–129
	>60 yr, F	5.5–10.5	71–135
	4–9 mo pregnant	6.1–17.6	79–227
Transferrin (S)		mg/dL	g/L
	Adult	220–400	2.20–4.00
	>60 yr	180–380	1.80–3.80

Triglycerides (S)		mg/dL		mmol/L	
		M	F	M	F
	12–15 yr	36–138	41–138	0.41–1.56	0.46–1.56
	16–19 yr	40–163	40–128	0.45–1.84	0.45–1.45
	20–29 yr	44–185	40–128	0.50–2.09	0.45–1.45
	30–39 yr	49–284	38–160	0.55–3.21	0.43–1.81
	40–49 yr	56–298	44–186	0.63–3.37	0.50–2.10
	50–59 yr	62–288	55–247	0.70–3.25	0.62–2.79
	Desired, Adult	<150		<1.69	

TEST/SPECIMEN	AGE GROUP OR OTHER FACTOR	Conventional	International Units
Triiodothyronine Resin Uptake (S)		% of Total	Fraction of Total
(T₃RU)	Adult	24–34	0.24–0.34
	>60 yr, M	24–32	0.24–0.32
	>60 yr, F	22–32	0.22–0.32
Triiodothyronine, Total (S)		ng/dL	nmol/L
(T₃)	10–15 yr	80–210	1.23–3.23
	Adult	120–195	1.85–3.00
	>60 yr, M	105–175	1.62–2.69
	>60 yr, F	108–205	1.66–3.16
Urea Nitrogen (S)		mg/dL	mmol/L urea
(BUN)	Child	5–18	0.8–3.0
	Adult	7–18	1.2–3.0
	>60 yr	8–21	1.3–3.5
Uric Acid (S)		mg/dL	mmol/L
(Uricase Method)	Child	2.0–5.5	0.12–0.32
	Adult, M	3.5–7.2	0.21–0.42
	Adult, F	2.6–6.0	0.15–0.35

URINE, RENAL FUNCTION TESTS

TEST/SPECIMEN	AGE GROUP OR OTHER FACTOR	REFERENCE RANGE	
		Conventional	International Units
Catecholamines, 24-hr (U)		<110 µg	<650 nmol
Creatinine, 24-hr (U)		*mg/kg*	*µmol/kg*
	Child	8–22	71–195
	Adolescent	8–30	71–265
	Adult, M	14–26	124–230
	Adult, F	11–20	97–177
	Decreases with age to 10 mg/kg/day at age 90.		
Creatinine Clearance (S, P, and U)		*mL/min/1.73 m²*	*mL/sec/m²*
	<40 yr, M	97–137	0.93–1.32
	<40 yr, F	88–128	0.85–1.23
	Decreases with age >40 yr.		

Inulin Clearance (S and U)		*mL/min/1.73 m²*		*mL/sec/m²*	
		M	F	M	F
	20–29 yr	90–174	84–156	0.87–1.68	0.81–1.50
	30–39 yr	88–168	82–150	0.85–1.62	0.79–1.44
	40–49 yr	78–162	82–146	0.75–1.56	0.79–1.41
	50–59 yr	68–152	66–142	0.65–1.46	0.63–1.37
	60–69 yr	57–137	58–130	0.55–1.32	0.56–1.25
	70–79 yr	42–122	45–121	0.40–1.17	0.43–1.17
	80–89 yr	39–105	39–105	0.38–1.01	0.38–1.01

TEST/SPECIMEN	AGE GROUP OR OTHER FACTOR	Conventional	International Units
pH (U)		4.5–8	4.5–8
Protein, Total (U)		1–14 mg/dL	10–140 mg/L
	At Rest	50–80 mg/day	50–80 mg/day
Specific Gravity, Random (U)		1.002–1.030	1.002–1.030
Uric Acid, 24-hr (U)		250–750 mg	1.48–4.43 mmol

HEMATOLOGY

TEST/SPECIMEN	AGE GROUP OR OTHER FACTOR	REFERENCE RANGE	
		Conventional	*International Units*
Bleeding time		3–9 min	180–540 sec
Erythrocyte Count (WB)		$\times 10^6/\mu L$	$\times 10^{12}/L$
	M	4.6–6.2	4.6–6.2
	F	4.2–5.4	4.2–5.4
Erythrocyte Indices (WB)			
Mean Corpuscular Volume		80–96 μm^3	80–96 fL
Mean Corpuscular Hemoglobin		27–31 pg	27–31 pg
Erythrocyte Sedimentation Rate (WB)		*mm/hr*	*mm/hr*
	M	1–13	1–13
	F	1–20	1–20
Fibrinogen (P)		200–400 mg/dL	2.00–4.00 g/L
Hematocrit (WB)		**% Packed RBC Volume**	**Volume Fraction**
	6–12 yr	35–45	0.35–0.45
	12–18 yr, M	37–49	0.37–0.49
	12–18 yr, F	36–46	0.36–0.46
	18–49 yr, M	41–53	0.41–0.53
	18–49 yr, F	36–46	0.36–0.46
Hemoglobin (WB)		*g/dL*	*mmol/L*
	6–12 yr	11.5–15.5	1.78–2.40
	12–18 yr, M	13.0–16.0	2.02–2.48
	12–18 yr, F	12.0–16.0	1.86–2.48
	18–49 yr, M	13.5–17.5	2.09–2.71
	18–49 yr, F	12.0–16.0	1.86–2.48
Hemoglobin A_{1c} (WB)		5.3–7.5% of total Hb	0.053–0.075
Leukocyte Count (WB)		$4.5–11 \times 10^3/\mu L$	$4.5–11 \times 10^9/L$
	Segs	31–71%	31–71%
	Bands	0–12%	0–12%
	Lymphocytes	15–50%	15–50%
	Monocytes	0–12%	0–12%
	Eosinophils	0–5%	0–5%
	Basophils	0–2%	0–2%

(continued)

HEMATOLOGY (*continued*)

TEST/SPECIMEN	AGE GROUP OR OTHER FACTOR	REFERENCE RANGE	
		Conventional	*International Units*
Absolute Neutrophil Count (ANC)			
ANC = (% Segs + % Bands) × Leukocyte Count			
Partial Thromboplastin Time, Activated (WB) (aPTT)		25–37 sec	25–37 sec
Platelets (WB)		$150–440 \times 10^3/\mu L$	$0.15–0.44 \times 10^{12}/L$
Prothrombin Time (WB)		Less than 2-sec deviation from control.	
Reticulocytes (WB)		0.5–1.5% of erythrocytes	0.005–0.015

REFERENCES

1. Burtis CA, Ashwood ER, eds. *Tietz textbook of clinical chemistry.* 2nd ed. Philadelphia: WB Saunders; 1994.
2. Henry JB, ed. *Clinical diagnosis and management by laboratory methods.* 18th ed. Philadelphia: WB Saunders; 1991.
3. Preventing lead poisoning in young children: a statement by the Centers for Disease Control. 4th rev. ed. Atlanta: Centers for Disease Control; 1991.
4. Système International (SI) units conversion table for common laboratory tests. *Ann Pharmacother* 1995;29:100–7.
5. Tietz NW, ed. *Clinical guide to laboratory tests.* 2nd ed. Philadelphia: WB Saunders; 1990.
6. Wallach J. *Interpretation of diagnostic tests: a synopsis of laboratory medicine.* 6th ed. Boston: Little, Brown; 1996.

David G. Dunlop

The following table lists common clinical laboratory tests and drugs that can interfere with those tests. Drugs can interfere with laboratory tests through pharmacological or toxic effects or through actual chemical interference with the testing process. Either effect can lead to an altered value of the laboratory test, resulting in an inappropriate diagnosis or treatment. It is therefore essential that clinicians recognize possible drug–laboratory interactions and use this information in the overall assessment of a patient's clinical status.

The table lists drug interferences with the most common laboratory tests. For detailed information on laboratory tests not covered here, see references 1–3 at the end of this section. Also, it should be noted that drugs can interfere with laboratory tests by many different mechanisms. The reader should refer to the references cited in the table and other relevant sources to obtain more information about a specific test.

The following abbreviations are used in the table:

(B)   — Blood
(CSF) — Cerebrospinal Fluid
(I)   — Analytical Interference of Drug
(P)   — Pharmacological/Toxic Effect of Drug
(S)   — Serum

■ DRUGS THAT CAN AFFECT RESULTS AND CAUSE OF INTERFERENCE

BLOOD, SERUM, PLASMA CHEMISTRY

Alkaline Phosphatase (S). *Elevated* by acetaminophen (P), acetohexamide (P), albumin (I), alitretinoin (P), allopurinol (P), aluminum salts (P), aminoglycosides (P), amiodarone (P), amphotericin B (P), anabolic steroids (P), azathioprine (P), barbiturates (P), bromocriptine (P), carbamazepine (P), cephalosporins (P), chenodiol (P), clofibrate (P), cyclophosphamide (P), cyclosporine (P), cytarabine (P), danazol (P), dantrolene (P), dapsone (P), disulfiram (P), docetaxel (P), erythromycin (P), estrogens (P), filgrastim (P), flucytosine (P), glycopyrrolate (P), gold salts (P), griseofulvin (P), haloperidol (P), hepatotoxic drugs (P), HMG-CoA reductase inhibitors (P), hydralazine (P), ibuprofen (I,P), isoniazid (P), isotretinoin (P), ketoconazole (P), lithium salts (P), meprobamate (P), mercaptopurine (P), methyldopa (P), mitomycin (P), nafarelin (P), niacin (P), nitrofurantoin (P), non-steroidal anti-inflammatory drugs (P), papaverine (P), penicillamine (P), penicillins (P), phenazopyridine (P), phenothiazines (P), phenytoin (P), pindolol (I), probenecid (P), propylthiouracil (P), pyrazinamide (P), quinidine (P), rifampin (P), sulfonamides (P), sulfonylureas (P), tetracyclines (P), thiabendazole (P), ticlopidine (P), topotecan (P), trimethoprim (P), troleandomycin (P), valproic acid (P), zidovudine (P).[1,3,4]

Decreased by bisphosphonates (P), calcitriol (P), carvedilol (P), citrate salts (I), clofibrate (P), cyclosporine (P), danazol (P), EDTA (I), estrogens (P), fluoride salts (I), phosphate salts (I), prednisolone (P), prednisone (P), tamoxifen (P), theophylline (I), tricyclic antidepressants (P), ursodiol (P), zinc (I).[1,3]

Aminotransferases (ALT [SGOT] or AST [SGPT]) (S). *Elevated* by abacavir (P), acarbose (P), acetaminophen (I,P), acetohexamide (P), acyclovir (P), albendazole (P), alitretinoin (P), allopurinol (P), amiodarone (P), ampicillin (I), anabolic steroids (P), anastrozole (P), asparaginase (P), azathioprine (P), aztreonam (P), barbiturates (P), carbamazepine (P), cephalosporins (P), chenodiol (P), chloral hydrate (P), chloramphenicol (P), chlordiazepoxide (I,P), cholestyramine (P), cholinergic agents (P), clopidogrel (P), COX-2 inhibitors (P), cyclophosphamide (P), cytarabine (P), danazol (P), dantrolene (P), delavirdine (P), denileukin diftitox (P), disulfiram (P), diuretics (thiazide) (P), docetaxel (P), efavirenz (P), erythromycin (I,P), estrogens (P), etoposide (P), fenofibrate (P), fluconazole (P), flucytosine (P), flutamide (P), fomepizole (P), ganciclovir (P), gemcitabine (P), gemtuzamab ozogamicin (P), gentamicin (I,P), glycopyrrolate (P), gold salts (P), griseofulvin (P), haloperidol (P), heparin (P), hepatotoxic drugs (P), HMG-CoA reductase inhibitors (P), hydralazine (P), IM injections (P), indinavir (P), interferon alfa-2a (P), interferon beta-1a (P), interferon beta-1b (P), irinotecan (P), isoniazid (P), isoproterenol (I), isotretinoin (P), ketoconazole (P), leflunomide (P), levodopa (I,P), meprobamate (P), mercaptopurine (P), methotrexate (P), methyldopa (I), mirtazapine (P), nafarelin (P), naltrexone (P), narcotics (I,P), nevirapine (P), niacin (P), nilutamide (P), nitrofurantoin (P), nonsteroidal anti-inflammatory drugs (P), olanzapine (P), penicillamine (P), penicillins (I,P), pentosan polysulfate sodium (P), phenazopyridine (P), phenothiazines (P), porfimer (P), probenecid (P), propylthiouracil (P), pyrazinamide (P), quetiapine (P), quinidine (P), quinupristin/dalfopristin (P), rifabutin (P), rifampin (P), rifapentine (P), riluzole (P), ritonavir (P), salicylates (I,P), sulfonamides (P), sulfonylureas (P), tacrine (P), temozolomide (P), tetracyclines (P), thiabendazole (P), ticlopidine (P), tolcapone (P), topotecan (P), total parenteral nutrition (P), troleandomycin (P), valproic acid (P), vidarabine (P), vinorelbine (P), vitamin C, zafirlukast (P), zalcitabine (P), zidovudine (P).[1–4,6]

Decreased by acetaminophen (I), aspirin (I), cyclosporine (I), fluoride salts (I), interferons (P), metronidazole (I), naltrexone (I), pindolol (I), rifampin (I), tricyclic antidepressants (P), ursodiol (P), vitamin C (I), zalcitabine (P).[1]

Ammonia (B). *Elevated* by acetazolamide (P), alcohol (P), ammonium chloride (P), asparaginase (P), barbiturates (P), carbamazepine (P), diuretics (loop, thiazide) (P), isoniazid (P), parenteral nutrition (P), smoking (P), valproic acid.[1,2,4,7]

Decreased by cefotaxime (I), kanamycin, oral (P), *Lactobacillus acidophilus* (P), lactulose (P), MAO inhibitors (P), neomycin, oral (P), phosphate salts (I), potassium salts (P), tetracycline (P).[1,2,4]

Amylase (S). *Elevated* by alcohol (P), angiotensin II receptor blockers (P), ACE inhibitors (P), asparaginase (P), azathioprine (P), chloride salts (I), cholinergic agents (P), cisplatin (P), contraceptives, oral (P), corticosteroids (P), denileukin diftitox (P), didanosine (P), diuretics, loop and thiazide (P), erythromycin (P), estrogens (P), fluoride salts (I), indinavir (P), lamivudine (P), metronidazole (P), narcotics (P), nitrofurantoin (P), opioids (P), pancreatotoxins (P), potassium iodide (P), rifampin (P), ritonavir (P), sulfonamides (P), valproic acid (P), vinorelbine (P), zalcitabine (P).[1,3,5,7]
Decreased by anabolic steroids (P), cefotaxime (I), citrate salts (P), fluoride salts (I), somatostatin (P).[1]

Bilirubin, Total (S). *Elevated* by acarbose (P), acetaminophen (P), acetohexamide (P), allopurinol (P), amiodarone (P), amphotericin B (I,P), anabolic steroids (P), asparaginase (P), azathioprine (P), barbiturates (P), capecitabine (P), carbamazepine (P), cephalosporins (P), chloramphenicol (P), cholinergics (P), colchicine (P), cyclophosphamide (P), cyclosporine (P), cytarabine (P), danazol (P), dantrolene (P), dapsone (P), dextran (I), disulfiram (P), diuretics, thiazide and loop (P), docetaxel (P), epinephrine (I), erythromycin (P), estrogens (P), etoposide (P), flutamide (P), gemtuzamab ozogamicin (P), glycopyrrolate (P), gold salts (P), haloperidol (P), hemolytic agents (P), hepatotoxic drugs (P), HMG-CoA reductase inhibitors (P), hydralazine (P), indinavir (P), interferon beta-1b (P), irinotecan (P), isoniazid (I), isoproterenol (I), isotretinoin (P), ketoconazole (P), levodopa (I), meprobamate (P), mercaptopurine (P), methimazole (P), methotrexate (I,P), methyldopa (I,P), narcotics (I), niacin (P), nitrofurantoin (I,P), nonsteroidal anti-inflammatory drugs (P), papaverine (P), penicillamine (P), penicillins (P), phenazopyridine (I), phenothiazines (P), phenelzine (I), probenecid (P), propranolol (I), propylthiouracil (P), pyrazinamide (P), quinidine (P), quinupristin/dalfopristin (P), rifampin (I,P), rifapentine (P), riluzole (P), salicylates (I,P), sulfonamides (P), sulfonylureas (P), theophylline (I), thiabendazole (P), topotecan (P), troleandomycin (P), valproic acid (P), vitamin C (I), zafirlukast (P), zidovudine (P).[1–3,5]
Decreased by amikacin (I), barbiturates (especially in newborns) (P), carbamazepine (P), corticosteroids (P), cyclosporine (P), fexofenadine (P), isotretinoin (P), levodopa (I), nitrofurantoin (I), phenazopyridine (I), phenytoin (P), pindolol (I), sulfonamides (P), temozolomide (P), theophylline (I), ursodiol (P), vitamin C (I).[3,4]

Calcium (S). *Elevated* by alitretinoin (P), amifostine (P), anabolic steroids (P), androgens (P), basiliximab (P), calcitriol (P), calcium salts (P), cefotaxime (I), chlorpropamide (I), diuretics, thiazide (P), estrogens (P), hydralazine (I), interferons (I), iron salts (I), lithium salts (P), magnesium salts (I), phenobarbital (P), progestins (P), sevelamer (P), tamoxifen (P), toremifene (P), thyroid (P), vitamin A (P), vitamin D (P).[1–5,7]

Decreased by acetazolamide (P), albuterol (P), asparaginase (P), aspirin (I), bisphosphonates (P), calcitonin (P), carbamazepine (P), cisplatin (P), citrate salts (P), contraceptives, oral (P), corticosteroids (P), diuretics, loop (P), EDTA (I), ethanol (P), fluoride salts (I,P), foscarnet (P), glucagon (P), heparin (I), laxatives (P), magnesium salts (P), phenobarbital (P), phenytoin (P), phosphate salts (P), plicamycin (P), sodium polystyrene sulfonate (P), sulfisoxazole (I), zalcitabine (P).[1-5]

Carbon Dioxide (B). *Elevated* by bicarbonate salts (P), diuretics (loop, thiazide) (P), respiratory depressants (P).[1,3]

Decreased by acetazolamide (P), aspirin overdose (P), nephrotoxic drugs (P), theophylline (P).[1,3]

Chloride (S). *Elevated* by acetazolamide (P), anabolic steroids (P), aspirin (I,P), carbamazepine (I), cefotaxime (I), cholestyramine (P), corticosteroids (by salt retention) (P), COX-2 inhibitors (P), cyclosporine (P), diuretics, carbonic anhydrase inhibitor, thiazide—chronically by alkalosis (P), estrogens (P), guanethidine (P), halogens (eg, bromides, fluorides) (I), methyldopa (P), nonsteroidal anti-inflammatory drugs (P), sodium phenylbutyrate (P).[1,3]

Decreased by allopurinol (P), bicarbonates (P), cefotaxime (metabolite) (I), chlorpropamide (P), corticosteroids (by alkalosis) (P), diuretics, loop, thiazide—by acute diuresis (P), fluoride salts (I), laxatives, long-term use (P), mannitol (P), mineralocorticoids (by alkalosis) (P), trimethoprim (P).[1,3]

Cholesterol, Total (S). *Elevated* by acetohexamide (P), β-adrenergic blocking agents (P), alitretinoin (P), amiodarone (P), amphotericin B (I), amprenavir (P), anabolic steroids (by cholestasis) (P), aspirin (I), basiliximab (P), carbamazepine (P), cefotaxime (I), chenodiol (P), clopidogrel (P), contraceptives, oral (P), corticosteroids (I,P), cyclosporine (P), danazol (P), dextran (I), diclofenac (P), disulfiram (P), diuretics, loop, thiazide (P), ethanol (P), fibrates (P), gold salts (P), hepatotoxic drugs (cholestatic effect) (P), ibuprofen (P), imipramine (P), isotretinoin (P), meprobamate (P), methotrexate (I), mirtazapine (P), mycophenolate (P), nafarelin (P), phenobarbital (P), phenothiazines (I,P), phenytoin (I,P), protease inhibitors (P), quetiapine (P), ritonavir (P), rosiglitazone (P), sirolimus (P), smoking (P), sorbitol (P), sotalol (P), spironolactone (P), sulfadiazine (P), tamoxifen (P), tetracycline (I), thiabendazole (P), ticlopidine (P), vitamin A (I), vitamin C (I,P), vitamin D (I,P).[1-5]

Decreased by acarbose (P), acebutolol (P), α-adrenergic blockers (P), allopurinol (I,P), aluminum salts (P), amiloride (P), amiodarone (P), ampicillin (I), anabolic steroids (by inhibiting synthesis) (P), ACE inhibitors (P), asparaginase (P), azathioprine (P), calcium channel blockers (P), carvedilol (P), chlorpropamide (P), cholestyramine (P), citrate salts (I), clofibrate (P), clomiphene (P), colchicine (P), colestipol (P), diuretics, thiazide (P), estrogens (P), fenofibrate (P), fluoride salts (I), haloperidol (P), hepatotoxic drugs (decreased synthesis) (P), HMG-CoA reductase inhibitors (P), hydroxychloroquine (P), insulin (P), isoniazid (P), isotretinoin (P), kanamycin, oral (P), ketoconazole (P), levothyroxine (P), MAOIs (P), metformin (P), methyldopa (I,P), metronidazole (P), neomycin, oral (P), niacin (P), nitrates (I), orlistat (P), penicillamine (I), pentamidine (P), phenytoin (P), pindolol (P), psyllium (P), raloxifene (P), rifampin (I), sevelamer (P) tamoxifen (P), tetracyclines (P), thyroid (P), ursodiol (P), valproic acid (P), vitamin C (I,P).[1-5]

Coombs' [Direct] (S). *Positive* by aztreonam (P), captopril (P), cephalosporins (P), chlorpromazine (P), chlorpropamide (P), ethosuximide (P), hemolytic agents (P), hydralazine (P), imipenem/cilastatin (P), indomethacin (P), isoniazid (P), levodopa (P), mefenamic acid (P), melphalan (P), methyldopa (P), nitrofurantoin (P), penicillamine (P), penicillins (P), phenytoin (P), procainamide (P), quinidine (P), quinine (P), rifampin (P), sulfasalazine (P), sulfonamides (P), sulfonylureas (P), tetracyclines (P), tolmetin (I).[1,3,4,6]

Creatine Kinase (S). *Elevated* by alcohol (chronic) (P), aminocaproic acid (P), amphotericin B (P), barbiturates (P), cefotaxime (I), clofibrate (P), cyclosporine (P), danazol (P), fenofibrate (P), HMG-CoA reductase inhibitors (P), gemfibrozil (P), IM injections (P), lithium salts (P), niacin (P), succimer (I), saquinavir (P), zidovudine (P).[1,2,4,5]

Decreased by amikacin (I), anesthetic agents (P), ascorbic acid (I), aspirin (I), dantrolene (P), phenothiazines (P), pindolol (I), succinylcholine (P), sulfamethoxazole (P), zalcitabine (P).[1]

Creatinine (S). *Elevated* by acebutolol (P), acetaminophen (I,P), acetohexamide (I), acyclovir (P), amiloride (P), aminoglycosides (P), amiodarone (P), amphotericin B (P), ACE inhibitors (P), antacids (P), asparaginase (P), aztreonam (P), carvedilol (P), cephalosporins (Jaffe method) (I,P), chloroquine (P), cidofovir (P), cimetidine (P), cisplatin (P), clofibrate (P), colistin (P), co-trimoxazole (P), cyclosporine (P), demeclocycline (P), denileukin diftitox (P), dextran (P), diuretics (P), dopamine (I), doxycycline (P), flucytosine (I,P), foscarnet (P), furosemide (I), ganciclovir (P), hydroxychloroquine (P), lactulose (I), levodopa (I), lidocaine (I), lithium (I,P), methicillin (P), methyldopa (P), mitomycin (P), nalidixic acid (P), nephrotoxic drugs (P), nifedipine (P), nitrofurantoin (I), nonsteroidal anti-inflammatory drugs (P), penicillamine (P), penicillin (I), pentamidine (P), phosphate salts (P), radiocontrast agents (P), ritonavir (P), salicylates (P), sirolimus (P), sulbactam (I), sulfamethoxazole (I), tacrolimus (P), tetracycline (P), vancomycin (P), vitamin C (I), vitamin D (P).[1-4,7]

Decreased by amikacin (I), cephalosporins (I), citrate salts (I), dopamine (I), ibuprofen (P), interferon alfa-2a (P), methyldopa (I), sulfonylureas (P), vitamin C (I).[1,5]

Glucose (S). *Elevated* by abacavir (P), acetaminophen (SMA 12/60 method) (I), acetazolamide (P), β-adrenergic blocking agents (also mask hypoglycemia) (P), albuterol (P), amiodarone (P), antidepressants (heterocyclic) (P), asparaginase (P), basiliximab (P), bicalutamide (P), cefotaxime (I), cholestyramine (P), citrate salts (I), clonidine (P), clozapine (P), corticosteroids (P), cyclosporine (P), daclizumab (P), dextran (I), dextroamphetamine (P), diazoxide (P), diclofenac (I), diltiazem (P), diuretics, loop and thiazide (P), epinephrine (I,P), ephedrine (P), estrogens (P), fosphenytoin (P), gemfibrozil (P), glucagon (P), interferon alfa-2a (P), iron dextran (I), isoniazid (P), isoproterenol (I), labetalol (I), lactose (I), levodopa (SMA 12/60 method) (I), lipids (P), lithium salts (P), mercaptopurine (I), methyldopa (I), metronidazole (I), mycophenolate (P), nalidixic acid (I), niacin (I,P), nifedipine (P), octreotide (P), olanzapine (P), pentamidine (IV, paradoxical effect) (P), perphenazine (P), phenothiazines (P), phenytoin (P), pravastatin (P), progestins (P), propranolol (P), propylthiouracil (I), protease inhibitors (P), reserpine (P), rifampin (I,P), salicylates (acute toxicity) (I,P), somatostatin (P), sorbitol (P), tacrolimus (P), terbutaline (P), tetracyclines (P), thiabendazole (P), thyroid (P), tolbutamide (P), vitamin C (neocuproin method) (I), zalcitabine (P).[1–5]

Decreased by acarbose (P), acetaminophen (GOD-Perid method) (I,P), acetazolamide (P), β-adrenergic blocking agents (nonselective) (P), alcohol (P), allopurinol (P), amikacin (I), anabolic steroids (P), antihistamines (P), chloroquine (P), chlorpropamide (I,P), cimetidine (P), clofibrate (P), disopyramide (P), doxazosin (P), erythromycin (P), estrogens (P), gemfibrozil (P), interferon beta-1b (P), hydralazine (I), insulin (P), isoniazid (I), levodopa (glucose oxidase and other methods) (I), lipids (I), MAO inhibitors (P), metformin (P), methyldopa (P), metronidazole (I), miglitol (P), niacin (P), octreotide (P), pentamidine (IV) (P), phenazopyridine (I), phosphorus (P), psyllium (P), repaglinide (P), salicylates (acute and chronic toxicity) (P), saquinavir (P), SSRIs (P), sulfonamides (P), sulfonylureas (P), tetracyclines (I), thiabendazole (P), tolazolmide (I), tolbutamide (I,P), verapamil (P), vitamin C (GOD-Perid method) (I,P).[1–3,6]

Iron (S). *Elevated* by cefotaxime (I), chloramphenicol (P), cisplatin (P), contraceptives (oral) (P), estrogens (P), ferrous salts (I), iron, parenteral (I,P), methyldopa (P), miglitol (P), rifampin (I).[1,3,5]

Decreased by allopurinol (P), aspirin (large doses) (P), cholestyramine (P), colchicine (P), deferoxamine (I,P), entacapone (P), metformin (P), penicillamine (P), pyrazinamide (I,P).[1,3,5]

Iron Binding Capacity, Total (S). *Elevated* by contraceptives, oral (P), propylthiouracil (P).[1,3,5]

Decreased by chloramphenicol (P), corticotropin (P), corticosteroids (P).[1,3,5]

Magnesium (S). *Elevated* by cefotaxime (I), diuretics, potassium-sparing (P), lithium salts (P), magnesium salts (P), pentamidine (P).[1,3,4,6]

Decreased by albuterol (P), alcohol (P), amifostine (P), aminoglycosides (P), amphotericin B (P), bisphosphonates (P), calcium salts (I), cefotaxime (I), cisplatin (P), citrate salts (I), contraceptive, oral (P), cyclosporine (P), digitalis (toxic concentrations) (P), diuretics, loop, and thiazide (P), foscarnet (P), glucagon (P), insulin (P), tacrolimus (P).[1,3,4,6]

Osmolality (S). *Elevated* by alcohol (ADH suppression) (P), citrate salts (I), corticosteroids (P), demeclocycline (ADH inhibition) (P), glucose (I), lithium salts (ADH inhibition) (P), mannitol (I,P).[1,4]

Decreased by antidepressants, tricyclic (P), carbamazepine (P), chlorpropamide (P), clonidine (P), cyclophosphamide (P), cytarabine (P), diuretics, thiazide (P), haloperidol (P), interferon alfa (I), MAOIs (P), phenothiazines (P), SSRIs (P), sulfonylureas (P), vasopressin (P), vinca alkaloids (P).[1,4]

Phosphate (S). *Elevated* by anabolic steroids (P), basiliximab (P), cefotaxime (I), contraceptives, oral (P), foscarnet (P), mannitol (I), methicillin (I,P), pindolol (P), rifampin (I,P), sodium phenylbutyrate (P), vitamin D (excessive) (P).[1,4]

Decreased by acetazolamide (P), antacids (phosphate binding; eg, aluminum, calcium, and magnesium salts) (P), bisphosphonates (P), calcitonin (P), carbamazepine (P), cidofovir (P), citrate salts (I), foscarnet (P), insulin (P), lithium salts (P), mannitol (I), mycophenolate (P), parenteral nutrition (P), phenobarbital (P), phenothiazines (P), phenytoin (P), sevelamer (P), sirolimus (P), sorbitol (P), sucralfate (P), tacrolimus (P).[1,4–6]

Potassium (S). *Elevated* by aminocaproic acid (P), angiotensin II receptor blockers (P), ACE inhibitors (P), β-adrenergic blockers (P), antineoplastic agents (cytotoxic effect) (P), basiliximab (P), cefotaxime (I), cisplatin (I), cyclosporine (P), COX-2 inhibitors (P), diuretics, potassium-sparing (P), fluconazole (P), fluoride salts (I), heparins (P), iodide salts (I), isoniazid (P), lithium salts (P), low-molecular-weight heparins (P), mannitol (P), mycophenolate (P), nephrotoxic drugs (P), nonsteroidal anti-inflammatory drugs (primarily indomethacin) (P), pentamidine (P), potassium penicillin (P), procainamide (I), salt substitutes (P), succinylcholine (P), tacrolimus (P), trimethoprim (P), tromethamine (P).[1–6]

Decreased by acetazolamide (P), β-adrenergic agonists (P), aminoglycosides (P), ammonium chloride (P), amphotericin B (P), basiliximab (P), bicarbonate salts (P), bisphosphonates (P), cisplatin (P), corticosteroids (P), diuretics (loop, thiazide) (P), fenoldopam (P), foscarnet (P), glucose (P), insulin (P), laxatives (P), levodopa (P), mineralocorticoids (P), mycophenolate (P), ondansetron (P), penicillins (extended-spectrum) (P), phosphate salts (P), salicylates (P), sirolimus (P), sorbitol (P), sodium polystyrene sulfonate (P), sodium phenylbutyrate (P), sulfasalazine (P), tacrolimus (P).[1–6]

Protein, Total. *Elevated* by anabolic steroids {S} (P), aspirin {CSF} (I), cephalothin {S} (I), chloramphenicol {S} (I), corticosteroids {S} (P), dextran {CSF/S} (I), imipramine {CSF} (I), lidocaine {CSF} (I), mannitol {CSF} (I), methotrexate {CSF} (I), penicillins {S/CSF} (I), phenazopyridine {S} (I), phenothiazines {CSF} (I), progestins {S} (I), radiocontrast agents {S} (I), rifampin {S} (I), sulfonamides {CSF} (I), tetracyclines {CSF} (I), thyroid {S} (P), vancomycin {CSF} (I), vitamin C {CSF} (I).[1–3]

Decreased by acetaminophen {CSF} (I), cefotaxime {CSF} (I), contraceptives, oral (from estrogen) {S} (P), cytarabine {CSF} (P/I), dexamethasone {CSF} (P), dextran {S} (I,P), estrogens {S} (P), hepatotoxic drugs {S} (P), pyrazinamide {S} (P), rifampin {S} (P).[1–3]

Sodium (S). *Elevated* by anabolic steroids (P), bicarbonate salts (P), carbamazepine (I,P), cefotaxime (I), cisplatin (I), clonidine (P), contraceptives, oral (P), corticosteroids (P), COX-2 inhibitors (P), diazoxide (P), estrogens (P), fluoride salts (I), lactulose (P), mannitol (P), methyldopa (P), mineralocorticoids (P), nitrofurantoin (P), nonsteroidal anti-inflammatory drugs (P), sodium phenylbutyrate (P), tetracycline (P).[1,3,5]

Decreased by acetazolamide (P), ammonium chloride (P), amphotericin B (P), antidepressants, tricyclic (P), bicarbonate salts (I), carbamazepine (P), chlorpropamide (P), cisplatin (P), clonidine (P), cyclophosphamide (P), cytarabine (P), diuretics, loop and thiazide (P), haloperidol (P), indomethacin (P), interferons (P), laxatives (P), lithium salts (P), mannitol (P), MAOIs inhibitors (P), miconazole (P), nifedipine (P), nonsteroidal anti-inflammatory drugs (P), phenothiazines (P), SSRIs (P), somatostatin (P), spironolactone (P), sulfonylureas (P), vasopressin and analogues (P), trimethoprim (P), vinca alkaloids (P).[1,3-5,7]

Thyroxine (S). *Elevated* by amiodarone (I,P), clofibrate (P), contraceptives, oral (from estrogen) (P), estrogens (P), fluorouracil (P), heparin (I), insulin (P), levodopa (P), prazosin (P), propranolol (P), propylthiouracil (P), prostaglandins (P), radiocontrast agents (I,P), tamoxifen (P).[1-6]

Decreased by anabolic steroids (P), asparaginase (P), barbiturates (P), carbamazepine (P), chlorpropamide (P), cholestyramine (P), clofibrate (P), colestipol (P), corticosteroids (P), danazol (I,P), diazepam (P), heparin (I), interferon alfa-2a (P), iodide salts (P), iron salts (P), lithium salts (P), penicillamine (P), phenytoin (P), propylthiouracil (P), reserpine (P), salicylates (P), sulfonamides (P), sulfonylureas (P), thyroid (P).[1-5]

Triglycerides (S). *Elevated* by β-adrenergic blockers (P), alitretinoin (P), amiodarone (P), amprenavir (P), aspirin (I,P), cholestyramine (P), colestipol (P), contraceptives, oral (P), cyclosporine (P), danazol (P), didanosine (P), diuretics, loop and thiazide (P), estrogens (P), fomepizole (P), interferon alfa-2a (P), isotretinoin (P), itraconazole (P), lipids (P), low-molecular-weight heparins (P), HMG-CoA reductase inhibitors (P), mirtazapine (P), nitroglycerin (I), olanzapine (P), protease inhibitors (P), quinidine (P), ritonavir (P), sirolimus (P), tamoxifen (P).[2-5]

Decreased by acarbose (P), α-adrenergic blockers (P), amiodarone (P), ACE inhibitors (P), asparaginase (P), aspirin (I), chenodiol (P), citrate salts (P), clofibrate (P), danazol (P), fenofibrate (P), gemfibrozil (P), HMG-CoA reductase inhibitors (P), hydroxychloroquine (P), hydroxyurea (I), ketoconazole (P), metformin (P), methotrexate (I), methyldopa (I), naproxen (I), niacin (P), nifedipine (P), orlistat (P), probucol (P), psyllium (P), rifampin (I), spironolactone (P), sulfonylureas (P), verapamil (P), vitamin C (I,P).[1-4]

Urea Nitrogen (S). *Elevated* by ACE inhibitors (P), acetazolamide (P), acetohexamide (I), aminoglycosides (P), anabolic steroids (P), antacids (prolonged use) (P), asparaginase (P), busulfan (P), carbamazepine (P), chloral hydrate (I), chloramphenicol (Nesslerization method) (I), cisplatin (P), clonidine (P), colistin (P), co-trimoxazole (P), cyclosporine (P), dexamethasone (P), dextran (I,P), diuretics, loop and thiazide (P), flucytosine (P), gold salts (P), hydralazine (P), hydroxyurea (P), ifosfamide (P), iron salts (P), methotrexate (P), methyldopa (P), methysergide (P), mitomycin (P), nalidixic acid (P), nephrotoxic drugs (P), nitrofurantoin (P), nonsteroidal anti-inflammatory drugs (P), penicillamine (P), pentamidine (P), radiocontrast agents (P), salicylates (P), sulfonamides (I), tacrolimus (P), tetracyclines (I,P), vancomycin (P), vitamin D (P).[1,3-5]

Decreased by amikacin (I), ascorbic acid (I), cefotaxime (I), chloramphenicol (Berthelot method) (I), fluoride salts (I), levodopa (P), phenothiazines (P), streptomycin (I).[1,3-5]

Uric Acid (S). *Elevated* by acetaminophen (I), acetazolamide (P), anabolic steroids (P), antineoplastics (P), azathioprine (P), basiliximab (P), caffeine (Bittner method) (I), cisplatin (P), citrate salts (P), cyclosporine (P), cytarabine (P), diazoxide (P), diuretics (carbonic anhydrase inhibitor, loop, thiazide) (P), epinephrine (I), ethambutol (P), filgrastim (P), hydralazine (I), isoniazid (I,P), levodopa (I,P), mercaptopurine (P), methyldopa (I), niacin (P), phenytoin (P), pyrazinamide (P), propranolol (P), propylthiouracil (P), rifampin (I), ritonavir (P), salicylates (low doses) (I,P), sodium phenylbutyrate (P), spironolactone (P), tacrolimus (P), theophylline (I,P), triamterene (P), vitamin C (I), zalcitabine (P).[2–5]

Decreased by acetohexamide (P), allopurinol (P), cefotaxime (I), cidofovir (P), clofibrate (P), corticosteroids (P), diflunisal (P), fenofibrate (P), glucose infusions (P), griseofulvin (P), guaifenesin (P), hydralazine (I), indomethacin (P), levodopa (I), lithium (P), losartan (P), mannitol (P), methyldopa (P), nonsteroidal anti-inflammatory drugs (P), phenothiazines (P), radiocontrast agents (P), salicylates (large doses) (P), spironolactone (P), sulfonamides (P), uricosurics (eg, probenecid, sulfinpyrazone) (P), verapamil (P), vitamin C (by Seralyzer) (I,P).[2–5]

URINE TESTS

Bilirubin. *Elevated* by acetohexamide (P), etodolac (I), hepatotoxic drugs (P), mefenamic acid (I), phenazopyridine (I), phenothiazines (I,P).[1,5]

Catecholamines. *Elevated* by acetaminophen (I), α_1-adrenergic blockers (P), alcohol (P), aspirin (I), atenolol (P), caffeine (P), chloral hydrate (I), chlorpromazine (I), dopamine (I,P), epinephrine (I), erythromycin (I), hydralazine (I), insulin (P), isoproterenol (I), labetalol (I), levodopa (I), methenamine (I), methyldopa (I), niacin (I), nifedipine (P), nitroglycerin (P), prochlorperazine (P), quinidine (I), reserpine (P), tetracyclines (I,P), triamterene (P).[1,2,4,5]

Decreased by α_2-adrenergic blockers (P), bromocriptine (P), clonidine (P), disulfiram (P), guanethidine (P), methenamine (destroys catecholamines in bladder urine) (P), radiocontrast agents (I), reserpine (P).[1,2,4]

Color. (*See* Drug-Induced Discoloration of Feces and Urine, page 1024.)

Creatinine. *Elevated* by anabolic steroid (increased muscle mass) (P), asparaginase (I), cephalosporins, except cefotaxime and ceftazidime; (Jaffe method) (I), corticosteroids (P), levodopa (I), methotrexate (P), methyldopa (I), nephrotoxic drugs (P), nitrofurantoin (I), reserpine (P), vitamin C (I).[1,4,5]

Decreased by anabolic steroids (anabolic effect) (P), captopril (P), cimetidine (P), diuretics, thiazide (P).[1,4,5]

Glucose. *Elevated or False Positive* by aspirin (copper reduction) (I,P), aminosalicylic acid (copper reduction) (I), cephalosporins, except cefotaxime (copper reduction) (I), chloral hydrate (copper reduction) (I), cidofovir (P), corticosteroids (P), dextroamphetamine (P), diuretics, loop and thiazide (P), glucagon (P), isoniazid (P), levodopa (copper reduction) (I), lithium salts (P), nalidixic acid (I), niacin (P), penicillins (I), pentamidine (P), phenazopyridine (Tes-Tape) (I), phenothiazines (P), probenecid (I), reserpine (P), sulfonamides (I), vitamin C (copper reduction).[1–6]

Decreased or False Negative by aspirin (glucose oxidase) (I,P), bisacodyl (I), chloral hydrate (glucose oxidase) (I), diazepam (I), digoxin (I), ferrous salts (I), flurazepam (I), furosemide (I), insulin (P), levodopa (glucose oxidase) (I), phenazopyridine (glucose oxidase) (I), phenobarbital (P), prednisone (glucose oxidase) (I), secobarbital (I), tetracycline (I), vitamin C (glucose oxidase).[1–6]

Gonadotropins (Pregnancy Test). *False Positive* by methadone (I), phenothiazines (I).[1,5]

Ketones. *Elevated* by acetylcysteine (I), albuterol (P), captopril (I), cephalosporins (I), dimercaprol (I), insulin (P), isoniazid (P), levodopa (Labstix) (I), mesna (I), metformin (I), methyldopa (I), niacin (P), penicillamine (I), phenazopyridine (I), phenothiazines (I), pyrazinamide (I), salicylates (acidotic effect) (I,P), succimer (I), valproic acid (I).[1,2,4,5]

Decreased by aspirin (oxidation of ketone bodies) (P), phenazopyridine (I).[1]

Protein. *Elevated* by acetaminophen (P), acetazolamide (I), aminoglycosides (I,P), asparaginase (P), bacitracin (P), bicarbonate salts (I), captopril (P), carbamazepine (P), cephalosporins (I,P), chlorpromazine (I), cidofovir (P), cisplatin (P), cyclosporine (P), delavirdine (P), dihydrotachysterol (I,P), diuretics, thiazide (P), gemcitabine (P), gold salts (P), griseofulvin (P), hydralazine (P), interferon beta-1b (P), iron salts (P), isoniazid (P), lithium salts (P), nephrotoxic drugs (P), nonsteroidal anti-inflammatory drugs (P), penicillamine (P), penicillins (I), pentamidine (P), phenazopyridine (I), radiographic agents (I), rifapentine (P), salicylates (I), sulfonamides (I), tetracycline (P), tolbutamide (I), vancomycin (P), vitamin C (I).[1,5]

Decreased by ACE inhibitors (P), cyclosporine (P), diltiazem (P), interferon alfa-2a (P), prednisolone (P).[1]

Specific Gravity. *Elevated* by dextran (P), diuretics (P), isotretinoin (P), mannitol (P), radiographic agents (P), sucrose (P).[1,4,5]

Decreased by colistin (P), lithium (P).[1]

HEMATOLOGY

Erythrocyte Sedimentation Rate (B). *Elevated* by contraceptives, oral (P), cyclosporine (P), dextran (P), isotretinoin (P), methyldopa (P), methysergide (P), nitrofurantoin (P), procainamide (P), theophylline (P), vitamin A (P).[1,5]

Decreased by corticosteroids (P), cyclophosphamide (P), infliximab (P), fluoride salts (I), gold salts (P), methotrexate (P), nonsteroidal anti-inflammatory drugs (P), penicillamine (P), quinine (P), salicylates (P), sulfasalazine (P), tamoxifen (P), trimethoprim (P), drugs that cause hyperglycemia (P).[1,5]

Prothrombin Time (B) [Does not include anticoagulants or drugs which potentiate or antagonize them]. *Elevated* by acetaminophen (P), antibiotics (gut sterilizing) (P), asparaginase (P), cephalosporins (P), chloramphenicol (P), chloral hydrate (P), chlorpromazine (P), chlorpropamide (P), cholestyramine (P), colestipol (P), cyclophosphamide (P), hepatotoxic drugs (P), laxatives (P), mercaptopurine

(P), metronidazole (P), niacin (P), propylthiouracil (P), quinidine (P), quinine (P), salicylates (P), sulfonamides (P).[1,4,5]

    Decreased by anabolic steroids (P), azathioprine (P), estrogens (P), vitamin K (P).[1,3,5]

REFERENCES

1. Young DS. *Effects of drugs on clinical laboratory tests.* 5th ed. Washington: AACC Press; 2000.
2. Salway JG editor. *Drug-test interaction handbook.* 1st ed. New York: Raven Press; 1990.
3. Sher PP. Drug interferences with clinical laboratory tests. *Drugs* 1982;24:24-63.
4. McEvoy GK, editor. *AHFS drug information 2001.* Bethesda: American Society of Health-System Pharmacists; 2001.
5. Wallach J. *Interpretation of diagnostic tests.* 7th ed. Philadelphia: Lippincott, Williams, & Brown; 2000.
6. Aronson JK ed. *Side effects of drugs annual.* 22nd ed. Amsterdam: Elsevier; 1999.
7. Burtis CA, Ashwood ER, eds. *Tietz textbook of clinical chemistry.* 3rd ed. Philadelphia: WB Saunders; 1999.

Pharmacokinetic Equations

5

James R. Lane, Jr.

Abbreviations used in this appendix:

Alb_{meas} = measured serum albumin
Alb_{nl} = normal serum albumin
α = fraction of drug unbound to albumin
C_{adj} = adjusted serum concentration
C_{des} = desired serum concentration
Cl = serum drug clearance
C_{meas} = measured serum concentration
ΔCp = desired increase in serum concentration
Cp_t = serum concentration at time t
C_{ss} = steady-state serum concentration
$C_{ss\ ave}$ = average steady-state serum concentration
$C_{ss\ max}$ = maximum (peak) steady-state serum concentration
$C_{ss\ min}$ = minimum (trough) steady-state serum concentration
C_{ti} = initial serum concentration
D = dose
F = fraction of dose absorbed
k_0 = infusion rate (dose/t_{inf})
ka = absorption rate constant
kd = elimination rate constant
km = Michaelis–Menten constant in mg/L
S = salt fraction
τ = dosage interval in hours
$t_{1/2}$ = elimination half-life
t_{inf} = duration of infusion
t_{max} = time of peak serum concentration
$t_{max\ ss}$ = time of peak serum concentration at steady state
V_d = apparent volume of distribution
V_m = maximum rate of metabolism in mg/day

■ ONE-COMPARTMENT EQUATIONS

$$kd = \frac{Cl}{Vd}$$

$$t_{1/2} = \frac{0.693 \times Vd}{Cl}$$

$$kd = \frac{0.693}{t_{1/2}}$$

$$kd = \frac{\ln (Cp_1 / Cp_2)}{t}$$

Where t = time between serum concentrations Cp_1 and Cp_2.

SINGLE-DOSE EQUATIONS

Concentration at time t (IV bolus):

$$Cp_t = \frac{S \times D}{Vd} \times e^{-kd \times t}$$

Concentration at time t (during IV infusion):

$$Cp_t = \frac{S \times k_0}{Cl} \times (1 - e^{-kd \times t_{inf}})$$

Concentration at time t (after the end of an IV infusion):

$$Cp_t = \frac{S \times k_0}{Cl} \times (1 - e^{-kd \times t_{inf}}) \times e^{(-kd \times [t - t_{inf}])}$$

Concentration at time t (PO or IM):

$$Cp_t = \frac{S \times F \times D \times ka}{Vd \times (ka - kd)} \times (e^{-kd \times t} - e^{-ka \times t})$$

Time to Peak (PO or IM):

$$t_{max} = \frac{\ln (ka/kd)}{ka - kd}$$

Loading Dose (negligible drug loss during administration):

$$LD = \frac{\Delta Cp \times Vd}{S \times F}$$

Loading Dose (IV loading dose when drug is lost during administration):

$$LD = \frac{Cl \times t_{inf} \times (C_{des} - [C_{ti} \times e^{-kd \times t_{inf}}])}{S \times (1 - e^{-kd \times t_{inf}})}$$

Loading Dose (IM or PO):

$$LD = \frac{Vd \times (C_{des} - [C_{ti} \times e^{-kd \times t_{max}}])}{S \times F \times (1 - e^{-kd \times t_{max}})}$$

STEADY-STATE EQUATIONS

Peak Concentration (IV):

$$C_{ss\,max} = S \times k_0 \times \frac{1 - e^{-kd \times t_{inf}}}{Cl \times (1 - e^{-kd \times \tau})}$$

Peak Concentration (PO or IM):

$$C_{ss\,max} = \frac{S \times F \times D \times e^{-kd \times t_{max\,ss}}}{Vd \times (1 - e^{-kd \times \tau})}$$

Trough Concentration (IV):

$$C_{ss\,min} = C_{ss\,max} \times e^{-kd \times (\tau - t_{inf})}$$

Trough Concentration (PO or IM):

$$C_{ss\,min} = \frac{S \times F \times D \times ka}{Vd \times (ka - kd)} \times \left[\frac{e^{-kd \times \tau}}{1 - e^{-kd \times \tau}} - \frac{e^{-ka \times \tau}}{1 - e^{-ka \times \tau}} \right]$$

Average Concentration (IV, PO, or IM):

$$C_{ss\,ave} = \frac{S \times F \times D}{Cl \times \tau}$$

Time to Peak (PO or IM):

$$t_{max\,ss} = \frac{\ln (ka \times [1 - e^{-kd \times \tau}]) / (kd \times [1 - e^{-ka \times \tau}])}{ka - kd}$$

Dosage Interval:

$$Interval = T + \frac{(\ln [C_{max} / C_{min}])}{kd}$$

where T = infusion time for IV doses and t_{max} for PO and IM doses.

■ MICHAELIS–MENTEN EQUATIONS

$$\text{Daily Dosage} = \frac{Vm \times C_{ss\ ave}}{S \times F \times (km + C_{ss\ ave})}$$

$$C_{adj} = \frac{C_{meas}}{\left([1-\alpha] \times \dfrac{Alb_{meas}}{Alb_{nl}}\right) + \alpha}$$

$$C_{ss\ ave} = \frac{S \times F \times \text{Dosage}/\text{day} \times km}{Vm - (S \times F \times \text{daily dosage})}$$

Index